PEDIATRIC SURGERY

Volume 1

PEDIATRIC SURGERY

Edited by

MARK M. RAVITCH, M.D., F.A.C.S.

Professor of Surgery, The University of Pittsburgh School of Medicine
Surgeon-in-Chief, Montefiore Hospital, Pittsburgh, Pennsylvania

KENNETH J. WELCH, M.D., F.A.C.S.

Associate Clinical Professor of Surgery, Harvard Medical School
Senior Associate in Surgery, Children's Hospital Medical Center
Boston, Massachusetts

CLIFFORD D. BENSON, M.D., F.A.C.S.

Professor of Clinical Surgery, Wayne State University School of Medicine
Emeritus Surgeon-in-Chief, Children's Hospital of Michigan
Surgeon, Harper Hospital, Detroit, Michigan

EOIN ABERDEEN, M.D.

Professor of Surgery, Acting Director of Pediatric Surgery
New Jersey Medical School, Newark, New Jersey

JUDSON G. RANDOLPH, M.D., F.A.C.S.

Professor of Surgery, George Washington University School of Medicine
and Health Sciences
Surgeon-in-Chief, Children's Hospital, Washington, D.C.

THIRD EDITION
Volume 1

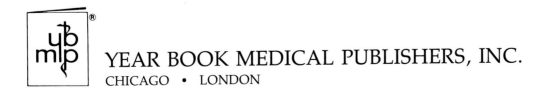

YEAR BOOK MEDICAL PUBLISHERS, INC.
CHICAGO • LONDON

The editors gratefully acknowledge the courtesy of the publishers who have granted permission to reprint the following material from their publications in this work: Fig. 35–2, Radiology 112:175–176, 1974; Figs. 37–4 and 37–5, R. T. Soper, *Synopsis of Pediatric Surgery*, Georg Thieme Verlag, Stuttgart, 1975; Fig. 43–24, Journal of Thoracic and Cardiovascular Surgery 66:333–342, 1973; Fig. 46–8, Pediatrics 54:4, 1974; Fig. 58–1, Little, Brown & Co., Boston, and Annals of Thoracic Surgery 23:378, 1977; Fig. 81–3, Surgery 78:76–86, 1975; Fig. 81–5, Surgery, Gynecology and Obstetrics 140:952, 1975; Fig. 81–9, Surgery, Gynecology and Obstetrics 108:9, 1959; Fig. 81–12, Surgery 75:664–673, 1974; Table 95–4, Acta Paediatrica Scandinavica 60:209–215, 1971; Fig. 95–5, Archives of Disease in Childhood 41:454, 1966; Fig. 95–9, Surgical Clinics of North America 50:1151, 1970; Fig. 95–18, New England Journal of Medicine 293:685, 1975; Fig. 95–19, New England Journal of Medicine 285:17, 1971; Fig. 95–21, New England Journal of Medicine 289:1099, 1973; Figs. 98–3, 98–4 and 98–6, Surgical Clinics of North America 56:385, 1976; Fig. 98–7, Surgical Clinics of North America 56:385, 1976, and Journal of Pediatric Surgery 2:106, 1967; Fig. 100–5, Surgery 64:834, 1968; Fig. 110–2, Williams & Wilkins Co., Baltimore, and Journal of Urology 109:888, 1973; Figs. 126–1 and 126–2, Journal of Pediatric Surgery 9:446–447, 1974; Fig. 126–3, The C. V. Mosby Co., St. Louis, and Surgery 62:967–973, 1967.

Library of Congress Cataloging in Publication Data
Main entry under title:

Pediatric Surgery

    Includes bibliographies and index.
    1. Children—Surgery.   I. Ravitch, Mark M., 1910-
RD 137.P42 1979   617′.98   78-25865
ISBN 0-8151-7107-2

Preface to the Third Edition

A RATHER LONGER PERIOD OF TIME has elapsed between the Second and Third Editions than between the First and Second Editions, in part because of the changes in the Editorial Board and in part because of the magnitude of the task involved in a complete rewriting of the book. Bill Snyder died on June 1, 1974. The editors and publishers have lost a warm friend, a surgeon of great scholarship, an editor of rare discernment and a colleague whose wisdom and stability had much to do with the success of the First and Second Editions. Bill Mustard insisted on retiring simultaneously from both his clinical and editorial responsibilities, and no amount of persuasion could budge him. He was a leading force in the book from its inception, a brilliant and original contributor, and enlivened the meetings of the Board.

The book has been almost totally rewritten and in several areas sharply reoriented, as a result of the increasing importance of some facets of pediatric surgery, the obsolescence or universal acceptance of others. By the same token, not only has the Editorial Board undergone a major change, but the passage of time, the entrance into the field of men making major new contributions, and the retirement of some of our contributors have led to a major change in the list of contributing authors. One hundred and six new authors appear in the Third Edition. There are 31 new chapters representing either treatment of subjects, or phases of subjects, for the first time, or elevation of the status of the brief treatments previously afforded. Among the 31 new chapters are those on Total Parenteral Nutrition, Radiation Therapy for Solid Tumors, Children as Accident Victims, Emergency Management of the Severely Injured Child, Skin and Subcutaneous Tissue Injuries, Musculoskeletal Injuries, Snakebite, Spider Bites, Craniofacial Abnormalities, Hodgkin's Disease, Surgical Pulmonary Complications of Cystic Fibrosis, Volvulus of the Stomach, Necrotizing Enterocolitis, Inflammatory Bowel Disease, Enuresis, Cystic Disease of the Kidney, Renal Fusions and Ectopy, Renal Vein Thrombosis, Pyeloureteral Obstruction, Bifid Ureters, Vesicoureteral Reflux, Abnormalities of the Urethra, Urinary Undiversion, Abnormalities of the Penis, Rhabdomyosarcoma, von Recklinghausen's Disease, Infections of Bones and Joints, Tumors of Bone, and Deformities of the Spinal Column.

There is a new part on Trauma, collecting together the sections on trauma that appeared in scattered places in the previous editions and adding several new chapters. The organization of the Cardiac, Urologic and Musculoskeletal sections has been radically revised.

In response to the plea of many of our readers, the book has been rearranged so that all of the portion of abdominal surgery is in one volume.

The editors are grateful to the contributors for their support, cooperation and industry, and the quality of their contributions. The allocation of areas of principal editorial responsibility is unchanged. Doctor Randolph took on the previous responsibilities of Doctor Snyder, adding to his responsibilities the Trauma section, and Doctor Aberdeen took on the previous responsibilities of Doctor Mustard. Doctor Ravitch functioned as chairman of the Board. Our secretaries, Margaret Shandor, Suzanne Danais, Geraldine Bush, Dolores Bigger and Linda Bowersock, have put in long and arduous hours in typing and retyping the manuscripts. We are grateful to them for their patient and sustained efforts, and to those in our offices who carried the burden in such a dedicated manner.

It is a pleasure to express our warm appreciation to the staff at Year Book Medical Publishers for their support, counsel and tolerance, and for their willingness to undertake the publication of what is, in most respects, a new book, and to do it with the high level of performance in the publishers' art that has characterized the previous editions. It is a source of some regret that the inclusion of much new material has necessarily led to some increase in the size.

THE EDITORS

v

Preface to the First Edition

PEDIATRIC SURGERY today is one of the most vigorously growing fields in surgery. The establishment of chairs, divisions and departments of pediatric surgery in university centers attests to an increasing awareness of the special problems in this field. Several societies have been founded to promote knowledge in this area, and special sections exist in others. Two journals are devoted entirely to pediatric surgery, a third has a special department and others publish special issues concerned with its problems.

In June of 1959, an editorial board was formed to enroll the services of recognized authorities in writing a complete textbook of pediatric surgery that would reflect the best thoughts of men from representative institutions, covering a wide geographic area in the United States, Canada and England. As in any branch of surgery, during a period of rapid development and experimentation, much of the material is new, and much of it is as yet unpublished elsewhere in any form.

Our colleagues in many countries are contributing importantly to the growth of pediatric surgical knowledge. They will find repeated references to their published material. We regret that we could not enlist the services of many worthwhile contributors from Australia, Scandinavia and Continental Europe.

This project was conceived to meet the need for a comprehensive work on pediatric surgery presented from as broad a point of view as possible. There was agreement that all aspects of pediatric surgery would be covered, although, in order to limit the work to a reasonable size, it was necessary to restrict the space allotted to such specialty fields as ophthalmology, otolaryngology, orthopedics and neurosurgery. The heaviest concentration is in the traditional fields of general, thoracic and urologic surgery.

Particular emphasis has been laid on appropriate treatment of the physiologic, anatomic and embryologic aspects of specific surgical problems. Because we feel that the current state of knowledge is best understood in the light of its development, we have prefaced many subjects with an historical résumé.

Contributors have been urged to express their own feelings clearly on controversial points, to draw particularly on their own experience and, in addition, to evaluate and comment upon the work of others. To this end, we have encouraged extensive bibliographic lists, with annotations in the text. Particular attention has been paid to the illustrations and the publishers have been generous concerning the number included.

Our contributors have been cooperative, prompt and patient with our editorial suggestions, and we are grateful to them. Some duplication of coverage will necessarily occur in a multiauthor textbook, and we think this not undesirable. Differences of opinion are expressed in some areas, and such differences will be found to exist. In details of treatment, and in other matters, in a variety of aspects of pediatric surgery, the editors do not hold uniform opinions—nor do the contributors. It was felt important only that an individual contribution present a valid and supportable point of view and a satisfactory method of treatment.

It is hoped that the various sections are developed in a manner systematic enough to make them useful to the student or house officer interested in the field of pediatric surgery, that the presentations are broad enough and sufficiently free from surgical minutiae to be useful to the pediatrician and yet detailed enough to convey to the informed general surgeon each author's assessment of current knowledge in his field and his own recommendations.

We have felt strongly that the value of this presentation would be increased in direct proportion to the briefness of time between the preparation of the manuscript and publication. In a multiauthor work, a good deal of time is necessarily expended in the transmission of manuscripts from authors to editors, in circulation among editors, and resubmission to authors for consideration of joint editorial suggestions. Six months were spent by the editorial board in organizing the form of the work, the division of subject matter, the matter of presentation, the division of editorial responsibilities and the assignment of subjects to the editors and contributors. The actual writing, editing and publication have been accomplished in less than two years.

The editorial board has functioned in a coordinated effort. While the editors were individually responsible for given Parts, each contributed Sections to Parts for which others were editorially responsible. Every chapter has been reviewed by several members of the board. The distribution of a model chapter, prepared by Doctor Mustard, greatly simplified the problem of achieving uniformity. Doctor Welch served as chairman of the board and was editorially responsible for PART I: *General*, PART II: *Head and Neck*, and PART V: *Genitourinary System*. Doctors Mustard and Ravitch were responsible for PART III: *The Thorax*, Doctor Mustard for PART VI: *Integument and Musculoskeletal System*, and Doctor Ravitch for PART VII: *Nervous System*. Doctors Benson and Snyder prepared PART IV: *Abdomen*. The selection of contributors was a joint editorial effort. Mrs. Muriel McL. Miller was responsible for the uniform pen and ink illustration concept.

We wish to acknowledge our gratitude to our secretaries, Mrs. Ralph Conjour, Miss June Gerkens, Mrs. Grace Crabbe, Mrs. Josephine Dyer and Miss Linda Morse, for their tolerance and patience, and their willingness to type and retype manuscripts at a rapid pace and make early publication a reality.

We are grateful also to the staff of Year Book Medical Publishers for their enthusiasm and cooperation. The many meetings of the editorial board have been made possible through their generous support.

THE EDITORS

List of Contributors

ABERDEEN, EOIN, M.D.: Professor of Surgery, Acting Director of Pediatric Surgery, New Jersey Medical School, Newark, New Jersey

ADELMAN, SUSAN E., M.D.: Assistant Professor of Clinical Surgery, Wayne State University School of Medicine; Assistant Attending Active Staff, Children's Hospital of Michigan, Detroit, Michigan

ADKINS, JOHN C., M.D.: Assistant Professor of Pediatric Surgery, Department of Surgery, University of Pittsburgh School of Medicine, Children's Hospital of Pittsburgh, Pittsburgh, Pennsylvania

ALLEN, GEORGE S., M.D.: Assistant Professor, Department of Neurosurgery, The Johns Hopkins University School of Medicine, The Johns Hopkins Hospital, Baltimore, Maryland

ALTMAN, R. PETER, M.D., F.A.C.S.: Professor of Surgery and Child Health and Development, George Washington University School of Medicine and Health Sciences; Senior Attending Surgeon, Children's Hospital National Medical Center, Washington, D.C.

ANDERSON, KATHRYN D., M.D., F.A.C.S.: Associate Professor of Surgery, George Washington University School of Medicine and Health Sciences; Senior Attending Surgeon, Children's Hospital National Medical Center, Washington, D.C.

ARCINIEGAS, EDUARDO, M.D.: Associate Clinical Professor of Surgery, Wayne State University School of Medicine; Chief, Department of Cardiovascular Surgery, Children's Hospital of Michigan, Detroit, Michigan

ASHCRAFT, KEITH W., M.D., F.A.C.S.: Associate Clinical Professor of Surgery, University of Missouri School of Medicine; Chief, Section of Urology, Children's Mercy Hospital, Kansas City, Missouri

BAHNSON, HENRY T., M.D., F.A.C.S.: George Vance Foster Professor of Surgery, Chairman, Department of Surgery, University of Pittsburgh School of Medicine, Pittsburgh, Pennsylvania

BECKER, JERROLD M., M.D., F.A.C.S.: Clinical Professor of Surgery, State University of New York at Stony Brook Health Sciences Center School of Medicine; Chief of Pediatric Surgery, Long Island Jewish-Hillside Medical Center, New Hyde Park, New York

BEHRENDT, DOUGLAS M., M.D.: Professor of Surgery, Section of Thoracic Surgery, University of Michigan, University Hospital, Ann Arbor, Michigan

BELMAN, A. BARRY, M.D., M.S., F.A.C.S., F.A.A.P.: Associate Professor of Urology and Child Health and Development, George Washington University School of Medicine and Health Sciences; Chairman, Department of Pediatric Urology, Children's Hospital National Medical Center, Washington, D.C.

BENSON, CLIFFORD, D., M.D., F.A.C.S.: Professor of Clinical Surgery, Wayne State University School of Medicine; Emeritus Surgeon-in-Chief, Children's Hospital of Michigan; Surgeon, Harper Hospital, Detroit, Michigan

BHARATI, SAROJA, M.D., F.A.C.C.: Research Associate Professor, Department of Medicine, Abraham Lincoln School of Medicine, University of Illinois; Associate Professor, Departments of Pediatrics and Pathology, Rush Medical College; Associate Director, Congenital Heart Disease Research and Training Center, Chicago, Illinois

BILL, ALEXANDER H., JR., M.D., F.A.C.S.: Clinical Professor of Surgery, University of Washington School of Medicine; Attending Surgeon, Director of Surgical Department Emeritus, Children's Orthopedic Hospital and Medical Center, Seattle, Washington

BLACK, PERRY, M.D.: Associate Professor of Neurological Surgery, The Johns Hopkins University School of Medicine, The Johns Hopkins Hospital, Baltimore, Maryland

BOLES, E. THOMAS, JR., M.D.: Professor and Director, Division of Pediatric Surgery, Department of Surgery, Ohio State University College of Medicine; Chief, Department of Pediatric Surgery, Montefiore Hospital and Medical Center, Bronx, New York

BOLEY, SCOTT J., M.D., F.A.C.S., F.A.A.P. (S): Professor of Surgery, Albert Einstein College of Medicine; Director of Pediatric Surgery, Montefiore Hospital and Medical Center, Bronx, New York

CASTANEDA, ALDO R., M.D., F.A.C.S.: William E. Ladd Professor of Surgery, Harvard Medical School; Cardiovascular Surgeon-in-Chief, Children's Hospital Medical Center, Boston, Massachusetts

CATLIN, FRANCIS I., M.D.: Professor of Otorhinolaryngology and Communicative Sciences, Baylor College of Medicine, Houston, Texas

CHISHOLM, TAGUE C., M.D., F.A.C.S.: Clinical Professor of Surgery, University of Minnesota Medical School, Minneapolis, Minnesota

COLODNY, ARNOLD H., M.D.: Associate Clinical Professor of Surgery, Harvard Medical School; Associate Director, Division of Urology, Senior Surgeon, Children's Hospital Medical Center, Boston, Massachusetts

COOLEY, DENTON A., M.D., F.A.C.S.: Surgeon-in-Chief, Texas Heart Institute of St. Luke's Episcopal and Texas Children's Hospitals; Clinical Professor, University of Texas Medical School, Houston, Texas

CORAN, ARNOLD G., M.D.: Head, Section of Pediatric Surgery, Professor of Surgery, University of Michigan Medical School; Chief of Pediatric Surgical Services, Mott Children's Hospital, Ann Arbor, Michigan

CRAWFORD, JOHN S., M.D., C.M., D.O.M.S. (Eng), F.R.C.S. (C): Professor of Ophthalmology, University of Toronto Faculty of Medicine; Ophthalmologist-in-Chief, Hospital for Sick Children, Toronto, Ontario

CROCKER, DEAN, M.D., C.M.: Director, Department of Respiratory Therapy, Children's Hospital Medical Center; Clinical Associate in Anesthesia, Harvard Medical School, Boston, Massachusetts

D'ANGIO, GIULIO J., M.D.: Director, Children's Cancer Research Center, Children's Hospital of Philadelphia, Philadelphia, Pennsylvania

DANIELSON, GORDON K., M.D.: Professor of Surgery, Mayo Medical School; Consultant in Thoracic and Cardiovascular Surgery, Mayo Clinic, Rochester, Minnesota

DAUM, FREDRIC, M.D.: Chief of Gastroenterology, North Shore University Hospital–Cornell University Medical College, New York, New York

DEAN, RICHARD H., M.D.: Associate Professor of Surgery, Vanderbilt University School of Medicine, Nashville, Tennessee

DIBBINS, ALBERT W., M.D.: Assistant Clinical Professor of Surgery, Tufts University School of Medicine, Boston, Massachusetts; Director, Division of Pediatric Surgery, Maine Medical Center, Portland, Maine

DINARI, GABRIEL, M.D.: Chief of Pediatric Gastroenterology, Beilinson Hospital, Israel

DONAHOE, PATRICIA K., M.D., F.A.C.S.: Assistant Professor of Surgery, Harvard Medical School; Assistant Surgeon, Massachusetts General Hospital, Boston, Massachusetts

DONAHOO, JAMES S., M.D.: Associate Professor of Surgery, The Johns Hopkins University School of Medicine, The Johns Hopkins Hospital, Baltimore, Maryland

DOWNES, JOHN J., M.D.: Professor, University of Pennsylvania School of Medicine; Director, Department of Anesthesia, Children's Hospital of Philadelphia, Philadelphia, Pennsylvania

DUCKETT, JOHN W., JR., M.D., F.A.C.S.: Associate Professor of Urology, University of Pennsylvania School of Medicine; Director of Pediatric Urology, Children's Hospital of Philadelphia, Philadelphia, Pennsylvania

EATON, RICHARD G., M.D., F.A.C.S.: Associate Clinical Professor of Surgery, Columbia University College of Physicians and Surgeons; Co-Director, Hand Service, The Roosevelt Hospital, New York, New York

EDGERTON, MILTON T., JR., M.D.: Professor and Chairman, Department of Plastic and Maxillofacial Surgery, University of Virginia School of Medicine, Charlottesville, Virginia

EPSTEIN, MELVIN, M.D., F.A.C.S.: Associate Professor of Neurosurgery, Associate Professor of Emergency Medicine, The Johns Hopkins University; Director of Pediatric Neurosurgery, The Johns Hopkins Hospital, Baltimore, Maryland

EXELBY, PHILIP R., M.D., F.A.C.S.: Associate Professor of Surgery, Cornell University Medical College; Attending Surgeon and Chief, Pediatric Surgical Service, Memorial Sloan–Kettering Cancer Center, New York, New York

FARMER, ALFRED W., M.B.E., M.D., F.R.C.S. (C): Professor of Surgery Emeritus, University of Toronto Faculty of Medicine; Honorary Staff, Hospital for Sick Children; Staff, Sunnybrook Hospital, Toronto, Ontario

FERGUSON, COLIN C., M.D., F.R.C.S. (C), F.A.C.S.: Professor, Department of Surgery, University of Manitoba Medical Faculty; Head, Section of Paediatric General and Cardiopulmonary Surgery, Health Sciences (Children's) Centre, Winnipeg, Manitoba

FILLER, ROBERT M., M.D.: Professor of Surgery, University of Toronto Faculty of Medicine; Surgeon-in-Chief, Hospital for Sick Children, Toronto, Ontario

FILMER, R. BRUCE, M.D., F.R.A.C.S., F.R.C.S. (Eng), F.A.C.S.: Pediatric Urologist, Royal Alexandra Hospital for Children, Sydney, Australia; Wade House Consulting Rooms, Royal Alexandra Hospital for Children, Camperdown, Australia

FISHER, JOHN H., M.D., F.A.C.S.: Associate Clinical Professor of Surgery, Harvard Medical School; Senior Associate in Surgery, Children's Hospital Medical Center, Boston, Massachusetts

FOLKMAN, M. JUDAH, M.D., F.A.C.S.: Julia Dyckman Andrus Professor of Pediatric Surgery, Harvard Medical School; Surgeon-in-Chief, Children's Hospital Medical Center, Boston, Massachusetts

FONKALSRUD, ERIC W., M.D., F.A.C.S.: Professor and Chief of Pediatric Surgery, UCLA School of Medicine, Los Angeles, California

FOSTER, JOHN H., M.D., F.A.C.S.: Professor of Surgery (Retired), Vanderbilt University School of Medicine, Nashville, Tennessee

GROSFELD, JAY L., M.D.: Professor and Director, Section of Pediatric Surgery, Indiana University School of Medicine; Surgeon-in-Chief, James Whitcomb Riley Hospital for Children, Indianapolis, Indiana

HALL, JOHN E., M.D.: Professor of Orthopedic Surgery, Harvard Medical School; Chief of Clinical Orthopedic Services, Children's Hospital Medical Center, Boston, Massachusetts

HALLER, J. ALEX, JR., M.D.: Robert Garrett Professor of Pediatric Surgery, The Johns Hopkins University School of Medicine; Children's Surgeon-in-Charge, The Johns Hopkins Hospital, Baltimore, Maryland

HARDY, BRIAN E., M.D.: Associate Professor, University of Toronto Faculty of Medicine; Staff Urologist, Hospital for Sick Children, Toronto, Ontario

HENDREN, W. HARDY, M.D., F.A.C.S.: Professor of Surgery, Harvard Medical School; Chief of Pediatric Surgery, Massachusetts General Hospital, Boston, Massachusetts

HERTZLER, JACK H., M.D., F.A.C.S.: Associate Professor of Surgery, Wayne State University School of Medicine; Chairman of Surgical Services, Children's Hospital of Michigan, Detroit, Michigan

HOLDER, THOMAS M., M.D., F.A.C.S.: Clinical Professor of Surgery, University of Missouri School of Medicine; Chief, Section of Thoracic and Cardiovascular Surgery, Children's Mercy Hospital, Kansas City, Missouri

HOWARD, RICHARD J., M.D., Ph.D.: Assistant Professor of Surgery, University of Minnesota Medical School, Minneapolis, Minnesota

JAFFE, NORMAN, M.D.: Division Chief, Division of Solid Tumors, Pediatrician and Professor of Pediatrics, M.D. Anderson Hospital and Tumor Institute, Houston, Texas; formerly Chief, Pediatric Solid Tumor Service, Sidney Farber Cancer Institute, Boston, Massachusetts

JEWELL, PATRICK, M.D., F.A.C.S., F.A.A.P.: Clinical Assistant Professor, Department of Surgery, Wayne State University School of Medicine; Attending Surgeon, Children's Hospital of Michigan; Senior Attending Surgeon, Saint John Hospital, Detroit, Michigan

JEWETT, THEODORE C., JR., M.D.: Professor of Surgery, State University of New York at Buffalo School of Medicine; Chief, Department of Surgery, Buffalo Children's Hospital, Buffalo, New York

JOHNSON, DALE G., M.D., F.A.C.S.: Professor of Surgery and Professor of Pediatrics; Head, Division of Pediatric Surgery, University of Utah College of Medicine; Chairman, Department of Surgery, Primary Children's Medical Center, Salt Lake City, Utah

JOHNSTON, J. HERBERT, M.D.: Lecturer in Paediatric Urology, University of Liverpool; Urological Surgeon, Alder Hey Children's Hospital, Liverpool, England

JONES, PETER G., M.D., M.S. (Melb), F.R.C.S. (Eng), F.R.A.C.S., F.A.C.S.: Senior Surgeon, Royal Children's Hospital, Melbourne, Australia

KABAN, LEONARD B., D.M.D., M.D.: Assistant Professor of Oral Surgery, Harvard School of Dental Medicine; Associate in Surgery, Children's Hospital Medical Center; Associate in Surgery, Peter Bent Brigham Hospital, Boston, Massachusetts

KEVY, SHERWIN W., M.D.: Associate Professor of Pediatrics, Harvard Medical School; Director of Transfusion Service, Children's Hospital Medical Center, Boston, Massachusetts

KIDD, B.S. LANGFORD, M.D., F.R.C.P. (Edinburgh and Canada): Harriet Lane Home Professor of Pediatric Cardiology, The Johns Hopkins University School of Medicine; Director, Division of Pediatric Cardiology, The Johns Hopkins Hospital, Baltimore, Maryland

KIESEWETTER, WILLIAM B., M.D., F.A.C.S.: Professor of Pediatric Surgery, University of Pittsburgh School of Medicine; Surgeon-in-Chief, Children's Hospital of Pittsburgh, Pittsburgh, Pennsylvania

KING, LOWELL R., M.D., F.A.C.S.: Professor of Urology and Surgery, Northwestern University Medical School; Surgeon-in-Chief, Children's Memorial Hospital, Chicago, Illinois

KIRKLIN, JOHN W., M.D.: Fay Fletcher Kerner Professor and Chairman, Department of Surgery; Surgeon-in-Chief, University of Alabama School of Medicine and Medical Center, Birmingham, Alabama

KLEINHAUS, SYLVAIN, M.D., F.A.C.S.: Associate Professor of

Surgery, Albert Einstein College of Medicine; Associate Professor of Surgery, Montefiore Hospital and Medical Center, Bronx, New York

KOTTMEIER, PETER K., M.D., F.A.C.S.: Professor of Surgery, Chief, Pediatric Surgical Service, State University of New York Downstate Medical Center College of Medicine, Brooklyn, New York

KROOVAND, R. LAWRENCE, M.D.: Assistant Professor of Urology, Wayne State University School of Medicine; Associate Director of Pediatric Urology, Children's Hospital of Michigan, Detroit, Michigan

LATTIMER, JOHN K., M.D., Sc.D., F.A.C.S.: Professor and Chairman, Department of Urology, Columbia University College of Physicians and Surgeons; Director, Squier Urological Clinic, New York, New York

LEAPE, LUCIAN L., M.D., F.A.C.S.: Professor of Surgery, Tufts University School of Medicine; Chief of Pediatric Surgery, New England Medical Center, Boston, Massachusetts

LEBOWITZ, ROBERT L., M.D.: Assistant Professor, Department of Radiology, Harvard Medical School; Senior Associate in Radiology, Assistant in Urologic Surgery, Children's Hospital Medical Center, Boston, Massachusetts

LEV, MAURICE, M.D., F.A.C.C.: Distinguished Professor, Departments of Pediatrics, Internal Medicine and Pathology, Rush Medical College; Director, Congenital Heart Disease Research and Training Center, Chicago, Illinois

LILLY, JOHN R., M.D., F.A.C.S.: Professor of Surgery; Chief, Pediatric Surgery, University of Colorado School of Medicine, Denver, Colorado

LINDESMITH, GEORGE G., M.D.: Associate Clinical Professor of Surgery, University of Southern California School of Medicine; Head, Division of Thoracic and Cardiovascular Surgery, Children's Hospital of Los Angeles, Los Angeles, California

LINDSAY, WILLIAM K., M.D., F.R.C.S. (C), F.A.C.S.: Professor of Surgery, University of Toronto Faculty of Medicine; Chief, Division of Plastic Surgery, Hospital for Sick Children, Toronto, Ontario

LLOYD, JAMES R., M.D., F.A.C.S., F.A.A.P.: Assistant Clinical Professor of Surgery, Wayne State University School of Medicine; Attending Surgeon and Director, Burn Center, Children's Hospital of Michigan, Detroit, Michigan

LONG, DONLIN M., M.D., Ph.D.: Professor and Chairman, Department of Neurosurgery, The Johns Hopkins University School of Medicine, The Johns Hopkins Hospital, Baltimore, Maryland

LYNN, HUGH B., M.D., F.A.C.S.: Professor of Surgery, University of Alabama School of Medicine and Medical Center, Children's Hospital, Birmingham, Alabama

MALM, JAMES R., M.D.: Professor of Clinical Surgery, Columbia University College of Physicians and Surgeons, New York, New York

MARTIN, LESTER W., M.D., F.A.C.S. Professor of Surgery and Pediatrics, University of Cincinnati College of Medicine; Director of Pediatric Surgery, Children's Hospital, Cincinnati, Ohio

MAUER, S. MICHAEL, M.D.: Associate Professor of Pediatrics, University of Minnesota Medical School, Minneapolis, Minnesota

McGOON, DWIGHT C., M.D.: Stuart W. Harrington Professor of Surgery, Mayo Medical School; Section of Thoracic, Cardiovascular and General Surgery, Mayo Clinic, Rochester, Minnesota

McPARLAND, FELIX A., M.D.: Clinical Professor of Surgery, University of Minnesota Medical School, Minneapolis Children's Health Center, Minneapolis, Minnesota

McQUEEN, J. DONALD, M.D., F.R.C.S. (C), F.A.C.S.: Professor of Clinical Neurological Sciences, University of Saskatchewan College of Medicine, Saskatoon, Saskatchewan

MELICOW, MEYER M., M.D.: Given Professor Emeritus of Uropathology Research and Special Lecturer in Uropathology,

Columbia University College of Physicians and Surgeons, New York, New York

MICHELI, LYLE J., M.D.: Instructor of Orthopedic Surgery, Harvard Medical School; Director, Division of Sports Medicine, Children's Hospital Medical Center, Boston, Massachusetts

MILLER, RICHARD C., M.D., F.A.C.S., F.A.A.P.,: Associate Dean, Professor of Pediatric Surgery, University of Mississippi School of Medicine, Jackson, Mississippi

MULLIKEN, JOHN B., M.D., F.A.C.S.: Associate Professor of Surgery, Harvard Medical School; Assistant in Surgery, Children's Hospital Medical Center; Junior Associate in Surgery, Peter Bent Brigham Hospital, Boston, Massachusetts

MUNRO, IAN R., M.B., F.R.C.S. (C): Assistant Professor, Department of Surgery, University of Toronto Faculty of Medicine; Staff Plastic Surgeon, Hospital for Sick Children; Staff Plastic Surgeon, Sunnybrook Hospital, Toronto, Ontario

MURRAY, JOSEPH E., M.D., F.A.C.S.: Professor of Surgery, Harvard Medical School; Chief of Plastic Surgery, Children's Hospital Medical Center and Peter Bent Brigham Hospital, Boston Massachusetts

MYERS, NATHAN A., M.D.: Professorial Associate, University of Melbourne; Chairman, Department of Surgery, Royal Children's Hospital, Melbourne, Australia

NAJARIAN, JOHN S., M.D.: Professor and Chairman, Department of Surgery, University of Minnesota Medical School, Minneapolis, Minnesota

NOBLETT, HELEN, M.D., F.R.A.C.S.: Consultant Paediatric Surgeon, Bristol Royal Hospital for Sick Children, Bristol, England

NORWOOD, WILLIAM I., M.D., Ph.D.: Assistant Professor of Surgery, Harvard Medical School; Senior Associate in Cardiovascular Surgery, Children's Hospital Medical Center, Boston, Massachusetts

O'NEILL, JAMES A., JR., M.D., F.A.C.S.: Professor and Chairman, Department of Pediatric Surgery, Vanderbilt University School of Medicine, Nashville, Tennessee

PACIFICO, ALBERT D., M.D., F.A.C.S.: Professor of Surgery, University of Alabama School of Medicine and Medical Center, Birmingham, Alabama

PASHBY, ROBERT C., M.D., F.R.C.S. (C): Clinical Teacher, University of Toronto Faculty of Medicine; Staff Ophthalmologist, Hospital for Sick Children, Toronto, Ontario

PERLMUTTER, ALAN D., M.D., F.A.C.S.: Professor of Urology, Wayne State University School of Medicine; Chief, Department of Pediatric Urology, Children's Hospital of Michigan, Detroit, Michigan

PHILIPPART, ARVIN I., M.D., F.A.C.S.: Associate Professor of Surgery, Wayne State University School of Medicine; Chief of Pediatric General Surgery, Children's Hospital of Michigan, Detroit, Michigan

PITTS, R. MARSHALL, M.D.: Clinical Assistant Professor of Surgery, University of Alabama School of Medicine and Medical Center; Staff, Children's Hospital, Birmingham, Alabama

PITTS, WILLIAM J., M.D.: Chairman, Department of Plastic and Reconstructive Surgery, St. Vincent's Hospital, Birmingham, Alabama

RANDOLPH, JUDSON G., M.D., F.A.C.S.: Professor of Surgery, George Washington University School of Medicine and Health Sciences; Surgeon-in-Chief, Children's Hospital, Washington, D.C.

RAPHAELY, RUSSELL C., M.D.: Assistant Professor of Anesthesia and Medical Director, Pediatric Intensive Care Unit, Children's Hospital of Philadelphia, Philadelphia, Pennsylvania

RAVITCH, MARK M., M.D., F.A.C.S.: Professor of Surgery, University of Pittsburgh School of Medicine; Surgeon-in-Chief, Montefiore Hospital, Pittsburgh, Pennsylvania

RECTOR, FREDERICK E., M.D.: Attending Surgeon, Memorial Mission Hospital and St. Joseph Hospital, Asheville, North Carolina

REED, JOSEPH O., M.D.: Clinical Professor of Radiology, Wayne State University School of Medicine; Chief of Radiology, Children's Hospital of Michigan, Detroit, Michigan

RETIK, ALAN B., M.D., F.A.C.S.: Associate Professor of Urologic Surgery, Harvard Medical School; Chief, Division of Urology, Children's Hospital Medical Center, Boston, Massachusetts

RISEBOROUGH, EDWARD J., M.D.: Senior Associate in Orthopaedic Surgery, Children's Hospital Medical Center, Boston, Massachusetts

ROSENTHAL, ROBERT K., M.D., F.A.C.S.: Instructor in Orthopaedic Surgery, Harvard Medical School; Associate in Orthopaedic Surgery, Children's Hospital Medical Center, Boston, Massachusetts

ROWE, MARC I., M.D., F.A.C.S.: Professor of Surgery and Pediatrics, Chief, Division of Pediatric Surgery, University of Miami School of Medicine, Miami, Florida

RUSH, BENJAMIN F., JR., M.D., F.A.C.S.: Johnson and Johnson Professor of Surgery, Chairman, Department of Surgery, New Jersey Medical School, Newark, New Jersey

SABISTON, DAVID C., JR., M.D.: James B. Duke Professor and Chairman, Department of Surgery, Duke University School of Medicine, Durham, North Carolina

SANTULLI, THOMAS V., M.D., F.A.C.S.: Professor of Surgery, Columbia University College of Physicians and Surgeons; Attending Surgeon, Columbia-Presbyterian Medical Center; Chief, Pediatric Surgical Service, Babies Hospital, New York, New York

SCHNEIDER, KEITH M., M.D.: Clinical Professor of Surgery and Pediatrics, Albert Einstein College of Medicine; Director, Pediatric Surgery, Hospital of the Albert Einstein College of Medicine, Bronx, New York

SCHUSTER, SAMUEL R., M.D., F.A.C.S.: Associate Clinical Professor of Surgery, Harvard Medical School; Associate Chief of Surgery, Children's Hospital Medical Center, Boston, Massachusetts

SCHWARTZ, MARSHALL Z., M.D.: Instructor in Surgery, Harvard Medical School; Assistant in Surgery, Children's Hospital Medical Center, Boston, Massachusetts

SCOTT, WILLIAM W., Ph.D., M.D., D.Sc.: David Hall McConnell Professor of Urology Emeritus, The Brady Urological Institute, The Johns Hopkins University School of Medicine, The Johns Hopkins Hospital, Baltimore, Maryland

SHAW, ANTHONY, M.D., F.A.C.S.: Professor of Surgery and Pediatrics, University of Virginia School of Medicine; Chief, Pediatric Surgical Division, Department of Surgery, University of Virginia Medical Center, Charlottesville, Virginia

SIEBER, WILLIAM K., M.D., F.A.C.S.: Clinical Professor of Surgery, University of Pittsburgh School of Medicine; Senior Staff, Surgery, Children's Hospital of Pittsburgh, Pittsburgh, Pennsylvania

SLOAN, HERBERT E., JR., M.D., F.A.C.S., F.A.A.P.: Professor and Head, Section of Thoracic Surgery, University of Michigan Hospital, Ann Arbor, Michigan

SOPER, ROBERT T., M.D.: Professor of Surgery, University of Iowa College of Medicine; Director of Pediatric Surgical Services, University of Iowa Hospitals and Clinics, Iowa City, Iowa

STARK, JAROSLAV, M.D.: Consultant Cardiothoracic Surgeon, Hospital for Sick Children, London, England

STEICHEN, FELICIEN M., M.D., F.A.C.S.: Professor of Surgery, New York Medical College; Director of Surgery, Lenox Hill Hospital, Valhalla, New York

STEPHENS, F. DOUGLAS, M.S. (Melb), F.R.A.C.S.: Professor of Surgery and Urology, Northwestern University Medical School; Urologist, Department of Urology, Children's Memorial Hospital, Chicago, Illinois; formerly Royal Children's Hospital, Melbourne, Australia

STONE, H. HARLAN, M.D. F.A.C.S., F.A.A.P., F.A.P.S.: Professor of Surgery, Emory University School of Medicine; Director of Pediatric Surgery, Burn, and Trauma Services, Grady Memorial Hospital; Director, Surgical Bacteriology Laboratory, Emory University School of Medicine, Atlanta, Georgia

SUBRAMANIAN, S., M.D.: Professor of Surgery, State University of New York at Buffalo School of Medicine; Chief, Division of Cardiovascular Surgery, Children's Hospital, Buffalo, New York

THOMPSON, J. S., M.D.: Professor of Anatomy, University of Toronto Faculty of Medicine, Toronto, Ontario

THOMPSON, MARGARET W., Ph.D.: Professor of Medical Genetics, University of Toronto Faculty of Medicine; Senior Staff Geneticist, The Hospital for Sick Children, Toronto, Ontario

THOMSON, HUGH G., M.D.: Associate Professor of Surgery, University of Toronto Faculty of Medicine, Plastic Surgeon, Hospital for Sick Children, Toronto, Ontario

THOMSON, SANDRA J., M.D.: Instructor in Orthopedic Surgery, Harvard Medical School; Associate in Orthopedic Surgery, Children's Hospital Medical Center, Boston, Massachusetts

TOULOUKIAN, ROBERT J., M.D., F.A.C.S.: Professor of Surgery and Pediatrics, Yale University School of Medicine; Chief, Pediatric Surgery, Yale–New Haven Hospital, New Haven, Connecticut

TROTT, ARTHUR W., M.D.: Clinical Instructor of Orthopedic Surgery, Harvard Medical School; Senior Associate in Orthopedic Surgery, Children's Hospital Medical Center, Boston, Massachusetts

TRUMP, DAVID S., M.D., F.A.C.S., F.A.A.P.: Chief, Section of Pediatric Surgery, Maricopa County Hospital; Pediatric Surgeon, St. Joseph's Hospital and Good Samaritan Hospital, Phoenix, Arizona

TRUSLER, GEORGE A., M.D., F.R.C.S. (C), F.A.C.S.: Associate Professor of Surgery, University of Toronto Faculty of Medicine; Chief, Division of Cardiovascular Surgery, Hospital for Sick Children, Toronto, Ontario

UDVARHELYI, GEORGE B., M.D., F.A.C.S.: Professor of Neurosurgery and Associate Professor of Radiology, The Johns Hopkins University School of Medicine; Neurosurgeon, The Johns Hopkins Hospital, Baltimore, Maryland

USON, AURELIO C., M.D., F.A.C.S.: Professor and Chairman, Department of Urology, San Carlos Hospital Medical School; Complutense University, Madrid, Spain

VON BERG, VOLLRAD J., M.D., F.A.C.S., F.A.A.P.: Clinical Assistant Professor, Department of Surgery, Wayne State University School of Medicine; Attending Staff, Children's Hospital of Michigan, Detroit, Michigan

WALKER, A. EARL, M.D.: Professor of Neurosurgery Emeritus, The Johns Hopkins University School of Medicine, The Johns Hopkins Hospital, Baltimore, Maryland

WALSH, PATRICK C., M.D., F.A.C.S.: Professor and Director, Department of Urology, The Johns Hopkins University School of Medicine; Urologist-in-Chief, Brady Urological Institute, The Johns Hopkins Hospital, Baltimore, Maryland

WATTS, HUGH G., M.D.: Assistant Professor of Orthopedics, Harvard Medical School; Senior Associate, Department of Orthopedics, Children's Hospital Medical Center, Boston, Massachusetts

WECHSLER, MICHAEL, M.D., F.A.C.S.: Assistant Professor of Clinical Urology, Columbia University College of Physicians and Surgeons; Assistant Attending Physician, Cancer Research Center, Harlem Hospital—Presbyterian Hospital, New York, New York

WELCH, KENNETH J., M.D., F.A.C.S.: Associate Clinical Professor of Surgery, Harvard Medical School; Senior Associate in Surgery, Children's Hospital Medical Center, Boston, Massachusetts

WELDON, CLARENCE S., M.D.: Professor of Surgery and Professor of Pediatrics, Washington University School of Medicine; Chief, Cardiothoracic Surgery, Barnes Hospital and St. Louis Children's Hospital, St. Louis, Missouri

WIENER, EUGENE S., M.D.: Clinical Assistant Professor of

Pediatric Surgery, University of Pittsburgh School of Medicine; Attending Staff, Children's Hospital of Pittsburgh, Pittsburgh, Pennsylvania

WILLIAMS, D. INNES, M.D., M. CHIR., F.R.C.S.: Senior Lecturer in Urology, Institute of Child Health, University of London; Consultant Urologist, Hospital for Sick Children, London, England

WILLIAMS, WILLIAM G., M.D.: Assistant Professor of Surgery, University of Toronto Faculty of Medicine; Staff Surgeon, Hospital for Sick Children, and Toronto General Hospital, Toronto, Ontario

WOOLLEY, MORTON M., M.D., F.A.C.S.: Professor of Surgery, University of Southern California School of Medicine; Surgeon-in-Chief, Children's Hospital of Los Angeles, Los Angeles, California

WOOLLEY, PAUL V., JR., M.D.: Professor of Pediatrics and Chairman Emeritus, Department of Pediatrics, Wayne State University School of Medicine; Pediatrician-in-Chief Emeritus and Director of the Growth and Development Clinic, Children's Hospital of Michigan, Detroit, Michigan

WUKASCH, DON C., M.D., F.A.C.S., F.A.C.C., F.A.C.C.P.: Associate Surgeon, Texas Heart Institute of St. Luke's Episcopal and Texas Children's Hospitals; Clinical Associate Professor, University of Texas Medical School, Houston, Texas

Table of Contents

VOLUME 1

PART I
General

PART II
Trauma

PART III
Head and Neck

PART IV
The Thorax
and
Cardiovascular
System

Table of Contents

PART VI
Genitourinary System

PART VII
Integument and Musculoskeletal System

PART VIII
The Nervous
System

Color Plates

PEDIATRIC SURGERY

Volume 1

PART I

General

1
Genetics M. W. Thompson / J. S. Thompson

MANY DISORDERS OF INTEREST to pediatric surgeons are caused at least in part by genetic factors. Among these conditions perhaps the most important are congenital malformations, which result from some disruption of the normal process of morphogenesis. The process of morphogenesis is determined at each step by genes, but the expression of the genes depends on environment; thus, dysmorphism can have an entirely genetic origin, can arise solely through certain environmental alterations even when the genetic potential itself allows for normal development or can be produced by gene-environment interaction. Understanding of the genetic background of a congenital malformation is a prerequisite for determination of the recurrence risk in the family members and the range of variability of the clinical expression. The genetic aspects of a number of pediatric disorders are described in the appropriate sections of these volumes; the purpose of this chapter is to describe briefly the general principles that underlie medical genetics and to point out how genetics may assist in the evaluation of patients with congenital malformations.

Three categories of genetic defect are recognized: single-gene, chromosomal and multifactorial. In *single-gene disorders*, the genetic basis is an abnormality in a major gene, in single or double dose. In *chromosomal disorders*, some gross abnormality of chromosome number or structure produces genetic imbalance, which leads to a relatively well-defined syndrome of congenital malformations, often associated with mental retardation. In *multifactorial disorders*, including many common congenital malformations, the defect is determined by many genes acting together, each with only a minor effect, and sometimes also in part by environmental factors. For completeness, a fourth category may be added: *birth defects of nongenetic origin*. There is a growing list of malformation syndromes in which an environmental insult to the fetus appears to play a role, but in many of these the fetal or maternal genotype may also have an effect.

Single-Gene Disorders

The genetic information of the human zygote and the individual developing from it is contained in its double set of chromosomes, one set from each parent. The individual in turn passes on to each offspring one complete chromosome set comprising one member of each chromosome pair. The double chromosome set of 46 includes 22 pairs of *autosomes* and one pair of *sex chromosomes* (XY in males, XX in females). Each gene has a specific position (*locus*) on a specific chromosome. The genes in the same locus on each of a chromosome pair are *alleles* of one another. With the exception of genes on the X and Y in males, all genes are present in pairs.

The gene has a double role: determination of the structure of a particular polypeptide chain and transmission of the genetic code for that polypeptide to subsequent generations. A gene may undergo a change or *mutation*, leading to the synthesis of an altered gene product, usually one that differs

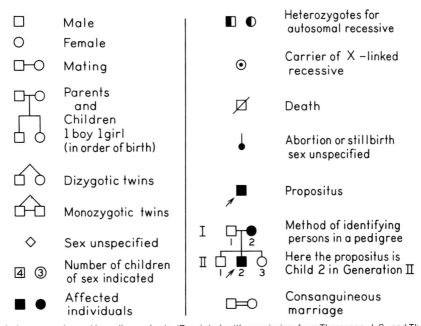

Fig. 1-1.—Symbols commonly used in pedigree charts. (Reprinted, with permission, from Thompson, J. S., and Thompson, M. W., *Genetics in Medicine* [2d ed.; Philadelphia: W. B. Saunders Company, 1973].)

from the normal polypeptide only in the substitution of one amino acid for another at some specific site on the chain. Although the biochemical difference at the level of the gene and its immediate product is slight, the ultimate consequences may be extensive, even catastrophic.

A gene is referred to as *autosomal* if it is on one of the 22 pairs of autosomes or *X-linked* if it is on the X. (The Y carries no mutant genes of clinical importance.) If a mutant gene is expressed in single dose (i.e., when present on only one member of a chromosome pair, matched with its normal allele on the other member of the pair), it is referred to as *dominant;* if it is expressed only when present in double dose, it is referred to as *recessive.* (As an exception, a recessive on the single X of males always is expressed, because it has no allelé to modify its expression.) If both alleles of a pair are alike, the individual is *homozygous* in that respect; if different, he is *heterozygous.* Note that dominance and recessivity refer only to the phenotypic expression of the gene and are not properties of the gene itself; at the molecular level, both alleles of any autosomal pair are active, but in heterozygotes the phenotypic expression may depend chiefly on one member of the pair, and that member then is said to be dominant. (In females, because of X-inactivation, only one of each pair of X-linked genes is active; this special situation is described in more detail later.)

McKusick[1] has enumerated more than 2300 single-gene

traits, with brief descriptions and key references. Such traits are said to be "Mendelian" because their transmission through families is in accordance with the laws of heredity discovered by Mendel in 1865. Typical pedigree symbols used as a shorthand method of presenting family history information are shown in Figure 1–1.

Autosomal Dominants

In clinical genetics, autosomal dominant disorders typically are seen in heterozygotes, i.e., in persons having a single dose of the abnormal gene paired with a normal allele. If an individual is homozygous for an autosomal dominant mutation, the expression of the defect usually is much more severe. The risk that any one child of an affected person will receive the gene is 50%. However, for some conditions, the probability that the disorder actually will be expressed in a clinically significant form may be lower than 50%, because there may be great variability in the expression of an autosomal dominant, even within a single family. The trait may be completely unexpressed (nonpenetrant) in some family members who have inherited the gene responsible for it or it may show variable expression, being severe in some members and milder in others. Autosomal dominant ectrodactyly, a developmental malformation of the hand and foot, is an example of a condition that may either be expressed as a

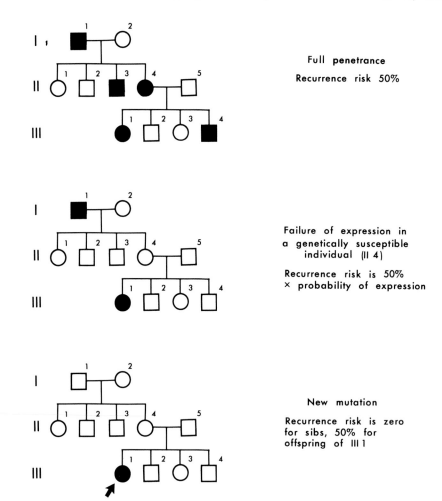

Full penetrance

Recurrence risk 50%

Failure of expression in a genetically susceptible individual (II 4)

Recurrence risk is 50% × probability of expression

New mutation

Recurrence risk is zero for sibs, 50% for offspring of III 1

Fig. 1-2. — Typical pedigrees of autosomal dominant inheritance.

severe defect or remain completely nonpenetrant. In contrast, neurofibromatosis is penetrant to some degree in almost all heterozygotes but widely variable in expression. For conditions with reduced penetrance or variable expressivity, it may be difficult to know on casual examination whether a family member who has no overt expression of the gene is heterozygous or a normal homozygote, although careful examination sometimes will reveal minor stigmata.

In the analysis of a suspected autosomal dominant disorder, it is of primary importance to know whether the defect has been inherited from a previous generation or whether the patient is a new mutant. New mutants are rare, but for certain types of genetic defect they may form a large proportion of the total patient group. As a general rule, the more severe the defect and the more it interferes with normal reproduction the higher the probability that a given patient is a new mutant. As an example, patients with Apert syndrome usually are new mutants and rarely reproduce, but when an Apert patient does have a child, that child has a 50% risk of the disorder. One probable, undesirable, result of the admirable advances that have been made in the surgical treatment of craniofacial disorders such as Apert syndrome in the past decade is that the cosmetic improvement will increase the patient's likelihood of having a child, who (if the defect is autosomal dominant) has a 50% chance of inheriting it. The long-range consequence then will be an increased population frequency of the defect. Because of the genetic risk, genetic analysis and genetic counseling always should be a part of the management of such patients.

For pediatric problems, genetic counseling usually involves parents of an affected child, who are primarily concerned about the recurrence risk for their subsequent children. In such cases, firm identification of a defect as a new mutation means that the parents can be assured that it is very unlikely that they could have another child with the same defect, although their affected child's chance of transmitting it is 50%. If the disorder is known to have variable expression, it is important to examine the parents, other children in the family and other relatives at risk to attempt to identify minor stigmata. It is also important to ensure that the defect is characterized as accurately and completely as possible, since defects that are superficially similar may have quite different genetic patterns.

Pedigrees illustrating autosomal dominant inheritance are shown in Figure 1–2.

Autosomal Recessives

Autosomal recessive disorders typically are seen in patients who have a double dose of a mutant gene, inherited from clinically normal parents, each of whom has a single dose of the gene matched with a normal allele, as shown in Figure 1–3. The risk that any subsequent child of the same parents will have the same gene pair and the same disorder is 25%. For any other relatives, the risk is much lower, because an autosomal recessive is expressed only when the abnormal gene is present in double dose, i.e., inherited from both parents, and the odds are against other heterozygotes marrying into the family, because heterozygotes are much less common than homozygous normals. When a disease frequency is known, the heterozygote frequency can be calculated as "double the square root of the disease frequency"; for cystic fibrosis, with a disease frequency of about 1/2000 in Caucasians, the heterozygote frequency is $2\sqrt{1/2000}$, or 1 in 22. The probability that both parents carry the same recessive mutant and thus can have a child with a double dose of the mutant is enhanced if the parents are related by descent, so parental consanguinity is strong evidence (although not proof) of recessive inheritance.

New mutation of either member of the gene pair in the patient is an unlikely finding in autosomal recessive pedigrees; simply on the basis of chance, it is much more likely that both mutant alleles have been inherited and that both parents are heterozygotes.

Autosomal recessives are more consistent in their expression than are autosomal dominants. This probably is because, in the homozygote, both alleles of a gene pair determine the same product whereas in the heterozygote, the two alleles have different products. Enzyme defects usually are autosomal recessive, suggesting that the product of a single normal allele in a clinically normal heterozygote is enough to produce an adequate functional level of the given enzyme, only the homozygous deficiency being functionally abnormal.

In discussing the evaluation of autosomal dominants, we noted the importance of distinguishing new dominant mutations from inherited ones with clinical expression so variable that recognition of the presence of the gene in the heterozygous parent is difficult. It is also often necessary to attempt to distinguish new dominant mutations from autosomal recessives. This distinction may be of serious practical

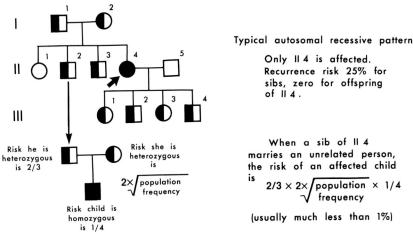

Fig. 1-3.—A pedigree of autosomal recessive inheritance, showing calculation of the recurrence risk for the subsequent generation.

significance. For example, in counseling for the numerous genetically diverse forms of dwarfism, if a disorder in the first affected child of clinically normal parents is due to a new dominant mutation, it is unlikely to recur in sibs but has a 50% risk for each child of the patient; but if it is an autosomal recessive there is a 25% risk for sibs but a very low probability that it will appear in offspring of the patient. For many rare types of dwarfism, the distinction between the two patterns can be made, if at all, only on the basis of the clinical and radiologic features and from previous experience with patients of the same phenotype. If there is no helpful information in the literature, a clue to autosomal recessive inheritance may be provided by parental consanguinity (or, less reliably, by closely similar ethnic or geographic background).

X-Linked Disorders

The definitions of dominance and recessivity that apply to autosomal disorders break down to some extent when applied to X-linked characteristics. This is because males, who have a single X chromosome, express any mutant gene on the X, whether that gene is dominant or recessive in female heterozygotes.

An X-linked recessive condition should be suspected when the patient is male and related to other affected males in the pedigree through unaffected females. As a general rule, as Figure 1–4 illustrates, X-linked recessive disorders

are expressed only in males and are transmitted in the family only through heterozygous females, who are unaffected. All the sons of an affected male are normal and all the daughters are carriers (heterozygotes). Each son of a carrier has a 50% risk of being affected and each daughter has a 50% risk of being a carrier. Hemophilia A is a classic example of this pattern of inheritance.

X-linked dominants, which are uncommon, are expressed in both male and female but can be distinguished from autosomal dominants by the pattern of transmission of the trait from affected males; a male with an X-linked dominant condition has no normal daughters and no affected sons. The transmission pattern by females cannot be distinguished from the autosomal dominant pattern.

Many X-linked traits, especially if they are severe and interfere with normal reproduction, frequently appear as new mutants in otherwise normal families. In such cases, genetic counseling can be difficult, because it involves determination of whether the patient's mother and any other females in the family are carriers. A common example in orthopedic surgery is Duchenne muscular dystrophy, in which an affected boy has a one-third probability of being a new mutant and another one-third chance of having a new-mutant mother; here, carrier detection tests and pedigree analysis with particular attention to the number of normal males in the history are of great importance (Murphy and Chase[2]).

In X-linked dominants, as noted above, affected males

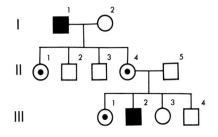

Typical X-linked recessive pattern

Recurrence risk is 50% for brothers of III 2; 50% risk that a sister will be a carrier

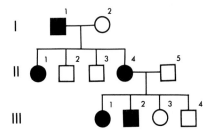

Typical X-linked dominant pattern

Recurrence risk is zero for brothers, 100% for sisters of II 4; 50% for offspring

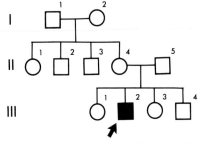

New mutation

Recurrence risk is zero in sibs, 50% in sons of daughters of III 2

Fig. 1-4. — Typical pedigrees of X-linked inheritance.

have no affected sons. However, the heterozygous daughters usually are less severely affected than the affected males in the family.

X-INACTIVATION AND MANIFESTATION IN HETEROZYGOTES. — The expression of X-linked genes is complicated by the fact that, in normal females, one X chromosome in each cell is inactive, appearing as the Barr body. The inactive X may be the one contributed to the female by the father (the paternal X) or the one contributed by the mother (the maternal X); the "decision" as to which X will be inactivated by a given cell appears to be made at random in a few-cell embryonic stage but to be permanent in the clonal descendants of the cell in which inactivation first occurred. Thus, females are mosaics with respect to their X chromosomes. As a consequence of the random nature of X-inactivation, some women heterozygous for X-linked genes actually may manifest the condition, although rarely as severely as do affected males. For example, the gene for hemophilia A may be clinically expressed, biochemically detectable or indistinguishable in heterozygous females, even within the same sibship (Graham et al.[3]), and a small proportion of carriers of Duchenne muscular dystrophy have enlarged calves or even muscle weakness (Kloepfer and Emery[4]).

Chromosomal Disorders

Errors of chromosome behavior at meiosis or in early mitotic divisions after formation of the zygote are a major cause of abnormal development. The abnormality results from the developmental confusion produced when the genes are not present in appropriate balance. Any discrepancy in chromosome number, whether excess or deficiency, or any aberration in chromosome structure resulting in an excess or deficiency of only a part of a chromosome may lead to abnormal development. On the whole, it is less damaging to have extra chromosomal material than to lack part of the double set and less damaging to have a sex chromosome anomaly than to have an autosomal anomaly. If the accident happens after the zygote has been formed, the resulting individual may be a *mosaic*, with a mixture of normal and abnormal cell lines, and in such cases the severity of the abnormality depends on what proportion of the cells have abnormal karyotypes.

About 1 in every 200 infants has a recognizable chromosomal abnormality. More than a quarter of these have Down syndrome (trisomy 21) and most of the remainder have some other form of trisomy. (Trisomy is the term used to describe the presence of one extra chromosome; consequently, three of one kind instead of the normal pair.) In abortuses, especially those that occur spontaneously in the first trimester, the proportion that are chromosomally abnormal is very much higher than in liveborns, approaching 50% of the abortuses and an estimated 4% of all pregnancies. The abnormalities that have been identified in abortuses include many that cause such severe damage that they rarely or never are seen in liveborns.

Not all chromosome abnormalities involve changes in chromosome number. A small proportion, about 2%, are structural changes resulting from chromosomal breakage.

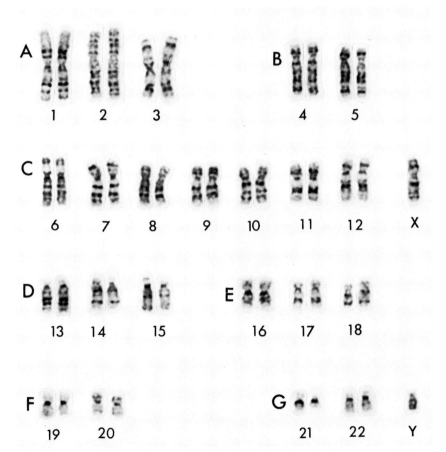

Fig. 1-5. — Normal male karyotype, with Giemsa stain, after pretreatment with trypsin. Analysis of "banding" patterns allows identification of individual chromosomes and permits identification of many previously undetectable lesions. An extra chromosome no. 21 is seen in most children with Down syndrome.

When a chromosome breakage occurs, a piece may be lost or there may be a rearrangement of the broken pieces in some abnormal configuration. Loss of part of a chromosome is termed *deletion*. The most common type of rearrangement is a *translocation*. When an individual carries a translocation in balanced form, he usually has an entirely normal phenotype. However, when he forms germ cells there is a high risk of an unbalanced gamete and consequently a chromosomally abnormal child. The phenotypes of such children are extremely variable, depending as they do on the specific chromosome segments involved.

The identification and characterization of syndromes determined by chromosomal abnormalities has been much improved in recent years by the development of a variety of special staining techniques that allow unequivocal identification of each chromosome of the set and permit recognition of many previously undetectable structural aberrations (Fig. 1–5).

Chromosome preparations can be made from any cell type that will divide in culture, but the usual sources are the leukocytes of peripheral blood, skin biopsies and, for prenatal diagnosis, cells in the amniotic fluid. For cultures set up from peripheral blood, the technique is to separate the white cells and grow them in culture for approximately 72 hours, then treat the culture with colchicine, which has the action of poisoning the mitotic spindle and thus accumulating metaphases in the culture. The cells then are subjected to treatment with hypotonic solution, which causes the two chromatids (of which any metaphase chromosome is composed) to swell and separate from each other, remaining attached, however, at the centromere. The chromosomes then are spread on slides, stained and photographed. Finally, the chromosomes are counted and analyzed.

When an abnormal number of X chromosomes is suspected, a buccal smear may be examined for sex chromatin bodies (Barr bodies). All but one of the X chromosomes present in the cell are represented in interphase cells as Barr bodies; thus, the number of Barr bodies is always one less than the number of X chromosomes in the cell. Chromosome analysis provides the same information, especially with the newer staining techniques, but buccal smears still can provide useful preliminary information.

Indications for Chromosome Analysis

Chromosome analysis forms part of the evaluation of two main types of patients: (1) those in whom a chromosome disorder is probable on the basis of the phenotype or is suspected because the child has multiple malformations and mental retardation and (2) patients with ambiguous genitalia or delayed sexual development. If a child is found to have a structural type of chromosomal abnormality, such as translocation, it then is necessary to test both parents to determine whether either one carries the abnormality in balanced form or whether the abnormality is a new occurrence in the patient. If one parent carries the abnormality, the recurrence risk is high and there is a need to extend chromosome studies in that parent's family to look for other carriers who may be at risk.

The use of chromosome analysis in prenatal diagnosis is discussed in a later section.

Abnormalities of structure arise when a chromosome, or two or even more, breaks and is reconstituted in an abnormal arrangement. Several of the possible rearrangements are not harmful to the individual, as they are balanced; i.e., all the chromosome material is present in normal amount, but it is arranged abnormally and thus there is a risk of producing an unbalanced offspring.

Autosomal Trisomies

There are three autosomal trisomies that can be compatible with postnatal life. These are trisomy 21 (Down syndrome, mongolism), trisomy 18 (E trisomy) and trisomy 13 (D trisomy). Trisomies of other autosomes have been seen in abortuses but only rarely in liveborn infants, and the corresponding monosomies are even more rare. The abnormalities associated with trisomy 18 and trisomy 13 are so severe that children with these defects are unlikely to be candidates for operative correction. However, Down syndrome children may be born with a number of types of operable defects, of which the most common are heart lesions (especially A-V canal defects, tetralogy of Fallot and ventricular septal defect), tracheoesophageal fistula, esophageal atresia and duodenal atresia. Because the affected children are mentally retarded and may have other associated defects, the ethical problem of whether or not to operate may be a difficult one for the surgeon and the parents alike. Decisions about surgical intervention require consideration of all the individual child's problems, not only the immediate operative indication.

Sex Chromosome Abnormalities

There are two common syndromes associated with sex chromosome abnormalities: the Turner syndrome, female phenotype with 45 chromosomes including a single X, and the Klinefelter syndrome, male phenotype with 47 chromosomes including two Xs and a Y. The XYY syndrome and the XXX syndrome also rate mention. XYY individuals perhaps are more notorious for violent behavior than they deserve, but rarely are severely abnormal; occasionally, radioulnar synostosis, cryptorchidism and hypospadias are seen. The XXX karyotype may be associated with retardation or infertility, but many XXX females are quite normal. Sex chromosome constitutions with greater numbers of X and/or Y chromosomes are found occasionally, and these present exaggerated degrees of physical and mental abnormality. Mosaicism is also common among individuals with karyotypes that differ from the standard 46,XX and 46,XY.

XO TURNER SYNDROME. – Patients with Turner syndrome may come to surgical attention for a variety of reasons, including cosmetic surgery for neck webbing, protruding auricles and prominent inner canthal folds. They frequently have cardiovascular problems, especially coarctation of the aorta. Although renal anomalies such as horseshoe kidney are frequent, they do not usually affect the patient's health. Short stature and ovarian dysgenesis are present in virtually all patients with Turner syndrome.

Apart from the classic XO karyotype, stigmata of Turner syndrome are seen in a number of structural anomalies of the X chromosome and in mosaics with more than one cell line, such as XO/XX. The recurrence risk for any of these anomalies within a family is quite low.

XXY KLINEFELTER SYNDROME. – Although Klinefelter syndrome is a common disorder, affecting about 1 in 500 males, it may not be diagnosed until puberty. The patients typically are tall and slender, intellectually slightly retarded, often with hypogonadism and hypogenitalism, but otherwise indistinguishable in the population until features of testosterone insufficiency become apparent at puberty.

The chief surgical problem is likely to be gynecomastia, seen in about 40% of cases. Cryptorchidism, hypospadias and scoliosis are seen occasionally.

Klinefelter syndrome has been known to recur in families and to appear in sibships with other trisomies.

Ambiguous Genitalia

Chromosome analysis is a necessary part of the evaluation of patients with ambiguous genitalia. Especially in newborns, the test should precede a decision as to sex of rearing. Some cases of ambiguous genitalia have their basis in a single-gene defect (e.g., congenital adrenal hyperplasia, Opitz syndrome of hypertelorism and hypospadias or feminizing testes syndrome). Others are associated with rare chromosomal abnormalities, such as XO/XY or XX/XY. Many are difficult to analyze. The chromosomal sex, the specific diagnosis and possibility of treatment and the anatomy of the child's external and internal genitalia must all be taken into account in determining the sex of rearing.

Because of the risk of malignancy, it is advisable to remove any intra-abdominal testicular tissue.

Discrepancy between chromosomal sex and phenotypic sex, although rare, is not unknown. Examples are phenotypic males with an XX karyotype and phenotypic females with an XY karyotype who also have the X-linked gene for feminizing testes. The presence of inguinal hernias containing testes in infants with female or ambiguous external genitalia is a useful clue to the feminizing testes syndrome.

Multifactorial Inheritance

Many normal characteristics are inherited by numerous genes individually of small effect, and sometimes under considerable environmental influence. Such characteristics typically follow a normal curve of distribution; examples include many of the quantitative characteristics commonly measured in routine tests, where the decision as to whether a particular measurement is "normal" depends on how it compares with values found in an appropriate control series. Thus, multifactorial traits behave genetically as though liability toward the trait shows continuous variation; but for malformations with this type of inheritance, the underlying variation is divided into two categories, normal and abnormal, by a *threshold* (Fig. 1–6).

The family history of a multifactorial condition shows no simple, consistent pattern of transmission, but *empirical recurrence risks* can be determined by analysis of large series of families. The recurrence risk varies with the population frequency of the malformation, the sex of the affected child, the number and sex of affected family members, the number and sex of normal family members and the severity of the malformation.

The risk declines sharply with more distant degrees of relationship. For a typical congenital malformation with a population frequency of about 1:1000, the risk is (very approximately) 5% in first-degree relatives or, more precisely, the square root of the population frequency. It is less than 1% in second-degree relatives (e.g., nephews, nieces, grandchildren) and only about 0.2% in third-degree relatives (e.g., first cousins).

Other significant points about the familial distribution of multifactorial malformations are:

1. The sex ratio may be uneven and, if so, the sex *less* likely to be affected is the sex *more* likely to have affected sibs or offspring.

2. The more severe the expression of the defect the more likely it is to recur.

3. When two children in a family, or parent and child, are affected, the risk for subsequent children rises from 5% to 10% or more.

PYLORIC STENOSIS.—Pyloric stenosis was the first congenital malformation in which multifactorial inheritance was demonstrated (Carter and Evans[5]). The risks of pyloric stenosis in first-degree relatives are approximately as follows:

Male relatives of male patients 1/25
Female relatives of male patients . . . 1/37
Male relatives of female patients . . . 1/11
Female relatives of female patients . 1/25

These figures show the influence of sex on recurrence risk, especially for a condition with a much greater frequency in one sex than the other. Pyloric stenosis is 5 times as common in males in the general population, and its recurrence risk is higher in males, but higher in relatives of affected females than in relatives of affected males.

CONGENITAL HEART DEFECTS.—Heart malformations, as a group, have low recurrence risks, the risk for any one defect in sibs of index patients being close to the square root of the population risk, as expected for multifactorial traits. Risk figures based on data of Nora[6] for several congenital heart

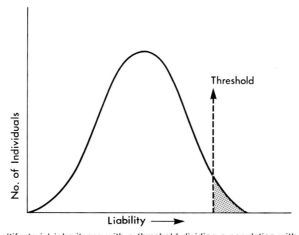

Fig. 1-6.—Model of multifactorial inheritance with a threshold dividing a population with underlying continuous variability into "normal" and "abnormal" classes.

TABLE 1-1.—CONGENITAL HEART DEFECTS:
POPULATION RISK AND EXPECTED
RECURRENCE RISK IN SIBS°

TYPE OF DEFECT	POPULATION RISK (p)	RECURRENCE RISK IN SIBS ($\sqrt{p}$)
Ventricular septal defect	1/400	1/20
Patent ductus arteriosus	1/800	1/28
Tetralogy of Fallot	1/1000	1/32
Atrial septal defect	1/1000	1/32
Pulmonic stenosis	1/1200	1/35
Aortic stenosis	1/2300	1/48
Coarctation of aorta	1/1700	1/41
Transposition of great vessels	1/2100	1/46
Atrioventricular canal	1/2500	1/50
Tricuspid atresia	1/5000	1/70
Ebstein's anomaly	1/20,000	1/140
Truncus arteriosus	1/20,000	1/140
Pulmonic atresia	1/10,000	1/100

°Based on data of Nora.[6]

lesions are given in Table 1-1. Much remains to be learned about the family patterns of heart defects, their concordance or group associations within families and their genetic heterogeneity.

NEURAL TUBE DEFECTS.—Anencephaly and spina bifida have been the subject of numerous investigations, in which exhaustive attempts have been made to identify environmental factors that might contribute to the wide variations in incidence shown by these etiologically related conditions in relation to geography, ethnic background, season of birth, parental socioeconomic background, dietary factors and other variables. Although it is not clear what part, if any, environmental factors play, the family patterns and empirical risks best fit multifactorial inheritance. Table 1-2 shows approximate risk figures based on data of Carter and Evans[7] for sibs of patients, indicating the increase in risk with an increase in the number of other affected family members and their degree of closeness of relationship.

Because the risk of recurrence is high and the handicap suffered by many surviving children with spina bifida is severe, it is fortunate that prenatal diagnosis of most neural tube defects now is practical (see later).

CLEFT LIP AND CLEFT PALATE.—The genetic aspects of cleft lip and cleft palate have been reviewed recently by Fraser.[8] As a general rule, cleft lip with or without cleft palate is etiologically different from isolated cleft palate. Both conditions are genetically heterogeneous. There are about

TABLE 1-2.—RECURRENCE RISK OF ANENCEPHALY AND
SPINA BIFIDA IN SIBS°

	PARENTS UNAFFECTED	ONE PARENT AFFECTED	BOTH PARENTS AFFECTED
No sibs	0.3%	5%	30%
One sib affected	4%	12%	38%
One sib and one second-degree relative affected	6%	16%	40%
Two sibs affected	10%	20%	40%

°Based on data of Carter and Evans.[7]

30 single-gene syndromes in which either cleft lip, cleft lip with cleft palate or isolated cleft palate is a regular or frequent finding. An autosomal dominant form is the *lip-pit syndrome,* in which mucous pits of the lower lip are associated with clefts of the primary and/or secondary palate. Cleft lip and palate is also a common finding in one chromosomal syndrome, trisomy 13, and an occasional observation in many other chromosomal defects, including Down syndrome. It is also a feature of a number of syndromes whose etiology is uncertain, e.g., Pierre Robin syndrome. Although there is little evidence for environmental etiology, at present there is some suspicion that anticonvulsant drugs taken by the pregnant mother increase the risk of cleft lip and palate in the child.

However, by far the majority of cases of cleft lip and cleft palate are believed to have a multifactorial basis. In these, the risk for relatives is about 4% for first-degree relatives (parents, sibs and offspring), somewhat higher for the more severe defects and lower for the milder ones, and much higher (about 9–15%) if more than one sib or parent and child are affected.

Thus, a birth defect that usually is multifactorial may also be produced by one of many single mutant genes, by an abnormal karyotype, possibly by prenatal environmental factors or by causes as yet unknown. The nature of the causal mechanism has implications not only for understanding the morphogenesis of the defect itself but also for predicting its recurrence risk within families.

Prenatal Diagnosis

An increasingly important aspect of the management of genetic disorders is the use of prenatal diagnosis of fetal disorders by amniocentesis, at a stage of pregnancy early enough to allow termination if indicated.

In many centers, the following situations are considered to be indications for amniocentesis:

1. Late maternal age (35 or older), which is associated with increased risk of a trisomic child.

2. Previous trisomic child; the recurrence risk of the same or a different trisomy is about 1%.

3. Chromosome translocation in either parent, with a significant risk of a chromosomally unbalanced child.

4. For women who are carriers of X-linked recessive defects (e.g., Duchenne muscular dystrophy) (fetal sex determination with abortion of male fetuses).

5. Certain rare biochemical defects (e.g., Tay-Sachs disease).

6. Neural tube defects.

For late maternal age, previous trisomy, translocation in a parent or fetal sex determination, the chromosomes of the fetus are determined from study of cultured amniotic fluid cells. Amniotic fluid can be obtained at about 16 weeks of gestation. It contains cells that will grow in culture, allowing analysis of the fetal chromosomes within about 2 weeks.

For rare recessive abnormalities such as Tay-Sachs disease, enzyme studies on cultured amniotic fluid cells can make the diagnosis of a defective fetus. Such tests are applicable at present only when both parents are known to carry a specific deleterious gene, either on the basis of population screening (as in Tay-Sachs disease) or because they already have had a child with a defect that is expressed in cultured cells.

For neural tube malformations, assay of alpha-fetoprotein, which is present in increased quantities in the amniotic fluid when an open neural tube defect is present, can be used to detect virtually all cases of anencephaly and about 80% of cases of spina bifida. These tests are given only to women known to be at increased risk of having a child with a neural tube defect; i.e., women who already have had such a child and women who (or whose husbands) have spina bifida or have a close relative who is affected. The development of an accurate alpha-fetoprotein assay on maternal serum gives hope of a more widely applicable diagnostic technique (Brock, Wald and Cuckle[9]).

Ultrasonography and direct visualization of the fetus by fetoscopy also offer approaches to detection of malformations.

Transplantation

Transplantation of tissues and organs is successful only when the donor and host are histocompatible; otherwise, the graft is rejected. Rejection is the general rule for allografts (grafts between genetically dissimilar individuals). Isografts (grafts exchanged between members of a monozygotic twin pair) are accepted.

The genetic system responsible for graft rejection or acceptance is the HLA system. HLA is a complex genetic locus on chromosome no. 6, within which at least four separate but closely linked genes have been defined. Each has numerous allelic forms; already, for the two major genes, A and B, 15 A alleles and 20 B alleles are known, allowing for 300 possible "haplotypes" (combinations of A and B alleles on a single chromosome) and, with two haplotypes per individual, 45,254 possible genotypes. The haplotypes are inherited as "codominants"; i.e., both haplotypes are fully expressed. Graft rejection occurs when donor and host are not HLA-compatible. Compatibility for the ABO blood group system is also very important.

The best source of an HLA-compatible donor is a sib of the patient. Any sib has a 25% chance of having the same two haplotypes as the patient and thus being histocompatible. Although monozygotic co-twins always are histocompatible, the normal twin may be genetically at risk of the same disease that necessitated the transplant in the affected twin.

Knowledge of the genetics and immunology of histocompatibility is increasing so rapidly that review articles and books appear at frequent intervals. A current review by noted authorities is that by Snell, Dausset and Nathenson.[10]

Management of the Genetic Aspects of Surgical Problems

If a disorder is genetic there is a responsibility to investigate the family history and to inform the patient or parents of the genetic implications. This is especially important when the patient is a child, because the parents may wish to limit their future childbearing, to have prenatal diagnosis or to complete their families using some other option such as adoption or artificial insemination.

The importance of accurate diagnosis as a prerequisite to genetic counseling cannot be overemphasized. Descriptions of dysmorphic syndromes (e.g., Smith,[11] and Gorlin, Pindborg and Cohen[12]) are invaluable diagnostic aids. Access to a cytogenetic laboratory with a full range of services is essential. If the malformation is so severe that it leads to stillbirth or early postnatal death, genetic advice often still can be provided if photographs are taken and a chromosome study and an autopsy are performed.

What use do parents make of genetic information? Studies have shown that they usually are reluctant to have another child if the recurrence risk is high (10% or more), but that in making the decision they also wish to take into account the burden of the disorder, i.e., its severity and duration, as well as the possibility of successful prenatal diagnosis. To help provide the answers to such questions, most major medical centers now have medical genetics units with staff who can assist either directly with the family or as consultants to the surgeon. In the last analysis, the surgeon who is aware of the genetic implications of his patient's problem may be the best person to provide genetic counseling as an integral part of his management of the case.

REFERENCES

1. McKusick, V. A.: *Mendelian Inheritance in Man. Catalogs of Autosomal Dominant, Autosomal Recessive and X-linked Phenotypes* (5th ed.; Baltimore: Johns Hopkins University Press, 1978).
2. Murphy, E. A., and Chase, G. A.: *Principles of Genetic Counseling* (Chicago: Year Book Medical Publishers, Inc., 1975).
3. Graham, J. B., Miller, C. H., Reisner, H. M., Elston, R. C., and Olive, J. A.: The phenotypic range of hemophilia A carriers, Am. J. Hum. Genet. 28:482, 1976.
4. Kloepfer, H. W., and Emery, A. E. H.: Genetic Aspects of Neuromuscular Disease, in Walton, J. N. (ed.), *Disorders of Voluntary Muscle* (3d ed.; New York: Churchill Livingstone, 1974).
5. Carter, C. O., and Evans, K. A.: Inheritance of congenital pyloric stenosis, J. Med. Genet. 6:233, 1969.
6. Nora, J. J.: Etiological factors in congenital heart diseases, Pediatr. Clin. North Am. 18:1059, 1971.
7. Carter, C. O., and Evans, K.: Spina bifida and anencephalus in Greater London, J. Med. Genet. 10:209, 1973.
8. Fraser, F. C.: The genetics of cleft lip and cleft palate, Am. J. Hum. Genet. 22:336, 1970.
9. Brock, D. J. H., Wald, N. J., and Cuckle, H.: Organization of maternal serum-α-fetoprotein screening for fetal neural-tube defects, Lancet 1:700, 1977.
10. Snell, G. D., Dausset, J., and Nathenson, S.: *Histocompatibility* (New York: Academic Press, 1976).
11. Smith, D. W.: *Recognizable Patterns of Human Malformation* (2d ed.; Philadelphia: W. B. Saunders Company, 1976).
12. Gorlin, R. J., Pindborg, J. J., and Cohen, M. M.: *Syndromes of the Head and Neck* (2d ed.; New York: McGraw-Hill Book Company, Inc., 1976).

2 JOHN J. DOWNES / RUSSELL C. RAPHAELY

Anesthesia and Intensive Care

Pediatric Anesthesia

GOOD PEDIATRIC ANESTHESIA requires adequate analgesia, life support, intensive surveillance and appropriate operating conditions for the surgeon. Preoperative and postoperative intensive care is an extension of this life support and surveillance appropriate for the patient's condition outside the operating room. The best use of the talents and skills of the anesthesiologist, surgeon and operating room nursing staff require definition of responsibilities, close communication and the spirit of a cohesive team that serves the patient throughout the entire surgical experience.

The major medical advances of the past 20 years affecting pediatric anesthesia include: the physiology and adaptation of the neonate to extrauterine life; the clinical pharmacology of nonflammable anesthetic agents and muscle relaxants in infants and children; improved technology of monitoring equipment; advances in the cannulation of small peripheral arteries and the maintenance of those catheters for extended periods; extensive improvement in intensive respiratory care; and ultramicro techniques for rapid analysis of arterial blood for pH, blood gas tensions and other biochemical measurements.[1-4] These advances have essentially reduced the mortality and morbidity associated with anesthesia and life-threatening illness in infants and children. The term "anesthetic death" can be applied when the administration of anesthesia was directly responsible for or a major and obvious contributing factor in the death of a patient. Surveys prior to 1964 indicate an over-all anesthesia death rate of 3.3 per 10,000 anesthetics in infants and children, and more than half of the pediatric anesthesia deaths occurred in apparently healthy children.[5] Anesthetic mortalities tend to be lower in major pediatric centers. For the decade prior to 1968, the anesthesia death rate at Children's Hospital Medical Center of Boston was 1.6 per 10,000 anesthesias, less than half the rate observed with pooled data from many hospitals in a large metropolitan area.[6] Although a comparable survey has not been completed for anesthesia death rates in infants and children between 1964 and 1976, indications are that this rate has been reduced. At The Children's Hospital of Philadelphia in the past 12 years, more than 50,000 anesthetics have been performed with an over-all mortality rate of 0.2 per 10,000 patients. These deaths occurred in critically ill children. During the most recent decade there has also been a significant reduction in the mortality at Children's Hospital Medical Center of Boston.[7]

Principles of Pediatric Anesthesia

PREANESTHETIC EVALUATION.—Information provided to the anesthesiologist by the parents, the surgeon and the pediatrician may be vital to the child's welfare. For example, a recent upper respiratory infection or a previous history of laryngotracheitis (croup) predisposes the child to postintubation subglottic edema. A familial history of prolonged respiratory depression following anesthesia suggests the possibility that the patient may be that 1 in 3000 individuals who has atypical plasma pseudocholinesterase and could develop prolonged apnea if succinylcholine were used as a muscle relaxant.[8] A history of unexplained sudden deaths during general anesthesia in healthy young members of a family raises the question of malignant hyperthermia as a cause of death.[9] Hyperthermia might occurr without warning during anesthesia in any of the relatives, including children.

Parents must be questioned specifically regarding: (1) recent upper respiratory infections, (2) asthmatic episodes or wheezing during respiratory infections, (3) previous laryngeal stridor or laryngotracheitis (croup), (4) recent exposure to the exanthemata, (5) abnormal reactions to drugs, including anesthetic agents, (6) blood transfusion reactions, (7) previous administration of corticosteroids, (8) medications currently being given, (9) emotional reactions of the child to the proposed operation and (10) familial history of major problems associated with anesthesia.

Prior to emergency operation, parents should be asked when and what the child last ate. However, most anesthesiologists regard the unprepared ambulatory child as having a full stomach and take appropriate precautions. In the child who has sustained acute trauma, gastric emptying ceases at the time of injury, so that the stomach may be full even if anesthesia is delayed many hours.[10]

The preanesthetic physical examination should emphasize the upper airway, lungs and heart. Small, narrow nares filled with secretions, large tonsils and adenoids that necessitate open-mouth breathing or an underdeveloped mandible with protruding maxilla predispose to upper airway obstruction after sedation or induction of anesthesia. A high thyroid cartilage located within one or two fingerbreadths of the symphysis menti indicates that the larynx lies cephalad and anterior to its normal position, and tracheal intubation may prove difficult. The mouth always should be examined for the presence of loose teeth. The presence of a heart murmur, a cardiac dysrhythmia or rales in the chest requires investigation and consultation before the anesthesiologist proceeds. A rectal temperature greater than 38 C (100.4° F) constitutes a contraindication to elective anesthesia and operation.

The laboratory tests required prior to anesthesia consist of hemoglobin or hematocrit determination, white cell count and urinalysis. In the full-term infant, hematopoiesis resumes when the hemoglobin level reaches 11–12 gm/dl. This occurs between 6 weeks and 12 weeks of age, depending on the amount of hemoglobin present at birth. By the third to the sixth month, supplementary iron will be needed. Certain conditions (infection, renal disease, malignancy, etc.) interfere with hematopoiesis and may enhance iron-deficiency anemia or prevent the hematopoietic response to iron. If the infant has iron deficiency alone, the response to iron is seen in an increased reticulocyte count in a few days and a normal or near-normal hemoglobin level in a month or less. The mean lowest point of hemoglobin level in normal infants is about 11–12 gm/dl and the lowest level of the 95% range (two standard deviations below the mean) is 10 gm/dl. The minimal value of 10 gm/dl hemoglobin for elective surgery, therefore, eliminates only the lowest 2.5% of all apparently normal infants, a conservative approach indeed.[11] In patients with serious systemic disease or those about to undergo an extensive operation, a preoperative chest roentgenogram, arterial pH, Pa_{O_2} and Pa_{CO_2} and serum electrolytes, including ionized calcium, will provide data that often prove to be extremely valuable during and after anesthesia.

The anesthesiologist must correlate the history, physical findings and laboratory results to make an assessment of the child's physical status. The American Society of Anesthesiologists' classification provides a useful numerical scale of physical status[12]:

Class 1. No organic, physiologic, biochemical or psychiatric disturbance.

Class 2. Mild to moderate systemic abnormalities, caused either by the disease to be treated surgically or by another pathophysiologic process.

Class 3. Severe systemic abnormality from any cause.

Class 4. Immediately life-threatening, severe systemic disorder.

Class 5. Moribund patient who is submitted to operation in desperation.

Emergency Operation (E). Any patient in one of the classes above who is operated on as an emergency receives the letter E beside the numerical classification, e.g., 2E.

The total "risk" of anesthesia and operation includes consideration not only of the child's physical status but also of the skill and experience of the anesthesiologist and surgeon in treating infants and children. The presence in the hospital of pediatric subspecialty consultants, pediatric nurses and allied health personnel, pediatric respiratory therapy equipment, monitoring systems designed for infants and children and laboratory facilities with ultramicro methods serves to decrease the total risk of a given procedure.

PREANESTHETIC PREPARATION.—Normal children, especially those between 1 and 4 years of age who are unable to understand the purpose of hospitalization, experience fear when forced to leave the security and familiarity of home to stay in the hospital. Terrifying experiences during induction of anesthesia or in the immediate postoperative period can produce disturbing psychologic changes manifested by night terrors, enuresis and temper tantrums.[13, 14] Certain steps will minimize the psychic trauma. Parents must be encouraged to display confidence and cheerfulness, since their tension is readily transmitted to the child.

A medical social worker trained to orient parents and children and act as their advocate can do a great deal to allay anxiety.[15] The anesthesiologist always should visit the child prior to operation, with the parents present, and discuss the proposed anesthesia and related events in a manner that both the child and parents can comprehend.[16] In this way, the child will regard the anesthesiologist as a friend who will be caring for him. Appropriate preanesthetic sedation permits the child to be transported to the operating room lightly asleep, allows induction of anesthesia without awakening (a "steal induction") and provides some analgesia in the immediate postoperative period.

Numerous drugs in a variety of combinations have been used in children for preanesthetic sedation.[17, 18] Intramuscular barbiturates in combination with an opiate and belladonna alkaloid produce suitable preanesthetic sedation in most children. Table 2–1 gives the dosage schedule for this type of sedation, which has been subjected to a systematic double-blind study[17] and subsequently used in more than 50,000 infants and children at The Children's Hospital of Philadelphia. Up to 6 months of age, only a belladonna derivative is required. Atropine provides more effective abolition of vagal reflexes than does scopolamine, particularly in infants.[19] Scopolamine appears to be more effective than atropine in drying upper airway secretions[20] and it adds to the sedative effect of a barbiturate, but when used with only a barbiturate it increases the incidence of postanesthetic excitement.[17]

The child's stomach should be empty prior to anesthesia, yet it is important to interrupt fluid intake for only a minimal period. No milk or solids should be given within 12 hours of induction of anesthesia. Clear liquids with glucose must be given up to 4 hours prior to induction in infants to age 6 months, 6 hours prior to induction from age 6 months to 3 years and 8 hours prior to induction after 3 years of age. Children to be operated on in the afternoon should receive clear liquids in the morning up to 4–6 hours prior to the scheduled time for anesthesia induction. In children with a full stomach, orally administered antacids may elevate gastric pH above 3.0, so reducing acidity and thereby reducing the risk of an intense chemical pneumonitis should pulmonary aspiration of gastric contents occur during the induction of anesthesia.[21]

The febrile, dehydrated child who requires an emergency operation, such as appendectomy, should receive rapid, at least partial, rehydration with intravenous fluids as well as correction of any concomitant metabolic acidosis with intravenous sodium bicarbonate. Under general endotracheal anesthesia with neuromuscular blockade and controlled ventilation, surface cooling with circulating cold water mattresses should be used until the rectal or esophageal temperature drops to 39° C (102° F). Operation then can be started and cooling continued to a body temperature of 38° C (100° F).

TABLE 2-1.—PREANESTHETIC MEDICATION[17]

AGE (Months)	DRUGS
0–6	Atropine only
6–12	Atropine + pentobarbital
Over 12	Atropine + pentobarbital + morphine

DOSAGE	
Atropine or scopolamine	0.02 mg per kg—minimum 0.10 mg; maximum 0.60 mg
Pentobarbital	3.0–4.0 mg per kg—maximum 120 mg
Morphine	0.05–0.10 mg per kg—maximum 10 mg
Meperidine	1.0–2.0 mg per kg—maximum 100 mg

INTRAOPERATIVE ANESTHETIC MANAGEMENT.—All of the common inhalation agents and techniques have been used in children, but in the past decade halothane and nitrous oxide with neuromuscular blockade have become the principal agents in pediatric anesthesia. Flammable anesthetics such as cyclopropane and diethyl ether are used in relatively few pediatric centers today. Their removal occurred as the result of the widespread use of electrocautery by surgeons as well as the proliferation of electrical equipment for patient monitoring, maintenance of body temperature and heated humidification of anesthetic gases. Low dead space, low resistance anesthetic systems have greatly facilitated the administration of anesthesia to infants and small children.[22] For induction of anesthesia, most anesthesiologists prefer gravity flow of nitrous oxide with or without halothane over the face of the patient, and application of a mask after the child loses consciousness.

Clinical experience and pharmacologic studies in man have shown that muscle relaxants such as succinylcholine,[23, 24] pancuronium[25] and d-tubocurarine[26, 27] can be used effectively and safely, even in the newborn, and provide for optimal gas exchange. Neostigmine preceded by atropine will restore neuromuscular transmission at the termination of anesthesia.

Tracheal intubation is indicated in: (1) operations of the head and neck, including intraoral procedures such as tonsillectomy; (2) intrathoracic and intraperitoneal procedures; (3) operations in the prone position; (4) most procedures in infants under 1 year of age; and (5) all emergency procedures where there is uncertainty about the contents of the stomach. Appropriate dimensions of endotracheal tubes for patients of various ages are present in Table 2–2. Ventilation should be controlled manually or mechanically in intrathoracic, intraperitoneal and intracranial procedures, and when the patient is in the prone position.

The minimum of monitoring aids for any pediatric patient undergoing general anesthesia should include: a precordial or esophageal stethoscope, a blood pressure cuff, an electrocardiogram and a temperature probe inserted into the rectum, esophagus or nasopharynx (axillary temperature is not sufficiently reliable). A Doppler transducer (in lieu of the conventional stethoscope) transmits Korotkoff sounds accurately with systolic arterial pressures as low as 40 mm Hg[28]; this device should be used in infants under 1 year of age and is useful in patients of all ages. An indwelling peripheral arterial cannula provides the key to cardiopulmonary monitoring and appropriate assessment of biochemical status. A modified Allen test to ensure patency of the ulnar artery and palmar arch can be performed readily with fingertip plethysmography.[29] A radial artery catheter (22 gauge) then can be inserted percutaneously[30] or under direct vision by a modified cutdown technique without ligation of the artery. If the radial artery cannot be utilized, a temporal[31] or dorsalis pedis artery can be cannulated. In the newborn, the umbilical artery may be used but has certain drawbacks (see below). All arterial lines should be attached to a transducer to monitor systemic arterial mean and systolic pressures as well as to warn of disconnection. To prevent clots from developing in the lumen of the catheter or in the proximal vessel, a continuous dilute heparin infusion (1 unit/ml) at the rate of 1 ml/hr should be provided by constant infusion pump through a small-bore flush system.° This fluid must be calculated into the daily fluid intake of the infant.

A right atrial catheter can be useful as an additional route of drug and fluid infusion, but it seldom provides informative blood gas tension data in the critically ill patient. The central venous line cannot serve as a substitute for a properly functioning systemic arterial line. A pulmonary artery catheter of the Swan-Ganz type, including the new 5 Fr quadrilumen catheter† with a thermodilution cardiac output sensor, can be inserted through the internal jugular or other large vein. This will provide pulmonary artery and wedge pressures (reflecting left heart filling pressure) as well as cardiac output in patients with severe cardiopulmonary disorders.

The degree of neuromuscular block can be assessed by

° Intraflo Continuous Flush System, Sorenson Research Company, Salt Lake City, Utah.
† Edwards Laboratories, Santa Ana, California.

TABLE 2-2.—DIMENSIONS OF ENDOTRACHEAL TUBES[1]

AGE	INTERNAL DIAMETER (I.D.) (mm)	CONNECTOR (I.D.)[2] (mm)	MINIMAL LENGTH (Oral)[3] (cm)
Premature	2.5–3.0	3.0	10–11
Full term	3.0–3.5	3.0–4.0	11–12
6 mo	4.0	4.0	13
12 mo	4.5	5.0	14
18–24 mo	5.0	5.0	15
4 yr	5.5	6.0	16
6 yr	6.0	6.0	18
8 yr	6.5	7.0	20
10 yr[4]	7.0	7.0	21
12 yr[4]	7.5	8.0	22
14 yr[4]	8.0	8.0	23
Adult[4]	8.5–9.5	9.0–10.0	24–26

[1]*Average* size for age. Occasionally a size 0.5 mm I.D. smaller or larger will be required in normal patients.
[2]We recommend only connectors with tapered 15-mm male machine end. Size refers to internal diameter of tube end.
[3]For nasal tubes, add 2–3 cm length.
[4]Patients age 10 yr and older vary widely in tracheal size. High-volume, low-pressure cuffs may be required for short-term use (less than 24 hours). When using a cuffed tube, select size 0.5 mm I.D. smaller.
Note: Thin wall, uncuffed plastic Magill or Murphy tubes that conform to ANSI Standard Z.79.1 and the USP animal implant test are recommended for infants and children under 10 yr. Such tubes will be labeled "Z.79.I.T." with internal and external diameter in mm.
References: (a) ANSI Standard Z.79.1 "Tracheal Tubes and Cuffs," American National Standards Institute, 1430 Broadway, New York, N.Y. 10018.
(b) Guess, W. L.: Tissue testing of polymers, Int. Anesthesiol. Clin. 8:787, 1970.
(c) United States Pharmacopoeia, Vol. 17, p. 905.

battery-operated nerve stimulators, which provide transcutaneous single twitch and tetanic[32] or train-of-four[33] stimulation to the ulnar nerve at the wrist or posterior tibial nerve at the ankle. A urinometer collection system with a bag applied over the perineum enables the anesthetist to assess hourly urine output, the best continuous indicator of organ perfusion and renal function. The volume of blood aspirated from the operative field can be measured more accurately by using short suction lines of small internal volume and 100-ml traps in the suction line. Fluid losses other than blood and urine, such as aspirated gastric fluid, should also be measured. Serial determinations of Pa_{O_2}, pH, Pa_{CO_2}, glucose, electrolytes, osmolarity, ionized calcium, total protein and hematocrit at frequent intervals provide the data essential for appropriate ventilatory and biochemical support.

Ionized calcium measurements will detect hypocalcemia (Ca^{++} less than 2.0 mEq/l) that can produce low cardiac output and systemic hypoperfusion.[34] Hypocalcemia frequently occurs during and after transfusion of citrated blood in volumes exceeding more than half the patient's estimated blood volume. Serum total protein is the major contributor to plasma oncotic pressure and should be maintained at 6 gm/dl or higher, thereby reducing the tendency for transudation of fluid into the extravascular spaces of the lung and other major organs.

In modern air-conditioned operating rooms with ambient temperatures of approximately 20° C, hypothermia (rectal temperature < 36° C) frequently develops in infants undergoing even short, superficial procedures[35] and is also common in older children during long operations with an open thorax or abdomen. Heat loss can be minimized by: a warming mattress on the operating table maintained at 40–41° C water temperature[35]; heating the humidified anesthetic gases to a temperature of 36° C at the trachea[36]; warming the patient's skin with an overhead radiant warmer providing a temperature of 36° C; elevation of the operating room temperature; warming of all intravenous fluids; and covering an infant's trunk and proximal extremities with a plastic drape.*[37]

Malignant hyperthermia, the abrupt and unexplained rise in body temperature above 40° C (104° F) during administration of inhalation anesthesia, occurs in children and adults of all ages but most commonly in children over the age of 2 years and in young adults. The syndrome appears to be related to a hypermetabolic state in skeletal muscle induced by inhalation anesthetic agents and depolarizing muscle relaxants (e.g., succinylcholine) in a predisposed patient.[38] This predisposition may occur through familial genetic transmission, although many cases are nonfamilial. The incidence of this syndrome has been reported to be 1:15,000 anesthesias in children, with an over-all mortality of 65%.[38a] Since a high probability exists that every major pediatric surgical center will encounter this syndrome, monitoring of rectal, esophageal or nasopharyngeal temperature, heart rate and ECG continually in *all* patients undergoing anesthesia will be necessary for early diagnosis. When the syndrome has been detected at the outset and an appropriate therapeutic program immediately initiated, the incidence of cardiac arrest and permanent central nervous system damage as well as the mortality rate can be substantially reduced.[39, 40] The criteria for diagnosis and a plan of treatment for malignant hyperthermia are outlined in Table 2–3. Certain drugs (procaine, procainamide, dexamethasone, dantrolene) have been recommended as specific for the metabolic disorder

---

*Steri-Drape, 3M Company, St. Paul, Minnesota.

TABLE 2-3.—MANAGEMENT OF
MALIGNANT HYPERTHERMIA

DETECTION
  History of hyperthermia—patient
                      —family
  Unexplained tachycardia (*early sign*)
  Rigidity after succinylcholine
  Sudden, unexplained temperature rise
THERAPY
  Immediate
    Cessation of anesthesia
    Hyperventilation with 100% oxygen
    Initiation of cooling:
      —immersion in ice
      —lavage of stomach, body cavities with iced saline
    Intravenous sodium bicarbonate (3–5 mEq/kg)
    Intravenous *iced* 5% dextrose in Ringer's lactate
      (3–5 times maintenance rate)
    Diuretics—mannitol, furosemide
    Monitoring—ECG
              Rectal, esophageal *and* nasopharyngeal
                temperature
              Arterial cannula (blood pressure, pH, P_{CO_2}, P_{O_2})
              CVP catheter
              Urinary catheter—urine ml/hr
  Later
    Correction of coagulopathy
    Partial cardiopulmonary bypass (if needed)
    Intravenous dextrose with insulin
    Control of intracranial pressure (if needed)
      subdural bolt
      corticosteroids
      hyperventilation
      mannitol
      pentobarbital (intravenous)
      moderate hypothermia (30–32° C)

---

occurring in the skeletal muscles; although these drugs have been effective under certain conditions in swine with induced malignant hyperthermia, their effectiveness in man remains highly questionable, and they should be reserved for use in patients in whom other measures have failed to reverse the syndrome. Procainamide and procaine can induce severe systemic hypotension unresponsive to catecholamine infusion. If regional or local anesthesia has been chosen for a patient predisposed to the syndrome, local anesthetics of the "ester" class (procaine, tetracaine and chloroprocaine) should be selected because agents of the "amide" class (lidocaine, prilocaine, etidocaine, mepivacaine, bupivacaine) have been implicated in triggering hyperthermia.

INTRAOPERATIVE FLUID THERAPY.—Intraoperative fluid therapy with crystalloid and colloid fluids and blood products follows the general guidelines described in Table 2–4.[41] In infants and small children undergoing extensive procedures, fluids given in continuous infusion should be administered by a calibrated infusion pump and those given intermittently by manual syringe injection, in specific volumes. Gravity-dependent infusion systems introduce unacceptable variations due to imprecise tube clamp adjustments and fluctuations of venous pressure in relation to the height of the drip chamber above the heart. Provided that the patient has a normal cardiovascular system, blood loss due to acute surgical bleeding up to 10% of the estimated blood volume can be satisfactorily replaced with Ringer's lactate solution. Blood losses between 10% and 20% of the estimated blood volume should be replaced with 25% salt-poor albumin diluted with Ringer's lactate to a protein con-

TABLE 2-4.—FLUID AND BLOOD MANAGEMENT

MAINTENANCE FLUIDS

5–10% dextrose in 0.22% saline
- 100 ml/kg/24 hr
- 1000 ml plus 50 ml/kg (10–20 kg)/24 hr
- 1500 ml plus 20 ml/kg (> 20 kg)/24 hr

"THIRD SPACE" FLUID

5% dextrose in Ringer's lactate
- 3–10 ml/kg/hr during operation depending on location of surgery; maximum 40 ml/kg

COLLOID REPLACEMENT

Fresh-frozen plasma
5% albumin in Ringer's lactate } 10–20 ml/kg

BLOOD REPLACEMENT

Assume normal blood volume: 80–90 ml/kg newborn
75 ml/kg infant
70 ml/kg child

Assume normal hematocrit: 40 vol% newborn, child
30–35 vol% infant to 6 mo

Replace 10–20 ml/kg with 5% albumin in Ringer's lactate or with fresh-frozen plasma

Losses > 20 ml/kg replace with blood to maintain hematocrit at
35–40 vol% newborn,
30–35 vol% older infants and children

TECHNIQUE

Warm fluids and blood
Use calibrated syringe pump for maintenance fluids
Use manual syringe injection for colloid solutions, blood

centration of 5% or with fresh-frozen plasma, if supplemental clotting factors are required. Losses in excess of 20% of the blood volume should be replaced with whole blood or packed red blood cells and appropriate volumes of 5% albumin or fresh-frozen plasma. Serial hematocrits may serve as a reasonable guide for replacement of blood.[42] In infants less than 1 week of age, the hematocrit should be maintained at 40 vol% or higher and in older infants and children at 30–35 vol%.

Rapid transfusion of cold bank blood can produce cardiac arrest. Therefore, blood should be warmed to at least 30° C before infusion. Warming blood not only reduces the hypothermic stress to the heart and other organs but also reduces the hyperkalemia present in cold bank blood. Bank blood (ACD or CPD) older than 7–10 days will have serum potassium levels of 15–20 mEq/l at 4° C,[43] a pH less than 7.00 and a low level of ionized calcium.[34] Intravenous calcium chloride (50–100 mg/100 ml blood given) will help restore ionized calcium toward normal, thereby enhancing myocardial function and reducing the toxic effects of hyperkalemia.[34] If hypoperfusion accompanies the need for massive transfusion, intravenous sodium bicarbonate (2 mEq/kg initially) will help correct the metabolic acidosis that occurs.

Although "third space" losses have not been proved to exist in young infants undergoing extensive operative procedures, clinical experience indicates that sequestration of fluid appears to occur with extensive dissection and manipulation of major organs. During such operative procedures, 5–10 ml/kg/hr with a maximum of 40 ml/kg additional fluid as Ringer's lactate solution will restore that volume lost to the interstitial tissues. Replenishment of third space losses must proceed cautiously in patients with cardiopulmonary disease, since interstitial pulmonary edema can result. In patients with marginal cardiac function, maintenance fluids should be reduced for 48 to 72 hours postoperatively while this sequestered fluid is being reabsorbed into the circulation. Serial determination of hematocrit, serum osmolarity,

serum total protein, urine output per hour and Pa_{O_2} (at a constant FI_{O_2}) provide necessary guides to fluid therapy.

Patients with sepsis, especially those in septic shock, require large volumes of colloid infusion to maintain an adequate intravascular volume early in the disease process. Infusion of salt-poor albumin will help maintain plasma oncotic pressure, thereby retaining fluid in the intravascular space. Later, when capillary leakage may develop, continued infusion of albumin will only serve to raise the oncotic pressure of the interstitial fluid and aggravate the loss of fluid into the interstitial spaces.

Coagulopathies commonly accompanying gram-negative sepsis involve multiple defects in coagulation.[44] In our clinical experience, the most effective treatment for disseminated intravascular coagulopathy has been platelet transfusions, fresh-frozen plasma and fresh whole blood (less than 24 hours old). Coagulopathies induced by massive transfusion require the same fundamental therapy as well as the infusion of calcium.

Postanesthetic Recovery

Recovery room facilities and experienced nurses in adequate numbers must be available to provide surveillance of airway patency, adequacy of ventilation and circulatory stability following anesthesia. Postanesthetic excitement (emergence delirium) is the most common complication of the recovery period in children over 2 years of age. The incidence appears to be greatest (13%) between the ages of 3 and 9 years and tends to be more frequent in healthy children who have undergone tonsillectomy or have received barbiturate-scopolamine sedation.[16, 45] Morphine in the preanesthetic sedation significantly reduces the incidence of excitement.[17] Intravenous diazepam (0.1–0.2 mg/kg) usually quiets the excited child and produces a state of light sleep for 20–30 minutes, after which the child usually awakens peacefully. If considerable incisional pain exists, a short-acting narcotic such as fentanyl (1 μg/kg intravenously or intramuscularly) often will be required to control the child's agitation.

Children with a history of repeated episodes of infectious laryngotracheitis may develop stridor due to subglottic edema following tracheal intubation. A tight-fitting endotracheal tube and long procedures involving movement of the head and neck (e.g., cerebral angiography or tonsillectomy) also increase the risk of postintubation subglottic edema. A high-humidity environment, epinephrine aerosol inhalation by mask every 1–3 hours[46] and intravenous fluids for 6–12 hours usually will relieve the partial airway obstruction. Corticosteroids have been shown in double-blind studies to be of no value in postintubation or infectious subglottic edema.[47] Rarely, nasotracheal intubation or tracheostomy for 2–3 days may be required to relieve airway obstruction.

Despite efforts to conserve body heat during anesthesia, a low body temperature frequently develops in infants or small children immediately after operation. Persistent hypothermia can cause respiratory depression, peripheral vasoconstriction, metabolic acidosis and delayed recovery of neuromuscular function following reversal of nondepolarizing relaxants.[48] A radiant heater and warm water mattress usually will restore body temperature to normal within an hour. Malignant hyperthermia can occur immediately following inhalation anesthesia, so careful temperature monitoring remains important during recovery, and techniques for controlled body cooling must be available.

Prolonged respiratory depression or apnea occurring in the recovery period may be associated with persistent effects of muscle relaxants, narcotics, anesthetic agents, airway obstruction, asphyxia (hypoxemia, acidemia), hypothermia or hypoglycemia. If narcotics have been used during anesthesia, naloxone (5 μg/kg intravenously or intramuscularly) will temporarily reverse respiratory depression and stupor; however, the effects of naloxone may disappear within 30–60 minutes and respiratory depression recur due to persistent effects of the narcotic. Naloxone also prolongs narcotic respiratory depression, perhaps by competing with the narcotic for metabolic sites.[49] Therefore, patients should be kept in the recovery room for at least 2 hours following injection of naloxone.

Muscle weakness resulting in respiratory depression most often can be attributed to an excessive dosage of depolarizing relaxants (e.g., succinylcholine) or inadequate reversal of nondepolarizing relaxants (e.g., pancuronium or d-tubocurarine) with intravenous atropine and neostigmine. Monitoring of the compound muscle action potential[26] or muscle twitch response[50] facilitates the management of such complications. In most cases involving nondepolarizing relaxants, adequate reversal will be obtained with a repeated dose of atropine and neostigmine.

A variety of factors may retard or prevent recovery of consciousness following anesthesia. Paramount among these is overdose with the anesthetic agent, a problem more commonly encountered with inhalation agents highly soluble in blood and water, such as halothane, enflurane and methoxyflurane. Preanesthetic sedatives may also delay awakening. Inadequate ventilation caused by drug-induced central nervous system depression, cardiopulmonary disease or muscle weakness can produce Pa_{CO_2} levels over 70 torr, which can result in loss of consciousness or coma.[51] A metabolic disorder such as severe hyponatremia or hypoglycemia also causes coma. Therefore, delayed recovery of consciousness calls for evaluation of arterial pH, Pa_{CO_2} and Pa_{O_2} as well as

blood sugar and serum sodium. Failure to regain consciousness after 1–2 hours despite adequate ventilation and circulation raises the possibility of central nervous system damage due to prolonged intraoperative hypoxia, which may not have been recognized, or air embolism. An immediate neurologic examination and electroencephalogram are required to establish a diagnosis and prognosis.[52, 53] Consideration then must be given to a therapeutic regimen for control of cerebral edema and intracranial pressure (see below).

Pulmonary aspiration of gastric or upper intestinal contents during induction or recovery constitutes the major anesthetic hazard of emergency operations in children. The endotracheal tube must remain in place until the child regains full consciousness and attempts to remove the tube himself. If aspiration occurs, the immediate treatment consists of ventilation with oxygen, tracheal intubation and tracheobronchial suctioning. For aspiration of solid material, bronchoscopy and tracheobronchial lavage with saline should be performed. Systemic corticosteroids and antibiotics may decrease inflammation induced by acid and bacteria, and intensive respiratory care usually will be required (see below).

Anesthesia for the Critically Ill Infant

Anesthetic management of a critically ill infant requires an understanding of: (1) the adaptation of the newborn to extrauterine life, and growth and development during the first year; (2) the support of vital system function in the ill infant; (3) the lesions requiring anesthesia and operation in infancy; and (4) the principles and techniques for administration of anesthetic and adjuvant drugs in infants. Although this section emphasizes the anesthetic management of the neonate (age 0–28 days), the principles and techniques described apply to infants up to 24 months of age. Because of the complexities of the lesions and of the techniques used in their treatment, we shall not discuss anesthesia for infants requiring cardiovascular surgery; the interested reader should consult the literature.[54]

PHYSIOLOGY OF ADAPTATION.—To survive, a newborn infant must meet 6 major obligations:

1. Expand the lungs to establish a functional residual capacity and initiate ventilation concomitant with absorption of fetal lung fluid by the pulmonary lymphatic system.[55]

2. Convert the fetal circulatory pattern, with the pulmonary and systemic circuits in parallel to the adult pattern with these circuits in series. This adaptation involves a marked and abrupt reduction in pulmonary vascular resistance and increased blood flow, and functional closure of the foramen ovale and ductus arteriosus.[56]

3. Recover from birth asphyxia and correct the arterial pH, Pa_{CO_2} and base deficit to normal neonatal levels, metabolize lactic acid and improve oxygen uptake and transport, resulting in Pa_{O_2} levels of 55 torr and higher.[57]

4. Maintain a core temperature of approximately 37° C despite the stress of a cool environment (<32° C). This requires that the infant increase his oxygen consumption in direct proportion to the temperature gradient between the skin and his immediate environment. The increase in metabolic rate, mediated through the sympathetic nervous system, will be minimal when the environmental temperature is 32–34° C, the abdominal skin 36° C and the colonic temperature 37° C, a condition known as the neutral thermal state.[58, 59]

5. Establish renal function and regulate fluid balance.

TABLE 2-5.—NORMAL PHYSIOLOGIC DATA IN INFANTS

A. PULMONARY FUNCTION (mean values)[1]

	NEWBORN	ADULT
Body wt (kg)	3	70
V_T (ml/kg)	6	6
f (breaths/min)	35	15
$\dot{V}_E$ (ml/kg/min)	210	90
$\dot{V}_A$ (ml/kg/min)	130	60
V_D Anat. (ml/kg)	2.5	2.0
V_D/V_T ratio	0.30	0.33
$\dot{V}_{O_2}$ (ml/kg/min)	6.4	3.5
$\dot{V}_{CO_2}$ (ml/kg/min)	6	3
Cal/kg/hr	2	1
FRC (ml/kg)	30	34
V.C. (ml/kg)	35	70
Tracheal length (mm)	57	120
Tracheal diameter (mm)	4	16

B. FLUID VOLUMES AND CHARACTERISTICS
(range or mean ± SD)

	AGE 1–30 days	1–24 mo
Urine volume (ml/kg/hr)[4]	1–4	2–4
Urine osmolarity (mOsm/l)[4]	100–600	50–1400
Extracellular volume (% body wt)[5]	42 (6)	34 (4)
Blood vol (% body wt)[6]	80–90	75

C. pH, BLOOD GAS TENSIONS, HEMATOCRIT
(mean ± SD)

	1 hr[2]	AGE 24 hr[2]	1–24 mo[3]
pH	7.33	7.37 (.03)	7.40 (.03)
Pa_{CO_2} (torr)	36 (4)	33 (3)	34 (4)
BE (mEq/l)	– 6.0 (1)	– 5.0 (1)	– 3.0 (3)
Pa_{O_2} (FI_{O_2} 0.21) (torr)	63 (11)	73 (10)	
Hct (vol%)	54 (5)	55 (7)	35 (2.5)

D. BLOOD CHEMISTRIES (normal range)[4]

	AGE 1–30 days	1–24 mo
Sodium (mEq/l)	139–150	139–146
Potassium (mEq/l)	5.0–6.5	4.1–5.3
Chloride (mEq/l)	93–112	95–110
Bicarbonate (mEq/l)[2]	18–24	17–25
Calcium ion (mEq/l)	2.0–2.6	2.0–2.6
Calcium, total (mg/dl)	7.4–14.0	10.4–12.0
Glucose (fasting)(mg/dl)	50–80	60–100
Total protein (gm/dl)	4.7–7.6	6.2–8.1
BUN (mg/dl)	5–15	10–20

E. CARDIOVASCULAR FUNCTION (mean and range or SD)

	AGE 1–30 days	1–24 mo
Heart rate (bpm)[4]	120 (90–180)	120 (80–160)
Systemic arterial pressure (torr)[7]	73 (8) / 50 (5)	96 (30) / 66 (25)
Cardiac index (L/Min/M²)[7, 8]	4.1 (1.3)	4.5 (.94)

[1]Adapted from Scarpelli, E. M. (ed.): *Pulmonary Physiology in the Fetus, Newborn, and Child* (Philadelphia: Lea & Febiger, 1975), p. 168.
[2]Koch, G., and Wendel, H.: Biol. Neonate 12:136, 1968.
[3]Albert, M. S., and Winters, R.: Pediatrics 37:728, 1966.
[4]Adapted from McKay, R. J., and Vaughn, V. C.: *Nelson's Textbook of Pediatrics* (10th ed.; Philadelphia: W. B. Saunders Company, 1975), pp. 1783–1799.
[5]Friis-Hansen, B.: Acta Paediatr. Scand. (supp.) 110:36, 1957.
[6]Mollison, P. L.: *Blood Transfusion in Clinical Medicine* (Philadelphia: F. A. Davis Company, 1967), p. 145.
[7]Emmanouilides, C. C., *et al.*: Biol. Neonate 15:186, 1970.
[8]Graham, T. P., and Jarmakani, M. M.: Pediatr. Clin. North Am. 18:1109, 1971.

The newborn kidney is immature compared to that of the older infant and child, particularly in its limited ability to concentrate urine when there has been excess fluid loss, and to dilute urine and excrete fluid in the face of fluid overload.[60]

6. Maintain adequate energy substrate levels to meet metabolic requirements. The brain and heart depend on glucose as the major energy substrate. However, limited glycogen stores, especially in the low birth weight infant (<2500 gm), and numerous other factors predispose a large number of neonates to hypoglycemia (serum glucose level <30 mg/100 ml).[61] Free fatty acids provide an important source of energy for the maintenance of body temperature. Again, the low birth weight infant possesses limited fat reserves for maintenance of adequate levels of this substrate.[61]

Physiologic data pertinent to the adaptation and care of the critically ill infant are presented in Table 2–5. In evaluating the success of adaptation achieved by an infant, a number of factors deserve consideration. The actual weight should be compared with the predicted weight for the patient's age. In the newborn, this requires comparison of birth weight with gestational age, thus providing quick identification of the infant who is small for gestational age and will require investigation to exclude various disorders.[62] Pulmonary status of the infant can be evaluated by physical examination, chest roentgenogram and arterial blood gas tension measurement at a known inspired oxygen concentration. Assessment of circulatory function includes determination of heart rate, systemic arterial pressure, pulses, urine flow rate, hematocrit and examination for murmurs. If a murmur other than that associated with a patent ductus arteriosus is found in the premature infant, an electrocardiogram and four-view chest roentgenogram with barium swallow should be performed to aid in excluding the common cardiovascular anomalies of infancy.[63] Bradycardia must be prevented because an adequate cardiac output depends on a high rate due to the relatively incompliant ventricles and small stroke volume of the infant.

The hematocrit is roughly proportional to the blood volume in the newborn[64] but decreases with age and becomes a less reliable index of blood volume after the neonatal period. Acid-base status should be determined in all newborns requiring anesthesia,[65] in older infants undergoing extensive surgical procedures and in infants whose ASA physical status is 3 or worse. This can be done reliably only by measurement of arterial pH, Pa_{CO_2} and base excess or plasma bicarbonate.

The patient's thermal adaptation can be assessed by determining the severity and duration of cold stress to which the infant has been subjected, as well as the type of treatment applied to restore body temperature. Proper evaluation requires the knowledge of colonic, skin and environmental temperatures. Infants subjected to environmental temperatures below 28° C frequently develop a nonrespiratory (metabolic) acidosis.[66] Infants under 1500 gm treated with radiant heat warmers may incur considerable increases in insensible water loss with resultant dehydration.[67]

Determination of serum glucose, bilirubin, sodium, potassium and ionized calcium will detect the common metabolic abnormalities of the immediate newborn period.[68-71] The infant's renal status can be evaluated simply by measurement of hourly urine volume. Severe oliguria in the face of adequate hydration and circulation calls for an evaluation to exclude major anomalies of the genitourinary system.

LESIONS REQUIRING EARLY CORRECTION IN INFANCY.— Thorough evaluation of a newborn or young infant facing anesthesia and operation requires consideration of the surgical lesion and its systemic effects, potential for blood loss, special requirements, such as the patient's position in relation to monitoring devices and vascular catheters, and the possible existence of associated anomalies.[72] Congenital cardiovascular malformations occur in 23% of infants with diaphragmatic hernia,[73] 20% with omphalocele,[74] 15% with esophageal atresia[75] and 12% with imperforate anus.[76] The common lesions requiring early correction in infancy and the special problems affecting anesthetic management are outlined in Table 2–6.

Controversy exists regarding the optimal time to undertake anesthesia and operation for lesions requiring early correction in the neonate. Advocates favoring immediate operation point to the advantage of prompt correction of the physiologic effects of the lesion, decreased likelihood of systemic infection prior to operation and the presence of a high hemoglobin concentration. Those favoring delay state that after 24 hours of extrauterine life the infant will have recovered from birth asphyxia and thermal stress, have more complete adaptation of circulation and ventilation and have had sufficient time to manifest other anomalies or disorders.

TABLE 2-6.—SURGICAL LESIONS AND ANESTHETIC
PROBLEMS IN THE INFANT

LESIONS	SPECIFIC PROBLEMS
Airway obstruction Choanal atresia Pierre Robin Neoplasm Laryngeal stenosis	Asphyxia—arrest Aspiration Pneumothorax
Diaphragmatic hernia Eventration	Asphyxia, shock Hypoplastic lung, pulmonary hypertension Gastric distention Congenital heart disease Pneumothorax Small abdomen
Esophageal atresia Tracheoesophageal fistula	Pneumonitis Gastric distention Airway secretions Congenital heart disease
Lobar emphysema	Air trapping Mediastinal shift
Congenital heart disease	Asphyxia Cardiac failure Shock Pulmonary edema
Omphalocele Gastroschisis	Hypothermia Hypovolemia Shock, asphyxia Congenital heart disease
Intestinal atresia Pyloric stenosis	Regurgitation Dehydration
GI perforation, peritonitis, other obstruction (volvulus, intussusception)	Hypovolemia Distention Shock Aspiration Sepsis Hypoventilation
Incarcerated hernia, imperforate anus, megacolon	Fluid deficit, loss Blood loss—occult
Sacrococcygeal teratoma	Blood loss Position Hypothermia

There can be no clear answer, and each case must be judged alone. Lesions with devastating physiologic consequences, such as diaphragmatic hernia, require immediate repair whereas a lesion such as imperforate anus may not require operation for 24 hours or longer. The decision as to when to operate must take into consideration the consequences of delay in repair of the surgical lesions, the degree of birth asphyxia or other stresses placed on the infant and the possible presence of associated anomalies or other disorders.

STABILIZATION OF THE INFANT.—Preparation of an infant for transport to a referral center[77] or for anesthesia and operation aims at stabilization of the cardiopulmonary system, metabolism and temperature, correction of birth asphyxia and provision of adequate energy substrates to meet immediate metabolic needs. A protocol for achieving this is outlined in Table 2–7 and appropriate drug dosages are given in Table 2–8. Proper preparation plays a major role in success during the operative and postoperative periods. The rush to transfer an infant or perform an operation at the expense of the time required to stabilize the patient properly can only increase morbidity and mortality.

The pharynx must be cleared of secretions and soft tissue obstruction. In the infant who is obtunded or has anomalies of the upper airway, this may be achieved most readily by orotracheal intubation (Table 2–2). The inspired oxygen concentration (FI_{O_2}) should be adjusted to maintain Pa_{O_2} within the normal range for the infant's age. In the newborn, a Pa_{O_2} of 50–75 torr will reduce pulmonary vascular resistance to a near minimal value and enhance cardiopulmonary adaptation; levels in excess of 75 torr may substantially increase the risk of retrolental fibroplasia in infants less than 44 weeks postconceptual age.[78, 79] Decompressing the stomach will reduce the likelihood of regurgitation and aspiration.

TABLE 2-7.—STABILIZATION

Clear airway
Oxygen—keep Pa_{O_2} 50–75 torr
Decompress stomach
Warm to 37° C (colonic), 36° C (skin)
Establish intravenous route
    Plastic cannula
    Cutdown
Correct acidosis if pH ≤ 7.30
Ventilate if Pa_{CO_2} ≥ 50 torr
Correct dehydration—Insensible losses
              —Other losses
Correct hypovolemia—Ringer's lactate, albumin,
                plasma, RBCs,
                whole blood
Correct hypoglycemia (≤ 30 mg/100 ml)—25% G/W
Atropine—0.04 mg/kg IV (≤ 4 kg)

Neutral thermal conditions should be provided to minimize oxygen consumption and metabolic stress.[58] An intravenous infusion route must be established for the correction of metabolic acidosis and the provision of maintenance fluids and energy substrates. This is best accomplished with a peripheral plastic cannula (20–22 gauge), of which several satisfactory types are marketed. An umbilical vein catheter inserted into the right atrium, with its location confirmed by x-ray, can serve as a central venous route but poses the hazard of periportal cirrhosis and other sequelae. An arterial pH less than 7.30 due to a base deficit over 6 mEq/l should be corrected with intravenous sodium bicarbonate (Table 2–8). Patients with a Pa_{CO_2} over 50 torr should undergo tracheal intubation and controlled ventilation to restore adequate ventilation in the preoperative period. Prior to tracheal intu-

TABLE 2-8.—INTRAVENOUS DRUG DOSAGES IN NEWBORNS AND INFANTS DURING ANESTHESIA

ADJUVANT DRUGS		NEWBORN	INFANT
Atropine		0.04 mg/kg (to 4 kg)	0.02 mg/kg (> 4 kg) minimum 0.16 mg
d-Tubocurarine	Initial:	0.3 mg + 0.3 mg increments to effect	0.6 mg/kg
	Maintenance:	25% initial total dose	25% initial dose
Pancuronium	Initial:	0.05 mg + 0.05 mg increments to effect	0.1 mg/kg
	Maintenance:	25% initial total dose	25% initial dose
Succinylcholine		4 mg/kg	2 mg/kg
Neostigmine		0.07 mg/kg	0.07 mg/kg
Thiopental (2.5%)		4 mg/kg	4 mg/kg
Ketamine		2 mg/kg	2 mg/kg
Fentanyl		1–2 μg/kg	1–2 μg/kg
Morphine		0.1–0.2 mg/kg	0.1–0.2 mg/kg

CARDIOVASCULAR DRUGS		DOSAGE
Sodium bicarbonate		1–3 mEq/kg (depending on arterial pH, base deficit)
Calcium chloride (10%)		10–20 mg/kg
Calcium gluconate (10%)		15–60 mg/kg
Epinephrine	Initial:	1–10 μg/kg
	Maintenance*:	0.1–1.0 μg/kg/min
Isoproterenol*		0.1–1.0 μg/kg/min
Dopamine†		1–10 μg/kg/min
Furosemide		0.5 mg/kg
Lidocaine (1%)		1.0 mg/kg

*Dilute in syringe to 1 μg/kg/ml; give with calibrated syringe pump.
†Dilute in syringe to 10 μg/kg/ml; give with calibrated syringe pump.

bation, all infants require intravenous atropine (Table 2–8) to prevent bradycardia.

Insensible and urinary fluid losses should be replaced before and during anesthesia; this may require infusion rates of 8–12 ml/kg/hr for a period of 2–3 hours. Patients with hypovolemia associated with sequestration of fluid containing proteins in the intestinal lumen or other body compartments will require infusion of 10–20 ml/kg of 5% albumin in Ringer's lactate, or fresh-frozen plasma in order to restore an adequate circulating blood volume. Infants with a blood sugar less than 30 mg/dl should receive initially 2–4 ml/kg of 25% glucose in water intravenously followed by 10–15% glucose in 0.2% saline at 4 ml/kg/hr in order to maintain adequate blood glucose levels.[61] Guidelines for fluid management are outlined in Table 2–4.

During this period of stabilization, an arterial line should be inserted in any critically ill infant. We prefer the radial or temporal artery for this purpose, although the umbilical artery is technically easier and relatively safe for 1–2 days if the catheter is properly inserted and maintained. An arterial catheter permits continual monitoring of systemic arterial pressure, which, in conjunction with heart rate, provides the most readily available estimate of cardiac output and blood flow in the neonate. ECG, respiratory rate (by impedance plethysmography) and skin and rectal temperatures should be monitored continually throughout the preoperative period.

ANESTHETIC MANAGEMENT. — *Preanesthetic medication.* — Intravenous atropine should be administered during the period of stabilization or immediately prior to anesthesia induction. In our opinion, narcotics, barbiturates and other sedatives are not required in the preanesthetic period for critically ill infants.

Equipment. — Appropriate anesthetic equipment constitutes an essential element in the safe and effective administration of anesthesia to small infants.[80] Currently available masks for infants are of a variety sufficient to enable the anesthetist to fit the mask adequately without producing excessive pressure on the skin, eyes or nose (with resultant airway obstruction). Infant metal and plastic Guedel oropharyngeal airways in a variety of sizes (000 to 1) and thicknesses should be available to permit relief from soft tissue upper airway obstruction during induction of anesthesia. Nasopharyngeal tubes have not been developed for infants, but an appropriate size of endotracheal tube can be cut to serve this purpose. Except in cases of anesthesia for very brief superficial operations, most pediatric anesthesiologists advocate tracheal intubation of all infants under the age of 1 year in order to ensure patency of the airway.

The Miller-0 laryngoscope blade for low birth weight infants, the Miller-1 for full-term infants up to 4 kg and the Wis-Hipple 1½ for infants between 4 and 10 kg have proved to be easy to use and provide adequate exposure. Uncuffed Magill or Murphy tracheal tubes are preferred by most pediatric anesthesiologists in the United States. The Cole tube has certain theoretic advantages that have not been borne out in clinical practice; bronchial intubation is not averted, airway resistance does not improve appreciably and the widened shoulder of the upper portion of the tube impinges on the delicate laryngeal tissues, resulting in greater trauma than occurs with the appropriate size of Magill tube.

The two systems most commonly used in pediatric anesthesia are: (1) the modifications of the Mapleson "T" piece system[80] and (2) the infant circle absorber system.[81] The Mapleson systems have the advantages of simplicity (require no valves), light weight, easy cleaning and sterilization, low cost and ease of adaptation for heated humidification and expired gas evacuation. Fresh gas flow requirements as a function of body weight have been determined for the various Mapleson modifications.[82] The recent Bain modification[83] provides an extraordinarily light, compact connection to the endotracheal tube for all procedures (but especially those on the head and neck) in infants as well as older children and adults, and the system can be adapted for convenient expired gas evacuation. Fresh inspired gas delivered through the internal tube is partially heated by expired gas passing through the outer tube.

Heated humidification of inspired gas is an essential element in the anesthetic management of infants. Dry gas inhaled for more than 1 hour causes definite abnormalities in the tracheal mucosal cells,[84] and failure to heat inspired gases will result in heat loss, further aggravating the thermal stress associated with anesthesia and operation. If the Bain tubing is not heated, a temperature of 42°C in a humidifier on the anesthesia machine will provide 28 mg of water per liter of gas flow (at 8 lpm) at a temperature of 28.5°C at the tracheal connection of the system.[85]

The infant circle system, when arranged so that fresh gas passes through the soda lime absorber prior to delivery to the patient, can provide reasonable heating and humidification of inspired gas. However, the infant must provide the initial calories and water vapor to convert the absorber into a humidifier. Heat and moisture exchangers (HME)[86] inserted at the tracheal connection provide approximately 19 mg/l of water vapor (in contrast to approximately 13 mg/l without humidifiers) at room temperature, increase dead space and can become plugged with secretions. Nonetheless, an HME should be used if other humidifying devices are not available. Adult circle absorber systems have been utilized in infants, but because of the excessive compressible gas volume within the system, subtle changes in resistance or compliance of the infant's lungs will not be detected.

Automatic mechanical ventilators can be utilized during anesthesia for infants with safety and effectiveness provided that one compensates for the internal compliance (compressible gas volume stated in ml/cm H_2O airway pressure)[87] in the anesthesia and ventilator delivery system. A finely adjustable pressure relief valve should be provided to prevent excessive pressure within the system. The major advantage of an automatic anesthesia ventilator is the consistent delivery of a preset minute volume, thus freeing the anesthetist's hands for other purposes. The major disadvantages are the loss of appreciation by the anesthetist of: (1) subtle changes in pulmonary compliance and resistance, thus precluding those fine adjustments in lung inflation that provide optimal operating conditions during intrathoracic procedures and (2) small, yet important, losses of tidal volume due to undetected leaks in the delivery system. Mechanical ventilation has proved to be most useful during anesthesia for nonthoracic procedures lasting more than 1 hour, cardiovascular procedures utilizing cardiopulmonary bypass and in thoracic procedures during periods when the lung is not manipulated. A pressure manometer in the delivery system will aid detection of small volume losses and alterations in total compliance or airways resistance. Whether automatic or manual ventilation is used, Pa_{O_2} and Pa_{CO_2} should be checked at least at 30-minute intervals in critically ill infants.

In addition to the mandatory oxygen fail-safe device, we advocate equipping every anesthesia machine used in the care of infants with a continuous-reading oxygen concentration monitor placed in the inspiratory line distal to the common gas outlet of the machine. A gas ratiometer providing oxygen concentrations from 21% to 100% blended with nitrous oxide provides additional assurance against delivery of mixtures that cause hypoxemia.[88] Because of the hazard of retrolental fibroplasia in infants under 44 weeks postconceptual age,[79] anesthesia machines should be equipped to provide oxygen concentrations as low as 21%, enabling the anesthetist to keep the Pa_{O_2} between 50 and 75 torr and thereby minimize the risk of retrolental fibroplasia. An easily adjustable and reliable pressure relief valve is required for safety when ventilating small infants, who need relatively high inflating pressures for lung expansion.

Anesthetic agents and adjuvant drugs. — Despite the lack of a discriminating response to pain, the newborn infant reacts with a mass reflex response to all sudden stimuli and develops tachycardia, hypertension and considerably increased skeletal muscle tone in response to pain. In the first 6 months of extrauterine life, the infant achieves more discrete pain perception with appropriate withdrawal defenses. However, for many years pediatric anesthesiologists have appreciated that the infant under 6 months of age requires a relatively higher delivered concentration of anesthetic agents to achieve satisfactory surgical anesthesia than does an older child or an adult. Higher blood levels of cyclopropane are required to achieve comparable levels of anesthesia in infants under 6 months of age as compared with adults.[89] The medial effective dose (ED_{50})[90] and minimal alveolar concentration (MAC)[91] for halothane are significantly higher in infants under 6 months of age than in older children and adults. Although other anesthetic agents, including intravenous agents, have not been evaluated in this manner, clinical observations suggest that infants under 6 months of age require a higher dosage for a comparable effect with all agents.

Nitrous oxide, in combination with nondepolarizing muscle relaxants and/or halothane, has become the most widely utilized agent. In inspired concentrations of 65–70%, nitrous oxide provides analgesia adequate for most operations, has minimal cardiovascular depressant effects and has no known adverse effects on the newborn liver or kidneys. However, muscle relaxants must be used to prevent gross movement during the procedure. The uptake and excretion of nitrous oxide and halothane occur more rapidly in the newborn and small infant than in the adult.[92] This is related to numerous physiologic differences, including the infant's increased cardiac output, greater alveolar ventilation, smaller functional residual capacity and proportionately larger compartment of well-perfused tissues relative to body mass. Thus, more rapid achievement of surgical planes of anesthesia and more rapid emergence from anesthesia induced by nitrous oxide will occur in healthy infants as compared with healthy adults.

Halothane appears to be a more potent depressant of cardiovascular function in the infant than in the adult. A higher incidence of systemic arterial hypotension at ED_{50} with halothane has been observed in the infant under 6 months of age.[90] Thus, for halothane, the margin of safety is narrowed; i.e., the effective dose is closer to the toxic (or hypotensive) dose. As a consequence of this and of the rapid uptake of halothane, severe arterial hypotension and cardiac arrest occur more commonly in the young infant during induction of anesthesia with halothane than with other agents. Anesthesia may be induced with intravenous thiopental in infants with normal cardiovascular function or with ketamine in infants predisposed to decreased cardiac output and arterial hypotension.

With nitrous oxide-relaxant anesthesia, additional analgesia may be required during intra-abdominal or intrathoracic operations. Fentanyl will reduce the hypertension and tachycardia that accompany painful stimulation, yet permit return of adequate unassisted ventilation after approximately 2 hours, provided that the total dose does not exceed 2 micrograms per kilogram. The pharmacokinetics and side-effects of fentanyl in the newborn and young infant have not been studied. However, the drug appears to have no additional adverse effects on the infant other than respiratory depression as observed in adults.[93] Morphine and meperidine also provide additional analgesia but will produce a much longer period of postoperative respiratory depression. These drugs should be reserved for the infant who will require postoperative mechanical ventilation for a period of many hours.

Neuromuscular blocking drugs play an extraordinarily important role in the anesthetic management of young infants, since they enable the anesthetist to provide optimal operating conditions while utilizing minimal dosages of toxic anesthetic or analgesic agents. A single intravenous dose of succinylcholine can facilitate rapid tracheal intubation; a larger dose per unit weight is required to achieve paralysis in the neonate and young infant compared with older children and adults.[23, 24] The nondepolarizing relaxants *d*-tubocurarine[26, 27] and pancuronium[25] will provide complete neuromuscular blockade for periods of 20–45 minutes, after which they can be reversed with atropine and neostigmine (Table 2–8). Pancuronium does not cause release of histamine as does curare, and therefore will not cause the arterial hypotension observed occasionally with *d*-tubocurarine in infants.

The neonate manifests a much broader range of response to nondepolarizing muscle relaxants than do older patients[27]; therefore, one should use approximately 25–50% of the calculated initial dose at 2–3-minute intervals until appropriate relaxation is achieved (Table 2–8), which may or may not require the full calculated initial dose. Subsequent maintenance doses should be approximately 25% of the total initial dose. Problems with reversal of the nondepolarizing relaxants appear to be more common in infants than in older children, but often this is due to hypothermia, hypocalcemia or central nervous system immaturity rather than the direct effect of these drugs.

Monitoring. — Conditions change more rapidly, with less warning, and more readily deteriorate into disaster during anesthesia in infants than in any other age group.[94] Proof of this can be seen in the significantly higher cardiac arrest rate[95] and anesthetic mortality[1] observed in these patients. For this reason, more extensive monitoring must be utilized in relation to the patient's physical status and the planned operative procedure than might otherwise be necessary in older patients. Monitoring guidelines for infants and older patients are presented in Table 2–9.

In infants under 1500 gm, peripheral arterial cannulation[31] may prove to be technically more difficult, and an umbilical artery catheter inserted to the level of the bifurcation of the aorta (as confirmed by x-ray) will suffice.[96] However, the umbilical artery catheter samples blood below the ductus arteriosus and may not reflect the higher Pa_{O_2} that can occur above that level (in the retinal artery) when the ductus is patent.[97] Thus, the anesthetist may not be aware of the increased hazard of producing retrolental fibroplasia that results from hyperoxemia in the retina. The duration of hyper-

TABLE 2-9.—MONITORING

Breath sounds ⎫ Heart tones ⎬	Precordial, esophageal stethoscope
ECG	—Lead 2
Systemic arterial pressure	—Infant cuff —Oscillometer —Doppler transducer —Direct
Arterial catheter	—Radial —Temporal
CVP catheter	—Umbilical vein —Internal jugular
Temperature	—Colonic —Esophageal —Nasopharyngeal
Ventilation	—Breath sounds —Airway pressure —FI_{O_2}, Pa_{O_2} —Pa_{CO_2}
Blood loss	—Small volume suction traps —Weight sponges —Serial Hct
Urine volume	—1–2 ml/kg/hr minimum

oxemia necessary to increase the risk of retrolental fibroplasia remains uncertain, but may be only a few hours.[79]

Induction of anesthesia.—The technique and agents used to induce anesthesia and permit tracheal intubation will vary with: (1) the age and size of the infant, (2) the relative hazard of regurgitation of gastrointestinal contents and (3) the physical status. In all instances, induction of anesthesia should be preceded by intravenous atropine to prevent bradycardia. Within 6 hours after birth, the pH of gastric contents falls from alkaline levels to a mean of 2.5.[98] Pulmonary aspiration of gastric secretions poses the same hazard for infants as for adults. Thus, most pediatric anesthesiologists prefer awake tracheal intubation without neuromuscular blockade in infants less than 4.0 kg and 4 weeks of age, especially in cases of gastrointestinal obstructive lesions. Although all such patients should have their stomachs emptied by nasogastric suction, one must not assume that the risk of vomiting has been eliminated. In critically ill infants, especially those with serious cardiopulmonary disease, mass reflex responses and struggling associated with laryngoscopy may be detrimental to the maintenance of adequate ventilation; in such instances, intravenous succinylcholine in association with gentle cricoid pressure to prevent reflux of gastric contents will facilitate tracheal intubation. Succinylcholine does not cause fasciculations or an increase in intragastric pressure in infants,[99] eliminating the need for an antifasciculating dose of *d*-tubocurarine. The inspired oxygen concentration (FI_{O_2}) should be maintained at 100% for at least 2 minutes prior to and for at least 1 minute following tracheal intubation. Intravenous thiopental or ketamine can be used in infants over 1 month of age in a rapid-sequence intravenous induction.

During induction of anesthesia and at the time of tracheal intubation, maintenance of the proper head position reduces the incidence and severity of soft tissue airway obstruction that commonly occurs in the small infant. This position involves moderate flexion of the cervical spine with extension of the occipitoatlantal joint ("sniffing position").[100] A 3–4-cm-thick pad placed under the occiput, with the infant's shoulders flat on the operating table, achieves the appropriate degree of cervical flexion; adequate extension of the occipitoatlantal joint then can be acomplished by simply elevating the infant's chin.

In infants over 1 month of age who are not at risk for regurgitation or critically ill, anesthesia can be induced with nitrous oxide followed by a nondepolarizing muscle relaxant given intravenously to permit tracheal intubation and provide conditions for the operative procedure. Physical status 1 and 2 infants (p. 13) over 10 kg undergoing short, superficial procedures not involving the airway may be safely anesthetized with nitrous oxide-oxygen-halothane by mask. The systemic arterial pressure must be checked at 1–2-minute intervals during induction with halothane to detect the unpredictable onset of hypotension.

Nitrous oxide diffuses rapidly into closed spaces[101] and may cause increased intraluminal pressure in obstructed segments of bowel. For this reason, in infants with intestinal obstruction, nitrous oxide should be withheld until the peritoneum has been opened. Anesthesia for tracheal intubation and skin incision can be provided by intravenous ketamine or thiopental.

Intraoperative anesthetic management.—In all but the briefest superficial procedures, endotracheal anesthesia with controlled ventilation using nitrous oxide and *d*-tubocurarine or pancuronium appears to be the safest, effective technique. This avoids the problems of cardiovascular depression from halothane and inadequate ventilation or upper airway obstruction, which occur commonly in infants during spontaneous ventilation without tracheal intubation. Additional analgesia can be provided by narcotics or low inspired concentrations (0.2–0.5%) of halothane. Infants unable to tolerate nitrous oxide can be ventilated with oxygen and have adequate analgesia with intermittent doses of intravenous ketamine or narcotics (Table 2–8).

Heat loss poses one of the major intraoperative hazards for the infant, particularly the low birth weight and/or premature infant.[102] Although temperature regulation in the newborn receiving various anesthetic agents has not been studied, clinical experience indicates that anesthesia may impair the expected increase in metabolic rate and utilization of free fatty acids in response to thermal stress. Methods for maintaining body temperature were presented above.

Termination of anesthesia.—At completion of the operation, a decision must be made whether or not to reverse neuromuscular blockade prior to transfer of the infant to the recovery room or an infant intensive care unit. Systemic arterial hypotension, hypothermia or hypocalcemia ordinarily contraindicates an attempt to reverse the nondepolarizing muscle relaxants. Infants who have undergone extensive intrathoracic or intra-abdominal procedures are transported to an infant intensive care unit prior to reversal of relaxants and tracheal extubation. During transport, heart tones, ECG, systemic arterial pressure and body temperature are monitored continually. The time between termination of anesthesia and stabilization in the infant intensive care unit constitutes a most hazardous period. Airway obstruction, inadequate ventilation, arterial hypotension and cold stress pose threats to the infant's welfare. Thus, the infant should be moved in a heated infant transport incubator[77] equipped with oxygen, suction, appropriate monitoring devices and with manually assisted ventilation.

Reversal of neuromuscular blockade can be undertaken when at least 25 minutes has elapsed since the last dose of the relaxant and some spontaneous movement or twitch response to nerve stimulation has returned. Atropine should immediately precede the administration of neostigmine (Table 2–8). If the infant does not breathe spontaneously and exhibits a vigorous response to stimulation, including facial grimacing and leg movement, within 5 minutes after administration of neostigmine, one of the complicating factors cited above may be present. However, the most common cause for inactivity is a Pa_{CO_2} level below 30 torr. A timed 30–60-second trial of apnea, following 1 minute of ventilation at normal tidal volumes and frequencies with 100% oxygen, often will result in an increase in Pa_{CO_2} sufficient to initiate spontaneous breathing. Other causes for delayed return of activity were discussed above.

In the critically ill infant, a 30–60-minute trial of spontaneous breathing with a T piece, continuous positive airway pressure at 2 cm H_2O (which mimics the natural expiratory resistance of the nose and pharynx)[103] and an appropriate FI_{O_2} to maintain the Pa_{O_2} within acceptable limits provide time to evaluate the cardiopulmonary system. An arterial blood sample analyzed for pH, Pa_{CO_2} and Pa_{O_2} will confirm the status of ventilation. If the Pa_{CO_2} exceeds 50 torr, the Pa_{O_2} is less than 60 torr ($FI_{O_2} > 0.60$), the mean respiratory frequency exceeds 60 or if systemic arterial hypotension and/or tachycardia occur, the tracheal tube should remain in place and intensive cardiopulmonary care be instituted (see below).

When the infant appears to be fully conscious and has vigorous neuromuscular activity and cardiopulmonary stability, the tracheal airway may be removed. The stomach, oropharynx and nares should be aspirated. After cardiopulmonary operative procedures, or if tracheobronchial secretions are audible on auscultation, sterile tracheobronchial toilet with saline will serve to clear the airways prior to extubation. Hyperventilation of the infant's lungs with 100% oxygen before extubation of the trachea minimizes the risk of postextubation hypoxemia. Removal of the tube while the lungs are inflated to a point near the maximal inspiratory capacity ensures that on withdrawal of the tube a rapid exhalation simulating an effective cough will occur. This tends to expel secretions from the larynx and reduces the likelihood of laryngospasm or aspiration.

POSTANESTHESIA CARE.—In the immediate postanesthetic period, meticulous attention must be directed to patency of the infant's airway and maintenance of adequate ventilation. Monitoring of respiratory rate by the impedance method is essential for early detection of respiratory distress, breathing dysrhythmias and apneic episodes. These are more prone to occur in the infant less than 2500 gm and 36 weeks gestational age, but may occur in any newborn or young infant in the postanesthetic period. Infants between 2 weeks and 6 months of age who are predisposed to the sudden infant death syndrome (SIDS),[104] such as those with a history of premature birth, intermittent apneic episodes or upper respiratory infection, may have unpredictable apneic episodes with severe bradycardia in the first 1–2 hours following anesthesia. An inspired oxygen concentration required to keep the Pa_{O_2} between 50 and 75 torr, to maintain adequate oxygenation while minimizing the risks of retrolental fibroplasia, should be provided with heated humidification in a small plastic hood. Alveolar ventilation can be

presumed to be adequate when the Pa_{CO_2} is below 40 torr.

Whenever respiratory distress (tachypnea, retractions and cyanosis) develops in the postanesthetic period, a chest roentgenogram should be obtained to exclude pneumothorax, atelectasis and aspiration syndrome. Persistent effects of narcotics or volatile anesthetics, hypothermia or residual partial neuromuscular blockade can cause subtle upper airway obstruction and hypoventilation. If these occur, assisted ventilation by bag and mask or reintubation of the trachea and mechanical ventilation will be required.

Cardiovascular monitoring, including ECG, heart rate and systemic arterial pressure (through an indwelling line or by frequent determination with a Doppler device), along with hourly urine output provide the essential information to evaluate the adequacy of organ perfusion. Provision of neutral thermal conditions (see above) will minimize metabolic stress. An arterial pH maintained between 7.30 and 7.45 aids cardiopulmonary adaptation in the postoperative period.

Intravenous fluid management in the postanesthetic period follows the guidelines utilized for the preoperative and intraoperative period. The infant's daily weight, determined each time under identical conditions, will warn of excess fluid intake or loss that might not otherwise be appreciated.

One of the most common causes of death and severe morbidity in the postanesthetic period of the infant is acute respiratory failure (ARF). The general criteria for the diagnosis of ARF include:

$Pa_{O_2} < 60$ torr (at an $FI_{O_2} > 0.60$).

$Pa_{CO_2} > 50$ torr.

Recurrent apneic episodes and bradycardia.

Arterial hypotension.

Persistent clinical signs of respiratory distress despite tracheal intubation.

Any two of these signs indicate the presence of life-threatening impairment of pulmonary gas exchange. These criteria for diagnosis of ARF are less stringent than some may propose for infants with respiratory distress syndrome and other cardiopulmonary disorders of infancy, yet experience suggests that to delay until further deterioration occurs in an infant after operation will lead to an unacceptable incidence of cardiopulmonary arrest.[105, 106]

Infants predisposed to develop acute respiratory failure in the postanesthetic period include: low birth weight and premature infants, infants with severe cardiopulmonary disease in the preoperative period and infants with diaphragmatic hernia, tracheoesophageal fistula, omphalocele, congenital cardiac lesions and vascular rings. Once a diagnosis of ARF is made, intensive respiratory care must be instituted to re-establish adequate pulmonary gas exchange. The elements of intensive respiratory care[105-108] are presented below.

RESULTS.—One might ask what an intensive, complex effort by a group of physicians and nurses working with ill infants who have severe anomalies ultimately accomplishes. The answer is that a great deal can be accomplished. In the past 10 years, the first-year mortality rate due to all congenital anomalies has declined from 3.6 to 2.8 per 1000 live births, a 22% reduction.[109] This has been due in part to the advances in pediatric anesthesia and infant intensive care, which have permitted the technical surgical advances to develop and succeed.

An example of this can be seen with esophageal atresia (EA) and tracheoesophageal fistula (TEF), lesions that were uniformly fatal 40 years ago. In the past 13 years at The Children's Hospital of Philadelphia, all of the 50 full-term newborns with EA and TEF who had no associated major anomalies or pneumonitis before operation have survived,[110] as has been observed in other pediatric surgical centers (see Chap. 43).

Special Problems in Older Infants and Children

Children with major systemic diseases such as congenital cardiovascular anomalies, asthma or cystic fibrosis obviously require special evaluation and care when undergoing any type of anesthesia and surgery. However, certain disorders may produce complications associated with anesthesia that one would not ordinarily anticipate. A number of such disorders are listed in Table 2–10 along with the major problem to be anticipated during anesthesia.

Over the past 20 years, halothane has become the most frequently used inhalation anesthetic in pediatric practice.

The National Halothane Study[123] failed to document a greater incidence of hepatic toxicity following halothane anesthesia than with other inhalation agents. However, case reports suggest that the rare individual can incur hepatic necrosis following halothane or cyclopropane anesthesia. This complication is seen less frequently in children, but when it occurs it may be fatal.[2] Unexplained fever following inhalation anesthesia is a warning sign that the patient may have developed a hepatic toxic reaction. In such a patient, the relative advantages of halothane for anesthesia in the future must be weighted against the possibility of fatal hepatic damage.

Comment: Although firm national statistics do not exist, the best available current estimate for an over-all pediatric anesthesia death rate is approximately 2 per 10,000 anesthetics. A significant reduction in this figure will depend on a better understanding of the normal and pathologic physiolo-

TABLE 2-10.–SPECIAL PROBLEMS IN PEDIATRIC ANESTHESIA

DISORDER	SPECIFIC PROBLEM	REFERENCE
Asthma	Bronchospasm with curare; adrenal insufficiency after withdrawal of corticosteroids	111
Cystic fibrosis	Impacted bronchial secretions with positive airway pressure; postoperative hypercapnia, hypoxemia	112
Reye syndrome	Elevated intracranial pressure	113
Sickle cell anemia	Sickling crisis with decreased Pa_{O_2}, pH; thromboses (CNS, renal) with dehydration	114
Extensive burns or trauma	Sudden severe hyperkalemia and cardiac arrest after succinylcholine	115
Renal tubular disease	Prolonged neuromuscular blockade after gallamine (muscle relaxant) due to delayed excretion	116
Inherited atypical plasma cholinesterase	Prolonged neuromuscular blockade after succinylcholine due to atypical plasma cholinesterase	117
Myasthenia gravis	Prolonged neuromuscular blockade after nondepolarizing relaxants, e.g., *d*-tubocurarine; resistant to depolarizing relaxants	118
Myotonia congenita, myotonia atrophica	Severe, intractable muscle spasm after succinylcholine; malignant hyperthermia	112
Neuroblastoma, pheochromocytoma	Severe hypertension with tumor manipulation requiring adrenergic blockade	119, 120
Familial dysautonomia (Riley-Day syndrome)	Circulatory instability with hypertension or hypotension and vomiting during anesthesia; hyperpyrexia; recurrent bronchopneumonia	112
Acute porphyria	Extreme sensitivity to barbiturates	121
Hurler, Pierre Robin, Treacher Collins syndromes	Severe upper airway obstruction when unconscious; difficult tracheal intubation	122
Glycogen storage disease	Metabolic acidosis, hypoglycemia during anesthesia	112

gy and pharmacology of the infant, further insight into the effects of anesthetic drugs on the infant and child, wider use of available monitoring techniques and an approach to all major pediatric surgical problems that involves close, direct communication among anesthesiologist, pediatrician and surgeon.

Pediatric Intensive Care

The major objective of intensive care is to provide maximal surveillance and support of vital systems in patients with acute, but reversible, life-threatening disease. In pediatric patients, the reversal of life-threatening conditions and the preservation of essential functions, especially those of the brain, may result in many years of useful life. For example, in the United States, a 3-year-old white female child has a life expectancy of 78 years and a 1-year-old black male child, although less favored, still has an expectancy of 61 years.[124] However, if brain function becomes permanently impaired as a result of delayed or improper care, both the patient and society will suffer for many years. In this section, we cite the elements and the special considerations involved in the intensive care of critically ill pediatric patients, including the common causes of acute major organ failure, cardiopulmonary resuscitation and the management of acute respiratory failure.

Elements of Pediatric Intensive Care

The elements of intensive care have been defined[125] as: (1) geographic full-time physician specialists in anesthesiology, medicine (pediatrics), general surgery and its subspecialties; (2) a full-time physician director of intensive care; (3) nursing and allied health personnel specially trained in care of the critically ill; (4) availability of resuscitation and respiratory therapy equipment and drugs; (5) monitoring and alarm systems for continuous assessment of vital functions; (6) a 24-hour laboratory service for the rapid determination of pH and blood gas tensions, oxygen content, hemoglobin, blood sugar and plasma sodium, potassium, calcium, osmolarity and total protein; (7) a 24-hour radiology service responsive to the needs of the critically ill; (8) location of these facilities in one area of the hospital. Pediatric intensive care involves these elements as they apply to critically ill patients ranging in age from the newborn to the late adolescent. This requires that the personnel involved be thoroughly familiar with pediatric anatomy, physiology, pharmacology, pathology, psychology and appropriate technical maneuvers.

Causes of Acute Major Organ Failure

The common disorders resulting in acute major organ failure in infants and children are outlined in Table 2–11 according to the primary systems involved.

NERVOUS SYSTEM.—Acute central nervous system failure poses an immediate threat to life due to: (1) coma, with upper airway obstruction or pulmonary aspiration of gastric contents; (2) disturbed respiratory control secondary to medullary depression; (3) increased intracranial pressure, causing brain stem and cortical compression.

TABLE 2-11.—COMMON PEDIATRIC DISORDERS RESULTING IN ACUTE MAJOR SYSTEM FAILURE IN OLDER INFANTS AND CHILDREN

NERVOUS SYSTEM
  Central
    Trauma to the head
    Cerebral hypoxia
    Encephalitis
    Cerebral hemorrhage
    Drug ingestion poisoning
    Hydrocephalus
    Tumor
    Reye syndrome
    Status epilepticus

  Peripheral
    Polyneuritis (Guillain-Barré syndrome)
    Myasthenia gravis
    Tetanus
    Poliomyelitis

CARDIOVASCULAR SYSTEM
  Congenital cardiac lesions
  Myocarditis
  Septic shock
  Blood loss
  Fluid overload

RENAL SYSTEM
  Acute tubular necrosis
  Renal vein thrombosis
  Hemolytic uremia syndrome
  Goodpasture's syndrome

HEMATOPOIETIC SYSTEM
  Sickle cell anemia
  Leukemia

The clinical signs of increasing intracranial pressure include decreased consciousness and response to pain, papilledema, increasing systemic arterial pressure, bradycardia and irregular breathing. Unfortunately, the increase in intracranial pressure may exceed considerably the normal upper limit of 20 torr before these clinical signs are recognized. Therefore, in patients at risk from increased intracranial pressure, a subdural bolt[126] should be fastened into a bur hole to provide access for direct measurements. With the bolt attached to a transducer and slow-speed recorder, and simultaneous recording of systemic arterial pressure and heart rate, the intermittent intracranial pressure waves that precede development of a continually raised pressure can be detected and treated. Also, a continuous estimate of the cerebral perfusion pressure may be made. Appropriate therapy with oxygen, hyperventilation, maintenance of normal body temperature and intravenous corticosteroids, barbiturates and mannitol can be instituted before irreversible brain damage occurs.[127] Reye syndrome is a bizarre encephalopathy of childhood associated with cerebral edema and fat deposition in the liver and other viscera.[128] The monitoring and treatment of increased intracranial pressure due to cerebral edema appear to be rewarding in this syndrome.[113] Disorders such as the Guillain-Barré syndrome and myasthenia gravis that produce peripheral neuromuscular failure may pose a threat to life because of respiratory depression and impairment of upper airway reflexes.[107]

CARDIOVASCULAR SYSTEM.—Congenital cardiovascular lesions are among the leading causes of death in infants less than 1 year of age. Lesions associated with cyanosis, such as tetralogy of Fallot and transposition of the great arteries, cause severe tissue hypoxemia and eventual myocardial and central nervous system failure. In addition, these lesions are associated with polycythemia and increased blood viscosity. Hematocrits in excess of 60% may result in widespread vascular thrombosis, especially in the brain. Many of these children require intensive care and surgical correction or palliation in the first year of life to prevent irreversible hypoxic damage.[129] Infants and young children with acyanotic heart disease often have congestive cardiac failure, pulmonary edema[130] or pulmonary artery hypertension.[131] These infants are particularly susceptible to pulmonary infections, especially pneumonitis caused by gram-negative organisms, which may be the precipitating factor in the development of congestive cardiac failure.

Myocarditis, most often viral in origin, can cause congestive cardiac failure with pulmonary edema, as well as potentially lethal arrhythmias. Sepsis caused by gram-negative organisms in infants less than 1 year of age commonly causes severe arterial hypotension, necessitating administration of large volumes of intravenous fluids and infusion of catecholamines to maintain adequate organ perfusion.

RENAL SYSTEM.—Acute renal failure may be associated with bacterial or uremic pneumonitis or with pulmonary edema in infants and children.[132] The hyperkalemia that usually occurs can produce lethal arrhythmias and eventual myocardial depression with systemic arterial hypotension unless controlled by peritoneal dialysis. Goodpasture's syndrome is an uncommon disorder of unknown etiology affecting the basement membranes of the lungs and kidneys, with consequent diffuse intra-alveolar hemorrhage and glomerulonephritis; it occurs in older children.[133] Survival is possible if the pulmonary hemorrhages can be controlled.[134]

HEMATOPOIETIC SYSTEM.—Two of the most common pediatric hematologic disorders, sickle cell anemia and leukemia, may produce acute life-threatening conditions that are reversible with appropriate care. Children with sickle cell anemia can manifest severe high-output congestive cardiac failure, and respond to transfusions of erythrocytes, digitalis, diuretics and control of the associated pulmonary edema.[114] These patients may also develop cerebrovascular thromboses, from which they can recover with appropriate control of intracranial pressure, hydration and erythrocyte transfusions. With modern chemotherapy, children seldom die from the direct effects of leukemia, but rather from sepsis, pneumonitis or unrecognized expanding intracerebral metastatic lesions. Most often, the pneumonitis is caused by gram-negative organisms such as Pseudomonas or by the parasite *Pneumocystis carinii*, to which these children become susceptible because of the immunosuppressant effects of chemotherapy. Fortunately, many leukemic children have recovered from prolonged respiratory failure and returned to normal childhood activities for a number of years.

Cardiopulmonary Resuscitation

DIAGNOSIS OF CARDIOPULMONARY ARREST.—The cardinal signs of cessation of effective ventilation and circulation are: (1) gasping or apnea; (2) pallor; (3) severely diminished or absent peripheral pulses (carotid and femoral); (4) faint or absent heart tones; and (5) dilatation of the pupils. The appearance of dilated pupils indicates cessation of cerebral circulation for a period of at least 3 minutes; this sign does not imply that resuscitation should not be initiated, especially in infants and children, whose central nervous system has a remarkable capacity to recover.

MANAGEMENT OF CARDIOPULMONARY ARREST.—The American Heart Association has fostered a useful alphabetic mnemonic using the letters A through F.[135] Basic resuscitation consists of (A) airway management, (B) breathing and (C) cardiac massage. Advanced resuscitation includes (D) drugs, (E) electrocardiogram, endotracheal intubation, evaluation and (F) fibrillation treatment. A cart with the items outlined in Table 2–12 should be available at all times in emergency rooms, hospital ward treatment rooms and intensive care units caring for infants and children. These items should be used in conjunction with a bedside ECG writer and oscilloscope, measurement of systemic arterial pressure and temperature monitors.

Basic resuscitation.—The patient should be in the supine position and placed on a firm surface with ready access to the head and thorax for the personnel performing resuscitation. This may require placement of a board of appropriate size underneath the patient's body.

A. AIRWAY. The airway is cleared by turning the head to one side and aspirating secretions as well as solid material from the oropharynx; if a suction apparatus is not available, the oropharynx should be wiped with a finger. The head then is returned to the face-up position and the occiput maximally extended while the cervical spine is slightly flexed. The mandible is drawn forward to open the pharyngeal airway and bring the tongue anterior. If attempts to ventilate are unsuccessful because of airway obstruction, an oropharyngeal or nasopharyngeal airway of appropriate size should be inserted. If a foreign body is lodged in the larynx or trachea, sudden external compression of the epigastrium by the resuscitator may expel the foreign body.[136]

B. BREATHING. Ventilation by the mouth-to-mouth, mouth-to-nose or bag and mask method should be initiated as soon as the airway is cleared. Four large tidal volumes delivered rapidly will serve to increase alveolar oxygen ten-

TABLE 2-12.—RECOMMENDED CONTENTS FOR A
PEDIATRIC RESUSCITATION CART

AIRWAY EQUIPMENT
1. Bag and masks (infant, child, adult) with nonrebreathing valve that has
  universal 15-mm female adaptor for male 15-mm endotracheal tube connectors

2. Oropharyngeal airways (Guedel sizes 00, 0, 1, 2, 3, 4)

3. Orotracheal uncuffed tubes (complete sterile set of 2 of each size 2.5 mm
  I.D. to 8.0 mm I.D.) with appropriate size straight 15-mm male connectors;
  cuffed tubes 6.0–8.0 mm I.D.; lengths cut to minimal length plus 2 cm

4. Laryngoscope
  Adult handle, pediatric handle
  Blades: Miller—premature
       Wis-Hipple 1 and 1½
       Flagg—child
       Macintosh—adult (nos 3, 4)
       2 extra batteries
       1 extra light
       1 extra light for each blade

5. Aspiration equipment
  Metal tonsil aspirator (Yankauer)
  Disposable sterile plastic suction catheters,
    sizes (Fr) 5, 8, 10, 14

6. Magill forceps

7. Stylets (Teflon coated for tubes size 2.5–8.0 mm I.D.

DRUGS
Sodium bicarbonate (1 mEq/ml)   Dopamine (0.2 μg/ml)
Epinephrine (1.0 mg/ml)   Dextrose (500 mg/ml)
Isoproterenol (0.2 mg/ml)   Diazepam (5 μg/ml)
Calcium chloride (100 mg/ml)   Heparin (1000 units/ml)
Calcium gluconate (100 mg/ml)   Saline (for dilution)
Atropine sulfate (400 μg/ml)

DEFIBRILLATOR
Direct current with range of 20–400 watt-seconds
  Saline-soaked 4×4 gauze pads stored with external paddles
  Infant (3 cm diameter), pediatric (5 cm diameter) and adult (8
    cm diameter) external paddles

MISCELLANEOUS
Intracardiac needles: 20 and 22 ga, 6–8 cm length
Plastic intravenous cannulae (16 ga, 18 ga, 20 ga, 22 ga) and scalp vein sets
Sterile cutdown tray with pediatric instruments
Tongue blades   Scissors
Alcohol swabs   Syringes (plastic disposable)
Sterile hemostat   Needles
                Sterile 4×4 gauze sponges

sion prior to the institution of cardiac massage. Thereafter, the respiratory frequency in infants and children under 3 years of age should be approximately 20 breaths per minute. An inspiratory/expiratory ratio of 1:1 is appropriate. The hallmark of effective ventilation is a synchronous rise of the thorax and abdomen during the inspiratory phase. One may also listen for exhaled air through the nose or mouth. A resuscitator's exhaled air contains approximately 17% oxygen, which will raise the alveolar oxygen tension to approximately 80 mm Hg. If supplementary oxygen is available, it should be used in order to further elevate the alveolar oxygen tension and increase the uptake of oxygen from the lungs. The delivered inspired oxygen concentration will vary from 30% to 80% with self-inflating resuscitator bags at oxygen flows of 5–15 liters[137]; an inspired oxygen concentration of 100% is

ideal and can be delivered by a modified "T" piece system with a mask or endotracheal tube.[80]

C. CARDIAC MASSAGE. This is achieved by downward displacement of the sternum and ventricular compression against the thoracic vertebrae at a rate of 100 per minute in infants and 60–80 per minute in children and adults. The middle third of the sternum should be depressed 2–3 cm in infants and 5–6 cm in adults. The sternum should be held depressed for 0.2–0.3 second to produce a pulse contour and mean arterial pressure that approach normal.[138] This can be achieved in the infant by the two-thumb chest-encircling midsternal method.[139] In older infants, 2 or 3 fingers and in a child over 2 years of age the heel of one hand placed over the midsternum are effective. In children over 6 years of age, the two-hand adult method should be used. The hallmarks of effective circulation are a palpable carotid or femoral pulse and a decrease in the size of the pupils.

In children, with their yielding chest wall, closed chest cardiac massage is so effective that it may be questioned whether open chest massage is ever justified except during a thoracotomy or in cardiac tamponade.

Advanced cardiopulmonary resuscitation.—Once the airway has been opened, ventilation of the lungs initiated and reasonably effective cardiac compression with systemic perfusion achieved, the next phase in cardiopulmonary resuscitation can be undertaken. An intravenous infusion must be established with an indwelling plastic cannula inserted percutaneously or by cutdown in the largest accessible vein. In the event of intense vasoconstriction, a butterfly needle can be inserted in any peripheral vein until such time as a large vein can be cannulated. However, a small metal needle in a peripheral vein is not a safe lifeline for a patient who requires cardiopulmonary resuscitation. The proper intravenous fluid regimen will depend on the etiology of the arrest. The patient's weight, or a reasonable estimate, must be assessed in order to select the appropriate fluid infusion and drug dosages.

D. DRUGS. The fundamental drug administered in cardiopulmonary resuscitation is *oxygen*. Oxygen (100%) should be given by mask as soon as possible. The other drugs in recommended concentrations and dosages are presented in Table 2–13. Sodium bicarbonate in an initial intravenous dose of 2–4 mEq/kg serves to correct partially the inevitable metabolic acidosis associated with the severe tissue hypoxemia that results from ineffective ventilation and circulation. In the presence of cardiac standstill that is refractory to ineffective ventilation, closed chest massage and intravenous sodium bicarbonate, intravenous epinephrine should be administered and if that fails, the epinephrine may be injected directly into the heart (diluted to a volume of 2–5 ml with saline, depending on the size of the patient). A conservative alternative to intracardiac injection is intratracheal instillation of epinephrine, in the intracardiac dosage, diluted to a volume of 2–5 ml with *distilled water*.[140] Uptake from the lungs will occur if pulmonary perfusion is maintained by effective closed cardiac massage.

Intracardiac injection should be reserved for those instances in which repeated intravenous or intratracheal injections of drugs have proved to be ineffective. This will occur when the circulating blood volume is inadequate or closed chest massage is not effective because of congenital aortic outflow tract obstruction. Intracardiac injection should be performed with a syringe and 10-cm, 22-gauge needle inserted in the notch between the xiphoid and left costochondral margin, with the needle aimed at the acromion process of the left shoulder. The needle then is advanced through the diaphragm into the base of the left ventricle, exerting slight negative pressure on the syringe until a free flow of blood is obtained. The drug should be injected rapidly and the needle withdrawn. The classic position for intracardiac injection in the fourth intercostal space to the immediate left of the sternum will produce a very high incidence of pneumothorax and less reliable entrance into the left ventricle.

TABLE 2-13.—DRUGS FOR RESUSCITATION

DRUG	CONCENTRATION	INTRAVENOUS DOSE	INTRACARDIAC DOSE	FREQUENCY OF DOSE
Sodium bicarbonate	1 mEq/ml	2–4 mEq/kg, up to 200 mEq	½ intravenous	5–10 min°
Epinephrine	1:10,000 (0.1 mg/ml)	0.01 mg/kg., up to 0.5 mg	Same as intravenous	5–10 min
	µg/ml numerically equal to wt in kg†	0.2–2.0 µg/kg/min	—	Continuous infusion
Isoproterenol	1:10,000 (0.1 mg/ml)	0.01 mg/kg, up to 0.5 mg	—	Single dose
	µg/ml numerically equal to wt in kg	0.2–2.0 µg/kg/min	—	Continuous infusion
Dopamine	µg/ml numerically equal to wt in kg†	2.0–20.0 µg/kg/min	—	Continuous infusion
Atropine sulfate	400 µg/ml	10–20 µg/kg	—	30 min
Calcium chloride	10% (100 mg/ml)	20 mg/kg	—	10 min
Calcium gluconate	10% (100 mg/ml)	60 mg/kg	—	10 min

Defibrillation: 2–5 watt-seconds/kg (external)

°Obtain arterial sample for pH, P_{CO_2}, base excess, as soon as possible to guide alkali therapy.
†See text.

The inhibitory effect of an acidotic pH on the chronotropic and inotropic action of catecholamines should be kept in mind if the initial injection of epinephrine proves to be ineffective. It may be necessary to administer an additional dose of sodium bicarbonate immediately prior to the injection of epinephrine. Atropine intravenously can be used for recurring bradycardia and can be repeated twice in a 1-hour period. Calcium chloride administered through a central vein should be reserved for those instances in which an increase in myocardial contractility beyond that achieved with epinephrine is required.[141] Intravenous calcium increases the hazard of ventricular arrhythmias in patients who have been receiving digitalis.

Once spontaneous cardiac activity is restored, cardiac output still may be insufficient to maintain adequate tissue perfusion. Closed chest cardiac massage should be continued temporarily and consideration given to a constant infusion of an inotropic drug. Epinephrine increases stroke volume, peripheral vascular resistance (in higher doses) and the cardiac rate even in the presence of a diminished circulating blood volume. If the circulating blood volume is adequate or excessive and a decrease in systemic vascular resistance is desirable, isoproterenol will provide an increased stroke volume and heart rate with a decrease in peripheral vascular resistance. Dopamine in low doses has minimal effects on systemic vascular resistance, increases stroke volume with a small increase in heart rate and is useful in patients who have a tachycardia but require increased cardiac output.[142] These drugs should be provided in an initial concentration according to the following formula:

$$\text{Concentration} = \text{micrograms per ml numerically}$$
$$\text{equivalent to body weight (kg),}$$
e.g., 20-kg child = concentration of
20 micrograms per ml

With this concentration, the number of milliliters per minute equals the micrograms per kilogram per minute (μg/kg/min).

E. ELECTROCARDIOGRAM, ENDOTRACHEAL INTUBATION, EVALUATION. As soon as possible, a continuous-writing electrocardiogram (ECG) and oscilloscope monitor should be attached. The standard lead 2 usually will provide the best assessment of cardiac rhythm. The four common ECG dysrhythmias seen are: standstill, ventricular fibrillation, multifocal ventricular tachycardia and idioventricular bradycardia. The intravenous injection of epinephrine usually will facilitate the correction of ventricular fibrillation by electrical defibrillation. Multifocal ventricular tachycardia usually will respond to an intravenous injection of lidocaine (Xylocaine) in an initial dose of 1.0 mg/kg.

Tracheal intubation should be performed as soon as basic resuscitation has become effective, or previously if the airway cannot be maintained as described under A. Evaluation of the cause of the arrest and a written record must be initiated at this point. The few moments spent ultimately may save the patient's life. The record should include: (1) the time that the cardiopulmonary arrest was diagnosed, resuscitation begun and restoration of breathing and cardiac activity achieved; (2) the drugs, routes and doses utilized, as well as other maneuvers performed; and (3) the names of all actively participating personnel.

Hypothermia with core temperatures below 36° C can develop during resuscitation and have disastrous effects: apnea, progressive metabolic acidosis, decreased cardiac output with persistent arterial hypotension and ventricular arrhythmias. During the period of resuscitation it is important to maintain the patient's core temperature with external heating devices such as water blankets and overhead radiant heaters. Mild hypothermia does nothing to protect the brain against hypoxemia and creates conditions that retard or prevent successful resuscitation.

F. FIBRILLATION—TREATMENT. Electrical defibrillation ordinarily is required to convert the heart with ventricular fibrillation to a standstill or regular rhythm. A direct-current defibrillator should be utilized with appropriate sized paddles (3–4 cm diameter in infants; 4–5 cm diameter in the child; 8 cm diameter in the adult). The initial external defibrillation energy dose should be 2 watt-seconds per kg.[143] If this is not successful, the shocks can be increased to 5–10 watt-seconds per kg with a maximum of 400 watt-seconds. The risk of skin burns increases with increasing dosages; saline-soaked gauze pads provide a good conductor that will minimize the hazard of burns. Severe acidosis, extreme hyperkalemia or hypokalemia or a Pa_{O_2} less than 30 torr may make the fibrillating ventricle refractory to defibrillation.

Postresuscitation care.—Immediately following successful resuscitation, treatment must be directed at two problems: the underlying cause of the cardiopulmonary arrest and the sequelae of cardiopulmonary arrest. This can be executed best in an intensive care unit. The immediate common sequelae of cardiopulmonary arrest are: (1) metabolic acidosis (rebound acidosis) secondary to increased perfusion and removal of lactic acid from peripheral tissues that had been ischemic during the period of inadequate circulation; (2) hyperkalemia secondary to extreme metabolic acidosis; (3) acute renal tubular failure secondary to extreme hypotension; (4) cerebral edema with possible increased intracranial pressure secondary to extreme hypoxemia; and (5) cardiovascular instability with arterial hypotension, dysrhythmias or recurrent arrest if the primary cause is not corrected.

Treatment of postresuscitation acidosis should be guided by repeated arterial pH and blood gas tension measurements. Hyperkalemia with serum potassium levels in excess of 6 mEq/l should be treated during continuous ECG monitoring by the intravenous infusion of: (1) calcium gluconate (50 mg/kg or 0.5 ml/kg of 10% solution); (2) 25% glucose (4 ml/kg) followed by regular insulin (0.3 unit/kg); and (3) sodium bicarbonate to keep arterial pH above 7.30.[143a] The treatment of acute renal tubular failure in the early phase involves the rapid infusion of intravenous fluids, followed by a single intravenous injection of mannitol (1 gm/kg) or furosemide (1 mg/kg) once cardiovascular stability has been achieved. If this fails to produce urine flow, the fluid challenge can be repeated. If urine flow remains less than 0.5 ml/kg/hour for 6 hours, the patient must be considered oliguric or anuric and be placed on a severely restricted fluid and electrolyte regimen; peritoneal dialysis can also be utilized.[143b]

The key to successful postresuscitation management is adequate monitoring. The ECG and heart rate must be assessed continually with high- and low-rate alarms. The systemic arterial pressure should be measured continually through a peripheral arterial cannula.

In patients who have suffered a severe anoxic episode, the continual monitoring of intracranial pressure through a subdural bolt provides the only effective early warning system of progressive cerebral edema and elevated intracranial pressure.[126] When the intracranial pressure exceeds 20 torr, whether or not decerebrate or decorticate posturing or convulsions occur, steps to decrease intracranial pressure should be undertaken immediately.[127] These include: (1) hyperventilation with oxygen to reduce the Pa_{CO_2} to a level between 25 and 30 torr, which, in turn, decreases cerebral blood volume; (2) intravenous infusion of mannitol (1.0 gm/kg) to decrease brain water content; (3) adrenocorticosteroids (dexamethasone 1.0 mg/kg/6 hr); and, rarely, (4) intravenous pentobarbital (2 mg/kg/3 hr)[144] and deliberate hypothermia (esophageal temperatures between 31° C and 33° C) to decrease brain oxygen consumption. In most cases, a hypothermia blanket will be necessary to prevent hyperthermia and maintain the patient's core temperature between 37° C and 38° C.

Complications.—The immediate common complications are pneumothorax, skin burns from the defibrillator paddles and metabolic sequelae (e.g., hypernatremia, hyperosmolarity and alkalosis). Fluid overload from excessive administration of intravenous fluids during resuscitation can manifest itself as pulmonary edema shortly after the resuscitation; this is best treated with diuretics such as furosemide, mechanical ventilation with continuous positive airway pressure and fluid restriction. A portable chest X-ray taken as soon as the patient is stable following successful resuscitation is necessary to rule out pneumothorax, to assess the proper placement of a tracheal airway and to exclude atelectasis or aspiration pneumonitis.

Laceration of the liver as a result of misplaced excessive pressure during closed chest cardiac massage is exceedingly rare. The most disastrous late sequelae are acute renal tubular necrosis and severe, permanent cortical brain injury due to delayed or ineffective therapy.

RESULTS.—Recent data indicate high success rates in cardiopulmonary resuscitation, especially in infants and children.[145] The ultimate survival rate of pediatric patients with arrest was 47% in a large university hospital with a well-organized pediatric resuscitation team; of the survivors, 88% had no evidence of brain damage. The message seems quite clear: in infants and children with cardiopulmonary arrest who are not afflicted with a terminal disease or anomalies incompatible with conscious, potentially enjoyable life, an all-out effort must be made to restore effective ventilation and circulation and to support life following resuscitation.

Acute Respiratory Failure

The majority of disorders requiring intensive care in infants and children are associated with impaired ventilation. When the impairment of ventilation is sufficient to pose an immediate threat to life, acute respiratory failure exists. The principal causes of acute respiratory failure are outlined in Table 2–14. The criteria for a diagnosis of acute respiratory failure vary with the age of the patient and the primary disease. Although clinical observations are of considerable importance, the diagnosis should depend on repeated physiologic measurements, particularly arterial pH and blood gas tensions. Specific criteria have not been developed for all of the causes of acute respiratory failure in the pediatric age group, but in children who have acute pulmonary disease, the general criteria outlined in Table 2–15 can be used to diagnose acute respiratory failure. In infants and children with infectious polyneuritis (Guillain-Barré syndrome), the criteria outlined in Table 2–16 can prove useful in the diagnosis of impending respiratory failure and determination of the need for an artificial tracheal airway and mechanical ventilation.

TREATMENT OF ACUTE RESPIRATORY FAILURE.—*Initial therapy.*—Once the diagnosis of acute respiratory failure is

TABLE 2-14.—COMMON PEDIATRIC DISORDERS RESULTING IN ACUTE MAJOR SYSTEM FAILURE OF THE RESPIRATORY SYSTEM

UPPER AIRWAY OBSTRUCTION
  Croup
    Infectious
    Postintubation
  Epiglottitis
  Congenital subglottic stenosis
  Foreign body
  Vocal cord paralysis
  Vascular ring
  Granuloma
  Burns

LOWER AIRWAY OBSTRUCTION
  Status asthmaticus
  Bronchopneumonia (bronchiolitis)
  Smoke inhalation
  Cystic fibrosis
  Aspiration syndrome
  Lobar emphysema

ALVEOLAR DISORDERS
  Pneumonia
    Infectious
    Chemical
  Pulmonary edema
  Pulmonary hemorrhage
  Trauma
  Oxygen toxicity

OTHER
  Pneumothorax
  Hemothorax
  Diaphragmatic eventration
  Pneumomediastinum
  Severe kyphoscoliosis

made, steps should be taken immediately to improve pulmonary gas exchange. Evidence of severe hypoxemia, bradycardia or systemic arterial hypotension calls for the use of 100% oxygen by bag and mask with assisted ventilation, aspiration of upper airway secretions, establishment of an adequate intravenous route with a plastic cannula, monitoring of precordial heart tones and electrocardiogram and use of intravenous sodium bicarbonate to restore the pH of arterial blood to 7.20 or higher.

Consideration should be given to forms of therapy that

TABLE 2-15.—CRITERIA FOR DIAGNOSIS OF RESPIRATORY FAILURE IN INFANTS AND CHILDREN WITH ACUTE PULMONARY DISEASE

CLINICAL
  Decreased or absent inspiratory breath sounds
  Severe inspiratory retractions and use of accessory muscles
  Cyanosis in 40% ambient oxygen
  Depressed level of consciousness and response to pain
  Poor skeletal muscle tone
PHYSIOLOGIC
  $Pa_{CO_2} \geqslant 75$ torr
  $Pa_{O_2} \leqslant 100$ torr in 100% oxygen*
  Three clinical and one physiologic criteria = acute respiratory failure

*In the absence of cyanotic congenital heart disease.

TABLE 2-16.—CRITERIA OF RESPIRATORY FAILURE
IN INFANTS AND CHILDREN WITH
INFECTIOUS POLYNEURITIS

CLINICAL
    Weak to absent cough reflex
    Incompetent swallowing mechanism
    Weak to absent gag reflex

PHYSIOLOGIC
    Vital capacity $\leq$ 12 ml/kg
    $Pa_{O_2} \leq$ 70 torr (in air)
    Inspiratory pressure < 20 cm H_2O

Two clinical and one physiologic criteria = impending respiratory
    failure

may improve gas exchange without an artificial tracheal airway or mechanical ventilation. However, unless a dramatic improvement in ventilation and blood gas tensions occurs as a result of the immediate resuscitative measures or other therapy, an orotracheal tube should be inserted and the lungs ventilated with 100% oxygen. Most of these patients have retained gastric secretions or food and must be treated with this in mind when inserting the tracheal tube (see above). Following orotracheal intubation and ventilation with oxygen, secretions in the trachea and bronchi should be aspirated, utilizing sterile techniques. If the patient's general condition permits, chest physiotherapy and tracheobronchial toilet and manual hyperinflation of the lungs performed with the patient in both lateral positions often will reinflate atelectatic segments.

Tracheal airway.—Nasotracheal intubation and tracheostomy are elective procedures, to be accomplished after initial orotracheal intubation. If an artificial tracheal airway will be needed for longer than 12 hours but less than 5–7 days, we prefer a nasotracheal rather than an orotracheal tube. A properly placed nasotracheal tube provides more stable fixation, less danger of accidental extubation, fewer oropharyngeal secretions and permits care of the mouth and oropharynx. With rare exceptions, a tube of the same diameter as that used for the oral route can be inserted nasally. Cuffed tubes are not necessary in infants and small children, whose narrow subglottic tracheal diameters ensure an adequate tracheal seal. Unless very high pressures are necessary for adequate mechanical ventilation, a tracheal tube permitting a slight leak at 40 cm H_2O airway pressure should be used to minimize trauma to the subglottic area. Children more than 8 years of age may require tubes with low-pressure, large-volume cuffs when high airway pressures are necessary to provide adequate alveolar ventilation (e.g., in status asthmaticus). Once the nasotracheal tube has been inserted, a roentgenogram of the chest must be obtained to exclude bronchial intubation and pneumothorax. The tube should be fixed by careful application of waterproof adhesive tape after drying and preparation of both tube and skin with tincture of benzoin. Meticulous attention to these details will protect the patient against the disaster of accidental extubation.

Tracheostomy is preferable to nasotracheal intubation when an artificial airway is needed for more than 7 days or in cases of intrinsic laryngeal disease, extremely thick tracheal secretions or pulmonary hemorrhage with blood clots. Appropriate surgical techniques for tracheostomy in infants and children have been described[146] (see Chap. 39). Experience with polyvinyl pediatric tubes,* proper humidification

and airway care has made the metal tube with a cannula obsolete. A flexible attachment† from the tracheostomy tube to a ventilator or T piece is essential. Cuffed tracheostomy tubes almost never are necessary in the care of infants and children. If a cuff must be used, it should be of a low-pressure, high-volume type inflated to the minimal pressure required to ensure a satisfactory seal.[147] Cuffed tracheostomy tubes can lead to severe tracheal stenosis, and their use in pediatric patients ought to be limited.

Airway care.—An artificial tracheal airway in a child requires expert care. Inspired gas should be humidified to provide 35–44 mg of water vapor per liter of gas flow at 37° C (80–100% relative humidity) in the trachea. Most commercial humidifiers fail to accomplish this; therefore, instillation of sterile saline solution (1–3 ml) at hourly intervals is necessary to prevent occlusion of the tracheal airway and bronchi by dried secretions. Secretions in the smaller bronchi and bronchioles can be mobilized and moved toward the trachea by changes in the patient's position and chest vibration and percussion every 1–2 hours. These maneuvers are followed by sterile tracheal aspiration utilizing a catheter with a proximal thumb hole and a molded-tip with an end hole and multiple distal side holes. The catheter is inserted to the maximal depth but pulled back 2–3 mm before applying vacuum. Vacuum pressure limited to 100–200 torr may decrease the extent of mucosal damage.[148] Artificial coughing, a technique involving manual inflation of the lungs with a bag, followed by application of manual pressure on the bag and in the airway can be very useful in raising thick secretions. Before and after tracheal aspiration, the patient's lungs should be intermittently inflated with oxygen to a volume near vital capacity for a period of 1–3 minutes to protect against hypoxemia and to re-expand atelectatic segments.

Continuous positive airway pressure (CPAP).—In the child who has a large venoarterial shunt through unventilated but perfused segments of lung resulting in Pa_{O_2} less than 100 torr at 50% inspired oxygen, the institution of tracheal intubation and continuous elevation of the end-expiratory pressure to 5–10 cm H_2O above atmospheric can substantially improve arterial oxygenation. This can be applied with the patient breathing spontaneously and unassisted (if Pa_{CO_2} $\leq$ 50 torr) or as an adjunct to mechanical ventilation. In a wide variety of patients who have diffuse alveolar collapse, continuous positive airway pressure (CPAP) or positive end-expiratory pressure (PEEP) during mechanical ventilation has been shown to increase functional residual capacity and decrease venoarterial shunt, apparently by the inflation of previously collapsed alveoli, which then can participate in gas exchange throughout the ventilatory cycle.[149] In normovolemic children, CPAP causes minimal or no depression of systemic arterial pressure. With CPAP, many patients increase the Pa_{O_2} sufficiently to permit reduction of the inspired oxygen concentration to lower, and potentially less toxic, levels.

Mechanical ventilation.—Once the tracheal airway has been established and secretions removed, mechanical ventilation can be instituted. A mechanical ventilator simply replaces the bellows function of the diaphragm and thoracic wall muscles. Positive-pressure mechanical ventilation, when applied properly, also tends to improve the distribution of gas within the lung and expand atelectatic segments. The ultimate test of a mechanical ventilator is its ability to provide adequate ventilation under conditions of increased airway resistance and decreased lung compliance. In the

---

*Aberdeen pediatric tubes, Harlake Co., Cleveland, Ohio.

†Pediatric Swivel, Clarence B. Smith Company, Arlington, Massachusetts.

presence of adverse changes in pulmonary mechanics, volume preset ventilators are far more effective than those that are pressure preset.[150] Although pressure preset ventilators can compensate to a limited extent for minor leaks in the tracheal airway, this advantage is of minimal importance when an airway of the proper size has been inserted. The assist mode (a mechanism that allows the patient to initiate a breath) is provided with most pressure preset ventilators but is of minimal practical value in infants and small children. The volumes that an infant must inspire in order to trigger the device vary widely from model to model.[151] In the management of acute respiratory failure in infants and children, including the period when the patient is being "weaned" from the ventilator, the control mode has proved to be effective and adequate.

A major problem associated with the use of most commercially available volume preset ventilators in infants and children is their large internal compliance (compression volume).[87] Internal compliance can be defined as the volume of gas compressed in the ventilator system per unit mean airway pressure; this gas does not participate in the minute ventilation of the patient. For example, if the internal compliance is 4 ml per cm H_2O pressure and an infant is ventilated with a tidal volume that results in a mean airway pressure of 15 cm H_2O, 60 ml of gas are compressed within the ventilator, tubing, humidifier, water trap and alarm system. Thus, a volume setting of 60 ml would result in virtually no inspired gas passing through the tracheal tube to the patient's lungs. The ventilator volume setting must be increased to compensate for this internal compliance. Apparatus dead space has received considerable attention in the past but is not of critical importance in clinical care, and can be readily compensated for by an appropriate increase in the tidal volume. The patient's minute volume requirement may be difficult to predict unless the amount of wasted ventilation is known. Frequently one must rely on visual and auscultatory evidence of ventilation during the initial adjustments and readjust the tidal volume and respiratory frequency according to serial Pa_{CO_2} and Pa_{O_2} determinations. Initial tidal volumes of 10–15 ml/kg at a respiratory frequency approximately two-thirds normal for the patient's age will serve to correct arterial blood gas tensions toward normal.

Coordination of the patient with the mechanical ventilator often can be achieved merely by providing adequate alveolar ventilation and oxygenation. Diazepam (0.1 mg/kg intravenously) or morphine (0.1 mg/kg intravenously), in repeated doses or continuous infusion, will produce adequate sedation and depression of the respiratory drive in the restless infant or child. In patients who have severe bronchospasm and air trapping (e.g., status asthmaticus or bronchiolitis) or in whom severe pneumonia has resulted in a marked reflex tachypnea, neuromuscular blockade by continuous infusion of pancuronium provides minimal chest wall resistance to ventilation and appears to reduce the hazards of pneumothorax or pneumomediastinum. When muscle relaxants are used, the patient must be cared for by personnel who have considerable experience in handling apneic, paralyzed infants and children. We prefer the continuous infusion of sedatives and neuromuscular blockers for evenness of effect. However, infusions should be stopped daily and not restarted until signs of recovery from pharmacologic effects are evident.

Discontinuing mechanical ventilation.—A program for discontinuing mechanical ventilation in stages generally can be initiated when the Pa_{CO_2} remains less than 50 torr and Pa_{O_2} more than 100 torr at 50% inspired oxygen concentration

with peak inflating pressures less than 25 cm H_2O. In children who have cyanotic congenital heart disease, a Pa_{O_2} of more than 35 torr appears adequate. Unfortunately, there are no reliable physiologic criteria by which one can predict whether a patient can surely have ventilator support withdrawn. For that reason, and not because of psychic dependence on the ventilator, a program of intermittent mandatory ventilation (IMV), or progressively longer intervals without mechanical ventilation, usually must be carried out. IMV[152] is a technique in which the gas flow through the ventilator system is sufficient to prevent rebreathing during spontaneous ventilation. Mandatory lung inflations, provided by the ventilator at preset tidal volumes, are delivered 1–20 times per minute, depending on the patient's ability to maintain adequate minute ventilation. During this period, frequent determinations of arterial blood gas tensions and pH and daily roentgenograms of the chest are essential. A progressively rising Pa_{CO_2} or falling Pa_{O_2}, even though not to levels considered diagnostic of respiratory failure, indicates that the patient has not recovered sufficiently and continued mechanical ventilation is necessary. Clinical evidences of excessive work of breathing—tachypnea and tachycardia—frequently are seen prior to changes in blood gas tensions, and in themselves may be an indication for increased support of ventilation.

Once the patient can tolerate spontaneous ventilation for at least 12–24 hours, consideration should be given to removal of the tracheal airway. It is preferable to maintain 2–3 cm H_2O CPAP while the tracheal tube is in place to achieve optimal Pa_{O_2} levels.[103] Extubation should not be done until secretions are minimal and of thin consistency, the chest roentgenogram shows continuing improvement and the patient's general condition is stable. For at least 12 hours prior to and 24 hours after removal of a nasotracheal tube, oral intake should be restricted and hydration maintained with intravenous fluids. Because of the temporary incompetence of the larynx and impaired subglottic ciliary function following removal of a nasotracheal tube, tracheobronchial suction with a sterile catheter under direct laryngoscopy may be needed once or even twice daily for 1 or 2 days.

Supportive therapy.—Normal body temperature should be maintained by utilizing automated heating and cooling blankets, as well as vasodilating drugs such as chlorpromazine. Appropriate intravenous fluids and electrolytes, calories to prevent further catabolism and antibiotic therapy for infection are essential to the recovery of the child with respiratory failure. Caloric deprivation is a common consequence of critical illness. Since 5% intravenous glucose can provide only a fraction of the basal caloric needs, supplementary gastrointestinal feedings or intravenous alimentation must be utilized. Careful attention to washing and general care of the skin, frequent changes of position, passive range of motion exercises and judicious use of orthopedic splints will prevent skin breakdown and contractures.

Extracorporeal membrane oxygenation.—Extracorporeal membrane oxygenation (ECMO) has been the subject of laboratory investigation for more than 20 years and has been used for cardiopulmonary bypass in open heart operations for more than 10 years. Since 1970, considerable effort has been expended in a number of centers to develop ECMO for life support of patients with reversible pulmonary lesions who have acute respiratory failure with hypoxemia unresponsive to conventional therapy, including mechanical ventilation and positive end-expiratory pressure (PEEP). The objective of ECMO for this purpose is to provide a period of cardiopulmonary stability during which the lungs can recover sufficiently to meet the body's requirements for gas exchange. Presumably, recovery will be enhanced by minimizing the lung injury associated with high inflation pressures, high levels of PEEP and inspired oxygen concentrations greater than 50%. The ECMO technique consists of diversion of a major portion (usually 80%) of the patient's cardiac output through cannulae in large vessels to an artificial membrane lung, the control of blood flow regulated by a roller pump.

ECMO has proved to be an effective means of oxygenation and life support with the potential for intact survival and recovery of patients.[152a] However, the state of the art at present is analogous to that of hemodialysis 20 years ago. At that time, hemodialysis was associated with an 85% mortality, and today the mortality associated with ECMO in 300 patients worldwide is between 85% and 90%.[152b] These statistics do not include patients under the age of 12 years, although ECMO has been utilized, on occasion successfully, in children.

Numerous problems and disadvantages attend the use of ECMO. Extraordinary manpower is required to provide safe and effective perfusion over a period of days, and in most intensive care units this will tend to detract from the care of other patients. Anticoagulation must be continued throughout the period of perfusion, with the hazard of extensive bleeding; hemorrhage has been responsible for approximately 25% of the deaths. The reversibility of a lung lesion in a given patient cannot be predicted with certainty, yet one must presume that the lesion can resolve substantially within a few days if ECMO is to be used. Failure of the lungs to improve sufficiently to support life has led to perfusion for as long as 2 weeks, with an eventual fatal outcome. The efficiency of the membrane oxygenator tends to decrease, and the hazards to increase, with the duration of perfusion in both experimental animals and patients. Thus, most clinicians will wait until the patient's situation becomes desperate before using ECMO. The dilemma becomes more acute when one considers the available data, which indicate that earlier use of ECMO has been associated with shorter perfusion time and higher survival rates.

The major problem with ECMO in the neonate and young infant has been access to arteries and veins sufficiently large to accept cannulae that will permit adequate systemic blood flow and effective oxygen uptake in the extracorporeal membrane lung. Otherwise, infants and children would appear to be the best candidates to meet the objectives of ECMO. The lungs and central nervous system of infants and small children show a remarkable capacity to recover from severe tissue injury, and many of the disorders producing acute respiratory failure in this age group are reversible. Effective perfusion with ECMO has been accomplished in infants as small as 1100 gm with idiopathic respiratory distress syndrome and in larger neonates, infants and young children.[152c] ECMO may also improve tissue perfusion in children with low cardiac output unresponsive to conventional therapy. However, the effectiveness of ECMO in comparison with mechanical ventilation, PEEP, IMV and appropriate use of inotropic and vasodilator drugs has not been evaluated in pediatric patients.

The 3-year National Heart and Lung Institute collaborative extracorporeal membrane oxygenation study was completed in June of 1977. The 9 collaborating centers throughout the United States evaluated a total of 89 patients between the ages of 12 and 65 years (mean 36 years) with acute respiratory failure due to a reversible cardiopulmonary disorder. All patients faced a 90% or higher mortality with conventional therapy. The patients were prospectively random-

ized into two groups: (1) patients to receive continuing conventional therapy, including mechanical ventilation and PEEP; (2) patients to receive ECMO. None of the patients in the study were breathing spontaneously with IMV and high levels of PEEP (above 25 cm of water). The most common disorder producing respiratory failure was pneumonia. The over-all mortality in both groups was 90%, thus demonstrating no superiority of ECMO over conventional therapy under the conditions of this study.

In the future, improved ECMO devices and technique may result in a greater survival rate, especially in infants and children who have failed to respond to conventional techniques or to IMV with high levels of PEEP. Collaborative, prospective randomized studies must be carried out in children, including neonates, in order to evaluate objectively the benefits and risks of ECMO and to define its appropriate use in the critically ill infant and child. Despite the lack of more definitive criteria, we can say that, for the present, ECMO should be reserved for infants and children with acute, reversible cardiopulmonary failure that does not respond to conventional therapy, in whom the risk of dying is greater than the risk of ECMO itself.

Complications

AIRWAY COMPLICATIONS.—Accidental tracheal extubation or occlusion of the lumen of the tracheal airway by secretions usually can be prevented by attention to the details of airway care described above and proper humidification of the inspired gas. Prolonged nasotracheal intubation has been associated with postextubation subglottic stenosis, granuloma formation and fibrotic bands,[153] although the incidences vary considerably with different diseases and from one institution to another. Subglottic obstruction has been reported in 3–5% of children intubated for more than 24 hours. These subglottic complications cause partial upper airway obstruction and may appear as late as 6 weeks after extubation. However, with atraumatic insertion, proper fit and the use of polyvinylchloride tubes that are implant tested and not sterilized with ethylene oxide, such complications have become relatively rare.[154]

Tracheostomy may lead to granuloma formation distal to the end of the tracheostomy tube and at the cephalad margin of the tracheostomy incision. Difficulties in extubation of small infants following tracheostomy can result from instability of the anterior tracheal wall. Tracheal stenosis secondary to tracheostomy is extremely rare in infants and children because cuffed tracheostomy tubes are not ordinarily necessary and the surgical technique should not involve excision of cartilage (see Chap. 39).

PULMONARY COMPLICATIONS.—The major intrapulmonary complications are caused by retention of tracheobronchial secretions, contamination of the airways with pathogenic organisms, overdistention of the lungs associated with maldistribution of gas at high airway pressures, excessive pulmonary extravascular water[155] and oxygen toxicity.[156] Sudden deterioration in the circulatory status or blood gas tensions in a patient receiving mechanical ventilation necessitates an immediate roentgenogram of the chest to exclude tension pneumothorax. The hazard of pneumothorax probably is increased when the peak airway pressure exceeds 40 cm H_2O or when CPAP exceeds 10 cm H_2O.

In a number of children undergoing prolonged mechanical ventilation, we have seen decreases in urinary output and water retention, with or without radiographic evidence of interstitial pulmonary edema, and a decreasing

Pa_{O_2} similar to that observed in adults. Fluid restriction and diuretics such as furosemide often will result in a brisk diuresis, an increase in Pa_{O_2} and radiographic evidence of improvement. Most of these patients also require large tidal volumes and CPAP to maintain an optimal Pa_{O_2}. The etiology of the fluid retention remains obscure. Ultrasonic nebulizers should not be used with mechanical ventilation because they can provide a water content in gas in excess of 100% humidity at 37° C,[157] resulting in uptake of an unpredictable volume of water from the lungs.

Oxygen has the ability to damage human alveolar tissue with prolonged exposure at high concentrations.[158] Exposure to concentrations of less than 50% for many days does not appear to harm the normal human lung,[159] but the effect on diseased lungs remains uncertain. The most sensitive indicator of impaired lung function due to oxygen toxicity is a decrease in Pa_{O_2} during breathing of 100% oxygen. Arterial hypoxemia does not appear to protect the lungs against injury from high alveolar oxygen tensions.[160] However, fear of pulmonary oxygen toxicity should not preclude the use of sufficiently high inspired oxygen concentrations to maintain the Pa_{O_2} at a level compatible with adequate oxygenation of the brain and other organs. The term "respirator lung" has been incorrectly applied to fatal pulmonary oxygen toxicity or to other pulmonary conditions.[161] Mechanical ventilation itself, when properly applied to *normal* mammalian lungs, does not result in serious physiologic dysfunction or histologic damage.[162]

INFECTION.—Infection poses one of the major risks involved in the treatment of acute respiratory failure. Trauma to the tracheal mucosa associated with catheter aspiration[163] and breaks in aseptic technique account for the high incidence of tracheitis, associated with pathogenic bacteria found on smear and culture. Because of the danger of emergence of virulent gram-negative pathogens or antibiotic-resistant strains, we do not advocate the use of antibiotics unless there is evidence of associated bronchopneumonia, fever not readily explained by other causes, leukocytosis or the development of copious, thick, purulent secretions. Gram-negative septicemia often occurs in critically ill patients in whom the airway and multiple intravascular catheters represent the probable routes of contamination, and the hands of professional personnel the major vectors.[164] Careful hand washing with a bactericidal agent by physicians and nurses, limited examination of the patient by personnel not immediately involved with patient care, rigid aseptic practice in the handling of the patient's airway and vascular catheters, frequent changing or chemical decontamination of respiratory therapy equipment, proper care of the patient's skin and the meticulous handling of airway connections can reduce substantially the incidence of infection.

MECHANICAL COMPLICATIONS.—Complications associated with the mechanical aspects of respiratory care can be virtually eliminated by detailed attention on the part of the nurses and physicians to the ventilator system itself and by the use of reliable, tested equipment. Mechanical complications are quite common when a team of physicians and nurses first embarks on a program of intensive respiratory care; as they gain experience, these become much less frequent and the complications mentioned previously emerge as the most difficult problems to solve.

OTHER COMPLICATIONS.—The circulatory consequences of mechanical ventilation seldom are a serious problem in infants and children. Hypocapnia ($Pa_{CO_2} < 28$ torr) and alkalosis (pH > 7.45) may decrease cerebral blood flow[165] and cardiac output,[166] although quantitative data in infants and children are lacking. Our clinical experience indicates that induced respiratory alkalosis produces little harm, even when tetany has occurred, whereas inadequate alveolar ventilation has dire consequences. Overheating of inspiratory gas resulting in fever, or muscular work associated with dyscoordination of the patients and ventilator, will increase the patient's metabolic rate. Vigorous treatment of fever, regardless of the cause, and careful attention to coordination of the patient with the ventilator serve to minimize metabolic stress.

Results of Pediatric Intensive Care

A survey of 8 major pediatric intensive care units admitting all types of critically ill infants and children indicates an average survival rate of 88%.° The detailed statistics for survival rates associated with acute respiratory failure from various causes are not available. During the years 1976–1977, in the Pediatric Intensive Care Unit at The Children's Hospital of Philadelphia, acute respiratory failure from all causes treated with mechanical ventilation was associated with an 82% *survival* rate. The major causes of death were irreversible central nervous system damage and irreparable congenital heart disease.

Intensive care services are extremely expensive and should not be duplicated in every hospital. Therefore, a pressing need for regional distribution of pediatric intensive care centers exists. These centers should be serviced by an effective and safe transportation network to facilitate the transfer of patients from other hospitals. With this type of system we can provide every critically ill or injured child an optimal chance for full recovery at the least cost to his family and community.

REFERENCES

1. Rackow, H., and Salanitre, E.: Modern concepts in pediatric anesthesiology, Anesthesiology 30:208, 1969.
2. Downes, J. J., and Nicodemus, H. F.: Preparation for and recovery from anesthesia, Pediatr. Clin. North Am. 16:601, 1969.
3. Downes, J. J., and Raphaely, R. C.: Pediatric intensive care, Anesthesiology 43:238, 1975.
4. Edmunds, L. H., Jr., and Downes, J. J.: Assisted Ventilation in Infants, in Sabiston, D. C., Jr., and Spencer, F. C. (eds.), *Gibbon's Surgery of the Chest* (Philadelphia: W. B. Saunders Company, 1976).
5. Graff, T. D., Phillips, O. C., Benson, D. W., and Kelly, E.: Baltimore anesthesia study committee: Factors in pediatric anesthesia mortality, Anesth. Analg. 43:407, 1964.
6. Smith, R. M.: *Anesthesia for Infants and Children* (3d ed.; St. Louis: The C. V. Mosby Company, 1968), pp. 504–507.
7. Smith, R. M.: Personal communication, 1976.
8. Ernst, E. A., and Smith, J. C.: A pharmacogenetic study of a family exhibiting atypical and silent genes for plasma cholinesterase, Anesthesiology 28:1085, 1967.
9. Denborough, M. A., Forster, J. F. A., Lovel, R. R. H., Maplestone, P. A., and Villiers, J. D.: Anaesthetic deaths in a family, Br. J. Anaesth. 34:395, 1962.
10. Smith, R. M.: *Anesthesia for Infants and Children* (3d ed.; St. Louis: The C. V. Mosby Company, 1968), pp. 384–387.
11. Rackow, H., and Salanitre, E.: Modern concepts in pediatric anesthesiology. Review article, Anesthesiology 30:208, 1969.
12. Saklad, M.: Grading of patients for surgical procedures, Anesthesiology 2:281, 1941.
13. Eckenhoff, J. E.: Relationship of anesthesia to postoperative personality changes in children, Pediatrics 86:587, 1953.
14. Jackson, K., Winkley, R., Faust, O., Cermak, E. G., and Burtt, M. M.: Behavior changes indicating emotional trauma in tonsillectomized children, Pediatrics 12:23, 1953.

° Downes, J. J.: Unpublished data.

15. Amend, E.: Orientation for the Short Term Surgical Patient, in Bergersen, B. S., *Current Concepts in Clinical Nursing* (St. Louis: The C. V. Mosby Company, 1970).
16. Korsch, B. M.: The child and the operating room, Anesthesiology 43:251, 1975.
17. Freeman, A., and Bachman, L.: Pediatric anesthesia: An evaluation of preoperative medication, Anesth. Analg. 38:429, 1959.
18. Keller, M. L., Sussman, S., and Rochberg, S.: Comparative evaluation of combined preoperative medications for pediatric surgery, Anesth. Analg. 47:199, 1968.
19. Bachman, L., and Freeman, A.: The cardiac rate and rhythm in infants during induction of anesthesia with cyclopropane, J. Pediatr. 59:922, 1961.
20. West, J. S., and Papper, E. M.: Preanesthetic medication for children, Anesthesiology 11:279, 1950.
21. Lahiri, T. A., Thomas, A., and Hodgson, R. M. H.: Single dose antacid therapy for prevention of Mendelson's syndrome, Br. J. Anaesth. 45:1143, 1973.
22. Dorsch, J. A., and Dorsch, S. E.: *Understanding Anesthesia Equipment* (Baltimore: The Williams & Wilkins Company, 1975), pp. 221–230.
23. Nightingale, D. A., Glass, A. G., and Bachman, L.: Neuromuscular blockade by succinylcholine in children, Anesthesiology 27:736, 1966.
24. Cook, D. R., and Fisher, C. G.: Neuromuscular blocking effects of succinylcholine in infants and children, Anesthesiology 42:662, 1975.
25. Goudsouzian, N. G., Ryan, J. F., and Savarese, J. J.: The neuromuscular effects of pancuronium in infants and children, Anesthesiology 41:95, 1974.
26. Long, G., and Backman, L.: Neuromuscular blockade by *d*-tubocurarine in children, Anesthesiology 28:723, 1967.
27. Goudsouzian, N. G., Donlon, J. V., Savarese, J. J., and Ryan, J. F.: Re-evaluation of dosage and duration of action of *d*-tubocurarine in the pediatric age group, Anesthesiology 43:416, 1975.
28. McLaughlin, G. W., Kirby, R. R., Kemmerer, W. T., and de-Lemos, R. A.: Indirect measurement of blood pressure in infants utilizing Doppler ultrasound, Pediatrics 79:300, 1971.
29. Brodsky, J. B.: A simple method to determine patency of the ulnar artery intraoperatively prior to radial artery cannulation, Anesthesiology 42:626, 1975.
30. Adams, J. M., and Rudolph, A. J.: The use of indwelling radial artery catheters in neonates, Pediatrics 55:261, 1975.
31. Gauderer, M., and Holgerson, L. O.: Peripheral arterial line insertion in neonates and infants: A simplified method of temporal artery cannulation, J. Pediatr. Surg. 9:875, 1974.
32. Katz, R. L.: A nerve stimulator for continuous monitoring of muscle relaxant action, Anesthesiology 26:832, 1965.
33. Ali, H. H., Uhing, J. E., and Gray, C.: Stimulus frequency in the detection of neuromuscular block in humans, Br. J. Anaesth. 42:967, 1970.
34. Drop, L. J.: Interdependence between ionized calcium and hemodynamic performance. Doctoral thesis published by Massachusetts General Hospital (Printing Office), Boston, 1974.
35. Goudsouzian, N. G., Morris, R. H., and Ryan, J. F.: The effects of a warming blanket on the maintenance of body temperatures in anesthetized infants and children, Anesthesiology 39:351, 1973.
36. Rashad, K. F., and Benson, D. W.: Role of humidity in prevention of hypothermia in infants and children, Anesth. Analg. 46:712, 1967.
37. Bennett, E. J., Patel, K. P., and Grundy, E. M.: Neonatal temperature and surgery, Anesthesiology 46:303, 1977.
38. Gordon, R. A., Britt, B. A., and Kalow, W.: *International Symposium on Malignant Hyperthermia* (Springfield, Ill.: Charles C Thomas, Publisher, 1973).
38a. King, J. O., and Denborough, M. A.: Anesthetic-induced malignant hyperpyrexia in children, Pediatrics 83:37, 1973.
39. Saidman, L. J., Harvard, E. S., and Eger, E. I.: Hyperthermia during anesthesia, JAMA 190:1029, 1964.
40. Relton, J. E., Britt, B. A., and Steward, D. J.: Malignant hyperpyrexia, Br. J. Anaesth. 45:269, 1973.
41. Holliday, M. A., and Segar, W. E.: Maintenance need for water in parenteral fluid therapy, Pediatrics 19:823, 1957.
42. Furman, E. B., Roman, D. G., Lemmer, L. A. S., *et al.*: Specific therapy in water, electrolyte and blood-volume replacement during pediatric surgery, Anesthesiology 42:187, 1975.
43. Mollinson, P. L.: *Blood Transfusion in Clinical Medicine* (Philadelphia: F. A. Davis Company, 1967), pp. 627–628.

44. Hathway, W. E.: Coagulation problems in the newborn infant, Pediatr. Clin. North Am. 17:929, 1970.
45. Eckenhoff, J. E., Kneale, D. H., and Dripps, R. D.: The incidence and etiology of postanesthetic excitement, Anesthesiology 22:667, 1961.
46. Jordan, W. S., Graves, C. L., and Elwyn, R. A.: New therapy for postintubation edema and tracheitis in children, JAMA 212:585, 1970.
47. James, J. A.: Dexamethasone in croup. A controlled study, Am. J. Dis. Child. 117:511, 1969.
48. Cannard, T. H., and Zaimis, E. J.: Effect of lowered muscle temperature on the action of neuromuscular blocking drugs in man, J. Physiol. 149:112, 1959.
49. Romagnoli, A., and Keats, A. S.: Respiratory depression by fentanyl and morphine: Duration, cumulation and antagonism, ASA Abstracts, p. 261, 1975.
50. Katz, R. L.: Comparison of electrical and mechanical recording of spontaneous and evoked muscle activity, Anesthesiology 26:204, 1965.
51. Kilburn, K. H.: Neurologic manifestations of respiratory failure, Arch. Intern. Med. 116:409, 1965.
52. Bellville, J. W., and Howland, W. S.: Prognosis after severe hypoxia in man, Anesthesiology 18:389, 1957.
53. Pampiglione, G., and Harden, A.: Resuscitation after cardiocirculatory arrest: Prognostic evaluation of early electroencephalographic findings, Lancet 1:1261, 1968.
54. Glover, W. J.: Management of cardiac surgery in the neonate, Br. J. Anaesth. 49:59, 1977.
55. Avery, M. E., and Fletcher, B. D.: *The Lung and Its Disorders in the Newborn Infant* (3d ed.; Philadelphia: W. B. Saunders Company, 1974).
56. Pang, L. M., and Mellins, R. B.: Neonatal cardiorespiratory physiology, Anesthesiology 43:171, 1975.
57. Auld, P. A. M.: Pulmonary Physiology of the Newborn Infant, in Scarpelli, E. M. (ed.), *Pulmonary Physiology in the Fetus, Newborn, and Child* (Philadelphia: Lea & Febiger, 1975), p. 147
58. Adamsons, K., and Towell, M. E.: Thermal homeostasis in the fetus and newborn, Anesthesiology 26:531, 1965.
59. Silverman, W. A., Sinclair, J. C., and Scopes, J. W.: Regulation of body temperature in pediatric surgery, J. Pediatr. Surg. 1:321, 1966.
60. Kenney, R. A.: Renal function, Pediatr. Clin. North Am. 23:651, 1976.
61. Cornblath, M., and Schwartz, R.: *Disorders of Carbohydrate Metabolism in Infancy* (Philadelphia: W. B. Saunders Company, 1966).
62. Sweet, A. Y.: Classification of the Low Birth Weight Infant, in Klaus, M. H., and Fanaroff, A. A. (eds.), *Care of the High Risk Neonate* (Philadelphia: W. B. Saunders Company, 1973), p. 36.
63. Rowe, R. D., and Mehrizi, A.: *The Neonate with Congenital Heart Disease* (Philadelphia: W. B. Saunders Company, 1968).
64. Faxelius, G., Raye, J., Gutberlet, R., *et al.*: Red cell volume measurements and acute blood loss in high-risk infants, J. Pediatr. 90:273, 1977.
65. Srouji, M.: The acid-base status of the surgical neonate on admission to the hospital, Surgery 62:958, 1967.
66. Gandy, G. M., Adamsons, K., Cunningham, N., *et al.*: Thermal environment and acid-base homeostasis in human infants during the first few hours of life, J. Clin. Invest. 43:751, 1964.
67. Wu, P. Y. K., and Hodgman, J. E.: Insensible water loss in preterm infants: Changes with postnatal development and non-ionizing radiant energy, Pediatrics 54:704, 1974.
68. Oh, W.: Disorders of fluid and electrolytes in newborn infants, Pediatr. Clin. North Am. 23:601, 1976.
69. Walk, M. K.: Problems in Chemical Adaptation, in Klaus, M. H., and Fanaroff, A. A. (eds.), *Care of the High Risk Neonate* (Philadelphia: W. B. Saunders Company, 1973), p. 168.
70. Odell, G. B., Poland, R. L., and Ostrea, E. M.: Neonatal Hyperbilirubinemia, *Ibid.*, p. 183.
71. Tsang, R. C., Donovan, E. F., and Steichen, J. J.: Calcium physiology and pathology in the neonate, Pediatr. Clin. North Am. 23:611, 1976.
72. Greenwood, R. D.: Patterns of gastrointestinal and cardiac malformations, J. Pediatr. Surg. 11:1023, 1976.
73. Greenwood, R. D., Rosenthal, A., and Nadas, A. S.: Cardiovascular malformations associated with congenital diaphragmatic hernia, Pediatrics 57:92, 1976.
74. Greenwood, R. D., Rosenthal, A., and Nadas, A. S.: Cardiovascular malformations associated with omphalocele, J. Pediatr. 85:818, 1974.

75. Greenwood, R. D., and Rosenthal, A.: Cardiovascular malformations associated with tracheoesophageal fistula and esophageal atresia, Pediatrics 57:87, 1976.
76. Greenwood, R. D., Rosenthal, A., and Nadas, A. S.: Cardiovascular malformations associated with imperforate anus, J. Pediatr. 86:576, 1975.
77. Hackel, A.: A medical transport system for the neonate, Anesthesiology 43:258, 1975.
78. James, S. L., and Lanman, J. T. (eds.): History of oxygen therapy and retrolental fibroplasia, Pediatrics (suppl.) 57:591, 1976.
79. Betts, E. K., Downes, J. J., Schaffer, D., and Johns, R.: Retrolental fibroplasia and oxygen administration during general anesthesia, Anesthesiology 47:518, 1977.
80. Dorsch, J. A., and Dorsch, S. E.: *Understanding Anesthesia Equipment* (Baltimore: The Williams & Wilkins Company, 1975), p. 221.
81. *Ibid.*, pp. 159–173.
82. Nightingale, D. A., Richards, C. C., and Glass, A.: An evaluation of rebreathing in a modified T-piece system during controlled ventilation of anaesthetized children, Br. J. Anaesth. 37:762, 1965.
83. Bain, J. A., and Spoerel, W. E.: Flow requirements for a modified Mapleson D system during controlled ventilation, Can. Anaesth. Soc. J. 20:629, 1973.
84. Chalon, J., Lowe, D., and Malebranche, J.: Effects of dry anesthetic gases on tracheobronchial ciliated epithelium, Anesthesiology 37:338, 1972.
85. Weeks, D. B.: Provision of endogenous and exogenous humidity for the Bain breathing circuit, Can. Anaesth. Soc. J. 23: 185, 1976.
86. Weeks, D. B.: Humidification of anesthetic gases with an inexpensive condenser-humidifier in the semiclosed circle, Anesthesiology 41:601, 1974.
87. Haddad, C., and Richards, C. C.: Mechanical ventilation of infants: Significance and elimination of ventilator compression volume, Anesthesiology 29:365, 1968.
88. Heath, J. R., Anderson, M. M., and Nunn, J. F.: Performance of the Quantiflex monitored dial mixer, Br. J. Anaesth. 45:216, 1973.
89. Deming, M. V.: Agents and techniques for induction of anesthesia in young children, Anesth. Analg. 31:113, 1952.
90. Nicodemus, H. F., Nassiri-Rahimi, C., Bachman, L., and Smith, T. C.: Median effective doses (ED_{50}) of halothane in adults and children, Anesthesiology 31:344, 1969.
91. Gregory, G., Eger, E. I., and Munson, E. S.: The relationship between age and halothane requirement in man, Anesthesiology 30:488, 1969.
92. Salanitre, E., and Rackow, H.: The pulmonary exchange of nitrous oxide and halothane in infants, Anesthesiology 30: 388, 1969.
93. Downes, J. J., Kemp, R. A., and Lambertsen, C. J.: The magnitude and duration of respiratory depression due to fentanyl and meperidine in man, J. Pharmacol. Exp. Ther. 158:416, 1967.
94. Salem, M. R., Bennett, E. J., Schweiss, J. F., *et al.*: Cardiac arrest related to anesthesia, JAMA 233:238, 1975.
95. Rackow, H., Salanitre, E., and Green, L. T.: Frequency of cardiac arrest associated with anesthesia in infants and children, Pediatrics 28:697, 1961.
96. Vidyasagar, D., Downes, J. J., and Boggs, T. R.: Respiratory distress syndrome of newborn infants. II. Technique of catheterization of umbilical artery and clinical results of treatment of 124 patients, Clin. Pediatr. 9:332, 1970.
97. Murdoch, A. I., Burrington, J. B., and Swyer, P. R.: Alveolar to arterial oxygen tension difference and venous admixture in newly born infants with congenital diaphragmatic herniation through the foramen of Bochdalek, Biol. Neonate 17:161, 1971.
98. Harries, J. T., and Fraser, A. J.: The acidity of the gastric contents of premature babies during the first fourteen days of life, Biol. Neonate 12:186, 1968.
99. Salem, M. R., Wong, A. Y., and Lin, Y. H.: The effect of suxamethonium on the intragastric pressure in infants and children, Br. J. Anaesth. 44:166, 1972.
100. Stark, A. R., and Thach, B. T.: Mechanisms of airway obstruction leading to apnea in newborn infants, J. Pediatr. 89:982, 1976.
101. Eger, E. I., II: *Anesthetic Uptake and Action* (Baltimore: The Williams & Wilkins Company, 1974), pp. 171–183.
102. Bennett, E. J., Patel, K. P., and Grundy, E. M.: Neonatal temperature and surgery, Anesthesiology 46:303, 1977.
103. Berman, L. S., Fox, W. W., Raphaely, R. C., and Downes, J. J.: Optimum levels of CPAP for tracheal extubation of newborn infants, J. Pediatr. 89:109, 1976.
104. Beckwith, J. B.: The Sudden Infant Death Syndrome in *Current Problems in Pediatrics* (Chicago: Year Book Medical Publishers, Inc., June, 1973).
105. Downes, J. J.: Respiratory care of the newborn, ASA Refresher Courses in Anesthesiology 2:65, 1974.
106. Gregory, G. A.: Respiratory care of infants, ASA Refresher Courses in Anesthesiology 3:81, 1975.
107. Downes, J. J., Fulgencio, T., and Raphaely, R. C.: Acute respiratory failure in infants and children, Pediatr. Clin. North Am. 19:423, 1972.
108. Downes, J. J., and Goldberg, A. I.: Airway Management, Mechanical Ventilation, and Cardiopulmonary Resuscitation, in Scarpelli, E., and Auld, P. A. M. (eds.), *Pulmonary Disease in the Fetus, Newborn and Child* (Philadelphia: Lea & Febiger, 1978).
109. Wegman, M. E.: Annual summary of vital statistics – 1975, Pediatrics 58:793, 1976.
110. Koop, C. E., Schnaufer, L., and Broennle, A. M.: Esophageal atresia and tracheoesophageal fistula: Supportive measures that affect survival, Pediatrics 54:558, 1974.
111. Woo, S. W., Malhotra, I. V., and Hedley-Whyte, J.: Anesthetic Considerations, in Weiss, E. B., and Segal, M. S. (eds.), *Bronchial Asthma – Mechanisms and Therapeutics* (Boston: Little, Brown and Company, 1976), pp. 999–1006.
112. Brown, B. R., Walson, P. D., and Taussig, L. M.: Congenital metabolic diseases of pediatric patients, Anesthesiology 43: 197, 1975.
113. Berman, W., Pizzi, F., Schut, L., Raphaely, R., and Holtzapple, P.: Effects of exchange transfusion on intracranial pressure in patients with Reye syndrome, J. Pediatr. 87:887, 1975.
114. Murphy, S.: Difficulties in Sickle-Cell States, in Cooperman, L. H., and Orkin, F. K. (eds.), *Complications in Anesthesiology* (Philadelphia: J. B. Lippincott Company). (In press.)
115. Tolmie, J. D., Joyce, T. H., and Mitchell, G. D.: Succinylcholine danger in the burned patient, Anesthesiology 28:467, 1967.
116. Churchill-Davidson, H. C., Way, W. L., and deJong, R. H.: The muscle relaxants and renal excretion, Anesthesiology 28: 540, 1967.
117. Whittaker, M.: Genetic aspects of succinylcholine sensitivity, Anesthesiology 32:143, 1970.
118. Foldes, F. F.: Myasthenia gravis: A guide for anesthesiologists, Anesthesiology 23:837, 1962.
119. Ortiz, F. T., and Diaz, P. M.: Use of enflurane for pheochromocytoma removal, Anesthesiology 42:495, 1975.
120. Farman, J. V.: Neuroblastoma and anaesthesia, Br. J. Anaesth. 37:866, 1965.
121. Dundee, J. W., McCleery, W. N. C., and McLaughlin, G.: The hazard of thiopental anesthesia in porphyria, Anesth. Analg. 41:567, 1962.
122. Vaughn, V. C., and McKay, R. J. (eds.): *Nelson's Textbook of Pediatrics* (10th ed.; Philadelphia: W. B. Saunders Company, 1975), pp. 788, 796–797, 1479.
123. Subcommittee on the National Halothane Study, National Academy of Sciences-National Research Council: Summary of the national halothane study, JAMA 197:775, 1966.
124. Vaughn, V. C., and McKay, R. J. (eds.): *Nelson's Textbook of Pediatrics* (10th ed.; Philadelphia: W. B. Saunders Company, 1975), pp. 2–5.
125. Guidelines for Organization of Critical Care Units. Report of the Committee on Guidelines. J. J. Downes, Chairman, JAMA 222:1532, 1972.
126. James, H. E., Bruno, L., Schut, L., *et al.*: Intracranial subarachnoid pressure monitoring in children, Surg. Neurol. 3: 313, 1975.
127. Mickell, J. J., Reigel, D. H., Cook, D. R., *et al.*: Intracranial pressure: Monitoring and normalization therapy in children, Pediatrics 59:606, 1977.
128. Reye, R. D., Sydney, M. D., Morgan, G., *et al.*: Encephalopathy and fatty degeneration of the viscera: A disease entity in childhood, Lancet 2:749, 1963
129. Waldhausen, J. A., Friedman, S., Tyers, G. F. O., *et al.*: Ascending aorta-right pulmonary artery anastomosis: Clinical experience with 35 patients with cyanotic congenital heart disease, Circulation 38:463, 1968.
130. Downes, J. J., Nicodemus, H. F., Pierce, W. S., *et al.*: Acute respiratory failure in infants following cardiovascular surgery, J. Thorac. Cardiovasc. Surg. 59:21, 1970.
131. Park, C. D., Nicodemus, H. F., Downes, J. J., *et al.*: Changes

in pulmonary vascular resistance following closure of ventricular septal defects, Circulation 39(Supp. 1):193, 1969.

132. Dobrin, R. S., Larsen, C. D., and Holliday, M. A.: The critically ill child: Acute renal failure, Pediatrics 48:286, 1971.

133. Benoit, F. L., Rulon, D. B., Theil, G. B. P., *et al.*: Goodpasture's syndrome, a clinicopathologic entity, Am. J. Med. 37:424, 1964.

134. Munro, J. F., Geddes, A. M., and Lamb, W. L.: Goodpasture's syndrome: Survival after acute failure, Br. Med. J. 2:95, 1967.

135. AMA: Standards for Cardiopulmonary Resuscitation (CPR) and Emergency Cardiac Care (ECC), JAMA 227:165, 1973.

136. Heimlich, H. J.: A life-saving maneuver to prevent food-choking, JAMA 234:398, 1975.

137. Carden, E., and Bernstein, M.: Investigation of the nine most commonly used resuscitator bags, JAMA 212:589, 1970.

138. Falsetti, H. L., and Greene, D. G.: Technique of compression in closed chest cardiac massage, JAMA 200:793, 1967.

139. Todres, I. D., and Rogers, M. C.: Methods of external cardiac massage in the newborn infant, J. Pediatr. 86:781, 1975.

140. Redding, J. S., Asuncion, J. S., and Pearson, J. W.: Effective routes of drug administration during cardiac arrest, Anesth. Analg. 46:253, 1967.

141. Schaer, H.: Effects on ionized calcium of acidosis with alkalinizing agents: A rational basis for the administration of calcium in cardiac resuscitation, Br. J. Anaesth. 48:327, 1976.

142. Goldberg, L. I.: Dopamine—clinical uses of an endogenous catecholamine, N. Engl. J. Med. 291:707, 1974.

143. Gutgesell, H. P., Tacker, W. A., Geddes, L. A., *et al.*: Energy dose for ventricular defibrillation of children, Pediatrics 58:898, 1976.

143a. Williams, G. S., Klenk, E. L., and Winters, R. W.: Acute Renal Failure in Pediatrics, in Winters, R. W. (ed.), *The Body Fluids in Pediatrics* (Boston: Little, Brown and Company, 1973), pp. 548–549.

143b. *Ibid.*, pp. 551–555.

144. Shapiro, H. M. Wyte, S. R., and Loeser, J.: Barbiturate augmented hypothermia for reduction of persistent intracranial hypertension, J. Neurosurg. 40:90, 1974.

145. Ehrlich, R., Emmet, S. M., and Rodríquez-Torres, R.: Pediatric cardiac resuscitation team: A 6 year study, J. Pediatr. 84:152, 1974.

146. Aberdeen, E., and Downes, J. J.: Artificial airways in children, Surg. Clin. North Am. 54:1155, 1974.

147. Magovern, G. J., Shively, J. G., Fecht, D., *et al.*: The clinical and experimental evaluation of a controlled-pressure intratracheal cuff, J. Thorac. Cardiovasc. Surg. 64:747, 1972.

147a. Jung, R. C., and Gottlieb, L. S.: Comparison of tracheobronchial suction catheters in humans, Chest 69:179, 1976.

147b. Hill, J. D., O'Brien, T. G., Murray, J. J., Dontigny, L., Bramson, M. L., Osborne, J. J., and Gerbode, F.: Prolonged extracorporeal oxygenation for acute post-traumatic respiratory failure, N. Engl. J. Med. 286:629, 1972.

147c. Bartlett, R. H., Gazzaniga, A. B., Fong, S. W., Jeffries, M. R., Roohk, V., and Haiduc, N.: Extracorporeal membrane oxygenator support for cardiopulmonary failure, J. Thorac. Cardiovasc. Surg. 73:375, 1977.

148. Jung, R. C., and Gottlieb, L. S.: Comparison of tracheobronchial suction catheters in humans, Chest 69:179, 1976.

149. Abboud, N., Rehder, K., Rodarte, J. F., *et al.*: Lung volumes and closing capacity with continuous positive airway pressure, Anesthesiology 42:138, 1975.

150. Fairley, H. B., and Hunter, D. D.: The performance of respirators used in treatment of respiratory insufficiency, Can. Med. Assoc. J. 90:1397, 1964.

151. Epstein, R. A.: The sensitivities and response times of ventilatory assistors, Anesthesiology 34:321, 1971.

152. Downs, J. B., Klein, E. F., Desautels, D., *et al.*: Intermittent mandatory ventilation, Chest 64:331, 1973.

152a. Hill, J. D., O'Brien, T. G., Murray, J. J., Dontigny, L., Bramson, M. L., Osborne, J. J., and Gerbode, F.: Prolonged extracorporeal oxygenation for acute post-traumatic respiratory failure, N. Engl. J. Med. 286:629, 1972.

152b. Zapol, W. M., and Qvist, J. (eds.): *Artificial Lungs for Acute Respiratory Failure* (New York: Academic Press, 1976), pp. 465–479, 513–524, 525–530, 531–549.

152c. Bartlett, R. H., Gazzaniga, A. B., Fong, S. W., Jeffries, M. R., Roohk, V., and Haiduc, N.: Extracorporeal membrane oxygenator support for cardiopulmonary failure, J. Thorac. Cardiovasc. Surg. 73:375, 1977.

153. Striker, T. W., Stool, S., and Downes, J. J.: Prolonged nasotracheal intubation in infants and children, Arch. Otolaryngol. 85:210, 1967.

154. Allen, T. H., and Steven, I. M.: Prolonged nasotracheal intubation in infants and children, Br. J. Anaesth. 44:835, 1972.

155. Sladen, A., Laver, M. B., and Pontoppidan, H.: Pulmonary complications and water retention in prolonged mechanical ventilation, N. Engl. J. Med. 279:448, 1968.

156. Winter, P. M., and Smith, G.: The toxicity of oxygen, Anesthesiology 37:210, 1972.

157. Hayes, B., and Robinson, J. S.: An assessment of methods of humidification of inspired air, Br. J. Anaesth. 42:94, 1970.

158. Clark, J. M., and Lambertsen, C. J.: Pulmonary oxygen toxicity. A review, Pharmacol. Rev. 23:37, 1971.

159. Barber, R. E., Lee, J., and Hamilton, W. K.: Oxygen toxicity in man, N. Engl. J. Med. 283:1478, 1970.

160. Miller, W. W., Waldhausen, J. A., and Rashkind, W. J.: Comparison of oxygen poisoning of the lung in cyanotic and acyanotic dogs, N. Engl. J. Med. 282:943, 1970.

161. Nash, G., Bowen, J. A., and Langlinais, P. C.: Respirator lung: A misnomer, Arch. Pathol. 91:234, 1971.

162. Lee, C. J., Lyons, J. H., Konigsberg, S., *et al.*: Effects of spontaneous and positive-pressure breathing of ambient air and pure oxygen at one atmosphere pressure on pulmonary surface characteristics, J. Thorac. Cardiovasc. Surg. 53:759, 1967.

163. Sackner, M. A., Landa, J. F., Greeneltch, N., *et al.*: Pathogenesis and prevention of tracheobronchial damage with suction procedures, Chest 64:284, 1973.

164. Lowbury, E. J. L., Thorn, B. T., Lilly, H. A., *et al.*: Sources of infection with *Pseudomonas aeruginosa* in patients with tracheostomy. J. Med. Microbiol. 3:39, 1970.

165. Smith, A. L., and Wollman, H.: Cerebral blood flow and metabolism: Effects of anesthetic drugs and techniques, Anesthesiology 36:378, 1972.

166. Prys-Roberts. C., Kelman, G. R., Greenbaum, R., *et al.*: Circulatory influences of artificial ventilation during nitrous oxide anaesthesia in man. II: Results: The relative influence of mean intrathoracic pressure and arterial carbon dioxide tension, Br. J. Anaesth. 39:533, 1967.

3 Marc I. Rowe

Preoperative and Postoperative Management: The Physiologic Approach

This chapter discusses three major problem areas in the care of the pediatric surgical patient before and after operation: energy balance, fluid and electrolyte management and gram-negative sepsis and shock.

These three subjects were chosen primarily because, along with respiratory difficulties, they account for the bulk of the morbidity and mortality that occur on a pediatric surgical service. In addition, a detailed discussion of three problems rather than a broad survey of the multitude of preoperative and postoperative difficulties provides an opportunity to illustrate and emphasize a physiologic approach to management that is flexible and can be applied to a wide spectrum of pediatric surgical patients. Rigid "cookbook" methods of patient care are not effective in pediatric surgery because there are no typical patients. Management must be based on understanding physiologic and pathophysiologic mechanisms and then utilizing this knowledge to tailor treatment to meet the unique and constantly changing needs of a variety of patients.

Energy Balance

Carbohydrates, proteins, fats, vitamins, minerals and trace elements are essential for proper nutritional balance in the pediatric surgical patient. The space allotted precludes discussion of all aspects of nutrition. As a compromise, I have emphasized primarily energy balance. At all ages, fuel must be available to supply energy for the vital processes of the body and to maintain body temperature at a level that will enable these processes to operate effectively. Surgical patients may have markedly increased energy requirements over basal needs as a result of disease, infection, operation or injury. If energy demands are not met, eventually the individual will die. Long before death by starvation, body defenses and functions will be altered profoundly. The pediatric surgical patient, compared to the adult, is at a disadvantage in energy balance, because the young patient has a greater basal energy expenditure, must expend more energy to maintain thermal stability, requires calories for growth and development and often has strikingly reduced energy reserves.

Basal Energy Needs

Infants and children have a higher basal metabolic rate than adults.[1-11] The minimal rate in babies depends on the length of gestation, the relationship of body weight to gestation and the time from birth. A full-term, full-size infant at birth has the lowest metabolic rate he will have until he is an adult—32 cal/kg/24 hr (adult average basal metabolic rate 24 cal/kg/24 hr). The rate rises significantly during the first day of life, and gradually over the next 2 weeks, to reach a peak level of 48 cal/kg/24 hr. This level remains essentially un-changed until the early teens, when there is a fall to adult levels. The metabolic rate of low birth weight babies in the first few hours of life, depending on the length of gestation, is slightly above or below that of the full-term infant. Pre-term infants tend to increase their metabolic rate only gradually, but this increase continues, reaching very high levels by 6 weeks of age—59 cal/kg/24 hr. Small-for-dates, compared to pre-term, infants tend to be hypermetabolic, increasing their basal rate more rapidly in the first 10 days of life and then at a more gradual rate.

Energy Requirements for Growth and Development

An estimate of the caloric needs for growth and development can be arrived at by calculating the energy values of the protein and fat mass at different ages. These values are only approximate and do not take into account the energy cost of growth. Using these rough calculations, the energy needs vary significantly at different ages. The greatest caloric expenditure for growth occurs in infancy—33 cal/kg/24 hr. By 3 months, energy needs for growth and development have fallen to 18 cal/kg/24 hr and by 6 months to 4 cal/kg/24 hr. Energy expenditures remain fairly constant at this level until the age of 12–13 years in girls and 15–16 years in boys, when the intense pubertal growth period usually occurs.[12]

Energy Cost of Staying Warm

Individuals of all ages must expend energy above basal levels in order to maintain a normal body temperature when exposed to a cool environment. A baby, within a few hours of birth, is a thermally active individual and, responding to cold exposure by an almost threefold increase in metabolic activity, can maintain normal body temperature.[13] The small-for-date infant's homeothermic response closely resembles the full-size baby's. Pre-term infants have the same response, but it is quantitatively less than the full-term and small-for-date infant.[14] In comparison to the adult, babies of any gestational age and size are at a disadvantage when exposed to a cool environment. The infant lacks the quantity of fat of older individuals to serve as insulation and has a large surface area to body mass ratio, which results in increased heat loss by radiation and evaporation. The range of thermal neutrality for the adult is 28–30° C. Between these temperatures, metabolic activity and heat production are at a basal level. At about 27° C, the naked adult must increase his metabolic activity in order to prevent a drop in body temperature.[15, 16] In contrast, the zone of thermal neutrality in the infant varies with size and postnatal age but is much warmer.[17] At 5 days of age, the thermally neutral ambient environmental temperature for a 1-kg baby is 34.7° C and for a 3-kg baby 33.4° C. At 30 days of age, the smaller infant's thermal neutral zone is about 33.3° C and the larger baby's 32.5° C, still considerably higher than the adult's. For this reason, unless utmost care is taken to provide a controlled environment at close to thermal neutrality, the increased metabolic work that the baby must perform to maintain normal body temperature will result in exhaustion of energy supplies and a huge energy debt.

Energy Losses as a Result of Surgical Factors

Pediatric and adult surgical patients all suffer significant energy losses because of the surgical illnesses that brought them to the hospital. Inactivity and semistarvation, often associated with the hospitalized surgical patient, tend to reduce the energy expenditure, but operation and injuries may increase metabolic work by 10–25% for as long as 3 weeks.[18] Sepsis greatly increases energy demand—as much as 50% above predicted normal levels.[19, 20] The caloric cost of infection is discussed in more detail in the section on Gram-Negative Sepsis. One of the most striking examples of hypermetabolism occurs in the burn patient. Energy losses may increase 125% over predicted normal levels. This hypermetabolic state extends from the third post-burn day until the burns are healed.[21]

Energy Reserves

The pediatric surgical patient has an increased basal metabolic rate, pays a high energy price to stay warm, must expend additional calories to provide for growth and development and, like all surgical patients, may have excess energy losses because of surgical illnesses. In addition, the baby often has meager energy stores in comparison to the adult. The most immediate source of energy is stored in the liver as glycogen. Glycogen rapidly accumulates just before birth. However, if the infant is born prematurely, these stores may not have had time to accumulate. Intrauterine malnutrition may lead to inadequate reserves. Hypoxia and other types of intrauterine stress may result in consumption of hepatic glycogen before birth. Even in infants who are born with significant stores of glycogen, the energy demands at birth are intense, since the maternal supply of glucose is cut off and rapid glycogenolysis occurs. Almost all the hepatic glycogen may be utilized in the first 3 hours of life. Fat forms the largest source of available energy supply in the body and also serves as an efficient insulator against cold. Here again, the smallest and the youngest infants are at a disadvantage in relationship to older children and adults. The small premature infant has only about 1% fat per gram of body weight whereas the full-term infant has about 16% fat. After birth, fat stores accumulate rapidly over the first 2 months of life to reach a level of 22% of the body weight. By 3–12 months this has reached 24%. During the next 4 years there is a fall in the percentage of fat, so that at about 5 years fat makes up about 12.5% of the body weight. The percentage of fat then increases until adolescence, when there is a leveling-off period. The adult male has about 12.3% fat stores, females 24%. In the average adult male, fat represents approximately 135,000 calories of energy reserve. Heird and his coworkers[22] graphically illustrated the vulnerability of the small infant because of his increased energy demands and inadequate reserves. They calculated the theoretic time of death from energy depletion of small premature infants, large pre-term infants, term infants, 1-year-old children and adults. They made these calculations on the basis of the mass of fat and protein available as potential energy. Small pre-term infants would die in approximately 4 days, larger

pre-term infants in 10 days. The term infant would survive 32 days, the child as long as a month. An infusion of 10% glucose and water at maintenance volumes would prolong life by only 7 days in the small infant and 18 days in the large pre-term infant. These calculations point out the rapidity of energy depletion in tiny infants.

Effects of Undernutrition

When a patient's nutritional demands are greater than his intake and reserves, the effects are not solely acute energy deficits that eventually may lead to cell failure and death. Changes also take place that may permanently affect body and intellectual growth and alter the organism's defenses against infection. Normal fetal and neonatal growth involves an increase in the number of cells in the body. Further growth only involves increase in the size of the cells. Undernutrition at an early age inhibits cell division, and the resulting decrease in the number of cells leads to a nonrecuperable deficit in the number of cells in various organs.[23] This may result in permanent stunting of body growth. In 1962, McCance and Widdowson[24] observed that older animals suffering from undernutrition had temporary restriction of growth. With resumption of an adequate intake, these deficits were made up and growth proceeded at a normal rate. However, undernutrition early in life prevented the full predicted genetic stature. Winick[25, 26] concluded, as a result of his animal and human DNA and RNA studies, that undernutrition during the period of cell division in the brain may lead to retardation of brain growth and have a permanent deleterious effect on intellectual function. He found that cell division in the human brain appears to continue only until 5 months of age and then permanently ceases.

Since primitive times it has been known that there is an association between undernutrition and infection. Studies of infants and children suffering from caloric and protein malnutrition suggest that there is an increased susceptibility to and severity of diseases caused by bacteria, viruses, parasites and other organisms. Studies have shown defects of antibody response, serum transferrin and skin and gut defenses. Cell-mediated immunity, the major defense system against intracellular organisms, appears to be severely affected.[27] Douglas and Schopfer[28] have demonstrated impairment of intracellular bacterial digestion by white blood cells of undernourished children. Serum complement generally is low in starved children and this may affect the opsonization of bacteria. Experimental evidence also suggests that the reticuloendothelial system may be affected by acute starvation.[29]

Clinical Implications

A nutritional program must be devised for each pediatric surgical patient. Some may require only simple fluid maintenance with 5% dextrose, water and electrolytes. Other patients, such as those who sustain a major body burn, need an excess quantity of nutrients simply to maintain balance. Some patients, because of pre-existing deficits, meager energy reserves and high demands, may require vigorous nutritional therapy on an urgent basis. Others, for example, older children with adequate reserves, may be closely observed over a period of days before a decision for therapy need be made. To evaluate the energy needs of each individual patient, answers to the following questions will be helpful: (1) What are the basal energy needs of this particular patient? (2) How adequate is this patient's thermoregulatory system and has this patient undergone or will he undergo significant cold stress that will result in a metabolic debt? (3) What are his energy requirements for growth and development? (4) Are there special factors present, such as infection or trauma, that will produce a hypermetabolic state? (5) Does this patient have adequate energy reserves? (6) Is there already an energy deficit? (7) Will the surgical condition or his therapy make it difficult or impossible for the patient to receive adequate nutrition? (8) How long will a state of inadequate intake exist?

To meet the specific requirements of each patient there is available a variety of formulas that can be administered through the gastrointestinal tract to provide an excess of essential nutrients, and effective and relatively safe techniques for total parenteral nutrition and intravenous hyperalimentation. These special methods for supplying energy will be discussed in Chapter 4.

Fluid and Electrolytes

The management of fluid and electrolyte problems in the pediatric surgical patient should be approached realistically. The physician must acknowledge that none of the formulas, rules or complex physiologic principles can ever accurately predict the fluid and electrolyte needs of an individual patient during a specific time. He must accept the fact that his fluid and electrolyte plan is, at best, a rough estimate of the needs of the patient and must be subject to continuous evaluation and readjustments. The initial calculations are important only because they help the surgeon to put together a trial program that can be modified as the patient's responses are measured. Effective fluid and electrolyte management, regardless of age, level of maturation or size of the patient, involves four basic steps: (1) The supply of water and electrolytes needed by the body to maintain vital functions is calculated. These are the estimated maintenance requirements. (2) The losses of fluid and electrolytes are measured and estimated and the pre-existing deficits are estimated. (3) Once the tentative program is initiated, specific methods are systematically utilized to monitor the patient's responses. (4) The information derived from the monitoring is analyzed and then used to modify the program. This is a feedback system.

Maintenance Needs

ESTIMATING MAINTENANCE NEEDS.—Maintenance needs can be met if losses from the skin, lungs and gastrointestinal tract are replaced and there are no abnormal losses of body fluids. Many rules of thumb, and formulas, have been developed for computing maintenance needs. For many years, physicians have sought one unifying concept based on physiologic principles that will allow calculation of maintenance requirements for patients of all ages, weight and maturity. Unfortunately, this goal has never been fully achieved.

The simplest concept would be that fluid and electrolyte maintenance is directly proportional to body weight. A moment's reflection will immediately reveal that a close relationship between body weight and fluid needs for all ages does not exist. For example, a 1500-gm small-for-date infant requires approximately 150 ml of fluid per kilogram of body weight per 24 hours.[30] This adds up to 225 ml of fluid per day. A 70-kg adult weighs 47 times as much as this infant. If fluid requirements were governed by body weight alone, the adult would need 10,500 ml of fluid daily to remain in balance. Weight, then, is helpful only as a guide to maintenance requirements for specific, narrow age and weight

groups. Table 3–1 gives examples of maintenance requirements for patients of different ages and weights.

A more unifying concept that applies to most age groups is based on the fact that fluid and electrolyte needs are fundamentally related to energy expenditure—the amount of calories necessary for the body to perform its vital functions. If fluid and electrolyte requirements are proportional to how fast the individual turns over water, electrolytes and substrate—his metabolic rate—the critical question is: How do we find each individual's metabolic rate? Unfortunately, there are no simple measuring devices currently available that will accurately and simply measure metabolic activity in the clinical setting. Therefore, we are forced to utilize various systems to calculate metabolic activity and then relate these estimates to fluid and electrolyte quantities.

Rubner[31] first noted a relationship between surface area and metabolic rate of 1000 cal/m^2/24 hr over a wide range of body size. Utilizing the theoretic relationship between metabolic rate, surface area and water and solute requirements, maintenance water requirements were calculated as 1200–1500 ml/m^2/24 hr. As more information became available, multiple violations of this general rule served to undermine the idea that the surface area law was physiologically valid. A striking example was the finding that the small-for-date infant's metabolic rate, expressed as calories per kilogram, was 2.5 times that of the adult. However, when calculated by surface area, it was 140 cal/m^2/24 hr less than the same adult (Table 3–2). In 1956, Holliday and Segar[32] published a concise monograph entitled *Parenteral Fluid Therapy*. In it, they clearly demonstrated that the surface area method led to many inaccuracies in calculating metabolic rate. They proposed that the high metabolic rate per kg of body weight of the infant versus the adult could be explained by the infant's predominance of metabolically active organs, such as the brain, per unit body weight. In 1961, Kleiber,[33] in his book, *The Fire of Life*, pointed out that four of the six ideas related to surface area and metabolic rate are invalid, and that the derivation of body surface is vague and inaccurate. Kinney *et al.*[18] stated that it is reasonable to express basal metabolic rate in units of active mass rather than in terms of the gross mass of the body or the body surface area.

TABLE 3-1.—APPROXIMATE MAINTENANCE WATER REQUIREMENTS FOR VARIOUS WEIGHTS AND AGES

AGE	WEIGHT (KG)	WATER REQUIREMENTS (ML/KG/24 HR)
2 days	800 gm	175 ml
3 days	1100 gm	130 ml
4 days	2200 gm	110 ml
3 months	5.5 kg	82 ml
18 months	10.8 kg	68 ml
10 years	32 kg	52 ml
Adult	70 kg	36 ml

TABLE 3-2.—PARADOX OF SURFACE AREA LAW IN LOW BIRTH WEIGHT BABY

	CAL/KG/24 HR°	CAL/M²/24 HR†
1.5-kilo baby	59	760
70-kilo adult	24	900

°Cal/kg/24 hr—energy requirement of *baby* 2.5 times adult.
†Cal/M²/24 hr—energy requirement of *adult* 1.5 times baby.

TABLE 3-3.—ENERGY EXPENDITURE AND ITS
RELATIONSHIP TO WEIGHT°

0-10 kg	100 cal/kg
10-20 kg	1000 cal + 50 cal/kg for each kg over 10
20 kg and up	1500 cal + 20 cal/kg for each kg over 20

°From Holliday and Segar.[32]

The failure of the surface area law led to its replacement by the caloric method. Total caloric expenditures of an individual infant or child are determined from a graph developed by Holliday and Segar.[32] This graph plots the body weight of individuals weighing 3-70 kg against calories burned in 24 hours under basal conditions, bed rest and during full activity. Most clinicians memorize rules derived from Holliday and Segar's middle curve to determine caloric expenditures (Table 3-3). Total water maintenance then is generally summed up as 100 ml/100 cal metabolized per 24 hours and electrolytes as sodium and potassium 1-3 mEq/100 cal/24 hr.

MODIFYING FACTORS IN CALCULATING MAINTENANCE NEEDS. — *Insensible water loss.* — Insensible water loss primarily consists of water evaporated from the skin and lungs. Water molecules actually diffuse through the cells of the skin and then are evaporated from the external surface. The characteristics of the skin surface may markedly affect insensible water loss. For example, evaporated water loss in the small 1000-gram pre-term infant has been measured to be as high as 64 ml/kg/24 hr, almost 6½ times that of the adult.[30] This discrepancy probably is due to certain characteristics of the premature infant's skin surface—his large surface area in relation to body size, a thinner epidermis and increased water content, permeability and blood supply of the skin.[34-36] Infants placed in radiant heat warmers have an increased evaporated water loss. In small babies, this may represent an increase in insensible water loss of as much as 191%.[37, 38] Phototherapy similarly intensifies evaporated water loss.[39, 40] The mechanism for loss in phototherapy is not known but may be related to changes in surface blood flow. Water is lost from the lungs through the expired air. Inspired air becomes totally saturated with moisture to a vapor pressure of 47 mm Hg. Since the vapor pressure of the environment usually is far less, water is lost to the atmosphere. Changes in the humidity have a profound effect on insensible water loss. Hey and Katz[41] were able to lower evaporated water loss by 30% in infants by increasing humidity to a vapor pressure of 26 mm Hg. The reduction in evaporated water loss with increased relative humidity is more marked with respect to the lungs than to the skin.

Increased metabolic activity as a result of either physical work or medical conditions such as trauma and sepsis markedly affects evaporated water losses. Crying may double insensible water loss in a baby. About 25% of the metabolic heat produced by the body is carried away by water evaporated from the skin and lungs. To dissipate 1 calorie of heat, 1.70 gm of water must be evaporated, or, for every 100 calories, 43 ml of water.[41] As metabolic rate increases in order to maintain normal body temperature, the volume of water evaporated must increase.

A hot environment also intensifies insensible water loss. Much of this increase is due to sweating. Sweating is lacking in the infant of less than 30 weeks' gestation and only a limited sweat response is found in infants of 36 weeks' gestation. Most full-term infants have an adequate sweat response.[42-44]

Renal water requirements. — One of the major functions of the kidney is the excretion of the end products of metabolism—such compounds as urea, creatinine, uric acid, sulfate and phenols. As metabolic activity increases, more substrate is burned and more solute is presented to the kidney for excretion. One of the key goals of maintenance therapy is to provide an adequate volume of fluid to allow the excretion of the solute load at a urine concentration that will not tax the diluting or concentrating ability of the kidney.

Calculating the renal water requirement necessary to reach this goal is particularly difficult in young patients because of the differences in renal function between the newborn and the more mature individual.[45] The neonatal kidney is characterized by a low glomerular filtration rate and decreased tubular function. However, since both are reduced, it appears that the over-all pattern is one of glomerular-tubular balance. The diluting ability of the infant's kidney appears to be adequate but the concentrating ability is reduced. There is definite evidence that the low birth weight infant loses a relatively large amount of sodium in the urine, even in the face of hyponatremia, probably on the basis of reduced sodium reabsorption from the distal tubules. Paradoxically, the capacity of infants to respond to a sodium load is not as great as that of the older child or the adult. The evidence to date suggests that, taking the above factors into consideration, it appears that the kidneys are not fully mature until about 1 year of age, but the control mechanisms for maintaining homeostasis are operative and perfectly adequate for most of the infant's needs. Perhaps the regulatory mechanisms are not as finely tuned as in the older individual, and, as a result, may not effectively handle conditions brought on by extreme stress.

A precise recommendation as to how much water should be administered to a patient in order to cover renal water loss cannot be made, because of the variability in renal function of the pediatric patient and the difference in solute load that is presented to the kidneys of different individuals. Most maintenance systems attempt to provide enough water to maintain a urine flow rate in the newborn of about 40-100 ml/kg/24 hr and a urine osmolality of between 75 and 300 milliosmoles.[3, 30] In the older infants and children, flow rates of 30 ml/kg/24 hr or 55 ml/100 cal/24 hr and osmolalities of 100-320 mOsm/kg are the goal.[32]

COMMENT ON MAINTENANCE REQUIREMENTS. — The greatest variability in metabolic activity and insensible water loss occurs in the newborn period, particularly among low birth weight babies. For this reason, it probably is safer to estimate maintenance needs by body weight in this age group and then readjust the program as the feedback information from the patient's responses is studied. In older patients, the caloric or meter square methods usually are sufficient to calculate safe maintenance needs.

Losses and Deficits

Administration of fluid and electrolytes in quantities sufficient to meet maintenance needs will keep the patient in balance only if there are no ongoing losses or previous deficits. Losses of body fluids can be roughly divided into two categories: measurable losses, losses that reach the external surfaces of the body and can be collected and measured, and immeasurable or hidden losses, the so-called third-space losses.

The body fluids usually lost in pediatric surgical patients are: gastric, small bowel, biliary, pancreatic, ascitic and diarrheal. Usually these can be collected and the volume measured every 6–8 hours. If losses continue for only brief periods and are in relatively small volumes, the electrolyte concentration can be estimated by referring to one of the many published tables. Minor electrolyte adjustments usually will be made by the kidney. It is important to realize, however, that there is a good deal of variability in the electrolyte content of body fluid drainage. For example, it is rare that nasogastric drainage represents only gastric juice; when ileus or intestinal obstruction is present, it may contain large quantities of duodenal or small bowel contents and, at various times, large amounts of saliva. For this reason, when losses are massive or prolonged, the patient's reserves are meager or depleted; when renal or cardiovascular function is compromised, the lost fluids must be sampled and analyzed frequently. An aliquot is taken daily—in extreme cases more frequently—the fluid spun down and the supernatant sent to the laboratory for electrolyte determination. Replacement then is made on a milliliter for milliliter and milliequivalent for milliequivalent basis. Unlike measurable losses, the magnitude of immeasurable losses and existing deficits can be estimated only by utilizing clinical, laboratory and physiologic measurements. The methods of measurement will be discussed below.

Methods of Monitoring

The preceding discussion has stressed the fact that the calculated fluid program for an individual patient at best is an educated guess and requires constant reassessment and modification. An important objective, then, is for us to evaluate the existing fluid and electrolyte status of the patient and repeatedly assess the effectiveness of our fluid and electrolyte program. Ideal characteristics for such methods include: simplicity, rapidity, safety and availability.

CLINICAL OBSERVATION.—The most common abnormality of fluid and electrolyte balance in the pediatric surgical patient is isotonic dehydration. The acute loss of relatively isotonic body fluid such as gastric or intestinal juices is followed by a significant decrease in the extracellular fluid volume and little change in the intracellular fluid volume. Fluid will not be transferred from the intracellular space to fill the depleted extracellular space, since the tonicity remains the same in the two compartments. Careful clinical examination gives important clues as to the severity of the volume deficit. With a massive reduction in extracellular fluid volume, central nervous system and cardiovascular signs are present. The patient usually is lethargic and his activity is reduced. Signs of shock or of impending shock may be present. The skin is cool and mottled, with poor capillary filling. Peripheral veins frequently are collapsed. The mucous membranes often are dry, skin turgor is reduced and the anterior fontanelle sunken. When these findings are present, the situation is critical and reduction in body water is approximately 9% in a child and 14% in an infant. Moderate signs of dehydration without cardiovascular changes usually suggest about 6% dehydration in a child and about 10% in an infant. Patients with hypotonic dehydration, in contrast, have a greater loss of extracellular volume. Fluid is passed from the extracellular space into the intracellular space in an effort to increase extracellular tonicity. Blood volume is markedly reduced and clinical signs of dehydration and cardiovascular impairment may be more marked than in a comparably volume-depleted patient who is isotonically dehydrated.

With hypertonic dehydration there usually is only a minimal reduction in the intravascular space as water moves from the intracellular and interstitial space in an effort to establish normal osmolality. Patients suffering from severe hypertonic dehydration have had as much as a 20% reduction in body weight with only a 7% reduction in blood volume. As a result, the degree of volume deficit may be underestimated. Signs of shock occur late. The skin often is flushed and feels doughy. Body temperature is elevated. The tongue may be red and swollen. Central nervous system signs predominate. The patient often is lethargic and may be stuporous. The cry is high pitched and seizures may be present.

URINE OUTPUT.—Measurement of the urine output as a means of monitoring fluid and electrolyte balance in the infant and child often is neglected. Pediatric patients, like adults, produce significant volumes of urine when well hydrated and scant urine when underhydrated. But it is important to keep in mind what is a large and what is a small volume of urine, particularly in the infant. What is necessary for each patient is a urine flow that will allow the excretion of the expected solute load at a reasonable concentration. In most pediatric surgical patients, a reasonable concentration of solutes in the urine would be equal to 260 milliosmoles ± 30 milliosmoles. For a child, a urine flow rate of approximately 500–600 ml of urine/m²/24 hr or about 55–56 ml of urine/100 calories metabolized per 24 hr is necessary to excrete the solute load at this osmolality.[32] In newborn infants, the urine output often is proportionally higher and it is convenient to calculate flow in ml/kg/24 hr. For the full-term infant, 25 ml/kg/24 hr will allow adequate solute load. In the low birth weight infant, flow might be as high as 50–100 ml/kg/24 hr.[3, 30] In most infants, the urine can be collected for volume measurements by use of a plastic adhesive bag. In severely hypovolemic patients, a catheter or small feeding tube is passed into the bladder for accurate and frequent measurements.

URINE OSMOLALITY.—The infant and the child, like the adult, excrete a concentrated urine when dehydrated and a diluted urine when overhydrated. The urine osmolality measurements are a simple, rapid method of evaluating the renal excretion of solutes and water and a guide to the state of hydration of the patient. The solute load presented to the kidney is determined by the amount of energy utilized and the nature of the metabolic mixture from which the energy was derived. For example, patients whose energy is derived from a high-protein and fat mixture usually have a high solute excretion, as do patients with increased protein catabolism, such as burn or injured patients. The adult kidney can concentrate urine to an osmolality of 1200–1400 mOsm/kg of urine, the young child to 700 mOsm/kg but we have not encountered a urine osmolality above 500 milliosmoles in a markedly dehydrated newborn baby. Although the urine osmolality of 400 in an adult or older child would be considered normal, the same value in a 2-day-old infant suggests marked dehydration and maximal concentration of urine. We attempt to maintain a urine osmolality in surgical patients of 260 milliosmoles/kg or less, but the trend of serial measurements of urine osmolality, rather than the individual values, are most important in managing fluid therapy. Together, serial determinations of urine volumes and urine osmolality serve as an important guide to the quantity and rate of intravenous fluid to be administered.

BODY WEIGHT.—Serial measurements of body weight are an excellent guide to total body water in the pediatric patient. Fluctuations over a 48-hour period are primarily related to loss or gain of body fluids. Roughly 1 gm of weight loss or gain can be equated to a loss or gain of 1 ml of water. The scales must be kept accurate and calibrated frequently. Patients should be weighed naked and dressings removed or weighed. The weight of nasogastric and other tubes can be arrived at by weighing similar tubes and subtracting the weight of these from the body weight.

HEMATOCRIT AND REFRACTOMETER TOTAL PROTEIN. — Serial hematocrit determinations can be simply and rapidly done by the physician. They are a measure of the ratio of red blood cell mass to plasma volume. Serial changes in hematocrit over an 8–24-hour period in the absence of hemolysis or bleeding suggest a loss or gain in plasma water. Serum total protein serially determined by a Goldberg refractometer, like hematocrit, is a simple method of estimating plasma water. It actually measures the refractory index of serum or plasma. The deflection of light passing through a test solution is proportional to the total solutes in solution. The refractory index then is converted, by utilizing formulas, to total solids and total protein. The correlation between biuret measured total protein and refractometer total protein is close. The advantages of the refractometer are that it is inexpensive, the technique of measurement is rapid and the results are reproducible. The physician can do the determinations himself on a single drop of plasma or serum. In healthy low birth weight infants, average refractometer total protein is 5.04, the term infant's 6.25, babies up to 11 months 6.11, children 7 and adults 7.45. Over a 24-hour period, in the absence of massive protein loss, a fall in refractometer total protein suggests an increase in plasma water and a rise suggests a loss of plasma water.[46]

CENTRAL VENOUS PRESSURE. — The measurement of central venous pressure has been considered a simple, rapid and extremely valuable method of monitoring the hypovolemic patient. Low central venous pressure suggested a decrease in blood volume and in cardiac function. It was believed that the volume and rate of fluid therapy could be safely gauged by the initial reading and the response of central venous pressure to fluid and electrolyte infusions. Recently there has been disenchantment with this technique. Without x-ray confirmation, as many as 35% of catheters thought to be inserted into the central venous system are not central in location.[47] Unless the catheter lies in the superior vena cava system or the right atrium, pressure is not recorded reliably. The usual clinical method for monitoring central venous pressure is by the water manometer. The manometer can respond to only one or two variations per second whereas accurate representation of physiologic changes requires a frequency response of the system of at least 20 cycles per second. Since atrial pressure may vary considerably over a single cardiac cycle, the water manometer may reflect maximal pressure rather than mean central venous atrial pressure.[48] Falsely elevated central venous pressure readings can also be produced by respiratory distress, positive pressure ventilation and abdominal distention.

From a functional standpoint, central venous pressure accurately reflects right atrial pressure, but in the critically ill patient it may not reflect changes in the left atrium and left ventricle. As a result, central venous pressure probably is not a good measure of the competence of the heart. With the advent of bedside monitoring of pulmonary wedge pressure utilizing the Swan-Ganz catheter, it has been shown that there frequently is variation between pulmonary wedge pressure, which accurately reflects left atrial pressure, and central venous pressure in patients with multiple injuries, peritonitis and cardiac lesions. Right and left atrial pressure can be independent of each other and there can be a disparity between ventricular pressure and atrial pressure. For this reason, it is thought that measurements of pulmonary wedge pressure are a much more reliable indicator of end-diastolic pressure in the left ventricle.[49, 50] Recently, small Swan-Ganz catheters have become commercially available and can be utilized in large babies and children. These catheters have the added advantage of having a thermistor tip so that cardiac output can be measured by the thermodilution method. We have found that children usually show a close correlation between central venous pressure and pulmonary wedge pressure, since they generally do not have the frequent cardiac lesions of the adult. We reserve use of the Swan-Ganz catheter for patients in severe hypovolemic or septic shock and those on respirators who require high positive end-expiratory pressures.

Despite the inherent difficulties, we usually use central venous pressure to monitor most hypovolemic patients because it is a simple, rapid, inexpensive system that gives a rough index of an increase or decrease in blood volume, particularly in response to therapy. To use this monitor effectively, it is essential that the catheter be placed centrally and the position confirmed by x-ray and emphasis placed on changes in central venous pressure in response to therapy rather than on individual readings. Most important, changes in central venous pressure can be helpful only if they are interpreted in their relation to the over-all clinical condition of the patient.

COMMENT. — The above methods are helpful in arriving at the proper volume of fluid to be administered. A rough estimate of maintenance electrolyte requirements can be calculated by one of the methods, such as caloric or body surface. Electrolyte losses from sources such as the gastrointestinal tract can be determined by direct electrolyte analysis of samples. Pre-existing deficits and immeasurable losses must be estimated. There are several measurements that are helpful in arriving at these estimates and monitoring the adequacy of replacement therapy.

SERUM ELECTROLYTES. — Serum electrolytes — sodium, potassium and chloride — can be measured in small samples in most clinical laboratories. Combined with blood urea nitrogen and blood sugar determinations, this yields an excellent picture of the concentration of serum solutes. The use of serum electrolytes for monitoring requires a trained technician and a biochemistry laboratory, and factors of time and cost impose limits on the possible frequency of determinations.

SERUM OSMOLALITY. — Serum osmolality gives less information than serum electrolyte determination, but osmolality measurements have the advantage of requiring only 0.2 ml of serum; samples can be collected from a capillary puncture and, most important, a physician or a nurse rather than a trained technician can do the determinations. The nurses in our newborn surgical unit measure serum osmolality before the change of each shift on all babies who receive intravenous infusions. The results of the serum osmolality measurements are known immediately. A normal serum osmolality in infants and children is between 270 and 280 milliosmoles/kg.[51] Osmolality is a measure of the concentration — the number of particles in a kilogram of a solvent. In serum, the major determinant of osmolality is the sodium ion. To a lesser degree, sugar and urea nitrogen contribute to the total osmolality. We utilize the following formula[52] for calculating osmolality:

$$\text{Osmolality} = \text{Sodium} \times 1.86 \times \frac{\text{BUN}}{2.8} + \frac{\text{Glucose}}{18} + 5$$

Our approach to electrolyte therapy of patients who require intravenous therapy for more than a few days, those who are low birth weight or patients with a serious fluid and electrolyte problem is to obtain an initial measurement of serum electrolytes, blood urea nitrogen, sugar and serum osmolality. The tonicity of the patient's serum then is followed during intravenous therapy by frequent determinations of serum osmolality. A rise in osmolality suggests that too little water or too great a quantity of electrolytes, usually sodium, has been given. A fall in osmolality suggests that sodium replacement is inadequate or that too great a quantity of water is being administered. An unexpected change in osmolality, particularly an increase, requires a repeat determination of serum electrolytes, blood urea nitrogen and sugar and calculation of the osmolality by the formula. By studying each component that makes up osmolality it is possible to determine whether the rise in osmolality is due to an increase in serum sodium, hyperglycemia or high blood urea nitrogen. If the measured serum osmolality is higher than the calculated serum osmolality, it suggests that an unidentified osmolarly active substance is present in the serum. A measured osmolality higher than calculated has been found during the terminal phases of shock and after the injection of radiographic contrast material intravascularly or into the gastrointestinal tract.

Gram-Negative Sepsis

Overwhelming gram-negative infection is a significant cause of death in newborn surgical patients. Microorganisms are found in large numbers in the bloodstream, and progressive signs of shock and multiple sequential organ failure develop. Basically, there are two reasons for this predilection for the neonatal surgical patient to develop gram-negative septicemia: increased exposure to bacteria and reduced host defenses.

Before and after operation, newborn infants now frequently are managed in large neonatal units where infants suffering from septic and nonseptic conditions are housed together, allowing multiple opportunities for cross contamination. In the past, rigid control of baby contact and traffic was practiced in all neonatal nurseries. With the advent of sophisticated medical technology came an influx of specialized personnel who now work in infant care areas and frequently handle the baby and his equipment. The common use of intravascular catheters for monitoring and delivering fluids has introduced multiple direct portals of infection. Endotracheal tubes, ventilators and inhalation therapy equipment for the treatment of respiratory problems have increased the infant's exposure to bacteria, particularly waterborne bacteria. Total intravenous nutrition now is in widespread use. This technique requires a long-term intravascular foreign body and infusion of concentrated sugar solutions, a combination that intensifies the danger of bloodstream infection. The emergence of resistant bacterial strains probably is due to the common practice of administering multiple antibiotics to high-risk patients.

The concept that the newborn patient has reduced host defenses appears to be generally accepted. To evaluate host defenses and be able to determine where the baby stands in his ability to resist infection, it is necessary for the surgeon to understand basic immunobiologic mechanisms. The literature of the immunobiology of infection is complex and sometimes conflicting. For example, the terminology and symbols used to describe the complement system or the immunoglobulins are unfamiliar to most of us. The surgeon begins to believe that he has wandered into foreign and perhaps even hostile territory. At the risk of oversimplification, I will attempt to describe the body's defensive responses to invading bacteria and relate these responses to the newborn surgical patient.

Host Defenses

As bacteria enter the body, alarms are sounded and two basic mechanisms are activated to eliminate the invaders—the humoral and the cellular. Humoral defenses involve antibodies—immunoglobulins. B-lymphocytes develop into plasma cells, which, in turn, manufacture immunoglobulins. They can elaborate immunoglobulins rapidly in response to foreign antigens in cooperation with T-lymphocytes—"helper" cells. When a microorganism enters the body, it is recognized as a foreign antigen by processes still not fully understood and then may be bound to a specific immunoglobulin. Generally, the IgG immunoglobulins bind gram-positive organisms and the IgM bind gram-negative organisms. The complex that results when antibody and antigen combine activates the effector arm of the humoral defense mechanisms—the classic complement system. The complement system reacts in a specific sequence—a cascade of reactions beginning with C1, the first protein in the sequence, and ending with C9. The latter half of the sequence of complement interaction is a membrane attack phase. Products of the cascade (C5b6789 complex) insert themselves into the bacterial cell membrane and cause cell lysis and death. During the chain reaction of the complement system, biologically active peptides are broken off and released into the circulation and produce some of the systemic signs of infection.

Phagocytosis and intracellular killing of bacteria is the second and more important method to combat acute bacterial infection. The principal phagocytic cell against most bacterial invaders is the polymorphonuclear leukocyte. Phagocytosis involves several steps. The phagocytic cell is first led to the site of the microorganism by chemotaxis. Then, the bacteria must be recognized and processed for engulfment—opsonization. Next, the microorganism is engulfed by the phagocyte. After the bacteria is phagocytized it is killed and digested inside the phagocytic cell.

Leukocytes are attracted to the site of the bacterial invasion by elements of the complement system, particularly C3 and C5. These are chemotactic elements and must be in adequate supply for the white blood cell to migrate to the inflammatory area. The process of recognition and ingestion of the microorganism is facilitated by opsonization. Certain immunoglobulins and complement products serve as opsonins and bind themselves to the bacteria. The phagocyte now can recognize and ingest the microorganism. Opsonization and phagocytosis can take place sluggishly without complement, but it is only with an intact complement system that these mechanisms become effective. It appears that the alternate or properdin complement pathway rather than the classic complement pathway C1 through C9 is the principal method of production of opsonins. In the alternate pathway, the cascade of complement is activated at the C3 level. To re-emphasize, complement is necessary for efficient opsonization and phagocytosis and the complement particles are produced for opsonization as a result of activation of the alternate rather than the classic complement pathway. After opsonization, the final phase of phagocytosis is ingestion. The cytoplasmic processes of the white blood cell extend around the microorganism and alternately fuse to form a phagocytic vacuole or phagosome. Now, bacterial killing takes place. White blood cell respiration intensifies, energy is utilized, hydrogen peroxide production increases and the cytoplasmic granules fuse with the phagosome and empty their contents into it. The actual killing is a complex process involving hydrogen peroxide and myeloperoxidase to iodinate the cell wall of the bacteria, lactoferrin, lysosome enzymes, an acid medium and cation proteins.

In evaluating the infant surgical patient's defenses, we must ask a series of questions: (1) Does he have adequate antibodies and an intact classic complement system to bind bacteria and then lyse the invader? (2) Does he have a functioning alternate complement system so that there will be sufficient chemotactic agents present and sufficient opsonins to allow for attraction, recognition and preparation of the bacteria for ingestion by the polymorphonuclear white blood cell? (3) Does he have sufficient phagocytic cells present? (4) Are the polymorphonuclear white blood cells functionally adequate to ingest bacteria and then kill them?

The Adequacy of the Newborn Surgical Patient's Host Defenses

The infant's defenses may have certain deficiencies that make him vulnerable to gram-negative infections. Some are the result of his "immaturity" whereas others are directly related to his being a surgical patient—his exposure to trauma and the complications of his disease and therapy.

IMMUNOGLOBULINS.—IgG antibodies make up about 80% of all human immunoglobulins, and included among them are antibodies to gram-positive bacteria, viruses and some bacterial toxins. IgG is the only immunoglobulin that passes through the placental barrier to the fetus. As a result, the cord IgG levels at birth are as high as or higher than those of the mother. In contrast, IgM, the principal immunoglobulin for gram-negative organisms, is absent at birth under normal circumstances. The dowry of IgG from the mother and the lack of IgM may contribute to the infant's susceptibility to gram-negative organisms.[53-57]

What probably is more important to the infant, however, is not the presence or absence of IgM at birth but whether the baby, when exposed to a gram-negative antigen, can produce antibodies rapidly and in adequate numbers. The infant at delivery has his own immunologically competent system and can mount an immune response to antigenic challenges. By 3–5 months of gestation, the system is set to function against antigens.[58, 59] At birth, the B-lymphocytes are present and awaiting differentiation into plasma cells, which synthesize and secrete immunoglobulins. The B cells are driven to differentiate into plasma cells and produce immunoglobulins in response to the antigenic challenge of the extrauterine world. Much of the antigenic drive for gram-negative antigens arises from the gut flora. IgM antibodies to coliform organisms are present within the first week of life.[60] Probably the most important immunologic defect of the newborn is really the virginity of the lymphocytes rather than their inadequacy.[61] They just have not had the experience with the huge number of antigens that they are exposed to. They meet them for the first time at birth and then must make antibodies to deal with the present encounter and remember the antigens so that they are prepared for later exposure. In some cases, their antibody production is sluggish and delayed. For organisms such as *H. influenzae*

and meningococcus, this is particularly striking. It takes as long as 9–12 months to develop immunoglobulins to these antigens.[61]

THE COMPLEMENT PATHWAYS.—The complement system is a critical mechanism for adequate host defense. It permits lysis of bacteria already fixed by antibodies and produces chemotactic and opsonic elements essential for phagocytosis.[62-67] The newborn infant has decreased total complement activity. Most significant, the concentration of C3 is about one-half that of the adult, and the lower the total complement activity the lower the C3 level. The rate of bacterial opsonization is directly correlated to the C3 level in the serum. C3 along with C5 and C567 complex serve as chemotactic elements. These elements are reduced in neonatal serum.[68]

The classic complement pathway begins at C1 and goes through the 9 steps in sequence. This pathway requires antibody to activate it. It is logical that another method of activating the complement system that would not require antibodies should be available in the event that no specific antibodies are present. This appears to be the function of the alternate or properdin pathway. The alternate pathway can be activated by bacterial polysaccharides, such as endotoxin, without antibodies. It begins at the C3 level. For the bacterial products to activate the system, factor B, a beta-pseudoglobulin, and properdin, a beta-globulin, must be present in sufficient quantities. The newborn infant's serum is deficient in these elements. Concentrations are less than half that of the adult.[69, 70]

PHAGOCYTOSIS AND BACTERIAL KILLING.—Under normal conditions, studies of the white blood cell function of most term and moderately low birth weight infants demonstrate normal opsonization and chemotaxis as well as effective ingestion and killing. This is despite the recorded low concentrations of complement elements. However, some apparently normal infants and most stressed infants have reduced leucocyte function due to serum and cell factors.[67, 73, 74] Wright *et al.*[71] found in hypoxic and other sick infants that there was a killing defect of the white blood cells. Forman and Stiehm[72] reported that in very low birth weight infants below 1900 gm, killing ability was reduced and opsonization was markedly abnormal. They also found that sick full-term infants had reduced white blood cell function.

To summarize, the concentration of opsonic and chemotactic elements in the newborn serum is less than the adult's. Despite this, the white blood cells of most healthy full-size and moderately low birth weight babies have adequate metabolism and killing ability. The polymorphonuclear white cells of some apparently healthy full-size infants, many very small babies and most stressed and septic infants have reduced phagocytosis and killing ability. The defect more often is due to serum rather than cell factors.

SURGICAL FACTORS.—Unless specific measures are taken, most pediatric surgical patients undergo variable periods of starvation. In a preceding section I described the reduction of host defense that resulted from starvation. Protein-caloric malnutrition appears to be related to defects in serum and cellular host defense mechanisms. Copeland, MacFayden and Dudrick[75] found that cell-mediated immunity is reduced in malnutrition and can be restored by vigorous intravenous hyperalimentation. A specific deficiency of C3 proactivator recently has been documented in malnutrition.[76] A brief fast in normal adult subjects of 4–5 days has not been shown to produce any abnormalities of phagocytosis or white blood cell function.[77] Children with kwashiorkor type of protein-calorie malnutrition have reduction of the bactericidal capacity of their white blood cells.[27] Chandra[78] demonstrated that children under 8 years of age with iron-deficiency anemia also frequently had reduced bacterial killing capacity of their white blood cells. He found that this defect could be reversed in a week by parenteral iron replacement therapy. The trauma and infection associated with operation and injuries may affect the pediatric surgical patient's resistance to infection. Alexander, Hegg and Altemeier[77] found profound abnormalities of white blood cell function during the first week after thermal injury and mild dysfunctions immediately following physical injuries and operative trauma. The most profound deficits are the result of infection. Established sepsis affects the serum and cellular aspects of defense. Weinstein and Young[79] found that patients with gram-negative septicemia seldom had intrinsic white blood cell bactericidal defects but commonly had impaired opsonization. In a recent report, Alexander and his co-workers[80] discussed a consumptive opsoninopathy in patients with serious infections. C3 and properdin are consumed. These authors suggested that as these factors are consumed, the patient's ability to opsonize is severely compromised, leading to an increased susceptibility to superinfection or progression of the existing infection. Antibodies also are consumed in acute infections. During pseudomonas infection, type-specific antipseudomonas antibody is reduced. This defect can be corrected by giving a specific hyperimmune antibody.[81, 82]

Certain drugs that may be administered to pediatric surgical patients have an effect on the white blood cell itself and on phagocytosis. The most striking effect is produced by drugs that interfere with the bone marrow production of white blood cells and results in neutropenia. Chemotherapeutic agents used in tumor therapy are prime examples. When white blood cell count falls below 1000, the patient is in serious jeopardy of developing infection, and when the count falls below 500 there is a grave risk of developing a rapidly fatal infection.[83] Several of the steroid hormones—hydrocortisone, methylprednisolone and dexamethasone—reduce white blood cell chemotaxis and appear to affect intracellular killing of bacteria.[84-87]

Diagnosis of Neonatal Sepsis

The clinical signs of gram-negative septicemia in the newborn infant are subtle and nonspecific and may go unnoticed until deterioration is far advanced. At present, a definitive diagnosis must await a report of a positive blood culture. It takes between 24 and 48 hours for bacteria to be identified on the culture media. Because of the inherent delay before a positive blood culture can be reported there is continuing search for more rapid methods of diagnosing septicemia. The Limulus lysate assay described by Levin and Bang[88] in 1964 is a quick and sensitive method of detecting gram-negative bacteremia and endotoxemia. The test solution is prepared from the blood cells of the horseshoe crab—*Limulus polyphemus*. This material gels on exposure to minute quantities of endotoxin. Levin and his associates[89] found that the test was positive in 71% of patients with gram-negative septicemia. We[90] reported 64% positive tests in infant surgical patients suffering from gram-negative bacteremia. However, Feldman and Pearson[91] reported only a 7% positive limulus test in patients with gram-negative septicemia and Stumacher et al.[92] a 36% positive assay in patients with gram-positive bacteremia. The variability in results among investigators probably stems from the differences in extraction and preparation of the biologic material

and contamination of the specimen during collection and performance of the assay. We believe that this test is an effective method of identifying patients with significant gram-negative bacteremia, but it requires a skilled technician who has an interest in the method, a well-prepared supply of the lysate and personnel trained to obtain uncontaminated specimens from the patient.

It is believed that infants suffering from bacteremia have proportionally more organisms circulating in their blood than do adults. Probably as a result, 70% of infants with serious gram-negative septicemia have identifiable organisms seen when a Gram stain of the buffy coat of the blood sample is examined.[93] This is a simple, rapid method that can be done without sophisticated laboratory equipment. When bacteria are positively identified there is little chance for error in the diagnosis. This method also may help identify the infecting microorganisms. Changes in the total white blood cell count are of very limited value in the diagnosis of septicemia in the newborn patient. Elevations often are late and inconsistent.[94-96] In patients with positive blood cultures, white blood cell counts frequently remain normal. We have found that the white blood cell counts of surgical babies with gram-negative sepsis average 8596, with a range of 2050–29,400. Forty-two per cent of the infants had white blood cell counts below 5000 when they had advanced signs of septicemia.[90] In contrast to the total white blood cell count, elevation of the band neutrophil count appears to be a reliable means of indicating infants who may be suffering from bacteremia. Zipursky, Palko, Milner and Akenzua[96] found that 11 of 15 premature infants with proved infection had elevation of their band neutrophils. The rise occurred within 24 hours of the onset of clinical sepsis. These same authors also found that with proved sepsis there were significant changes in the appearance of the white blood cells. The most frequent findings were Döhle bodies, vacuolization and toxic granules.

We have found that the serial platelet count in the postoperative infant is another rapid method of screening patients for gram-negative septicemia.[90] Platelets react with endotoxin and complement, producing platelet aggregation, adherence of platelets to vascular endothelium and platelet destruction. A rapid and profound fall in platelet count results. One hundred per cent of infant surgical patients with blood cultures positive for gram-negative rods had platelet counts below 100,000. The average value was 67,000 in the septic patients and 280,000 in those without infection. With acute septicemia, we have observed falls as great as 222,000 in less than 24 hours.

Patients at risk of developing gram-negative septicemia should be monitored initially by serial platelet counts and careful clinical observation. A significant fall in platelet count suggests gram-negative septicemia, particularly a decrease below 150,000. Multiple blood cultures should be drawn and a blood smear examined. An increase in total band neutrophils or the appearance of many Döhle bodies, vacuoles or toxic granules in the white blood cells makes the diagnosis almost certain. If gram-negative bacteria are identified on a Gram stain of the buffy coat, the diagnosis of septicemia is confirmed.

Treatment of Host Defense Deficiencies

Neonatal surgical patients may have decreased white blood cells, leukocyte dysfunction and serum complement and antibody deficiencies. It is logical to consider replacement therapy of depleted host defense factors in the treatment of sepsis. The most direct method would be exchange transfusion. This has the theoretic value of reducing the concentration of circulating endotoxins as well as increasing circulating white blood cells, antibodies and the components necessary for opsonization and chemotaxis. Whole blood stored up to 21 days contains all the necessary opsonins, with only a slight reduction as compared to fresh whole blood.[80] Even if fresh blood is utilized, the survival of functioning white blood cells will be minimal—less than 5%. Although exchange transfusion has little if any value as a method of giving a patient a significant number of functioning leukocytes, it is an excellent method of supplying serum factors, particularly opsonins and antibodies. We believe that in patients rapidly deteriorating from sepsis, exchange transfusions should be attempted. There has been a recent report[97] of survival in newborn infants with overwhelming sepsis and sclerema after one or more exchange transfusions. This technique should also be considered if disseminated intravascular coagulation is present with infection.

For those patients who may not need exchange transfusions, it still is important to increase the level of serum factors. This can be done by transfusions of whole blood or by the infusion of fresh-frozen plasma. Blood or plasma can be used as part of the initial resuscitation fluid in the treatment of septic shock to replace low or consumed serum factors.

White blood cell transfusions appear to be an attractive technique for combating infection, particularly in patients with severe leukopenia. Bodey *et al.*[98] established the incidence of infection for various circulating neutrophil levels. Patients with white blood cell counts above 1000 are not at an increased risk of developing infection. The difficulties associated with successful white cell transfusions are multiple. Foremost is the fact that, unlike red blood cells, leukocytes are rich in histocompatibility antigens (HL-A). If transfusion is matched to the donor on all four HL-A loci, about 50% of the cells survive. If only one locus is matched, recovery is reduced to 3%.[99] Another limiting factor of successful white blood cell transfusions is the short life of the leukocyte. They remain in the circulation only about 10 hours and, with infection, the rate of disappearance is accelerated. Even during normal conditions, only 50% of the white blood cells actually are in the central vascular system; the rest adhere to small blood vessels and roll along vascular walls.[100-102] There now are methods available to harvest large amounts of viable white blood cells from donors and match the cells to the recipient. Under these ideal conditions, Graw and his associates[99] gave 96 granulocyte transfusions to 39 compatible donors with severe sepsis. There was a 46% survival vs a 30% survival in the control group. Other authors have reported similar results in adult patients.[103] Pole, Kershaw, Barter and Willoughby[104] reported a recent study in children. They gave unmatched granulocyte transfusions to infected neutropenic children. They reasoned that proportionately more cells would be received in children than in adults because of the small size of the young patient's blood volume. Twenty-five of 30 patients were treated successfully.

We believe that component blood therapy as well as exchange transfusion for the treatment of sepsis has a place, particularly in replacing depleted serum factors. At present, we believe that white blood cell transfusions should be utilized only in agranulocytic patients with infections, if conditions are ideal. The hospital facilities must be adequate for HL-A typing and white blood cell harvesting. The physician must have an active interest in this form of therapy and have techniques available to follow white blood cell survival and function of the infused white blood cells.

Gram-Negative Septicemic Shock

One of the most active and complex fields of clinical and animal research today concerns the pathophysiology and treatment of septic shock. Sadly, progress in this field has been made as a result of studies of the adult patient and animal. The pertinence of many of the important observations to the infant patient is yet to be proved. Despite this, we are forced to apply to the baby the knowledge currently available and wait hopefully for information from pediatric investigators concerning the septic process in the neonatal and young subject.

PATHOGENESIS AND PATHOPHYSIOLOGY.—It is not clear to what extent direct damage to the body results from invading microorganisms and their by-products, particularly endotoxin, and how much from the interaction of the invaders and the body's host defenses. Endotoxin may have a direct effect on cell function and the capillary membrane, but Hinshaw and his co-workers[105, 106] have not been able to demonstrate impairment of myocardial function by endotoxin. A large body of information has accumulated that suggests that many of the systemic changes seen in gram-negative shock are the direct result of the violent struggle between the body's defense mechanisms and bacteria and bacterial by-products.[107-111]

Endotoxin appears in increasing concentrations in the circulation as bacteria are killed by the host. It is a lipopolysaccharide found on the cell membrane of gram-negative bacteria. Platelets react with endotoxin and complement, causing platelet aggregation and destruction. The aggregates and platelet fragments, along with clumped white blood cell and leukocyte debris, are swept into the microcirculation and can produce microcirculatory blockade. This debris in the pulmonary microvasculature has been implicated in the pulmonary hypertension and failure that develops with gram-negative sepsis.[107, 112, 113] With platelet destruction, there is release of vasoactive substances—serotonin, ADP, ATP, prostaglandins E_2 and F_2 and histamine. When the complement system is activated by endotoxin through the alternate pathway, fragments of the complement system produce systemic effects. C3a and C5a are called anaphylatoxins and bind mast cells, triggering the release of histamine. Histamine produces vasodilatation and increases capillary permeability.[62] Peptidases released from injured tissues induce intravascular clotting and plasmin activity. In response to sepsis, a series of powerful vasoactive substances, the kinins, are activated. Bradykinin, one of the products of the kinin system, is elevated in 65% of the patients with infection and hypotension.[108, 109]

The role of the lysosome in shock still is not clear. In septic shock there is an increased level of acid hydrolysates. These enzymes are thought to be derived from cell lysosomes. With tissue damage, the lysosome membrane ruptures and these enzymes are released. It has been postulated that the hydrolase action of these agents may produce autolysis of the cell—cellular self-destruction, generalized cardiovascular reactions and remote tissue damage. Alho,[114] in a review of lysosomal function in circulatory shock, concluded that the role of lysosomes in cell autolysis during shock probably is not a significant factor contributing to the irreversibility of the shock state. He presented evidence that supports the concept that the lysosomal enzymes have general circulatory effects, including production of coagulation disorders, but also may have some protective functions by aiding the renal tubules and reticuloendothelial system in eliminating deleterious metabolic products of shock.

A prominent feature of septic shock is the development of hypovolemia. This appears to be on the basis of capillary leak and the loss of fluid into the interstitial space. Blood volume in adults can fall 20% or more. Moore and his group[115] found that extracellular water increased 130% and intracellular water fell 90%.

Several systems are prominently involved in the body's response to gram-negative septicemia. The pathogenesis of progressive pulmonary failure commonly seen with severe septic shock still is a subject of debate. Clowes, Farrington, Zuschneid, Cossetts and Saravis[116] discussed the progressive lung lesion that begins with interstitial pneumonitis and ends with extensive bronchopneumonia. Initially there is mild hypovolemia, alkalosis and moderate right-to-left shunting. Later, pulmonary vascular resistance increases, the PO_2 falls, microatelectasis is common, shunting increases and the compliance and functional residual capacity of the lung decrease.[117]

Cardiac function has been studied extensively in gram-negative and endotoxic shock. Myocardial dysfunction progressively develops as the shock state proceeds. A circulatory myocardial depressant factor responsible for this change has never been confirmed.[106, 118] Inadequate coronary perfusion and deficiencies of energy substrate seem the most likely primary factors in the cardiac failure of gram-negative sepsis. A major key to survival appears to be the cardiovascular system's ability to satisfy the increased cellular demands of the tissues for oxygen and nutrients. Survival and recovery is associated with elevations of the cardiac output, peripheral vasodilatation and opening up of arteriovenous shunts. In the adult, cardiac indices of 3.5–7 liters/m²/min are common. This is the so-called high output stage of septic shock. Patients unable to meet the elevated circulatory demands develop a falling cardiac output, hypotension, peripheral vasoconstriction, a rising lactic acidemia and death. Hypotensive patients with cardiac indices below 2.8 liters/m²/min have a mortality rate greater than 70%[119-122] As cardiac failure continues, both right-sided and left-sided failure are seen and central venous pressure and pulmonary wedge pressure increase.

The changes in energy metabolism with sepsis are profound.[123-127] For the purpose of this discussion, it is best to divide septic shock into two phases: the hyperdynamic and the hypodynamic. Initially, and persistently in patients who survive there is a hyperdynamic state, cardiac output and blood insulin are elevated and energy demands are strikingly elevated as the body attempts to combat infection. In the adult patient suffering from peritonitis, the energy expenditure may increase 60% or more. The metabolic rate far exceeds that predicted by the elevation of body temperature alone. Carbohydrate stores are rapidly depleted and serum insulin levels remain elevated. Increased insulin concentration inhibits the lipogenic response of adipose tissue. In other words, even if the patient has an adequate supply of body fat as an energy reserve, because of the high insulin level, this fat cannot be mobilized and utilized for energy. Muscle then becomes the prime energy provider and an intense proteolysis occurs.

In contrast, patients who cannot maintain the hyperdynamic state develop a decreased cardiac output and a decreased serum insulin. The low insulin levels may be the result of the accelerated activity of the sympathetic-adrenal system, with a large release of catecholamines. Carbohydrate stores are depleted, blood sugar falls and there is much less energy substrate available to the cells. Muscle appears to be resistant to insulin and does not provide large quantities of energy. The patient is energy depleted. There is, in addition, accumulating evidence that the low insulin levels have a direct effect on the myocardium and contribute significantly to the myocardial failure that develops in severe gram-negative septicemic shock.

TREATMENT.— Survival ultimately is determined by the successful eradication of the invading microorganisms. For this reason, high doses of antibiotics are administered intravenously. Multiple cultures are taken to isolate the pathogen and determine its antibiotic sensitivities. Physiologic monitors are essential to guide resuscitation. In the small infant, a line is passed into the superior vena cava system to measure central venous pressure. A catheter is placed in the radial or temporal artery to monitor arterial blood pressure, pH and blood gases. Cardiac rate is continually measured by pulse monitors. A small catheter is passed into the bladder for hourly urine output determinations. In larger patients, a Swan-Ganz catheter is utilized for repeated measurements of pulmonary wedge pressure and cardiac output. We attempt to gauge cardiac function in the newborn patient, since direct measurement of cardiac output is technically difficult, by central venous pressure readings, hourly urine output, the arterial blood pressure, pulse pressure and the shape of the pulse curve displayed on an oscilloscope.

The hypovolemia that develops as a result of translocation of fluid into the interstitial spaces in septic shock is corrected by rapid intravenous infusions. The rate and volume are determined by changes in the central venous pressure and urine output and the response of the blood pressure. We generally do not use albumin-containing solutions for fluid resuscitation. We believe that there is extensive capillary membrane damage during gram-negative shock and the albumin leaks out of the injured vessels, increasing fluid loss and edema.[128, 129] In pre-term infants, our initial fluid often is one-half strength Ringer's lactate solution, but in many full-term infants normal saline solution is infused. Despite our reluctance to administer colloid, in patients with overwhelming infection who may have marked reduction in opsonic and chemotactic serum factors we administer fresh whole blood or fresh-frozen plasma.

Although evidence of its effectiveness still is not conclusive, we inject a single bolus of 30 mg/kg of methylprednisolone to patients who have evidence of gram-negative septic shock. In 1962[130] and 1965,[131] Sambhi, Weil and Udhoji described the hemodynamic effects of pharmacologic doses of corticosteroids. In 1964, Lillehei, Longerbeam, Bloch and Manax[132] presented evidence of the beneficial effects of large doses of steroids in the treatment of refractory shock. Reports of improved survival in patients and animals suffering from endotoxic,[133-136] hemorrhagic,[137-139] traumatic,[140] epinephrine[141] and snake venom[142] shock followed. There have been conflicting reports of the direct inotropic effect of methylprednisolone. Sambhi and his associates[130, 131] and Sayers and Solomon[143] found that increased cardiac output with methylprednisolone injection probably was on the basis of a direct myocardial effect. Other investigators, including Gunnar[144] and Replogle and his co-workers,[145] found no inotropic effect of corticosteroids in patients and animals in shock.

Although the inotropic effect of corticosteroids still is being debated, it is generally agreed that these agents decrease peripheral resistance and improve microcirculatory flow.[146] Pharmacologic doses appear to reduce platelet aggregation and the sequestration of red blood cells in the microcirculation.[147] High doses may also protect the integrity of the capillary wall.[148] There is experimental evidence to suggest that, in high doses, corticosteroids have a stabilizing effect on the cell and lysosomal membranes.[148-153] Several investigators[154] believe that steroids have a protective effect by decreasing complement interaction and thereby preventing the release of vasoactive substances that produce the third-space fluid loss in septic shock.

Recently, Schumer[155] presented an 8-year prospective clinical study on the use of steroids in the treatment of septic shock. This was a double-blind study. One group received saline, the other a single bolus of 3 mg/kg of dexamethasone or 30 mg/kg of methylprednisolone. In the saline-treated group, the mortality was 38.4% and in the steroid-treated group it was 10.4%. Schumer also did a retrospective study of 328 patients. Mortality in the steroid-treated group was 14%, but patients without steroid treatment had a 42.5% mortality. This report, presented at the meeting of the American Surgical Association in New Orleans in 1976, seemed convincing, but many clinicians have challenged Schumer's findings. They report that they have not seen such striking results in their own experience. They question whether this was truly a double-blind study. Nevertheless, the bulk of the evidence suggests that a single large dose of methylprednisolone in patients who are suffering from septic shock does not appear to be detrimental and may be beneficial. For this reason, we utilize this agent.

Infant patients with gram-negative septicemia frequently are debilitated, depressed by the effects of anesthesia and have abdominal distention and peritonitis. As a result, respiratory acidosis and hypoxia develop due to inadequate ventilation. The respiratory failure encountered in the septic adult "shock lung" is also seen often in the infant with septicemia. Pulmonary arterial resistance increases, shunting occurs at the pulmonary and ductus arteriosus level and there is increasing pulmonary edema and diffused bronchopneumonia. Because of the extensive lung involvement, newborn surgical patients with sepsis should be maintained on a ventilator. The rate, pressures, volume and the concentration of inspired O_2 are determined by the arterial blood gas values. We have found that the progressive pulmonary failure with a falling Po_2 often can be reversed by adding positive end-expiratory pressure (PEEP). In the low birth weight infant, we have used pressures as high as 6 cm of water, and in the full-term infant a maximum of 8 cm of water. It is essential that cardiac function be monitored when positive end-expiratory pressure is used. At high pressures, venous return and cardiac output fall.

Despite correction of hypovolemia, treatment of respiratory failure and the administration of methylprednisolone, blood pressure may remain at a low level in the face of a normal or high central venous pressure. This suggests inadequate myocardial function. If cardiac output measurements are available, this impression can be confirmed. There are a number of therapeutic measures presently utilized to increase cardiac output in patients with septic shock. Dopamine, because it increases myocardial contractility, redistributes flow to essential viscera and can be titrated to attain different pharmacologic effects, has been suggested as the drug of first choice for the treatment of septic shock.[156-158] Dopamine has been characterized as having alpha and beta effects midway between isoproterenol and epinephrine. Wilson, Sibbald and Jaanimagi[158] studied the hemodynamic effects of dopamine in 20 septic hypotensive patients. Blood pressure rose as a result of an increase in cardiac output, peripheral resistance rose only slightly and pulmonary vascular resistance fell. They concluded that dopamine was a useful drug in treating cardiac failure with septic shock but that it should be used after large volumes of fluid have been administered. The dose schedules for infants have not been clearly established. In adults, an infusion of $2-5$ μg/kg/min increases cardiac output, renal blood flow and urine output. With larger doses up to 30 micrograms there is a further increase in cardiac output and presumably renal blood flow. At higher doses, peripheral vasoconstriction becomes a predominant action due to an adrenergic effect. In septic infants with low urine output and signs of failing circulation, after fluid replacement therapy, we begin an infusion of dopamine at a dose of 3 μg/kg/min and increase up to 20 μg/kg/min if urine output and hemodynamic functions do not improve.

A large group of investigators recently have stressed the role of glucose, potassium and insulin therapy in improving myocardial performance in the low-output phase of septic shock. They point out that serum insulin and blood sugar levels are markedly reduced in the low-output state. Infusion of hypotonic glucose alone has been found to increase cardiac output and left ventricular stroke work. Hinshaw *et al.*[126] noted a similar improvement with infusions of insulin. Weisul's group[125] demonstrated improved cardiac function with the infusion of glucose, insulin and potassium in patients suffering from septic shock. Clowes *et al.,*[123] in a clinical and experimental study of low-output septic shock, found that glucose, potassium and insulin infusions returned cardiovascular function from a low-output state to a high cardiac output state. The usual dose recommended for a bolus injection is: glucose 1 gm/kg, crystalline insulin 1.5 units/kg and 1 mEq of potassium chloride per kg.

REFERENCES

1. Sinclair, J. C.: Metabolic Rate and Temperature Control, in Smith, C. A., and Nelson, N. M. (eds.), *The Physiology of the Newborn Infant* (4th ed.; Springfield, Ill.: Charles C Thomas, Publisher, 1976), p. 354.
2. Scopes, J. W., and Ahmed, I.: Minimal rates of oxygen consumption in sick and premature newborn infants, Arch. Dis. Child. 41:407, 1966.
3. Sinclair, J. C., Driscoll, J. M., Heird, W. C., and Winters, R. W.: Supportive management of the sick neonate, Pediatr. Clin. North Am. 17:863, 1970.
4. Sinclair, J. C., and Silverman, W. A.: Intrauterine growth in active tissue mass of the human fetus, with particular reference to the undergrown baby, Pediatrics 38:48, 1966.
5. Brück, T.: Temperature regulation in the newborn infant, Biol. Neonate 3:65, 1961.
6. Adamsons, K., Jr., Gandy, G. M., and James, L. S.: The influence of thermal factors upon oxygen consumption of the newborn human infant, J. Pediatr. 66:495, 1965.
7. Levison, H., and Swyer, P. R.: Oxygen consumption and the thermal environment in newly born infants, Biol. Neonate 7:305, 1964.
8. Hill, J. R., and Rahimtulla, K. A.: Heat balance and the metabolic rate of newborn babies in relation to environmental temperature, and the effect of age and of weight on basal metabolic rate, J. Physiol. 180:239, 1965.
9. Hey, E. N.: The relation between environmental temperature and oxygen consumption in the newborn baby, J. Physiol. 200:589, 1969.
10. Brück, K., Parmalee, A. H., Jr., and Brück, M.: Neutral temperature range and range of "thermal comfort" in premature infants, Biol. Neonate 4:32, 1962.
11. Hill, J. R., and Robinson, D. C.: Oxygen consumption in normally grown small-for-dates and large-for-dates newborn infants, J. Physiol. 199:685, 1968.
12. Widdson, E. N.: Nutrition, in Davis, J. A., and Dobbins, J. (eds.), *Scientific Foundations of Pediatrics* (Philadelphia: W. B. Saunders Company, 1974), p. 46.
13. Brück, K.: Temperature regulation in the newborn infant, Biol. Neonate 3:65, 1961.
14. Sinclair, J. C.: Thermal control in premature infants, Annu. Rev. Med. 23:129, 1972.
15. Brody, S.: *Bioenergetics and Growth* (New York: Hafner, 1964), p. 61.

16. Erikson, H., Krog, J., Anderson, K. L., and Scholander, P. F.: The critical temperature in naked man, Acta Physiol. Scand. 37:35, 1956.
17. Hey, E. N., and Katz, G.: The optimum thermal environment for naked babies, Arch. Dis. Child. 45:328, 1970.
18. Kinney, J. M., Duke, J. H., Long, C. L., and Gump, F. E.: Carbohydrate and nitrogen metabolism after injury, J. Clin. Pathol. 23 (supp.) 4:65, 1970. (R. Coll. Pathol.)
19. Kinney, J. M.: Energy Demands in Septic Patients, in Hershey, S. G., Del Guercio, L. R. M., and McConn, R. (eds.), *Septic Shock in Man* (Boston: Little, Brown and Company, 1971).
20. Kinney, J. M., and Roe, C. F.: The caloric equivalent of fever: I. Patterns of postoperative response, Ann. Surg. 156:610, 1962.
21. Pruitt, B. A.: Postburn Hypermetabolism and Nutrition of the Burn Patient, in Committee on Pre and Postoperative Care, American College of Surgeons: *Manual of Surgical Nutrition* (Philadelphia: W. B. Saunders Company, 1975).
22. Heird, W. C., Driscoll, J. M., Schullinger, J. N., Grebin, B., and Winters, R. J.: Medical progress: Intravenous alimentation in pediatric patients, J. Pediatr. 80:351, 1972.
23. Winick, M., and Noble, A.: Cellular response in rats during malnutrition at various ages, J. Nutr. 89:300, 1966.
24. McCance, R. A., and Widdowson, E. M.: Nutrition and growth, Proc. R. Soc. Lond. (Biol.) 156:326, 1962.
25. Winick, M.: Changes in nucleic acid and protein content of the human brain during growth, Pediatr. Res. 2:352, 1968.
26. Winick, M., and Coombs, J.: Nutrition, environment and behavioral development, Annu. Rev. Med. 23:149, 1972.
27. Purtilo, D. T., and Connor, D. H.: Fatal infections in protein-calorie malnourished children with thymolymphatic atrophy, Arch. Dis. Child. 50:149, 1975.
28. Douglas, S. D., and Schopfer, K.: Phagocyte function in protein calorie malnutrition, Clin. Exp. Immunol. 17:121, 1974.
29. Scovill, W. A., and Saba, T. M.: Humoral recognition deficiency in the etiology of reticuloendothelial depression induced by surgery, Ann. Surg. 178:59, 1973.
30. Roy, R. N., and Sinclair, J. C.: Hydration of the low birth weight infant, Clin. Perinatol. 2:393, 1975.
31. Rubner, M. Über den Werth der Weizenkleie für die Ernährung des Menschen, Z. Biol. Munich 19:534, 1883.
32. Holliday, M. A., and Segar, W. E.: *Parenteral Fluid Therapy* (2d printing; Indianapolis: Indiana University Medical Center, 1956).
33. Kleiber, M.: *The Fire of Life—An Introduction to Animal Energetics* (New York: John Wiley & Sons, Inc., 1961).
34. Gleiss, J., and Stuttgen, G.: Morphologic and Functional Development of the Skin, in Stave, U. (ed.), *Physiology of the Perinatal Period* (New York: Appleton-Century-Crofts, Inc., 1970), Vol. III, pp. 889–906.
35. Nachman, R., and Esterly, N.: Increased permeability in preterm infants. Abstract presented at the meeting of the American Pediatric Society and Society for Pediatric Research, Atlantic City, New Jersey, April 28–May, 1, 1971.
36. Silverman, W. A.: General Considerations. Relationship between Length, Weight, Surface Area and Fetal Age, in *Dunham's Premature Infants* (3d ed.; New York: Harper & Row, Publishers, 1964), pp. 56–57.
37. Williams, P. R., and Oh, W.: Effects of radiant warmer on insensible water loss in newborn infants, Am. J. Dis. Child. 128:511, 1974.
38. Wu, P. Y. K., and Hodgman, J. E.: Insensible water loss in preterm infants: Changes with postnatal development and nonionizing radiant energy, Pediatrics 54:704, 1974.
39. Oh, W., and Karecki, H.: Phototherapy and insensible water loss in the newborn infant, Am. J. Dis. Child. 124:230, 1972.
40. Oh, W., Yao, A. C., Hanson, J. S., and Lind, J.: Peripheral circulatory response to phototherapy in newborn infants, Acta Paediatr. Scand. 62:49, 1973.
41. Hey, E. N., and Katz, G.: Evaporative water loss in the newborn baby, J. Physiol. 200:605, 1969.
42. Behrendt, H., and Green, M.: Nature of the sweating deficit of prematurely born neonates, N. Engl. J. Med. 286:1377, 1972.
43. Foster, K. G., Hey, E. N., and Katz, G.: The response of the sweat glands of the newborn baby to thermal stimuli and to intradermal acetylcholine, J. Physiol. 203:13, 1969.
44. Green, M., and Behrendt, H.: Sweating responses of neonates to local thermal stimulation, Am. J. Dis. Child. 125:20, 1973.
45. Edelman, C. M., and Spitzer, A.: The Kidney, in Smith, C. A., and Nelson, N. M. (eds.), *The Physiology of the Newborn Infant* (4th ed.; Springfield, Ill.: Charles C Thomas, Publisher, 1976), p. 416.

46. Rowe, M. I., Lankau, C., and Newmark, S.: Clinical evaluation of methods to monitor colloid oncotic pressure in the surgical treatment of children, Surg. Gynecol. Obstet. 139:889, 1974.
47. Civetta, J. M.: Instrumentation and the Monitoring of Patients in Shock, in Callahan, A. B., Malinin, T. I., Zeppa, R., and Drucker, W. R. (eds.), *Acute Fluid Replacement in Shock* (New York: Intercontinental Medical Book Corporation, 1974).
48. Civetta, J. M.: Pulmonary artery pressure determination: Electronic superior to manometric (Letter to Editor), N. Engl. J. Med. 285:1145, 1971.
49. Berglund, E.: Balance of left and right ventricular output: Relation between left and right atrial pressures, Am. J. Physiol. 178:381, 1954.
50. Rapaport, E., and Scheinman, M.: Rationale and limitations of hemodynamic measurements in patients with acute myocardial infarction, Mod. Concepts Cardiovasc. Dis. 38:55, 1969.
51. Rowe, M. I.: The role of serial serum osmolality measurements in the management of the neonatal surgical patient, Surg. Gynecol. Obstet. 133:93, 1971.
52. Mansberger, A. R. N., Boyd, D. R., Crowley, R. A., and Buxton, R. W.: Refractometry and osmometry in clinical surgery, Ann. Surg. 169:672, 1969.
53. Gally, A. J.: Structure of Immunoglobulins, in Sela, M. (ed.), *The Antigens* (New York: Academic Press, 1973), p. 161.
54. Henley, W. L.: The Immunoglobulins: Structure, Function, Immune Response, Synthesis and Genetic Regulation, in Schulman, I. (ed.), *Advances in Pediatrics* (Chicago: Year Book Medical Publishers, Inc., 1972), Vol. 19, pp. 281–318.
55. Morrell, A., Skvaril, F., Hitzig, W. H., and Barandum, S.: IgG subclasses: Development of the serum concentrations in "normal" infants and children, J. Pediatr. 80:960, 1972.
56. Rosen, F. S.: Neonatal Immunity, in Smith, C. A., and Nelson, N. M. (eds.), *The Physiology of the Newborn Infant* (4th ed.; Springfield, Ill.: Charles C Thomas, Publisher, 1976), p. 740.
57. Gitlin, D., Kumate, J., Urrusti, J., and Morales, C.: The selectivity of the human placenta in the transfer of plasma proteins from mother to fetus, J. Clin. Invest. 43:1938, 1964.
58. Gitlin, D., and Biasucci, A.: Development of γG, γA, $\beta_2 C/\beta_1 A_1$, C′1 esterase inhibitor, ceruloplasmin, transferrin, hemopexin, haptoglobin, fibrinogen, plasminogen, α_1-antitrypsin, orosomucoid, β-lipoprotein, α_2-macroglobulin, and prealbumin in the human conceptus, J. Clin. Invest. 48:1433, 1969.
59. Allansmith, M. R., McClellan, B. H., and Butterworth, M.: Individual patterns of immunoglobulin development in ten infants, J. Pediatr. 75:1231, 1969.
60. Smith, R. T., Eitzman, D. V., Catlin, M. F., Wirtz, E. O., and Miller, B. E.: The development of the immune response: Characterization of the response of the human infant and adult to immunization with Salmonella vaccines, Pediatrics 33:163, 1964.
61. Rosen, F. S.: Immunity in the Fetus and Newborn, in Gluck, L. (ed.), *Modern Perinatal Medicine* (Chicago: Year Book Medical Publishers, Inc., 1974), pp. 273–283.
62. Johnston, R. B., Jr., and Stroud, R. M.: Complement and host defense against infection, J. Pediatr. 90:169, 1977.
63. Fireman, P., Zuchowski, D. A., and Taylor, P. M.: Development of human complement system, J. Immunol. 103:25, 1969.
64. Sawyer, M. K., Forman, M. L., Kuplic, L. S., and Stiehm, E. R.: Developmental aspects of the human complement system, Biol. Neonate 19:148, 1971.
65. Feinstein, P. A., and Kaplan, S. R.: The alternative pathway of complement activation in the neonate, Pediatr. Res. 9:803, 1975.
66. Stossel, T. R., Alper, C. A., and Rosen, F. S.: Opsonic activity in the newborn: Role of properdin, Pediatrics 52:134, 1973.
67. McCracken, G. H., and Eichenwald, H. F.: Leukocyte function and the development of opsonic and complement activity in the neonate, Am. J. Dis. Child. 121:120, 1971.
68. Miller, M.: Chemotactic function in the human neonate: Humoral and cellular aspects, Pediatr. Res. 5:487, 1971.
69. Stossel, T., Alper, C. A., and Rosen, F. S.: Serum-dependent phagocytosis of paraffin oil emulsified with bacterial lipopolysaccharide, J. Exp. Med. 137:690, 1973.
70. Rosen, F. S.: Neonatal Immunity, in Smith, C. A., and Nelson, N. M. (eds.), *The Physiology of the Newborn Infant* (4th ed.; Springfield, Ill.: Charles C Thomas, Publisher, 1976), p. 744.
71. Wright, W. C., Jr., Ank, B. J., Herbert, J., and Stiehm, E. R.: Decreased bactericidal activity of leukocytes of stressed newborn infants, Pediatrics 56:579, 1975.
72. Forman, M. L., and Stiehm, E. R.: Impaired opsonic activity but normal phagocytosis in low-birth-weight infants, N. Engl. J. Med. 281:926, 1969.

73. Miller, M. E.: Phagocytosis in the newborn infant: Humoral and cellular factors, J. Pediatr. 74:255, 1969.

74. Coen, R., Grush, O., and Kauder, E.: Studies of bactericidal activity and metabolism of the leukocyte in full-term neonates, J. Pediatr. 75:400, 1969.

75. Copeland, E. M., MacFayden, B. V., Jr., and Dudrick, S. J.: Effect of intravenous hyperalimentation on established delayed hypersensitivity in the cancer patient, Ann. Surg. 183:60, 1976.

76. Sirisinha, S., Suskind, R., Edelman, R., *et al.:* Complement and C3 proactivator levels in children with protein calorie malnutrition, Lancet 1:1016, 1973.

77. Alexander, J. W., Hegg, M., and Altemeier, W. A.: Neutrophil function in selected surgical disorders, Ann. Surg. 168:447, 1968.

78. Chandra, R. K.: Reduced bactericidal capacity of polymorphs in iron deficiency, Arch. Dis. Child. 48:861, 1973.

79. Weinstein, R. J., and Young, L. S.: Neutrophil function in gram-negative rod bacteremia, J. Clin. Invest. 58:190, 1976.

80. Alexander, J. W., McClellan, M. A., Ogle, C. K., and Ogle, J. D.: Consumptive opsoninopathy: Possible pathogenesis in lethal and opportunistic infections, Ann. Surg. 184:672, 1976.

81. Alexander, J. W.: Emerging concepts in the control of surgical infection, Surgery 75:934, 1974.

82. Alexander, J. W., and Fisher, M. W.: Immunization against pseudomonas infection after thermal injury, J. Infect. Dis. 130(supp.): S152, 1974.

83. Quie, P. G.: Pathology of bactericidal power of neutrophils, Semin. Hematol. 12:143, 1975.

84. Chretien, J. H., and Garagusi, V. F.: Corticosteroids effect on phagocytosis and N.B.T. reduction by human polymorphonuclear neutrophils, J. Reticuloendothel. Soc. 11:358, 1972.

85. Mandell, G. L., Rubin, W., and Hook, E. W.: The effect of an NADH oxidase inhibitor (hydrocortisone) on polymorphonuclear leukocyte bacterial activity, J. Clin. Invest. 49:1381, 1970.

86. Olds, J. W., Reed, W. P., Eberle, B., *et al.:* Corticosteroids, serum, and phagocytosis. In vitro and in vivo studies, Infect. Immun. 9:524, 1974.

87. Fuenfer, B. A., Olson, G. E., and Polk, H. C.: Effects of various corticosteroids upon the phagocytic bactericidal activity of neutrophils, Surgery 78:27, 1975.

88. Levin, J., and Bang, F. B.: A description of cellular coagulation in the Limulus, Bull. Johns Hopkins Hosp. 115:337, 1964.

89. Levin, J., Poore, T. E., Zauber, N. P., and Oser, R. S.: Detection of endotoxin in the blood of patients with sepsis due to gram-negative bacteria, N. Engl. J. Med. 283:1313, 1970.

90. Rowe, M. I., Buckner, D. M., and Newmark, S.: The early diagnosis of gram-negative septicemia in the pediatric surgical patient, Ann. Surg. 182:280, 1975.

91. Feldman, S., and Pearson, T. A.: The Limulus test and gram-negative bacillary sepsis, Am. J. Dis. Child. 128:172, 1974.

92. Stumacher, R. J., Kovnat, M. J., and McCabe, W. R.: Limitations of the usefulness of the Limulus assay for endotoxin, N. Engl. J. Med. 228:1261, 1973.

93. Faden, H. S.: Early diagnosis of neonatal bacteremia by buffy-coat examination, J. Pediatr. 88:1032, 1976.

94. Akenzua, G. I., Hui, Y. T., Milner, R., and Zipursky, A.: Neutrophil and band counts in the diagnosis of neonatal infections, Pediatrics 54:38, 1974.

95. Cartwright, G. E., Athens, J. W., and Wintrobe, M. M.: The kinetics of granulopoiesis in normal man, Blood 24:780, 1964.

96. Zipursky, A., Palko, J., Milner, R., and Akenzua, G. I.: The hematology of bacterial infections in premature infants, Pediatrics 57:839, 1976.

97. Xanthou, M., Xypolyta, A., Anagnostakis, C., *et al.:* Exchange transfusion in severe neonatal infection with sclerema, Arch. Dis. Child. 50(pt. 2):901, 1975.

98. Bodey, G. P., Buckley, M., Sathe, Y. S., and Freineich, O. J.: Quantitative relationships between circulating leukocytes and infections in patients with acute leukemia, Ann. Intern. Med. 64:328, 1966.

99. Graw, R. G., Jr., Herzig, G., Perry, S., *et al.:* Normal granulocyte transfusion therapy: Treatment of septicemia due to gram-negative bacteria, N. Engl. J. Med. 287:367, 1972.

100. Athens, J. W.: Blood: Leukocytes, Annu. Rev. Physiol. 25:195, 1963.

101. Cartwright, G. E., Athens, J. W., and Wintrobe, M. M.: The kinetics of granulopoiesis in normal man, Blood 24:780, 1964.

102. Boggs, D. R.: The kinetics of neutrophilic leukocytes in health and in disease, Semin. Hematol. 4:359, 1967.

103. Boggs, D. R.: Transfusion of neutrophils as prevention or treatment of infection in patients with neutropenia, N. Engl. J. Med. 290:1055, 1975.

104. Pole, J. G., Davie, M. I., Barter, D. A. C., and Willoughby, M. L. N.: Granulocyte transfusion in treatment of infected neutropenic children, Arch. Dis. Child. 51:521, 1976.

105. Hinshaw, L. B., Greenfield, L. J., Owen, S. E., Black, M. R., and Guenter, C. A.: Precipitation of cardiac failure in endotoxin shock, Surg. Gynecol. Obstet. 135:39, 1972.

106. Hinshaw, L. B., Archer, L. T., Black, M. R., Elkins, R. C., Brown, P. P., and Greenfield, L. J.: Myocardial function in shock, Am. J. Physiol. 226:357, 1974.

107. Blaisdell, F. W., Linn, R. C., and Stallone, R. J.: The mechanism of pulmonary damage following traumatic shock, Surg. Gynecol. Obstet. 130:15, 1970.

108. Altar, S. M. A., Tingey, H. B., McLaughlin, J. S., and Cowley, R. A.: Bradykinin in human shock, Surg. Forum 18:46, 1967.

109. Colman, R. W., O'Donnell, T. F., Talamo, R. C., and Clowes, G. H. A., Jr.: Bradykinin formation in sepsis: Relation to hepatic dysfunction and hypotension, Clin. Res. 21:596, 1973.

110. Guenter, C. A., Ciorica, R., and Hinshaw, L.: Cardiorespiratory and metabolic responses to live *E. coli* and endotoxin in the monkey, J. Appl. Physiol. 26:780, 1969.

111. Lefer, A. M.: Blood-borne humoral factors in the pathophysiology of circulatory shock, Circ. Res. 32:129, 1973.

112. Davis, R. B., Meeker, W. R., and McQuarrie, D. G.: Immediate effects of intravenous endotoxin on serotonin concentrations and blood platelets, Circ. Res. 8:234, 1960.

113. Das, J., and Folkman, J.: The Limulus gelation test in the diagnosis of gram-negative sepsis (abst.), Proc. 3d Ann. Meeting, Am. Pediatr. Surg. Assoc., Hot Springs, Va., 1972, pp. 26–27.

114. Alho, A.: Lysosomal functions in circulatory shock, Ann. Chir. Gynaecol. Fenn. 60:159, 1971.

115. Moore, F. D., Olesen, K. H., McMurrey, J. D., Parker, H. V., Ball, M. R., and Boyden, C. M.: *The Body Cell Mass and Its Supporting Environment* (Philadelphia: W. B. Saunders Company, 1963).

116. Clowes, G. H. A., Jr., Farrington, G. H., Zuschneid, W., Cossetts, G. H., and Saravis, C. A.: Circulating factors in the etiology of pulmonary insufficiency and right heart failure accompanying severe sepsis (peritonitis), Ann. Surg. 171:663, 1970.

117. Clowes, G. H. A., Jr., Zuschneid, W., Turner, M., Blackburn, G. L., Rubin, J., Toala, P., and Green, G.: Observations of the pathogenesis of the pneumonitis associated with severe infection in other parts of the body, Ann. Surg. 167:630, 1968.

118. Lefer, A. M.: Role of a myocardial depressant factor in the pathogenesis of circulatory shock, Fed. Proc. 29(pt. 2):1836, 1970.

119. Clowes, G. H., Vucinic, M., and Weidner, M. G.: Circulatory and metabolic alteration associated with survival or death in peritonitis. Ann. Surg. 163:866, 1966.

120. MacLean, L. D., Mulligan, W. G., McLean, A. P., *et al.:* Patterns of septic shock in man—a detailed study of 56 patients, Ann. Surg. 166:543, 1967.

121. Siegel, J. M., Greenspan, M., DelGuercio, L. R. M.: Abnormal vascular tone, defective oxygen transport and myocardial failure in human septic shock, Ann. Surg. 165:504, 1967.

122. Wilson, R. F., Thal, A. P., Kindling, P. M., *et al.:* Hemodynamic measurements in septic shock, Arch. Surg. 91:121, 1965.

123. Clowes, G. H. A., O'Donnell, T. F., Ryan, N. T., and Blackburn, G. L.: Energy metabolism in sepsis: Treatment based on different patterns in shock and high output stage, Ann. Surg. 179:684, 1974.

124. Imamura, M., Clowes, G. H. A., Blackburn, G. L., O'Donnell, T. F., Trerice, M., Bhimjee, Y., and Ryan, N. T.: Liver metabolism and glucogenesis in trauma and sepsis, Surgery 77:868, 1975.

125. Weisul, J. P., O'Donnell, T. F., Jr., Stone, M. A., and Clowes, G. H. A.: Myocardial performance in clinical septic shock: Effects of isoproterenol and glucose potassium insulin, J. Surg. Res. 18:357, 1975.

126. Hinshaw, L. B., Archer, L. T., Benjamin, B., and Bridges, C.: Effects of glucose or insulin on myocardial performance in endotoxic shock, Proc. Soc. Exp. Biol. Med. 152:529, 1976.

127. Gump, F. E., Long, C., Killian, P., and Kinney, J. M.: Studies of glucose intolerance in septic injured patients, J. Trauma 14:378, 1974.

128. Rowe, M. I., and Arango, A.: The choice of intravenous fluid in shock resuscitation, Pediatr. Clin. North Am. 22:269, 1975.

129. Rowe, M. I., and Arango, A.: Colloid versus crystalloid resuscitation in experimental bowel obstruction, J. Pediatr. Surg. 11:635, 1976.

130. Sambhi, M. P., Weil, M. H., and Udhoji, V. M.: Pressor response to norepinephrine in humans before and after corticosteroids, Am. J. Physiol. 203:961, 1962.
131. Sambhi, M. P., Weil, M. H., and Udhoji, V. M.: Acute pharmacodynamic effects of glucocorticoids, cardiac output and related hemodynamic changes in normal subjects and patients in shock, Circulation 31:523, 1965.
132. Lillehei, R. C., Longerbeam, J. K., Bloch, J. H., and Manax, W.: The nature of irreversible shock: Experimental and clinical observations, Ann. Surg. 160:682, 1964.
133. Levitan, H., Kendrick, A., and Kass, E. H.: Effect of route of administration on protective action of corticosterone and cortisol against endotoxin, Proc. Soc. Exp. Biol. Med. 93:306, 1956.
134. Lillehei, R. C., and MacLean, L. C.: Physiological approach to successful treatment of endotoxic shock in experimental animals, Arch. Surg. 78:464, 1959.
135. Spink, W. W., and Vick, J.: Evaluation of plasma, metaraminol, and hydrocortisone in experimental endotoxic shock, Circ. Res. 9:184, 1961.
136. Thomas, C. S., and Brockman, S. K.: The role of adrenal corticosteroid therapy in *Escherichia coli* endotoxin shock, Surg. Gynecol. Obstet. 126:61, 1968.
137. Connolly, J. E.: The use of adrenal cortical compounds in hemorrhagic shock, Lancet 79:460, 1959.
138. Hakstian, R. W., Hampson, L. G., and Gurd, F. N.: Pharmacological agents in experimental hemorrhagic shock, Arch. Surg. 83:335, 1961.
139. Halpern, B. N., Benacerrof, B., and Briot, M.: The roles of cortisone, desoxycorticosterone, and adrenaline in protecting adrenalectomized animals against hemorrhagic, traumatic and histamine shock, Br. J. Pharmacol. 7:287, 1952.
140. Vander Nennett, K., and Schneewind, J. H.: The effect of steroids on mortality in experimental traumatic shock, Proc. Soc. Exp. Biol. Med. 109:674, 1962.
141. Fukunda, T., Ohuma, H., and Hata, N.: Epinephrine shock, its relation to plasma epinephrine level and the mechanism of its protection by glucocorticoid, Jpn. J. Physiol. 17:746, 1967.
142. Somani, P., and Arora, R. B.: Effect of hydrocortisone on capillary permeability changes induced by *Echis carinatus* (saw-scaled viper) venom in the rat, J. Pharm. Pharmacol. 14:535, 1962.
143. Sayers, G., and Solomon, N.: Work performance of a rat heart-lung preparation: Standardization and influence of corticosteroids, Endocrinology 66:719, 1960.
144. Gunnar, R. M.: Clinical Experience with Corticoids in Shock. Internal Medicine, in Schumer, W., and Nyhus, L. M. (eds.), *Corticosteroids in the Treatment of Shock* (Urbana: University of Illinois Press, 1970).
145. Replogle, R. L., Kundler, H., Schottenfeld, M., and Spear, S.: Hemodynamic effects of dexamethasone in experimental shock—negative results, Ann. Surg. 174:126, 1971.
146. Schumer, W., Moss, G. S., and Nyhus, L. M.: Metabolism of lactic acid in the macacus rhesus monkey in profound shock. Am. J. Surg. 118:200, 1969.
147. Pierce, C. H., Briggs, B. T., and Gutelius, J. R.: Methylprednisolone and Phenoxybenzamine in Experimental Cardiovascular Dynamics and Platelet Function, in Forscher, B. K., Lillehei, R. C., and Stubbs, S. S. (eds.), *Shock in Low Flow States* (Amsterdam: Excerpta Medica, 1972).
148. Motsay, G. J., Alho, A. V., Schultz, L. S., Dietzman, R. H., and Lillehei, R. C.: Pulmonary capillary permeability in the post-traumatic pulmonary insufficiency syndrome: Comparison of isogravimetric capillary pressures, Ann. Surg. 173:244, 1973.
149. Lefer, A. M., and Martin, J.: Mechanism of the protective effect of corticosteroids in hemorrhagic shock, Am. J. Physiol. 216:314, 1969.
150. Holden, W. D., DePalma, R. G., Drucker, W. R., and McKalen, A.: Ultrastructural changes in hemorrhagic shock: Electron microscopic study of liver, kidney and striated muscle cells in rats, Ann. Surg. 162:517, 1965.
151. Martin, A. M., and Hackel, D. B.: An electron microscopic study of the progression of myocardial lesions in the dog after hemorrhagic shock, Lab. Invest. 15:243, 1966.
152. Janoff, A., Weissmann, G., Zweifach, B. W., and Thomas, L.: Pathogenesis of experimental shock. IV. Studies on lysosomes in normal and tolerant animals subjected to lethal trauma and endotoxemia. J. Exp. Med. 116:451, 1962.
153. Jefferson, T., Glenn, T. M., and Lefer, A. M.: Cardiovascular and lysosomal actions of corticosteroid in the intact dog, Proc. Soc. Exp. Biol. Med. 136:276, 1971.
154. Schumer, W., Erve, P. R., and Obernolte, R. P.: Mechanism of steroid protection in septic shock, Surgery 72:119, 1972.
155. Schumer, W.: Steroids in the treatment of clinical septic shock, Ann. Surg. 184:333, 1976.
156. Reid, P. R., and Thompson, W. L.: The clinical use of dopamine in the treatment of shock, Bull. Johns Hopkins Hosp. 137:276, 1975.
157. Schwartz, R. H., and Aviado, D. M.: Drug action, reaction, and interaction: Dopamine for endotoxic shock, J. Clin. Pharmacol. 16:88, 1976.
158. Wilson, R. F., Sibbald, W. J., and Jaanimagi, J. L.: Hemodynamic effects of dopamine in critically ill septic patients, J. Surg. Res. 20:163, 1976.

4

Arnold G. Coran / Robert M. Filler

Total Parenteral Nutrition

HISTORICAL BACKGROUND.—The history of parenteral nutrition begins in 1658 with Sir Christopher Wren, who predicted that it should be possible to inject any liquid into the bloodstream. His friend, Dr. Robert Boyle, proved the possibility in 1659, when he injected opium into the veins of a dog. In 1664, Casper Scotus gave wine intravenously and, 1 year later, Sir Christopher Wren administered alcohol intravenously. The earliest intravenous injection of oil was given by Corten in 1679. The first parenteral administration of fat was in 1869 by Menzel and Perco, who carried out extensive animal experiments with injections of fat. Following the early unsuccessful attempts to give intravenous fat, the first systematic investigations on the role of intravenous fat emulsions were carried out in Japan during the 1920s and 1930s. However, the use of intravenous fat emulsions did not gain significant popularity because of the serious toxic reactions that occurred. One of the major breakthroughs in the use of fat emulsions intravenously came in the 1950s, when Lipomul was thoroughly investigated by the American Army Medical Services. Not long after its initial clinical use, significant toxic reactions were noted with this emulsion and it was removed from the market. The major breakthrough in the clinical use of intravenous fat emulsions came in 1962, when Wretlind introduced the soybean oil emulsion, Intralipid.[19]

The background of amino acid therapy dates back 75 years, when hydrolysis of protein, either chemically or enzymatically, was first utilized. In 1904, Abderhalden and Ronner administered an enzymatically digested protein intravenously and in 1913 Henriques and Anderson succeeded in maintaining normal weight in a goat by the infusion of a protein dialysate. Over the past 50 years, a wide variety of hydrolysates have been investigated, including those prepared from lactalbumin, bovine serum protein, human serum albumin and horse fibrin. Today, the most frequently used protein hydrolysates are prepared from casein and fibrin. More recently, the introduction of crystalline amino acid solutions, which are reasonably priced, has increased the use of such solutions over protein hydrolysates.[18]

The first documented report of successful total parenteral nutrition in an infant was published in 1944 by Helfrick and Abelson.[16] They administered a mixture of 50% glucose, 10% casein hydrolysate and homogenized olive oil-lecithin emulsions into a 5-month-old infant with success. During the next 20 years, total parenteral nutrition in infants and children was without success because the solutions could not be infused into peripheral veins and insufficient calories were provided to allow the administered amino acids to be anabolized. In 1968, Dudrick and his co-workers provided the major breakthrough that made total parenteral nutrition a practical reality.[9, 10] Dudrick devised a method by which a catheter could be implanted and maintained in the superior vena cava for prolonged periods. Using this delivery system, Dudrick showed that adequate growth and development could be achieved in beagle puppies and subsequently in an infant. This demonstration provided the stimulus for the current widespread use of total parenteral nutrition in pediatric and adult patients.

Insufficient caloric intake for a prolonged period contributes appreciably to the mortality of infants and children with lesions of the gastrointestinal tract. Not uncommonly, patients with persistent intestinal obstruction, bowel fistulas or short-bowel syndrome die of inanition and its complications before curative treatment or appropriate surgical procedures can be carried out. Experience from our institutions and others indicates the lifesaving potential of total parenteral nutrition (TPN) in infants and children with inadequate gastrointestinal tract function.

Success of this mode of treatment was brought about by the development of special techniques for the intravenous administration of adequate quantities of calories and nitrogen. Use of this life-sustaining system requires the careful selection of patients for therapy, constant surveillance for complications and attention to the minute details of procedures that minimize these dangers.

In recent years, an alternative approach to hyperalimentation in infants and children has been adopted in the United States and abroad. This technique involves the infusion of fat solutions, along with glucose and amino acids, into peripheral veins.[2-5] This program obviates the need for a central venous catheter, thereby eliminating certain complications. Because of the limited supply of intravenous fat solutions in the United States, peripheral hyperalimentation without lipid emulsions has been utilized more recently in a number of institutions.[13] In many clinical situations, the choice of a given technique involves individual patient consideration.

Indications

Central hyperalimentation has been used extensively at the Children's Hospital Medical Center of Boston since 1968. To date, more than 350 infants and children have been treated. During the 2½-year period from January, 1972 to June, 1974, 80 infants and children at the Los Angeles County-USC Medical Center and Los Angeles Childrens Hospital received intravenous feeding through peripheral veins using the fat emulsion Intralipid.° An additional 22 infants and children at the Mott Children's Hospital in Ann Arbor, Michigan have been so treated. In addition, from July, 1974 to the present, more than 60 infants and children at the Mott Children's Hospital, The University of Michigan Medical Center, have been treated with peripheral hyperalimentation composed of fat-free solutions.

TPN is reserved for those infants and children whose lives are threatened because feeding by means of the gastrointestinal tract is impossible, inadequate or hazardous. The goal

of treatment depends on the patient's underlying condition. In some instances, such as those infants with chronic nonspecific diarrhea, placing the gastrointestinal tract at rest for a prolonged period is curative. In others, the restoration and maintenance of adequate nutrition will permit a corrective operation.

The common conditions for which this treatment has been used include chronic intestinal obstruction due to adhesions or peritoneal sepsis, bowel fistulas, inadequate intestinal length, chronic severe diarrhea, extensive body burns and abdominal tumors treated by operation, irradiation and chemotherapy. Although TPN is used to replete the malnourished child, it may be started prophylactically in clinical situations where prolonged starvation is expected.

As confidence and experience with the method have grown, additional indications for its use have developed. For example, with certain modifications, we have utilized TPN in very small premature infants (less than 1 kg) who, despite an apparently normal gastrointestinal tract, constantly regurgitate feedings placed in the stomach by gavage or by gastrostomy. Dudrick *et al.*[8] have successfully treated uremia and hyperkalemia of acute renal failure with intravenous infusions of purified amino acids and glucose, thus reducing the need for dialysis.

The decision to begin a program of total intravenous alimentation requires mature clinical judgment. Such a decision can be made readily for an infant with complicated omphalocele or for one in whom a large portion of the midgut has been resected because of volvulus. In others, the decision may be more difficult. For example, in a child with chronic diarrhea and malnutrition, one must be certain that customary therapy has failed before beginning total intravenous therapy. Although anorexia, vomiting and diarrhea commonly accompany irradiation and chemotherapy, only the occasional patient becomes so debilitated that treatment is required.

One must weigh the need for improved nutrition to save life and reduce morbidity against the possibility of serious complications of TPN, especially sepsis. TPN should not be used in those children in whom nutrients can be safely delivered and absorbed from the gastrointestinal tract by oral feedings, gavage or gastrostomy. On the other hand, our experience indicates that when the technique is applied with the proper care, the threat of serious morbidity is sufficiently low to justify its use in an ever-increasing number of patients.

Composition of Solutions

Central Feeding

The composition of the basic solutions for TPN used at Children's Hospital Medical Center of Boston is noted in Table 4–1. Solution I contains 20% glucose, a solution designed for infusion through a central venous catheter. Solutions I and II are similar except for the lower vitamin, calcium and trace metal content of II. The infusion of 135 ml/kg/day of solution I into a central venous catheter provides an appropriate mixture of glucose, amino acids and other nutrients to meet the normal infant's need for tissue repair and growth. Even in the older child whose basic caloric requirements are less, 135 ml/kg/day may be administered safely. However, to avoid vitamin, calcium and trace metal excesses in these older patients, solution II should be given for nutritional needs in excess of 1000 ml/day. More dilute glucose solutions (basic formula diluted in half with 5% dextrose in water) are used during the first day or two of

---

°Manufactured by Vitrum Company, Stockholm, Sweden and kindly supplied by Cutter Laboratories, Berkeley, California.

TABLE 4–1.–SOLUTIONS FOR CENTRAL IV ALIMENTATION

SOLUTION I		
Each 1000 ml contains:		
Protein hydrolysate	(108 cal)	30.0 gm
Dextrose (hydrous)	(668 cal)	196.6 gm
Potassium		12.0 mEq
Sodium		15.0 mEq
Calcium	540 mg	(27.0 mEq)
Phosphorus (P)		155.0 mg
Magnesium	92 mg	(7.6 mEq)
Chloride		10.8 mEq
Folic acid		0.5 mg
Multivitamins (MVI)		5.0 ml
Vitamin K_1		0.2 mg
Vitamin B_{12}		6.6 μg
Trace element (Zn, Cu, I, F, Mn) sol		2.0 ml

Each 1000 ml contains approximately
4.1 gm nitrogen and 800 calories

SOLUTION II		
Each 1000 ml contains:		
Protein hydrolysate	(108 cal)	30.0 gm
Dextrose (hydrous)	(668 cal)	196.6 gm
Potassium		12.0 mEq
Sodium		15.0 mEq
Calcium	60 mg	(3.0 mEq)
Phosphorus (P)		155.0 mg
Magnesium	92 mg	(7.6 mEq)
Chloride		10.8 mEq
Folic acid		0.5 mg
Vitamin K_1		0.2 mg
Vitamin B_{12}		6.6 μg

Each 1000 ml contains approximately
4.1 gm nitrogen and 800 calories

MVI°	
Each 10 ml contains:	
Ascorbic acid (C)	500 mg
Vitamin A	10,000 IU
Vitamin D	1000 IU
Thiamine	50 mg
Riboflavin	10 mg
Pyridoxine	15 mg
Niacinamide	100 mg
Dexpanthenol	25 mg
Vitamin E	5 IU

°USV Pharmaceutical Corp.

TRACE ELEMENT SOLUTION
Each 1000 ml contains:
Zinc sulfate 800 μg
Copper sulfate 400 μg
Sodium fluoride 20 μg
Sodium iodide 118 μg
Manganese sulfate 400 μg

therapy. During this period, the child is adapting to the glucose load, and the high concentration of glucose may produce an osmotic diuresis, which will lead to hypertonic dehydration. As the patient's tolerance develops, judged by diminishing glycosuria, solution I or II may be used. The administration of insulin is not necessary in nondiabetic children.

In most patients, additional potassium and sodium chloride are necessary. Usually, the addition of 30 mEq of NaCl and 20 mEq KCl to a liter of the standard infusate will suffice and will not overburden the normal infant kidney or cardiovascular system. The electrolyte contents of different amino acid sources vary, a factor that must be considered if an amino acid preparation other than that listed in Table 4–1 is used. Children with normal renal function rarely have serum electrolyte abnormalities with this program. However, more caution is necessary for those with reduced renal function and other metabolic defects. Iron requirements are met either by weekly intramuscular injections of iron dextran or by blood transfusion. Trace elements are added to the basic mixture routinely (Table 4–1). Essential fatty acids can be supplied by the daily application of sunflower seed oil to the child's chest.[22]

Peripheral Feeding

The nonfat solution containing protein, glucose, electrolytes and vitamins is the same whether or not Intralipid is used. A stock solution of 10% protein hydrolysate is used to make up the infusate. The mixing is carried out in the hospital pharmacy under a laminar flow hood. The amino acid solution is diluted with glucose to make up a 2% protein hydrolysate in a 12% glucose solution. The final solution contains 0.56 cal per ml. Electrolytes are added to the

infusate to provide the recommended daily requirements plus additional needs based on the patient's clinical condition (Table 4–2). The electrolyte and vitamin concentrations are essentially the same as those recommended for central feeding. Heparin at 0.5 units/ml is added to the solution to minimize the likelihood of phlebitis. For infants, 200–250 ml/kg/24 hours is administered, providing 112–140 calories per day. In older children, the volume is reduced according to the caloric needs.

When Intralipid is used, 4 gm (40 ml) of fat/kg body weight/24 hours is administered to infants and the nonlipid solution is reduced to 120–160 ml/kg/24 hours (Table 4–3). This provides 111–134 calories/kg, which is more than adequate for infant weight gain and growth. In older children, the Intralipid is reduced to 2 gm/kg/24 hours and the nonlipid solution is further decreased according to the specific ca-

TABLE 4–2.–PERIPHERAL HYPERALIMENTATION WITHOUT FAT IN INFANTS

CONSTITUENT	AMOUNT PER KG PER 24 HR
Water	200–250 ml
Protein	4–5 gm
Glucose	24–30 gm
Calories	112–140
Heparin	100 IU°
Sodium	2–4 mEq
Potassium	2–3 mEq
Chloride	2–4 mEq
Magnesium	0.6 mEq
Calcium	1.0 mEq
Phosphate	3.5 mm

°International Units.

TABLE 4–3.—PERIPHERAL HYPERALIMENTATION
WITH FAT IN INFANTS

CONSTITUENT	AMOUNT PER KG PER 24 HR
Volume	160–200 ml
Intralipid	40 ml
Water	120–160 ml
Protein	2.4–3.2 gm
Glucose	14–19 gm
Fat	4 gm
Calories	111–134
Heparin	100 IU*
Sodium	2–4 mEq
Potassium	2–3 mEq
Chloride	2–4 mEq
Magnesium	0.6 mEq
Calcium	1.0 mEq
Phosphate	3.5 mm

*International Units.

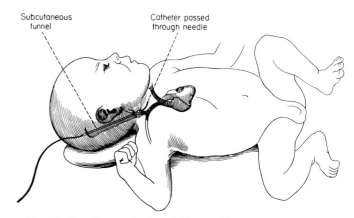

Fig. 4-1.—Insertion and fixation of silicone rubber central venous catheter in an infant. The catheter is passed through a hollow needle, which has created a subcutaneous tunnel from the venous cutdown site in the neck to the appropriate skin exit site behind the ear.

loric needs. Intralipid meets all the essential fatty acid requirements. For both peripheral venous methods of feeding, the administration of vitamins and iron is as described in the central feeding program. Trace metals are given as necessary.

Methods

Central Feeding

Hypertonic infusates must be delivered through a central venous catheter to avoid peripheral venous inflammation and thrombosis. For this purpose, a silicone rubber catheter is passed through the internal or external jugular vein to the superior vena cava. This procedure is best carried out in an operating room or cardiac catheterization laboratory where adequate exposure, proper instruments and strict aseptic conditions are available. To minimize bloodstream contamination, the venous catheter is tunneled from the vein entry point to a skin exit site, which is placed 2–4 inches away. In the infant, it is brought out on the scalp whereas in the older child the exit site may be the neck or upper extremity. Central venous intubation by percutaneous subclavian vein puncture can also be used. The silicone rubber venous line is left in place until the completion of therapy unless it becomes accidentally dislodged or septic complications develop. We have had a single catheter in place for as long as 120 days.

The central venous catheter can be inserted under local or general anesthesia. The head is turned to the side and the scalp shaved. A transverse incision, 1–2 cm long, is made over the sternocleidomastoid muscle at the junction of the middle and lower thirds of the neck. Ordinarily, the external jugular vein is preferred and usually can be cannulated successfully even in the premature infant. However, if either external jugular vein is unavailable because of previous use or small caliber, or if entrance of the catheter from the external jugular vein into the vena cava is not possible, the internal jugular vein can be used for cannulation. A long hollow needle with an obturator in place is passed beneath the skin of the neck from the incision to the scalp (Fig. 4–1). If the internal jugular vein is being used, the needle also pierces the belly of the sternocleidomastoid muscle. After the obturator is removed, the silicone rubber catheter (for an infant, the internal diameter is 0.025 in. and the outside diameter is 0.047 in.) is passed through the needle. When the needle is withdrawn, the catheter resides in its subcutaneous tract. Prior to cannulation, the vein is ligated distally and an incision is made between this point and a proximal controlling ligature. If the internal jugular vein has been selected, ligature of the vein sometimes can be avoided by passing the cannula into the vein through an incision made in the center of a pursestring suture. The jugular vein then is cannulated and the tubing advanced to the region of the right atrium (approximately 5 cm in an infant) (Fig. 4–2). Occasionally, some manipulation is necessary to obtain entry into the superior vena cava from the external jugular vein. The exact location of the catheter is confirmed radiographically by taking a single x-ray with the catheter filled with radiopaque contrast material.

The silicone rubber catheter slides easily and is soft and compressible. The ligature that holds it in the vein must be tied so that it neither occludes the lumen of the tube nor allows the catheter to slip out of the vessel. To fix the tube properly, we use a circular sleeve of silicone rubber to which Dacron wings have been bonded (manufactured by Medical Devices, Inc.). After venous cannulation, the sleeve of silicone rubber is opened and, at its entrance into the jugular vein, the venous catheter is placed within the lumen of the sleeve. The venous catheter is glued to the sleeve with silicone cement. The Dacron wings are sutured with nonabsorbable sutures to the surrounding tissues. To remove the central venous line, the sleeve and its Dacron attachments must be cut free by opening the neck wound under local anesthesia.

Antibiotics are administered only when indicated by the child's primary illness, but not specifically to prevent sepsis, which might occur from the presence of a central venous line.

An antibacterial ointment and sterile dressing are applied to the skin exit site, and, to avoid accidental displacement, a coil of catheter is included in the dressing. Every 2 days, the dressing is removed aseptically, the skin cleansed with an antiseptic and a sterile dressing and antibacterial ointment reapplied. Povidone-iodine (Betadine) ointment now is used routinely because of its effectiveness against both bacteria and fungi. Before the infusion is started, a Millipore filter (0.22 μ) is placed in line to remove particulate matter and/or microorganisms that may have contaminated the solution. A calibrated buret is placed in the circuit to monitor accurately the volume delivered. Injection tubing (T-connector, manu-

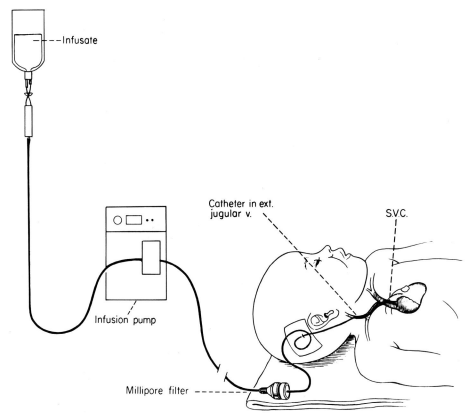

Fig. 4-2.—System for long-term central total parenteral nutrition. Amino acid-dextrose infusate flows through a calibrated buret. Infusion pump ensures uniform hourly flow rate. The Millipore filter in the circuit will remove any microorganisms that may have contaminated the system. The venous catheter enters the scalp behind the ear. The appropriate position of the catheter in the superior vena cava is confirmed radiographically.

factured by Abbott Laboratories) may also be added to the circuit so that intravenous drugs can be given aseptically above the filter. All intravenous tubings and the bottle of infusate are changed daily. Since the high sugar content of these infusates supports the growth of yeast, the external surfaces of all intravenous tubings should be washed with Betadine solution twice a day to remove traces of nutrient solution that may have inadvertently dripped from the bottle onto the tubing. Betadine ointment should also be applied to all joints in the circuit to prevent entry of microorganisms at these points.

The infusate must be delivered at a slow, uniform rate to ensure proper utilization of the glucose and amino acids. In a small infant, this is most readily accomplished by the use of a constant-infusion pump (see Fig. 4–2). In some centers, gravity drip is used for older patients.

In many institutions, patients on TPN are treated in one intensive care area. Because of our geographic and departmental structure and the diversity of disease states, we have found it more efficient to treat these children on the medical or surgical divisions where they would be ordinarily. To provide standardized optimal care, we utilize a nurse who oversees the care of every patient on TPN. This nurse makes rounds twice a day to check the intravenous tubings, pumps and infusates. She advises and instructs the floor nurse and house staff on proper techniques and management and is on call for any unforeseen mechanical problems that may develop. On alternate days, she changes the dressings over the central venous catheter and often is the only person who is permitted to draw blood from the central venous line to ob-

tain samples for routine weekly analysis or for additional studies that may be required by special protocol.

Peripheral Feeding with Fat

The technique of infusion is depicted in Figure 4–3. In infants, a 21–23-gauge scalp vein needle (sometimes even a 25-gauge needle) is inserted into a peripheral vein, usually in the scalp, and the intravenous tubing from the bottle containing the amino acids is connected to this needle. The tubing from the Intralipid bottle then is inserted into the rubber nipple at the end of the tubing from the first bottle ("piggy-backed") and secured to this tubing with tape. A calibrated buret is placed in each intravenous line and both bottles are infused over a 24-hour period using two separate constant-infusion pumps. The 24-hour infusion with two separate pumps is used to ensure proper utilization of the administered fat, glucose and amino acids. No filters are used, since these would block the infusion of the fat. The needle usually requires changing every 3–4 days because of infiltration. In children, the same technique is used except that the dorsum of the hand rather than the scalp is used.

Peripheral Feeding without Fat

The techniques involved here are no different from those used for routine intravenous infusions. The entire solution is contained in one bottle and is infused into a small needle placed into a peripheral vein in the scalp or extremity. A Millipore filter (0.22 μ) is placed in line and the infusion is run over 24 hours for the various reasons already discussed.

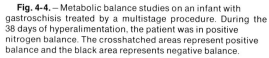

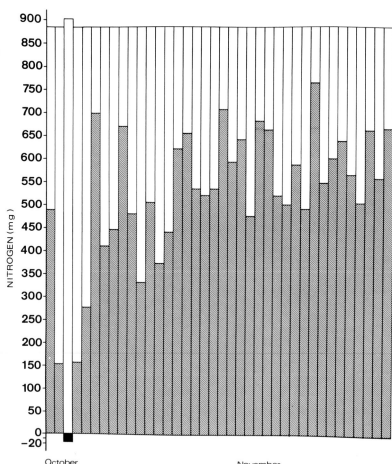

Fig. 4-3.—Technique of intravenous feeding with Intralipid. In infants, a needle is inserted into the scalp; in older children, the veins on the dorsum of the hand generally are used. See text for details.

Fig. 4-4.—Metabolic balance studies on an infant with gastroschisis treated by a multistage procedure. During the 38 days of hyperalimentation, the patient was in positive nitrogen balance. The crosshatched areas represent positive balance and the black area represents negative balance.

In infants, an infusion pump is used; in older children a pump is unnecessary. The intravenous sites last 24–48 hours and are changed promptly when signs of infiltration or phlebitis are noted. Warm soaks placed over the infiltrated skin reduce the swelling rather quickly. Rarely, a small skin slough results, which heals fairly rapidly with local care.

Metabolic Observations

Clinical measurements that are essential include daily body weight, accurate volume of urine and other body fluid losses. The urine sugar content is monitored at each voiding. The important blood tests and the frequency of study in the usual patient are given in Table 4–4. More frequent monitoring of some variables may be necessary in patients with specific metabolic abnormalities, such as those with renal or hepatic disease.

Weight changes during the period of intravenous feeding will vary with the patient's over-all clinical status. Weight gains comparable to those of normal infants may be expected in those children who are not malnourished at the time intravenous feedings are instituted or in whom sepsis is not a part of the clinical picture. In the patient with infection or another clinical problem that increases metabolic requirements, a flatter growth curve may be observed. A significant weight gain in the first 2 weeks of therapy is not usually seen in those infants and children who are severely depleted at the start of treatment. The weight gains observed with the three different techniques are comparable, averaging 20–30 gm per day in the neonate.

TABLE 4–4.—BLOOD VALUES MONITORED ROUTINELY DURING TOTAL PARENTERAL NUTRITION

FREQUENCY OF MONITORING		
At Start of Therapy and Weekly	At Start of Therapy and Every 2 Weeks	As Indicated
Na, K, Cl	SGOT, LDH, alkaline phosphatase	Copper
Urea	Bilirubin	Zinc
Glucose	Creatinine	Iron
Magnesium		Ammonia
Calcium, phosphorus		Osmolarity
Total protein		pH
Hgb, Hct, WbC		
Blood culture		
Candida precipitins		

Despite the variations in weight curves, positive nitrogen balance has been noted in all patients studied in detail (Figs. 4–4 and 4–5). Fecal loss of nitrogen usually is negligible, since stools are infrequent and scanty during periods of exclusively intravenous feeding. Urinary amino acid losses have been found to be negligible and not sufficient to produce osmotic diuresis except in infants weighing under 1 kg and in those children with severe renal disease.

In most patients, the large quantity of intravenous glucose is well tolerated without the addition of exogenous insulin. Blood sugar levels remain in the normal range, but urinary

CUMULATIVE NITROGEN BALANCE

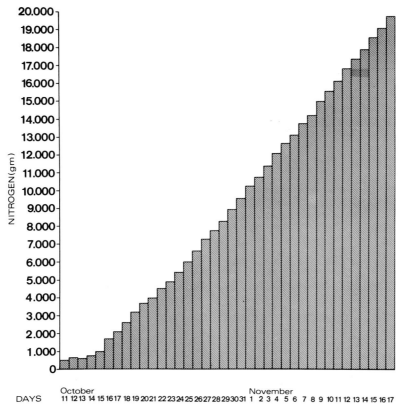

Fig. 4-5.—Cumulative nitrogen balance in the patient described in Figure 4-4.

sugar content usually varies between 0 and 3+ by the Clini-test method. Urinary sugar levels generally are highest during the first day or two of treatment. Qualitative urine sugars consistently above 3+ may cause an osmotic diuresis and often signal the likelihood of bloodstream infection, especially in the patient who has been treated for many days without glycosuria. A temporary decrease in hourly infusion rate or use of a more dilute solution usually corrects the problem if it is not due to sepsis.

Water balance is maintained even in infants weighing under 2.5 kg and in those following operation despite the infusion of this hypertonic solution. Urinary solute excretion of this intravenous diet usually is greater than that observed during oral feeding, but this increased load does not exceed the concentrating capability of the normal infant kidney.

Complications

Metabolic Complications

The metabolic complications that have occurred during TPN in infants and children are listed in Table 4–5. The potential complications are many, but most patients tolerate these intravenous mixtures quite well. Although some of the complications are unavoidable, most can be prevented by appropriate adjustments of the infusate based on careful clinical monitoring.

Glucose intolerance and hyperglycemia have been observed (in the absence of sepsis) only in low birth weight premature infants and others with severe renal and central nervous system abnormalities. In some of these cases, widely fluctuating blood sugar levels even with the use of insulin have forced us to abandon the intravenous feeding program.

Although hypoglycemia has been reported when TPN is stopped abruptly, we have not observed this complication despite the many accidental interruptions of the infusion. Nevertheless, when TPN no longer is needed and oral intake starts, we recommend a gradual weaning from the intravenous diet to avoid this potential complication.

Metabolic acidosis has occurred as a complication of TPN. Although the amino acids in all presently available TPN solutions challenge the patient with a large acid load, on our current formulas most patients do not become acidotic. The acidity and free water content of our mixtures is such that the acid-base regulatory mechanisms of the average infant and child are adequate to compensate for the acid load. When a more concentrated preparation (5.25% FreAmine and 25% glucose) was used in the past, smaller infants developed acidosis with serum pH as low as 7.0. In susceptible individuals, such as the low birth weight premature infant and those with renal or hepatic disease, frequent monitoring

TABLE 4–5.—METABOLIC COMPLICATIONS

Persistent hyperglycemia and glycosuria
Osmotic diuresis
Postinfusion hypoglycemia
Acidosis
Hyperammonemia
Amino acid toxicity
Hypomagnesemia
Hypocupremia
Essential fatty acid deficiency
Hypocalcemia, hypercalcemia, hypophosphatemia
Hepatic impairment (toxic)
Hypercholesterolemia
Hypertriglyceridemia

of blood pH is necessary to avoid acidosis even when using our present mixtures.

Hyperammonemia has been reported in infants, generally those less than 6 months of age.[14, 17] It has been postulated that it is due to one or a combination of the following factors: (a) infusion of large quantities of ammonia, present in protein hydrolysate solutions; (b) the administration of a diet that contains inappropriate proportions of amino acids; (c) subclinical liver disease or hepatic immaturity; and (d) arginine deficiency. We have measured blood ammonia at varying intervals after the institution of TPN in 23 infants. In 12 infants with elevated SGOT, LDH and bilirubin, blood ammonia levels were normal. In 11 others with normal liver function tests, blood ammonia was elevated (75 mg/100 ml) in 2 but normal in the others. Clinical signs of ammonia intoxication were never evident in any of these 23 patients or in any other patient whom we treated.

Plasma and urine amino acids were measured in a small group of children; in some, abnormal serum values were detected. Histologic examination of the central nervous system in children who died while on TPN did not reveal the hypothalamic lesions produced in mice by the administration of protein hydrolysate or acidic amino acids.[20]

Hypomagnesemia causing seizures was seen in several patients early in our experience. In each case, the patient had prolonged diarrhea prior to the institution of TPN. Typically, seizures occurred within the first week of TPN therapy. Seizures due to hypomagnesemia have been largely eliminated since the magnesium content of the standard infusate has been increased and additional magnesium has been administered at the start of therapy to patients with hypomagnesemia from chronic diarrhea.

Copper deficiency has been observed recently as a result of chronic diarrhea and diets with insufficient copper, such as TPN programs.[1, 18] Copper now is given routinely to all patients. The features that have been ascribed to lack of copper include anemia, neutropenia, hypoproteinemia, osteoporosis, deep pigmentation of skin and hair, hypotonia and psychomotor retardation. In the malnourished patient with depleted copper stores, overt signs of copper deficiency are most likely to develop when weight gain and growth occur on a high-caloric, high-protein diet low in copper. In the past 3 years, serum copper was measured in 76 infants and children on TPN. In 23 cases, serum copper was low and ranged from 20 to 75 μg/100 ml (normal 87–150 μg/100 ml). Nineteen of these 23 patients were on TPN because of chronic diarrhea and had a low serum copper at the onset of therapy. The other 4 were not depleted at the start but developed low serum copper before copper was added to the intravenous mixture routinely from 1 to 5 months after the start of therapy. Anemia, which was noted in 15 of these copper-deficient patients, was due at least in part to copper deficiency. Clinical evaluation for bone abnormalities was not performed. Increase in the serum copper was noted in depleted patients who were treated with small quantities of copper sulfate by mouth and in the others when oral feedings resumed.

Serum zinc was measured in conjunction with serum copper in these 76 patients. Low serum zinc was never observed (even after 6 months of TPN), even when the only source of zinc available was from transfusion. Nevertheless, zinc now is given to all patients in the trace metal solution.

Clinical signs of essential fatty acid deficiency were apparent in only 2 children on the central feeding program, although in our series and others,[21] serious abnormalities in serum lipids have been noted after prolonged fat-free therapy. Each of the 2 patients had been on TPN longer than 3 months when a severe generalized skin rash typical of essential fatty acid deficiency developed. Fortunately, at this stage of therapy, each infant was able to tolerate a small quantity of fat by mouth and the skin lesions soon disappeared. Essential fatty acid deficiency did not develop in any of the patients on Intralipid nor was this syndrome seen in the infants receiving sunflower seed oil cutaneously. Most of the patients on Intralipid had normal triglyceride and cholesterol levels in their serum; however, a few, who were on hyperalimentation for longer than 1 month, ran serum triglycerides in the range of 300–350 mg/100 ml (normal 150–250 mg/100 ml) and serum cholesterols of 150–250 mg/100 ml (normal 100–150 mg/100 ml). These mild elevations returned to normal once the Intralipid was stopped.[6]

Hypocalcemia, hypercalcemia, hypophosphatemia and hyperphosphatemia have all occurred in patients being fed solely by vein.[23, 24] Quantities of calcium and phosphorus in our present intravenous mixture appear sufficient to avoid these problems in the vast majority of patients treated. Weekly monitoring of serum calcium and phosphorus suffices to detect an abnormality that might require modification in the quantities of calcium and phosphorus infused.

Signs of abnormal liver function often have been observed during TPN. Transient hepatic enlargement, with or without abnormal liver function tests, was noted during the first week of therapy in most small infants. Variable and intermittent elevations of SGOT, LDH and bilirubin occurred throughout the course of treatment in many patients. The histologic appearance of the liver either by biopsy or autopsy fails to reveal a consistent pathologic alteration. Although the nature of the underlying clinical problems for which TPN is required offers sufficient explanation for the liver abnormalities noted in some of the patients, in others such a cause is not apparent. We must remain alert to the possibility that these liver abnormalities may be due to a harmful substance in the infusate or to a dietary imbalance. The liver abnormalities seen with and without Intralipid appear to be the same and disappear once the intravenous feeding is stopped. In addition, intravenous fat pigment usually is seen in the Kupffer cells of the liver in most patients on Intralipid for longer than 1 month. This pigment deposition appears to have no effect on liver function.

About 80% of the patients on Intralipid develop a peripheral eosinophilia in the range of 5–10% and in a few this may rise to 35%. There are no clinical manifestations of this abnormality, such as skin rashes, urticaria, etc.

Osmotic diuresis secondary to significant glycosuria occurs occasionally when the 20% glucose infusate is used. The premature infant with underdeveloped renal tubules is most susceptible to this complication. This phenomenon is not seen with peripheral hyperalimentation because of the lower tonicity of the infusate.

No instance of fluid overload in the form of pulmonary edema, peripheral edema or congestive heart failure was seen in any of the patients treated with the three various techniques. This is especially significant in the group managed with peripheral hyperalimentation without fats, in which the volume of fluid infused is quite high.

Technical Complications

Many of the early technical problems associated with the catheter have been either corrected or reduced in frequency. The use of polyvinyl catheters was associated with a high incidence of sterile inflammation and thrombosis; nonreactive silicone rubber catheters have minimized these haz-

ards. Transitory arrhythmias may occur during the insertion of the catheter, especially if the tip enters the heart. The position of the catheter tip must be checked radiographically to be certain that the irritating hyperosmolar solution is delivered into the superior vena cava and not into a smaller vein with a lower blood flow, such as the hepatic. Dislocation of the catheter is less frequent since a flange has been used to secure it.

Venous perforation, a complication reported in the literature, has not occurred in our patients. Thrombosis of the vein in which the catheter resides can occur, especially in the critically ill patient with sepsis and inadequate circulation. Thrombosis in the superior vena cava is better tolerated than in most other vessels. Although evidence of thromboembolism has been noted at autopsy in children dying with the central venous catheter in place, manifestations of this phenomenon in vivo are rare. Among the important factors in the prevention of venous complications are the use of jugular veins rather than femoral or umbilical veins for intubation, x-ray control of the catheter position, avoidance of sepsis and the use of a silicone rubber catheter.

No case of phlebitis was seen in the patients treated with Intralipid peripherally despite the fact that the entire infusate is slightly hypertonic. Intralipid in some fashion appears to protect the vein from phlebitis. When infiltration does occur, it usually is bland and the fluid is rapidly reabsorbed. Phlebitis is seen occasionally in the patients fed peripherally without fat but disappears when the infusion site is changed. In the 60 patients treated with peripheral hyperalimentation without fat, 3 cases of skin slough at the infusion site were seen; 2 healed spontaneously and 1 needed skin grafting.

Infection

Sepsis remains the major complication of central TPN in the pediatric patient. Long-term indwelling venous cannulas are a well-documented source of bloodstream infection. Organisms may enter the bloodstream along the catheter tract or in a contaminated intravenous solution. The catheter, a foreign body in the bloodstream, may act as a focus for growth of organisms entering from a distant septic site. To minimize the risk of sepsis, the following measures and precautions should be taken. Catheters should be placed under aseptic conditions in an operating room. Silicone rubber catheters rather than polyethylene or polyvinyl catheters should be used because they cause less tissue reaction and are less likely to produce a thrombus, which will support the growth of microorganisms along the wall of the intubated vein. The skin exit site for the catheter should be in an area that can be cleansed aseptically and meticulously. Proper care of this site and all the connectors and tubings between the intravenous bottle and the patient is essential. Use of the central venous catheter for necessary blood sampling should be performed only by properly trained personnel.

Any relaxation in strict adherence to the standard technique of catheter care is followed by a sharp rise in the incidence of infective complications. Some institutions[7] have reported such an extremely high incidence of fungal septicemia and death that treatment with TPN in such a hospital is unwarranted.

A review of the Children's Hospital Medical Center of Boston experience indicated that 42 of 264 patients (16%) had one or more septic complications. The incidence of sepsis was not related to the patient's age or diagnosis. Analysis of our septic complications reveals that the likelihood of sepsis was clearly related to the duration of therapy. For each week of therapy after the first week, the risk of sepsis increases by about 5%.

Fever, leukocytosis and/or unexplained glycosuria usually were the first clues to bloodstream infection. Infection was confirmed when microorganisms were cultured from blood obtained through the central venous line. Candida was isolated in 18 blood cultures, a variety of gram-negative bacteria in 9 cultures and staphylococcus, streptococcus or diphtheroids in 20. In 5 cases, more than one organism was found.

Infants with proved Candida bloodstream infection were treated by removal of the central venous line; chemotherapy usually was withheld because of the toxicity of amphotericin. In those with bacterial sepsis, the line usually was withdrawn and appropriate antibiotics were given. In 5 patients with bacterial infection, the venous catheter was left in place and antibiotic therapy alone was curative. Recovery from septicemia usually was evident within 24 hours. Forty of 42 patients survived the septicemia episode, although 6 eventually died of their primary disease. Two deaths could be attributed directly to catheter sepsis. One infant, a newborn with gastroschisis and intestinal obstruction, developed Candida septicemia on the sixteenth day of TPN and the line was removed. The central venous line was inserted 5 days later, but septicemia recurred and the infant died. The other death occurred in an 8-week-old infant with a complicated esophageal abnormality including tracheo-esophageal fistula and massive chalasia. The patient developed Candida septicemia on the twenty-second day of TPN. The line was removed, blood cultures became negative and a second line was inserted 10 days later. On the following day, bilateral overwhelming monilial pneumonia due to embolization of a septic thrombus in the superior vena cava resulted in the death of this infant. Despite the relatively high incidence of infection, the overwhelming majority of affected patients recover without serious sequelae.

Invasive sepsis related to hyperalimentation was not seen in any of the 102 patients treated with Intralipid nor in any of the infants and children managed with peripheral intravenous feeding without fat.

When patients are properly selected for treatment and appropriate precautions are exercised, the benefits far outweigh the risks. It has been most gratifying to see that parenteral nutrition has been responsible for the salvage of many children who in the past would have died of starvation.

REFERENCES

1. Ashkenazi, A., Levin, S., Djaldetti, M., Fishel, E., and Benvenisti, B.: The syndrome of neonatal copper deficiency, Pediatrics 52:525, 1973.
2. Borresen, H. C., Coran, A. G., and Knutrud, O.: Metabolic results of parenteral feeding in neonatal surgery: A balanced parenteral feeding program based on a synthetic L-amino acid solution and a commercial fat emulsion, Ann. Surg. 172:291, 1970.
3. Coran, A. G.: The intravenous use of fat for the total parenteral nutrition of the infant, Lipids 7:455, 1972.
4. Coran, A. G.: The long-term total intravenous feeding of infants using peripheral veins, J. Pediatr. Surg. 8:801, 1973.
5. Coran, A. G.: Total intravenous feeding of infants and children without the use of a central venous catheter, Ann. Surg. 179:445, 1974.
6. Coran, A. G., Edwards, B., and Zaleska, R.: The value of heparin in the hyperalimentation of infants and children with a fat emulsion, J. Pediatr. Surg. 9:725, 1974.
7. Curry, C. R., and Quie, P. G.: Fungal septicemia in patients receiving parenteral hyperalimentation, N. Engl. J. Med. 285:1221, 1971.
8. Dudrick, S. J., Steiger, E., and Long, J. M.: Renal failure in surgical patients: Treatment with intravenous essential amino acids and hypertonic glucose, Surgery 68:180, 1970.
9. Dudrick, S. J., Wilmore, D. W., Vars, H. M., and Rhoads, J. E.: Long-term parenteral nutrition with growth, development, and positive nitrogen balance, Surgery 64:134, 1968.
10. Dudrick, S. J., Wilmore, D. W., Vars, H. M., and Rhoads, J. E.: Can intravenous feeding as the sole means of nutrition support growth in the child and restore weight loss in an adult? An affirmative answer, Ann. Surg. 169:974, 1969.
11. Filler, R. M.: A new method of fixation of silicone rubber catheters for long-term hyperalimentation, J. Pediatr. Surg. 8:395, 1973.
12. Filler, R. M., Eraklis, A. J., Rubin, V. G., and Das, J. B.: Long-term parenteral nutrition in infants, N. Engl. J. Med. 281:589, 1969.
13. Fox, H. A., and Krasna, I. H.: Total intravenous nutrition by peripheral vein in neonatal surgical patients, Pediatrics 52:14, 1973.
14. Ghadimi, H., Abaci, F., Kumar, S., and Rathi, M.: Biochemical aspects of intravenous alimentation, Pediatrics 48:955, 1971.
15. Heird, W. C., and Winters, R. W.: Total parenteral nutrition: The state of the art, J. Pediatr. 86:2, 1975.
16. Helfrick, F. W., and Abelson, N. M.: Intravenous feeding of a complete diet in a child: Report of a case, J. Pediatr. 25:400, 1944.
17. Johnson, J. C., Albritton, W. L., and Sunshine, P.: Hyperammonemia accompanying parenteral nutrition in newborn infants, Pediatrics 81:154, 1972.
18. Karpel, J. T., and Peden, V. H.: Copper deficiency in long-term parenteral nutrition, Pediatrics 80:32, 1972.
19. Lee, H. A.: *Parenteral Nutrition in Acute Metabolic Illness* (New York: Academic Press, 1974).
20. Olney, J. W., Ho, O. L., and Rhee, B.: Brain-damaging potential of protein hydrolysates, N. Engl. J. Med. 289:391, 1973.
21. Paulsrud, J. R., Pensler, L., Whitten, C. F., Stewart, S., and Holman, R. T.: Essential fatty acid deficiency in infants induced by fat-free intravenous feeding, Am. J. Clin. Nutr. 25:897, 1972.
22. Press, M., Hartop, P. J., and Prottey, C.: Correction of essential fatty-acid deficiency in man by the cutaneous application of sunflower-seed oil, Lancet 1:579, 1974.
23. Shils, M. E.: Guidelines for total parenteral nutrition, JAMA 220:1721, 1972.
24. Travis, S. F., Sugarman, H. J., Ruberg, R. L., Dudrick, S. J., Papadopolous, M. D., Miller, L. D., and Oski, F. A.: Alterations of red-cell glycolytic intermediates and oxygen transport as a consequence of hypophosphatemia in patients receiving intravenous hyperalimentation, N. Engl. J. Med. 285:763, 1971.

5 SHERWIN V. KEVY

Surgical Implications of Hematologic Disorders

THE RAPID EVALUATION of the hemorrhagic state prior to, during and immediately following an operation and the refinement in blood component therapy in the past decade have resulted in an increased operative incidence in hematologic conditions. This chapter will present a practical approach to, and an overview of, the most commonly encountered hematologic problems in pediatric surgical patients. Those vexing hematologic problems that the surgeon may see once in a lifetime have been omitted.

Nonhemolytic Anemias

Blood-loss anemia, either acute or chronic, and iron-deficiency anemia are the most common forms of anemias encountered by the surgeon. In many instances, transfusion is required not only in the management of these conditions but also in preparation for elective operation. Despite its importance, there is less investigative information on the volumetric aspect of blood transfusion than on any other category of transfusion therapy. Overloading the circulation in the treatment of chronic anemia and either overtransfusion or undertransfusion at operation or for acute hemorrhage are responsible for many of the complications related to transfusion. These symptoms seldom are recognized and the symptoms that ensue usually are attributed to the anemia or to the trauma of operation and stress of anesthesia.

Acute Blood Loss

The net result of acute hemorrhage is a decrease in blood volume. Treatment is based on control of hemorrhage, signs of shock and the estimation of blood loss. A useful guide for suspecting hemorrhage of 30% or more of the blood volume for children 13–16 years of age is a systolic pressure of less than 65 mm Hg.[1]

The hemoglobin level or the hematocrit may not be a reliable index of the extent of hemorrhage until a period of 24–36 hours has elapsed, when sufficient hemodilution will have occurred to indicate the extent of blood loss. Only one-half the volumetric decrease is replaced within 24 hours after a loss of 10% of the blood volume. Significant reduction of hemoglobin concentration within 3–6 hours of hemorrhage suggests a blood loss greater than 20% of the blood volume.[2]

Chronic Blood Loss and Iron-Deficiency Anemia

Many anesthesiologists consider a hemoglobin level of 10 gm/100 ml the minimal safe level for anesthesia. The justification for this is that it provides a margin of safety in the event of unexpected acute hemorrhage. The child in whom anemia has developed gradually rarely will manifest symptoms or have insufficient erythrocytes for adequate oxygen transport, and a hemoglobin rise of 1.5 gm/100 ml per week can easily be achieved by adequate oral iron therapy.

If transfusion is indicated because of time factors, sedimented or packed red blood cells is the therapy of choice. To assess the amount of sedimented or packed red blood cells required to reach the hemoglobin concentration (hematocrit) desired, the following simple formula may be used: Volume of cells = patient's weight (kg) × increment in HCT desired.

Most transfusionists recommend the adoption of 10 ml/kg as a maximal pediatric transfusion, in the absence of hypovolemia, unless the initial hemoglobin level is less than 5 gm/100 ml, when the figure of 5 ml/kg should be used.[3]

Aplastic Anemia

The term aplastic anemia is used to describe a blood dyscrasia characterized by diminished production of red cells, granulocytes and platelets by the bone marrow. Aplastic anemia occurs idiopathically in approximately 50% of patients; most of the remainder of cases are caused by physical and chemical agents. In the pediatric population, chloramphenicol probably is the most frequent cause of idiosyncratic drug-induced aplastic anemia. Two different types of chloramphenicol-related suppression of bone marrow function have been observed. In one type, chloramphenicol interferes with erythropoiesis as shown by a rise in serum iron and the appearance of vacuoles in nucleated red cells. This effect is dose related and reversible when the drug is stopped. The second form of bone marrow suppression is unrelated to dose. There is some evidence that its occurrence in these situations is due to a genetic susceptibility.[4, 5]

Surgical consultation frequently is sought for the control of localized infection in the liver, lung and perirectal areas. Operation for this and unrelated diseases such as appendicitis should be undertaken only when extensive blood component support is available. These patients require preoperative and postoperative platelet transfusions. In the event of infection, white cell transfusions are of great benefit.[6]

The Hemolytic Anemias

Hemolytic anemia will result when red cell survival is reduced to one eighth of normal—a level at which complete compensation by the bone marrow is impossible. The etiologies of the hemolytic anemias involve complex metabolic processes in red cell production as well as abnormal hemoglobin catabolism. The surgeon must be cognizant of the fact that many of the children in this group have been chronically transfused and have a predilection for the development of irregular antibodies and may present a problem in crossmatching. In addition, 63% of all chronically transfused children develop leukoagglutinins, which are responsible for a significant number of febrile nonhemolytic reactions. This is by far more common in patients with thalassemia and other hemolytic anemias than in other patients. These patients will require granulocyte-poor blood using leukocyte filter (Leuko-Pak) or frozen red cells to alleviate or prevent the occurrence of such reactions preoperatively or during operation.

Hereditary Spherocytosis

Hereditary spherocytosis is the prototype of hemolytic anemia in which the abnormality in red cell shape leads to splenic entrapment and eventual hemolysis. The disease is an autosomal dominant disorder that may become clinically manifested at any time but usually between the ages of 4 and 10.

The presence of spherocytosis, a spleen palpable 2–3 cm below the costal margin, an increased osmotic fragility and a positive family history certainly suggest the diagnosis. Other conditions such as burns, liver disease, immune hemolysis and hypersplenism of any cause may be associated with spherocytosis.

In patients with spherocytosis, a lessening of jaundice will be due to a decrease of red cell production, with resultant severe anemia. These aplastic crises usually are self-limited and the patients do not require transfusion. However, if the episodes are severe and frequent enough, early splenectomy should be considered.

The spleen, through its dual role as a filter and as a major site of antibody recognition and antibody production, is an important part of the child's defense system.[7] Splenectomy before the age of 5 should be avoided if possible. If splenectomy cannot be delayed, these patients must thereafter be closely followed for any signs of sepsis. Since the organisms most often responsible for fulminant infection in these children are penicillin sensitive, prophylactic therapy is warranted even though controlled studies are not available.[8, 9]

There is also a group of patients in whom the hemolysis is so mild that some pediatricians and hematologists will advise not doing a splenectomy. However, the incidence of gallstones and secondary biliary tract disease is high enough in patients with this disorder to recommend splenectomy for all patients.

Sickle Cell Syndromes and Hemoglobin C Disease

The most frequent qualitative hemoglobinopathies seen in the United States are sickle cell anemia and hemoglobin C and their variants. The average incidence of the sickle gene among American blacks is approximately 8%.

Although the diagnosis of sickle cell anemia can be made at birth by agar gel electrophoresis, it is unusual for it to be made until a painful crisis occurs or progressive hemolytic anemia and splenomegaly develop. The blood picture characteristically is one of a severe normocytic anemia with sickle cells in the peripheral smear. The diagnosis can be confirmed by a positive sickling test with sodium metabisulfite and the zygosity determined by hemoglobin electrophoresis.

During the first 2 years of life, the patient experiences the onset of vaso-occlusive episodes, which are responsible for the painful crisis. Such crises will occur in association with an upper respiratory infection and are due to infarctions in the various organ systems. Most commonly, the painful crises involve the periosteum, bones and joints. In infants, the bones of the hands and feet are the most frequent sites of in-

farction, resulting in both swelling and tenderness, the so-called hand-foot syndrome.

Painful abdominal crises are common and represent a situation for which the surgeon frequently is consulted. When the abdominal pain is accompanied by increased jaundice, a common duct stone or acute cholecystitis must be considered. Acute appendicitis or bowel or splenic infarction must be ruled out. Many patients suffer abdominal catastrophes because of the hematologist's overconfidence in his diagnosis of a painful sickle cell abdominal crisis. The presence of bowel sounds supports the diagnosis of abdominal crisis rather than that of an acute abdomen. The white count and differential are of no help, since the granulocytes almost always are increased in patients with sickle cell disease after the age of 6. Most patients will follow a repeated symptom pattern with each crisis. Deviation from that pattern should suggest a more serious problem.

Hyposthenuria and infection are the major renal complications of sickle cell disease. The resulting obligatory water loss makes the patient more liable to dehydration and resultant crisis. This factor must be borne in mind by the surgeon when preparing the child for elective operation. In such instances, it is judicious to place the child on a slow intravenous infusion the evening prior to operation. Many hematologists also recommend that a patient being prepared for an elective major surgical procedure undergo a modified exchange transfusion with normal red cells to ensure the presence of at least 70% normal adult hemoglobin. This should prevent or alleviate the serious crisis in the event of unexpected anoxia during induction of anesthesia or intraoperatively.

Leg ulcers frequently occur in adults, since venous circulation is less competent, but are rare in childhood. Far more common and a very important problem is the occurrence of priapism in adolescence. This often is self-limited but can be severe enough to require treatment by exchange transfusion or surgical intervention. Patients who have had prolonged priapism and/or surgical intervention must be warned of consequent impotence.

The child with sickle cell trait usually will not manifest any symptoms and has a normal blood smear. A diagnosis is made either as part of a routine survey or as a genetic evaluation. The surgeon should be aware, however, that in the event that arterial oxygen saturation is decreased, the child with sickle cell trait may suffer a vascular occlusion.

Hemoglobin C disease is a relatively mild disorder characterized by hemolytic anemia, splenomegaly and target cells in the peripheral blood smear. Vaso-occlusive phenomena are rare but do occur, a fact that must be borne in mind if the patient is to be operated on.

The Thalassemia Syndromes

The term thalassemia is more familiar to most surgeons under the older terms of Cooley's anemia and Mediterranean anemia. At last accounting, there were some 22 disorders included in this syndrome complex.

Homozygous beta thalassemia or thalassemia major is the primary disorder in this group for which the surgeon is most likely to be consulted. The clinical course in virtually all instances is severe. Within several months after birth, the patient develops a hypochromic, microcytic, hemolytic anemia, which heralds the need for a regular transfusion program. This is the age when children frequently undergo elective herniorrhaphy. If an infant is found to be anemic, because of the similarity of the peripheral blood smear, care must be taken to differentiate thalassemia (major or minor) from iron-deficiency anemia.

With time, a thalassemic patient's spleen and liver become progressively enlarged and the child develops a typical facies. As with all chronically transfused patients, iron overload is responsible for damage to the heart, liver, pancreas and other endocrine organs.

Splenectomy has an important role in the management of thalassemic patients. If the child is maintained on a hypertransfusion program from an early age, extramedullary erythropoiesis is suppressed and splenomegaly is delayed or suppressed. However, most if not all patients ultimately develop true hypersplenism with evidence of destruction of red cells, white cells and platelets in the spleen. Splenectomy is recommended if there is increasing difficulty in maintaining adequate hemoglobin levels despite appropriate transfusion therapy. This rarely is necessary before the age of 5 or 6 years. Surgeons must be aware of the extreme hazards of overwhelming infection in this group of patients whose reticuloendothelial system is loaded with iron.[8, 9] Prior to operation, each patient should undergo evaluation of hepatic and cardiac function.

Glycolytic Enzyme Deficiencies

The most common hemolytic anemias due to a glycolytic enzyme deficiency are glucose-6-phosphate dehydrogenase (G-6-PD) and pyruvate kinase (PK) deficiency.

Hemolysis of red cells deficient in G-6-PD is triggered by the administration of reducing drugs. Among those commonly prescribed by surgeons are the sulfonamides and the nitrofurans. Its incidence is as high as 30% of Sephardic Jews, 35% of Sardinians, 11% of Greeks and 13% of American blacks. Full expression of the disease in females is rare and the abnormality, in most instances, is more severe in Caucasians than in blacks. Treatment consists of discontinuing the offending drug or compound. There is no indication for splenectomy.

Pyruvate kinase (PK) is a key enzyme in the glycolytic pathway of the red cell. Most patients with PK deficiency are of north European ancestry. The onset of symptoms occurs in early infancy or childhood. At times, it may even present in the newborn period so that exchange transfusion is required to treat the hyperbilirubinemia. Splenomegaly is more prominent in these children than in those with G-6-PD deficiency. Splenectomy has proved to be of value in occasional cases, and should be seriously considered if hemolysis is severe.[10]

Platelets

Platelet Function

The template bleeding time (TBT) is the most sensitive and reliable method for evaluating in vivo platelet function. The TBT becomes prolonged at platelet counts of 75,000–100,000 mm³, but significant prolongation occurs only at levels of 30,000 mm³ or less. Spontaneous hemorrhage is rare with counts above 30,000 mm³ and major surgical procedures usually can be carried out without platelet support.[11]

The role of platelets in the control of hemorrhage is related not only to their number but, even more important, to their stickiness or ability to aggregate. An enormous volume of literature has accumulated during the past 5 years relating a defect in this quality to various drugs and disease states.

Aspirin, probably the single most commonly used drug, has a marked effect on platelet function when measured by aggregometry and TBT. In a child, this effect will last for up to 5 days following ingestion of a single aspirin. A large number of the commonly used drugs such as diphenhydramine (Benadryl), glyceryl guaiacolate (found in proprietary cough mixtures) and chlorpromazine have been shown to cause abnormalities in platelet aggregation when added to platelet-rich plasma. The most definitive work in this field has been done by Buchanan and Handin,[12] who evaluated antiplatelet drugs and their effect on hemostasis in 30 normal subjects and 18 patients with severe hemophilia. They demonstrated that only aspirin has a significant in vivo effect on hemostasis. Based on these findings, it is strongly suggested that the question of aspirin ingestion be specifically included in every "surgical history" and elective operation be delayed for 5 days after aspirin intake. The presence of aspirin effect can be determined by demonstration of an abnormal bleeding time.

Idiopathic Thrombocytopenic Purpura

Platelet number and function are similar in children and adults with the exception of infants in the immediate newborn period. The term idiopathic thrombocytopenic purpura (ITP) is used to define a state that results when there is a marked reduction of circulating platelets in the presence of a normal bone marrow and the absence of associated systemic disease. In children, ITP may occur at any age but is most frequent between the ages of 2 and 6 years. In contrast to adults, in whom there is a 4:1 preponderance in females, ITP occurs with equal frequency in boys and girls.

Acute ITP is characterized by an abrupt onset with spontaneously developing petechiae and ecchymosis and platelet counts of less than 15,000 mm³. At least 80–85% of patients will achieve a complete and permanent recovery without any specific treatment. Of the patients who recover spontaneously, slightly more than half do so within 1 month of onset and 85% recover within 4 months. An additional 5–10% will recover within 1 year.[13] The decision to utilize steroid therapy is based on the drug's ability to decrease the bleeding tendency in the early phase of the disease by elevating the platelet count or by improving vascular integrity. Platelet therapy is virtually useless and unwarranted in this disease except in the very rare instances of central nervous system hemorrhage or in adolescence when emergency splenectomy is necessary. Platelet therapy under these conditions is effective only when given by constant infusion.

Any thought of splenectomy must take into consideration the natural history of ITP in childhood. Persistence of thrombocytopenia for 1 year is indicative of chronicity, and spontaneous recovery is rare. Splenectomy is the treatment of choice for chronic ITP. More than 70% of patients operated on recover completely; those who do not still exhibit significant improvement in their bleeding tendency. The peak platelet count usually is seen within 2 weeks following splenectomy. A good prognostic sign is the achievement of a platelet count of greater than 500,000 mm³ within 1 week of operation. One note of caution regarding splenectomy must be made at this time. There is an immune disorder in childhood (Wiskott-Aldrich) that is characterized by thrombocytopenia, eczema and recurrent infections. Splenectomy does not modify the course of the thrombocytopenia in this disease but does make overwhelming infection a virtual certainty.[14]

Hypersplenism

The diagnosis of hypersplenism must be considered when there is depression of one or more of the formed elements of the blood, a normal bone marrow with perhaps a slight increase in the number of precursor cells and splenic enlargement. The rare instances in which it is a primary disease in children occur when there is cystic transformation following trauma. Most often it occurs secondary to such varied conditions as portal hypertension due to liver disease or an extrahepatic block, rheumatoid arthritis, the lymphomatous diseases and many of the hematologic conditions described previously.

Splenectomy is the treatment of choice and is uniformly successful in correcting the hematologic abnormalities. Prior to undertaking this procedure, the prognosis and natural history of the underlying disease must be evaluated, as well as any future operative procedures contemplated to alleviate the underlying condition.

Nonthrombocytopenic Purpura

Anaphylactoid Purpura (Schönlein-Henoch)

This syndrome is a systemic vasculitis characterized by abdominal pain, periarticular swelling, nephritis and a skin rash, most often occurring in children under 7 years of age. The rash is pathognomonic. Initially it is urticarial but soon develops central red areas that eventually become hemorrhagic, almost exclusively involving the legs, buttocks and perineal areas. Abdominal colic is severe and almost always associated with gastrointestinal bleeding of varying degree. Intussusception, which usually is ileo-ileal in nature, can occur during the course of the abdominal phase of the disease.[15]

Intravenous administration of corticosteroids in high doses leads to dramatic improvement in the abdominal and joint symptoms. In my experience, none of the children so treated have ever developed an intussusception. However, corticosteroids do not alter the course of the disease, as evidenced by continuing appearance and disappearance of the skin rash. Thus, care should be taken to gradually taper the steroid therapy.

Coagulation

Physiology of Coagulation

Coagulation abnormalities tend to produce terror in the heart of even the boldest surgeon. However, the investigation of a bleeding diathesis becomes a straightforward diagnostic exercise once the basic elements of clot formation are understood. Hemostasis depends on three variables: (1) the state of the vasculature, (2) the quantity and functional capability of the platelets and (3) the activation of the coagulation factors in plasma.

The current schema of blood coagulation is diagrammatically presented in Figure 5–1. There are two basic mechanisms for generating coagulation. One is initiated when blood contacts tissue, as in the case of an injury, and is called the extrinsic clotting mechanism. The other is activated in plasma by exposure to a foreign surface and is known as the intrinsic clotting mechanism.

As shown in Figure 5–1, the intrinsic clotting mechanism is initiated when factor XII (Hageman factor) becomes activated and acquires enzymatic activity following interaction of normal plasma with an abnormal surface. This allows it to interact with factor XI (plasma thromboplastin antecedent) and a sequential series of cascading reactions occur. Activated factor XI interacts with factor IX (Christmas factor) in the presence of calcium. Ultimately, a complex is formed that is composed of activated factor IX, factor VIII, phospholipid and calcium. This, in turn, activates factor X (Stuart factor), which reacts with factor V (proaccelerin) to catalyze the conversion of prothrombin to thrombin.

In the event that tissues are injured, a shortcut is taken— thromboplastic material is released from the cells, activating the extrinsic clotting mechanism. As shown in Figure 5–1, a complex forms with factor VII (SPCA), calcium and phospholipid to react with activated factor X and ultimately catalyze the conversion of prothrombin to thrombin.

Preoperative Evaluation of Hemostatic Disorders

A bleeding disorder should be suspected when the child's history reveals (1) unexpected or unexplained bleeding associated with a surgical procedure, (2) bleeding that persists

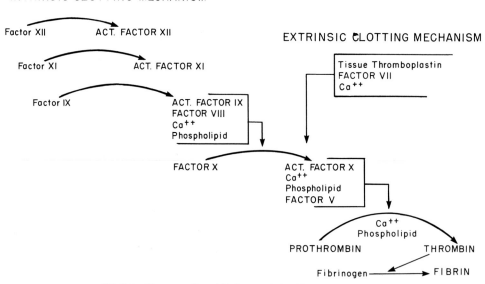

INTRINSIC CLOTTING MECHANISM

EXTRINSIC CLOTTING MECHANISM

Fig. 5-1. – The generation of fibrinogen during blood coagulation.

TABLE 5-1.—LABORATORY ABNORMALITIES OF COMMONLY OBSERVED COAGULATION DISORDERS

DEFECT	RED CELLS	PROTHROMBIN TIME (PT)	PARTIAL THROMBO-PLASTIN TIME (PTT)	BLEEDING TIME	PLATELETS	FIBRIN SPLIT PRODUCTS	EUGLOBULIN LYSIS TIME
Liver disease	Targeting	Prolonged	Normal	Normal	Normal or decreased	Normal or increased	Normal
Hemophilia (VIII)	Normal	Normal	Prolonged	Normal	Normal	Normal	Normal
Christmas disease (IX)	Normal	Normal	Prolonged	Normal	Normal	Normal	Normal
Von Willebrand's disease	Normal	Normal	Prolonged	Prolonged	Normal	Normal	Normal
Thrombocytopenia	Normal	Normal	Normal	Prolonged	Markedly decreased	Normal	Normal
Functional abnormalities of platelets (aspirin)	Normal	Normal	Normal	Prolonged	Normal	Normal	Normal
Intravascular coagulation	Fragmented	Prolonged	Prolonged	Normal or prolonged	Decreased	Increased	Normal
Primary fibrinolysis	Normal	Normal or prolonged	Normal or prolonged	Normal	Normal	Normal	Abnormal

for more than 2 hours after dental extraction, (3) bleeding that begins several hours after dental extraction or suturing of a laceration, (4) the presence of petechiae or ecchymoses larger than 5 cm in diameter or (5) a family history of a bleeding disorder. Characteristically, bleeding due to a capillary or platelet defect is superficial and begins immediately after trauma and is effectively stopped by local pressure, whereas clotting abnormalities should be suspected from such findings as large hematoma, bleeding into joints, delay in onset after trauma and only temporary stoppage by local pressure. There are four relatively simple tests that will confirm or exclude the existence of a bleeding disorder and indicate the area of further evaluation. They are the prothrombin time (PT), activated partial thromboplastin time (PTT), platelet count and template bleeding time (TBT).

The PT is abnormal in virtually all acquired coagulation defects. It is a measure of the over-all efficiency of the extrinsic pathway. Thus, an abnormal PT is indicative of a deficiency of factors that enter into the coagulation scheme at the level of factor X or later (see Fig. 5-1). The PTT, on the other hand, is a sensitive assessment of the intrinsic pathway and is abnormal when any coagulation factor is below 30% of its normal value. For example, a mild hemophiliac with a factor VIII level of 8% will bleed postoperatively and have a normal whole blood clotting time but a prolonged PTT. Both of these tests must be performed in parallel using normal plasma as a control, and the standard for each laboratory must be known, to evaluate the significance of any aberration from the norm. The TBT is the most sensitive test, not only for the quantitative aspect of platelets but their functional capability as well. Kits are available with calibrated templates that will enable the technician to perform this test with acceptable reproducibility. Table 5-1 summarizes the results of the laboratory abnormalities in the hemostatic disorders encountered most frequently by the surgeon.

Hemophilia (Factor VIII, AHF Deficiency)

Hemophilia, or factor VIII deficiency, the most common of the congenital coagulation defects, is transmitted as a sex-linked recessive trait. The baseline factor VIII level within the individual patient's plasma and within his kindred is constant and determines the severity of the disease. A severe hemophiliac will have a baseline factor VIII level of less than 0.5%. These children, except for the first year of life, will have a history of spontaneous bleeding into the joints and soft tissues and excessive bleeding following minor trauma. Mild to moderate hemophiliacs, whose baseline levels vary between 2% and 15%, may remain unsuspected until such time as a laceration occurs or operation is performed. All patients with mild hemophilia have a positive family history whereas one-quarter of the severe hemophiliacs do not.[16]

Major surgical procedures can be performed with relative ease on even a severe hemophiliac. However, they do require the availability of accurate measurement of the clotting factors. Prior to contemplating an elective operation, the patient must be evaluated for the presence of an inhibitor that would negate the clinical effectiveness of the factor VIII concentrate.

As shown in Table 5-2, the minimal factor VIII (AHF) level to ensure proper hemostasis for an operative procedure is 50% of normal. This can be achieved easily even in the smallest child using commercially available concentrates. Since factor VIII has a half-life of only 12 hours, the initial or priming dose calculated to achieve a level of 100% should be given at least 30 minutes prior to operation. Thereafter, one-half the initial dose is administered every 12 hours for a period of 7-10 days to ensure good wound healing. Lacerations, whether or not they require suturing, have to be treated in a similar manner initially but for a shorter duration of time to prevent the occurrence of a wound hematoma. Unfortunately, an operation frequently must be performed on a known hemophiliac in an emergency when complete laboratory services are not available. In those instances, a PTT should be obtained prior to and one-half hour following the infusion of enough factor VIII to raise the child's level to 100%. If the PTT is brought to normal, one can be sure that significant inhibitors can be excluded and the blood level is greater than 50% of normal.

Christmas Disease (Factor IX, PTC Deficiency)

Factor IX deficiency is identical to hemophilia in symptomatology, mode of inheritance and in the varying degrees of severity. The preoperative and postoperative management

TABLE 5–2.–THERAPY OF COMMONLY OBSERVED COAGULATION DISORDERS

DEFECT	PREPARATION TO USE	HALF-LIFE HOURS	LEVEL AFTER TRANSFUSION OF 1 u/KG	MINIMAL HEMOSTATIC LEVEL FOR SURGERY (% Normal)	GENERAL COMMENTS
Hemophilia (factor VIII, AHF)	Commercial AHF concentrate. Unitage stated on label	8–12	2%	50%	Therapy must be given every 12 hr for 7–10 days
Christmas disease (factor IX, PTC)	Factor IX concentrate. Unitage stated on label	24	1–1½%	30%	Concentrate administered daily up to the post-operative day. Thereafter, plasma administered in a dose of 3 ml/kg body weight for 3–4 days
	Fresh-frozen or bank plasma	24			
Von Willebrand's disease	Cryoprecipitate or fresh-frozen plasma	24–48	3%	50%	Administration of 2 bags of cryoprecipitate per 10 kg body weight will achieve this level. Daily therapy for 7–10 days
Factor V globulin	Fresh-frozen plasma, fresh plasma	36	1½%	15–25% needed for therapy	Administer in dose of 5–10 ml/kg body weight once daily
Liver disease. Low levels factor VII & X	Plasma or commercial factor IX concentrate	36–72	1%%	15–25%	Concentrate should not be used if fibrin split products are detected
Thrombocytopenia	Platelet concentrates stored at 22° C	72	100,000 mm³	25,000–40,000 mm³	

of the patient is analogous to that of hemophilia. As shown in Table 5–2, factor IX has a half-life of 24 hours, which allows the physician to administer either factor IX concentrate or plasma only once a day. It is our usual practice to administer factor IX concentrate for the first 4 postoperative days and then switch to plasma, since the hemostatic levels necessary are not as high as those required for hemophilia.

Von Willebrand's Disease

This is an autosomal dominant inherited disorder characterized by a low factor VIII (AHF) level in the plasma, a prolongation of the bleeding time and impaired platelet aggregation and/or adhesiveness. The typical clinical history is one of a mild bleeding tendency characterized by frequent epistaxis, easy bruising and prolonged bleeding from lacerations and dental extractions. The severity of the disease varies from one affected patient to another and, unlike patients with hemophilia, even within the same kindred.

When either normal plasma, stored plasma or plasma fractions rich in factor VIII are administered to patients with von Willebrand's disease, the factor VIII activity exceeds the level predicted from the amount administered and persists for a longer duration than it would in a patient with true hemophilia. This apparent induction of synthesis of factor VIII in vivo makes this condition relatively easy to treat but can make the diagnosis virtually impossible to prove in the bleeding surgical patient if a transfusion has been given.[17] In some patients, the factor VIII concentration will rise to almost normal levels without transfusion when they are stressed by infection, activity or hemorrhage. However, platelet aggregometry and the bleeding time remain abnormal. The patient then may have to be treated as one with von Willebrand's disease and the condition ultimately confirmed or refuted when a basal state is reached. If the diagnosis has been established preoperatively, therapy can be started 6–8 hours prior to operation, as indicated in Table 5–2. The prolonged bleeding time, even though only transiently corrected by factor VIII therapy, should not present problems in the postoperative period.[18]

Disseminated Intravascular Coagulation (DIC)

DIC is an acquired coagulation disorder resulting from widespread activation of the clotting mechanism that literally results in the conversion of plasma to serum within the circulation. In a majority of instances, DIC appears to be initiated by entry of thromboplastic substances into the circulation. Another significant group of cases results from damage to the endothelium of vessels with exposure of collagen and subsequent activation of factor XII (Hageman factor, see Fig. 5–1). A number of conditions are known to be associated with DIC. Among the more common are: (1) gram-negative sepsis, (2) anoxia, (3) tissue ischemia following injury or shock, (4) acidosis.

The diagnosis of DIC should be suspected in a patient with one of these underlying conditions who develops an acute deficiency of clotting factors. The laboratory findings depend on the stage of the disorder. Very early in the course, slight to modest thrombocytopenia develops (75,000–150,000 mm³). Fibrinogen levels, which ordinarily are increased to 3 times normal in the presence of infection or inflammation, are normal or low normal, indicating increased fibrinogen destruction. As the disorder progresses, factors V and VIII are destroyed. The PTT and PT become prolonged, the platelet count drops to very low levels, the red cells appear fragmented (microangiopathic changes) and fibrin split products usually are detectable in the circulation. The clinical picture in the later stages of the disorder is characterized by mucosal bleeding, generalized ecchymosis and oozing from venipuncture and wound sites. Treatment should be withheld until it is determined that the disorder is progressive or has reached a point where clinical manifestations are present.

Treatment should be directed toward amelioration of the condition that precipitated the episode of DIC. The use of heparin in doses of 50–75 units per kg intravenously is recommended by many hematologists. However, there are no controlled studies of its efficacy in the human. Replacement of clotting factors with fresh plasma (fresh-frozen plasma) and platelet transfusions may be given once the patient is heparinized.[19] Fibrinolysis always is a sequel of DIC and is the mechanism for removal of fibrin from the microcirculation.

Fibrinolysis

In fibrinolytic syndromes, plasminogen, the precursor of a fibrinolytic enzyme, is converted to its active form, plasmin, which has among its substrates fibrin, fibrinogen and several clotting factors (V, VIII and IX). A hemorrhagic diathesis due to primary fibrinolysis is extremely rare in pediatric surgery. It nearly always results as an aftermath of intravascular coagulation. However, there are very rare instances in which primary fibrinolysis does occur in pediatrics: (1) operative correction of scoliosis, (2) extracorporeal circulation, (3) operative repair of craniosynostosis. In such instances, the platelet count is normal unless there is evidence of dilutional thrombocytopenia. The euglobulin lysis time, a rapidly and easily performed test, will be less than 45 minutes and the thrombin time will be prolonged. Only in those instances in which one can determine that fibrinolysis is primary should epsilon-aminocaproic acid (EACA) be administered. EACA is contraindicated in defibrination.

Liver Disease

Liver disease probably is the most common cause of acquired hemostatic abnormalities. Moderate to severe hepatic insufficiency will result in the plasma levels of clotting factors being low, since the liver is the site of synthesis of the vitamin K-dependent clotting factors, factor V and fibrinogen. In addition, severe liver disease often is associated with hypersplenism and thrombocytopenia as well as intravascular coagulation. In the event of biliary tract obstruction, lipid absorption is impaired and, therefore, the vitamin K-dependent factors will be low. The prothrombin time is the most consistent abnormality observed in severe parenchymal hepatic disease.[20]

The use of commercially available concentrates of prothrombin complex in patients whose liver is unable to synthesize the vitamin K-dependent factors is a rational approach to ensuring adequate hemostasis. However, they should not be used in patients who have laboratory evidence of DIC. In the latter instance, the safest replacement therapy is a modified exchange transfusion with fresh whole blood or red cells resuspended in fresh-frozen plasma.

Massive Transfusion

A massive transfusion in pediatrics is defined as the rapid infusion of blood approaching or exceeding 30% of the patient's own blood volume in a short space of time. A review of 139,751 transfusions at the Children's Hospital Medical Center in Boston during an 11-year period revealed that 15.83% are in this category. Massive transfusion often results in dilutional thrombocytopenia, which is the most common acquired hemostatic defect intraoperatively or in the immediate postoperative period. Statistics reveal that its occurrence rate was 6% during the 11-year period studied.

A majority of such transfusions occur in the operating room in electively scheduled cases. In these instances, blood usage can be predicted based on the child's age and the operative procedure. Fresh blood is routinely made available for administration when the predicted operative blood loss is equivalent to 40% of the child's blood volume. This approach has decreased the incidence of dilutional thrombocytopenia to 0.3%. If fresh blood is not available, the administration of platelets in a dose of 1 unit of platelets per 7 kg of body weight should correct the existing thrombocytopenia. Except in cases of extracorporeal bypass procedures, we have never observed clinically significant dilution of clotting factors or acquired abnormalities of platelet function.

REFERENCES

1. Grant, R. T., and Reeve, E. G.: Observations in the general effects of injury in man, with special reference to wound shock, Spec. Rep. Ser. Med. Res. Counc. (Lond.) No. 277, 1951.
2. Howarth, S., and Sharpey-Schafer, E. P.: Low blood pressure phases following hemorrhage, Lancet 1:19, 1947.
3. Kevy, S. V.: Pediatric Transfusion Therapy, in *Transfusion Therapy, A Technical Workshop* (Washington, D.C.: American Association of Blood Banks, 1974).
4. Saidi, P., Wallerstein, R. D.: Effect of chloramphenicol on erythropoiesis, J. Lab. Clin. Med. 57:247, 1961.
5. Nagao, T., and Mauer, A. M.: Concordance for drug-induced aplastic anemia in identical twins, N. Engl. J. Med. 281:7, 1969.
6. Boggs, D. R.: Transfusion of neutrophils as prevention or treatment of infection in patients with neutropenia, N. Engl. J. Med. 290:1055, 1974.
7. Kevy, S. V., Taft, M., Vawter, G. F., and Rosen, F. S.: Hereditary splenic hypoplasia, Pediatrics 42:752, 1968.
8. Eraklis, A. J., Kevy, S. V., Diamond, L. K., and Gross, R. E.: The hazard of overwhelming infection after splenectomy in childhood, N. Engl. J. Med. 276:1225, 1967.
9. Eraklis, A. J., and Filler, R. M.: Splenectomy in childhood. A review of 1413 cases, J. Pediatr. Surg. 7:382, 1972.
10. Zuelzer, W. W., Robinson, A. R., *et al.*: Erythrocyte pyruvate kinase deficiency in nonspherocytic hemolytic anemia: A system of multiple genetic markers, Blood 32:33, 1968.
11. Harker, L. A., and Slichter, S. J.: The bleeding time as a screening test for evaluation of platelet function, N. Engl. J. Med. 287:155, 1972.
12. Buchanan, G. R., and Handin, R. I.: Effects of anti-platelet drugs in hemostasis in normal subjects and in patients with severe hemophilia, Abstr. Am. Soc. Hematology, December, 1976.
13. Lusher, J. M., and Zuelzer, W. W.: Idiopathic thrombocytopenic purpura in childhood, J. Pediatr. 68:971, 1966.
14. Pearson, H. A., and Shulman, N. R.: Platelet survival in Wiskott-Aldrich syndrome, J. Pediatr. 68:755, 1966.
15. Allen, D. M., and Diamond, L. K.: Anaphylactoid purpura in children (Schoenlein-Henoch syndrome), Am. J. Dis. Child. 99:147, 1960.
16. Ratnoff, O. D., and Bennet, B.: The genetics of hereditary disorders of blood coagulation, Science 179:1291, 1973.
17. Weiss, H. J.: Von Willebrand's disease—diagnostic criteria, Blood 32:668, 1968.
18. Ratnoff, O. D., and Bennet, B.: Clues to the pathogenesis of bleeding in von Willebrand's disease, N. Engl. J. Med. 289:1182, 1973.
19. Colman, R. W., and Robboy, S. J.: Disseminated intravascular coagulation (DIC): An approach, Am. J. Med. 52:679, 1972.
20. Spector, I., and Corn, M.: Relationship of laboratory tests of hemostasis to hemorrhage in liver disease, Arch. Intern. Med. 119:577, 1967.

6 H. HARLAN STONE

Surgical Infections

DESPITE MAJOR ADVANCES in the control of many communicable diseases and, more recently, the development of highly effective antimicrobial agents, infection has remained throughout the world the most frequent cause of death in children. Such statistics are especially significant during infancy, a time when the newly born individual develops his own specific immunity against those bacterial and viral pathogens that challenge his future existence. In the more developed countries, however, where appropriate community health measures are almost routinely implemented, life-threatening sepsis is primarily confined to the neonate and to those older children with disease or drug-induced malfunctions of their reticuloendothelial system.

Components of Infection

Three basic factors influence the development and progression of every infection: (1) an inoculum of pathogens, (2) nutrient media for initial microbial sustenance and (3) host resistance. It is the continuous interaction among these three components that, first, determines whether mere colonization or, instead, actual invasion by a given set of microorganisms will occur and, second, what the final outcome in the individual case will be, i.e., complete elimination of the infectious agent, parasitic tolerance or eventual death of the host.

Inoculum

The INFECTIOUS POTENTIAL of any given inoculum varies considerably and is reflected in the product of the absolute number of challenging microbes multiplied by the collective virulence of all participating pathogens. The MINIMAL INFECTIVE QUANTITY for most pathogenic species is somewhere between 10^3 and 10^6. Extreme examples are an infecting dose of less than 10 for some highly virulent species such as Group A beta-hemolytic streptococcus and, by contrast, the entirely innocuous challenge presented by *Bacillus subtilis* despite even a massive inoculation of greater than 10.[14] Even if the initial inoculum is below the critical amount required for infection by that particular organism, time, or neglect of the contaminated area, may permit a primary colonization and then subsequent increases in local microbial population to levels eventually capable of creating an invasive infection.

The sum VIRULENCE of individual species, subspecies or strains participating in the inoculum is the other major determinant of outcome in any specific case, i.e., infection, colonization or microbe eradication. EXOTOXINS account for most of the infectiveness. These are digestive enzymes elaborated by the invading pathogen in an effort to break down surrounding complex substrate into more absorbable and utilizable forms. Although the effect is essentially a local one, it does afford a means for microbial invasion (proteases, hyaluronidase, etc.). Some exotoxins are absorbed unaltered

into lymphatic and venous channels and can thereby inflict a more distant injury on the host (tetanus, diphtheria, etc.). ENDOTOXINS, on the other hand, are large chemical moieties that are normally present within the microbial cell proper, can become operative only if death of the pathogen has permitted their release, have no lytic or other adverse effect on local tissues but appear to produce damage pharmacologically on specific and more remote organ systems.

Recent studies, especially those related to the prevalence and role of anaerobic species in clinical sepsis,[1] have demonstrated that many infections are POLYMICROBIAL in nature; that is, these infections are due to a mixed bacterial flora with organisms having considerable variation in oxygen and pH requirements, nutrient demands, ability to degrade specific substrates and even tolerance to one another. The interactions between the several species within such an ecologic preparation are said to be indifferent, antagonistic or synergistic.

INDIFFERENCE is characterized by a relatively stable balance between individual members of a microbial mixture. The diverse aerobic bacterial population colonizing a chronically open wound represents a good example. Another is the very complex bacterial flora contained within the unaltered human colon.

ANTAGONISM between microbes is common and routinely culminates in the predominance of only a few species out of an initial multiplicity. Strains of a single species may even destroy one another, this being the basis for the pyocin method of typing *Pseudomonas aeruginosa*. The introduction of an artificial influence, such as antibiotics, can also upset a given microbial balance and accordingly lead to an entirely different set of dominant microorganisms. An example is the development of oral candidiasis (thrush) when an antimicrobial effective against the normal mouth flora has been given for an extended period.

SYNERGISM between bacterial species was first documented by Meleney.[2] Until recently, this was believed to be a relatively uncommon event. However, it now appears that the majority of intra-abdominal infections of gastrointestinal origin are of this type, especially those developing after contamination by contents of the colon or obstructed small bowel.[3] In these cases, observed virulence greatly exceeds the mere addition of all individual infectious factors. Participating in the mixed flora are two or more separate microbial groups, each having considerably different culture and growth characteristics and yet each contributing to the infectious process through specific roles in oxygen consumption, enzymatic tissue destruction, antibiotic neutralization, etc. In such peritonitis, the AEROBIC COMPONENT is one or more of the gram-negative rods, with or without the company of Enterococcus. The aerobic species, being in actuality facultative anaerobes, maintain the local oxygen tension at a greatly reduced level. Endotoxin appears to be the only other factor in gram-negative infections to share in direct

TABLE 6–1.–BACTERIAL SYNERGISM
(Laparotomy Contamination of the Rat Peritoneum)

ORGANISMS	DOSE	NUMBER OF RATS	DIED WITH SEPTICEMIA	LIVED, BUT INFECTED	NOT INFECTED
E. coli	10^8	10	–	1	9
E. coli	10^9	12	–	8	4
E. coli	10^{10}	14	9	3	2
E. coli	10^{11}	10	10	–	–
Bact. fragilis	10^9	10	–	–	10
Bact. fragilis	10^{10}	9	1	–	8
Bact. fragilis	10^{11}	10	–	–	10
E. coli and Bact. fragilis	10^6 10^6	10	1	2	7
E. coli and Bact. fragilis	10^8 10^8	14	5	8	1
E. coli and Bact. fragilis	10^{10} 10^{10}	10	10	–	–

The most common bacterial synergism seen clinically is that between *E. coli* and various anaerobic species, especially *Bacteroides fragilis*. This can be reproduced in a rat preparation whereby the virulence of the combination is much greater and accordingly demands significantly fewer organisms in the bacterial challenge for infection to be produced.

host destruction, serving as the precipitating agent immediately leading to death. The ANAEROBIC COMPONENT includes a vast multitude of different species, although *Bacteroides fragilis* may predominate later. It is the secretion of potent enzymes by the anaerobes that dramatically augments bacterial invasiveness and provides relatively digested substrate for the nourishment of both sets of pathogens. However, without the lowered redox potential created by metabolism of the aerobes, anaerobic life could not otherwise exist.

Such synergistic relationships can readily be quantitated by determination of minimal infective doses for single species alone and then in combination (Table 6–1).

Even though an absolute number of organisms in the inoculum is not the sole determinant of infection, it still is an exceedingly important consideration. It is for this very reason that aseptic precautions are practiced in the operating room and wherever else patients are made susceptible to infection because of an altered immune mechanism or exposure of deeper tissue planes. The SOURCE of any microbial challenge must also be taken into account if contamination is to be avoided or at least kept at levels below that necessary to cause infection.

Inoculation by EXOGENOUS microorganisms is a never-ending process, yet potential pathogens vary considerably in virulence. Microbes residing within the hospital environment are consistently the more dangerous, for they often are the ones that have survived the onslaught of cleaning compounds, human resistance factors and antibiotic therapy. Hospital personnel and the various instruments used by them to treat or monitor the patient then become vectors for transmission of these highly virulent and now antibiotic-resistant pathogens. Masks to cover the nose and mouth, short or covered hair, frequent hand washing and other appropriate isolation practices can never be overemphasized.

With the exception of aerobic-anaerobic mixtures, normally present in the mouth and large bowel, ENDOGENOUS flora is relatively innocuous. Nevertheless, if such microscopic ecologies are altered by the introduction of some potent and entirely foreign set of organisms, subsequent infection with highly virulent species can take place whenever normal protective barriers are lost or sufficiently impaired. An all-too-common example is the replacement of a relatively bland skin flora by resistant strains of *Staphylococcus aureus* during a prolonged preoperative hospital stay. The increase in clean wound infections then is directly proportional to the duration of hospitalization prior to operation and is almost entirely accounted for by incisional infections due to the

TABLE 6–2.–RELATIONSHIP OF INGUINAL HERNIORRHAPHY WOUND INFECTION TO LENGTH
OF PREOPERATIVE HOSPITAL STAY
(Pediatric Surgical Service – Grady Memorial Hospital – 1963 through 1966)

PREOPERATIVE STAY (Days)	NUMBER OF OPERATIONS	WOUNDS INFECTED	INCIDENCE OF INFECTION	INFECTIONS DUE TO STAPHYLOCOCCUS AUREUS	PROPORTION OF INFECTIONS DUE TO STAPHYLOCOCCUS
1	213	5	2.3%	2	40%
2	184	9	4.9%	7	78%
3	101	11	10.9%	10	91%
4	37	9	24.3%	8	89%
5	21	8	38.1%	8	100%
TOTAL	556	42	7.6%	35	83%

Acquisition of more virulent and antibiotic-resistant bacterial species as a part of the skin flora occurs with an increasing frequency as the duration of preoperative stay is prolonged, thereby producing a greater infection rate in the elective clean case.

newly acquired pathogen (Table 6-2). Such data lend further support to the concept of outpatient surgery and exceedingly brief preoperative stays.

Operations on the oropharynx and colon offer the only other significant threats by an endogenous set of microbes. It is for this reason that preoperative cleansing of the large bowel should without exception be accomplished by mechanical as well as antimicrobial means. For the latter, oral nonabsorbable agents effective against both components of the mixed flora should be used, i.e., neomycin or kanamycin for the aerobes, erythromycin base for the anaerobes.[4]

Nutrient Substrate

For growth of the initial inoculum there always must be some form of substrate from which the pathogens can derive nourishment. Accumulations of blood or its products, necrotic tissue or otherwise healthy areas with curtailed local resistance offer ideal nutrient media for the infecting microbes. The only other component necessary for pathogen existence is water, and that is generously provided by all open wounds and every mucosal surface. Thus, if infection is to be avoided, masses of nonviable tissue must be removed and any space with potential for the collection of blood or serum should be obliterated.

The chances of infection developing in a blood clot within an open wound or within a wound that has been drained are significantly greater than if an identical hematoma has been left undisturbed in a closed injury.[5] Seldom do infections arise in an ecchymosis, contusion or fracture unless the depths of the wound or its clot have been exposed to bacterial contamination by operation, attempts at aspiration or external communication through a drain. Likewise, the traumatic or surgically incised wound has a high risk of infection whenever a sizable clot is allowed to collect, regardless of whether wound closure was performed under the so-called sterile conditions of an operating room or without attention to such antiseptic details.

Host Resistance

There are three functional elements in host resistance: (1) external barriers, (2) a phagocytic system and (3) the immune mechanism. Although each has a different responsibility—prevention of initial invasion, the immediate local response to that invasion and a later mobilization of more specific anti-infectious factors, respectively—their activities overlap in regard to temporal relationships as well as in mutual support.

Effective BARRIERS to pathogen invasion are routinely provided by the skin and mucous membranes. Any disruption in continuity or failure in repletion of these surface linings immediately places the host in jeopardy. In addition, under certain physiologic conditions and at specific stages in life, the protection offered by these barriers is relatively incomplete. Examples are the skin of the neonate to aerobic gram-positive cocci; the intestinal mucosa of prematures to various gram-negative rods, especially after a hypoxic or ischemic insult to the bowel, thereby leading to necrotizing enterocolitis; and the penetrability of the small bowel lining to animate and inanimate objects, such as *Candida albicans* and starch at any age.[6] This almost unimpeded passage of matter across a mucosal barrier, as first described by Volkheimer and Schulz[7] and termed PERSORPTION by them, may well be the mechanism by which many instances of neonatal sepsis evolve.

PHAGOCYTES are generally classified according to their mobility and number of nuclei. The mononuclear tissue histiocytes are not fixed but roam freely throughout the extracellular fluid spaces. Any acute inflammatory process, however, increases both their local number and the intensity of their activity. On the other hand, chronicity of infection appears to favor the development of multiple nuclei. MONOCYTES behave similarly, yet always seem to maintain their mononuclear state. These, like the *polymorphonuclear granulocytes* (neutrophilic and eosinophilic), are blood borne and arrive at the site of infection by passage through the endothelial walls of congested capillaries. More fixed phagocytes, such as *Kupffer cells* in the liver, line vascular channels and eliminate circulating pathogens as well as foreign matter that have reached the bloodstream.

Phagocytes ingest particulate material in an ameboid fashion. Initially there is *chemotaxis*, that is, a chemical attraction of the phagocyte toward an infectious focus or autogenous waste product. Prior tagging to identify as foreign or for partial neutralization *(opsonization)* often is required prior to ingestion. Enzymatic digestion of such incorporated substances occurs in the intracellular vacuoles, final eradication of the infectious agent taking place on its absorption into the phagocyte's own cytoplasm. At times, however, ingested bacteria or their products are of sufficient potency to destroy the phagocyte prior to ingestion; or, if the vacuole wall has been disrupted, the release of contained lysozymes can lead to a destructive autodigestion.

Immune Mechanism

There are two major divisions to the immune system.[8] One, the HUMORAL MECHANISM, is thymic-independent and is based on bursal-cell lymphocytes and plasma cells. The other component is made up of thymic-dependent lymphocytes and is essentially a CELLULAR MECHANISM.

B-CELL SYSTEM.—Ehrlich repeatedly stressed the importance of humoral antibodies and their role in toxin neutralization, tagging of foreign matter for opsonization and actual lysis of invading cellular pathogens.[9] The reactive components of this system are produced by plasma cells and nonthymic-dependent lymphocytes that reside in the bone marrow and in the germinal centers and medullary cords of lymph nodes.[8] These account for most of the human immunity against extracellular bacterial species.

Immunity provided by the B-cell system consists of both (1) heat-stable, relatively specific antibodies and (2) heat-labile, relatively nonspecific complement. ANTIBODY reactor sites combine with antigen to form either soluble macromolecular compounds or insoluble complexes that precipitate or agglutinate. Although such humoral substances are actively circulating, they vary considerably in concentration, diffusibility, size and many other properties according to their own particular class of immune globulin (Table 6-3).

COMPLEMENT is consumed whenever the humoral system has been activated.[8] The classic reaction is a cascading system of at least nine complement components. However, endotoxin, properdin and other proteins are known to activate this sequence as well; that is referred to as the alternate pathway.

T-CELL SYSTEM.—The cellular component of immunity was first championed by Metchnikoff long before our present understanding of its thymic dependency.[9] The system is based on sensitized lymphocytes, probably of thymic origin, that are located in subcortical regions of lymph nodes

TABLE 6–3.—CHARACTERISTICS OF HUMAN IMMUNOGLOBULINS

	IgG	IgA	IgM	IgD	IgE
Origin	Plasma cell	Local lymphoid cells	–	Lymphocytes	Local lymphoid cells
Location	Intravascular & extravascular	Secretions	Intravascular	Intravascular	Intravascular and secretions
Half-life (days)	20–25	5–8	5	3	1–2
Molecular weight	150,000	175,000	900,000	150,000	200,000
Present in fetus	Transplacental	In colostrum	+++	+	?
Placental transfer	++	0	0	0	?
Complement binding	++	0	++	0	0
Average adult concentration (mg/100 ml)	1250	300	120	4	0.1

Human immunoglobulins are of five basic types, each having its own physiologic, molecular and longevity characteristics.

and in the periarterial spaces of the spleen that together form a part of the recirculating lymphocyte pool.[8] The T-cells are specifically responsible for immunity to viruses, most fungi and intracellular bacteria.

Host Deficiency States

An increased susceptibility to infection is regularly noted whenever some component of the host defense mechanism is absent, reduced in absolute numbers or significantly curtailed in function. Such derangements may have a congenital basis, although the majority are acquired as a direct result of drugs, radiation, endocrine disease, surgical ablation, tumors or bacterial toxins.

BARRIER DEFECTS.—Any alteration in timing, magnitude or quality of the host inflammatory response may permit the immediate invasion of pathogens. These defects in local reaction to injury are noted with extreme degrees of vasoconstriction (pheochromocytoma and shock), in thyroid excess as well as deficiency states and with both endogenous and exogenous hypercorticoidism (Cushing's syndrome). In addition, if the barrier has been injured by physical or chemical trauma (e.g., burns), fails to repair or loses its impenetrability (persorption), microbial invasion can occur. Apparently all three of these mechanisms are responsible for sepsis whenever a normal drainage system becomes obstructed (nephrolithiasis, cholangitis, etc).

PHAGOCYTE DEFICIENCY.—In diabetes mellitus there often is a failure of leukocytes to respond normally to chemotaxis. Measurable reductions in number of mature phagocytes are noted in leukemia, agranulocytosis and marrow dysplasia. Tumor, drugs (chloramphenicol and steroids), radiation or some other form of hematopoietic involution account for many of these derangements. Nevertheless, an impairment in phagocyte function as caused by various bacterial toxins can be just as dangerous to the host, if not more so.[6]

IMMUNE DEFICIENCIES.—Susceptibility to a specific infection in cases of an immune defect is based on which of the two systems is involved. B-CELL DEFICIENCIES are associated with extracellular bacterial sepsis, especially that due to pneumococci, *Hemophilus influenzae* and meningococcus. Often there is a fulminating course that rapidly ends in death despite timely and energetic anti-infectious measures.[10] Although congenital dysgammaglobulinemias have been the most publicized, other causes of these humoral defects include radiation, steroid and antimetabolite therapy, sepsis,[6] splenectomy[10] and starvation.[11]

T-CELL DEFICIENCIES are responsible for many viral, fungal and intracellular bacterial infections. Cutaneous candidiasis is a good example. DiGeorge's syndrome is a developmental anomaly whereby both thymic and parathyroid glands are deficient, thus explaining the combination of a propensity for infection and hypocalcemic tetany during infancy. Bacterial toxins,[6] immunosuppressive drugs, starvation[11] and radiation can also produce such defects.

Specific Types of Surgical Infection

Clinical infection presents in several different ways, each dependent on characteristics of the individual pathogens, area of the body infected, pre-existing local conditions (i.e., trauma, blood supply, etc.), the inflammatory response to injury and both general and specific resistance of the host to that infection. Chronologic age of the child, maturity of the newborn, state of nutrition, complicating diseases and concomitant drug therapy also influence manifestations of infection. Nevertheless, local signs of inflammation usually are present, even if late in their appearance, and are located within the site of infection proper, at its immediate periphery or both. These classically include pain and tenderness, increased local temperature, erythema and swelling or edema.

Systemic signs are not as specific, especially in the neonate. Although fever, tachycardia, irrational behavior and leukocytosis develop regularly in older children, the newborn seldom reveals such changes. Lethargy, refusal of feedings, jaundice and thrombocytopenia may be the only indications of life-threatening infection in the premature infant or term newborn. As a general rule, whenever any baby fails to suckle or performs abnormally in any way, sepsis should be suspected immediately.

Cellulitis

A diffuse inflammatory response in the absence of tissue necrosis or loculated pus is called CELLULITIS. In this case, the vascular component of inflammation is characteristically extreme. Complications reflect the natural course of the disease and include conversion of initial areas of inflammation to gangrene, development of isolated abscesses and eventually a bacteremia that can progress to lethal septicemia.

The usual cause of cellulitis is infection by beta-hemolytic streptococci or *Staphylococcus aureus*. Occasionally both species may be present in a symbiosis. In other types of infection there usually is a halo of cellulitis at the interface between active infection and unaffected host tissue. Cellulitis is relatively common. Its most virulent form, due to a streptococcal infection, generally is referred to as erysipelas. The SCALDED-SKIN SYNDROME in infants and children is a good example of how destructive staphylococcal enzymes can become. The resultant area of infectious cellulitis is almost indistinguishable from a partial-thickness burn.[12]

The treatment of cellulitis is almost entirely based on parenteral antibiotics specific for the presumed causative organisms. Preferred agents are the penicillins, cephalosporins and erythromycin macrolides. The intense erythema so characteristic of this infection guarantees a rapid delivery of antibiotic to the area of infection. Initial chemotherapy then should be maintained unless the clinical course does not improve or primary cultures grow antibiotic-resistant species. Continued observation is also warranted to detect any major complication, such as gangrene or abscess formation.

Phlegmon

If inflammation is relatively diffuse and yet there are small areas of necrosis and accumulated pus, the infection is referred to as a PHLEGMON. Initially, the process appears to be a cellulitis, but progression of the infection into innumerable small abscesses is followed by multifocal tissue destruction. This compartmentalization of the infection into multiple pockets is a result of normal tissue plane division by intersecting strands of collagen. Thus, the development of a phlegmon is somewhat tissue dependent, e.g., the carbuncle over the nape of the neck, transmural gastritis, etc.

Staphylococcus aureus, often in combination with a virulent strain of streptococcus, is the usual pathogen. Nevertheless, gram-negative rods in synergism with various anaerobes have also been incriminated.

Initial treatment is similar to that for cellulitis; that is, intravenously administered large doses of appropriate antibiotics. If significant necrosis develops, wide debridement usually is required. The more minute abscesses may be resorbed but conglomeration into one or more large pockets of suppuration requires drainage. In general, the phlegmon is a much more destructive, fulminant and refractory process than an uncomplicated cellulitis.

Abscess

When an infection is limited to a single anatomic space by an area of granulations, necrotic tissue and purulent exudate collect in one or more identifiable cavities. The inflammatory process then is said to have suppurated and thereby to have formed an ABSCESS. The purulent fluid contained within the abscess consists of partially degraded host tissues, both living and dead bacteria, various components of the phagocytic system (primarily neutrophilic granulocytes) and extracellular fluid. The process usually begins within an identifiable wound or in an area of established inflammation. There then is rapid progression from small locules of suppuration into larger and larger pockets. Surrounding this is an area of intense inflammation, represented as a confining wall of cellulitis. Debris of both host and pathogen collect in the central cavity and active and invasive infection occurs along the periphery in the confining wall of inflammation.

Although abscesses can be caused by almost any combination of bacterial species, the usual culprits are hemolytic *Staphylococcus aureus*, various gram-negative rods and certain anaerobic bacteria, especially *Bacteroides fragilis.*[3] A significant role is played by the multiplicity of bacterial species often producing a synergism between aerobic gram-

negative rods, and any number of anaerobic microorganisms.

The cardinal treatment of all abscesses is drainage. The tract provided for escape of pus must establish a direct dependent drainage of the abscess to the outside through a relatively wide opening. Otherwise, drainage will be incomplete and result in a persistence of the infection, with the possibility of an even greater destruction of local tissue. If dependent drainage cannot be gained, sump suction should be used to overcome the force of gravity.

Antibiotics play only a secondary role in the treatment of abscesses. Nevertheless, if infection due to an undrained abscess has produced signs of a more generalized sepsis, appropriate parenteral antibiotics serve to destroy those bacteria that already have reached or continue to seed the bloodstream. Antibiotics also protect the host against the same bacteria that can be massaged into vascular channels during drainage of an abscess and contaminate the healthy tissues exposed by that surgical dissection. Mechanical scrubbing, forceful irrigation or snug packing of any abscess cavity further increases the magnitude of the associated bacteremia.

Gangrene

INFECTIOUS GANGRENE is caused by the direct action of microbial enzymes on otherwise healthy tissues or by a septic thrombosis of nutrient blood vessels serving the area. Both processes can occur simultaneously. In any event, the destruction of tissue usually is sufficient to produce grossly evident necrosis. According to the species of bacteria, tissues involved and general resistance of the host, infectious gangrene varies considerably with respect to rapidity and depth of necrosis as well as to its systemic manifestations.

Infectious gangrene is best classified on the basis of oxygen requirements of the individual pathogens and multiplicity of invading species. AEROBIC GANGRENE usually is due to a virulent strain of hemolytic streptococcus. Such infections may become epidemic on a hospital ward, yet they are merely an advanced and extreme form of streptococcal cellulitis. Treatment should be identical to that for erysipelas.

Other types of monobacterial aerobic gangrene occur in infections due to isolated bacterial species—Pseudomonas burn wound necrosis or pyodermum gangrenosa, the necrotizing adenopathy of anthrax and *Pasteurella pestis*, tularemia, etc. However, with the exception of that due to *Pseudomonas aeruginosa*, these are, at present, infrequent. Regardless of the cause, treatment requires wide debridement, with removal of all necrotic tissue, parenteral antibiotics appropriate to the pathogen to protect both bloodstream and freshly exposed tissue planes and some form of delayed wound closure.

ANAEROBIC GANGRENE classically is represented by the gas bacillus *Clostridium welchii*. The onset of GAS GANGRENE usually is sudden and progression is rapid. Tissues become dark, cool, brawny and occasionally crepitant; areas of hemorrhage develop at the margin of the infection; local pain is intense; any discharge from the wound is exceedingly foul smelling, brackish and watery; the patient develops a sustained high fever, becomes irrational and frequently is jaundiced.

Treatment must include radical debridement of any devitalized tissue, a widely open wound in anticipation of delayed closure many days hence and massive doses of penicillin or, if the patient is allergic, a tetracycline or cephalosporin given intravenously in concentrations sufficient to protect exposed adjacent tissues from contamination in the open wound.[13]

SYNERGISTIC GANGRENE is produced by the symbiosis of two or more bacterial species, with the resultant infection being more severe than either pathogen could cause alone. A progressive and recalcitrant surface ulceration (MELENEY'S CELLULITIS) is due to the combination of aerobic *Staphylococcus aureus* and an anaerobic Peptostreptococcus.[2] Other symbiotic gangrenous infections include: a fusiform bacillus with a spirochete, the combination producing an ulcerative infection of the gingiva (TRENCH MOUTH); various combinations of gram-positive cocci, leading to destruction of tissues about the nose and mouth (CANCRUM ORIS or NOMA); and synergisms involving anaerobic species, especially *Bacteroides fragilis*, and aerobic gram-negative rods, the latter infections being called NECROTIZING FASCIITIS or CELLULITIS.[14]

Synergistic gangrene demands the same basic treatment as do other forms of necrotizing infection; i.e., immediate and wide debridement of all nonviable tissue, delayed wound closure, usually by skin grafting, and large intravenous doses of appropriate antibiotics begun prior to the operative excision. Less than complete debridement leads to a persistence of gangrenous infection and is followed by extension into previously uninvolved tissues.

Toxemias

Although most infections are mediated by toxin injury of host tissues locally, certain serious forms of sepsis maintain a relatively small primary focus; yet, their virulence factors (exotoxins) are absorbed into vascular channels and exert a significantly destructive and generally disruptive influence at some distant site. Accordingly, such infections are appropriately referred to as TOXEMIAS. The classic example is TETANUS, where the site of toxin production appears to be an otherwise innocuous minor wound. Nevertheless, systemic manifestations are profound and frequently lethal. In tetanus toxemia, the central nervous system is primarily affected with irritability; muscle spasm, convulsions, coma and respiratory arrest are the stages in clinical progression to death. Two other equally life-threatening toxemias are DIPHTHERIA, arising from infection of the pharynx by *Corynebacterium diphtheriae* (a cardiac toxin producer) and Pseu-domonas wound sepsis, toxin absorbed from the heavily colonized burn wound inhibiting the reticuloendothelial system.

Initial treatment of toxemias should include: massive doses of intravenously administered antibiotic, appropriate to the infecting species; correction of fluid and electrolyte deficits, to make general anesthesia safer; and the administration of specific antitoxin, preferably of human origin. Wide excision of the site of infection, when feasible, with delayed wound closure is the only reliable method of final control. Preventive measures are much more effective, and these have been especially well defined in the case of tetanus wound prophylaxis.[15]

Septicemia

When bacteria invade the bloodstream, either through infection or by contamination of some intravascular monitoring or treatment device, the condition is said to be a BACTEREMIA. Progression to actual multiplication of bacteria within the blood vascular compartment creates a SEPTICEMIA and poses one of the greatest threats to continued host survival. Live bacteria, bacterial enzymes and tissue breakdown products (especially of erythrocyte and leukocyte origin) then circulate and exert profound pharmacologic influences on various organ systems. Peripheral pooling of blood, heart failure, various coagulopathies and many other phenomena can develop. A characteristic vasomotor collapse secondary to gram-negative bacteremia or septicemia generally is referred to as ENDOTOXEMIA. Individual reactions to different bacterial toxins as well as to host catabolic products produce somewhat specific clinical syndromes that can be differentiated into gram-positive, gram-negative, anaerobic or fungal septicemia (Table 6-4).

Unless the focus of origin is eradicated, bacteremia will persist and may progress to septicemia. As soon as possible, abscesses must be drained, necrotic tissue excised and venous cannulas removed. Parenteral antibiotics with activity against the presumed pathogens should also be given in large doses.

Sepsis in the Newborn

With the event of birth, the newly born infant enters a pathogen-filled world from a relatively GERMFREE ENVIRON-

TABLE 6-4.—CLINICAL DIFFERENTIATION OF SEPTICEMIAS

	GRAM-POSITIVE	GRAM-NEGATIVE	ENDOTOXEMIA	ANAEROBIC	FUNGAL
Sensorium	Irrational	Rational	Irrational	Irrational	Rational
Temperature	Spiking 39–40° C	Sustained 38–39° C	Falling hypothermia	Spiking 39–40° C	Sustained 38–39° C
Blood pressure	Gradual fall	Gradual fall, to sudden shock	Sudden shock	Gradual fall	Gradual fall
Urine flow	Gradual oliguria	Oliguria until sudden anuria	Sudden anuria	Gradual oliguria	Gradual oliguria
Jaundice	Often	Rare	—	Common	Rare
White blood count	> 16,000	10–16,000	< 6000	> 14,000	> 14,000
Urine microscopic	—	—	—	—	Yeast
Wound appearance	Dissolution of granulations	Focal necrosis of granulations	Enlarging focal necrosis	Extensive gangrene	Occasional focal necrosis
Wound odor	Sour/sweetish	—	—	Putrid	—
Source of infection	Soft tissues IV site Respiratory tract	Abdominal Urinary Incision (wound) Pulmonary	Abdominal Urinary Burn wound	Abdominal Perineal Pulmonary	Alimentary Intravenous

The microbe responsible for a given septicemia often can be diagnosed with a fair degree of accuracy on purely clinical findings.

MENT. Less than 10% of babies are delivered from a contaminated uterus.[16] From that moment on, life is an ever-expanding challenge by the microscopic milieu. The skin, mouth and alimentary tract are initially colonized by microbes from the maternal introitus. Thereafter, the infant's endogenous flora is gradually supplanted by microorganisms from his immediate environment.

The HOST DEFENSE MECHANISM already has developed by term, although its full competence still must be gained through subsequent contact with pathogens. In the premature, on the other hand, many such defense mechanisms have not yet reached a maturity sufficient either to produce an effective nonspecific response or to permit the acquisition of more specific competence. For example, at birth, only maternal IgG antibodies that have crossed the placental barrier are present. These provide resistance to most viral infections but little against bacteria. Shortly thereafter, IgM levels are detectable; local intestinal antibodies, specifically those of the IgA fraction, are uniformly lacking until acquired orally from colostrum and maternal milk of the first several postpartum days.[17]

Normal BARRIERS to invasive infection are also poorly established. Skin and the intestinal tract are particularly vulnerable to penetration by some newly acquired pathogen. Breaks in the skin for intravenous feeding and monitoring as well as external conduits into the airway (endotracheal tubes) and urinary tract (catheters) offer ready access to the hospital microbial flora, especially since it is the premature infant or the neonate with a major congenital anomaly whose hospitalization is protracted. In this light, the increasing incidence of serious infection is not at all surprising.

The DIAGNOSIS of newborn sepsis usually is made by culture confirmation of a clinical suspicion.[16] Reduced activity (lethargy, rare spontaneous motion, refusal to suck, etc.), a depressed nervous system (absent or poor Moro reflex), paralytic ileus (refusal to feed, abdominal distention and eventually vomiting), respiratory distress (overt pneumonia, hypoxia, etc.), convulsions or coma (meningitis) and pallor can be ominous signs, even if occurring singly. Laboratory studies are of little value, although thrombocytopenia, acidosis or jaundice always makes sepsis a real possibility. Blood, spinal fluid and urine cultures, however, are the only

reliable tests, as these can be positive in the absence of essentially all physical signs. Fever and leukocytosis seldom if ever are seen before the tenth day of life. Until appropriate cultures have been reported, antimicrobial therapy is undertaken whenever sepsis is suspected. Antibiotics should be chosen for their reliable activity against the more common nursery pathogens as determined by almost monthly epidemiologic surveys[5, 16] and changed if necessary when the organism is identified. Gram-negative rods and gram-positive cocci are the usual isolates, although Listeria and other equally rare pathogens are noted occasionally. Anaerobes are also uncommon, even when a severe gastrointestinal infection such as necrotizing enterocolitis has perforated (Table 6–5).

DRUG TOXICITY must also be feared. More immediate reactions, such as those due to chloramphenicol, are obvious. It is late sequelae that might arise from aminoglycosides (deafness and renal failure) that present an uncertain future.

Postoperative Wound Infection

At some time during the postoperative course, children often become febrile. Certainly, infection does occur after operation or injury, but there are many other and perhaps more common causes of postoperative fever. Nevertheless, infection must be suspected and prime areas of involvement investigated. The common foci are the lungs, urinary tract, veins used for intravenous lines and the surgical wound.

The postoperative day on which a given wound infection becomes manifest and the local signs of sepsis vary according to the bacteria responsible for the infection and the concomitant use of specific antiseptic measures, such as parenteral antibiotics (Table 6–6). As a general rule, the earlier the onset of wound sepsis the more destructive and life-threatening the infection will become.

Treatment of the infected surgical incision is straightforward. The wound must be opened throughout its length and the patient positioned so as to obtain reliably dependent drainage; if tissue necrosis is extensive, careful debridement should be performed.[14] The wound then is allowed to close spontaneously by contracture, with split-skin grafts or through rotation of a pedicled flap—the specific technique selected being appropriate for the size, type and location of the surface defect.

Antibiotics

Different antimicrobial agents have different sites of action. Some destroy bacteria by "punching holes" in the cell wall (i.e., penicillins); others act as detergents and disrupt the cell membrane (i.e., polymyxin); still others interfere with nucleic acid replication during protein synthesis (aminoglycosides). Finally, several antimicrobials (primarily the sulfonamides) block one or more metabolic steps in the production of some critical substrate (i.e., folic acid). Resistance to these antimicrobial effects can develop along one of several lines: elaboration of an enzyme to block or destroy the antibiotic (i.e., penicillinase), passive transfer of chromosome-like resistance factors (R factors), actual mutation into a new and resistant strain, activation of latent biochemical mechanisms or acquisition of a critical substrate from the local environment rather than relying on self-production.

Antibiotics preferred for infections due to specific bacterial species are listed in Table 6–7. At times, therapy with a combination of antibiotics may be required, especially if infection is due to a polymicrobial flora. For example, an

TABLE 6–5.—PERITONEAL CULTURES FROM PERFORATED NECROTIZING ENTEROCOLITIS
(Grady Memorial Hospital—40 Consecutive Infants)

PATHOGEN	NUMBER	% OF TOTAL
Klebsiella enterobacter	33	83
E. coli	30	75
Ps. aeruginosa	8	20
Other gram negatives	14	35
Enterococcus	20	50
Streptococcus	7	18
Staph. aureus	9	23
Staph. epidermidis	9	23
Anaerobes	3	8
Candida albicans	1	3
Miscellaneous	7	18

The bacterial flora of the peritoneal cavity as noted in infants with perforated necrotizing enterocolitis is mixed, primarily gram negative and almost uniformly aerobic.

TABLE 6–6.—POSTOPERATIVE WOUND INFECTIONS
(Time of Onset, Usual Pathogen and Clinical Findings)

ONSET (PO Day)	USUAL PATHOGEN	WOUND APPEARANCE	OTHER SIGNS
1–3	*Clostridium welchii*	Brawny, hemorrhagic, cool Occasional gaseous crepitance Putrid "dishwater" exudate Intense local pain	High sustained fever (39–40° C) Irrational Leukocytosis >15,000/mm³ Occasional jaundice
2–3	Streptococcus	Erythematous, warm, tender Occasionally hemorrhagic with blebs Serous exudate	High spiking fever (39–40° C) Irrational at times Leukocytosis >15,000/mm³ Rare jaundice
3–5	Staphylococcus	Erythematous, warm, tender Purulent exudate	High spiking fever (38–40° C) Irrational at times Leukocytosis 12,000–20,000/mm³
>5	Gram-negative rod	Erythematous, warm, tender Purulent exudate	Sustained low-grade to moderate fever (38–39° C) Rational Leukocytosis 10,000–16,000/mm³
>5	Symbiotic (usually anaerobes plus gram-negative rods)	Erythematous, warm, tender Focal necrosis Purulent, putrid exudate	Moderate to high fever (38–40° C) Leukocytosis >15,000/mm³ Occasional jaundice Mentation variable

The bacteria responsible for a given postoperative wound infection usually can be predicted on the basis of time of onset of sepsis, wound appearance and systemic response.

aminoglycoside plus penicillin, with or without clindamycin, often is selected for treatment of peritonitis of colonic origin.

Risk of infection in the contaminated wound can be diminished considerably by use of delayed primary wound closure on the third to fifth postoperative day or with instillation of some topical antimicrobial directly into the wound prior to primary closure.[14] When wound contamination is predictable, however, an appropriate parenteral antibiotic can provide a moderate degree of protection against subsequent wound infection if such an agent is given before operation in time to establish bactericidal levels in the exposed tissues and local extracellular fluid. In any case, antibiotic use for prophylaxis must be selective, never indiscriminate, since even greater problems can be created by the evolution of antibiotic-resistant strains.

REFERENCES

1. Gorbach, S. L., and Bartlett, J. G.: Anaerobic infections, N. Engl. J. Med. 290:1177, 1237, 1289, 1974.
2. Meleney, F. L.: Hemolytic streptococcus gangrene, Arch. Surg. 9:317, 1924.
3. Stone, H. H., Kolb, L. D., and Geheber, C. E.: Incidence and significance of intraperitoneal anaerobic bacteria, Ann. Surg. 181:705, 1975.
4. Washington, J. A., II, *et al.*: Effect of preoperative antibiotic regimen on development of infection after intestinal surgery; prospective, randomized, double-blind study, Ann. Surg. 180:567, 1974.
5. Cruse, P. J. E., and Foord, R.: A five-year prospective study of 23,649 surgical wounds, Arch. Surg. 107:206, 1973.
6. Stone, H. H., *et al.*: Candida sepsis; pathogenesis and principles of treatment, Ann. Surg. 179:697, 1974.
7. Volkheimer, G., and Schulz, F. H.: The phenomenon of persorption, Digestion 1:213, 1968.
8. Bellanti, J. A., and Hurtado, R. C.: Immunology and Resistance to Infection, in Remington, J. S., and Klein, J. O. (eds.), *Infectious Diseases of the Fetus and Newborn Infant* (Philadelphia: W. B. Saunders Company, 1976).
9. Dubos, R.: The Evolution of Medical Microbiology, in Dubos, R. J., and Hirsch, J. G. (eds.), *Bacterial and Mycotic Infections of Man* (Philadelphia: J. B. Lippincott Company, 1968).
10. Likhite, V. V.: Immunological impairment and susceptibility to infection after splenectomy, JAMA 236:1376, 1976.
11. Copeland, E. M., MacFadyen, B. V., and Dudrick, S. J.: Effect of intravenous hyperalimentation on established delayed hypersensitivity in the cancer patient, Ann. Surg. 184:60, 1976.
12. Melish, M. D., and Glasgow, L. A.: The staphylococcal scalded-skin syndrome, N. Engl. J. Med. 282:114, 1970.
13. Altemeier, W. A., and Fullen, W. D.: Prevention and treatment of gas gangrene, JAMA 217:806, 1971.
14. Stone, H. H.: Prophylactic Measures for Wound Infection, in Varco, R. L., and Delaney, J. P. (eds.), *Controversy in Surgery* (Philadelphia: W. B. Saunders Company, 1976).
15. Committee on Trauma, American College of Surgeons: Prophylaxis against tetanus in wound management, Bull. Am. Coll. Surgeons 57:32, 1972.
16. Klein, J. O., Remington, J. S., and March, S. M.: An Introduction to Infections of the Fetus and Newborn Infant, in Remington, J. S., and Klein, J. O. (eds.), *Infectious Diseases of the Fetus and Newborn Infant* (Philadelphia: W. B. Saunders Company, 1976).
17. Editorial: Oral immunization and antibodies in milk, Lancet 1:77, 1976.

TABLE 6-7.—ANTIMICROBIAL DRUGS

INFECTING ORGANISM	ANTIMICROBIALS	
	First Choice	Alternatives
GRAM-POSITIVE COCCI		
Streptococcus pyogenes		
(Groups A, B, C and G)	Penicillin G	Erythromycin; cephalosporin
(Viridans group)	Penicillin G	Cephalosporin; erythromycin with streptomycin
Enterococcus	Penicillin G	Plus gentamicin or tobramycin
Streptococcus, anaerobic	Penicillin G	Tetracycline; erythromycin
Diplococcus pneumoniae	Penicillin G	Erythromycin; lincomycin; chloramphenicol
Staphylococcus aureus		
(Nonpenicillinase)	Penicillin G	Lincomycin; cephalosporin; gentamicin; tobramycin
(Penicillinase)	Penicillinase-resistant Penicillins	Lincomycin; cephalosporin; gentamicin; tobramycin
GRAM-NEGATIVE COCCI		
Neisseria meningitidis	Penicillin G	Chloramphenicol; tetracycline; erythromycin; sulfonamide
Neisseria gonorrhoeae	Penicillin G	Ampicillin; tetracycline
GRAM-POSITIVE BACILLI		
Bacillus anthracis (anthrax)	Penicillin G	Erythromycin; tetracycline
Listeria monocytogenes	Penicillin/ampicillin	Tetracycline; erythromycin
Clostridium welchii (gas gangrene)	Penicillin G	Erythromycin; tetracycline
Clostridium tetani	Penicillin G	Tetracycline
Corynebacterium diphtheriae	Penicillin G	Erythromycin
GRAM-NEGATIVE BACILLI		
Salmonella	Chloramphenicol	Ampicillin
Shigella	Ampicillin	Oral kanamycin; tetracycline; chloramphenicol
Escherichia coli	Gentamicin/tobramycin	Cephalosporin; ampicillin; kanamycin; tetracycline
Klebsiella pneumoniae	Gentamicin/tobramycin	Cephalosporin; kanamycin; chloramphenicol
Enterobacter (Aerobacter)	Gentamicin/tobramycin	Kanamycin; chloramphenicol
Serratia	Gentamicin/tobramycin	Kanamycin; chloramphenicol
Proteus		
(*Mirabilis*)	Ampicillin	Cephalosporin; gentamicin; tobramycin; kanamycin
(Other)	Gentamicin/tobramycin	Kanamycin; carbenicillin; chloramphenicol
Providencia	Gentamicin/tobramycin	Carbenicillin
Mima, Herellea	Kanamycin	Gentamicin/tobramycin
Pseudomonas aeruginosa		
(Urinary tract infection)	Carbenicillin	Gentamicin/tobramycin/amikacin
(Other infections)	Gentamicin/tobramycin	Plus carbenicillin/amikacin alone
Bacteroides		
(Respiratory strains)	Penicillin G	Clindamycin; chloramphenicol; lincomycin; ampicillin; tetracycline; erythromycin
(Gastrointestinal strains)	Clindamycin	Chloramphenicol; lincomycin
Actinobacillus mallei (glanders)	Streptomycin with tetracycline	Streptomycin with chloramphenicol
Pseudomonas pseudomallei (melioidosis)	Tetracycline	Chloramphenicol
Brucella (brucellosis)	Tetracycline	Chloramphenicol plus streptomycin
Pasteurella tularensis (tularemia)	Streptomycin	Tetracycline
Pasteurella pestis (bubonic plague)	Streptomycin	Tetracycline
Pasteurella multocida	Penicillin	Tetracycline
Hemophilus influenzae		
(Respiratory infections)	Ampicillin	Tetracycline; streptomycin; sulfonamide
(Meningitis)	Ampicillin (P)	Chloramphenicol; tetracycline
Hemophilus ducreyi (chancroid)	Tetracycline	Sulfonamide; streptomycin
Hemophilus pertussis (whooping cough)	Erythromycin	Tetracycline; ampicillin
Fusobacterium fusiforme (Vincent's infection)	Penicillin G	Tetracycline; erythromycin
Calymmatobacterium granulomatis (granuloma inguinale)	Tetracycline	Streptomycin; ampicillin
Vibrio cholerae (cholera)	Tetracycline	Chloramphenicol; erythromycin

INFECTING ORGANISM	ANTIMICROBIALS	
	First Choice	Alternatives
ACID-FAST BACILLI		
Mycobacterium tuberculosis	Isoniazid with ethambutol	Rifampin; para-aminosalicylic acid (PASA) plus streptomycin plus streptomycin
Atypical mycobacteria	Isoniazid with ethambutol	Rifampin; ethionamide; cycloserine plus streptomycin
Mycobacterium balnei (marinum)	Cycloserine	Isoniazid; rifampin
Mycobacterium leprae (leprosy)	Sulfone	Amithiozone
SPIROCHETES		
Spirillum minus (rat-bite fever)	Penicillin G	Erythromycin; streptomycin
Borrelia recurrentis (relapsing fever)	Tetracycline	Penicillin G
Treponema pallidum (syphilis)	Penicillin G	Tetracycline; erythromycin
Treponema pertenue (yaws)	Penicillin G	Tetracycline; erythromycin
Leptospira	Penicillin G	Tetracycline
ACTINOMYCETES		
Actinomyces israelii (actinomycosis)	Penicillin G	Tetracycline; erythromycin
Actinomyces muris-ratti (rat-bite fever)	Ampicillin	Erythromycin; streptomycin
Nocardia	Sulfonamide with streptomycin	Tetracycline with cycloserine; sulfonamide with ampicillin
RICKETTSIA (Rocky Mountain spotted fever; endemic typhus; Q fever)	Tetracycline	Chloramphenicol
FUNGI		
Histoplasma capsulatum	Amphotericin B	
Candida albicans	Oral nystatin	Amphotericin B; flucytosine
Aspergillus	Amphotericin B	Flucytosine
Cryptococcus neoformans	Amphotericin B	Flucytosine
Mucor	Amphotericin B	
Coccidioides immitis	Amphotericin B	
Blastomyces dermatitidis (N. Amer.)	Amphotericin B	Hydroxystilbamidine
Blastomyces brasiliensis (S. Amer.)	Amphotericin B	A sulfonamide
Sporotrichum schenckii	Iodide	Amphotericin B; griseofulvin
Fonsecaea (chromoblastomycosis)	Amphotericin B	
Dermatophytes (tinea)	Griseofulvin	
MISCELLANEOUS		
Mycoplasma pneumoniae	Erythromycin	Tetracycline
Psittacosis (ornithosis)	Tetracycline	Chloramphenicol
Lymphogranuloma venereum	Tetracycline	Chloramphenicol; sulfonamide
Chlamydia trachomatis (trachoma)	Tetracycline (tropical)	Erythromycin (oral); chloramphenicol (tropical); sulfonamide (oral)
Inclusion conjunctivitis	Tetracycline (oral or topical)	Chloramphenicol (topical)
Vaccinia	Methisazone	Plus vaccinia immune globulin
Herpes simplex (keratitis)	Idoxuridine (topical)	
Influenza A	Amantadine	

Until culture sensitivity tests have been reported and are available to guide antibiotic therapy more accurately, choice of an antimicrobial agent generally is based on known responsiveness of specific bacterial species.

Cancer Chemotherapy

THE EVOLUTION OF TREATMENT for childhood cancer has expanded areas of overlapping skill into multidisciplinary programs. At present, four major disciplines are in clinical use: surgery, radiation therapy, chemotherapy and, to a limited extent, immunotherapy. Prior to initiation of treatment, a plan for over-all care is formulated by interdisciplinary consultation. This chapter is concerned with the potential contribution of chemotherapy. outlines indications for chemotherapy and discusses agents commonly used in pediatric tumors.

Indications for Chemotherapy

The tactics and strategy for the application of chemotherapy must be individualized for each patient. The following represent circumstances in which chemotherapy has been found to be beneficial:

1. Preoperative administration with or without radiation therapy to facilitate removal of large tumors by reduction in tumor volume (for example, Wilms' tumor).
2. Concurrent with radiation therapy for lesions in surgically inaccessible sites (for example, rhabdomyosarcoma of the nasopharynx).
3. Concurrent with radiation therapy to avoid mutilative operative procedures (for example, rhabdomyosarcoma of the eye, genitourinary system and extremities).
4. Concurrent with radiation therapy to eradicate metastases (for example, pulmonary metastases from Wilms' tumor).
5. Palliation for disseminated disease.
6. "Adjuvant" therapy for micrometastases.

A large number of communications attest to the efficacy of chemotherapy administered for these indications. The rationale underlying its administration in "adjuvant" therapy deserves additional comment.

"Adjuvant" Chemotherapy

Operation and radiation therapy constitute the major weapons of primary treatment. They provide a rapid definitive attack on the primary lesion. These techniques, however, approach the limits of their utility, since they generally are useful only against localized disease. In most malignant disease, microscopic foci already are disseminated at presentation. Treatment for this complication is provided through systemic "adjuvant" chemotherapy and/or immunotherapy. Experimentally, such therapy is most effective if applied when the tumor burden is at its nadir, as achieved clinically with operation and/or radiation therapy. This has resulted in longer disease-free intervals, increases in survival times and high percentages of cures.[1-4] These principles have been successfully extrapolated to human cancer.[5-9]

Classification of Chemotherapeutic Agents

The chemotherapeutic armamentarium available to the clinician for the treatment of pediatric malignancies is conveniently classified into the following categories: antimetabolites, alkylating agents, plant extracts and miscellaneous types. The agents may produce a wide variety of acute and chronic complications and thus must be used with considerable caution. Many are also immunosuppressive. Some are used in association with radiation therapy, which not only enhances their therapeutic efficacy but also the potential for toxicity. For effective application, the physician should have a working knowledge of their specific antitumor activity, toxic side-effects and mechanism of action. These are outlined in Table 7–1.

Antimetabolites

An antimetabolite is an anticancer agent that is structurally similar to one of the normal components of the cell. As such, it binds to specific enzymes and decreases or blocks normal cellular activity. It may also be incorporated into cellular structures and inhibit activity because of its nonfunctional character.

METHOTREXATE.—This is the most common antimetabolite used for the treatment of solid tumors. It binds stoichiometrically and firmly to the enzyme dihydrofolate reductase. This interferes with the biochemical reduction of dihydrofolate to tetrohydrofolate, which is required for the synthesis of purines and pyrimidines (specifically, thymidylate). This results in inhibition of DNA synthesis and cell death.

The activity of methotrexate is modified by the following factors: ability to enter the cell, quantity of free intracellular methotrexate and rate of turnover of dihydrofolate reductase. Some of these factors may be responsible for the development of resistance. The antidote to methotrexate is folinic acid (citrovorum factor). This is the end product of the biochemical reaction inhibited by the antitumor agent. Thymidine and other deoxynucleoside bases have also been used experimentally to avert its toxic potential.

Clinically, methotrexate is administered either orally or parenterally and is excreted primarily by the kidneys. Methotrexate is used principally in the treatment of leukemia but in pediatric neoplasms it has also been utilized in the management of lymphomas and tumors containing trophoblastic elements. A more recent application has been in the treatment of osteogenic sarcoma. Here, massive doses of the drug are administered over several hours, followed, after a specified time interval, by the antidote, citrovorum factor (citrovorum factor "rescue").[10, 11] This form of treatment should be conducted only in specialized centers where pharmacologic facilities to measure the serum level of methotrexate are available.

Toxicity to methotrexate comprises myelosuppression, stomatitis, skin rashes and aberrations in liver and renal function. Alopecia is a rare complication. The chronic administration of methotrexate is associated with cirrhosis and osteoporosis. Prerequisites for treatment include a normal creatinine clearance, hemogram, hydration and liver function.

Alkylating Agents

Alkylating agents are compounds that directly or indirectly contribute an alkyl group (R-CH-) to other compounds, ions or elements. The anticancer effects of these substances probably result from the replacement of a hydrogen atom in the molecules of the DNA chain to be alkylated by the alkyl group. It is also possible that they affect RNA and protein synthesis. The drugs are classified into several categories: the nitrogen mustards (nitrogen mustard, chlorambucil and cyclophosphamide), methane sulfonates (busulfan), ethylene imines (thio-tepa and TEM) and epoxides (benzoquinone).

The parent alkylating agent is nitrogen mustard. It was developed as a by-product of a study on poisonous war substances and was one of the first agents to be used clinically. In pediatric practice, it is used principally in the lymphomas and neuroblastoma.[12, 13] Some degree of nausea and vomiting generally is observed after its administration. The dose-limiting toxicity is myelosuppression, with a nadir occurring approximately 2–3 weeks after administration. It is also utilized for intracavitary lesions. The drug must be administered intravenously immediately after reconstitution. Extravasation causes local ulceration and necrosis.

Cyclophosphamide has had more extensive application; it is used in soft tissue sarcomas, osteogenic sarcoma, neuroblastoma and the lymphomas.[14-16] The drug must be phosphorylated by the liver to its active compound. It has been administered by a variety of schedules either as daily oral or short intensive courses at more prolonged intervals. With large doses, nausea and vomiting will occur. Metabolites of the compound are excreted through the kidneys, and prolonged contact with the bladder mucosa will result in irreversible bladder fibrosis. This may present initially as hemorrhagic cystitis. Adequate hydration is, therefore, an important prerequisite for treatment. If hemorrhagic cystitis occurs, the drug should be interrupted until the urine returns to normal. With recurrent cystitis, the drug should be discontinued and an intravenous pyelogram should be obtained at regular intervals. Simultaneous administration of cyclophosphamide and radiation therapy to the pelvic area should be avoided, since this accentuates the possibility of hemorrhagic cystitis. Myelosuppression is a major dose-limiting toxicity. Large doses are also accompanied by nausea and vomiting and alopecia. Amenorrhea and aspermia have been noted in adults receiving cyclophosphamide. However, this may be reversible. Teratogenesis has also been reported with its administration.

Chlorambucil is an oral nitrogen mustard compound. It is used principally in the treatment of lymphomas. Its major dose-limiting toxicity is myelosuppression and blood counts should be obtained at frequent intervals. Diarrhea, dermatitis, nausea, vomiting and hepatic dysfunction have been noted occasionally.

The other alkylating agents are used rarely in modern pediatric practice. Busulfan is largely utilized in chronic myelogenous leukemia.

NITROSOUREAS.—This group of compounds is believed to possess moieties that act as alkylating agents. Their importance derives from their ability, because of their lipid solubility, to cross the blood-brain barrier in cytotoxic quantities. Consequently, they are used as investigational drugs in the treatment of brain neoplasms. They have also been administered to patients with lymphomas and Ewing's sarcoma.[17, 18] The major side-effects include nausea, vomiting and myelosuppression. BCNU is an intravenous preparation whereas CCNU and methyl CCNU may be administered by the oral route. They probably act by inhibiting DNA repair.

Antibiotics

A number of antibiotics with antitumor activity have been discovered. The majority demonstrate little or no effect against microorganisms.

ACTINOMYCIN D.—The actinomycins are a series of antibiotics originally derived from Streptomyces cultures by Waksman and Woodruff. The most commonly used is actinomycin D. It acts by intercalating between base pairs of DNA, thereby blocking DNA-directed RNA synthesis.

Clinical and experimental investigations have demonstrated that actinomycin D potentiates the action of radiation therapy, reactivates latent effects of radiation therapy in previously irradiated tissues (a "recall" phenomenon) and is tumoricidal. The drug is particularly effective in treating patients with Wilms' tumor. With localized disease, cure rates approaching 90% have been reported when the drug is used postoperatively in combination with radiation therapy.[5] In patients with disseminated disease, survival rates approaching 60% have been achieved. Actinomycin D is also used in combination with other agents for the treatment of rhabdomyosarcoma, Ewing's sarcoma and gonadal tumors.[7-9, 19, 20] In many of these tumors, disease-free survivals in the vicinity of 80% in patients with localized disease have been achieved.

Since actinomycin D enhances the lethal effects of radiation therapy, some reduction in the dose of irradiation may be required if sensitive structures are being irradiated. This applies particularly to the oral mucosa, liver and intestine. The drug is primarily excreted by the liver, and simultaneous administration of actinomycin D and radiation therapy to the liver may greatly enhance its toxicity. Accordingly, the dose should be modified in the presence of liver dysfunction. The principal side-effects include nausea and vomiting and myelosuppression. Less commonly encountered are alopecia, stomatitis, acneiform eruptions, rash and fever. The drug is administered intravenously. Perivascular extravasation produces a chemical cellulitis and ulceration.

DAUNORUBICIN AND ADRIAMYCIN.—These agents belong to the class of antibiotics known as the anthracyclines. They both are derived from Streptomyces peucetius. They have similar chemical and pharmacologic properties and probably exert their cytotoxic effects by intercalating in the major groove of the DNA helix, preventing both DNA transcription and replication. Daunorubicin was first described in Italy following discovery of the antibiotic daunomycin from cultures of Streptomyces peucetius. A product was independently isolated from Streptomyces coeruleorubidus in France and designated rubidomycin. The accepted generic name for both drugs is daunorubicin. Adriamycin, or 14-hydroxy-daunorubicin, was later isolated from Streptomyces peucetius caesius.

Adriamycin, rather than daunorubicin, appears to have major activity against most pediatric solid tumors. This includes Wilms' tumor, neuroblastoma, rhabdomyosarcoma, Ewing's sarcoma, osteogenic sarcoma and the lymphomas.[21-24]

The drugs must be administered intravenously. Extravasation results in vesication. The medication has a red color that may appear in the urine. The major organ of excretion, however, is the liver, and some degree of dose modification should be considered in the presence of major liver dysfunction. Other side-effects include stomatitis, alopecia, bone

TABLE 7–1.—CHEMOTHERAPEUTIC AGENTS

AGENT	DOSE FORMULATION AND ADMINISTRATION	RECONSTITUTION
Actinomycin D Dactinomycin Cosmegen	Available in 500-μg vials as lyophilized powder Doses per course vary from 10 to 15 μg/kg/day for 7 or 5 days, respectively Courses administered every 2–3 months	1.1 mg sterile water; discard unused portion
Adriamycin Doxorubicin	10- and 50-mg vials Variable dosage. Generally administered as 50–75 mg/m² every 3 weeks	Saline Stable for 48 hours at 4° C
BCNU Bischloroethylnitrosourea Carmustine	100 mg/vial White powder Stored under refrigeration Dosage under investigation	3 ml absolute alcohol, then 17 ml water. Dilute to 100 ml with 5% glucose water; discard remainder
Bleomycin Bleonoxane	15 units/vial White crystals Stored at room temperature Dosage under investigation	3 ml saline; dilute for subcutaneous and intravenous infusion Stable 28 days at 4° C
CCNU Lomustine	10-, 40-, 100-mg capsules Refrigerated Dosage under investigation	Stable in capsule form
Chlorambucil Leukeran CB-1348	2-mg tablets Stored at room temperature Generally administered as 0.1–0.2 mg/kg/day p.o. for 2–3 months Often given as courses with 1-month intervals	
Cyclophosphamide Cytoxan Endoxan	100, 200, 500 mg/vial White powder 25-, 50-mg tablets Stable at room temperature Generally administered as 3 mg/kg/day p.o. and interrupted if white blood count falls below 1500 per cu mm, or 300 mg/m² daily IV for 7–10 days every 6 weeks	Add 5 or 10 ml sterile water; use within 3 hours; discard unused portion
Daunorubicin Daunomycin Rubidomycin	20 mg/vial Orange red crystals Stored at room temperature Generally administered as 30 mg/m² or 1 mg/kg daily for 2–3 days q 3–4 wk	10 ml water; discard 6 hours after mixing; avoid extravasation
Imidazole carboxamide Dimethyltriazeno IC DTIC DIC Dacarbazine	100, 200 mg/vial White powder Stored under refrigeration Generally administered as 250 mg/m² daily for 5 days q 3 wk	5–10 ml water; dilute in 5% dextrose water; stable for 72 hours at 4° C
Methotrexate Amethopterin MTX	2.5-mg tablets 5, 50, 500 mg and 1 gm/vial Yellow powder or liquid Stored at room temperature Doses vary for different tumors	Sterile water. After reconstitution, may be diluted in dextrose water

ROUTE OF ADMINISTRATION	TOXICITY	INDICATIONS
Intravenous. Avoid extravasation	Bone marrow depression, mucositis, stomatitis, exacerbation of radiation effect ("recall" phenomenon), acne, alopecia. Extravasation results in ulceration	Wilms' tumor, gestational trophoblastic tumors, testicular tumors, soft tissue sarcoma, rhabdomyosarcoma, Ewing's sarcoma
Intravenous. Avoid extravasation	Myelosuppression, nausea, vomiting, diarrhea, mucositis, possibly exacerbated with hepatic dysfunction, alopecia, phlebitis, skin rash, cardiac toxicity, exacerbation of radiation effect Excreted in urine—red color	Soft tissue sarcoma, rhabdomyosarcoma, Ewing's sarcoma, osteogenic sarcoma, lymphoma
Intravenous. Avoid extravasation	Myelosuppression, hypotension with rapid infusion	Brain tumors Hodgkin's disease
Intravenous, intramuscular and subcutaneous	Pulmonary fibrosis, skin eruptions Hypersensitivity reactions	Lymphomas Nasopharyngeal carcinoma
Orally on empty stomach	Myelosuppression	Brain tumors
Oral	Marrow depression, hepatotoxicity, nausea, vomiting, diarrhea, dermatitis	Lymphomas, testicular tumors, histiocytosis
Intravenous; oral	Myelosuppression, nausea, vomiting, alopecia, hemorrhagic cystitis, aspermia	Soft tissue sarcoma Rhabdomyosarcoma Osteogenic sarcoma Neuroblastoma Ewing's sarcoma
Intravenous	Similar to adriamycin	Similar to adriamycin
Intravenous. Avoid extravasation	Myelosuppression	Generally used in combination with adriamycin for sarcomas Malignant melanoma
Oral, intravenous, intramuscular, intrathecal and intracavitary	Myelosuppression, stomatitis, renal toxicity, hepatic toxicity, exaggeration of toxicity with renal impairment, osteoporosis with prolonged use, nausea, vomiting, abdominal pain, skin rash, alopecia	Gestational trophoblastic tumors Testicular tumors. Osteogenic sarcoma (high dose)

(Continued)

TABLE 7-1.—*Continued*

AGENT	DOSE FORMULATION AND ADMINISTRATION	RECONSTITUTION
Mithramycin Mithracin	2.5 mg/vial White powder Stable at 4° C Refrigerated 15 μg/kg/dose q.o.d. intravenously up to 8 doses per course	4.9 ml water; infuse in 50–1000 ml 5% dextrose water slowly Use immediately
Methyl CCNU Semustine	10, 50, 100 mg/vial Stored at 4° C 100–120 mg/m² q 4–6 wk Dosage under investigation	Stable
Nitrogen mustard Mustargen HN₂ Mechloroethamine	10 mg/vial White powder Stored at room temperature 0.2–0.6 mg/kg q 2–3 wk	10 ml water; use immediately
Procarbazine Matulane	50-mg capsules Stored at room temperature 50–100 mg/m²/day × 7–14 days q month	
Vinblastine Velban	10 mg/vial White powder Stored under refrigeration 0.1–0.15 mg/kg intravenously weekly or every 2 wk	10 ml saline; stable 30 days if refrigerated
Vincristine Oncovin	1.5 mg/vial White powder Stored under refrigeration 2 mg/m² weekly or at more prolonged intervals	10 ml saline; stable 14 days if refrigerated
Ortho para-DDD Mitotane Lysodren	500-mg tablets Stored at room temperature 2–10 gm daily p.o. titrated individually for patient	

marrow suppression and gastrointestinal disturbances. The principal long-term dose-limiting toxicity is cardiomyopathy, manifested as arrhythmia, hypotension, electrocardiac changes, cardiomegaly and acute congestive cardiac failure. These complications usually are more likely to occur after cumulative doses of 500 mg/m². At the Sidney Farber Cancer Institute, the maximal cumulative dose is restricted to 450 mg/m². Since adriamycin also potentiates the action of radiation therapy, the dose is restricted to 300 mg/m² in patients receiving precordial irradiation.

BLEOMYCIN.—This is a relatively recent antitumor agent derived from a strain of *Streptomyces verticillus*. It probably exerts its anticancer effect by binding to DNA, causing scission and fragmentation of the DNA helix, and is used principally in the treatment of lymphomas and testicular tumors. Its major side-effect is irreversible pulmonary fibrosis. This generally has occurred without warning after cumulative doses in excess of 300 mg/m². Pulmonary function studies do not seem to be of any predictive value. Other forms of toxicity include induration and erythema of the fingers and hands, which may proceed to desquamation and ulceration. This complication is particularly likely to occur in previously irradiated sites. It may be exacerbated with a subsequent administration of other agents such as methotrexate and BCNU. The drug is administered by the intravenous, intramuscular or subcutaneous route.

MITHRAMYCIN.—This was isolated from *Streptomyces atroolivaceus*. It acts by binding to DNA and inhibits RNA synthesis. It is administered intravenously for treatment of testicular tumors. Its major side-effects comprise disturbances in coagulation, causing a hemorrhagic diathesis, myelosuppression and renal and hepatic dysfunction. A precipitous fall in the serum calcium levels has also been noted and has been utilized for the treatment of hypercalcemia in malignancy.

Vinca Alkaloids

The Vinca alkaloids are nitrogenous bases of natural origin derived primarily from plants. Two such alkaloids with anticancer activity are in clinical use: vincristine and velban obtained from the periwinkle plant, *Vinca rosea linn*. The mechanism of action of these agents has not been fully defined. It is possible that they selectively kill cells in DNA synthesis. Several workers also describe crystallization of microtubules and spindle protein. The microtubules are

ROUTE OF ADMINISTRATION	TOXICITY	INDICATIONS
Intravenous. Avoid extravasation	Hemorrhagic syndrome, hepatic damage, renal damage, marrow depression, nausea, vomiting, hypocalcemia, gastrointestinal toxicity, skin necrosis, fever	Embryonal carcinoma of testis, hypercalcemia
Orally on empty stomach	Myelosuppression	Brain tumors
Intravenous, intracavitary. Avoid extravasation. Avoid contact with skin and eyes	Nausea, vomiting, myelosuppression, acute contact vesicant, extravasation causes ulceration, phlebitis, thrombosis	Hodgkin's disease, reticulum cell sarcoma, neuroblastoma, retinoblastoma
Oral	Bone marrow depression, severe nausea and vomiting, lethargy, central nervous system depression, drug dermatitis, stomatitis, myalgia, alopecia (uncommon)	Hodgkin's disease, lymphomas, melanoma
Intravenous	Bone marrow depression, nausea, vomiting, stomatitis, alopecia, peripheral neuropathy, cellulitis on extravasation	Hodgkin's disease, lymphosarcoma, reticulum cell sarcoma, histiocytosis, choriocarcinoma
Intravenous. Avoid extravasation	Moderate abdominal pain, peripheral neuropathy, obstipation, cellulitis on extravasation, muscle pain, numbness and tingling, alopecia, bone marrow depression, jaw pain	Wilms' tumor, rhabdomyosarcoma, soft tissue sarcoma, Hodgkin's disease, neuroblastoma, Ewing's sarcoma, retinoblastoma, histiocytosis X
Oral	Hypoadrenalism, severe nausea and vomiting, vertigo, mental depression, diarrhea, somnolence, skin eruption, muscle tremors	Metastatic functional carcinoma of adrenal gland

concerned with nerve conduction, spindle formation with cytokinesis and chromosome replication. The periwinkle alkaloids cause metaphase arrest and random placement of chromosomes within the cell. Similar effects are produced by colchicine.

Vincristine and velban differ structurally from each other only in a single carbon atom (formyl or ethyl, respectively). However, they differ broadly in their clinical application. Vincristine is moderately effective in patients with rhabdomyosarcoma and Wilms' tumor.[7, 8, 25-27] Reduction in the size of primary tumor and disappearance of metastases from Wilms' tumor have been demonstrated. Vincristine also appears active in neuroblastoma and Hodgkin's disease. Velban has produced responses in patients with Hodgkin's disease, neuroblastoma, Letterer-Siwe disease and testicular tumors.

The toxic effects principally involve nerve tissue. These comprise jaw pain, loss of deep tendon reflexes, constipation, ileus, weakness, paralysis and convulsions. Constipation may be quite severe and therapy with vincristine should not be resumed until these signs disappear. If the complication recurs, subsequent doses of vincristine should be reduced. Vincristine has relatively little myelosuppressive activity in contrast to vinblastine. Both drugs cause alopecia. Severe hyponatremia has been observed with vincristine therapy, particularly in patients who have received an overdose. Both alkaloids apparently are excreted primarily by the liver and their administration to patients with liver dysfunction during irradiation to the liver or following partial hepatectomy should be considered with caution. Administration is by the intravenous route, and perivenous escape results in vesication and ulceration.

Miscellaneous Agents

Procarbazine is a methylhydrazine synthesized during investigations of monoamine oxidase inhibitors for tumor activity. Its exact mechanism of action is not known, although some of the biologic reactions resemble those of alkylating agents. Chromatid breaks and suppression of mitoses have been reported.

The drug has been shown to suppress immune defense mechanisms and possess teratogenic and carcinogenic properties in experimental animals. It crosses the blood-brain barrier.

Procarbazine is used principally in patients with Hodgkin's disease. Its side-effects comprise nausea, vomiting, dermatitis and central nervous system depression. The weak monoamine oxidase inhibitory properties may account for some of its neurotoxic effects. Acute reactions have been reported in association with ingestion of phenothiazine derivatives, barbiturates, alcohol and/or ripe cheeses.

ORTHO PARA-DDD.—This drug acts specifically on the mitochondria of adrenal cortical cells, resulting in decreased production of glucocorticoids and 17-ketosteroids. Aldosterone secretion remains unchanged. It is administered to patients with metastatic adrenal cortical cell carcinoma. Side-effects include nausea, vomiting, diarrhea, hypoadrenalism, vertigo, mental depression, somnolence and skin eruption.

DIMETHYL TRIAZENO IMIDAZOLE CARBOXAMIDE (DTIC). —This is an analogue of aminoimidazole carboxamide that originally was thought to exert its toxic effect by inhibiting nucleic acid synthesis. It may possibly behave as an alkylating agent. It appears that the drug is excreted primarily through the kidneys. Its principal dose-limiting effect is myelosuppression. Administration is also accompanied by nausea and vomiting. It generally is administered in combination with adriamycin for the treatment of soft tissue sarcomas.

Combination Chemotherapy and Protocol Treatment

A major saltation in the treatment of malignancy has been the effective application of combination chemotherapy. This involves treatment with combinations of agents possessing different modes of action and minimal overlapping toxicity. Such combinations decrease the potential for toxicity and the development of drug resistance. Selection of specific agents is based on their pharmacologic properties, a knowledge of their efficacy and the feasibility of their application in clinical practice. In view of the complexity of the pharmacokinetics and pharmacology, the selection and design of combination chemotherapy is a discipline in its own right. The administration of such chemotherapy and its application to the other disciplines are referred to as a "protocol." Inherent in its construction are guidelines for modification of dosage and interruption of therapy because of potential toxicity. For example, therapy generally is interrupted if the white blood count falls to 2000 or the platelet count to 100,000. Subsequent courses are administered with appropriate reductions in drug dosages.[28]

Protocols vary from center to center, are subject to comparative clinical trials and undergo periodic change. Many involve a complex administration of chemotherapeutic agents and are beyond the scope of this chapter. They generally are available on request from individual institutions or cooperative groups. In view of the potential for toxicity, protocol treatment is best administered under the supervision of a pediatric medical oncologist who has kept abreast of the latest advances.

REFERENCES

1. Wilcox, W. S.: The last surviving cancer cell—the chances of killing it, Cancer Chemother. Rep. 50:541, 1966.
2. Schabel, F. M., Jr.: Concepts for systemic treatment of micrometastases, Cancer 35:15, 1975.
3. Skipper, H. E., Schabel, F. M., Jr., and Wilcox, W. S.: Experimental evaluation of potential anticancer agents. XIII. On the criteria and kinetics associated with "curability" of experimental leukemia, Cancer Chemother. Rep. 35:1, 1964.
4. Laster, W. R., Jr., Mayo, J. G., Simpson-Herren, L., *et al.:* Success and failure in the treatment of solid tumor. II. Kinetic parameters and "cell cure" of moderately advanced carcinoma 755, Cancer Chemother. Rep. 53:169, 1969.
5. Farber, S.: Chemotherapy in the treatment of leukemia and Wilms' tumor, JAMA 198:826, 1966.
6. Wolff, J. A., D'Angio, G. J., Hartmann, J., *et al.:* Long-term evaluation of single versus multiple courses of actinomycin D therapy of Wilms' tumor, N. Engl. J. Med. 290:84, 1974.
7. Jaffe, N., Filler, R. J., Farber, S., *et al.:* Rhabdomyosarcoma in children. Improved outlook with a multidisciplinary approach, Am. J. Surg. 125:482, 1973.
8. Wilbur, J. R.: Combination chemotherapy for embryonal rhabdomyosarcoma, Cancer Chemother. Rep. 58:281, 1974.
9. Heyn, R. M., Holland, R., Newton, W. A., Jr., *et al.:* The role of combined chemotherapy in the treatment of rhabdomyosarcoma in children, Cancer 34:2128, 1974.
10. Jaffe, N., Frei, E., III, Traggis, D., *et al.:* Adjuvant methotrexate and citrovorum-factor treatment of osteogenic sarcoma, N. Engl. J. Med. 291:994, 1974.
11. Rosen, G., Tan, C., Sanmaneechai, A., *et al.:* The rationale for multiple drug chemotherapy in the treatment of osteogenic sarcoma, Cancer 35:936, 1975.
12. Traggis, D., Jaffe, N., Cassady, J. R., *et al.:* Advanced neuroblastoma: Treatment with combination chemotherapy: vincristine, adriamycin, nitrogen mustard and DTIC (VAM-DTIC), Proc. ASCO/AACR, Abstract No. 558.
13. DeVita, V. T., Jr., Serpick, A., and Carbone, P. P.: Combination chemotherapy in the treatment of advanced Hodgkin's disease, Ann. Intern. Med. 73:881, 1970.
14. Sutow, W. W., Sullivan, M. P., Fernbach, D. J., *et al.:* Adjuvant chemotherapy in primary treatment of osteogenic sarcoma. A Southwest Oncology Group Study, Cancer 36:1598, 1975.
15. Evans, A. E., Albo, V., D'Angio, G. J., *et al.:* Cyclophosphamide treatment of patients with localized and regional neuroblastoma. A randomized study, Cancer 38:655, 1976.
16. Ziegler, J.: Chemotherapy of Burkitt's lymphoma, Cancer 30:1534, 1972.
17. Young, R. C., DeVita, V. T., Serpick, A. A., *et al.:* Treatment of advanced Hodgkin's disease with [1,3 bis (2-chlorethyl)-1-Nitrosourea] BCNU, N. Engl. J. Med. 285:475, 1971.
18. Freeman, A. I., Sachatello, C., Gaeta, J., *et al.:* An analysis of Ewing's tumor in children at Roswell Park Memorial Institute, Cancer 29:1563, 1972.
19. Rosen, G., Wollner, N., Tan, C., *et al.:* Disease-free survival in children with Ewing's sarcoma treated with radiation therapy and adjuvant four-drug sequential chemotherapy, Cancer 33:384, 1974.
20. Wollner, N., Exelby, P. R., Woodruff, J. M., *et al.:* Malignant ovarian tumors in childhood—prognosis in relation to initial therapy, Cancer 37:1953, 1976.
21. Tan, C., Etcubanas, E., Wollner, N., *et al.:* Adriamycin—an antitumor antibiotic in the treatment of neoplastic diseases, Cancer 32:9, 1973.
22. Wang, J. J., Cortes, E., Sinks, L. F., *et al.:* Therapeutic effect and toxicity of adriamycin in patients with neoplastic disease, Cancer 28:837, 1971.
23. Ragab, A. H., Sutow, W. W., Komp, D. M., *et al.:* Adriamycin in the treatment of childhood solid tumors, Cancer 36:1567, 1975.
24. Cortes, E. P., Holland, J. F., Wang, J. J., *et al.:* Amputation and adriamycin in primary osteosarcoma, N. Engl. J. Med. 291:998, 1974.
25. Vietti, T. J., Sullivan, M. P., Haggard, M. E., *et al.:* Vincristine sulfate and radiation therapy in metastatic Wilms' tumor, Cancer 25:12, 1970.
26. Sullivan, M. P., Sutow, W. W., Cangir, A., *et al.:* Vincristine sulfate in management of Wilms' tumor. Replacement of preoperative irradiation by chemotherapy, JAMA 202:381, 1967.
27. D'Angio, G. J., Evans, A. E., Breslow, N., *et al.:* The treatment of Wilms' tumor. Results of the National Wilms' Tumor Study, Cancer 38:633, 1976.
28. Furman, L., Camitta, B. M., Jaffe, N., *et al.:* Development of an effective treatment program for childhood acute lymphocytic leukemia: A preliminary report, Med. Pediatr. Oncol. 2:157, 1976.

Radiation Therapy for Solid Tumors

General Principles*

BOTH NORMAL AND NEOPLASTIC CELLS are affected by irradiation. In most instances there is a differential, and cancer cells are destroyed more readily than the adjoining normal cells. The difference, called "the therapeutic ratio," can be defined as the dose required to destroy the cancer cell divided by the dose tolerated by normal tissue. The ratio must be less than 1 if radiation therapy is to be used successfully and with safety. Normal cells differ in their radiosensitivity. In general, the more actively dividing the cell, and the more immature it is, the more sensitive it is to radiation damage. Cells within the hair follicle and the bone marrow are examples. In children, many tissues are actively dividing and maturing; therefore, the therapeutic ratio tends to be narrow in the young. Damage after irradiation is expressed in five main areas.

1. GROWTH AND DEVELOPMENT. — This is most obvious in the bony skeleton, where modest doses given to infants can lead to severe curtailment of growth. The younger the child the higher the dose, and the more actively growing the part the greater the damage.

2. IMPAIRED FUNCTION. — Irradiation of such organs as the liver, kidney and lung can lead to both acute and late changes. Aberrations of function may be subtle and detected only on careful clinical and laboratory investigation. In other cases, especially after high doses given to younger children, late damage can be irreparable if not lethal. The tolerances of normal tissues for radiation therapy alone, given at a weekly dose rate of 1000 rads, 200 rads per fraction, are shown in Table 8–1.[1]

3. GONADAL EFFECTS. — These are of three types: impaired hormonal function, infertility and genetic consider-

TABLE 8–1. — TOLERANCE OF NORMAL TISSUES

	TOTAL DOSE (1000 RADS/WK)
Eye: Globe	5500 rads
Lens	200 rads*
Lungs	1800 rads
Liver	2400 rads
Kidneys	1500 rads
Intestine	3000 rads
Bone	7000 rads
Skin	6500 rads
Central nervous system, brain	5500 rads
Spinal cord	4500 rads

*Lowest single dose known to produce cataract. Higher doses, even though protracted, can lead to progressive lenticular opacities and loss of vision, the effect being strongly dose dependent.

*The interested reader is referred to the article by D. Pearson and G. D'Angio (ref. 1) for a more complete exposition of these points.

ations. Irradiation adversely affects endocrine activity of both the male and female gonads. The severity is related to dose and inversely related to the age at the time of treatment. Sexual maturation can be arrested completely. In other patients, hormonal function may be relatively normal but fertility is impaired or destroyed. Genetic considerations are extremely complex. It is unlikely that the genetic damage produced in survivors after irradiation of the gonad will have a significant impact on future generations.[2] Offspring of treated children also do not appear to have an excess frequency of congenital malformations.[3] The issue has relevance because of attempts being made by relocation of the ovaries to sites outside the treatment beam to preserve ovarian function in girls requiring irradiation of the pelvis. Concern regarding genetic effects, therefore, need not be an issue in making the decision to perform that procedure when thought necessary.

4. ONCOGENESIS. — Ionizing radiations, such as x-rays, are carcinogenic.[4] Long latent periods of 5–10 years are the rule before second malignant neoplasms develop in irradiated sites. Such tumors are not common but, with this probability in mind, careful follow-up of all long-term survivors is mandatory. (See Late Consequences, below.)

5. PSYCHOSOCIAL CONSEQUENCES. — Direct effects on the brain are possible when young children are irradiated for brain tumors. Mental retardation sometimes is the result. Pronounced skeletal and physical disabilities elsewhere in the body produced by irradiation may lead to psychosocial disturbances as the children grow older and recognize their handicaps, particularly in relation to their age peers. Early identification of potential problems such as these and the institution of hormonal replacement in patients having suppression of endocrine function help mitigate the impact on the patient and the family.

Treatment Modalities

Radiation therapy can be delivered by any of several means.

1. X-RAY MACHINES. — Roentgen apparatus for clinical use is available in a variety of energy ranges. Low kilovoltage (kV) machines are those running in the 10–100 kV range. These are used exclusively for extremely superficial lesions, and seldom are used in pediatric radiation therapy. Today, only apparatus delivering beams of millions of volts (megavolts) is considered suitable for the treatment of deep-seated lesions. Machines commonly used range in energy from 4 to 12 MV, and the "orthovoltage" unit of 200–300 kV seldom is utilized.

2. RADIOACTIVE ISOTOPES. — These are of two types: nat-

urally occurring radionuclides, such as radium and radon, and those produced artificially, such as cobalt-60. Radioactive materials can be inserted directly into tumors after having been encapsulated in needles and tubes, can be used in liquid form or can be gathered into sizable aggregates and used to project a beam at a distance. Cobalt-60 commonly is used in the last fashion. Housed in a suitably protected container in an appropriately designed machine, it is used for the treatment of deep-seated tumors, the beam having an equivalent energy of approximately 1 million volts.

3. PARTICULATE RADIATIONS. — These are of three types: (a) electrons, (b) positively charged particles and (c) neutral particles. Electrons are light, negatively charged fragments of the atom. They can be accelerated by machines of appropriate design and are useful for the treatment of surface lesions and those a few centimeters deep. Neutral and positively charged particles are bits of the atomic nucleus or the nucleus itself. These are under active investigation in many centers for their potential clinical applicability but are not available for routine use.

Radiation Modifiers

These substances are designed to modify the therapeutic ratio. They are of two types: those that afford protection and those that enhance effects. The latter are of greatest interest for clinical use.

RADIATION ENHANCEMENT. — Ambient oxygen is needed in order for ionizing radiations to be maximally effective at the locus of the molecular changes they induce. Most tumors contain foci of necrosis. These are believed to be due to undervascularization; therefore, cells within and adjacent to necrotic regions are at varying stages of hypoxia, yet they may remain viable. Such cells may require as much as $2\frac{1}{2}-3$ times the radiation dose to an oxygenated cell to produce the same damage. Three approaches are being taken to circumvent this difficulty: the use of heavy-particle irradiation, hyperthermia and chemicals. Specialized beams consisting of neutrons or positively charged fragments of the atom, under certain circumstances, are relatively oxygen independent. The use of certain chemical compounds (metronidazole)[5] and hyperthermia[6] are additional means of making the radiation more efficient in hypoxic regions. Chemicals, such as actinomycin D[7] and hyperthermia[6] augment radiation effects in oxygenated tissues as well. Active investigations are under way to determine whether these largely laboratory observations can be adapted to clinical use.

The Role of Radiation Therapy

Combined care of all children with malignant diseases is essential if maximal survival rates are to be obtained and damage to normal tissues kept at a minimum. The radiation therapist, therefore, must function as a member of an integrated team that includes the pediatric surgeon, the pediatric oncologist and the family physician. Coordinated care requires clear exposition of the role that each member of the team plays at a given moment in the clinical evolution of a given case. Radiation therapy can be used for several specific goals.

1. CURATIVE RADIATION THERAPY. — This requires careful planning with respect to dose and technique. A balance must be made between what is needed to produce total local control of the disease process while not causing irreparable and crippling damage to adjoining sensitive structures. Sometimes it is necessary, however, as it is in an operation, to run the risk of sacrificing a normal structure, such as a kidney, when protective measures compromise chances for cure.

2. PALLIATION. — Most tumors of childhood are sensitive to radiation, so that modest doses often suffice to produce relief from pain, disfigurement and the other consequences of advanced malignant disease. Often, single doses of moderate magnitude suffice for the purpose. Treatments often can be given on an outpatient basis, making it possible for the child to remain at home as he declines.

3. RADIATION THERAPY AS AN ADJUNCT. — Irradiation can be added to surgery or chemotherapy in attempts to increase the likelihood of bringing the local disease under total control. It may be used preoperatively or postoperatively, the latter being used more commonly in pediatrics. The margins of the tumor will have been identified with certainty, metallic clips being used to indicate sites of potential involvement that require irradiation.

The modern management of children with malignant disease almost always entails the addition of one or more antineoplastic therapeutic agents in the postoperative course. These are given with two objects in mind: to destroy microscopic nests of tumor cells lying remote from the primary site ("microablative therapy") and to accomplish the same purpose in the local region. Radiation therapy also is used locally; disproportionately pronounced reactions result when the chemotherapeutic agents used concomitantly are radiation enhancers.

4. MICROABLATIVE RADIATION THERAPY. — Radiation therapy can be given to areas at high risk for tumor involvement, even though there may be no palpable or visible evidence of the disease at the time. An example is the spinal canal in children with medulloblastoma. Irradiation of the entire cranio-spinal axis is used routinely in these patients because of the high frequency of "drop" metastases along the spinal cord, the cells originating from the primary tumor in the posterior fossa.

Late Consequences of Successful Therapy

Combined modality therapy has been responsible for revolutionary improvements in survival rates in children with cancer. Modern management entails the coordinated use of surgery, radiation therapy and chemotherapy, usually with more than one drug. The use of potent antineoplastic agents entails some morbidity and — at times — engenders long-term complications.[8] When certain of these agents are combined with radiation therapy, radiation damage is magnified, sometimes to unacceptable levels if more than modest doses of radiation therapy are used.[9] Some radiation-enhancing drugs and radiation reactivators in common use in pediatric oncology include cyclophosphamide and methotrexate when given in high dose, actinomycin D and adriamycin. Therefore, any irradiated part suffers damage not only at the time one of these agents is given concomitantly with radiation therapy but at each subsequent course of chemotherapy, whether or not radiation is added. Careful follow-up of these patients for life is mandatory so that corrective measures can be instituted, when necessary, to avoid late, crippling disabilities and deformities. These are particularly prone to occur in irradiated sites, which therefore deserve particular attention at follow-up examinations. An additional problem is oncogenesis. In a recent study, 102 second malignant neoplasms were encountered among long-term survivors of pediatric cancer.[10] Sixty-two of these were in irradiated fields. The most common tumor types were bone and soft tissue sarcomas, skin cancers, brain tumors and thyroid neoplasms. Periodic x-ray examination to detect early changes in skeletal structures underlying irradiated zones is therefore advisable. No increase in frequency of second malignant neoplasms could be attributed to the use of chemotherapy. Rather, actinomycin D appeared to have a protective effect against radiation-associated malignant tumor induction.[11]

Radiation Therapy of Specific Conditions

All doses to be cited are delivered at the rate of 200 rads per day, 5 days per week, unless otherwise specified, and are predicated on the use of megavoltage beams. No correction is applied when doses to the lung are stated. Treatment plans always include at least two portals, and all fields are treated each day, dividing the dose among them.

The widespread use of multiple chemotherapeutic agents in conjunction with surgical and radiotherapeutic management of these patients makes necessary major modifications of standard radiation therapy doses and techniques. These include particularly the following.

1. "SPLIT COURSES."—By this is meant a planned interruption of radiation therapy to allow enhanced radiation reactions to subside, or to avoid such reactions. Thus, in a typical plan, 3000 rads may be given in 3 weeks, a rest period of 2–3 weeks allowed and an additional 3000 rads given thereafter. This method permits the introduction of a course of chemotherapy during the rest period. It also allows for observation of any reactivation of latent radiation damage that might be produced by the chemotherapeutic agents, so that future planning can take such "flare reactions" into account.

2. "SHRINKING FIELD."—By this is meant the use of initial large fields designed to include the primary ("bulky") tumor with wide margins. Relatively modest doses are given to the large field because only small nests of cells are suspected at a distance from the primary site and because chemotherapy assists in the ablation of such small nests of cells. The field size then is reduced, but generous margins still are allowed around the primary site. An additional increment of dose then is delivered and the field may be reduced a second time. Here, the aim is to deliver a "coup de

TABLE 8-2.—NATIONAL WILMS' TUMOR STUDY GROUPING SYSTEM

Group I—Tumor limited to kidney and completely excised

The surface of the renal capsule is intact. The tumor was not ruptured before or during removal. There is no residual tumor apparent beyond the margins of excision

Group II—Tumor extends beyond the kidney but is completely excised

There is local extension of the tumor; i.e., penetration beyond the pseudocapsule into the perirenal soft tissues, or periaortic lymph node involvement. The renal vessels outside the kidney substance are infiltrated or contain tumor thrombus. There is no residual tumor apparent beyond the margins of excision

Group III—Residual nonhematogenous tumor confined to abdomen

Any one or more of the following occur: (1) The tumor has been biopsied or ruptured before or during operation; (2) there are implants on peritoneal surfaces; (3) there are involved lymph nodes beyond the abdominal periaortic chains; (4) the tumor is not completely removable because of local infiltration into vital structures

Group IV—Hematogenous metastases

Deposits beyond Group III; e.g., lung, liver, bone and brain

Group V—Bilateral renal involvement either initially or subsequently

grace" to the site of origin of the neoplasm by giving the highest dose to the region where the most malignant cells were present at the initiation of therapy.

Wilms' Tumor

The routine use of postoperative radiation therapy for Wilms' tumor has long been advocated. The recently reported results of the first National Wilms' Tumor Study (NWTS-1) have established more precise criteria as to both the indication for irradiation and the volume to be subtended.[12]

Patients entered into the NWTS-1 were divided among five groups, according to the extent of the disease found at the time of operation and on pathologic examination of the specimen. The grouping system is shown in Table 8-2. The

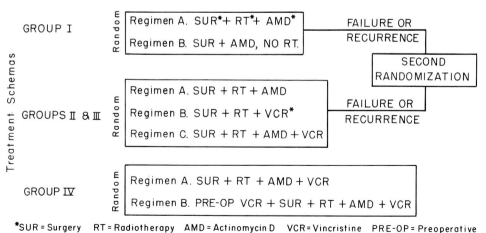

*SUR = Surgery   RT = Radiotherapy   AMD = Actinomycin D   VCR = Vincristine   PRE-OP = Preoperative

Fig. 8-1.—Design of the First National Wilms' Tumor Study. (From D'Angio, G. J., *et al.*, The treatment of Wilms' tumor, Cancer 38:633, 1976.)

TABLE 8–3.—WILMS' TUMOR:
RADIATION DOSE vs AGE

AGE	TOTAL TUMOR DOSE
Birth to 18 months	1800–2400 rads
18–30 months	2400–3000 rads
31–40 months	3000–3500 rads
41 months or more	3500–4000 rads

study design is shown in Figure 8–1. All Group I children received postoperative actinomycin D. This was given cyclically every 3 months for a total of 15 months. Half the patients received postoperative radiation therapy; the others did not. The doses used were adjusted according to age (Table 8–3). Anterior and posterior opposing fields were designed to include the entire affected kidney along with the tumor extent as delineated on the preoperative excretory urogram. The medial margin of the portal extended across the midline to include the entire width of the vertebral body. This was done to avoid asymmetric growth disturbances in the irradiated segments.

The 2-year relapse-free survival and 2-year survival rates for Group I children under 2 years of age were not significantly different for the irradiated and nonirradiated samples (Table 8–4). It therefore is safe to eliminate postoperative radiation therapy for young children qualifying as Group I. For children over 2 years of age, the situation is less clear. The nonirradiated patients developed more instances of intra-abdominal relapse, including 3 who developed recurrences in the operative bed. Although the eventual survival data are not significantly different between the irradiated and nonirradiated children, it would seem prudent to evaluate the primary lesions of older children with care. Children with findings suggesting possible local infiltration should receive postoperative radiation therapy along with chemotherapy. An example would be adherence to adjoining structures even though tumor penetration of the capsule cannot be identified grossly or microscopically.

The NWTS-1 also provides guidance for patients with more advanced stages of the disease. All children in Groups II and III were given postoperative radiation therapy along with actinomycin D, vincristine or both (Fig. 1). Good local control was achieved. There were only 5 instances of recurrent disease in the irradiated flank among 242 children studied.[13]

Fields and doses for Group II children were the same as

those for Group I. Group III children had portals of differing size, depending on the operative findings. In general, the portals were similar to those used for Groups I and II, but were extended to include the entire abdomen in patients with gross spillage of tumor into the peritoneal cavity or those with demonstrable widespread peritoneal implants. The boundaries of the portal extended from the domes of the diaphragm to the peritoneal floor and were shaped to exclude the proximal femora. The remaining kidney was protected by introducing heavy metal blocks so that the transmitted and scattered dose did not exceed 1500 rads. Similarly, the liver dose was adjusted so as not to be more than 2400 rads. It was found that large fields such as these are not needed for instances of minor and localized tumor spills nor in patients having had biopsies prior to interval nephrectomy.[14]

NWTS techniques for Groups II and III patients are recommended in view of the good results reported (Table 8–4).

Group IV patients almost invariably have pulmonary metastases as the first manifestation of disseminated disease. A single shaped field can be used to include the entire thoracic cavity and the affected kidney. The proximal humeri are excluded. Irradiation to the single field can be given at the rate of 150 rads per day until the midplane lung dose (uncorrected) is 1200 rads. Nephrectomy can be performed at this time and radiation therapy of the tumor bed resumed postoperatively. The dose to be added depends on the length of time treatment has been interrupted by the surgical procedure. The aim should be the delivery of doses equivalent to those shown in Table 8–3, using correction factors that take into account time, dose and fractionation.[15] The same general procedure outlined above can be followed should the patient have had a nephrectomy before irradiation is initiated.

Radiation therapy of these large fields is generally well tolerated even though actinomycin D is given concomitantly, although an occasional child will have prompt radiation enhancement necessitating interruption of treatment early in the course. The addition of vincristine should be delayed until radiation therapy is completed because double-agent chemotherapy increases the likelihood of complications when total abdominal irradiation is necessary because of the surgical findings.

Patients with bilateral disease (Group V) have excellent survival expectancy but require individualized care. In general, every attempt should be made to spare as much kidney parenchyma as possible by avoiding radical surgical pro-

TABLE 8–4.—FIRST NATIONAL WILMS' TUMOR STUDY:
TWO-YEAR RESULTS BY GROUP AND REGIMEN

GROUP	REGIMEN	NO. OF PTS.	RELAPSE-FREE RATE°	SURVIVAL RATE
I (<2 yr old)	Radiotherapy	38	90%	97%
	No radiotherapy	36	88%	94%
I (≥2 yr old)	Radiotherapy	39	77%	97%
	No radiotherapy	41	58%	91%
II & III	AMD†	63	57%	67%
	VCR	44	55%	72%
	Both	59	81%	86%
IV	Immediate surgery	13		83%
	Preop VCR	13		29%

°"Relapse-free" means continuously free from any tumor.
†AMD = actinomycin D; VCR = vincristine.

cedures, radiation or both. This can best be accomplished by following bilateral biopsies with a course of chemotherapy. Segmental resection thereafter at a "second look" with or without subsequent radiation therapy in modest dose (e.g., 1500 rads or less) is coupled with maintenance chemotherapy using actinomycin D and vincristine.[16]

Metastatic Disease

The lungs almost invariably are the first organs affected. Even though only a single focus is visible on the chest x-ray films, the vast majority of patients have microscopic deposits scattered elsewhere in the lungs. Therefore, both lung fields are irradiated and a total dose of 1200 rads is given. Combination chemotherapy is used. Surgical excision is recommended should one or more lesions fail to respond or reappear after pulmonary irradiation. Reirradiation of large segments of the lung leads to pulmonary damage that may prove lethal after the passage of some time, even though the recurrent tumor has been successfully eradicated.[17]

LIVER.—These lesions are very stubborn, and risks must be run in the attempt to secure cure. Surgical excision should be attempted first. If the lesions are too numerous or their location precludes resection, irradiation of the entire liver is indicated. A total dose of 3000 rads is delivered at the rate of 1000 rads per week, being sure to exclude the remaining kidney from the beam, especially when it is on the right side.

BONE AND BRAIN.—Metastases to these sites are very uncommon. Doses of not less than 3000 rads are recommended.

Comment

1. Combined modality care and radiation therapy techniques such as those outlined above give excellent results. The over-all 2-year survival rate can be expected to be better than 90% when the most effective NWTS regimens are used (Table 8-4).

2. Analyses of radiation therapy techniques used in the NWTS suggest that doses greater than 2400 rads probably are not necessary in most cases.[13] Therefore, it is recommended that doses of more than 2400 rads be used only when there is gross tumor present or when older patients (i.e., those in their teens or later) are to be treated. Tumors in such patients appear to be more aggressive, although the paucity of cases makes this difficult to document.

3. Selective, pronounced thrombocytopenia can result when large segments of the liver are irradiated in patients receiving actinomycin D. Frequent complete blood counts should be obtained in all such patients.[12]

Neuroblastoma

Effective chemotherapeutic management of these patients, comparable to that for Wilms' tumor, for example, has yet to be developed. Reliance therefore must be placed on an understanding of the natural history of the disease and on surgery and radiation therapy for definitive management. The special qualities of this tumor must be recognized. Age and stage (Table 8-5) are important prognostic factors.[18] Infants with this tumor in its early stages have a high chance for cure that is not clearly dependent on medical management. The older child, and the one with more advanced disease, has a poorer outlook, which—once again—is not nec-

TABLE 8-5.—NEUROBLASTOMA STAGING SYSTEM

Stage I:	Tumors confined to the organ or structure of origin
Stage II:	Tumors extending in continuity beyond the organ or structure of origin but not crossing the midline. Homolateral lymph nodes may be involved
Stage III:	Tumors extending in continuity beyond the midline. Bilateral regional lymph nodes may be involved
Stage IV:	Dissemination with metastases in skeleton, organs, soft tissue, distant lymph nodes, etc.
Stage IV-S:	Patients who would be in Group I or II were it not for the fact that they show dissemination in liver, skin, or bone marrow, but without radiographic evidence of bone metastases

essarily modified by treatment in the individual case. Concrete proposals with respect to radiation therapy, therefore, are difficult to give. The following recommendations are based on recent experience and the collected data from cooperative clinical trials as well as from the records of The Children's Hospital of Philadelphia.[19, 20]

STAGES I AND II.—Although there are no randomized clinical trial data available on this point, there is evidence to indicate that postoperative radiation therapy does not add to survival experience.[20] This is true even in patients with incomplete excision of Stage II disease who do not receive postoperative irradiation. Postoperative radiation therapy, therefore, is not recommended for children with Stage I tumors nor for those with Stage II disease who have complete surgical excision. This applies particularly to infants only a few days or months of age. If radiation therapy is withheld from those with incomplete removal of Stage II tumors, careful observation, including a "second look" in 3-6 months, would seem prudent. Irradiation then can be added depending on the clinical evolution of the case. It is difficult to recommend specific dosage should radiation therapy be indicated either initially or after a period of observation. This is because of the lack of clear relationship between irradiation and outcome. The dosage regimen utilized by one of the national study groups is the same as for Wilms' tumor and is shown in Table 8-3. The doses cited, which are varied according to age, are delivered at the rate of 1000 rads per week. These recommendations no doubt will be altered as increasing experience is accumulated. One modification that is suggested is a lowering of dose for very young infants—only a few days or weeks of age. Should radiation therapy be thought indicated, 800-rad increments can be given (200 rads for 4 days). Periods of 4 weeks can be allowed to intervene so as to observe responses. The total dose can be determined on the basis of the clinical response, but always kept below 3000 rads total.

STAGE III.—Postoperative radiation therapy appears to be of value.[20] Portals are adjusted to suit the extent of the disease as identified by the surgeon. Doses shown in Table 8-3 are given, with the same proviso for the extremely young patient.

STAGE IV.—The tumor metastasizes widely to the bony skeleton, the lungs being affected relatively rarely. Moderately large single doses (e.g., 300-500 rads) can be given to children with multiple painful sites. This technique is used for patients in the last stages of the disease so as not to protract the period of treatment. Otherwise, higher doses in the 1500–2500 rad range are given in 1½–2½ weeks to children whose life expectancy can be measured in terms of 6 months or more. The fields are designed to encompass the local region with adequate margins except in the case of retro-orbital metastases, with or without proptosis. These children almost invariably have extensive calvarial involvement as well. Therefore, shaped fields are used to include the posterior orbit and all the bones of the skull.

Soft Tissue Sarcomas[21]

Rhabdomyosarcoma

The role of surgery has been reevaluated in recent years, and procedures designed to preserve function as well as the part are being used with increasing frequency.[22] These developments have been coupled with improved survival rates now that effective multiple agent chemotherapeutic regimens are being introduced into the postoperative management of these children. Radiation therapy can be used in support of these general policies; that is, it can add a measure of protection after conservative surgical procedures, and in some cases can be used instead of surgical removal of the affected part. An example of the latter is rhabdomyosarcoma of the orbit.

High doses of radiation therapy, i.e., 5000 rads or more, have been found to be necessary in order to achieve local control of bulky lesions when radiation therapy is given alone. Since all patients with these tumors should be receiving chemotherapy, and most of the multiple agent regimens contain radiation enhancers, it no longer is necessary or possible to give doses of this kind without running the risk of incurring severe complications when large volumes are included in the beam. Also, recent studies have indicated that lower doses may suffice for control when only microscopic disease is present, although attempts to attain higher values are indicated when gross tumor is present.[22a]

Based on these considerations, the following treatment recommendations can be made.

1. No postoperative radiation therapy is given to patients without apparent residual disease on gross and microscopic inspection after wide excision.

2. Microscopic residual disease. A dose of 4000 rads is given to a wide field, designed to include the operative site and wide margins. The margins should extend from the origin to the insertion of the affected muscle. An additional 500–1000 rads is given to the region believed to harbor residual tumor cells.

3. Gross residual disease. Treatment is initiated with chemotherapy. Prompt and gratifying reduction of tumor mass often follows, making it possible to use more precise fields and thus irradiate less normal tissue. High-dose radiation therapy is planned but is administered in "split" courses (v.s.). These can be arranged according to the cycles of chemotherapy. For example, 3000 rads in 3 weeks through wide fields is delivered, followed by an interval of 2–3 weeks, during which a course of chemotherapy can be administered. An additional 3000 rads then is given for a total of 6000 rads in 8–9 weeks. A modification is to couple "shrinking" fields with a "double split." That is, two rest periods are allowed and the field is reduced for each successive course of therapy. An example would be the delivery of 3000 rads in 3 weeks to a large field. An additional

1500–2000 rads is given after a rest period, and a third increment of 1500–2000 rads, as tolerated, is delivered after a second rest interval. When using this method, careful treatment planning beforehand is necessary, because the bulk of the tumor will be gone by the time the last stage of treatment is reached.

TREATMENT OF SPECIFIC TUMOR SITES. — *Nasopharynx.* — These tumors usually are not resectable, and radiation therapy is the treatment of choice. High doses to large volumes are necessary for control. The portal thus extends from the base of the skull superiorly to the angle of the mandible inferiorly and from the tip of the mastoid posteriorly to the anterior nares anteriorly. The eyes, tongue and anterior mandible are excluded from the treatment portal by appropriately shaped lead blocks. The technique described above for "bulky" tumors can be followed and doses in the 5000–6000 rad range delivered using the shrinking field technique. Aggressive treatment of this kind can be successful even when there is evidence of bone destruction or cranial nerve involvement at the time of diagnosis. Seventeen of 19 patients reported by Donaldson and co-workers[23] achieved good control, with a survival rate in these patients of 74% (14 of 19 patients treated).

The complications of this kind of treatment, which entails concomitant chemotherapy, are considerable. Severe mucositis of all the irradiated surfaces is almost invariable when actinomycin D is included in the chemotherapy regimens. Intravenous fluids and nasogastric feeding tubes may be necessary in order to maintain hydration and nutrition during this uncomfortable period. If "split course" treatment has not been planned, it almost certainly will be imposed by intolerable local reactions, and the total dose delivered must be adjusted upward in such an event.

Middle ear and mastoid. — The outlook for these patients has been poor in the past. Radical surgical procedures seldom are successful in themselves. Multimodal therapy appears to have altered this outlook. Radical removal of the tumor and adjoining structures is followed by irradiation combined with chemotherapy. Specialized methods (e.g., "wedge pair" technique) are used to deliver high doses to the affected portions while avoiding high doses to the adjoining brain. The dose is adjusted according to whether gross or only microscopic disease remains (v.i.).

In general, results with rhabdomyosarcoma in other sites suggest that radical surgical procedures may be avoided in these cases by approaching them with aggressive chemotherapy and high-dose local radiation therapy.

Orbit. — These tumors tend to remain localized, so that the prognosis is better than for other primary sites. When present, metastases often are confined to the regional lymph node echelons. More distant deposits are not common.

Radical surgical exenteration of the orbital contents has been the traditional surgical procedure for these tumors. Postoperative radiation therapy is not indicated if the margins of the specimen are found to be free. Recent evidence suggests that radical operations can be avoided in these patients. Sagerman and his colleagues[24] have reported good results using high doses of radiation therapy alone. Good local control can be achieved with doses of 5000–6000 rads, and an 18-month survival rate of 67% (10 of 15) was reported by them. The technique is associated with local complications, which include not only bone growth disturbance but also cataract induction and damage to the globe. However, useful vision is preserved in a high proportion of cases. Should radiation therapy be used, the portal must include all the bony margins of the orbit and then be extended posteriorly to the level of the optic chiasm in patients with large tumors or when there is roentgen evidence of enlargement of the natural foramina and fissures. The opposite eye is protected by suitable blocks and beam angles. The dose and technique used depend on the size of the tumor and whether concomitant chemotherapy is being administered (v.i.).

Genitourinary tract.—Tumors of the prostate gland have a poor outlook; in other urogenital tract sites, the prognosis is relatively good.[21] Radical surgical procedures have been the mainstay of treatment, and postoperative radiation therapy is not given when the margins are free from tumor. Extreme care must be used in planning treatment when gross or microscopic disease remains after operation; therefore, radiation therapy is necessary. It is of material assistance if the operating surgeon will identify areas of known or suspected disease with radiopaque metallic clips. Treatment portals are shaped to accommodate the known or suspected sites of involvement. For example, for patients known to have unilateral or bilateral involvement of the iliac lymph node chains, the portal is designed to include one or both sides of the pelvis as indicated, and—narrowed—is extended to the L4–5 level. Total doses are adjusted as described above, but in view of the high probability of complications because of adherent bowel loops within the treatment beam, split course regimens are highly desirable. "Second look" surgical procedures may be of benefit, because areas of residual disease can be identified with greater certainty, allowing the use of small beams. Additionally, it may be possible to implant residual foci with radioactive sources, thus bringing the local tumor dose up to the requisite value while sparing adjoining structures.

It should be noted that the need for radical surgical procedures in these patients is coming under serious question. Attempts are being made to preserve function and integrity by combining less radical surgical procedures with combined chemotherapy and radiotherapy.[22]

Testicular and paratesticular origin.—Inguinal orchiectomy with high ligation of the spermatic cord and retroperitoneal lymph node dissection are indicated in these patients. Postoperative radiation therapy is given only in the face of identified disease. The methods used are similar to those for testicular tumors (v.i.) except that doses of 4500 rads should be used.

Uterus and vagina.—Treatment is much the same as that outlined for bladder and prostate.

Extremities.—The same general principles as those outlined above apply, wide fields and high doses being necessary, with supplemental doses given to the central region in children with bulky tumors. (See also Chapter 134.)

Comment.—There is increasing evidence that the use of chemotherapy alone in these patients will reduce tumor masses, and—in a few cases—result in prolonged local control. Radical surgical procedures, therefore, are being reserved in some centers for those tumors that fail to respond to chemotherapy with or without radiation therapy. Certainly every effort should be made to preserve the integrity of the affected part and amputation or exenterative procedures as part of primary management rarely resorted to.

Other Soft Tissue Tumors

FIBROSARCOMA, DESMOID TUMORS, THE FIBROUS PROLIFERATIVE DISORDERS AND NEUROFIBROSARCOMA.—Radiation therapy seldom is indicated in these patients. It is used in cases of fibrosarcoma with aggressive histologic patterns and with known residual tumor at the resection margins. The doses and techniques are as for rhabdomyosarcoma. Radiation therapy seldom is indicated in cases of the desmoid tumor but has been found to be of value in juvenile fibromatosis. Six thousand rads in 7½ weeks combined with multiple-agent chemotherapy resulted in gradual, total disappearance of a large mass in a patient so treated.[21] Radiation therapy may be attempted as a last resort for neurofibrosarcoma; the well-differentiated tumor is among the most radioresistant of lesions.

SYNOVIAL SARCOMAS.—Effective treatment methods remain to be defined. Meanwhile, the tumors would appear to be managed best by approaches similar to those used for rhabdomyosarcoma. Wide surgical excision is coupled with multiple-agent chemotherapy. Radiation therapy is given according to the indications outlined for rhabdomyosarcoma (q.v.).

ALVEOLAR SOFT PART SARCOMA.—This is not to be confused with the alveolar type of rhabdomyosarcoma. It is a specific tumor that affects younger patients. All but 1 of 12 patients under 16 years of age were girls. Slow in growth, they nonetheless are aggressive tumors, tending to recur locally and metastasize distantly. The lungs are affected most commonly. Lieberman et al.,[25] reporting the results in 50 cases of all age groups, record a 5-year survival rate of 60%. However, late relapses—sometimes decades later—appear to be the rule, and the lesion must be considered lethal in virtually all cases.

The role of radiation therapy in these patients is ill defined. The general precepts outlined for rhabdomyosarcoma (q.v.) can be followed.

Gonadal Tumors

OVARY.—These tumors in girls seldom are of the classic adult types. They commonly are teratomas and embryonal carcinomas. The latter category, for this discussion, includes the so-called yolk-sac tumor (Teilum tumor or tumor of the endodermal sinus).

All malignant ovarian tumors in girls are extremely aggressive, except for the dysgerminoma and theca-granulosa cell types, and require radical surgery, chemotherapy and radiation therapy. A recent review of patterns of failure in these cases demonstrates that whole abdominal irradiation is necessary. The field extends from the domes of the diaphragms to the pelvic floor, and doses of 4500 rads are delivered. The liver and kidneys are excluded from the beam so that no more than 3000 rads is given to the former and 1500 rads to the latter.[26] Such wide field treatment is necessary even in patients with what appears to be early-stage disease.

The treatment of the more radiosensitive dysgerminomas need not be so aggressive.[27] Simple surgical excision of the affected ovary suffices for cure in a high percentage of cases. Postoperative radiation therapy can be avoided in cases with negative lymphangiograms and no evidence of spread at the time of operation if the patient can be followed carefully. Otherwise, it seems prudent to add postoperative radiation therapy. The lesions are extremely radiosensitive and radiocurable. The field includes the ipsilateral pelvic lymph nodes and para-aortic chains up to the level of T9–10. The opposite ovary is shielded, and every attempt is made to preserve function. Patients with proved lymph node involvement are treated similarly, but the portal extends to include the mediastinum and the left supraclavicular region. The dose is 3000–3500 rads to areas of involvement, depending on bulk. Otherwise, 2000–2500 rads suffices for control of these sensitive lesions.

Treatment of granulosa-theca cell tumors consists of simple surgical excision and careful follow-up. Routine postoperative radiation therapy would not appear to be warranted in these cases, but is added to patients with ruptured or residual tumor, those with ascites or those of the sarcomatoid type.[27]

TESTIS.—Most of these tumors are of the embryonal cell type, the latter including the yolk-sac designation. Other tumor types are rare. The rhabdomyosarcoma is usually paratesticular rather than testicular but is treated in the same way.

Inguinal orchiectomy with high cord ligation and ipsilateral retroperitoneal lymph node dissections are indicated, because lymphangiograms are difficult to perform in these young patients. Lymph nodes seldom are involved, and postoperative radiation therapy is not given unless there is microscopic or lymphangiographic evidence of metastatic disease in the inguinal or para-aortic lymph nodes. When positive, 3000 rads is given to the ipsilateral pelvic nodes and para-aortic chain to the T9–10 level. Inclusion of the mediastinum in these patients would not appear to be warranted in view of the pronounced growth deformity produced by total axial irradiation in what usually are young boys. In view of the probability of left supraclavicular lymph node involvement when disease in para-aortic chains has been identified, a small field can be used to treat this region. A dose of 1500–2000 rads would appear reasonable under the circumstances.

Bone Tumors

Ewing's Tumor

The development of effective multiple-agent chemotherapy regimens for the control of remote micrometastases has markedly improved the outlook for patients with this hitherto almost uniformly lethal neoplasm.[28] The mainstay of control of the primary tumor remains radiation therapy. Regimens including high doses of cyclophosphamide, adriamycin and actinomycin D can markedly augment radiation reactions in the affected bone and overlying soft tissues. Therefore, modifications of radiation therapy technique as to both volume and dose are necessary in patients receiving radiation-enhancing drugs.

The entire bone from epiphyseal plate to epiphyseal plate in the case of long bones is included in the original beam. The joint surfaces can be excluded because Ewing's tumor rarely penetrates the epiphyseal plate, and an eventual better articulation will be procured if the joint can be eliminated from the high-dose portal. In the past, high doses in the 6000 rad range were given to the entire bone, perhaps with 500–1000 rad supplements to the bulky region. These doses are not tolerated in the face of radiation-enhancing agents; therefore, the "shrinking field" technique should be used.[29] Four thousand five hundred rads are given to the entire bone, the volume is reduced and an additional 1000–1500 rads directed to the site of the original tumor with wide margins. The primary site then is given a final supplement of approximately 500–1000 rads through a relatively small field. The doses and field sizes are governed by the volume of the original tumor. When large, higher doses and larger ports are used for each portion of the staged treatment. Therapy is protracted over several weeks in any case, the total of 6000 rads or more being delivered over 7–8 weeks. This technique is difficult to use when flat bones of the pelvis are affected because of the adjoining gut. Beam direction and rest periods are advised so as not to exceed the tolerance of these structures. One technique under investigation is the temporary surgical introduction of inert material into the iliac fossa to displace adjoining bowel from the direct beam, thus permitting high doses to be given with relative impunity.[30]

SPECIAL CONSIDERATIONS.—1. Field margins always should be adjusted so that a strip of overlying normal skin is left unirradiated, particularly when long bones are being treated. Otherwise, an encircling cicatrix is produced, which results in edema of the distal part.

2. Build-up or "bolus" material should be placed over the original biopsy site so as to bring the skin up to full dose and prevent implantation of tumor in the scar.

3. When the lesion is in one of the minor bones such as a rib or fibula, total removal of the bone may be preferable to radiation therapy as a method of management.

4. Radiation therapy should not be used for the definitive treatment of lesions of the small bones of the hands or feet (e.g., the metatarsal). The high doses of radiation therapy necessary are not well tolerated by these small parts, especially the weight-bearing foot, where pronounced secondary effects can be produced. Radiation therapy in moderate dose can be used as a surgical adjunct; e.g., to reduce tumor bulk and make subsequent removal easier.

5. The total dose delivered should be modified downward to about 5000 rads when one of the vertebral bodies or bones of the skull is affected because of the sensitivity of the underlying central nervous system structures.

6. "Prophylactic" irradiation of the lungs is under active investigation in a national trial. The results are awaited with interest. Meanwhile, the technique is not recommended.

METASTATIC DISEASE.—Ewing's tumor is markedly radioresponsive, so that modest doses result in prompt disappearance of pain and swelling. However, doses of not less than 4500 rads to bony metastases are recommended, when they are few in number. This policy ensures a prolonged recurrence-free period, which is important for these patients, who sometimes have a lengthy and indolent clinical course despite the presence of secondary deposits. "Pulmonary bath" techniques are used for lung metastases even though only a few may be visible on the original film. The fields are shaped to exclude the proximal humeri but are designed to include all the pulmonary parenchyma. Total doses of from 1500 to 1800 rads are given under these circumstances. The dose is modulated according to age, the lower dose being used for young children, i.e., those under 5 years of age. Supplementary doses for totals of up to 3000–4000 rads may be given to local lesions if of considerable size. Long-term survival can be obtained in a rare case with aggressive management of metastatic disease. However, any treatment plan must take into account the potentially lethal complications of combined treatment, such as pulmonary fibrosis, if high doses of radiation therapy are given to large volumes of the lung in combination with radiation-enhancing chemotherapeutic agents.

Osteogenic Sarcoma

The role of radiation therapy in osteogenic sarcoma is palliative. These tumors are markedly radioresistant, and high doses are needed for the relief from pain and disfigurement produced by metastatic foci.

Recent advances in combined treatment have given encouraging results.[28] Repeated surgical attacks on pulmonary metastases and the use of newly developed multiple-agent chemotherapy regimens have improved the survival expectancy in impressive fashion. Many varied attempts are being made to avoid amputation of the affected part by the use of internal prostheses, etc. The role of radiation therapy to the primary site is being re-examined in this light. Doses hitherto ineffectual have contributed to ablation of tumor in the irradiated volume when coupled with antineoplastic drugs.[28] Results in this important field are awaited with interest.

Liver Tumors

BENIGN.—Hemangiomas of the liver sometimes are so large as to produce high-output heart failure in infants. This complication can be life-threatening; therefore, modest doses of radiation therapy are given to accelerate regression of the lesion. Doses of perhaps 400 rads (200 rads q.d. × 2) are given in increments separated by a few weeks and the clinical course of the patient assessed to determine what total dose should be given. This rarely should exceed 1200 rads.

MALIGNANT.—Malignant tumors are of two main types: hepatocarcinoma and hepatoblastoma. In either case, treatment is surgical. Radiation therapy is given when the margins of resection are not clear or when the lesion is so large or so situated that surgical resection is impossible. Postoperative radiation therapy should be delayed after massive partial hepatectomy until regeneration of the liver has taken place. Usually 4–6 weeks' rest suffices for this purpose; liver scans can be obtained at frequent intervals to check the progress of regeneration and to allow more accurate timing for the radiation therapy. A total dose of not more than 4500 rads then can be given to the margin of resection.

In cases in which removal has not been possible, the "shrinking field" technique can be used in an attempt to control the primary lesion. Three thousand rads is given to the large volume, the margins are reduced and an additional 1500 rads given to the site of the bulky tumor.

Results have been poor in the past; multiple-agent chemotherapy is producing encouraging results in a small group of patients entered in a national trial.[31]

Teratomas

The most frequent site of origin is the sacrococcygeal region. Many teratomas are found in newborn girls and usually are benign. For the malignant lesions, work-up should include myelography, because the lesion commonly extends through neural foramina into the spinal canal. Radiation therapy is used postoperatively when the margins of excision are not clear. Total doses of 4500 rads are given. The smallest fields possible should be used so as to reduce bone growth disturbance and the damage to adjoining pelvic viscera. Because of this, "second look" surgical procedures are advisable prior to initiating radiation therapy when its value is in doubt for a particular case. Thus, after a course of chemotherapy, a second surgical procedure to explore the original operative site can be performed in 3–6 months. This permits the identification of any tumor that might be present, its accurate localization with radiopaque metallic clips and the use of smaller and more precisely oriented beams.

REFERENCES

1. Pearson, D., and D'Angio, G. J.: Radiation Therapy, in Bloom, H. J. G., Lemerle, J., Neidhardt, M. K., and Voute, P. A. (eds.), *Cancer in Children. Clinical Management* (New York and Berlin: Springer-Verlag, 1975), pp. 29–47.
2. Brent, R. L.: Discussion: Radiation therapy, Cancer 37:1121, 1976.
3. Li, F. P., and Jaffe, N.: Progeny of childhood cancer survivors, Lancet 2:707, 1974.
4. Hutchinson, G. B.: Late neoplastic changes following medical irradiation, Cancer 37:(supp.)1102, 1976.
5. Urtasun, R., *et al.*: Radiation and high-dose metronidazole in supratentorial glioblastomas, N. Engl. J. Med. 294:1364, 1976.
6. Hahn, E. W., *et al.*: The interaction of hyperthermia with fast neutrons or x-rays on local tumor response, Radiat. Res. 68:39, 1976.
7. D'Angio, G. J.: Clinical and biologic studies of actinomycin D and roentgen irradiation, Am. J. Roentgenol. 86:1092, 1961.
8. Meadows, A. T., *et al.*: Oncogenesis and other late effects of cancer treatment in children: Report of a single hospital study, Radiology 114:175, 1974.
9. Tefft, M., *et al.*: Acute and late effects on normal tissues following combined chemo- and radiotherapy for childhood rhabdomyosarcoma and Ewing's sarcoma, Cancer 37:(supp.)1201, 1976.
10. Meadows, A. T., *et al.*: Patterns of second malignant neoplasms in children, Cancer 40:1903, 1978.
11. D'Angio, G. J., *et al.*: Decreased risk of radiation-associated second malignant neoplasms in actinomycin D-treated patients, Cancer 37:(supp.)1177, 1976.
12. D'Angio, G. J., *et al.*: The treatment of Wilms' tumor. Results of the National Wilms' Tumor Study, Cancer 38:633, 1976.
13. D'Angio, G. J., Tefft, M., Breslow, N., and Meyer, J.: Radiation therapy of Wilms' tumor, Int. J. Radiat. Oncol. Biol. Phys. (in press).
14. Tefft, M., D'Angio, G. J., and Grant, W.: Postoperative radiation therapy for residual Wilms' tumor. Review of Group III patients in National Wilms' Tumor Study, Cancer 37:2768, 1976.
15. Orten, C. G., and Ellis, F.: Simplification in the use of the NSD concept in practical radio-therapy, Br. J. Radiol. 46:529, 1973.
16. Bishop, H., *et al.*, Survival in bilateral Wilms' tumor, J. Pediatr. Surg. 12:631, 1977.
17. Cassady, J. R., *et al.*: Considerations in the radiation therapy of Wilms' tumor, Cancer 32:598, 1973.
18. Evans, A. E., D'Angio, G. J., and Randolph, J.: A proposed staging for children with neuroblastoma, Cancer 27:374, 1971.
19. Evans, A. E., *et al.*: Cyclophosphamide treatment of patients with localized and regional neuroblastoma. A randomized study, Cancer 34:655, 1976.
20. Koop, C. E., and Johnson, D. G.: Neuroblastoma: An assessment of therapy in reference to staging, J. Pediatr. Surg. 6:585, 1971.
21. D'Angio, G. J., and Evans, A.: Soft Tissue Sarcomas, in Bloom, H. J. G., Lemerle, J., Neidhardt, M. K., and Voute, P. A. (eds.), *Cancer in Children. Clinical Management* (New York and Berlin: Springer-Verlag, 1975), pp. 217–241.
22. Clatworthy, H. W., Braren, V., and Smith, J. P.: Surgery of bladder and prostatic neoplasms in children, Cancer 32:1157, 1973.
22a. Jereb, B., *et al.*: Local control of embryonal rhabdomyosarcoma in children by radiation therapy when combined with concomitant chemotherapy, Int. J. Radiat. Oncol. Biol. Phys. 1:217, 1976.
23. Donaldson, S. S., *et al.*: Rhabdomyosarcoma of head and neck in children; combination treatment by surgery, irradiation and chemotherapy, Cancer 31:26, 1973.
24. Sagerman, R. H., Tretter, P., and Ellsworth, R. M.: The treatment of orbital rhabdomyosarcoma of children with primary radiation therapy, Am. J. Roentgenol. 114:31, 1972.
25. Lieberman, P. H., *et al.*: Alveolar soft-part sarcoma, JAMA 198:1047, 1966.
26. Cham, W. C., *et al.*: Patterns of extension as a guide to radiation therapy in the management of ovarian neoplasms in children, Cancer 37:1443, 1976.
27. D'Angio, G. J., and Tefft, M.: Radiation therapy in the management of children with gynecologic cancers, Ann. N. Y. Acad. Sci. 142:675, 1967.

28. Rosen, G.: Management of malignant bone tumors in children and adolescents, Pediatr. Clin. North Am. 23:183, February, 1976.

29. Sutow, W. W., Suit, H. D., and Martin, R. G.: Bone Tumors, in Bloom, H. J. G., Lemerle, J., Neidhardt, M. K., and Voute, P. A. (eds.), *Cancer in Children. Clinical Management* (New York and Berlin: Springer-Verlag, 1975), pp. 200–216.

30. D'Angio, G. J., *et al.:* Protection of certain structures from high doses of irradiation, Am. J. Roentgenol. 122:103, 1974.

31. Evans, A. E.: Personal communication.

PART II

Trauma

9 Judson Randolph
Children as Accident Victims

In 1974, 26,826 children died who were from 1 to 14 years of age. Of this number, 12,448 were victims of accidents. By far the leading offender in these accidental deaths was the automobile, accounting for 5796 dead children. Two thousand four hundred forty drowned, 1218 died of burns, 533 were injured fatally by firearms and 214 died after ingesting various poisons. When the nearly 12,500 children lost by accident are compared to the 2961 deaths in children from cancer, the magnitude of accidental death in childhood comes clearly into focus. Although infants under a year of age are less vulnerable to accidents, 1691 of approximately 5,500 deaths in this age group were caused, in order of frequency, by poisoning, suffocation and automobile collisions.[1] If an infectious disease caused such death and destruction among our children, the public outcry would demand protection and treatment. It is ironic that preventive measures that could alter these statistics in a major way go unheeded.

These stark facts demonstrate the urgency of reducing accidental injury to children. The surgeon's traditional role, the immediate care of accident victims, is well defined. Great gains have been realized in understanding the nature of bodily injury and its metabolic consequences. Coupled with technologic advances in life support systems and monitoring devices, this has produced steady improvement in the surgical salvage of injured children. Yet, the pediatric surgeon may have an even more important role to play on behalf of the injured child. Familiar as they are with the mechanisms as well as the consequences of trauma, surgeons have an obligation to the cause of accident prevention. Much can be done to eliminate existing hazards in the child's environment. This is best accomplished by modifying the environment of the child and by improving the education of all citizens with respect to safety practices.

A major portion of childhood accidents occur in the home. It is of the utmost importance, therefore, to teach adults about the avoidable causes of injuries. Children cannot be left alone, or in the care of other children. Young mothers must learn how to "childproof" the home. Matches must be kept hidden (Fig. 9–1). The busy, young, inexperienced mother must be taught how to handle boiling water, gas ovens and fireplaces with safety and common sense. The pot handles on the stove and the coffee pot on the breakfast table must be placed out of the toddler's reach (Fig. 9–2). Hot water heaters must be carefully regulated. Caustic materials cannot be placed in floor cabinets where toddlers can reach them. Electrical appliances must be built, maintained, used and stored according to predefined standards (Fig. 9–3).

Legislation, heightened public awareness and nationwide acceptance of family safety practices are essential if the annual toll of injured children is to be reduced by a major increment. Excellent examples of favorable modification of the child's environment against health threats are to be found in the control of lead poisoning and in the Flammable Clothing Act. Once it became obvious that peeling lead-based paint was being eaten by children, particularly in ghetto-urban settings, laws were enacted that eliminated the use of lead-based paint. This progressive action has materially reduced a major threat to children. The Flammable Clothing Act has had widespread importance for youngsters, and, as its effect spreads, greater protection will be realized, although the recent discovery of the carcinogenic nature of the flame retardant indicates the complexity of the problem.

Protection for children riding in automobiles has long been neglected. Shelness and Charles,[4] writing about children as passengers in automobiles, state that "it is ironic that a nation that ranks the welfare of children as priority is in the process of mandating the use of seat belts for parents, but does not insist on the same right for children." More small children are killed inside motor vehicles than outside.[3] For example, a review of automobile accidents and seat belt usage in 1970 disclosed that only 2880 (15%) of 19,061 children under 5 years of age in collisions were restrained. None of these restrained were killed but 82 of the 16,181 unrestrained children lost their lives. The committee on Accident Prevention of the American Academy of Pediatrics has stressed the need for special restraint systems for young children who do not fit in the customary lap and shoulder straps. Tennessee is the first state to enact legislation requiring that young children be restrained while riding in automobiles. Known as the Child Passenger Protection Act, this law requires all children under 4 to wear federally approved restraint systems while riding in an automobile.

The immediate care of the injured child has improved dramatically in the past decade. Study of the metabolic consequences of trauma in the child has led to important gains in treatment of injured youngsters. Progress in the transportation of the injured victim has been noteworthy. With regionalization of pediatric trauma facilities, the concept of rapid transportation of the injured victim to the nearest hospital has, in forward-thinking communities, given rise to a network of metropolitan and rural transportation programs that interact with designated primary, secondary and tertiary trauma treatment centers. The effectiveness of transportation networks has been augmented in many instances by radio and television communication systems. Proper triage of the injured victims ensures expeditious transfer of those children with severe or multiple injuries to tertiary centers.

Under ideal circumstances, basic life support for any accident victim should be initiated at the scene. Bystanders will be helpful only if they are prepared. Courses in basic cardiopulmonary resuscitation and emergency care might well be part of the curriculum for high school students. Such study should be mandatory for teachers, police, firemen and athletic coaches. Cardiopulmonary resuscitation courses such as those offered by the American Heart Association should be required of all persons providing immediate care for critically ill children. Traumatologists have pointed out many facets of care planning that could be implemented nation-

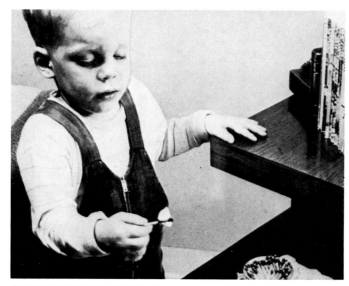

Fig. 9–1 (left). – Child with a lighted match. The fascination of fire and matches for the 5- or 6-year-old child is universal. All matches in the home must be kept sequestered from children.

Fig. 9–2 (below left). – The vulnerability of 2-, 3- and 4-year-old children to boiling liquids on the stove.

Fig. 9–3 (below). – Electrical plugs, wires and appliances are dangers inviting curious exploration by an unwatched child. (Photographs courtesy of Dr. A. M. Margileth.)

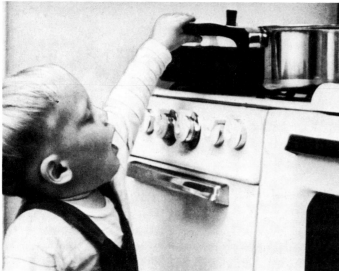

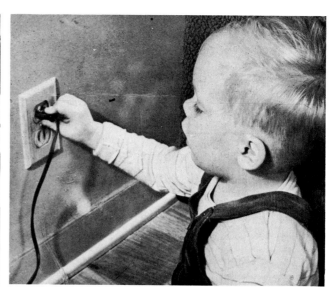

wide. Some of these elements are: (a) the universal establishment of the emergency 911 telephone service; (b) the creation of interconnected regional communications systems and emergency medical services operations centers (EMSOC); (c) the upgrading of all land and air ambulances to sophisticated, mobile intensive care units (MICU); (d) the upgrading of all ambulance attendants to emergency medical technicians (EMT) so that they can render advanced life support at the scene of the accident and during transportation; (e) the absolute control and continued monitoring of these emergency "beachheads" (EMT-MICU) by physicians and surgeons well versed in emergency care; and (f), most important, the regionalization and categorization of hospital emergency facilities for the care of children.[2]

When an injured child arrives in a hospital emergency facility, a trauma team should be on hand. Such a team may be headed by a pediatric surgeon and should include pediatricians, emergency nurses, an orthopedist, a neurosurgeon and a urologist. Resuscitation, stabilization, diagnosis and treatment should merge together smoothly.

It is especially important in children that critical assis-

tance be rendered in a calm, compassionate and reassuring manner. Indeed, the entire process of transportation, diagnosis in an emergency facility, treatment, hospitalization and recovery demands strong support of the psyche of any injured patient, and this need is magnified in younger subjects. Psychiatrists, psychiatric social workers and psychologists have become indispensable members of the pediatric trauma team.

All adults have a responsibility to modify the environment on behalf of children and thereby minimize the potential for accidents. When accidents occur in the home, on the playground or in the street, bystanders should have enough training that they can function as emergency personnel because of their preparedness through public education. The transport system should incorporate accurate appraisal and prompt triage to an emergency unit or a regional care center. Once in the system, the child should move smoothly and swiftly from appropriate emergency care to an operating suite or to a pediatric intensive care unit. Throughout this course, the child's psychologic needs should be considered and supported. Only when the foregoing elements have been provided can we begin to control accidents, which remain the number one threat to the health and life of all children.

REFERENCES

1. Garfinkel, J., Chabot, J. J., and Pratt, M. W.: Infant, maternal and childhood mortality in the U. S. DHEW publication no. (HSA) 75-5013 (Rockville, Md.: Health Services Administration, 1968–1973).

2. Haddon, W., and Baker, S. P.: Injury Control, in Clark, D., and MacMahon, B. (eds.), *Preventive Medicine* (2d ed.; Boston: Little, Brown and Company, 1977).
3. Harding, R. M.: Safety Belt Usage in Cars. DOT:NHTSA Survey, n43-31, July, 1974.
4. Shelness, A., and Charles, S.: Children as passengers in automobiles, Pediatrics 56:271, 1975.
5. Scherz, R. G.: Restraint systems for the prevention of injury to children in automobile accidents, Am. J. Public Health 66:451, 1976.
6. Steichen, F. M.: Personal communication.

10 Felicien M. Steichen

Emergency Management of the Severely Injured Child

INJURIES occur suddenly, most often to the unprepared, usually healthy, individual. The senseless, brutal character of trauma is especially revolting in the carefree child or teen-ager unaware or oblivious of the many physical dangers at home, in school, at play and in sports.

In the United States, trauma is the leading cause of death in children 1 year of age and over, and in teen-agers. Prevention or successful treatment of injuries in the young is followed by an average survival of 50–60 years of what should become a productive individual, given the usual opportunities of education, health and the pursuit of happiness.

Through their own, almost unavoidable, inexperience at various stages of development, the child and teen-ager usually are the passive victims of accidents of neglect, inattention, lack of education and thoughtlessness. Active children succumb to "booby traps" built into their environment. Rarely does a child search out danger for danger's sake.

The sources of childhood injuries are well recognized and, therefore, much could be done in the way of *prevention* and *education*—prevention of potential for home accidents by builders and parents alike, creation of safer toys, clothes and cars,[26] education in traffic hazards, teaching of safety rules in play and sports and, finally, education, support and counseling of parents and other adults given to child abuse. The list of what can be accomplished with a minimal investment of time, effort and thought by adults responsible for children is endless. Children are largely educated by example. A simple proof of this is seat belts.[2, 26] They are in every car, require a negligible amount of time and energy to use and, yet, how many children are shown the good example?

Hospital Emergency Service Organization

No child who arrives at a hospital Emergency Room alive should die in the E.R. To accomplish this, institutional planning, professional organization, architectural layout, material resources and specialized know-how should be adapted to the management of the injured child and his or her companion, most often an anxious parent.

If the emergency facility is part of a general hospital center (in many ways the best solution, because of easier accessibility as well as greater availability and rational use of emergency resources), a special area should be reserved and organized as a children's Emergency Room, if possible under the same roof with the adult facility. In freestanding children's hospitals, a specialized emergency facility usually is available to take care of pediatric trauma.

To the American public, visits to the Emergency Room have become synonymous with routine medical care after office hours to the point that only 2–5% of all Emergency Room patients suffer from life-threatening conditions and another 15–20% have true emergency problems. This is especially true in children, where the dividing line between what is acute and what is not often is difficult to define. The "common cold"—usually shrugged off by an adult—may be more spectacular in a child because of rhinorrhea and cough; it may be the hallmark of a strep throat or it may be the cause of severe croup and respiratory distress. It always is an acute emergency in the mind of the parent.

However, in order to reserve all of the needed human and material resources for the care of the injured and acutely ill child, an integral part of the organizational pattern of all busy children's Emergency Rooms should be triage of the pediatric patient, who may be examined and treated in a more leisurely fashion in a special "walk-in" facility, adjacent to the E.R., separately staffed and equipped and open from 9:00 A.M. to midnight, for instance. This triage is best accomplished by experienced and specially trained nurses or physicians' assistants, supervised and backed up by pediatricians. Triage should take place on arrival of the child, before the usual time-consuming collection of data for bureaucratic purposes. Following triage and proper identification, the child is immediately sent to the appropriate facility—either E.R. or walk-in clinic—while the parents or companions are occupied with the necessary paper work. If it is in the interest of good and efficient care—mostly in true emergencies—that the parents remain in the E.R. waiting room, the triage staff member(s) can double as a public relations officer, reassuring the parents and keeping them generally informed until such time as a physician is free to explain matters to parents.[6] Rooms and interpreters should be available for parent-physician consultations. In ambulance cases, triage starts at the scene of pickup and continues during transportation by two-way radio contact between the ambulance crew and the E.R. physicians so as to mobilize space, personnel and material for the management of an injured or acutely ill child.

Functional Emergency Room Plan (Including Trauma Center, Fig. 10–1)

Planning of the Emergency Room should include the following considerations: Easy accessibility on ground floor level; rational traffic coordination outside and inside; clear identification of separate entrances for children, adults and ambulance patients in the case of a combined facility; horizontal or vertical proximity to a walk-in clinic and major portions of the Outpatient Department; functional versatility allowing for the exchange and concentration of professional and material resources, such as triage, resuscitation, minor and major operating rooms; incorporation of diagnostic facilities; and areas for observing patients following their postoperative recovery, and even dispensing intensive care on a temporary basis. The master plan should be flexible to permit adaptation to special local and regional needs as well as to specific circumstances, such as a combined facility in a general hospital, a freestanding center affiliated with one or several hospitals, a specialized Emergency Room in a children's hospital.

The traffic inside the Emergency Room should be organized so that patients and their families only rarely, if ever, have to return to a given station. Time spent in the waiting room should be used to educate patients and their escorts on matters of trauma and emergency medicine by such techniques as are used by Mr. Rogers, Sesame Street and The Electric Company.

The inclusion in the over-all plan of a Central Core, containing not only areas for minor surgical procedures and re-

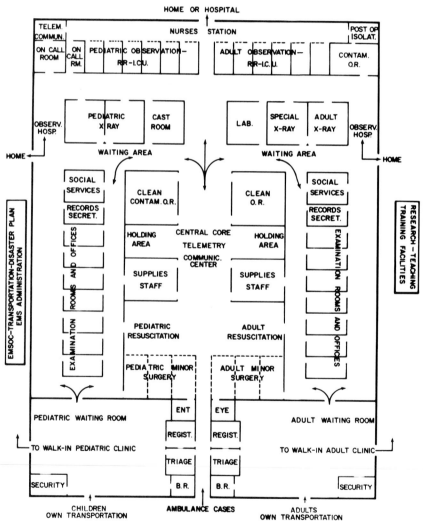

Fig. 10–1.—The "ideal" Emergency Room. This should include facilities for care of the severely injured as well as the acutely ill patient, since the immediate care and intensive diagnostic work-up are similar in both groups. A combined facility will make for a more rational use of resources but is not a must. In the present plan, for instance, a line drawn down the middle would produce two equivalent facilities. All the desirable features described in the text are shown in this plan. As an added feature, the minor surgery suites are divided into cubicles by curtains; these can be drawn and a large area including the resuscitation rooms will result, useful in the management of mass casualties.

suscitation that every Emergency Room should have but also regular operating rooms and the main two-way radio and telemetry station, will justify the concentration of professional talent of the highest caliber in sufficient numbers in this area. Response to the most simple as well as to the most challenging of conditions in the field and *intra muros* would be prompt, efficient and expert. The lag time that often exists between a brilliant resuscitation by the emergency team and the badly needed operation by a new, in-hospital, "elective" team in a distant operating room—if indeed the new team and operating room are free—will become a thing of the past. Finally, the same surgeons, having the best knowledge of a given patient from the moment of ambulance pickup through resuscitation, diagnostic work-up and operation, will be able to follow "their" patient during his earlier recovery period in a combined observation-recovery room-

intensive care unit located within the confines of the Emergency Room. If, through foresight and planning, the general operating rooms and recovery room-intensive care areas are horizontally or vertically contiguous to the Emergency Room, these facilities may not need duplication in the Emergency Room, provided that space always is reserved for emergency purposes and that the initial Emergency Room team continues to care for the patient. Although such an arrangement might result in savings of hard-to-get funds, it would have the disadvantage of removing from the communications area the most experienced members of the team for prolonged periods.

Since work in even the busiest Emergency Room fortunately is not a continuous parade of make-or-break problems, time ordinarily would be available for senior members of the team to supervise, teach and train their junior associates

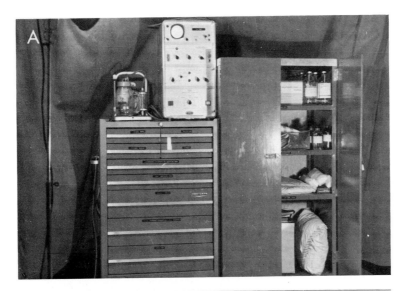

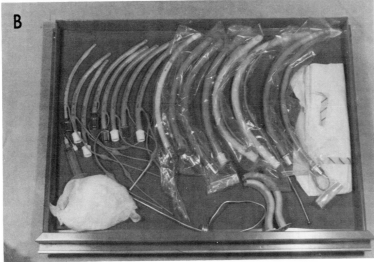

Fig. 10–2. – **A,** mobile auxiliary emergency cart. Besides the compact MAX cart containing drugs and instruments needed in CPR, we have used with great success a mobile homemade backup truck consisting of a platform mounted on swivel wheels and provided with a long electric extension cord. The platform carries a Sears-Roebuck tool chest and a homemade cabinet; a suction apparatus and ECG-defibrillator monitor are mounted on the tool chest and oxygen cylinders are attached to the side of the cabinet (not seen here). The drawers of the Sears cabinet contain all the instruments needed in CPR; the larger chest contains reserves of IV fluids, IV administration sets, laboratory tubes, venous cutdown-tracheostomy-thoracotomy-suture sets and mask-bag ventilators. Because of its great mobility and the long extension cord, this truck can be wheeled into any area of the Emergency Room where a patient requires resuscitation. **B,** the drawer containing all sizes of endotracheal tubes is shown. A similar variety of sizes should be available for laryngoscopes, bronchoscopes, bag-valve masks, oropharyngeal airways, defibrillator pedals and surgical instrument trays.

and indeed participate in the education and training of emergency physicians who plan a career in hospitals serving major emergency needs without the help of a house staff.

It is not my purpose to describe in detail all of the equipment needs that exist in a pediatric Emergency Room (Fig. 10–2, A).[1, 1a] However, it is obvious that all instruments for resuscitation in children should be available in sizes adapted to the various ages[24] (Fig. 10–2, B,). A running inventory should be kept, instantaneously replacing equipment as it is used, with absolute interdiction of removal of anything for use in other areas of the hospital.[16] Large charts, placed on walls and readable from afar, should feature dosages of the most frequently used drugs for various ages and weight levels.[1a, 24] The resuscitation areas should be equipped with timed audio equipment and possibly a television camera, so that a record superior to the faulty and harassed memory of the Emergency Room team becomes available. All trauma victims should be placed on a stretcher with a radiolucent top; built-in or mobile x-ray equipment should be available in all resuscitation areas and operating rooms. The MAX cart developed by Nobel[16] has been of invaluable help to us in the immediate resuscitation and in the moving of patients requiring continued CPR.

If and when regionalization of emergency care and categorization of emergency facilities become a reality, all major, optimally equipped Emergency Rooms should have the necessary programs and space for research related to trauma and acute illness and for continuing education of their own staff and emergency physicians from other hospitals, as well as for teaching and training of lay people.[1] Emergency Medical Services Operations Centers should be conveniently associated with major emergency facilities; control of all land and air ambulances will originate from such a center. Finally, regional and local disaster plans would be established and revised from this base.

Hospital Emergency Care

Attention to all the details of this initial response is only a beginning; the ultimate success depends on the constant availability and advanced expertise of a well-organized emergency team. The Emergency Room team should be led by a general surgeon, mature in his experience and understanding of the severely injured child, enthusiastic in his pursuit of the challenge posed by major trauma, free from all other major responsibilities. A senior resident or junior attending will best fill this bill. The ready availability of emergency consultation by general and specialty house and attending staffs, and of leadership by senior attendings, will harmoniously complete this basic standby team.

In addition to careful planning and a meticulous organization, the sudden and dramatic appearance of an injured child requires a cool response, almost reflex in nature, acquired through teaching but mostly through "on-the-job" training provided by repeated participation in "emergency actions" at various, progressive levels of responsibility. Basic to this response is the understanding that in the critically injured child, the routine of diagnosis first and treatment next has to be altered through the recognition of certain emergency clinical conditions that require immediate treatment before time is taken to establish a specific etiologic diagnosis. This immediate treatment is based on the perception of major physical findings characteristic of a given emergency condition and on the knowledge of priorities that should be respected in the management of the child with multiple injuries.[23]

A. Priorities

Beware of Cervical Spine!

Highest Priority
1. Cardiorespiratory impairment by maxillofacial, neck and chest injuries.
2. Severe external hemorrhage.

The possibility—often only suspected—of a cervical spine injury takes precedence over all other early considerations, since the usual maneuvers of cardiopulmonary resuscitation may seriously complicate a cervical spine fracture.[6] However, suspicion of a cervical spine injury should not prompt neglect of the obstructed airway. Modified maneuvers to open the airway, maintaining longitudinal traction on the head, must be undertaken in the apneic and partially obstructed patient[1a] and will be discussed later.

The highest priorities are those problems incompatible with life if the underlying conditions are not remedied at once. They include maxillofacial, neck and chest injuries resulting in respiratory and cardiac impairment, airway obstruction from a nontraumatic cause and deep wounds producing severe external hemorrhage.

High Priority
3. Retroperitoneal injury.
4. Intraperitoneal injury.
5. Craniocerebral, spinal injury.
6. Severe thermal injury.
7. Extensive soft tissue injury.

High priority is given to conditions that are also incompatible with life if the causative factors are not attended to or reversed promptly. In general, more time, even a short period of intense observation, is available for a more deliberate approach to problems in this group.

Retroperitoneal and intraperitoneal injuries are most serious because of their potential for hypovolemia due to hidden or open (GI bleeding, hematuria) hemorrhage and for peritonitis due to continued contamination from an open viscus. The presence of a penetrating wound—most often a stab wound, very rarely a gunshot wound—without signs of retroperitoneal or intraperitoneal damage is not any more an automatic indication for urgent laparotomy in itself.[5, 19, 22]

Injuries to the brain, the spinal cord and their bony envelopes follow next, since they do not threaten death as rapidly as do thoracic and abdominal injuries. Open wounds require early debridement and reliable closure of the dura; contamination is of the secondary type and not continuous as it is in visceral injuries. Most closed injuries tolerate and often benefit from a period of observation to evaluate progressive localizing signs and the state of consciousness, albeit the "golden time" of evaluation in acute extradural bleeding is very short.[10]

Severe thermal injuries and extensive soft tissue wounds and contusions close the list, because of their early potential for hypovolemic shock and all of its complications and their delayed potential for overwhelming sepsis due to secondary bacterial invasion of massively destroyed tissues, often void of protective skin.

Low Priority
8. Injury to lower male GU system.
9. Injury to peripheral vessels, nerves, locomotor system.
10. Limited soft tissue injury.

Low-priority injuries are not life-threatening by themselves. However, if neglected, they may result in loss of function, limb or both. In injuries to the lower genitourinary system, essentially the male urethra and the scrotum, the treatment of hemorrhage takes precedence over that of extravasation. Injuries to the bladder are part of the management of retroperitoneal and intraperitoneal injuries (Priorities 3 and 4).

Peripheral vascular injuries that do not result in external hemorrhage (Priority 2), peripheral nerve injuries and trauma to extremity bones, joints, tendons and muscles, as a group allow for a more deliberate approach, often after special studies have been obtained, provided that repair is completed within the accepted limits of tissue survival. Wounds require debridement and closure even if the underlying injury, as in some specific nerve and tendon injuries for instance, is left for secondary, elective repair after complete wound healing.

Soft tissue injuries limited to skin, subcutaneous tissue and superficial muscle layers close the list of priorities, although some of the superficial wounds, as in the head and neck area, may be very spectacular. The management of wounds takes precedence over contusion and hematoma. Primary wound healing and good cosmesis without excessive scar formation, especially in facial and neck wounds, are the leading considerations here, realizing that the best chances for an excellent result are present at the first wound repair.

Remember!

Limbs with fractures and dislocations should be *temporarily immobilized* as soon as the over-all course of emergency management permits, without jeopardizing lifesaving maneuvers. Reduction of fractures and dislocations and application of permanent casts, traction devices and the like should be performed after the patient is stable, often during or following an abdominal, thoracic or cranial operation in a regular operating room. Judgment should be exercised, especially by the newcomer to emergency care, to whom, for example, an obvious extremity fracture may seem more important than a still subtle head injury. While this physician is busy applying a cast, the head injury may progress from its subtle stage to an avoidable, more serious level, and to the now semiconscious, thrashing patient, the heavy weight of a cast will become a cause of great irritation, with straining and increasing cerebral edema adding to the original head injury. A simple, light immobilization device and early attention to the respiratory care of the patient (endotracheal, transtracheal, nasogastric tubes) would avoid this deterioration.[10]

In wounds exposed to secondary contamination and in suspected visceral injuries with continuous contamination, the need for *antibiotic prophylaxis* should be evaluated and the status of *tetanus prophylaxis* should be ascertained. Measures indicated in these two areas should be started before the child leaves the E.R. or the O.R., as the case may be.[20]

Pre-existing conditions, such as juvenile diabetes, sickle cell anemia, hemophilia, allergic reactions and congenital malformations, may complicate the basic injury and require special steps in the treatment in order to avoid a cascade of therapeutic insults adding to the original injury. In children especially, the history of injury may not be compatible with the seriousness of the findings because of misleading information from parents in cases of child abuse or because of

serious traumatic changes within an unsuspected lesion, such as liver hamartoma, renal neoplasm, bone cyst, hydronephrosis, horseshoe kidney or hydrocephalus.[6, 14]

Finally, the child's fright can either exaggerate or hide part or all of the pertinent history and physical findings; the strange and rigorously efficient atmosphere of an Emergency Room will only add to this fright and produce reactions that might be difficult to interpret for a moment. Therefore, early and continued reassurance of the child on arrival, and as various procedures are in progress, should be part of all pediatric emergency management.[6, 14]

B. Sequence of Emergency Management

The sequence and intensity of emergency management of the severely injured child depends on the level of emergency measures taken on the scene of the accident and during transportation as well as on the clinical condition at the time of admission to the E.R.

The severely injured child, often with multiple organs involved, may arrive at the Emergency Room apparently lifeless and unresponsive. A well-organized, decisive approach to this kind of problem is the sine qua non of success.

In a second group of patients, conscious on admission but with a history of severe trauma and findings to substantiate the history, the management should be expert and deliberate.

In a third group of patients in whom a history of severe trauma is contradicted by an apparent benign clinical picture, the risk of misjudgment is very high. Before the child is casually considered to live a fantasy or dream worthy of Baron von Münchhausen or Walter Mitty, it should be realized that he may just be a true disciple of Evel Knievel. Urgent treatment should be started on mere suspicion, so as to avoid or at least be prepared for a sudden collapse should the initial history turn out to be true after all. If it is not true, little is lost and the child may have learned a sobering lesson.

All drugs administered should be strictly dose controlled for a given estimated or known patient weight. Blood up to 20 ml/kg of body weight is tolerated without problems if the blood loss cannot be estimated accurately during the early phase of resuscitation.

I. "LIFELESS," UNRESPONSIVE
   Beware Cervical Spine!
   1. RESPIRATORY RESUSCITATION
      Airway patency—ventilation:
         mask—endotracheal—transtracheal.
   2. CARDIAC RESUSCITATION
      Closed massage 5 minutes.
      Open massage: No response—
         heart wound—spinal injury.
   3. MONITORING
      Chest—pulse—ECG.

Following severe trauma, the conditions that result in an immediate threat to the patient's life are respiratory impairment, resulting in inadequacy of oxygenation and ventilation as well as cardiac arrest, asystole or ventricular fibrillation. Airway patency is established by clearing and opening the patient's airway, and oxygenation and ventilation are ensured by breathing for him with a face mask, attached resuscitator bag with an oxygen reservoir and inflowing supplemental oxygen.

Endotracheal intubation is the next step in airway management, oxygenation and ventilation. The airway is secured and, with the cuff of the tube inflated, aspiration of gastric contents is prevented. Endotracheal intubation facilitates both oxygenation and ventilation by circumventing problems of securing a face mask fit. The correct insertion of an endotracheal tube requires adequate psychomotor skills and should be performed only by those who have been trained and can insert the tube rapidly and without trauma.[25]

An alternative method of oxygenation and ventilation is transtracheal jet ventilation (Fig. 10–3) using a large-bore plastic catheter (#14 or #16) and oxygen injected under pressure (30–50 psi).[11, 12, 21] This technique can be replaced by a tracheostomy at a later period. Transtracheal jet ventilation is a useful technique for patients with (a) brain injuries, because straining on an endotracheal tube will produce venous hypertension and increased brain edema; (b) cervical spine injuries, because extension of the head and neck in order to open the upper airways can precipitate or aggravate a cervical cord injury; and (c) maxillofacial injuries with severe oropharyngeal hemorrhage that prevents efficient mask-to-airway breathing and forbids adequate visualization in the pharyngolaryngeal area. Complications include subcutaneous and mediastinal emphysema, hemorrhage and perforation of the posterior tracheal wall into the esophagus.

While respiratory resuscitation is in progress, the circulation is maintained or restored by external cardiac compression. If there is no femoral or carotid pulsation with each closed chest compression, if the heart fails to show any response within 5 minutes,[3, 25] if a penetrating wound of the heart is suspected or if a cervical spine injury is evident, open chest cardiac massage is used.[1a] The use of primary open chest cardiac massage in suspected wounds of the heart and in proved cervical spine injuries is based on the fact that closed massage may be harmful. In the patient with a cardiac wound, it further empties an already empty pump and in the patient with cervical spine injury, it produces repeated flexion and extension movements of the cervical spine.

In order to assess the efficiency of the respiratory and cardiac resuscitation, chest movements and peripheral pulses are monitored, ECG leads are applied and connected to the ECG monitor.

4. INTRAVENOUS LINES
    Site – catheter – cutdown.
5. LABORATORY WORK
    Type/X-match, hematocrit,
        blood gases, chemistries,
        Hypaque IV, PRN.
6. VOLUME REPLACEMENT
    Lactated Ringer's – D5 N/S.

The placement of intravenous lines should be given some thought. For thoracic injuries, the lower extremities are used; for abdominal injuries, the upper extremities are preferred.[20] Subclavian vein placement, very popular in adults, is less so in children because of the increased seriousness of potential complications (pneumothorax, hemothorax, infusion hydrothorax). The internal jugular vein is preferred if a large vein is required for fluid administration. In the newborn with head and chest trauma, umbilical vessels may be used.

Intravenous catheters are preferred to needles, although many a well-placed scalp needle has saved the day during the early course of resuscitation. Following the placement of a needle, a cutdown can be performed with precision; cutdowns are used with greater frequency in children than in adults.

With one or several intravenous portals open, blood is drawn for the usual laboratory determinations. Blood gases, rarely needed this early, may be drawn by direct arterial puncture if there is a palpable pulse. However, even venous blood or capillary blood gases may give an approximation of ventilatory and acid-base status.

If there is reason or evidence to suspect a urinary tract injury, a "one shot" intravenous pyelogram can be performed with the injection of Urografin or Hypaque as soon as intravenous portals are established. As the patient's vital signs improve, and if x-rays are taken (in E.R., Radiology Department *or* O.R.), an "incidental" outline of the normal or both kidneys can be obtained.

Volume replacement is ensured with crystalloid solutions at this stage before quick typed or typed and cross matched blood becomes available. As with drugs and blood, volume replacement with crystalloids should be done on a patient weight basis. Microdip sets, especially in infants, represent an added safety against fluid overload.

7. CARDIAC RESUSCITATION
    Na bicarb – epinephrine – Ca chloride.
    Defibrillation PRN.
8. RESPIRATORY RESUSCITATION
    Endotrach. tube – tracheostomy.
    N/G tube – chest tube PRN.
9. VOLUME REPLACEMENT
    Typed blood – filter.
10. MONITORING
    Urine collect./analysis.
    Arterial – CV – PA pressures.
    Diuretic PRN.

Sodium bicarbonate (1 mEq/kg) is used in order to revert the acidosis of hypovolemia and hypoxia and to make the heart receptive to electrical and pharmacologic stimulation. However, excessive infusions of hypertonic sodium bicarbonate may lead to alkalosis, K imbalance, hyperosmolality and hypercarbia. As soon as circulation is restored, alkalinizing drugs are not needed. In asystole, myocardial contractility is stimulated with epinephrine and fine ventricular fibrillation is converted to coarse fibrillation, which facilitates countershock (0.1 ml/kg of 1:10,000 dilution IV). Calcium chloride 10% 10–20 mg/kg IV is an adjunct drug during asystole. Intracardiac injections of epinephrine and calcium can be used but constitute hazards, i.e., pneumothorax or damage to coronary vessels. If ventricular fibrillation is present, defibrillation by closed or open technique is initiated, depending on the route used for heart massage. Using a DC defibrillator with paddles on the chest wall, defibrillation is achieved with a countershock of 5 watt seconds/kg.

The state of respiratory resuscitation is re-examined and if endotracheal intubation could not be established safely before, mask-bag ventilation now may be replaced by an endotracheal tube. Simultaneous ventilation and inspection through a bronchoscope in children suspected of having aspirated a foreign body obstructing the trachea or a main bronchus can be lifesaving. For this purpose, several sizes of ventilating bronchoscopes should be available. Alternatively, the jet ventilator equipped with a long catheter (Fig. 10–3) can be used through a regular rigid bronchoscope. The instrument itself is positioned in the trachea like an endotracheal tube with the help of an anesthesia laryngoscope. Tracheostomy will replace a transtracheal approach if

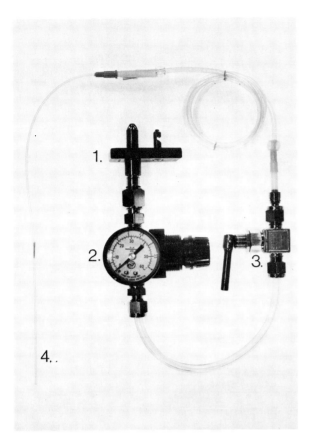

Fig. 10–3.—The transtracheal needle jet ventilator. Oxygen line connector *(1)*, a manometer and reducing valve *(2)*, a manual valve to control volume and frequency of oxygen jets *(3)* and a #16 angiocath *(4)*. Shown here is a long angiocath used in conjunction with a bronchoscope. For emergency transtracheal ventilation, a short #16 angiocath is introduced percutaneously between the first and second tracheal rings. (Courtesy of Dr. Miroslav Klain.)

the reasons for using the latter initially still persist. It must be realized that tracheostomy is a major operative procedure in a child and should be attempted only in the operating room[14] on a child who still is unconscious or has been anesthetized through the transtracheal needle jet ventilator.[11, 12, 21] Only after the trachea has been shielded by an endotracheal or tracheostomy tube should a nasogastric tube be used to empty the stomach. Clinically recognizable (needle aspiration) pneumothorax or hemothorax should be treated by tube thoracostomy without waiting for x-ray confirmation.[6]

As it becomes available, typed blood is administered if the primary volume deficit is due to persistent blood loss. If large blood volume replacements are anticipated, micropore blood filters should be used immediately. For large blood volume replacement, 2 ml of Na bicarbonate and 50 mg of Ca chloride should be used for each 100 ml of blood.

With control of life-threatening conditions, the monitoring of the patient becomes more complete. Urine is obtained for analysis by a gentle Credé maneuver and, if this is unproductive, by catheterization; quantity and specific gravity are to be followed precisely. Later on, the method of urine collection should become noninvasive (urine bag), as feasible, in order to avoid urinary infection and trauma to the child's urethra. Arterial pressure may be measured by cuff and manometer or by intra-arterial line (radial, ulnar, dorsa-

lis pedis, temporal, artery cutdown) and continuous display. The intra-arterial line is especially indicated if serial blood gas determinations are required.[20] Central venous pressures are followed via the transjugular route or a long catheter advanced centrally from a peripheral upper extremity venous cutdown.[20] Pulmonary artery and wedge pressure readings may be indicated during operation and especially during intensive postoperative trauma care as part of the total cardiopulmonary profile determinations.[4, 13]

Central venous and pulmonary artery pressures can be readily obtained only in the older child. If volume replacement is adequate and arterial pressure and central venous pressure or pulmonary artery pressure start to rise and urine output still does not improve, a diuretic should be used.

Although a resuscitative effort of this intensity will have given the physicians and nurses involved ample opportunity to find and record individual physical signs, time can and now should be taken to assemble the puzzle by capsule history and brief but thorough physical examination.

II. *CLINICAL SHOCK, RESPONSIVE*
 1. H & P, BP – P – R.
 2. INTRAVENOUS LINES
 3. LABORATORY WORK
 4. VOLUME REPLACEMENT
   Lactated Ringer's – D5 N/S
   Typed blood – filter.
 5. TUBES
   Tracheal – N/G – chest.
 6. MONITORING
   Urine collect./analysis.
   ECG – CVP – AP – PAP.
   Diuretic PRN.

Children admitted to the Emergency Room in shock but conscious and breathing represent the largest segment of all the children seen with severe trauma. Time is available for a short history and rapid, thorough examination; vital signs are recorded and monitored from the time of E.R. admission. Intravenous portals are established using the same guidelines, and blood is drawn for the laboratory studies. If the injury involves the abdomen, a "one shot" intravenous pyelogram is prepared with the injection of Hypaque intravenously. Volume replacement is, first with crystalloid solutions, then with typed blood as it becomes available. If transfusions are anticipated, filters should be used.

Nasogastric intubation is performed almost routinely in children with severe trauma, since the fright of the accident and injury makes them swallow large amounts of air.[6] Since the child is conscious, the danger of tracheal aspiration is lessened, although the frightened and weakened child may fight for air if vomiting does take place. In the obtunded child, therefore, the trachea should be isolated first. Tracheal intubation is also indicated in chest injuries. Transtracheal ventilation continues to be of help in brain, cervical spine and maxillofacial injuries, for the reasons given previously. If a pneumothorax and/or hemothorax is clinically apparent, chest drainage should be established without waiting for radiographic confirmation.[6]

Techniques and reasons for monitoring urinary output and specific gravity, electrocardiogram and central venous pressure are the same as were described previously. An indwelling arterial line is used only if continuous arterial pressure readouts and repeated blood gas determinations are necessary. Pulmonary artery and wedge pressures are measured in order to determine the over-all cardiopulmonary profile and to guide the management of fluids and drugs in the very critically injured and poorly responsive older child.[4, 13]

III. "STABLE" VITAL SIGNS
1. PERTINENT H & P
   BP — P — R — ECG.
2. INTRAVENOUS LINES
   CVP PRN.
3. LABORATORY WORK
4. MAINTAIN IV PATENCY
5. TUBES PRN
   N/G — Foley — chest,
   endotracheal.

The child's resilient body may incur injuries due to severe thoracic and abdominal compression, falls from impressive heights, ejection from an automobile, etc., with only minimal physical findings. On the other hand, minor injuries, usually well tolerated by the adult, such as a localized blow to the abdomen transmitted entirely through the lean abdominal wall, may result in rupture of the spleen, intestine, pancreas, full bladder, more rarely the liver or at least produce very worrisome signs of peritoneal irritation with no underlying organ injury. Finally, some children overreact to their injury and some parents are intentionally misleading.[14]

Whatever the ultimate conclusion may be, the surgeon should be wary and prepared in the "stable" child in whom the history does not agree with the findings or vice versa.[6] Time should be taken for a good history and physical examination, and vital signs and ECG should be monitored as a cautious routine.

Intravenous portals should be established and laboratory studies performed, as described previously. If there is any thought that it may be useful, a central venous pressure line should be introduced. Venous patency is maintained by the administration of crystalloid solutions; their rate of administration and the possible need for blood transfusion are determined by the initial findings and the continued monitoring.

Nasogastric aspiration and bladder drainage are established as needed. Basic radiographic studies then may be obtained — with a physician in attendance — and the findings on chest x-ray will determine the need for thoracostomy tubes and/or endotracheal intubation with respiratory stabilization in the case of multiple rib fractures in what usually would be a more discreet injury, not readily apparent clinically earlier.

If, on the other hand, the early impression of minor trauma is substantiated by minor findings, the intensity of emergency management is geared down and the child is admitted for observation or sent home, as the case may be.

NOTE: *Although intense and sophisticated monitoring is highly desirable in the injured and acutely ill child, all of the invasive techniques depend on patient size. Arterial line and pressure recordings are possible in any age group and represent the best way of monitoring treatment in the small child.* Central venous pressures rarely are possible before the age of 8 years and pulmonary artery and wedge pressures are difficult to obtain before the age of 10 years. Both of these measurements may be helpful in the assessment of treatment results, the need for therapy changes and the calculation of other cardiopulmonary parameters. In comparison to the case in adult trauma victims, the information obtained by central venous and pulmonary artery pressure measurements is less useful in the early phases of resuscitation, since most children have had normal cardiac and pulmonary systems prior to their accidents.

Disposition from Emergency Room

While resuscitation is in progress and long before success or failure can be ascertained, thought should be given to the next step in the patient's management and the necessary staff and material resources should be mobilized even though ultimately they may not be needed. A decision should be made as to:

1. Immediate transfer to an operating room because the condition can be controlled only by early operation. (In patients with well-defined chest injuries, immediate thoracotomy on arrival in the Emergency Room will be necessary.)

2. Continued diagnostic work-up to decide if urgent operation or if intensive observation and care are indicated, provided that the patient has a good response to all the resuscitative measures taken.

3. Transfer to an intensive care unit for observation and continued acute care of a stable patient who does not require operation at this point.

Continued diagnostic work-up will depend on the type and location of injury. In *abdominal stab wounds,* the mere presence of a wound is not an indication for routine operation, but the need for exploration can be determined by injection of the wound sinus with contrast material and radiographic examination to see if there is penetration into the cavity, or by continued clinical observation of signs of peritoneal irritation, such as quadrant or generalized tenderness and guarding, absent bowel sounds, all indicative of intra-abdominal injury. In some abdominal *gunshot wounds* where penetration is not suspected, contrast injection of the sinus tract or clinical observation may also be used, but in the vast majority of abdominal gunshot wounds, the evidence of intra-abdominal injury and the need for urgent laparotomy are quite clear.[5, 19, 22]

In *blunt injuries of the abdomen* where history and findings are equivocal, paracentesis with dialysis catheter and peritoneal lavage are very helpful. Although a negative examination does not rule out intra-abdominal trauma with absolute certainty, a high degree of proficiency with the technique and accuracy in its interpretation can be obtained through the frequent use of this examination and absolute adherence to all of its technical details.[17, 18] It should be noted that sinograms and peritoneal aspiration and irrigation should not be used in patients with possible adhesions from a previous laparotomy and should be preceded by a baseline radiographic examination, since air introduced iatrogenically may confuse the picture. Ideally, the responsible surgeon should also be present, since the penetration of the abdominal wall by Hypaque or a dialysis catheter produces a change in the clinical signs.

Intravenous pyelography and arteriography should be performed only in patients with a normal blood pressure in order to obtain a reliable result. If IVP is indicated and the "one shot" examination was not successful, an infusion pyelogram should be obtained in order to demonstrate a still functioning but severely contused kidney, for instance.[15] The increasing edema within the confining renal capsule will preclude a satisfactory concentration of contrast material if the conventional IVP is done late after admission. This may result in the erroneous diagnosis of a nonfunctioning kidney and in all of the potential conclusions that might result from such an error.

Arteriography, conventional scintigraphy and echography have an application in abdominal trauma only secondarily, in those patients who have stabilized with or without operation and in whom deep and subcapsular liver or spleen injury, pancreatic pseudocyst, amputation of a kidney pole and subphrenic abscess (to name but a few) need confirmation.

An exception to this is the suspected avulsion of the renal vascular pedicle in patients arriving in deep shock, showing signs of continued blood loss despite adequate blood replacement and in whom an IVP would have indicated a nonfunctioning kidney. Total body scanning will come to play a role in the diagnostic approach to a stable trauma victim. This role will be defined by experience as more and more CAT scanners are installed.

In the final analysis, it should be realized that in abdominal trauma, the indications for operation are largely based on the patient's clinical presentation. These indications are mandatory in the patient admitted in shock, having gastrointestinal bleeding or showing free air under the diaphragm in both penetrating and blunt injuries. In addition to that in penetrating injuries, the indications for operation are absolute in patients with evisceration, wound hemorrhage and hematuria. We do not operate on patients with blunt trauma thought to be limited to the retroperitoneum, especially when there is an associated pelvic fracture, since venous retroperitoneal hemorrhage due to blunt trauma is best treated by maintaining the patient's blood volume and allowing the posterior peritoneum to tamponade the bleeding.

In contrast to abdominal trauma, in *thoracic* injuries, open operation is indicated only rarely (in some 2–5% of patients). Airway patency and ventilation will be maintained by either endotracheal intubation or tracheostomy.

Diagnostically, percussion and auscultation of the thorax are extremely important, as is routine chest radiography. Thoracentesis will quickly establish the presumptive diagnosis of pneumothorax or hemothorax or a combination of both, often before a chest x-ray is taken, and, if positive, should be replaced by tube thoracostomy. Pericardiocentesis, under electrocardiographic control, will help in the diagnosis of cardiac tamponade and in the temporary or permanent decompression of the heart. Angiography is indicated in those patients with suspected injuries to the major vessels. Again, it should be stressed that contrast studies of the arterial vascular tree should be performed only with a patient who has a normal or near-normal blood pressure; this is especially important in penetrating injuries. Endoscopy with a flexible instrument is indicated in all patients with a suspected rupture of main or lobar bronchus or esophagus. Finally, it should be stressed that *immediate* thoracotomy is indicated and is both diagnostic and therapeutic in all patients who arrive at the Emergency Room with a chest injury and are lifeless or apparently lifeless. If the patient's condition turns out not to be due to an injury of the heart, the great vessels, the pulmonary hilus or the intercostal and internal mammary artery, immediate thoracotomy represents simply a better, more efficient way of cardiac resuscitation.

A more planned but still urgent, at times early (within 24 hours), thoracotomy is indicated for the following conditions: continued bleeding through the pleural drainage tubes or through pericardial intracaths and deteriorating vital signs; progressive cardiac tamponade or continued cardiogenic shock despite adequate cardiovascular resuscitation; wide mediastinum with falling vital signs and evidence on angiography of an injury to the large vessels; loss of 5% of estimated blood volume per hour for 2 or 3 hours; signs of acute herniation through the diaphragm; continued air leak with persistent lung collapse and/or subcutaneous emphysema; accumulated loss of 30% of estimated blood volume in 24 hours; and clotted hemothorax with mediastinal shift.

Of special concern are *combined injuries* of the thorax and abdomen or neck and chest or any variation of these basic injuries. We do explore all deep penetrating wounds of the neck. In combined injuries, the choice of incision is very important and, hence, the positioning of the patient becomes important. A detailed description of all the various incisions that can be used is beyond the scope of this presentation. However, it should be realized that the ideal incision for laparotomy is a midline incision and, hence, the surgeon never should be caught with the patient positioned in such a fashion that the abdomen cannot be approached. This means, in most cases, that the patient should be in dorsal decubitus or one side should be elevated sufficiently to permit an anterolateral thoracotomy. The abdominal midline incision then may be associated with an anterolateral thoracotomy, a bilateral anterior thoracotomy or may be extended through a median sternotomy, as the case may be. In cervical or thoracic injuries, the anterolateral thoracotomy may be associated with a separate neck incision, or a clearly indicated mediastinotomy may be extended obliquely into the neck on one side or the other. Chest tubes should be placed in such a fashion that they do not interfere with the ultimate need for an anterolateral thoracotomy, for instance. Because of this, we prefer the second interspace in the midclavicular line for pneumothorax and the seventh or eighth interspace in the midaxillary line for hemothorax, occasionally using both locations if much air and blood have to be evacuated continually.

Conclusion

As the severely injured child is successfully piloted through this early and intermediate phase of emergency care, there should be a means to evaluate success or failure in the individual case as well as to assess the value of the over-all emergency response system. These evaluations should be based on the review of reliable records by audio and visual monitoring as well as on the data accumulated by a review of complications and deaths. A computerized trauma registry in which all the data pertaining to the entire regional and local emergency response system, including the hospital Emergency Room and Trauma Center, will bring to the care of the trauma victim the same potential for rigid control of quality care that the record library does to the electively admitted patient.[6, 7] At the end of each individual case, and of each year, we have to ask the following three questions: Were the right steps taken? In correct sequence? With sufficient speed?

REFERENCES

1. American College of Surgeons Committee on Trauma: Optimal Hospital Resources for Care of the Seriously Injured, A. C. S. Bull. 61:15, 1976.
1a. American Medical Association: Standards for Cardiopulmonary Resuscitation (CPR) and Emergency Cardiac Care (ECC), JAMA (supp.) 227:833, 1974.
2. Braunstein, P. W., Moore, J. O., and Wade, P. A.: Preliminary findings of the effect of automotive safety design on injury patterns, Surg. Gynecol. Obstet. 105:257, 1957.
3. Cohn, J. D., and DelGuercio, L. R. M.: Cardiorespiratory analysis of cardiac arrest and resuscitation, Surg. Gynecol. Obstet. 123:1066, 1966.
4. Cohn, J. D., Angler, P. E., and DelGuercio, L. R. M.: The automated physiological profile, Crit. Care Med. 3:51, 1975.
5. Cornell, W. P., Ebert, P. A., and Zuidema, G. D.: X-ray diagnosis of penetrating wounds of the abdomen, J. Surg. Res. 5:142, 1965.
6. Fallis, J. D.: Initial Assessment of the Injured Child, in *Care for the Injured Child* (Baltimore: The Williams & Wilkins Company, 1975).
7. Frey, R., *et al.*: Recommendations of the International Symposium on Mobile Intensive Care Units and Advanced Emergency Care Delivery Systems, J. Am. Coll. Em. Physicians 4:60, 1975.

8. Haller, J. A., *et al.*: Use of a trauma registry in the management of children with life-threatening injuries, J. Pediatr. Surg. 11:38, 1976.

9. Hartong, J.: Personal communication.

10. Humphreys, R. P., Hendrick, E. B., and Hoffman, H. J.: Head Injuries, in *Care for the Injured Child* (Baltimore: The Williams & Wilkins Company, 1975).

11. Jacobs, H. B.: Needle catheter brings oxygen to the trachea, JAMA 222:1231, 1972.

12. Klain, M., Smith, R. B., and Rock, J. J.: Fluidic oxygen jet ventilator for emergency use, Crit. Care Med. 4:112, 1976.

13. Klain, M., Hirsch, S., and Sladen, A.: Automated physiological profile in the evaluation of critically ill patients, Crit. Care Med. 4:124, 1976.

14. Kottmeier, P. K.: What the Pediatrician Should Know About Pediatric Trauma, in *Current Problems in Pediatrics* (Chicago: Year Book Medical Publishers, Inc., June, 1976).

15. Morse, T. S.: Personal communication.

16. Nobel, J. J.: Mobile emergency life support and resuscitation system, Arch. Surg. 92:879, 1966.

17. Perry, J. F., Jr.: Blunt and Penetrating Abdominal Injuries, in *Current Problems in Surgery* (Chicago: Year Book Medical Publishers, Inc., May, 1970).

18. Root, H. D., Keizer, P. J., and Perry, J. F., Jr.: The clinical and experimental aspects of peritoneal response to injury, Arch. Surg. 95:531, 1967.

19. Rysoff, R. H., Shaftan, G. W., and Herbsman, H.: Selective conservation in penetrating abdominal trauma, Surgery 59:650, 1966.

20. Shandling, B.: Hemorrhage and Shock, in *Care for the Injured Child* (Baltimore: The Williams & Wilkins Company, 1975).

21. Spoerel, W. E., Narayanan, P. S., and Singh, N. P.: Transtracheal ventilation, Br. J. Anaesth. 43:932, 1971.

22. Steichen, F. M., *et al.*: Radiographic diagnosis versus selective management in penetrating wounds of the abdomen, Ann. Surg. 170:978, 1969.

23. Steichen, F. M.: The emergency management of the severely injured, J. Trauma 12:786, 1972.

24. Stephens, C. A., and Fallis, J. C.: Multiple Injuries, in *Care for the Injured Child* (Baltimore: The Williams & Wilkins Company, 1975).

25. Williams, W. G., and Brummitt, W. M.: Cardiac Arrest, in *Care for the Injured Child* (Baltimore: The Williams & Wilkins Company, 1975).

26. Wolf, R. A.: Four facets of automotive crash injury research, N.Y. State J. Med. 66:1798, 1966.

11 Hugh G. Thomson

Skin and Subcutaneous Tissue Injuries

PATIENTS WITH INJURIES to the skin, subcutaneous fat, fascia and muscle represent a large portion of the problems seen in the surgical division of a pediatric emergency department. These injuries may occur alone or in association with trauma to large vessels, nerves, tendons, ligaments and bones.

Primary wound healing is the aim of most treatment programs. Occasionally, due to the specific nature of the wound, the surgeon's plan is for healing by secondary intention. It is the purpose of this chapter to outline the general principles of management of soft tissue wounds commonly seen in the pediatric population of a hospital emergency department.

General Considerations

History

Obtain a detailed history of the injury. Relatives, or even friends and baby-sitters, usually can recreate the traumatic incident. All factors, regardless of apparent insignificance, frequently are important to the diagnosis, assessment and treatment. For example, consider a washing machine wringer injury of the extremity. Was the machine new or used? With automatic or manual release? Was the limb between the rollers for a short or long duration? With or without a piece of fabric acting as a shim? The information derived from these factors assists the surgeon in assessing the severity of the injury and determines the approach to treatment.

Do not overlook associated injuries! In addition, have respect for the small wound, as its size can be misleading! A small wound in a child can have a deep devastating effect and its significance can be overlooked unless a careful clinical examination is made (Fig. 11–1). Additional contamination during the initial examination of the wound prior to repair should be avoided. The examiner should wear a cap and mask. Avoid palpation with unscrubbed hands. The wound should remain covered with a sterile dressing before and after examination. Too often, wounds are left exposed in the emergency department. The child's tetanus immunization program must be determined and a decision made regarding the need for active and/or passive immunization—or none at all!

The injured part is examined for bleeding (rate and type of flow and color of blood), swelling that is increasing (possibly an expanding hematoma), color changes (redness or whiteness, ecchymosis, cyanosis and tattooing) and tenderness. The location, size and depth of any wound is noted. Anatomic structures in the immediate vicinity are examined for concomitant injury. Assessment of sensory and motor function, distal to the appropriate wound, must be completed.

General anesthesia often is necessary to complete the examination of a wound in a child. Such is the case when the bottom of the wound cannot be seen clearly or when the wound is close to an important structure; e.g., the eye. Nerves and vessels often are close to one another. If the wound is bleeding freely, injury to other structures, particularly nerves, should be suspected.

The concept of the "tidy" and the "untidy" wound is useful and involves considering several criteria. The untidy wound usually is produced by a contusing or avulsing force, may have ragged edges, may contain gross foreign material, or nonviable tissue such as muscle, and the time lapse from injury is greater than 6 hours. The experienced civilian sur-

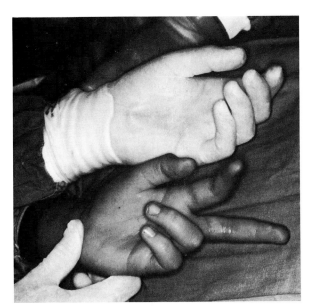

Fig. 11–1.—Tendon injury. Distal palmar laceration (hidden by fingertips) has transected flexor superficialis indicis and flexor superficialis and profundus to middle finger. Comparison with surgeon's hand demonstrates attitude of the hand as important clinical sign.

geon frequently can convert an apparently "untidy" wound to a "tidy" wound and effect a successful primary closure (Fig. 11–2). If this is not possible, the wound should be left open and closed at a later date (Fig. 11–3).

Parents are greatly concerned, regardless of the severity of the trauma. They are justified in requesting detailed information about the nature and severity of their child's injury. The treatment plan, the result normally expected and the probable complications should be discussed with the parents. This should be done as realistically, but as delicately, as possible, trying not to aggravate the feelings of guilt that the parents probably are already experiencing. For example, a laceration of the red lip frequently heals with an element of fullness or a "blob." If forewarned, parents will be more accepting of their child's treatment. Explanation is appreciated, develops understanding and avoids future disappointment.

Antibiotics

SYSTEMIC.—The use of prophylactic antibiotics is a controversial issue. If the wound is treated early and in a proper manner, there probably is no need for routine prophylactic antibiotic administration. The history may hint at the probability of infection. In addition, the child may be suffering from a concurrent active infection, such as impetigo, furunculosis, paronychia or acute tonsillitis. Depending on the circumstances, a limited and/or broad-spectrum systemic antibiotic may be indicated for 3 or 4 days.

LOCAL.—I commonly use an antibiotic in the depth of a wound. This technique is followed when contamination is likely, 4–8 hours have elapsed from the time of injury and the wound will remain open for an hour or more during repair. In such cases, the wound is flushed with a solution containing 10,000 units of bacitracin in 300 ml of Ringer's lactate solution. The effectiveness of this technique is difficult to establish.

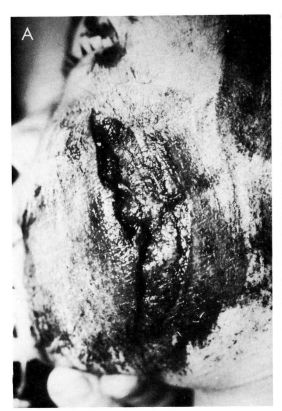
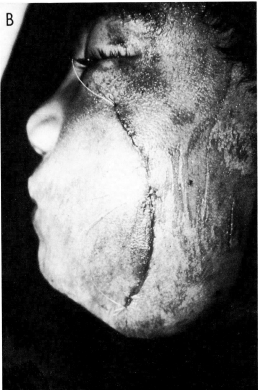

Fig. 11–2.—Untidy cheek wound. Contaminated, 8 hours old, abraded, filled with dirt, it is converted to a tidy surgical wound and closed with a subcuticular suture.

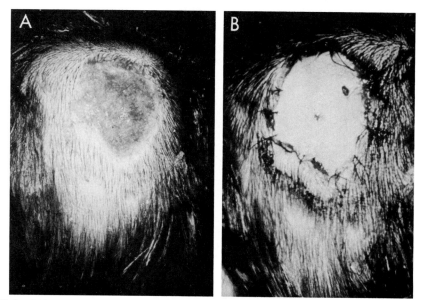

Fig. 11–3. — Untidy laceration — avulsion of the occiput. **A,** it is permitted to granulate. **B,** healing by secondary intention is hastened with a split-thickness skin graft.

Control of Initial Bleeding

Direct pressure on the wound with a sterile dressing, together with elevation when possible, usually will control hemorrhage. Arterial bleeding occasionally requires direct digital pressure in the wound. An open forceps should not be closed in a wound without direct and adequate surgical exposure of the wound depth.

Occasionally a tourniquet is necessary to control profuse bleeding from an extremity. Either a commercial tourniquet or a blood pressure cuff may be used. Inflation above arterial pressure is necessary to be effective. Pressures lower than this cause increased bleeding. The time of application and removal must be documented. It should not remain pressurized longer than 1 hour without careful reconsideration.

Preparation of Wound

SEDATION AND ANESTHESIA. — The cooperation of young patients under local anesthesia is somewhat limited. A general anesthetic may be indicated, particularly if significant inspection, manipulation or repair in the depth of a wound is imperative. Frequently it is necessary to extend wounds in order to provide adequate surgical exposure, which also limits the scope of local anesthesia. If local anesthesia is chosen, the use of preoperative Valium intramuscularly (0.2–0.5 mg/kg) or rectal Nembutal (2–3 mg/kg) prior to skin preparation may be worthwhile to provide additional comfort to the disturbed child. We perform a regional block or local infiltration of 0.5–1% Xylocaine, often through the wound itself, using a no. 25 needle. The amount of Xylocaine given should not exceed 3 mg/kg. If it is used with epinephrine (1/100,000), a larger amount (5 mg/kg) may be used because of slower absorption. Epinephrine is not normally used in the fingers or toes because of reported cases of associated ischemic necrosis. At this point, wound preparation can be achieved without unnecessary pain.

FLUID IRRIGATION. — Small superficial wounds are washed with normal saline or Ringer's lactate solution. Large or deep wounds are irrigated with copious amounts of the same fluids, usually with a large syringe.

MECHANICAL DEBRIDEMENT. — 1. Foreign bodies of all types are removed. Some can be removed individually with forceps. Others are embedded and must be cut away. It may be a technical impossibility to remove all visible foreign bodies without producing damage to vital structures. If this is the case, they must be left in the wound.

2. Potentially nonviable skin edges, which will not heal, are removed. This includes ragged, beveled and skived edges. Such removal must be done judiciously to avoid such problems as unnecessary lengthening of facial lacerations, tightening of finger and hand wound closures or the loss of key landmarks around eyelids, eyebrows and lips. Wound edge debridement usually is accomplished with a scalpel.

Closure of Wound

DEEP CLOSURE. — One or two layers of interrupted sutures of either plain, chromic catgut or Dexon are used for deep closure. The number of layers is determined by the depth of the wound and the ease with which the wound can be drawn together. It is important to eliminate all potential "dead space." If a suture heavier than 4-0 is required, the wound likely is complicated rather than simple and will require a modified type of closure.

SUPERFICIAL CLOSURE. — The use of landmarks on the skin surface makes wound closure more accurate. Match skin creases, orient hair direction, fit an irregularity on one skin edge into its proper place on the opposing edge.

Use 5-0 or 6-0 nonabsorbable suture material on a fine needle for skin closure. Simple interrupted sutures usually are best. They should be placed 2 or 3 mm from the wound margins. Straight wounds may be closed with a subcuticular or intradermal suture, which has the advantage of avoiding needle marks and provides for simple suture removal. Short superficial wounds may be closed by gauze strips held by skin glue or USP collodion or Steri-strip.

Problems Associated with Specific Wounds

Minor Skin Loss

Minor tissue loss may be difficult to differentiate from the normal spreading that occurs when an incision is made in skin. The former will require an abnormally increased tension at the time of wound closure. However, minor tissue loss usually can be treated by direct edge-to-edge closure, perhaps after judicious undermining. If suture material heavier than 4-0 is necessary, additional tension-reducing measures or treatment, as for major skin loss, is indicated. Simple tension reduction at the suture line can be achieved by using wire and buttons placed at a distance from the skin edges.

Major Skin and Soft Tissue Loss

If the wound demonstrates a significant soft tissue loss and is considered "tidy," a partial-thickness or full-thickness skin graft should be considered. Use the buttocks for partial-thickness graft donor sites and the lower left quadrant or inner arm for free full-thickness skin grafts. Donor site scars are prone to hypertrophy in children and may present as a late concern. Local or distant skin flaps may be necessary to cover important deep structures to achieve primary wound healing. This permits primary repair of the deep structures, but, on occasion, they must be left for secondary repair at a later date after satisfactory skin and soft tissue healing has occurred.

Avulsions

There are many types of avulsion wounds. All demonstrate a problem in wound healing.

WRINGER INJURY. — A limb caught in a wringer commonly suffers some avulsion of skin from underlying tissue. This type of injury is produced by a combination of compression, shear and friction forces (Fig. 11–4). There will be contused and avulsed tissue, abrasions, friction burns and, occasionally, a laceration of the thumb web. Fractures should be suspected but are rare. An expanding hematoma may develop under the avulsed skin. Rarely is there an associated subfascial muscle contusion that produces a secondary ischemia requiring a fasciotomy.

Treatment usually consists of cleansing, application of a sterile pressure dressing, elevation and observation within 24 hours for signs of vascular compromise. If skin death is apparent at a later date, a skin graft will be required.

BICYCLE SPOKE INJURY. — It usually is the pillion seat rider's or the bar rider's foot that is caught between the wheel and the frame. Deep abrasions, contusions and some avulsion occur. Treatment usually consists of cleansing, the application of an occlusive dressing and elevation. Healing usually is slow but satisfactory after 4 – 6 weeks, with no inconvenience to the patients, who can assume their day-to-day activities. This and other types of avulsion injuries may be associated with viable skin flaps, which may be sutured directly or, if the circulation appears inadequate, removed,

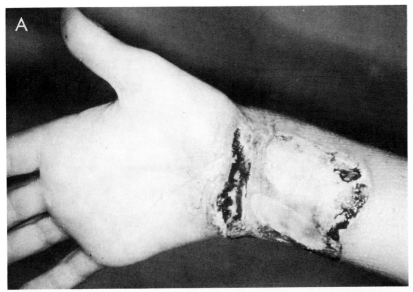

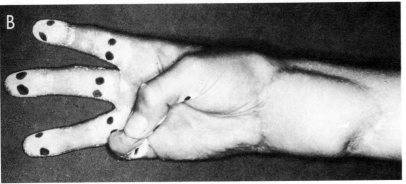

Fig. 11–4. — Wringer injury of wrist. **A,** there is a depressed third degree friction burn. **B,** this area of eschar or necrosis was excised primarily and a pedicle flap replacement closed the wound. Starch and iodine test and position of thumb demonstrate that median nerve is intact.

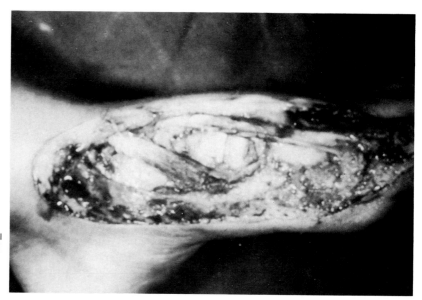

Fig. 11–5.—Tire injury of foot. The metatarsal-tarsal joints, tendon and bone are exposed, with associated skin loss.

defatted and returned as free full-thickness skin grafts. If the flaps are badly damaged, they may be discarded and replaced by partial-thickness grafts.

TIRE INJURY.—This is produced by a moving tire dragging the limb, frequently against the curb. Soft tissue injury is more pronounced and avulsion usually is more extensive. Exposure of bone, joints, tendons and nerves is common and should stimulate the need for primary wound closure (Fig. 11–5). Treatment methods outlined in spoke injury may be satisfactory. Occasionally local or even distant pedicle flaps are necessary.

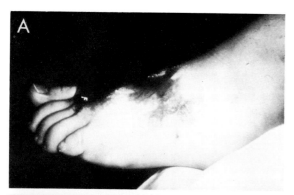

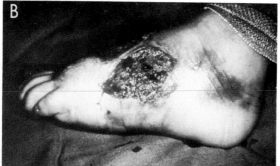

Fig. 11–6.—Crush injury of foot. **A,** zone of eschar and thinning of the skin; diffuse swelling obstructing distal vascular supply. **B,** increased swelling after escharectomy-fasciotomy.

CRUSH INJURY.—Strong compression-bursting forces produce superficial and deep damage that can involve all structures in the area. Late swelling is extensive. Necrosis of superficial and deep tissues is common, often becoming apparent a few days after injury. Serious consideration must be given to releasing tension by evacuating hematomas, excising inelastic dead skin (escharectomy) or performing a fasciotomy if the circulation to the area shows impairment (Fig. 11–6).

SHARP AVULSION.—This type of avulsion results from a force that separates the skin and subcutaneous fat from the fixed deeper structures in a clean, tidy manner.

The main consideration in the emergency department is whether the flap is likely to survive. This depends on the blood supply to the region, the relationship of the flap base to the axial blood flow, flap width, length and thickness. If the flap is of questionable viability, this is an ideal injury for total removal, defatting and replacement as a free full-thickness skin graft. This decision can be difficult!

DEGLOVING INJURIES.—This type of wound often is much worse than it appears in the emergency department, for reasons somewhat similar to those in sharp avulsions but on a greater scale. Both the laceration and the degree of avulsion or undermining are extensive. The tissues usually have suffered extensive crushing, abrasion and burning. Degloving injuries may be partial or total.

In partial degloving injuries, some of the tissues can be salvaged by excising the avulsed tissue and converting it to a free full-thickness or partial-thickness skin graft. Severely damaged tissues may be discarded and replaced by partial-thickness grafts from carefully selected donor sites.

Total degloving injuries are more extensive. The whole part is completely denuded of soft tissue cover. There usually are injuries to such deeper structures as joint, bone, tendons, nerves and vessels. Salvage is possible in some of these conditions. The flap may be replaced with success (Fig. 11–7). However, we sometimes are in error, and the assessment of the injury proves to be inaccurate, as evidenced by subsequent flap necrosis. If this occurs, patience and skin graft replacement are the best treatment (Fig. 11–8).

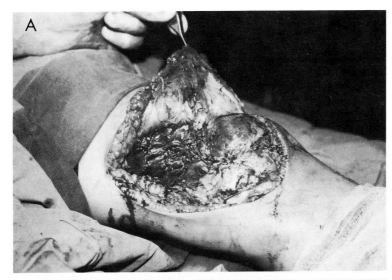

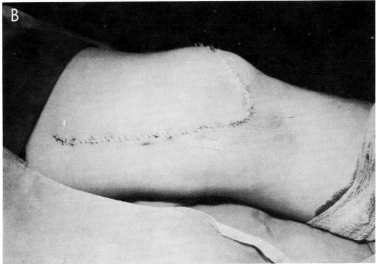

Fig. 11–7.—Avulsed flap, thigh. The flap, including vastus lateralis, was replaced with no evidence of ischemia.

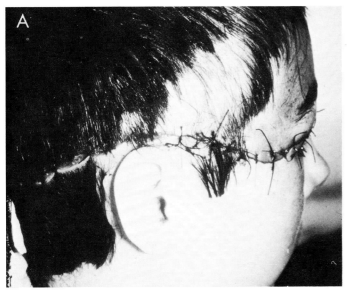

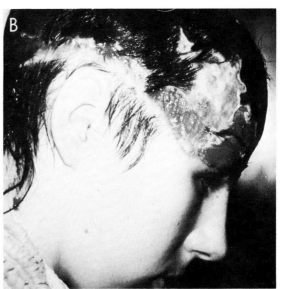

Fig. 11–8.—Degloving avulsion of scalp from car accident. **A,** the flap was thought viable and was replaced. **B,** an obvious zone of frontotemporal necrosis developed, showing granulation tissue and eschar.

In some severe degloving injuries there is such extensive injury to the deep structures as to bring into question the survival or future usefulness of the extremity. In such cases, amputation may be required rather than attempt at soft tissue replacement or skin graft coverage. The decision for amputation should be made in consultation, and the basis for it documented in writing.

Common Specific Lacerations

SCALP.—A convenient alternative to shaving around the periphery of the wound and suture closure can be used. Strands of the patient's hair adjacent to the laceration margins are tied on themselves. A chromic suture then is passed under this tie and it, in turn, is tied on itself. This will hold the edges firmly together.

MUCOUS MEMBRANE.—Through-and-through wounds of the lower lip, such as those produced by the central incisor teeth, should be closed by three layers of sutures, only after fastidious fluid and mechanical debridement. This reduces the dead space and the potential amount of red lip "blob" that will result.

TONGUE.—Some simple tongue lacerations may be left unsutured if bleeding has stopped. The tongue has amazing powers to heal and recontour itself. Jagged, skived and deep lacerations require suturing. Either chromic or Dexon 3-40 muscle sutures must be used. Chromic catgut or Dexon 3-40 is suitable for both layers. This will reduce the incidence of hematoma and wound breakdown!

ANIMAL BITES.—The most common bite is caused by the dog. There are two types of lacerations that are seen: (1) puncture wounds and (2) sharp avulsion lacerations. It is the patient with the multiple puncture wounds who can develop acute fulminating cellulitis within 24 hours. The obvious explanation for this complication is the surgeon's inability to complete an adequate wound toilet on the puncture laceration. No attempt is made to close the wound margins.

On the other hand, the avulsion laceration can be closed in exactly the same manner as any other laceration after excellent wound debridement (Fig. 11–9).

The use of prophylactic systemic penicillin on a short-term basis is advocated. This is particularly true with puncture wounds complicated by acute cellulitis. The common pathogen is *Pasteurella septica*, which is sensitive to penicillin. Concern about rabies is geographically endemic and primarily involves specific animals in these areas. The most accurate source of information on risk and treatment is the local Department of Health official.

Dressings

The aims of an ideal dressing are to prevent infection, restrict movement, prevent dehiscence, reduce pain, reduce

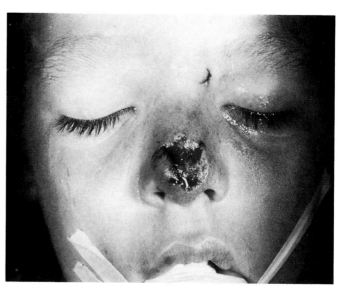

Fig. 11–9.—Dog-bite laceration—avulsion of the nasal tip. After surgical and fluid debridement, free full-thickness skin graft can be used to close the clean wound.

swelling and lessen the collection of fluid in the wound. A dressing is not necessary to eliminate the serosanguineous crust that accumulates along the wound margins. This can be accomplished by cleansing with simple solutions or application of ointments such as sterile petrolatum to the wound margins. Dressings can contribute to the successful management of many serious soft tissue repairs. Make dressings functional and neat. Sloppy dressings usually mean sloppy surgery. For children, the use of skin glues often helps to prevent dressings from slipping, particularly on the extremity. Dressings may be firm but not tight. Elastic bandages are a danger to children unless closely supervised to prevent circulatory embarrassment.

RECOMMENDED READING

1. McGregor, I. A.: *Fundamental Techniques of Plastic Surgery* (6th ed.; Edinburgh: Churchill Livingstone, 1975).
2. Mustarde, J. C.: *Plastic Surgery in Infancy and Childhood* (Edinburgh: E. & S. Livingstone, 1971).
3. Paletta, F. X.: *Pediatric Plastic Surgery.* Vol. 1, *Trauma* (St. Louis: The C. V. Mosby Company, 1967).
4. Peacock, E. E., and van Winkle, W.: *Surgery and Biology of Wound Repair* (Philadelphia: W. B. Saunders Company, 1970).
5. Stark, R. B.: *Plastic Surgery* (New York: Harper & Row, Publishers, 1962).
6. Thomson, H. G.: Soft Tissue Injuries, in *Children's Fractures* (Philadelphia: J. B. Lippincott Company, 1974).
7. Thomson, H. G.: Skin and Subcutaneous Tissue Injuries, in *Care for the Injured Child* (Baltimore: The Williams & Wilkins Company, 1975).
8. Grabb, W. G., and Smith, J. W.: *Plastic Surgery. A Concise Guide to Clinical Practice* (2d ed.; Boston: Little, Brown and Company, 1973).

12 K. J. WELCH

Thoracic Injuries

HISTORY.—The history of management of thoracic injuries traces the gradual understanding of the pathophysiology of the flail chest, open or sucking wounds, closed injuries with volume displacement by air or blood, tension pneumothorax, hemothorax and other phenomena. These subjects are adequately covered in other works.[4, 23, 37, 38] The following contributions are more pertinent to the present discussion. Blalock (1934) first repaired a wounded aorta.[5] Burford and Burbank (1945) described traumatic wet lung, common in children.[7] Harken (1946) removed a wide range of missile fragments from the cardiac chambers.[16] Lampson (1948) treated traumatic chylothorax by ligation of the thoracic duct above the diaphragm.[22] Carter et al. (1951) classified diaphragmatic hernias due to blunt trauma.[8] Avery et al. (1956) first used a volume respirator for internal pneumatic stabilization of the flail chest.[2] Hood and Sloan (1959) performed emergency thoracotomy for injuries of the trachea and major bronchi.[19] Reul et al. (1973) reported an incredible experience involving 1202 patients over one decade; mortality was 11.7%.[26]

Introduction

Thoracic injuries in children are relatively uncommon in our experience—44 patients compared to 600 patients with abdominal trauma. Of the 44 patients, 35 (79%) were due to blunt injury and 9 (20%) had penetrating injuries (Table 12–1); 28% had abdominal and thoracic injuries. Other experience includes 73 children reported by Kilman and Chamok[2]; 56 had blunt injury, 17 penetrating injury. Bellinger[3] reported 14 Vietnamese children with penetrating injuries. Most early deaths in the hospital result from failure to diagnose thoracic injury accurately and failure to take appropriate action once the diagnosis has been estab-

TABLE 12–1.—THORACIC INJURIES IN CHILDREN
(Boston City Hospital, 1968[35]; 44 Patients, Children's Hospital
Medical Center, 1977)

	BLUNT	PENETRATING	DEAD
Lungs and Pleural Cavity			
Hemopneumothorax	15	6	1
Contusion pneumonitis	4		2
Pneumothorax	3		
Traumatic lung cyst	1		
Trapped lung, clotted hemothorax	1		
	24	6	3
Trachea and Bronchi			
Ruptured bronchus	2		1
Ruptured trachea	1		
	3	0	1
Esophagus			
Rupture	1		
Laceration		1	
Tracheoesophageal fistula	1		
	2	1	0
Diaphragm			
Rupture	3		
Laceration		1	
	3	1	0
Heart and Great Vessels			
Heart		1	
Aorta	1		1
	1	1	1
Miscellaneous			
Fat embolism	2		
Traumatic chylothorax		1	
	2	1	0
TOTALS	35	10	5 (14%)

lished. Treatment of most injuries in children is relatively straightforward and, in most instances, identical to therapy recommended for adults. There are some differences: (1) Infrequency in the elastic developing thorax of rib and sternal fractures; indeed, devastating injuries may occur in the absence of any fractures. The child's thorax may be grossly deformed by blunt force and then return to normal configuration, leaving little or no external evidence of trauma. (2) Flexibility and easy displacement of the mediastinum; in tension pneumothorax, the mediastinum is driven far to the opposite side, interfering with cardiac filling and ejection and reducing the volume of the only functioning lung. (3) Absence of pre-existing cardiopulmonary disease in children makes for great power of recovery. Pulmonary and cardiac reserve is enormous, with excellent response to appropriate surgical measures. When isolated chest injury is encountered, mortality is low (6%). When it is combined with abdominal, intracranial or skeletal injuries, mortality triples. Penetrating wounds in 9 patients were due to impalement or knives; gunshot, inadvertent or accidental, occurred in 3 patients. The more serious blunt injury occurred in 35 patients; over-all mortality was 14%.

Diagnosis

Whenever thoracic injury is suspected, one must rapidly seek out, identify and treat any of the several conditions that cause severe cardiorespiratory malfunction. These conditions are open pneumothorax, airway obstruction, flail chest, tension pneumothorax, hemothorax or hemopneumothorax and cardiac tamponade. Other conditions, fortunately rare but often fatal, include injury to the heart or great vessels, diaphragmatic rupture, injuries of the trachea and main stem bronchi, ruptured esophagus and unilateral or bilateral pulmonary crush. Together, these have been called the dirty dozen.

Injuries to the chest wall, except from impalement, are encountered seldom in children. Multiple rib fractures are infrequent. Gunshot, especially at close range, tears away the chest wall, scatters bone fragments and injures all structures from entry to exit. Such injuries are rare in civilian pediatric experience. A reasonably accurate diagnosis can be made from the history and physical examination alone. Sucking wounds are self-evident from sound and inspection; they are treated with petrolatum gauze and tube thoracostomy well away from the site of injury. Stridor, crowing and labored respirations, absence of breath sounds, coarse breath sounds with rhonchi unilaterally or bilaterally all provide evidence of a major airway problem. This may be compounded by circulatory impairment, with hypovolemia and shock. Mixed lesions common in children are more likely to present as cardiorespiratory rather than ventilatory impairment. It is not a statement of personal defeat to admit that although much can be learned from observation, auscultation and percussion, the key to diagnosis lies in properly exposed chest x-ray films taken in the anteroposterior, lateral and upright positions. X-ray films should be inspected for rib fractures, abnormal collections of air in the subcutaneous tissues, pleural cavity or mediastinum, shift of mediastinal structures and opacities in either hemithorax. Widening of the mediastinum, or left hemothorax, implies injury to the heart or great vessels, especially when there is a fracture of the first rib. Air in the mediastinum usually is bronchial or esophageal in origin. Initially with pulmonary contusions, the lung fields are clear. Soon, flocculent opacities develop, progressing from base to apex until there is no visible aerat-

ed lung on one or both sides. This most serious condition must be recognized and treated properly from the start. Diaphragmatic contours must be inspected to be sure that they are at an equal and appropriate level; shift downward means tension pneumothorax on the involved side whereas "upward shift," with the loss of outline, suggests diaphragmatic rupture.

Management

As with other major injuries, one must insert a line for massive volume replacement, a bleed-off line for arterial blood gas determination and a central venous pressure line to run the tightrope between the underfill and overfill in children with functionally incompetent lungs.[36] Provision of an adequate airway requires suctioning of excess or abnormal tracheobronchial secretions, thoracentesis for diagnosis or initial treatment and most often tube thoracostomy, which one seldom regrets even if required high and low on one or both sides. Stabilization of the chest wall generally is not a consideration in children. Should it be necessary, tracheostomy and positive-pressure ventilation for internal pneumatic stabilization of the chest wall, as recommended by Avery et al.,[2] is instituted. We no longer use external traction.

Most conditions can be managed initially with tracheal intubation, ventilatory support and tube thoracostomy. In certain cases, thoracotomy will be required. In a few, partial and then full cardiopulmonary bypass is needed.

Chest Wall

Injuries to soft tissues, ribs, costal cartilages and sternum usually are of a minor nature. Gunshot in patients 15 years and younger in our area is rare. Pendelluft or to-and-fro movement of the chest with inefficient respiration, flail chest, is virtually never seen in children.[11] This requires at least 5–8 in-line rib fractures. The child is more likely to have destroyed lungs through pulmonary crush, but with a stable chest wall. Sternal fractures are not encountered because the sternum is mostly cartilaginous, except for the ossification centers, and segmented. The costal cartilages are flexible and have not yet calcified. Subcutaneous emphysema is common, unimportant and self-limited following treatment of the underlying condition. Open pneumothorax is rare in children and usually results from knife wounds or impalement. The sucking wound is debrided, covered with petrolatum gauze and tube thoracostomy is established at the appropriate level. Pleural cavity and wound infections are rare, provided that the lung remains satisfactorily expanded.

Lungs and Pleural Space

Injuries involving the lungs and pleural space are grouped together because of the interplay of factors affecting one or the other. Hemothorax without pulmonary air leak is seen in adults with penetrating injury to the great vessels. The source of the bleeding usually is the intercostal artery adjacent to rib fractures, the internal mammary artery in anterior crush or the pulmonary veins with whiplash of the pulmonary hilus. In children, a force sufficient to produce bleeding into the chest usually results in laceration of the ipsilateral lung, with air and fluid accumulation. An x-ray film of the chest taken in the supine position will fail to demonstrate 5 dl of blood. Upright anteroposterior and lateral x-ray films of the chest are required; even in the upright position, as much

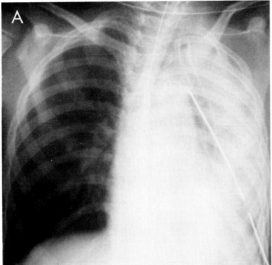

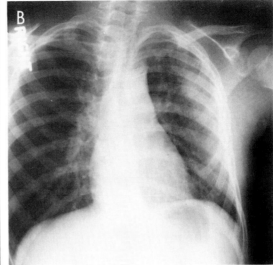

Fig. 12–1.—Hemopneumothorax in a 7-year-old boy due to blunt trauma. **A,** the left hemithorax is obscured by free blood in the pleural cavity. Two thoracostomy tubes have been placed, one reaching the apex and the other directed inferiorly and anteriorly. Approximately 500 ml of blood was aspirated from the chest, air leak gradually diminished and ceased at 72 hours.

The upper tube was removed first and then 48 hours later the lower tube was removed as drainage fluid gradually cleared. **B,** roentgenogram of the same patient 2 weeks later shows complete expansion of the left lung, with normal lung markings, normal position of the diaphragm and mediastinal structures as seen in the air tracheogram.

as 1.5 dl may not be detected, yet be recovered on thoracentesis.[34] As much as 40% of the calculated blood volume can be lost into one hemithorax. In one 35-kg child 1700 ml was removed. Blood loss of this magnitude usually is associated with injuries to the great vessels or structures at the pulmonary hilus; immediate thoracotomy is required. Physical findings indicative of hemopneumothorax include diminished motion of the involved hemithorax, dullness to percussion, absent breath sounds and usually some degree of displacement of mediastinal structures. Surgical treatment in most children consists of low thoracentesis for diagnosis and aspiration immediately followed by tube thoracostomy (Fig.

12–1). The catheter is attached to water seal drainage at 20 cm negative pressure.* Since 80% of children with hemothorax have hemopneumothorax, this essentially treats both conditions.[35] The sequestrated blood must be removed early and prior to clotting, and the lung must be fully expanded. If one fails to diagnose hemothorax, the lung will remain atelectatic and become enveloped in clotted blood, trapping the lower lobe, which then cannot be re-expanded (Fig. 12–2). In rare cases, thoracotomy will be necessary to free up the trapped lobe, remove the fibroclot and perform a parietal pleurectomy in order to ensure permanent full expansion of the lung. Great vessel injuries usually present as left-

---

* Pleurevac Deknatel.

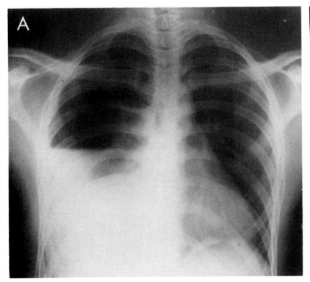

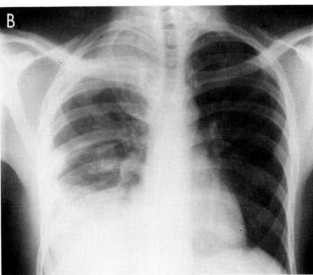

Fig. 12–2.—Classic right hemopneumothorax with air-fluid level. **A,** this patient was treated initially by thoracentesis, with reaccumulation of blood in the chest. **B,** after high and low tube thoracostomy, expansion of

the upper lobe was achieved but the lower lobe still was trapped in the clotted hemothorax. Thoracotomy and parietal pleurectomy were necessary in this instance for release of the right lower lobe to permit expansion.

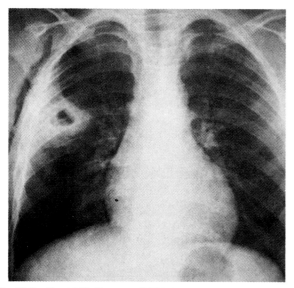

Fig. 12–3.—Traumatic "lung cyst." This has been reported in 8 children, 1 in our series. Usually a central lesion without pneumothorax, it probably represents a central contusion with temporary blocking of the segmental bronchus. The lesion appears quite similar to lung abscess but infection is not usually associated with this condition. All such lesions clear in 1–3 months, although the ring shadow may persist for some time. (Reproduced, with permission, from Ellis, R., Traumatic lung cysts, JAMA 236:1976, 1976.)

sided hemothorax; right-sided cases more likely are due to pulmonary hilus injury. Twenty-one children were encountered with hemopneumothorax; 15 sustained blunt injury and 6 penetrating injury. Thoracotomy was required in 3 patients with penetrating injury but in only 1 with blunt injury; decortication was required for clotted fibrothorax with persistent atelectasis.

Traumatic "lung cyst," as reported by Ellis,[14] has been encountered in 6 other children.[15, 20, 29, 31] The lesion is either a central laceration with cavitation or a cavitating hematoma. In all cases, the lesion cleared spontaneously, although a ring persisted for several months; none required operation (Fig. 12–3).

Tension Pneumothorax

Tension pneumothorax is much less common than hemopneumothorax and usually is due to blunt trauma. Our 3 patients all survived. With crush injury, the air leak may be substantial, rapidly accumulating and potentially lethal. With tension pneumothorax, in addition to volume displacement, displacement of the mediastinal structures and encroachment on the contralateral lung there is the problem of reduced perfusion and AV shunting. Arterial blood gas determinations are essential. On physical examination there is hyperresonance to percussion. Breath sounds are absent or, if there is partial function, distant with coarse rhonchi. In children, the trachea usually is displaced to the contralateral side and there may be interference with venous drainage at the base of the neck (Fig. 12–4). The pulse is elevated and soft in quality. The patient is tachypneic, usually with gray cyanosis, and appears anxious. Positive identification of the condition, once again, is by chest x-ray. Treatment consists of immediate tube thoracostomy, inserting a 28–34 F Argyle catheter into the fifth interspace. Initially, this is attached to water seal drainage to determine the size of the leak. As the leak diminishes, 20 cm negative suction is begun to ensure full expansion (Fig. 12–5). A second reason for tube thoracostomy rather than thoracentesis is that often many children are placed on volume ventilators as part of the over-all management of multiple injuries, reopening a leak that had sealed. This may occur unrecognized during anesthesia, and deaths have resulted. Rutherford[38] believes that death in children due to tension pneumothorax is more circulatory than ventilatory because of the soft, yielding and unstable mediastinum, similar to that in monkeys and dogs.

Pulmonary Contusion

Pulmonary contusion, traumatic wet lung or crushed lung is seen commonly in children. Kilman and Chamok[21] reported 13 children, with 1 death. We have encountered 4 patients; 2 died. In both, injury was caused by an automobile wheel passing transversely across the chest above the diaphragm. On admission, each child was ashen and hypovolemic and yet the chest x-ray film looked normal; no other injuries

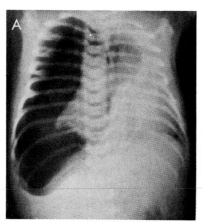
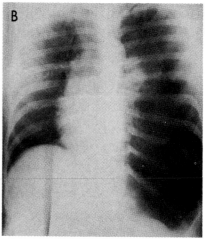

Fig. 12–4.—Tension pneumothorax in a child and an adult. **A,** roentgenogram of a child with tension pneumothorax showing the displacement of the right leaf of the diaphragm, shift of mediastinal structures to the left and ballooning of the right upper lobe well over into the left hemithorax, further compromising function of the left lung. **B,** left tension pneumothorax in an adult showing again depression of the diaphragm but no shift of mediastinal structures and an essentially normally expanded and functioning right lung. (Reproduced, with permission, from Ballinger, W. F., Rutherford, R. B., and Zuidema, G. D. [eds.], *The Management of Trauma* [Philadelphia: W. B. Saunders Company, 1973].)

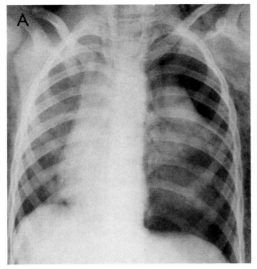

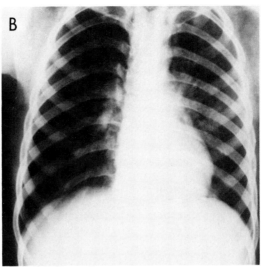

Fig. 12–5.—Tension pneumothorax. **A,** the left lung is compressed, with mediastinal shift compromising function of the right lung. In children, AV shunting and interference with caval return probably are more significant than problems of lung volume displacement. **B,** roentgenogram of the same patient 1 week later, following treatment by tube thoracostomy for 72 hours, shows normal mediastinal position and diaphragmatic leaves at the same level and full expansion of left lung.

could be identified. Within a few hours, fluffy exudates appeared throughout both lungs, maximal at the base and rising slowly to obliterate all lung markings, with an ultimate whiteout. Despite tracheostomy, ventilatory support using the Bennett MA-I volume respirator with peak end-expiratory pressure (PEEP) and inflationary hold (IH), the child succumbed (Fig. 12–6, *A*). In the second child, this experience was dismally repeated. In 2 other patients, damage was less severe and involved one lung predominantly; treatment was successful with gradual rise in PA_{O_2} and gradual weaning by the fifth day (Fig 12–6, *B*). With bilateral lung crush, the only hope for improved treatment would be through use of the membrane oxygenator. This device has been used successfully in 3 cases to date, 2 with semidrowning and 1 with *Pneumocystis carinii* infection. Theoretically, if one could provide extracorporeal support for 2–3 days, enough

areas of the lung not directly involved in the crush might recover to support life.

Pulmonary contusion has been studied by Roscher *et al.*[28] and Burford and Burbank.[7] The over-all picture is one of pulmonary edema and bronchospasm, rapid progression of signs and symptoms, worsening x-rays and a vicious circle of anoxia and lactic acidosis. The condition can be more accurately appraised today by serial blood gas determinations and pulmonary scans. Functioning components can be identified or the progression of pulmonary dysfunction can be documented. Depending on progression or improvement, one can determine the need for and type of treatment that must be initiated if the patient is to survive. Ventilatory assist devices, their variations, versatility and use are fully discussed in Chapter 2. Treatment over-all is quite similar to that required for white lung, pump lung, fat embolism,

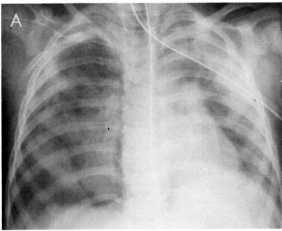

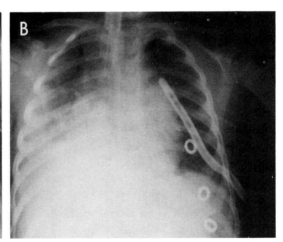

Fig. 12–6.—Contusion pneumonitis. **A,** with rupture of main stem bronchus. The child was run over by a car, the wheels traveling across her chest. Note the displaced fracture of the right scapula, the pneumothorax and compressed opacified lung on the right, the air in the mediastinum, the diffuse patchy consolidation of the left lung and the undisplaced esophagus. Emergency right thoracotomy showed avulsion of the lung root. Efforts at reconstruction were unavailing. The child died in 24 hours of progressive pulmonary insufficiency. **B,** right contusion pneumonitis with flocculation in the right lung field extending from base to apex progressively. There was an associated left hemopneumothorax treated by tube thoracostomy. The re-expanded left lung shows little radiographic evidence of injury. The child survived but required nearly 10 days of ventilatory support, with ultimate return of full function in both lungs as determined by xenon scan and roentgenogram.

smoke inhalation, semidrowning and damage due to hyper-oxygenation.

Trachea and Bronchi

Injuries to the trachea or main stem bronchi are rare and usually rapidly lethal without immediate surgical intervention. Inability to expand the involved lung, massive air leak and unresponding anoxia permit accurate diagnosis.[24] Such injuries usually are due to high-energy, blunt impact from a rapidly moving car, fall from a great height or shearing forces resulting from crush between a moving and a fixed object. Since the trachea and bronchi are adjacent to the heart and great vessels, which are likely to be injured at the same time, most children die at the site of injury or en route to the hospital. Provided that the injury is such as to avoid mortal injury, a child may present with avulsion of the main stem bronchus or an injured trachea. Action must be prompt and positive. All require immediate operation. Tube thoracostomy to water seal is followed by insertion of a cuffed endotracheal tube via tracheostomy into the contralateral bronchus leading to the only functioning lung. In older children, a Carlin bifid catheter may be used, but this is difficult to position. Even with a variety of catheters and techniques, one may not be able to achieve adequate ventilation, in which event partial and then full cardiopulmonary bypass is urgently needed. In the right-sided cases there usually is no injury to the contralateral hemithorax, improving the possibility of successful intervention. We have encountered 3 children with bronchial avulsion at the junction with the carina; anatomically, the surgeon knows exactly where to go. Bronchoscopy to identify the site of injury is not required. Repair may consist of linear closure of a tear extending into the trachea, partial circumferential repair of partial avulsion or end-to-end anastomosis for anatomic transection, using 4-0 proline or fine wire horizontal mattress sutures. Of our 3 patients, 1 had a crushed and partially transected trachea, with surviv-al; 1 had transection of the right main stem bronchus with avulsion of the lung root; she died despite heroic efforts to identify and repair the injury. One patient had 75% avulsive transection of the right main stem bronchus; direct repair was successful. Sinclair and Moore[30] encountered bronchial avulsion in 3 children; 2 died. Sperling[32] reported late repair of the left main stem bronchus in 1 child.

Esophagus

Esophageal injuries usually occur just above the carina. They can be suspected from the pneumomediastinum and rapidly developing shock. Occasionally there is left pneumothorax as well.[10, 25] Diagnosis must be made early by esophagoscopy and barium contrast study. There usually is escape of contrast material at the site of injury, at least for a few hours after injury. Later cases may be difficult to demonstrate because of the severe inflammatory reaction. Treatment in the case of a very small leak usually consists of upright position, one or more chest tubes and broad-spectrum antibiotics. With a larger rent, right thoracotomy through the bed of the fourth rib is required with direct repair. When there is injury to the esophagus and adjacent trachea, a traumatic tracheoesophageal fistula may develop, as reported by Antkowiak *et al.*[1] We encountered 3 children with esophageal injuries. In 1 instance there was a small leak treated conservatively and in 1 a knife laceration of the esophagus and pulmonary hilus; both were repaired via right thoracotomy. The third case appeared late, with aspiration difficulties and pneumonitis due to a traumatic tracheoesophageal fistula. Dissection and repair was relatively easy; a flap of mediastinal pleura was placed between the adjacent suture lines.

Diaphragm

Injuries to the diaphragm usually are due to blunt force. The position and outline of the dome of each diaphragm

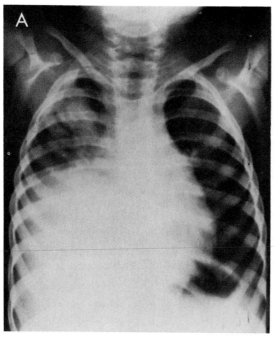
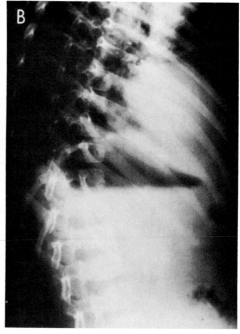

Fig. 12–7.—Traumatic diaphragmatic hernia. **A,** anteroposterior chest film shows the hernia extending to the fourth interspace, containing stomach and liver. **B,** lateral view. At operation, the blood supply of the stomach was found to be seriously compromised. A laceration of the dome of the liver was repaired, as was the diaphragmatic defect. The concept of urgent operation is supported by the findings in this case.

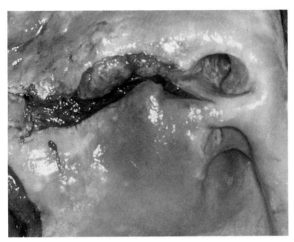

Fig. 12–8.—Traumatic rupture of the thoracic aorta due to a fall. The transverse disruption of the intima is readily seen. There was ragged disruption of the adventitia. The patient died at the site of injury from exsanguinating hemorrhage.

must be determined in every patient with suspected injuries of the chest or abdomen. A massive force must be applied to rupture this tough tendinomuscular structure, most frequently on the left side.[8, 9, 13] Tears usually are radial but at times they are circumferential. On the left side, abdominal viscera extrude into the chest, collapsing the left lung. When the right diaphragmatic leaf is ruptured, the liver moves through the defect, its ligamentous attachments usually torn completely away. There may be injury to the right lobe and displacement and traction interfere with venous return through the inferior vena cava. The stomach usually prolapses through the defect as well and there may be a vascular compromise of one or both organs. The condition can be readily diagnosed by x-rays, by insertion of a nasogastric tube that proceeds into the thorax or by contrast material injected through the nasogastric tube. Some have advocated pneumoperitoneum to show the transposed viscera in more detail. Immediate surgical intervention is required and recommended[18] (Fig. 12–7). We have encountered 4 children with diaphragmatic rupture. In 3 instances, the rupture was due to blunt force, 2 on the left side, 1 on the right; all

survived. One patient had a laceration of the right diaphragm due to a tenpenny nail thrown 60 feet by a power lawn mower. The nail entered the right chest, produced a linear laceration of the diaphragm and became buried deep in the substance of the right lobe of the liver. The patient had right thoracotomy, peripheral detachment of the diaphragm by the Waterston maneuver, removal of the missile, repair of the liver lobe by suturing and appropriate repair of the diaphragm.

Heart and Great Vessels

Injuries involving the heart and great vessels are common in adults,[17, 27, 33] largely due to gunshot, knives or steering posts. Children usually are involved in accidents as pedestrians. Gunshot is rare and usually due to mishandling of firearms. We have encountered 2 patients with injury to a great vessel or the heart. A 16-year-old boy fell from a ladder approximately 30 feet and was brought to the hospital dead on arrival. Autopsy revealed rupture of the thoracic aorta just distal to the origin of the left subclavian artery (Fig. 12–8). A 14-year-old boy had successful repair for a knife injury of the heart. He presented with tamponade, which reaccumulated after pericardiocentesis. Repair of the injury to the ventricular wall was carried out via sternal split; a pericardial window was made with Hemovac drainage.

Traumatic Chylothorax

This condition often arises as a post-thoracotomy complication, presenting particularly after operations involving dissection of the aorta, as a left-sided accumulation, more rarely on the right, with injury to the terminal segment of the thoracic duct. Treatment consists of closed tube thoracostomy and water seal suction. The condition has been discussed by Decancq[12] and Lampson.[22] The vast majority of such fistulas will close spontaneously unless due to malignant obstruction or high superior vena cava pressure. Several liters of chyle may be lost each day and replacement then becomes a problem because of the nutritional loss. The site of injury can be localized by peripheral lymphangiography in any child over 2 years of age. The site of injury can be recognized at thoracotomy through the left chest by injection of vegetable blue dye into the wall of the esophagus just above the diaphragm. Surgical treatment, if necessary, con-

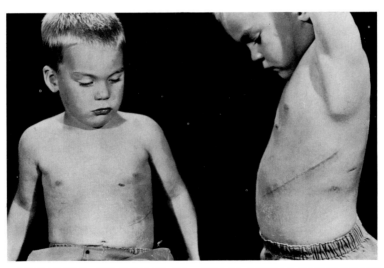

Fig. 12–9.—Penetrating thoracoabdominal injury. This 7-year-old boy shot himself with a .38 caliber revolver. The bullet passed through the left lung, diaphragm, stomach and spleen. The wounds of entrance and exit are readily seen. Nine of 34 such injuries were penetrating.

sists of ligation of the thoracic duct above the diaphragm as recommended long ago by Lampson.[22] We have encountered traumatic chylothorax due to a knife injury in 1 patient; management was conservative.

Fat Embolism

Fat embolism has been encountered twice, once in an obese 12-year-old boy with bilateral proximal femoral fractures and once in a child with avulsive crush injuries of the buttocks and lower extremities. The clinical picture is similar to contusion pneumonitis. Fat globules can be identified on Sudan III stain of sputum and urine sediment. Treatment is essentially that of traumatic pneumonitis. The lungs clear in 3–5 days. Fat embolism has not received much attention in the recent pediatric literature. We suspect that the condition is underdiagnosed and overlaps with white lung in trauma cases.[39]

Conclusions

Thoracic injuries are rare by comparison to abdominal injuries in children—approximately 10%. Seventy-five per cent are due to blunt trauma, 25% will have thoracoabdominal injuries and 50% will have injury of a third system (Fig. 12–9). As combined injuries accumulate, mortality rises from 6% to 14% as encountered by us in 44 patients, with 5 deaths. Injuries involving the lungs and pleural space were encountered in 28 patients. Most thoracic injuries reported in adults were encountered in children. Deaths occurred in 3 patients with crushed lung, injuries to the trachea and bronchi in 2 and rupture of the thoracic aorta in 1; 37 patients survived. Tube thoracostomy was required in 29 patients; 18 required thoracotomy.

REFERENCES

1. Antkowiak, J. G., Cohen, M. L., and Kyllonen, A. S.: Tracheoesophageal fistula following blunt trauma, Arch. Surg. 109:529, 1974.
2. Avery, E. E., Mörch, E. T., and Benson, D. W.: Critically crushed chests; new method of treatment and continuous mechanical hyperventilation to produce alkalotic apnea and internal pneumatic stabilization, J. Thorac. Surg. 32:291, 1956.
3. Bellinger, S. B.: Penetrating chest injuries in children, Ann. Thorac. Surg. 14:635, 1972.
4. Blair, E., Topuzlu, C., and Deane, R. S.: Major Blunt Chest Trauma, in *Current Problems in Surgery* (Chicago: Year Book Medical Publishers, Inc., May, 1969).
5. Blalock, A.: Successful suture of a wound of the ascending aorta, JAMA 103:1617, 1934.
6. Bugden, W. F., Chu, P. T., and Delmonico, J. E.: Traumatic diaphragmatic hernia, Ann. Surg. 142:851, 1955.
7. Burford, T. H., and Burbank, B.: Traumatic wet lung; observations on certain physiologic fundamentals of thoracic trauma, J. Thorac. Surg. 14:415, 1945.
8. Carter, B. N., Giusetti, J., and Felson, B.: Traumatic diaphragmatic hernia, Am. J. Roentgenol. 65:56, 1951.
9. Chamberlain, J. M.: Diaphragmatic hernia produced by indirect violence, Surg. Clin. North Am. 33:1505, 1953.
10. Chapman, N. D., and Braun, R. A.: The management of traumatic tracheoesophageal fistula caused by blunt chest trauma, Arch. Surg. 100:681, 1970.
11. Cullen, P.: Treatment of flail chest. Use of intermittent mandatory ventilation and positive end-expiratory pressure, Arch. Surg. 110:1099, 1975.
12. Decancq, J. G.: The treatment of chylothorax in children, Surg. Gynecol. Obstet. 121:509, 1965.
13. Desforges, G., *et al.*: Traumatic rupture of the diaphragm, J. Thorac. Surg. 34:799, 1957.
14. Ellis, R.: Traumatic lung cysts, JAMA 236:1976, 1976.
15. Greening, R., Kynette, A., and Hodes, P. J.: Unusual pulmonary changes secondary to chest trauma, Am. J. Roentgenol. 77:1059, 1957.
16. Harken, D. E.: Foreign bodies in, and in relation to, the thoracic blood vessels and heart, Surg. Gynecol. Obstet. 83:117, 1946.
17. Hewitt, R. L., *et al.*: Penetrating vascular injuries of the thoracic outlet, Surgery 76:715, 1974.
18. Hood, R. M.: Traumatic diaphragmatic hernia, Ann. Thorac. Surg. 12:311, 1971.
19. Hood, R. M., and Sloan, H. E.: Injuries of the trachea and major bronchi, J. Thorac. Cardiovasc. Surg. 38:458, 1959.
20. Jount, G. H. C., and Jaffe, F. L.: Solitary pulmonary hematoma, J. Thorac. Surg. 43:291, 1962.
21. Kilman, J. W., and Chamok, E.: Thoracic trauma in infancy and childhood, J. Trauma 9:863, 1968.
22. Lampson, R. S.: Traumatic chylothorax. A review of the literature and report of a case treated by mediastinal ligation of the thoracic duct, J. Thorac. Surg. 105:404, 1948.
23. Maloney, J. V., Jr., and MacDonald, L.: The treatment of blunt trauma to the thorax, Am. J. Surg. 105:404, 1963.
24. Munnell, E. R.: Fracture of major airways, Am. J. Surg. 105:511, 1963.
25. Nolan, J. J., and Ashborn, F. S.: Tracheoesophageal fistula as an isolated effect of steering wheel injury, Med. Ann. D. C. 24:384, 1960.
26. Reul, G. J., Jr., *et al.*: Recent advances in the operative management of massive chest trauma, Ann. Thorac. Surg. 16:52, 1973.
27. Reul, G. J., Jr., *et al.*: The early operative management of injuries to the great vessels, Surgery 74:862, 1973.
28. Roscher, R., Bittner, R., and Stockmann, U.: Pulmonary contusion: Clinical experience, Arch. Surg. 109:508, 1974.
29. Schwartz, A., and Borman, J. B.: Contusion of the lung in childhood, Arch. Dis. Child. 26:557, 1961.
30. Sinclair, M. C., and Moore, T. C.: Abdominal and thoracic trauma in childhood and adolescence, J. Pediatr. Surg. 9:155, 1974.
31. Sorsdahl, O. A., and Powell, J. W.: Cavitary pulmonary lesions following nonpenetrating chest trauma in children, Am. J. Roentgenol. 95:118, 1965.
32. Sperling, V. E.: Zur Problematik der kindlichen Bronchus ruptur, Z. Kinder Chir. 5:333, 1968.
33. Stallone, R. J., Ecker, R. R., and Samson, P. C.: Management of major acute thoracic vascular injuries, Am. J. Surg. 128:249, 1974.
34. Sturm, J. T.: Hemopneumothorax following blunt trauma of the thorax, Surg. Gynecol. Obstet. 141:539, 1975.
35. Welch, Kenneth J.: Abdominal and Thoracic Injuries, in Mustard, W. T., *et al.* (eds.), *Pediatric Surgery* (2d ed.; Chicago: Year Book Medical Publishers, Inc., 1969), vol. 1, pp. 708–731.
36. Wise, A., *et al.*: The importance of serial blood gases in blunt chest trauma, J. Thorac. Cardiovasc. Surg. 56:520, 1968.
37. Cave, E. F., Burke, J. F., and Boyd, R. J. (eds.): *Trauma Management* (Chicago: Year Book Medical Publishers, Inc., 1974).
38. Ballinger, W. F., Rutherford, R. B., and Zuidema, G. D. (eds.): *The Management of Trauma* (Philadelphia: W. B. Saunders Company, 1973).
39. Weisz, G. M.: Fat embolism, Curr. Probl. Surg. Nov. 1974.

13 K. J. WELCH

Abdominal Injuries

TRAUMA in all of its aspects is an increasing problem in children in a highly industrialized society. In the United States in 1974, accidents accounted for 10,919 deaths (44.3%) among children aged 1–14, both sexes. Death rate per 100,000 population was 21.6.[166] A Canadian survey revealed that accidents result in more deaths than all other causes combined, with 1 death in every 300 children.[32] Berfenstam et al.[14] reported 25,000 major injuries in Swedish children in 1 year; 463 involved abdominal viscera (1.8%). In all countries there is an alarming rise in deaths due to vehicular accidents. The most discouraging aspect is that few such children arrive at the hospital alive. Perry[121] reviewed 99 autopsies performed on children who arrived in extremis or dead on admission (DOA). Sixty-one children were DOA and 38 reached the hospital alive but died in the Emergency Room. Either the injuries were so complex and massive as to thwart treatment, the seriousness of the situation was not appreciated or sophisticated techniques were not available to deal with the more complex injuries. Velcek et al.[164] arrived at a similar conclusion in surveying traumatic death in urban children in the city of New York. They reported 911 children; 54% were less than 4 years of age, 50% were DOA. Eighty-two per cent of children with combined thoracoabdominal injuries were DOA or in extremis. Of these, 28% died after admission to the hospital without successful or attempted treatment. Van Wagoner[163] reviewed 600 deaths in the hospital after trauma; 18% of deaths would have been avoidable with the correct diagnosis and an equal number avoidable had the correct action been taken. There is considerable room for improvement in accident prevention and equal opportunity for improvement in the management of the most severely injured children once they arrive at the hospital. Boyd et al.[20] were innovators of the Trauma Registry, using computer methods to analyze the multiple factors in major injuries. They stressed the need for a statewide plan for trauma management with computer links. Haller et al.[60] began a Trauma Registry for children with life-threatening injuries.

Nine institutions reported on abdominal injuries in children during the period 1968–1976. Feix et al.[45] reported 47 laparotomies for abdominal trauma in children, with 4 deaths. Touloukian[157] reported 96 operations, with 3 deaths, all 3 due to liver injuries. Levey and Luder[87] reported 74 operations, with 7 deaths; 2 had ruptured livers. Richardson et al.[125] reported 40 operations, with deaths of 4 patients, of whom 1 had required hepatic resection and 1 had extensive pancreatic and duodenal injury. Hood and Smythe[71] reported 130 cases; death occurred in 14 of 33 patients with liver injury (42%), 3 deaths resulted from gastrointestinal injury, 7 of 29 patients died following splenectomy but none of the deaths was related to the splenic injury alone. Thus, death occurred in 20 of 130 cases (15%), higher than in other recent series. Sinclair and Moore[137] reported 199 patients; however, the age range was extended to 19. They encountered 100 penetrating injuries caused equally by knives and guns, much higher than in other pediatric series. There were no deaths following splenectomy in 43 patients; 6 of 22 patients with liver injuries succumbed (3 had injury to the inferior vena cava). Davis[26] reported 437 patients, with an overall mortality of 13%; again, 5 of 8 deaths were due to liver injuries. In our own experience during the period 1954–1977, 627 children were treated for abdominal injuries (Table 13–1). Of these, 93.5% were due to blunt trauma and 6.5% were due to penetrating or perforating wounds, in marked contrast to adult experience, in which the two groups are about equal. Where information is available in other children's series, 391 patients were operated on for blunt and 140 for penetrating abdominal trauma; however, the series is heavily weighted by Sinclair and Moore's cases.[137] The true incidence of penetrating abdominal injuries in children less than 15 years of age is about 10%. Stalowsky[142] came to the same conclusion on reviewing German children with abdominal injuries.

As in adult experience, the pendulum has swung to more conservative management of blunt and penetrating abdominal injuries. Jordan[77] recently has recommended conservatism in the management of abdominal trauma. There is an increasing trend toward conservative management of stab wounds and even some gunshot wounds whereas there is a trend toward more aggressive resection for injuries to the liver and pancreas, which he decries. The final outcome of this thesis has yet to be determined for children. We agree that it is appropriate to manage some solid organ injuries conservatively when accurately identified through special studies. Such patients must be kept under close observation and followed to healing. Nance et al.[112] selectively observed 393 patients with knife wounds, reducing the need for laparotomy from 53% to 11%, with an over-all mortality of 1.4%. In 1032 gunshot cases, 80% had multiorgan injury, with an over-all mortality of 12.5%; 52 patients were observed. The indication for operation in patients with penetrating injuries due to knives includes evidence of peritoneal irritation,

TABLE 13–1.—ABDOMINAL INJURIES
IN CHILDREN
(Boston City Hospital, 1968[175];
Children's Hospital Medical Center, 1968[152a];
Children's Hospital Medical Center, 1977)

172	Miscellaneous observed
171	Spleen
94	Genitourinary
89	Gastrointestinal
43	Liver
34	Pancreas
17	Pelvic crush
7	Major vascular
TOTAL 627	

hypovolemia and shock or evisceration. Thavendran[155] came to a similar conclusion in the management of 226 patients; 160 required operation. There were no deaths among patients treated by observation. X-rays were not helpful, pneumoperitoneum was seen seldom and wound injection studies seldom were of value. Local exploration of the wound under local anesthesia was condemned. Freeark[50] estimates that 33% of patients with stab wounds of the torso require surgical intervention. Systemic antibiotics are used routinely in patients who are selected for conservative management.

Male predominance in children with all types of injuries is widely recognized. Of our group, 420 were boys (68%) and 198 were girls (32%), maintaining the proportions of our earlier series (Fig. 13–1). Age ranged from the neonatal period to 15 years, with a peak incidence at 8 years (Fig. 13–1). At this age, youngsters in a crowded metropolitan area escape parental supervision and extend their range into accident-producing situations. Accidents occur near the home. Children with the most severe injuries die at the site of injury, in transit to the hospital or within minutes after arriving in the emergency room. This preselection of patients accounts for the relatively low mortality reported for in-hospital admissions of children following abdominal injury. One has a suspicion that things are not nearly as good as reported, nor as we have thought in the past.

A major factor in success of treatment for in-hospital patients is the extent and severity of associated injuries. Fifty-seven per cent of our patients sustained complicating craniocerebral, thoracic and/or musculoskeletal injury.

Etiology

The etiology of abdominal injuries, in our series, probably is typical of any area where economically substandard communities are served by a large children's hospital (Fig. 13–2).

Forty-one per cent of the patients were involved as pedestrians in motor vehicle accidents. Another 30% fell from a great height or against a fixed object. Others were occupants of motor vehicles or were injured at play or by assault. Velcek *et al.*[164] found 41% vehicular accidents and 27% caused by falls in 911 children. Parental assault, unfortunately, is common. Lauer *et al.*[85] reviewed 130 battered children under the age of 10 years during a 6-year period, 1965–1971. Forty-four per cent were abused previously; 6 children died. Sixty-three per cent were less than 2 years of age. The battered child is discussed further in Chapter 21.

Diagnosis and Management

Children with multisystem injuries should be admitted to a general pediatric surgical service and should remain under the supervision of individuals familiar with the problems of diagnosis, the patterns of organ injury and alternative methods of treatment. Such an administrative plan is not difficult to inaugurate and implement provided that realistic and prompt consultation with appropriate specialty services is requested.

Initial management begins with a carefully taken history, which foretells the type of injury, and an orderly physical examination. Extra-abdominal injuries may be overlooked initially and appear later to complicate operative management. Vital signs are recorded on a close time schedule and blood is drawn for appropriate laboratory studies, type and crossmatch. Urinary volume provides a useful guide to effective visceral perfusion. A Foley catheter is inserted, central venous and radial arterial lines are established and arterial blood gases are determined.

Certain lesions are associated with profound blood loss. With rapidly developing hypovolemia, notably in liver injuries, pelvic crush and combined abdominal and thoracic injuries, a central venous pressure line is established and venous pressure kept at 10–15 cm. Swan-Ganz wedge pressure is a more accurate guide to left ventricular filling.[27] Pancreatic injuries are common. The serum amylase level is measured initially and repeated on the third and fifth days after injury, matched against urinary amylase levels. A nasogastric tube is inserted and gastric contents are examined for blood or bile.

Anteroposterior and lateral upright chest films are obtained. We have seen hemopneumothorax 15 times, and it must be treated by tube thoracostomy prior to the induction of anesthesia. Flat, upright, left lateral and supine films of the abdomen are taken. Additional exposures of the skull

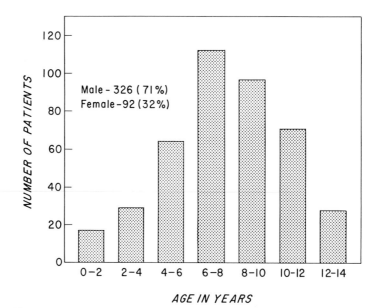

Male – 326 (71%)
Female – 92 (32%)

AGE IN YEARS

Fig. 13–1.—Age and sex distribution of children operated on for abdominal injuries.[175]

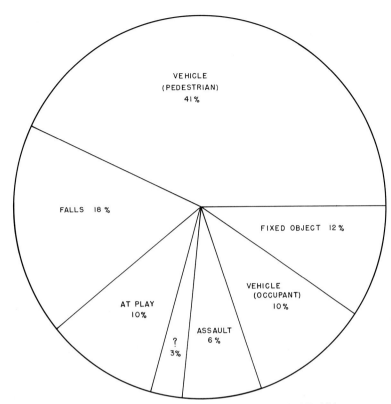

Fig. 13–2. — Etiology of abdominal injuries encountered in 627 children.

and extremities are obtained as needed. Renografin (1 ml/kg to 40 ml) is injected intravenously in all cases of abdominal injury whether or not hematuria is observed. A cystourethrogram is obtained in all cases of pelvic fracture or predominantly lower abdominal findings. On occasion, selective transfemoral retrograde arteriography is performed. The study is valuable in cases of solid organ injuries and also in pelvic or thoracic crush. Radionuclide scanning using technetium-99 sulfur colloid (20–40 μC/kg), a noninvasive technique, has supplanted arteriography for most suspected injuries to the liver, spleen and pancreas. Bedside scanning is possible with the rapid gamma camera and the use of Polaroid film. When conditions permit, it is best used in combination with arteriography with a high degree of correlation. Arteriography demonstrates the course and origin of the hepatic arteries, useful knowledge if a major hepatic resection is required.

Abdominal paracenteses in 4 quadrants is obsolete and less informative than peritoneal lavage. Root et al.[129] were the first to report on the use of diagnostic peritoneal lavage, subsequently improved by Olsen et al.,[116] who added quantitation, determining the degree of turbidity. Experience has been largely with adults. Thal and Shires[154] reported on 287 cases. There were 3.5% false positives and 3.1% false negatives. There were 4.5% complications, mostly puncture of large and small bowel and mesenteric vessels. Thal prefers quantitative counts. A positive test requires greater than 100,000 RBCs per ml. Ahmad and Polk[2] reported on 315 patients with 97% accuracy. They considered the test to be invaluable in patients with altered consciousness and equivocal physical findings. Parrin et al.[118] reported on 500 patients. Sixty-eight had major injuries identified (14%). The test was equivocal in 10% and negative in 335 patients who

were observed with no complications. Gill[55] reported on 299 patients; 44% of the tests were positive and 90% of the patients had major injuries identified. There were 3 negative laparotomies. False positives and false negatives were less than 1%. The only childhood experience is that of Powell et al.,[122a] who studied 52 of 500 patients less than 14 years of age. In 20 cases, the test was strongly positive; all patients had major injuries identified at operation; 10 tests were equivocal and the patients were observed after scan and arteriography. The test was negative in 22 patients observed, with no complications. Laparotomy for positive findings on physical examination resulted in 22% negative laparotomies; of those managed conservatively based on physical findings there was a false negative rate of 15%, subsequently proved at operation. There were no complications.

Peritoneal lavage requires the insertion of a peritoneal dialysis catheter in the midline below the umbilicus using a #14 Intracath with additional side holes. The bladder is decompressed by Foley catheter drainage. Ringer's solution (15 ml/kg) is instilled into the abdominal cavity, following which the drainage bottle is lowered and the liquid is removed by siphonage. The qualitative method of Olson requires that the fluid be estimated as clear, mildly opacified to permit the reading of newsprint or markedly opacified. Thal prefers quantitative counts of cellular elements.

The role of laparoscopy in closed abdominal injury in children is uncertain. Doletsky et al.[31] reported on use of the technique in children and confirmed injuries to the liver and spleen that were minor; patients were observed to healing Gazzaniga[53] reported laparoscopy in 37 adults, all with equivocal findings on physical examination, negative x-ray study and peritoneal lavage. Examination is conducted with CO_2 insufflation. Early in the study, all patients were operated on immediately after laparoscopy, 23 in all. Later, 12 patients were observed. Twenty-five laparotomies were thought to be necessary based on the findings at laparoscopy. Tostivint *et al.*[156] have also reported experience in adults.

All experts in the field of abdominal trauma have stressed that repeated physical examinations at intervals by a skilled observer is of primary importance. The regression or progression of signs from hour to hour in combination with highly selective studies foretells the severity and nature of visceral injuries and the need for surgical intervention.

Abdominal Contusions

The diagnosis of abdominal contusion has been reserved for patients who have a history of injury to the abdomen with abdominal pain, tenderness, rigidity and vomiting; bowel sounds are diminished to absent. Most patients had leukocytosis with a shift to the left. Many have extra-abdominal contusions, abrasions or assorted injuries to complicate interpretation (Fig. 13–3). More recently, peritoneal lavage and radionuclide studies lend support to the diagnosis of abdominal contusion without major visceral injury. Abdominal contusion is a distinct entity and in all probability represents injury to the musculature of the abdominal wall, pro- or retroperitoneal hemorrhage. One cannot rule out subserosal or mesenteric hematomas or subcapsular bleeding. Clinical findings are maximal within a few hours of injury, followed by rapid improvement 8–12 hours later. A rigid abdomen mimicking an abdominal catastrophe becomes soft with return of peristalsis. Localized tenderness in the specific area of abdominal wall injury persists. In a previous report,[175] I reported exploration in 12 of 172 such patients (7%). In 5, only minor findings were encountered; in 7, laparotomy was negative. The possibility of overlooking major injury in this group is much less today because of lavage, scanning and selective arteriography. Laparoscopy might be utilized in selected cases. It is unlikely that the now 20-year-old experience of Allen and Curry[3] will be repeated. They encountered 18 children at autopsy with major organ injury; all died without laparotomy.

Splenic Injuries

The diagnosis of isolated splenic rupture is suggested by a history of a major or relatively minor blow to the left upper quadrant or lower chest. The classic example is the sledding accident. The impact is immediately or soon followed by pain, pallor, collapse and sometimes vomiting. Later, there is gradual improvement. There is tenderness in the left upper quadrant and moderate rigidity. Many patients, 24–55%,[106, 175] have referred pain to the left shoulder on bimanual compression of the left upper quadrant (Kehr's sign). The children usually are not in shock while supine, although pressure falls as they assume the erect position. Systolic blood pressure usually is over 100 and pulse rate is in the same range. The hematocrit is around 30. There may be a drop of several points in serial hematocrit determinations over a period of several hours or days. Peritoneal lavage is performed in borderline cases. The study is of particular value in obtunded patients and others with multisystem injuries.

Radionuclide scanning using technetium-99 sulfur colloid is a valuable and accurate study when surveyed in several projections. Difficulties occur in cases with previous splenic injury, infarct or abnormal lobation. Usually the study will demonstrate a transverse linear defect with diminished uptake extending out from the hilus. Areas of splenic tissue deprived of blood supply account for diminished technetium uptake. Projections off the surface of the spleen represent perisplenic hematomas.

Lutzker *et al.*[93] assessed the relative value of scan and arteriography in splenic trauma in 16 patients (Fig. 13–4). They found high reliability with scanning and recommended arteriography only if the scan was equivocal or negative and there were clinical indications of splenic rupture. Villarreal-Rios and Mays[165] studied selective splenic arteriography in 10 patients; 8 were positive, confirmed at operation, and 2 were negative and observed. The most common patterns were extravasation, fragmentation, intrasplenic hematoma, stretched-out vessels and AV shunting proximal to the injury. Awe and Eidemiller[7] reported on selective angiography in 21 patients with splenic trauma; 19 were positive, confirmed at operation, but there were 2 negative laparotomies, a false positive rate of 10%. There were no false negatives. Nebesar *et al.*[114] reported on 32 patients. The scan was positive in 11 of 12 patients; all underwent splenectomy. There were no false positives. The study was negative in 16; 1 ultimately required splenectomy.

X-ray examination of the abdomen was helpful in establishing an accurate diagnosis of splenic rupture in only 5 of 74 cases (7%) in our early experience,[175] explained by the short interval (6.8 hours) between the time of injury and surgical exploration.

Wang and Robbins[168] described the cardinal x-ray signs of splenic rupture. In order of frequency, they are: loss of splenic outline, increased size of splenic shadow, loss of renal outline, loss of psoas shadow and serration of the greater curvature of the stomach, with medial displacement. Rib fractures lend support to the diagnosis, as does fixation of the diaphragm on fluoroscopy. Scoliosis has been described. Review of our cases, even in retrospect, revealed little such evidence. In a child, the spleen is essentially a thoracic organ. If one can see the sharp outline of a small or normal spleen there is little likelihood of splenic rupture; this rule is not infallible.

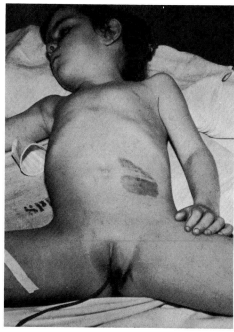

Fig. 13–3.—Abdominal contusion. Unconscious patient with superficial left upper quadrant abrasion and perineal laceration.

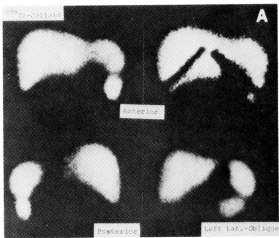
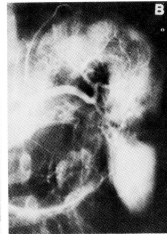
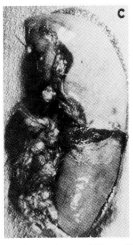

Fig. 13–4.—Ruptured spleen. Complete correlation between technetium-99 sulfur colloid splenic scan, selective splenic artery angiography and the removed specimen is seen in this patient, a 6-year-old boy with isolated splenic trauma. (Reproduced, with permission, from Lutzker et al.[93])

Treatment

In the early part of this series (Boston City Hospital, 1968; Children's Hospital Medical Center, 1968), 126 patients had splenectomy for traumatic rupture (Fig. 13–5). All spleens but 1 were previously normal; 1 had lymphoma. There were 2 instances of delayed rupture (2%) (adult series at that time averaged 15%). Shirkey et al.[134] reported on delayed rupture in 12 of 64 patients with blunt splenic injury (19%). Bollinger and Fowler,[18] in 248 cases, found delayed rupture in 21.5%. Over-all mortality for adults was 15%. More recently, Benjamin[12] has reported on rupture of the spleen in 332 adults. There were 47 deaths (14%). Delayed rupture was encountered in 6 patients (2%). Beal reported on 229 splenectomies for trauma; mortality was 13%. Delayed ruptures were 3.5%. There were 2 deaths in our 3 consecutive series involving 171 patients (Table 13–2). Both children had extra-abdominal injuries that were untreatable by today's techniques. One had a grossly lacerated brain and the other a torn-apart pelvis with complex vascular injury. This low mortality is not unusual for splenic injury in children. Boley et al.[17] reported on 33 consecutive splenectomies for trauma, with no deaths. Miller and Kelly[106] reported on splenic trauma in 56 children, with no deaths. There were no delayed ruptures and no patient developed postoperative infection. Two factors permit a higher salvage rate than in adults. First is the relative ease of diagnosis of splenic rupture in children; second, the spleen in young children can be literally avulsed without exsanguinating hemorrhage. The small muscular splenic artery and its branches contract and are occluded by a lifesaving thrombus. In one instance, the spleen was found free in the abdomen; the splenic vessels were occluded by a thrombus. Widmann and Laubscher[177] have reported splenosis following traumatic rupture in 70 patients. The condition seldom is troublesome and may even be beneficial. Zachary and Emery[180] have reported splenosis in a child. Many of our patients had associated pancreatic injury, renal contusion or perforation of the small bowel; two thirds of patients had extra-abdominal injuries. Average age was 8 years; the youngest were 3 newborn in-

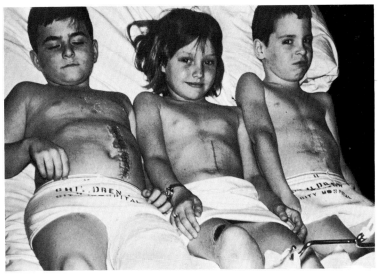

Fig. 13–5.—Splenic rupture. Three patients operated on in a 1-week period. The boy at the left had associated left hemopneumothorax and a complex knee fracture. The girl had multiple deep abrasions and fracture of the left femur. The boy at the right had a cerebral contusion and hematuria. The left paramedian rectus-splitting or midline incision is preferred.

TABLE 13-2.—SPLENIC INJURIES IN CHILDREN

SERIES	NO. CASES	SPLENECTOMY	DELAYED RUPTURE	SPLENIC REPAIR	PARTIAL SPLENECTOMY	OBSERVED TO HEALING
BCH, 1968[175]	71*	71	2			
CHMC, 1968[152a]	55	55	1			
CHMC, 1977	45	22	—	5	3	14
Totals	171	148	3	5	3	14

*2 deaths.
168 blunt injury, 3 penetrating.

fants. Sieber and Girdany[136] reported splenic rupture in a newborn, thought to be due to lateral flexion of the spine, often associated with breech extraction. The technique of splenectomy for rupture, which is similar for children and adults, is illustrated in Figure 13–6.

Overwhelming Postsplenectomy Sepsis

The argument for splenectomy in the management of traumatic rupture has been the almost routine success in children, with no mortality related to splenectomy per se; this is in sharp contrast to adult experience, where mortality still hovers around 15%. In the Boston City Hospital experience to 1968, 71 splenectomies were performed for traumatic rupture. Follow-up of these patients to 1969 disclosed no patient with postsplenectomy infection.[175] Tank et al.,[152a] reporting Children's Hospital cases to 1968, reached the same conclusion in 55 children, with no deaths. MacKinnon reported 26 children, again without identifying postoperative sepsis; all survived.[175] Orlando and Moore[117] reported 36 patients with no problem of late infection.

In favor of conservative management of splenic rupture is the strong case that can be developed for vulnerability to sepsis following removal of the spleen for any reason, including trauma. Attention was first called to susceptibility to infection following splenectomy in infancy by King and Schumacher in 1955.[82] Vulnerability is generally agreed to exist in patients undergoing splenectomy for hematologic disorders, notably thalassemia.[41] Lethal pneumococcal septicemia following Sulamaa intrathoracic splenic transposition for Chiari disease was reported by Stranch,[150] presumably because of devitalization. Overwhelming postsplenectomy infection (OPSI syndrome) is characterized by abrupt onset, exuberant bacterial growth, intravascular coagulopathy and death within hours of onset, with a mortality greater than 80%. The etiology in most instances is *D. pneumoniae* followed by *H. influenzae, B. meningitidis* and *E. coli*. Patients usually are less than 4 years of age and within 2–8 years of splenectomy. Vulnerability has been estimated to range from 60 to 200 times the normal expectation of major sepsis following any other operative procedure. The cause is not certain but several etiologies have been suggested. Constantoupoules et al.[24] identified a tuftsin deficiency with defective phagocytosis. Others have incriminated reduced IgM or decreased properdin. Most agree that there is relatively more of the reticuloendothelial system in the spleen of infants and children than in later life. Grosfeld and Ranochak[57] have demonstrated in animal models that splenectomy for trauma followed by challenge with type 2 pneumococcus resulted in a death rate of 35% as compared to controls without injury of 6.6%.

Infection following splenectomy for trauma in infants and children has been reported by Foward and Ashmore,[48] Robinson and Sturgeon[128] and Horan and Colebatch.[72] Hodam[68]

has established that adults are at risk as well at any age following splenectomy for any condition, including trauma. In a review of 310 cases, 2 were found with OPSI syndrome. One, an 11-year-old boy, developed major sepsis 5 years after splenectomy for blunt trauma. A 35-year-old male died 8 months following splenectomy for trauma, with grampositive cocci identified on smear and *D. pneumoniae* identified on blood culture. There was no response to penicillin. Reports of OPSI syndrome in children for conditions other than trauma are those by Ellis and Smith,[39] Erickson et al.[42] and Finland.[46] Haller[61] erroneously concluded that removal of the spleen in patients older than 1 year of age was acceptable. Erickson et al.[42] encountered an additional OPSI case in a child. Haron[61a] encountered a case in an infant. Eraklis and Filler,[40] in a survey of 1413 cases of splenectomy in childhood, encountered 342 operated on for trauma. There were 3 late deaths due to OPSI syndrome (0.9%). Singer[138] reviewed the literature to 1973 and encountered serious infection in 10 of 688 children who underwent splenectomy for trauma (1.5%); 4 died (0.58%). Balfanz et al.[9] identified patients who developed OPSI syndrome up to 15 years after splenectomy. The youngest patient was age 7 with splenectomy at age 4 and the oldest was 50 years of age; vulnerability is not limited to children. Thirteen were identified with OPSI syndrome following trauma; 9 died. Seven were less than 15 years of age. Typically, they described an 8-year-old female who underwent splenectomy for trauma and developed OPSI syndrome 4 months later. She died within 10 hours of onset. The portal of entry was right otitis media; *D. pneumoniae* was grown on blood culture. At autopsy there were bilateral adrenal hemorrhages. An accessory spleen apparently was of little use in defending against infection. Others subscribing to the concept of postsplenectomy sepsis include Coler,[23] Kiesewetter and Patrick[81] and Maron and Maloney.[95]

Conservative Management

The possibility of nonoperative management of splenic rupture following trauma was suggested by Upadhyaya and Simpson[161] in 1968. During the period 1956–1965, 52 children with suspected splenic rupture were encountered among 123 children with blunt abdominal trauma in Toronto. In Group I, 30 patients were operated on because of large volume blood loss. In Group II, 10 patients with suspected splenic trauma were operated on because of other major injuries. In Group III, 12 patients, no operation was performed. Patients were observed in the hospital for 8–10 days. All did well. Upadhyaya and Simpson predicted that the present policy of splenectomy for trauma soon would be revised in favor of conservative operation on the spleen or nonintervention. They postulated that splenic tears usually are in an anatomic transverse plane that promotes spontaneous healing (Fig. 13–7). The spleen has an unusually

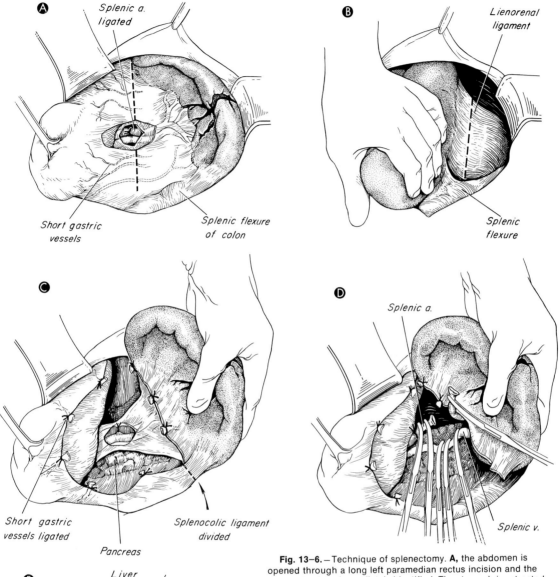

Fig. 13–6. — Technique of splenectomy. **A,** the abdomen is opened through a long left paramedian rectus incision and the ruptured spleen immediately identified. The stomach is retracted medially with a Babcock clamp, and the splenic vessels are identified at the superior border of the pancreas in the gastrolienal ligament. This is opened vertically and a 2-0 silk tie placed around the renal artery to control significant bleeding. **B,** the surgeon then sweeps his hand over the superior pole of the spleen and shifts the organ medially. This discloses the lienorenal ligament, which is divided. The splenic flexure of the colon may be mobilized in the process and displaced inferiorly to avoid injury to it. **C,** the splenocolic ligament is divided and the short gastric vessels are ligated. A transfixion suture should be used, grasping the seromuscular coat of the stomach and incorporating the vessels in the ligature. **D,** attention now is directed to the splenic artery and vein proximal to their branching at the hilus. The artery is divided first between double clamps, and an additional ligature and transfixion suture are placed to provide secure hemostasis. An identical technique is used in dividing, ligating and transfixing the splenic vein. Blunt dissection must be used to separate both structures from the tail and superior surface of the pancreas to avoid pancreatic injury and creation of a fistula. **E,** the raw bed is inspected for bleeding. The abdomen is closed without drainage if there are no other injuries.

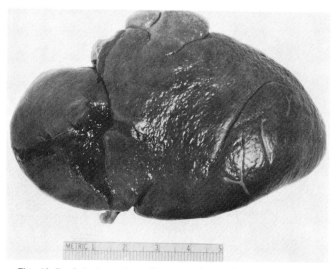

Fig. 13–7.—Splenic rupture. Gross specimen shows a typical transverse laceration in the plane of segmental vascular supply.

elaborate blood supply with 3 separate circulations, making infarction unlikely in damaged segments. Upadhyaya *et al.*[160] studied the effect of splenic trauma in monkeys. Splenic tears occurred segmentally and transversely for reason of blood supply in most instances. They observed healing by primary union in the vast majority. Vertical lacerations were poorly tolerated. In 1971, Douglas and Simpson,[34] pursuing the original concept, observed 25 of 32 patients with suspected splenic rupture. All were observed in the hospital to healing and without complications. The certainty of diagnosis in this series is far from established. Radionuclide scans and arteriography were not performed; the patients had no abdominal taps or peritoneal lavage. Diagnosis of splenic rupture in this series was largely a matter of clinical impression, typical history, positive physical findings, reduced hematocrit and occasional positive plain x-rays. The advisability of conservative management of splenic injury has been discussed by Welch *et al.*[172] One alternative to conservative management by splenectomy is some type of primary splenic repair. This was first suggested by Wojinar *et al.*, in 1964 and subsequently elaborated on by Orda *et al.* and by Deboer.[161] Various tissue adhesives were recommended,

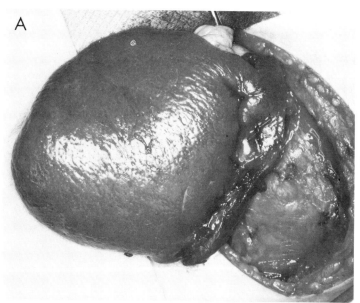

Fig. 13–8.—Partial resection of ruptured spleen. **A,** operative photograph showing resected lower pole with preservation of two-thirds of the spleen. Suturing is accomplished with catgut mattress sutures tied over bolsters. **B,** the resected specimen removed by completing the transverse fracture. **C,** preoperative and postoperative splenic scan showing the initially markedly diminished function returning to full splenic competence in the postoperative scan.

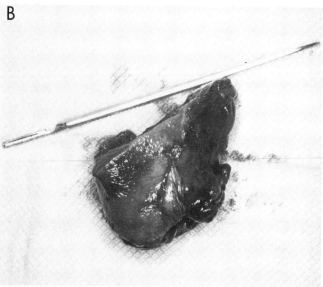

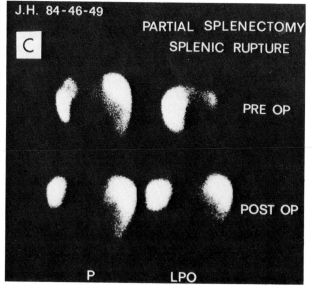

including cyanoacrylate monomer adhesive. Mishalny[107] recently has applied this to patients, recommending repair of the ruptured spleen rather than removal. Earlier experience was reported by Mazel[99] and Foster and Prey.[47] Mishalny sutured the spleen in 8 of 10 patients operated on for splenic trauma, including an 8-year-old boy who was followed to healing by scan and arteriography. Foster and Prey reported splenic repair in 6 patients, including a 13-year-old boy; however, there were 2 deaths. We have carried out successful splenic repair in 5 patients; all were followed to healing by scan with no loss of splenic substance. Segmental resection of the spleen for trauma was reported by Campos Christos[21] in 1962, with 8 patients treated in this manner. We have performed partial splenectomy in 3 children (Fig. 13–8).

The fourth possibility in management of splenic injury in children is nonintervention and observation in patients with splenic trauma diagnosed accurately by modern techniques. Egley[37] has reported splenic injury due to diagnostic amniocentesis. The lesion was identified by radionuclide scan and managed conservatively. In the past 3 years we have elected to observe and not intervene operatively in instances of isolated splenic trauma in children or when associated with other visceral injuries of a minor nature that did not of themselves require surgical intervention.[129a] The policy is as follows: The patient must be under observation in the hospital for 8–10 days. Lesions requiring surgical intervention must be excluded. Positive diagnosis must be established by radionuclide ^{99}Tc scan and/or arteriography. Peritoneal lavage has not been used consecutively to date but would serve to differentiate scan abnormalities due to recent trauma from pre-existing splenic conditions. Blood volume must be monitored accurately; patients are maintained in a hematocrit range of 25–30. If the hematocrit falls below 25, patients are transfused with packed cells in relatively small amounts to a total of 1 blood volume over a period of 24–72 hours. With these guidelines, 15 consecutive children with proved splenic injury have escaped operation. The patients ranged in age from 1 year, an infant who sustained splenic rupture

due to parental abuse, to 15 years, a patient who had a 1 volume transfusion over a 3-day period. All patients were followed to healing, usually in 3 months, through serial scanning (Fig. 13–9). Late rupture has not been encountered to date. One patient observed to healing had hemophilia.

From 1968 to 1974, 22 additional children underwent splenectomy for trauma, bringing our total experience to 171 patients, with 2 deaths; OPSI syndrome was not encountered in this series, although follow-up is weak (see Table 13–2).

Liver Injuries

History

There are several footnotes to the history of hepatic injury on which most current principles of management are based. Pringle (1908) conducted animal studies involving blunt hepatic injury, later translated to experience with patients. He demonstrated that major resections were possible through transient control of blood supply to the liver by cross-clamping of the hepatoduodenal ligament—the Pringle maneuver. A 15-minute period of interruption was recommended. Kuznetzoff was the first to use interlocking mattress sutures proximal to the line of hepatic resection, utilizing special needles. The method no longer is used. Lortat-Jacob (1952) was the first to perform total right hepatic lobectomy for neoplasm and trauma.[90] Further technical refinement of right hepatic lobectomy was contributed by the Quattlebaums.[124] Goldsmith and Woodburne[56] improved the accuracy of major resections through careful studies of surgical anatomy. The solution to the problem of uncontrollable intraoperative bleeding due to retrohepatic injuries to the hepatic veins and inferior vena cava was suggested by Schrock, who was the first to recommend use of an intracaval shunt, subsequently endorsed by Timmons.[94, 133] Merendino recommended routine common duct drainage following major hepatic resections.[94] This has proved to be controversial and counterproductive, among other reasons because of the high incidence of postoperative hemobilia, as reported by Lucas and Walt.[92] The value of hypothermia in protecting the liver during periodic cross-clamp ischemia was demonstrated by Bernhard[16] in animals and later applied to children with major hepatic injuries by Welch.[174] General guidelines to the management of liver injuries have been recorded by Madding and Kennedy.[94] The height of enthusiasm for hepatic resection for blunt injury was during the period 1965–1970. However, in large, mostly adult experience, this has not reduced the mortality for major liver injuries, which still hovers around 30–50%. Recently there has been a shift to more conservative management of most hepatic injuries, hepatic resection being reserved for the pulverized right lobe, persistent hemobilia and retrohepatic injuries of the hepatic veins and inferior vena cava.[36, 77, 89] Mays[96-98] has demonstrated that selective dearterialization reduces the need for hepatic resection as primary therapy in selected cases.

Diagnosis

Much recent attention has focused on new diagnostic aids. The popularity and usefulness of peritoneal lavage has been discussed. Nahum and Levesque[111] studied 87 patients by selective celiac arteriography, demonstrating the major types of liver injury, and recommended conservative management in some and resection in others. Levin et al.[88] recommend routine celiac angiography and venacavography in all patients except those with life-endangering hemorrhage.

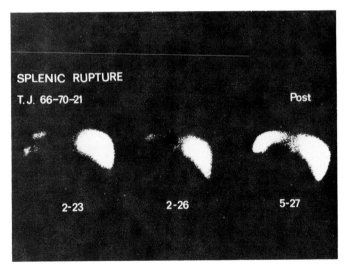

Fig. 13–9.—Splenic rupture—nonoperative treatment. This 8-year-old boy sustained traumatic rupture of the spleen. There were no associated injuries requiring operation. During the initial period of observation the child required one transfusion of packed cells. In the first scan there is an obvious concentration of radionuclear material at the upper and lower poles of the spleen, with diminished uptake centrally. Three days later there was virtually no uptake (slight in the upper pole) and 3 months following injury there was complete healing of the spleen with normal uptake of the technetium-99. Splenic competence is ensured.[129a]

Correlation between anatomic injury and operative findings was 90%. Popovsky et al.[122] have reported on radionuclide imaging for hepatic injuries using ^{99m}Tc sulfer colloid. They demonstrated high correlation with celiac arteriography. Selected cases could be observed without operation. Higher correlation was seen when radionuclide studies were combined with sonography. Richie and Fonkalsrud[126] reported 4 patients managed conservatively to complete healing demonstrated through serial scans, one a 12-year-old girl and one a 10-year-old boy. These studies play only a minor role in patients with massive bleeding due to juxtahepatic venous injury.

Clinical Experience

Most experience with liver injuries is in adults, with cases about equally divided between blunt injuries and penetrating injuries due to knives or guns. There are relatively few reports of hepatic injury in children; usually these are small series when compared to adult experience, where several thousand recent cases have been reported.[27, 110, 158]

CHILDHOOD EXPERIENCE.—Kaufman and Burrington[80] reported 40 cases of liver trauma in children; 37 were blunt and 3 were penetrating injuries. In 34 patients, the right lobe was involved. Twenty-eight patients had liver lacerations; in 20, the injury was considered to be major and life-endangering. There were 7 right hepatic ruptures, with 3 deaths from exsanguination, 2 intraoperatively. Five patients had minor injury, such as marginal laceration or subcapsular hematoma. Resection was performed in only 1 patient, a partial left hepatic lobectomy. Of 5 (12%) deaths, 3 were due to isolated liver injury. Morton et al.[109] reported 13 major hepatic resections in children for blunt trauma, with 1 death (8%). Stone[146] reported 16 children with hepatic trauma and 2 deaths (13%). Fifteen children underwent resection. Stone and Ansley[148] reported 203 children 16 years or younger with liver injuries, an extraordinary experience, from 1968 to 1975. At variance with other reports, 171 (mortality 3.4%) were penetrating whereas only 31 (mortality 19%) were caused by blunt trauma. Minor injury occurred in 137. Concentrating on blunt experience, 17 patients (54%) required hepatic resection previously reported.[147] In 12 recent cases, the traumatic fissure was packed with an omental graft—no resections were performed. Three patients died from uncontrollable hemorrhage. The authors did not use caval bypass, the Pringle maneuver or hypothermia. For associated injury to the inferior vena cava or hepatic veins, they used periodic taping of the inferior vena cava above the diaphragm and above the renal veins, plus occlusion of the abdominal aorta, using a special device. Suson et al.[152] reported 35 children, 31 with blunt and 4 with penetrating injuries. There were 7 deaths (20%). They did not use intracaval shunts. Cavitary hypothermia using iced Ringer's solution was used as recommended by Cooley.[94] Control of liver hemorrhage was achieved through elaborate cross-clamping. Major vessel injury was encountered in 5 fatal cases. Hepatic resection was performed in 8 patients; 6 survived. Two had total right hepatic lobectomy, 4 partial right hepatic lobectomy and 2 partial left hepatic lobectomy. Like Stone, they do not recommend T-tube drainage of the common hepatic duct. Srouji et al.[141] have reported on rupture of the liver in a neonate, identified by radionuclide scan, sutured and followed to healing. Mercadier et al.[102] reported 1 child, age 14, among 10 right hepatic lobectomies for blunt trauma, with a mortality of 40%.

ADULT EXPERIENCE.—Among the many reports of adult experience is that by Carroll et al.,[22] who reported 254 patients with liver wounds in Vietnam. They concluded that common duct drainage did not reduce the incidence of complications (16%), notably abscess, pulmonary problems, gastrointestinal bleeding and biliary fistula. Donovan et al.[33] reported hepatic lobectomy in 35 patients; 29 had right lobectomy, 6 left lobectomy. Eight patients had vascular isolation; 4 died intraoperatively. Over-all mortality was 43%. With associated venous injury, 12 patients, mortality rose to 67%. Faris and Dudley,[44] in animal studies, proved conclusively that CBD drainage did not reduce intrahepatic pressure, even with a common duct ligated distally. Bowen and Fleming[19] reviewed 81 liver injuries, focusing on whether T-tube (CBD) drainage predisposes to gastrointestinal hemorrhage. Seventy-nine patients who survived operation for liver injury had CBD drainage. Gastrointestinal hemorrhage occurred in 7 of 22 patients drained but in only 1 of 54 who were not drained. Faris[43] reported on 65 patients with blunt hepatic injury; 10 died intraoperatively (15%). Defore[27] reported 1600 consecutive liver injuries; 860 were due to gunshot, 490 to knives and 240 to blunt trauma. There were 49 hepatic resections; common duct drainage was used infrequently. Intracaval shunts were used in 15 patients; over-all mortality was 13.1%. Deaths in 209 patients were due to hemorrhage, 122 patients, multiple trauma 23, respiratory insufficiency 17, renal failure 15 and miscellaneous causes 23. Cross-clamping of the thoracic aorta was utilized in 50 patients, the Pringle maneuver in 17. Trunkey et al.[158] reported 811 consecutive patients, noting that mortality still hovers around 50% in the complicated group. There were 34 deaths (4%). A midline exploratory incision was used routinely with sternal split whenever vascular isolation or intracaval shunt was contemplated. Fifty-three patients (6.5%) required sublobar or lobar resections, 11 required hepatic vein repair and 15 had associated extrahepatic duct portal vein or hepatic artery injury. Mortality among 53 patients who required resection was 47%. Drezner[35] reported 57 patients; 16 underwent resection, 7 died (12%), 3 intraoperatively. Bleeding parameters were monitored, fresh-frozen plasma was given, 1 unit for every 5 units of whole blood. Platelet packs were given with counts below 50,000 and calcium levels were monitored. Morton et al.[110] reported 1068 patients, with 171 deaths; only 32% of cases were due to blunt trauma. In their most recent experience with 428 patients, mortality was 11.7%; 13 resections were performed and 8 patients had Schrock[133] caval catheter bypass. Adjunct hypothermia is not mentioned in recent adult experience.

Discussion

Liver injuries are said to be second only to head injuries in autopsy trauma material and are rapidly fatal[104]; they are more common in children than in adults. These injuries involve the right lobe in 80%; convex surface injuries are about twice as common as other types. Injuries fall in four anatomic groups (Fig. 13-10): A, convex surface and dome, usually not evident when the abdomen is first opened. B, anterior surface and margin, left or right lobe. C, inferior or concave surface, usually the right lobe and most likely to be associated with injuries to the extrahepatic bile ducts. D, posterior surface or contrecoup, usually the right lobe, most likely to be associated with injury to the hepatic veins or the retrohepatic segment of the inferior vena cava; with A, these account for most cases of traumatic hemobilia.[131]

Hepatic rupture is the major unsolved problem in the management of nonpenetrating wounds of the abdomen. Mikeskey et al.[104] reported 596 patients who sustained blunt

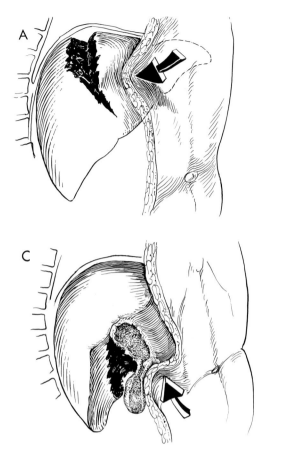

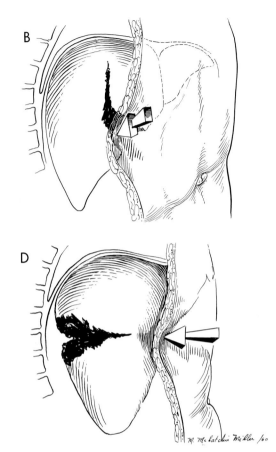

Fig. 13–10.— Mechanics of hepatic rupture. Right lobe and convex surface injuries account for 80% of these cases. Prompt debridement lateral to the traumatic fissure is advocated in dealing with a pulverized lobe or retrohepatic venous injury to avoid late sepsis, hemorrhage and hemobilia.

hepatic injury; 67% died before or after entering the hospital. The problem is all the more devastating in children (Fig. 13–11). Mortality was 40% for blunt injuries in the first decade of life, higher than for any other decade, including patients aged 60 or older.

Review of the problem after 10 years shows slow but gradual reduction of mortality (43–50%) resulting from complex blunt liver injuries.[27, 110, 158] Success or failure seems to depend on the location and extent of liver injury, presence or absence of injury to juxtahepatic vessels and the institutional setting. Most superficial lacerations of the liver can be dealt with by observation and transfusion or by simple surgical techniques and are not of themselves lethal.

Seven of 44 cases of major hepatic injury we treated were fatal (16%) (Table 13–3). In 2, no operation was performed; both were proved at autopsy. There were 3 intraoperative deaths due to inability to control massive hemorrhage; 2 died of late complications. Similarity in the appearance of these youngsters at the time of admission to the hospital has led us to believe that in the absence of an extensively fractured pelvis or injury to extra-abdominal great vessels one can suspect hepatic rupture with exsanguination by exclusion.

Surgical Management

When the diagnosis of hepatic rupture is made, the following steps should be taken. Two of the largest possible refill lines are established above the diaphragm, including a line for the measurement of central venous pressure or wedge pulmonary pressure, utilizing the Swan-Ganz catheter and a separate cephalic line for massive transfusion. A radial arterial line is established in the opposite upper extremity, with direct measurement of arterial blood pressure on digital strain gauge read-out. Blood is drawn for type and crossmatch, estimation of peripheral values and determination of

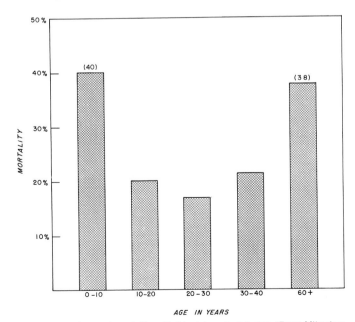

Fig. 13–11.—Age and mortality with blunt hepatic injuries. (From Mikeskey et al.[104])

TABLE 13–3.–LIVER INJURIES IN CHILDREN

SERIES	NO. CASES	MAJOR RESECTION	R. LOBE	L. LOBE	SUTURE	OBSERVED	DEATHS
BCH, 1968[175]	21	7	6	1	10	4	4
CHMC, 1968[152a]	8	2	1	1	6		2
CHMC, 1977	15	5	5		7	3	1
Totals	44°	14	12	2	23	7	7 (16%)

°3 penetrating, 41 blunt.

arterial blood gas levels. The always-present hypovolemic shock is treated initially with 5% albumin, single-donor AB plasma or Plasmanate. Within 15 minutes, a reliable rapid crossmatch can be obtained. Fresh whole blood transfusion is started as soon as possible, using a warming coil. Availability of ionized calcium is ensured by adding 0.5 gm of calcium as calcium gluconate for each unit of whole blood administered. Equally important is the monitoring of pH, with buffering as indicated. As in all low perfusion states, anoxic lactic acidosis should be anticipated and treated. Bleeding and clotting times plus prothrombin and PTT and platelets are measured for future reference.

With hypovolemia and shock, one must replace total calculated blood volume in the first hour. Estimates of blood volume range from 8% of total kg weight in older children to 10% in infants. When a reasonable blood pressure can be established there may be time for further diagnostic tests, notably peritoneal lavage and technetium scan. Arteriography is of little value in the emergency management of major liver injuries. The child is intubated, given succinylcholine, lightly anesthetized and then placed on a cooling mat (Davol) with ice bags, reducing body temperature to the range of 92–90 F (33–32 C). Bernhard[16] demonstrated that hepatic cellular activity, as measured by glucose, glycogen and lactose metabolism, ceases at 85–88 F (27–30 C). For this reason, moderate hypothermia is proposed as an adjunct to management of hepatic injuries where resection or venous repair may be required.[174] Wangensteen[169] showed that intermittent clamping of the blood supply to the liver could be carried out in intact animals for periods up to 15 minutes without causing hepatic necrosis. At normothermic levels in man, occasional and unpredictable liver necrosis has occurred with this period of clamping. With the protection of moderate hypothermia, the period of clamping probably can be safely doubled in quinidinized children with a previously normal liver. It is essential to accomplish hemostasis during the period of temperature reduction. A cold heart combined with any degree of anoxia due to uncorrected shock or anesthesia will result in extreme irritability and probable fibrillation. Howland *et al.*[74] showed that hypothermic patients are particularly vulnerable to cardiac irregularities with massive cold whole blood replacement. Electrocardiographic monitoring and apparatus for defibrillation are essential. On transfer to the operating room, anesthesia is deepened with Fluothane or with morphine and nitrous oxide to permit electrosurgery, for both resection and control of bleeding. The abdomen is entered through an exploratory midline incision extending from the manubrium to below the umbilicus, removing the xiphoid (Fig. 13–12). The hand is gently passed across the dome of the liver. If a deep rupture is identified, with little bleeding, the incision is carried across the costal margin into the fifth interspace. Alternatively or for injuries involving the medial segment of the left lobe, the incision is extended superiorly through

sternal split to the level of the manubrium, as recommended by Miller and Kelly[106] and Fullen *et al.*[52] If major venous injury to the retrohepatic segment of the inferior vena cava or hepatic veins is suspected, usually by the release of a massive amount of intra-abdominal liquid and clotted blood, a caval catheter is inserted and secured. If lateral thoracic extension is used, the diaphragm is cut down to the vena cava and hepatic vein junction. To avoid air embolism, the right hepatic vein should be positively identified and ligated as early as possible for right lobe injuries. Active bleeding can be greatly reduced by manual compression of the liver at the line of transection and by the Pringle maneuver. If right hepatic lobectomy or venous repair is required, vena cava flow must be ensured by inserting a shunt via the right atrium or inferior vena cava above the renal veins[94, 133] (Fig. 13–13). The placement of an intracaval shunt should be anticipated in the management of children with the major and complex forms of hepatic injury. A complete range of Portex tubes of suitable length must be available at all times and altered to suit the technique of insertion. A vascular noncrushing clamp is applied, incorporating all the structures in the hepatoduodenal ligament, and the clamp time noted. A bulldog clamp is placed on the superior mesenteric artery to prevent splanchnic sequestration. The decision is made between suturing the laceration with heavy catgut or resection if the lobe is hopelessly pulverized. If resection is considered appropriate, all liver tissue lateral to the injury is removed by the finger-fracture technique of Lin as rapidly as possible.[94] The vessels and bile ducts exposed on the retained liver surface are ligated with nonabsorbable transfixion sutures. Three periods of clamping not in excess of 15 minutes are permissible during the course of resection. The level of hypothermia can be adjusted intraoperatively by peritoneal lavage with cold or warm Ringer's solution, as reported by Suson *et al.*[152] Associated injuries to the inferior vena cava and hepatic vein roots are dealt with. The caval catheter, filled with blood or saline to avoid air embolism, is removed. The venotomy site or incision in the right atrium is closed appropriately.

Many materials have been proposed for covering the extensive raw liver surface following hepatic lobectomy. A plasma coagulum has been used[132] and Ivalon sponge has been recommended.[76] Freese *et al.*[51] advocated the use of acrylic adhesive; in our experience, none of these is necessary. McDermott and Ottinger[100] suggested a practical technique of detaching the falciform ligament from the anterior abdominal wall and applying it to the raw liver surface, in essence reperitonealizing the raw surface. Decompression of the biliary tract with T-tube drainage is controversial. Tank *et al.*,[152a] Suson *et al.*[152] and Stone[146] properly conclude that CBD drainage is not indicated in children. It fails to reduce intrahepatic pressure and indeed may promote late hepatic hemorrhage because of acid regurgitation into the biliary radicles. Because of failure of bile to enter the duode-

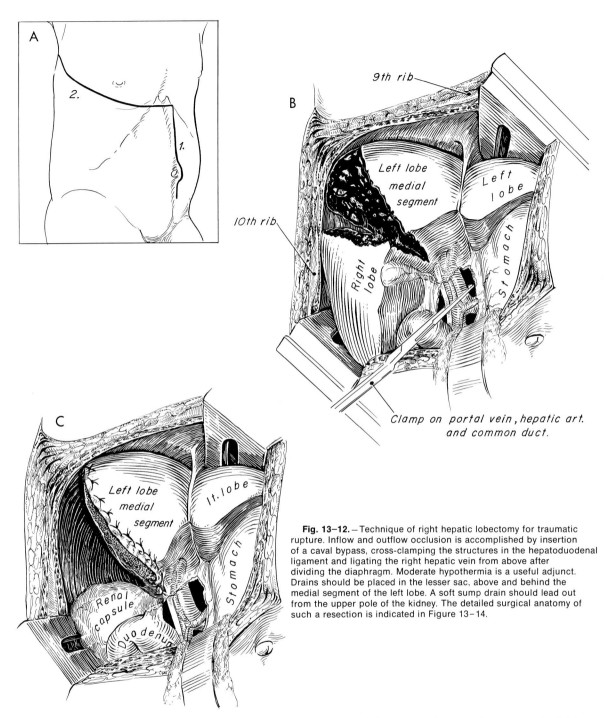

Fig. 13–12. — Technique of right hepatic lobectomy for traumatic rupture. Inflow and outflow occlusion is accomplished by insertion of a caval bypass, cross-clamping the structures in the hepatoduodenal ligament and ligating the right hepatic vein from above after dividing the diaphragm. Moderate hypothermia is a useful adjunct. Drains should be placed in the lesser sac, above and behind the medial segment of the left lobe. A soft sump drain should lead out from the upper pole of the kidney. The detailed surgical anatomy of such a resection is indicated in Figure 13–14.

num, pepsin stimulation occurs. We are in agreement with Lucas and Walt,[92] who conducted the only prospective randomized study, that CBD drainage is irrational. Multiple soft drains are placed in the subdiaphragmatic and subhepatic spaces and in the lesser sac. A sump drain is added. The right thorax is placed on water seal drainage for 48 hours if the pleural cavity has been entered; otherwise, the mediastinum is closed with Hemovac drainage lateral to the median sternotomy incision.

Experience and Results

Our total experience with hepatic injuries in children is limited to 44 patients, with 7 deaths (16%), small by comparison to adult series. Thirty-eight patients had blunt trauma, with 6 deaths; 5 had penetrating, with 1 death. There is much room for improvement in the management of this most serious organ injury.

We should like to enter a plea for more accurate reporting of resection for trauma in children. The present view of liver anatomy (Fig. 13–14) suggests that the right hepatic lobe includes 70% of the tissue to the right of the falciform ligament and always to the right of the portal vein and vena cava. Resection of the medial segment of the left lobe will be necessary only rarely in trauma. Resection of the lateral segment of the left lobe may be total or subsegmental. To date, we have performed 14 hepatic resections for trauma,

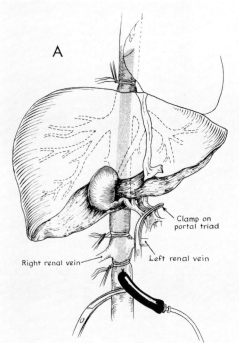
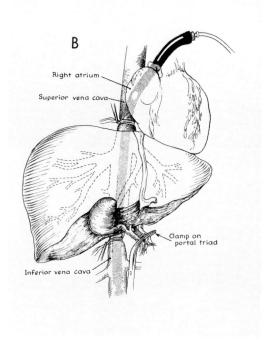
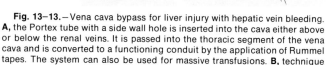

Fig. 13–13.—Vena cava bypass for liver injury with hepatic vein bleeding. **A,** the Portex tube with a side wall hole is inserted into the cava either above or below the renal veins. It is passed into the thoracic segment of the vena cava and is converted to a functioning conduit by the application of Rummel tapes. The system can also be used for massive transfusions. **B,** technique of caval bypass inserting the Portex tube through the right atrium. It is taped above the diaphragm and above the renal veins. The Pringle maneuver is demonstrated. (Reproduced, with permission, from Blaisdell, F. W. and Lim, Re.[94])

with 3 deaths (21%). Twelve involved the right lobe; 7 had total right hepatic lobectomy and 5 had right sublobar or segmental resection. The left lobe was resected on 2 occasions, in 1 sublobar and in the other an extended left lobectomy. Twenty-three patients were treated by suturing of the liver laceration, 7 patients were observed and 4 had minor injuries identified on scan and followed to healing.

Hemobilia

Traumatic hemobilia is a known and important complication of liver injury. The term was coined by Sandblom[131] in 1948, although Owing had described the condition a century before. Hemobilia is largely due to failure to resect pulverized liver tissue. It usually occurs with rupture of the central convex and anterior surfaces of the right lobe, requiring suture. The main clinical features are biliary colic followed by hematemesis and melena and frequently jaundice. The bleeding tends to be massive and episodic and in the instances due to trauma occurs days to weeks after injury. Selective hepatic arteriography and Tc scan are helpful in locating the site of bleeding and determining treatment.

Few cases of hemobilia in children have been reported.[175] We have encountered 4 cases. The first patient was untreated and died (Fig. 13–15). The second had right hepatic artery ligation.[175] The third mistakenly had "blind gastrectomy" after "negative gastric and duodenal exploration." The fourth had delayed right lobectomy; all 3 survived. Hendren *et al.*[65] reported nonoperative management of 5- and 6-year-old boys with traumatic hemobilia, with healing documented by serial angiography. Both bled massively 2 weeks after suturing of a laceration of the right lobe. The condition was observed and treated by transfusion. Two months later, arteriography in each case showed the lesion to be healed;

there was no further bleeding. Hemobilia in 3 children has been reported by Stone and Ansley.[148] Treatment consisted of unroofing the hematoma, vessel ligation and packing. Attiyeh *et al.*[6] reported on traumatic hemobilia as a complication of needle liver biopsy in a 15-year-old boy undergoing staging for Hodgkin's disease. McGehee *et al.*[101] reported on traumatic hemobilia in 2 cases and surveyed the literature. They were able to identify 69 adult patients; 58 of the cases were due to blunt trauma, with 12 deaths. Hepatic artery ligation was carried out in 12 patients; 3 rebled, with no deaths. Resections were carried out in 14 patients; 1 rebled, with 4 deaths. Vallidis[162] reported double hepatic artery ligation. Surgical treatment may consist of observation with transfusion, resection or ligation of the appropriate major hepatic artery branch. Proximal ligation must be done to either the left or the immediate right of the gastroduodenal artery.[98] Selective embolization is feasible but has not been reported to date. Our best estimate from the literature is that there now are approximately 75 cases involving 10 children and 65 adults. The subject has been reviewed extensively by Sandblom in a recent monograph.[130] Most cases have been due to blunt trauma, more commonly in children.

Injuries of the Extrahepatic Biliary Tract

Extrahepatic duct injuries in children have been reported sporadically[13, 66, 67, 171] as single cases. Such injuries can occur with or without associated liver injury. It is unforgivable for a surgeon to fail to diagnose and treat a ruptured or divided hepatic or common duct at the time of laparotomy for trauma. Our 2 patients had successful direct repair of the common hepatic duct. The gallbladder was electively removed in 7 patients undergoing right hepatic lobectomy. Stone and Ansley[148] encountered 11 children with extrahe-

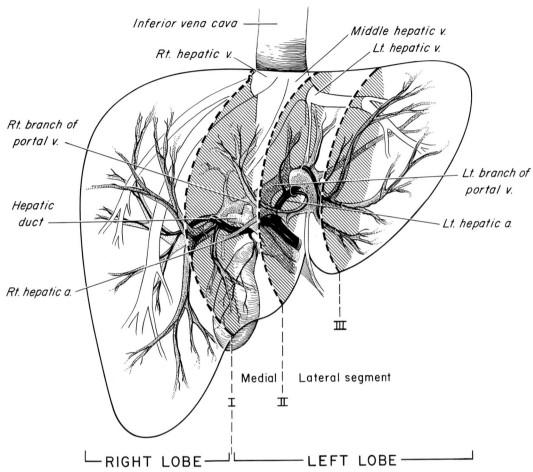

Inferior vena cava

Middle hepatic v.

Rt. hepatic v.

Lt. hepatic v.

Rt. branch of portal v.

Lt. branch of portal v.

Hepatic duct

Lt. hepatic a.

Rt. hepatic a.

III

Medial | Lateral segment

I

II

└─ RIGHT LOBE ─┘ └─ LEFT LOBE ─┘

Fig. 13–14.—Surgical anatomy of the liver. In addition to the three planes for lobar segmental or subsegmental resection, this drawing shows in detail the distribution and course of the hepatic artery, portal vein and the hepatic veins. The hepatic ducts are intimately associated with the branches of the portal vein and have been left out for purposes of clarity. Hepatic resections in children should be repaired anatomically.

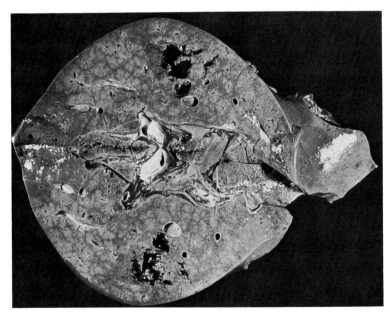

Fig. 13–15.—Hemobilia results from deep cavitation with arteriovenous fistula. This patient, a 4-year-old boy, died without surgical treatment. Death was a result of exsanguinating hemorrhage and intestinal gangrene due to mesenteric avulsion.

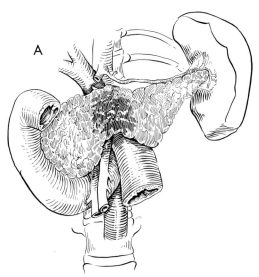
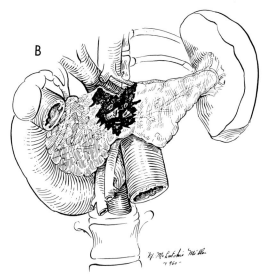

Fig. 13–16.—Pancreatic injuries. **A,** contusion of the body of the pancreas as it crosses the vertebral column. The lesser peritoneal sac should be opened, followed by the Kocher maneuver, and the degree of injury estimated by direct inspection. **B,** anatomic transection of the pancreatic body. Such injuries should be treated by distal pancreatectomy without splenectomy and with adequate drainage.

patic duct injuries. Cholecystectomy was required in 8 penetrating cases, direct repair of the common duct in 2 and repair of the left hepatic duct with shunt was successful in 3 children. Hartman and Greaney[63] have called attention to the syndrome of anorexia, weight loss, biliary ascites, jaundice and acholic stools in 5 children 2–7 years of age. Two patients had transection of the left hepatic duct, 1 had a split at the junction of the hepatic ducts, 1 had complete division of the common duct at the duodenal wall and 1 had a perforated gallbladder. All injuries were due to blunt force, once again in contrast to adult experience. Dietrich *et al.*[30] reported 6 adults with biliary tract injuries due to blunt trauma. Longmire and McArthur[89] reported 12 cases of common duct rupture or laceration. Five were treated successfully by choledochojejunostomy. Three had successful direct repair with T-tube drainage; 4 had miscellaneous procedures tailored to the anatomic injury. The injury was uniformly identified at the superior border of the pancreas at the duodenal wall. Direct repair of such injuries at the time of initial laparotomy is recommended. The technique of repair will vary.

Pancreatic Injuries

Pancreatitis in the acute or chronic form is a common disease in adults. The etiology is poorly understood; fewer than 4% of cases are thought to be due to trauma. Kinnaird[84] reviewed 1973 cases of pancreatitis in adults and found 56 due to trauma.

In contrast, pancreatitis is uncommon in childhood. It occurs in small infants after protracted vomiting and in association with severe dehydration. Rarely, it is due to a viral infection. Of known causes, the most common is direct blunt injury to the central portion of the pancreas as it crosses the vertebral column (Fig. 13–16). Blumenstock *et al.*[16a] collected 36 cases of pancreatitis in childhood; 7 were due to trauma. Our attention was directed to this entity in the postoperative management of certain children following splenectomy for trauma. Some had a protracted course with ileus, back pain and fever. Amylase determination in 1 such patient was 560 Somogyi units/dl. This child formed a pseudocyst, as did 10 of 34 children with traumatic pancreatitis encountered by us (Table 13–4). Thirty-one were due to blunt injury and 3 to penetrating injury.

Serum amylase levels are measured routinely on the first, third and fifth days in all patients admitted with the diagnosis of abdominal trauma. Twenty-eight had significantly elevated serum amylase levels—over 300 Somogyi units/dl. Six were excluded because of postoperative ileus, persistent vomiting or an open lesion in the gastrointestinal tract. Direct absorption of enzymes from the peritoneal surface following gut perforation and any condition resulting in increased intraduodenal pressure will cause elevated serum pancreatic enzyme levels. We do not agree that levels twice normal or higher are explained by stress. In a control group, 10 had exploratory laparotomy for other cause, 10 had isolated craniocerebral injury and 10 had isolated musculoskeletal injuries. All had levels within the normal range for our laboratory (80–140 Somogyi units/dl). This is in agreement

TABLE 13–4.—PANCREATIC INJURIES IN CHILDREN

SERIES	NO. CASES	BLUNT	PENE-TRATING	LAPA-ROTOMY	RESEC-TION	DRAINED	PSEUDO-CYST	C/G	ROUX	EXC.	OBSERVED
BCH, 1968[175]	20	18	2	11	2	9	4	2	1	1	9
CHMC, 1968[152a]	5	5		5	0	5	3	2	1		
CHMC, 1977	9	8	1	7	2	5	3	1		1	2†
TOTALS	34°	31	3	23	4	19	10	5	2	2	11

°1 death, gunshot.
†Observed to healing by scan and sonography.

with findings of Howard *et al.*[73] with pancreatic injury. Some elevations occurred the first day; others did not peak until the third or fifth day. Simultaneous urinary amylase determinations are helpful. In combination, the 2 tests ultimately are 90% accurate in establishing the diagnosis of pancreatic injury.[108, 171] Nardi and Lees[113] suggested that serum trypsin levels more accurately reflect the transudation of pancreatic enzymes. In our experience, laboratory data supported the diagnosis of pancreatic injury in 19 of 23 cases (83%) proved by operation. In 4 cases, the serum amylase level was normal and failed to identify the pancreatic injury.

White and Benfield[176] found serum amylase elevation in only 26% of 63 patients preoperatively; however, the urinary amylase was found to be elevated in 96% of patients postoperatively, a useful indicator of organ injury and the need for further medical or surgical treatment. Moretz *et al.*[108] found serum amylase determination of little or no value immediately after injury in 51 patients; however, 90% of patients with amylase levels above 300 SU were found at operation to have pancreatic injury. The test failed to identify 3 of 5 patients with major pancreatic injury requiring resection. Olsen,[115] in a prospective study, found only 8% of patients with increased amylase and pancreatic injury; conversely, 33% of patients with elevated amylase were found to have no significant injury at the time of laparotomy. This is counter to our own and to other reported experience.

Ekengren and Soderlund[38] described the radiologic features in 17 children with pancreatic trauma. Edema with duodenal atony in the acute stage was uniformly encountered with or without organ displacement.

Pancreatic injury in 30 children has been reported by Stone.[147] Twenty had penetrating injuries and 10 had blunt trauma. All were drained; there were no resections and 5 deaths. When both the pancreas and duodenum were injured, mortality rose by several percentage points. He encountered 3 pseudocysts; 2 were treated with cystogastrostomy and 1 with Roux-en-Y. Of our 23 patients with pancreatic injury identified at operation, 19 were drained and 4 were resected. Eleven patients not explored had classic symptoms of pancreatitis that responded to colloid, nasogastric suction and atropine derivatives,

more recently with adjunct central or peripheral total hyperalimentation. Cummins *et al.*[25] recommend total peripheral parenteral alimentation for children with severe pancreatic injuries. Of 10 patients encountered, 3 had total central hyperalimentation and 1 had rupture of the duodenum and pancreatic head, with survival. Adwers and Davis[1] have also reported on adjuvant hyperalimentation in animals. Much lower amylase values were found after induced pancreatic injury in animals treated with Ringer's solution. If volume requirements are met, there is reduced pancreatic response to injury. Pancreatic pseudocyst following trauma is reported in detail in Chapter 88. We encountered 10 such cases; 5 were treated with cystogastrostomy, 2 by Roux-en-Y, 2 were excised and 1 was observed to healing by serial sonography. Chylous ascites is a rare complication of blunt abdominal injury. Hoffman[69] was able to find 4 cases; 2 additional cases have been reported recently.[167] None had an associated pseudocyst, such as is illustrated in Figures 13–17 and 13–18.

Surgical Treatment

Operative treatment consists of complete exposure of the pancreas by widely opening the lesser sac, dividing the gastrocolic omentum and mobilizing the head of the gland through a Kocher maneuver. It is most important to assess the location, extent and distribution of pancreatic injury and in all instances to identify complete or partial division of the pancreatic duct. In most cases, treatment will consist of drainage using a single sump and multiple soft empty Penrose drains. Distal pancreatectomy is the treatment for actual or near transection of the pancreatic body as it crosses the second lumbar vertebra. Up to 90% resection of the pancreas for trauma has the support of Steele *et al.*[144] and Yellin *et al.*[179] Endocrine or exocrine deficiency has not been reported following resections of this magnitude (see Chapter 88). Total pancreatectomy, when (rarely) indicated, is preferable to pancreatoduodenectomy.

The most difficult problems occur in patients with injury to the pancreatic head, as it lies in close proximity to the inner curve of the duodenum. There often is associated duodenal injury that must be dealt with by a variety of tech-

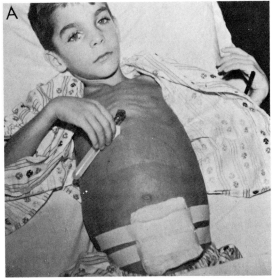 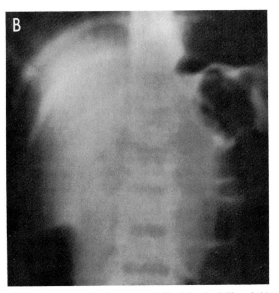

Fig. 13–17.—Pancreatic pseudocyst. **A,** in this 10-year-old boy, a pseudocyst developed after nonpenetrating abdominal injury. He also had chylous ascites and severe malnutrition. After Roux-en-Y cystojejunostomy, the ascites promptly disappeared. **B,** abdominal film of this patient. (See also Fig. 13–18.)

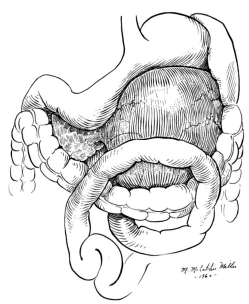

Fig. 13–18.—Pancreatic pseudocyst; artist's conception of the pseudocyst in Figure 13–17. A segment of jejunum was firmly attached to the cyst wall. Posterior cystogastrostomy or Roux-en-Y cystojejunostomy would be optional in this instance.

niques. There are several options: (1) Direct repair of the duct of Wirsung for complete division of the duct adjacent to the intact duodenum. Fine nonabsorbable sutures are used in constructing the anastomosis over a Silastic splint, which is brought to the skin surface through the duodenal wall after division of the sphincter of Oddi, as recommended by Sulamaa and Vitanen.[151a] (2) Extended (90%) pancreatic resection in cases in which the duct is uninjured in its most proximal portion and enters the duodenum normally. (3) In instances in which the head of the gland is pulverized, major vessel injuries coexist, with resultant devitalization of the duodenum. Treatment consists of pancreatoduodenectomy and appropriate reconstruction; 4 children requiring pancreatoduodenectomy have been reported recently.[151, 178] (4) "Diverticulization of the duodenum," as reported by Berne *et al.*[15] (5) Some variation of the Puestow operation, as reported by Balsano and Reynolds.[10] (6) Total pancreatectomy, leaving the duodenum intact, may be possible in selected cases. (7) Repair of the duodenum adjacent to repair of the duct of Wirsung utilizing the Thal patch[153] is suggested when the lateral duodenal wall has been destroyed, making direct repair technically impossible.

There is no clear road to the management of these complex conditions. Treatment must be highly individualized, at times settling for less than an ideal solution of the problem. A more desirable anatomic reconstruction can be accomplished at a later date.

Discussion

Fortunately, in children most pancreatic injuries are due to blunt trauma with maximal impact to the midbody segment. Drainage or conservative resection will cover most situations. In occasional patients, penetrating injury, usually due to gunshot, will require more extensive procedures, with a high mortality.

Multiple organ injury occurred in 17 of 34 patients in our experience, in contrast to Ekengren and Soderlund's[38] report of isolated pancreatic injury. Reports of experience in adults

provide useful information and stress the greater frequency of penetrating injuries.[11, 144] In general, the principles of surgical management are the same in any age group. Berne *et al.*[15] ignored the injured pancreas and performed a Billroth II resection with tube duodenostomy, vagotomy and common duct drainage. They reported 50 patients with 16% mortality; all pancreatic and duodenal fistulas closed spontaneously. Anderson *et al.*[5] reported 70 patients with few resections, promoting sump and soft tube drainage. Yellin *et al.*[179] reported 60 patients with distal pancreatectomy. All patients had disruption of the pancreatic duct; 90% resection was required in 15 patients. Mortality was 12%. There were 5 children. Anane-Sefah[4] reported 40 penetrating and 10 blunt injuries of the pancreas; mortality was 14%. Resections were carried out in 3 patients for blunt trauma and 16 for penetrating trauma, with 2 deaths. Drainage rather than resection was recommended for injuries of the head with an intact duct encountered in 9 patients; pancreatoduodenectomy was carried out in 4 patients, with no deaths. Steele *et al.*[144] reported 85 cases, two-thirds due to penetrating injury, with 23 deaths (27%). They recommend drainage only if the duct is intact, resection if the duct is divided. Subtotal pancreatectomy, up to 90%, was carried out in 26 patients, with 6 deaths. Diabetes or exocrine insufficiency was not observed. Belasegaren[11] reported 91 patients with pancreatic injury, 54 due to blunt trauma; mortality was 21%. Complete transection was encountered in 13, injuries of the duodenum and head of the pancreas in 12 and complete destruction of the pancreas and duodenum in 6. Thirty-five partial pancreatectomies were carried out, with 1 death; 8 patients had pancreatoduodenectomy, with 5 deaths. Strum *et al.*[151] reported 5 pancreatoduodenectomies, including one in a 14-year-old; the transected descending duodenum was avulsed from the pancreas. A 12-year-old boy with injury of the pancreatic head, duodenum and IVC due to gunshot required total pancreatectomy. Pancreatoduodenectomy was performed by Yellin[178] in 8 patients; mortality was 40%. Thal and Wilson[153] were the first to perform pancreatoduodenectomy for trauma. Subsequently, 60 patients have been reported, with 39 survivors. A disturbing note was added by Warren and Wagner.[170] In a study of long-term results following treatment of nonpenetrating pancreatic trauma, 20 patients followed 2–28 years had a high incidence of chronic pancreatitis, ulcers and recurrent cysts.

Conclusions

Because of the frequency of traumatic pancreatitis in children, it is important to expose the lesser peritoneal cavity and perform a Kocher maneuver in every patient undergoing exploration for abdominal injury. There may be diffuse contusion requiring only adequate drainage or there may be anatomic transection requiring resection (see Fig. 13–16). In the latter instance, one should not hesitate to perform a distal or extended pancreatectomy, closing the stump with nonabsorbable sutures after ligation of the pancreatic duct. Failure to remove this damaged segment results in prolonged illness, with eventual reoperation for removal of necrotic material or treatment of a pseudocyst. Combined pancreatic and duodenal injuries require great innovation and selective management, with uncertain results.

Gastrointestinal Injuries

Reports of exclusively gastrointestinal injuries are rare. Kakos *et al.*[78] reported on small bowel injuries in children after blunt abdominal trauma; 13 involved the duodenum,

TABLE 13–5.—GASTROINTESTINAL INJURIES IN CHILDREN

	B	P	B	P	B	P	TOTALS	B	P
	BCH, 1968		CHMC, 1968		CHMC, 1977				
Stomach	1	2	1°		1	1	6	3	3
Duodenum									
Perforation	2		3	2	1		8	6	2
TIHD	4		8		5		17	17	
Jejunum	9	3	4		2	2°	20	15	5
Ileum	6°	2	4		1	3	16	11	5
Colon	1	3	2	1	1	1	9	4	5
Mesentery	5				3	2	10	8	2
Vascular	1					2°	3	1	2
TOTALS	29	10	22	3	14	11	89	65	24

°Deaths:

Stomach	12 days	Dropped
Jejunum, colon, liver	2 yr	Gunshot
Ileum, mesentery	4 yr	Kicked
SMV, jejunum, pancreas	7 yr	Knifed

10 the jejunum and 3 the ileum. Mortality was 8%. Kaufer and Wulfing[79] have reported 9 children with gastrointestinal injuries; all survived. Dickenson *et al.*[29] reported on gastrointestinal injuries due to blunt trauma; of 26 patients, 19 had isolated gut injury, 7 with pneumoperitoneum (37%); 8 patients had traumatic intramural hematoma of the duodenum (TIHD) or duodenal perforation; 12 had simple perforations closed; 5 required resection. Lee[86] reported repair of transection of the duodenum with avulsion of the common duct and pancreatic head, with successful outcome. Jones *et al.*[75] reported on the use of a serosal patch for injuries involving the pancreatic head and duodenum, with many variations in 10 cases, 5 for trauma. The patch usually was applied as a Roux-en-Y. A fistula did not develop in any patient, a major contribution to the management of the more complex forms of duodenal injury.

Experience and Results

In our own experience, 89 patients sustained injuries of the gastrointestinal tract (Table 13–5). Sixty-five were due to blunt trauma and 24 to penetrating injuries. Most commonly, these injuries involved the jejunum or ileum (36 patients). In this group, 26 were blunt injuries and 10 penetrating. Of the blunt injuries, perforation of the antimesenteric surface of the small bowel was the most common finding. Such perforations may occur after the most trivial blow or with high-energy bursting injury with involvement of adjacent solid organs. Typical of the first group is the 4-year-old youngster who goes out to play after a noon meal with an overdistended subparietal segment of jejunum. As the result of a slight blow to the midabdomen, unprotected because of inadequate muscle development, the jejunum is ruptured 2 or 3 feet beyond the ligament of Treitz (Fig. 13–19) or the ileum 2–3 feet proximal to the ileocecal valve. Twenty-six ruptures were in this category. In 15 cases, the jejunum was involved and in 11 the ileum. Rupture with loss of continuity occurred twice, once in the proximal jejunum and once in the terminal ileum. In the proximal injury, transection was due to whiplash whereas the distal lesion was due to a shearing crush, with amputation of the ileocecal angle (Fig. 13–20). Both injuries were treated by primary anastomosis, with a satisfactory outcome. The 26 patients with blunt injury to the jejunum and ileum survived. Ten patients had penetrating injuries of the jejunum or ileum equally divided. Nine patients survived and 1 died as a result of gunshot of the midabdomen involving jejunum, colon and liver. On many occasions, antimesenteric rupture of the small bowel was unsuspected but identified in the process of examining the entire gastrointestinal tract as a routine in surgical exploration for blunt abdominal trauma. Associated solid organ injury to the liver, pancreas, spleen or kidney occurred in 50%. Abdominal x-rays are of little value in demonstrating bowel injuries. Pneumoperitoneum was observed in 6 of 36 cases (17%) despite at times extensive injury (Fig. 13–21). In others there was at most an abnormal collection of gas in a sentinel loop, with early obstruction.

Duodenal injury occurred in 8 patients, 6 blunt and 2 penetrating, both knife wounds. Of the 6 blunt injuries with perforation, the most common site of involvement was the

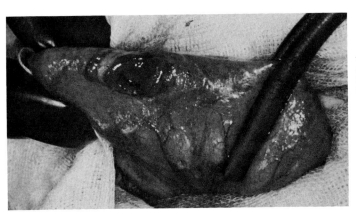

Fig. 13–19.—Traumatic perforation of the jejunum. Such injuries typically involve the antimesenteric surface and present a pouting mucosal layer with no tendency to spontaneous closure. This patient was unconscious for 4 days; laparotomy was performed on the seventh day after injury because of a subhepatic abscess.

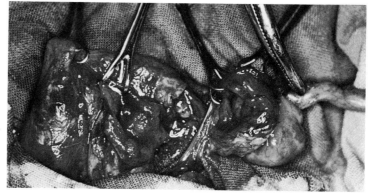

Fig. 13–20.—Avulsed cecum. Such injuries are rare and occur adjacent to fixed points such as the ligament of Treitz and the ileocecal angle.

second portion of the duodenum. In 4 there was associated pancreatic injury; all were treated by primary duodenal repair, 1 with a Thal patch. Pancreatoduodenal resection was not required. One patient was operated on for suspected appendicitis only to find a normal appendix and bile staining of the retroperitoneum.

Stomach injury occurred in 6 patients, 3 blunt and 3 penetrating. All but 1 were repaired successfully by suturing the perforation, in 3 located on the anterior surface, in 2 the posterior surface identified after widely opening the lesser sac. One patient died, a 12-day-old infant who allegedly was dropped.

Colon injury was encountered in 9 patients, in 4 due to blunt trauma, with 1 death. Three of 4 blunt injuries were associated with massive pelvic crush. Patients were treated by proximal colostomy in 2 instances and exteriorization of the perforation in 2. Three of 5 colon perforations due to knife wound were treated by primary repair without colostomy; 2 required proximal colostomy and repair.

Patients with injury to the small bowel mesentery or vessels of the mesenteric axis (13 in our series) are of considerable interest. Of the mesenteric injuries encountered in 10 patients, 8 were due to blunt trauma. Blunt mesenteric injuries tended to be minor, consisted of partial tears or hematomas at the base of the mesentery and generally required ligation of the injured vessel, with evacuation of the hematoma. Avulsion of the mesentery, reported by Penberthy,[120] can be fatal either because of immediate exsanguinating hemorrhage or because of subsequent necrosis and perforation of the devitalized segment. In 3 patients it was necessary to resect a segment of small intestine corresponding to the breach of mesenteric supply. In another, involving a 4-year-old boy, there was avulsion of the mesentery from several feet of ileum, with gangrene and perforation. The injury resulted from a kick to the midabdomen (Fig. 13–22). He died without operation. The condition was discovered at autopsy.

Three patients had an injury to the origin of the celiac artery or superior mesenteric vessels. Direct repair of a mesenteric arterial injury is possible. Ulvestad[159] reported successful repair of a lacerated superior mesenteric artery. We have repaired a lacerated superior mesenteric artery due to blunt injury in 1 patient, a 13-year-old boy.[175] Circulation was satisfactorily restored, with no late clinical or x-ray evidence of bowel ischemia. In addition, the patient suffered a pancreatic transection and jejunal transection 15 cm beyond the ligament of Treitz. The distal pancreas was resected and the jejunal injury repaired by direct anastomosis. One pa-

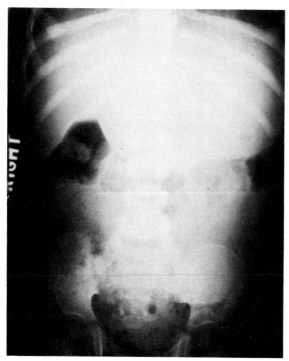

Fig. 13–21.—Blunt rupture of the jejunum. Upright abdominal x-ray film. There is evident pneumoperitoneum in a subhepatic location. The patient required sleeve resection and anastomosis.

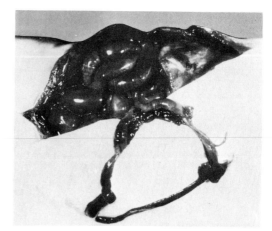

Fig. 13–22.—Avulsion of the small bowel mesentery (ileum) due to assault. This child was kicked in the abdomen and died of hemobilia and gram-negative septicemia, without operation.

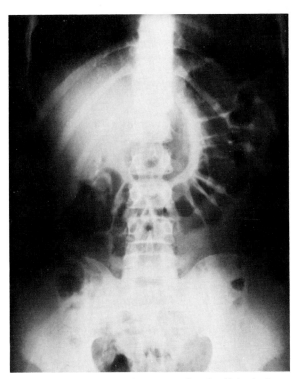

Fig. 13–23.—Division of superior mesenteric vein. Abdominal x-ray film showing a diffuse abnormality of gas pattern in the entire small bowel reminiscent of patients with the mesenteric ischemic syndrome. In this instance, a 9-year-old girl sustained knife injuries of the pancreas and jejunum. The superior mesenteric vein was completely transected at its origin. Repair was unsuccessful. She died ultimately of midgut infarction.

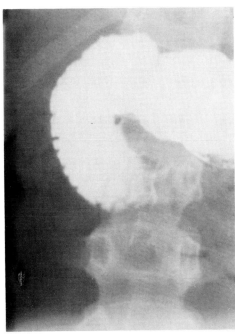

Fig. 13–24.—Traumatic intramural hematoma of the duodenum. Barium study of the stomach and duodenum shows an abrupt cutoff at the third portion of the duodenum as it crosses over the second lumbar vertebra. The obstruction was due to tamponade resulting from the hematoma.

tient had successful repair of a pseudoaneurysm of the celiac artery. Injury to the superior mesenteric vein is far more serious. There are no reports of successful repair, although several attempts have been made. The high failure rate usually is attributed to the low pressure and flow in the portal venous system. Our patient, a 9-year-old girl, the victim of multiple knife wounds of the midabdomen, had complete anatomic transection of the superior mesenteric vein at its root, with associated injuries to the jejunum and pancreas. Vascular repair was attempted but was unsuccessful. The entire midgut infarcted and the patient ultimately died (Fig. 13–23).

Traumatic intramural hematoma of the duodenum (TIHD).—This interesting and unique lesion is encountered most commonly in children as the result of contusion of the retroperitoneal portion of the duodenum, with resulting obstruction. Tamponade obstruction usually occurs in the fixed or retroperitoneal portion of the duodenum, at times extending into the proximal jejunum (Fig. 13–24). The radiographic signs of edema of the second and third portions of the duodenum, with complete or near complete obstruction, a history of trauma and often mild tenderness, make the diagnosis. Mestel *et al.*[103] reported 19 cases from the literature, 16 in children. Three cases were reported previously by Robarts.[127] Dickenson[29] recently has encountered 8 children; 3 were observed and 5 required operation. Holgerson and Bishop[70] reported 9 children; 8 were managed conservatively, with obstruction lasting 8–20 days. We have encountered 20 such patients, 15 reported previously, all due to blunt trauma.[145, 152a, 175] Most commonly, treatment has consisted of laparotomy, identification of the condition, evacua-

tion of clot and meticulous fulguration of bleeding points. The submucosa always is intact and bleeding occurs from bridging vessels between the muscularis and the submucosa (Fig. 13–25). In other cases, the true nature of the situation was not appreciated and some type of bypass was mistakenly performed. Izant[175] first recommended conservative treatment of such injuries; of 4 patients encountered, 3 were observed to spontaneous relief from obstruction in 7–10 days and 1 required operation. Tank *et al.*[152a] encountered 4 cases in children; 1 was observed and 3 required evacuation of a hematoma. Stewart *et al.*[145] treated 1 patient conservatively; 5 required evacuation of a hematoma and 2 had bypass. In our recent experience 2 patients have been managed nonoperatively and 3 required operation. In our total experience with 20 patients, 4 were managed without operation and 14 had evacuation of a hematoma. In 2 early cases, a jejunal bypass was performed. These were later taken down and anatomic continuity restored. Of 71 children with TIHD, 11 had some type of jejunal bypass, 40 had evacuation of a hematoma and 20 were managed nonoperatively (Table 13–6).

It is likely that these hematomas ultimately would be absorbed and patency of the intestinal tract would be restored without operation. To shorten the period of complete duodenal obstruction with its attendant dangers, laparotomy is indicated in most cases. The lesion should be treated by evacuation of the hematoma and hemostasis. One should not perform jejunal bypass or be tempted to resect the grossly deformed and discolored segment. Provided that associated organ injuries do not coexist, a case might be made for observation with sonography for a reasonable period of time, not in excess of 1 week. This must be matched against the danger of aspiration and nutritional depletion resulting from the massive fluid losses that occur with total mid-duodenal obstruction. Laparotomy and proper attention to the lesion seem to be dictated by common sense.

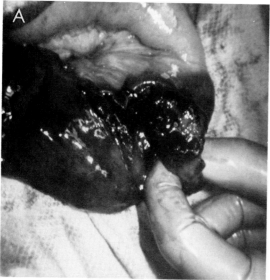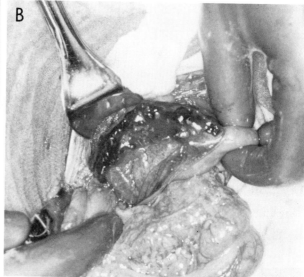

Fig. 13–25.—Traumatic intramural hematoma of the duodenum. **A,** operative photograph showing the hematoma extending into the proximal jejunum. The segment is grossly deformed and discolored. The serosa has been fractured with the finger and the hematoma is being evacuated. It may be liquid or clotted. **B,** evacuation of the hematoma has been completed. Note the entirely healthy appearing submucosa. Multiple small bleeding points are disposed of with pinpoint coagulation. No further treatment is required. The serosa can be lightly reapproximated. Gastrostomy with transduodenal jejunal feeding tube or other bypass procedures are not required.

Conclusions

Eighty-nine children with gastrointestinal injuries have been encountered; 65 were due to blunt trauma and 24 to penetrating injuries. Four died (4.4%). For the most part, these injuries are treated by conventional general surgical techniques. The most troublesome and complex injuries are those involving the duodenum and juxtaposed pancreatic head. No standard rules can be laid down for management. The problem always will be uniquely resolved with considerable innovation and selection from a wide range of operative procedures. Penetrating wounds of the abdomen when due to gunshot always should be explored and knife injuries of the epigastrium must be dealt with promptly if one is to have an opportunity to successfully repair mesenteric and other major vascular injuries. To date, complete transection of the superior mesenteric vein is untreatable. A unique problem resulting from blunt trauma is traumatic intramural hematoma of the duodenum (TIHD). Experience permits ready recognition of the lesion and its appropriate treatment, which, in most instances, will consist of evacuation of the hematoma and nasogastric drainage, with appropriate parenteral support. A prevalent injury, probably more common in children because of relatively poor muscle development, is perforation of the jejunum or ileum following minor local impact. Simple closure of such perforations usually suffices and resections seldom are required. Colonic injuries tend to be in association with penetrating trauma or massive crush injuries of the pelvis and lower abdomen. High-velocity impact injuries are encountered seldom in this age group and seem to be reserved for the adolescent who is injured as an occupant of a moving vehicle rather than as a pedestrian, as is the case with younger children.

TABLE 13–6.—TRAUMATIC INTRAMURAL HEMATOMA OF THE DUODENUM (TIHD) IN CHILDREN

| | YEAR | NO. OF CASES | TREATMENT | | |
			Cons.	E. H.	Bypass
Robarts, F.	1957	3		2	1
Mestel, A.	1959	16		9	7
Welch, K.	1962	3		3	
Izant, R.	1962	4	3	1	
Bailey, W.	1965	5		4	1
Derroede, G.	1966	3		3	
Babbitt, D.	1968	3	2	1	
Stewart (CHMC)	1969	8	1	5	2
Tank, E.	1968	4	1	3	
Dickenson, S.	1970	8	3	5	
Hólgerson, S.	1977	9	8	1	
Welch (CHMC)	1977	5	2	3	
TOTALS		71	20	40	11

Cons. = observation only; E. H. = evacuation of hematoma; Bypass = gastroenterostomy or Enteroenterostomy.

REFERENCES

1. Adwers, J. R., and Davis, W. C.: Adjuvant treatment of blunt pancreatic trauma, Surg. Gynecol. Obstet. 139:514, 1974.
2. Ahmad, W., and Polk, H. C.: Blunt abdominal trauma. A prospective study with selective peritoneal lavage, Arch. Surg. 111:489, 1976.
3. Allen, R. B., and Curry, G. J.: Abdominal trauma. A study of 297 consecutive cases, Am. J. Surg. 93:398, 1957.
4. Anane-Sefah, J.: Operative choice and technique following pancreatic injury, Arch. Surg. 110:161, 1975.
5. Anderson, C. B., *et al.:* Drainage methods for pancreatic injuries, Surg. Gynecol. Obstet. 138:587, 1974.
6. Attiyeh, F. F., McSweeney, J., and Fortner, J. G.: Hemobilia complicating needle liver biopsy. Radiology 118:559, 1976.
7. Awe, W. C., and Eidemiller, L.: Selective angiography in splenic trauma, Am. J. Surg. 126:171, 1973.
8. Bailey, W. C., and Akers, D. R.: Traumatic intramural hematoma of the duodenum in children, Am. J. Surg. 110:695, 1965.
9. Balfanz, J. R., *et al.:* Overwhelming sepsis following splenectomy for trauma, J. Pediatr. 88:458, 1976.
10. Balsano, N. A., and Reynolds, B. N.: Rupture of the common duct and ampulla of Vater due to blunt trauma, Ann. Surg. 178:200, 1973.
11. Belasegaren, M.: Surgical management of pancreatic trauma, Am. J. Surg. 131:536, 1976.
12. Benjamin, C. I.: Delayed rupture or delayed diagnosis of rupture of the spleen, Surg. Gynecol. Obstet. 142:171, 1976.

13. Benson, C. D.: Traumatic injury to the liver, gallbladder and biliary tract, Surg. Clin. North Am. 33:1189, 1953.

14. Berfenstam, R., *et al.:* Accident cases in Stockholm in 1955, Sven. läkartidn. 54:1950, 1957.

15. Berne, C. J., *et al.:* Duodenal "diverticulization" for duodenal and pancreatic injury, Am. J. Surg. 127:503, 1974.

16. Bernhard, W. F.: Feasibility of partial liver resection under hypothermia, N. Engl. J. Med. 253:159, 1955.

16a. Blumenstock, D. A., Mithoefer, J., and Santulli, T. V.: Acute pancreatitis in children, Pediatrics 19:1002, 1957.

17. Boley, S. J., MacKinnon, M. P., and Marpel, J.: Rupture of the spleen in children, Surg. Gynecol. Obstet. 109:78, 1959.

18. Bollinger, J. A., and Fowler, E. F.: Traumatic rupture of the spleen with special reference to delayed splenic rupture, Am. J. Surg. 91:561, 1956.

19. Bowen, J. C., and Fleming, W. H.: Upper gastrointestinal bleeding associated with biliary diversion after hepatic injury, Ann. Surg. 177:402, 1973.

20. Boyd, D. R., *et al.:* Trauma registry: New computer method for multi-factorial evaluation of a major health problem, JAMA 223:422, 1973.

21. Campos Christos, M.: Segmental resection of the spleen, report on first 8 patients operated upon, Hosp. Rio 3:575, 1962.

22. Carroll, C. P., Cass, K. A., and Whelan, T. J.: Wounds of the liver in Vietnam. A critical analysis of 254 cases, Ann. Surg. 177:385, 1973.

23. Coler, R. S.: Postsplenectomy sepsis. A review of the literature and two new cases, Northwest Med. 62:865, 1963.

24. Constantoupoules, A., Najiar, V. A., and Smith, J. W.: Tuftsin deficiency. A new syndrome with defective phagocytosis, J. Pediatr. 80:564, 1972.

25. Cummins, C. E., Grace, A. E. N., and Beardmore, H. E.: Supportive use of total peripheral parenteral alimentation in children with severe pancreatic injuries, J. Pediatr. Surg. 6:961, 1976.

26. Davis, J. J.: Diagnosis and management of blunt abdominal trauma, Ann. Surg. 183:672, 1976.

27. Defore, W. W., Jr.: Management of 1,590 consecutive cases of liver trauma, Arch. Surg. 111:493, 1976.

28. Devroede, G. J., *et al.:* Intramural hematoma of the duodenum and jejunum, Am. J. Surg. 112:947, 1966.

29. Dickenson, S. J., Shaw, A., and Santulli, T. V.: Rupture of the G.I. tract in children by blunt trauma, Surg. Gynecol. Obstet. 130:655, 1970.

30. Dietrich, E. B., *et al.:* Traumatic injuries to the extrahepatic biliary tract, Am. J. Surg. 112:756, 1966.

31. Doletsky, S. Y., Okulov, A. B., and Shpringralda Udris, S.: Laparoscopy in closed injury of the abdomen in children, Khirurgiia 42:112, 1971.

32. Dominion Bureau of Statistics: Death from Selected Causes, 1–14 Years (Ottawa, Canada, 1965).

33. Donovan, A. J., Michaelian, M. J., and Yellin, A. E.: Anatomical hepatic lobectomy in trauma to the liver, Surgery 73:833, 1973.

34. Douglas, G. J., and Simpson, J. S.: The conservative management of splenic trauma, J. Pediatr. Surg. 6:566, 1971.

35. Drezner, A. D.: Decreasing morbidity after liver trauma, Am. J. Surg. 129:483, 1975.

36. Editorial: Liver Injury, Br. Med. J. 3:558, 1975.

37. Egley, C. C.: Laceration of fetal spleen during amniocentesis, Am. J. Obstet. Gynecol. 116:582, 1973.

38. Ekengren, K., and Soderlund, K.: Radiological findings in traumatic lesions of the pancreas in childhood, Ann. Radiol. 9:279, 1966.

39. Ellis, E. F., and Smith, R. T.: The role of the spleen in immunity with special reference to the postsplenectomy problem in infants, Pediatrics 37:111, 1966.

40. Eraklis, A. J., and Filler, R. M.: Splenectomy in childhood. A review of 1413 cases (AAP Survey), J. Pediatr. Surg. 7:382, 1972.

41. Eraklis, A. J., Kevy, S. V., and Diamond, L. K.: Hazards of overwhelming infection after splenectomy in childhood, N. Engl. J. Med. 276:1225, 1967.

42. Erickson, W. D., Busgert, E. O., Jr., and Lynn, H. B.: The hazard of infection in children following splenectomy, Am. J. Dis. Child. 116:1, 1968.

43. Faris, I.: Extrahepatic biliary drainage in experimental liver injury, Br. J. Surg. 59:136, 1972.

44. Faris, I. B., and Dudley, H. A. F.: Closed liver injury: An assessment of prognostic factors, Br. J. Surg. 60:227, 1973.

45. Feix, F., *et al.:* The management of blunt trauma to the abdomen in infancy and childhood, Surg. Clin. North Am. 48:1265, 1968.

46. Finland, M.: Serious infection in splenectomized children, Pediatrics 27:689, 1961.

47. Foster, J. M., and Prey, D.: Rupture of the spleen, Am. J. Surg. 47:487, 1940.

48. Foward, A. D., and Ashmore, P. G.: Infections following splenectomy in infants and children, Can. J. Surg. 3:229, 1960.

49. Fowler, R., and Hiller, H. G.: Selective hepatic arteriography in the management of traumatic hemobilia, J. Pediatr. Surg. 2:253, 1967.

50. Freeark, R. J.: Penetrating wounds of the abdomen, N. Engl. J. Med. 291:185, 1974.

51. Freese, P., Heinrich, P., and Hinze, M.: Care of traumatic liver wounds with acrylic adhesives, Chirurg 36:483, 1965.

52. Fullen, W. D., *et al.:* Sternal splitting approach for major hepatic or retrohepatic vena cava injury, J. Trauma 14:903, 1974.

53. Gazzaniga, A. B.: Laparoscopy in the diagnosis of blunt and penetrating injuries to the abdomen, Am. J. Surg. 131:315, 1976.

54. Giedion, A.: Die geburtstraumatische Rupture parenchymatöser Bauchorgane (Leber, Milz, Nebenniere und Niere) mit massivem Blutverlust und ihre radiologische Darstellung, Helv. Paediatr. Acta 18:349, 1963.

55. Gill, W.: Abdominal lavage in blunt trauma, Br. J. Surg. 62:121, 1975.

56. Goldsmith, N. A., and Woodburne, R. T.: The surgical anatomy pertaining to liver resection, Surg. Gynecol. Obstet. 105:310, 1957.

57. Grosfeld, J. L., and Ranochak, J. E.: Are hemisplenectomy and/or primary splenic repair feasible?, J. Pediatr. Surg. 11:419, 1976.

58. Hakami, M., Mosavy, S. H., and Vakilzadeh, Gh.: Splenosis: A rare complication of trauma to the spleen, Abdom. Surg. 10:15, 1977.

59. Haller, J. A.: Role of the spleen and experimental neonatal infections in transplantation, J. Pediatr. Surg. 5:172, 1970.

60. Haller, J. A., *et al.:* Use of a trauma registry in the management of children with life-threatening injuries, J. Pediatr. Surg. 11:381, 1976.

61. Haller, J. A.: In discussion of Douglas, G. J., and Simpson, J. S.[34]

61a. Haron, M., and Calebetch, J. H.: Splenectomy and subsequent infection, Arch. Dis. Child. 32:398, 1962.

62. Harris, B. H., *et al.:* Radioisotope diagnosis of covert splenic injury. Presented at the Annual Meeting, American Academy of Pediatrics, Chicago, October 18, 1976.

63. Hartman, S. W., and Greaney, E. M.: Traumatic injuries to the biliary system in children, Am. J. Surg. 108:150, 1964.

64. Hendren, W. H., Jr., Greep, J. M., and Patton, A. S.: Pancreatitis in childhood. Experience with 15 cases, Arch. Dis. Child. 40:132, 1965.

65. Hendren, W. H., *et al.:* Traumatic hemobilia: Non-operative management with healing documented by serial angiography, Ann. Surg. 174:991, 1971.

66. Hicken, N. F., and Stevenson, V. L.: Traumatic rupture of the choledochus associated with an acute hemorrhagic pancreatitis, Ann. Surg. 128:1178, 1948.

67. Hicks, J. H.: A case of traumatic perforation of the gallbladder in a child of three years, Br. J. Surg. 31:305, 1944.

68. Hodam, R. P.: The risk of splenectomy, Am. J. Surg. 119:709, 1970.

69. Hoffman, W.: Collective review: Free chyle in the acute abdomen, Surg. Gynecol. Obstet. 98:209, 1954.

70. Holgerson, L. O., and Bishop, H. C.: Nonoperative treatment of duodenal hematomata in children, J. Pediatr. Surg. 12:11, 1977.

71. Hood, J. M., and Smythe, B. T.: Nonpenetrating abdominal injuries in children, J. Pediatr. Surg. 9:69, 1974.

72. Horan, M., and Colebatch, J. H.: Relation between splenectomy and subsequent infection, Arch. Dis. Child. 37:398, 1962.

73. Howard, J. H., *et al.:* Plasma amylase activity in combat casualties, Ann. Surg. 141:338, 1955.

74. Howland, W. S., *et al.:* Physiologic alterations with massive blood replacement, Surg. Gynecol. Obstet. 99:478, 1955.

75. Jones, S. A., Gazzaniga, A. B., and Keller, T. B.: The serosal patch: A surgical parachute, Am. J. Surg. 126:186, 1973.

76. Jones, T. W., Nyhus, L., and Harkins, H. N.: Formalinized polyvinyl alcohol (Ivalon) sponge in repair of liver wounds, Arch. Surg. 76:583, 1958.

77. Jordan, G. L., Jr.: Conservatism in the management of abdominal trauma, Am. J. Surg. 126:581, 1973.

78. Kakos, G. S., Grosfeld, J. L., and Morse, T. S.: Small bowel injuries in children after blunt abdominal trauma, Ann. Surg. 174:238, 1971.

79. Kaufer, C., and Wulfing, D.: Darmverletzungen bei Kindern als Folge stumpfer Bauchtraumen, Z. Kindechir. 6:55, 1968.

80. Kaufman, J. M., and Burrington, J. D.: Liver trauma in children, J. Pediatr. Surg. 6:586, 1971.

81. Kiesewetter, W. B., and Patrick, D. B.: Childhood splenectomy. Indications for and results from, Am. Surg. 37:135, 1971.

82. King, H., and Schumacher, H. B., Jr.: Susceptibility to infection after splenectomy in infants, Am. Surg. 36:239, 1952.

83. King, H., and Schumacher, H. B., Jr.: Susceptibility to infection after splenectomy performed in infancy, Ann. Surg. 136:239, 1955.

84. Kinnaird, D. W.: Pancreatic injuries due to nonpenetrating abdominal trauma, Am. J. Surg. 91:552, 1956.

85. Lauer, B., Broeck, E. T., and Grossman, M.: Battered child syndrome: Review of 130 patients with controls, Pediatrics 54:67, 1974.

86. Lee, D.: Primary repair in transection of duodenum with avulsion of the common duct, Arch. Surg. 111:592, 1976.

87. Levey, J. L., Jr., and Luder, L. H.: Major abdominal trauma in children, Am. J. Surg. 120:55, 1970.

88. Levin, D. C., et al.: Angiography in blunt hepatic trauma, Am. J. Roentgenol. 119:95, 1973.

89. Longmire, W. P., Jr., and McArthur, M. S.: Occult injuries of the liver, bile duct, and pancreas after blunt abdominal trauma, Am. J. Surg. 125:661, 1973.

90. Lortat-Jacob, U. L., and Roberts, L. G.: Hepatectomie droite réglée, Presse Med. 60:549, 1952.

91. Lucas, C. E., and Ledgerwood, A. M.: Controlled biliary drainage for large injuries of the liver, Surg. Gynecol. Obstet. 137:585, 1973.

92. Lucas, C. E., and Walt, A. J.: Critical decisions in liver trauma, Arch. Surg. 101:277, 1970.

93. Lutzker, L., et al.: The role of radionuclide imaging in spleen trauma, Radiology 110:419, 1974.

94. Madding, G. F., and Kennedy, P. A.: *Trauma to the Liver* (Philadelphia: W. B. Saunders Company, 1971).

95. Maron, B. J., and Maloney, J. R.: Septicemia following traumatic or incidental splenectomy, Johns Hopkins Med. J. 130:366, 1972.

96. Mays, E. T.: Hepatic trauma, N. Engl. J. Med. 288:402, 1973.

97. Mays, E. T.: Lobar dearterialization for exsanguinating wounds of the liver, J. Trauma 12:397, 1972.

98. Mays, E. T.: Hepatic Trauma, in *Current Problems in Surgery* (Chicago: Year Book Medical Publishers, Inc., November, 1976).

99. Mazel, M. S.: Traumatic rupture of the spleen, J. Pediatr. 28:82, 1945.

100. McDermott, W. V., Jr., and Ottinger, L. W.: Elective hepatic resection, Am. J. Surg. 112:376, 1966.

101. McGehee, R. N., et al.: Traumatic hemobilia, Ann. Surg. 179:311, 1974.

102. Mercadier, M. P., Clot, J. P., and Cady, J. P.: Right hepatectomy in the treatment of liver trauma, Am. J. Surg. 124:353, 1972.

103. Mestel, A. L., et al.: Acute obstruction of small intestine secondary to hematoma in children, Arch. Surg. 78:25, 1959.

104. Mikeskey, W. E., Howard, J. M., and DeBakey, M. E.: Collective review: Injuries of the liver in 300 consecutive patients, Surg. Gynecol. Obstet. 103:323, 1956.

105. Miller, D. R.: Sternotomy extension of abdominal incision for hepatic lobectomy, Ann. Surg. 175:193, 1972.

106. Miller, D. W., Jr., and Kelly, D. L.: Splenic trauma: Surgical management in children, Arch. Surg. 105:561, 1972.

107. Mishalny, H.: Repair of the ruptured spleen, J. Pediatr. Surg. 9:175, 1974.

108. Moretz, J. A., et al.: Significance of serum amylase level in evaluating pancreatic trauma, Am. J. Surg. 130:739, 1975.

109. Morton, C. E., Holcomb, G. W., and Foster, J. H.: Major hepatic resections in children, J. Pediatr. Surg. 10:195, 1975.

110. Morton, J. R., Roys, G. C., and Bricker, D. L.: The treatment of liver injuries, Surg. Gynecol. Obstet. 134:298, 1972.

111. Nahum, H., and Levesque, M.: Arteriography in hepatic trauma, Radiology 109:557, 1973.

112. Nance, F. C., et al.: Surgical judgment in the management of penetrating wounds of the abdomen: Experience with 2212 patients, Ann. Surg. 179:639, 1974.

113. Nardi, G. L., and Lees, C. W.: A new diagnostic test for pancreatic disease, N. Engl. J. Med. 258:797, 1958.

114. Nebesar, R. A., Rabinov, K. R., and Potsaid, M. S.: Radionuclide imaging of the spleen in suspected splenic injury, Radiology 110:609, 1974.

115. Olsen, W. R.: The serum amylase in blunt abdominal trauma, J. Trauma 13:200, 1973.

116. Olsen, W. R., Redman, D. H., and Hildreth, D. H.: Quantitative peritoneal lavage in blunt abdominal trauma, Arch. Surg. 104:536, 1972.

117. Orlando, J. C., and Moore, T. C.: Splenectomy for trauma in childhood, Surg. Gynecol. Obstet. 134:94, 1972.

118. Parrin, S., et al.: Effectiveness of peritoneal lavage in blunt abdominal trauma, Am. J. Surg. 181:255, 1975.

119. Pedersen, B., and Vidibach, A.: On the late effects of removal of the normal spleen, Acta Chir. Scand. 131:89, 1966.

120. Penberthy, G. C.: Avulsion of mesentery with adjacent necrosis, Surg. Clin. North Am. 33:1179, 1953.

121. Perry, J.: In discussion of Tank, E., et al.[152a]

122. Popovsky, J., et al.: Liver Trauma: Conservative management and the liver scan, Arch. Surg. 108:184, 1974.

122a. Powell, R. W., et al.: Peritoneal lavage in children with blunt abdominal trauma, J. Pediatr. Surg. 6:973, 1976.

123. Pringle, J.: Notes on the arrest of hepatic hemorrhage due to trauma, Ann. Surg. 48:541, 1908.

124. Quattlebaum, J. K., and Quattlebaum, J. K., Jr.: Technique of hepatic lobectomy. Ann. Surg. 149:648, 1959.

125. Richardson, J. D., Belin, R. P., and Griffen, W. O., Jr.: Blunt abdominal trauma in children, Ann. Surg. 176:213, 1972.

126. Richie, J. P., and Fonkalsrud, E. W.: Subcapsular hematoma of the liver, Arch. Surg. 104:781, 1972.

127. Robarts, F. H.: Traumatic intramural haematoma of the proximal jejunal loop. Presented at the Annual Meeting, British Association of Pediatric Surgeons, Edinburgh, 1957.

128. Robinson, T. W., and Sturgeon, P.: Post splenectomy infection in children, Pediatrics 25:941, 1960.

129. Root, H. D., et al.: Diagnostic peritoneal lavage, Surgery 57:633, 1965.

129a. Rosello, P., and Eraklis, A. J.: Conservative management of splenic rupture. Presented at the Annual Meeting, American Pediatric Surgery Society, Boca Raton, Fla., April, 1976.

130. Sandblom, P. H.: *Hemobilia* (Springfield, Ill.: Charles C Thomas, Publisher, 1972).

131. Sandblom, P.: Hemorrhage into the biliary tract following trauma: "Traumatic hemobilia," Surgery 24:571, 1948.

132. Sano, M. E., and Holland, C.: Coagulum technique in traumatic rupture of the liver in dogs, Science 98:524, 1943.

133. Schrock, T., Blaisdell, W., and Matthewson, C.: Management of blunt trauma to the liver and hepatic veins, Arch. Surg. 96:698, 1968.

134. Shirkey, A. L., et al.: Surgical management of splenic injuries, Am. J. Surg. 108:630, 1964.

135. Shohl, T.: Hepatic artery ligation for massive hemobilia, Surgery 56:855, 1964.

136. Sieber, W. K., and Girdany, B. R.: Rupture of the spleen in newborn infants, N. Engl. J. Med. 259:1074, 1959.

137. Sinclair, M. C., and Moore, T. C.: Abdominal and thoracic trauma in childhood and adolescence, J. Pediatr. Surg. 9:155, 1974.

138. Singer, D. B.: Postsplenectomy Sepsis, in Rosenberg, H. J., and Bolande, R. P. (eds.), *Perspectives in Pediatric Pathology* (Chicago: Year Book Medical Publishers, Inc., 1973), Vol. 1, pp. 285–311.

139. Sokol, D. M., Thompkins, D., and Izant, R. J.: Rupture of the spleen and liver in newborn, J. Pediatr. Surg. 9:227, 1974.

140. Spector, N.: Ligation of the right hepatic artery in hemobilia: Report of a case with recovery, Ann. Surg. 145:244, 1957.

141. Srouji, M. N., Williams, M. L., and Werner, J. H.: Neonatal rupture of the liver, use of exchange transfusions, J. Pediatr. Surg. 6:56, 1971.

142. Stalowsky, H. J.: Stumpfes Bauchtrauma und Darmruptur in Kindesalter, Chirurg 36:4, 1965.

143. Steele, M., and Lim, R. C.: Advances in management of splenic injuries, Am. J. Surg. 130:159, 1975.

144. Steele, M., Sheldon, G. F., and Blaisdell, F. W.: Pancreatic injuries. Methods of management, Arch. Surg. 106:544, 1973.

145. Stewart, D. R., Byrd, C. L., and Schuster, S. R.: Intramural hematomas of the alimentary tract in children, Surgery 68:550, 1970.

146. Stone, H. H.: Major hepatic resections in children, J. Pediatr. Surg. 10:127, 1975.

147. Stone, H. H.: Pancreatic and duodenal trauma in children, J. Pediatr. Surg. 7:670, 1972.

148. Stone, H. H., and Ansley, J. D.: Management of liver trauma in children, J. Pediatr. Surg. 12:3, 1977.

149. Stormo, A. C.: Traumatic chylous ascites, Arch. Surg. 92:115, 1966.

150. Stranch, G. O.: Lethal pneumococcal septicemia following splenic transposition for Chiari's disease, J. Pediatr. Surg. 8:63, 1973.

151. Strum, J. T., *et al.*: Patterns of injury requiring pancreatoduodenectomy, Surg. Gynecol. Obstet. 137:629, 1973.
151a. Sulamaa, M., and Vitanen, I.: Treatment of pancreatic rupture, Arch. Dis. Child. 39:187, 1964.
152. Suson, E. M., Clats, D., and Kottmeier, P. K.: Liver trauma in children, J. Pediatr. Surg. 10:411, 1975.
152a. Tank, E., Eraklis, A. J., and Gross, R. E.: Blunt abdominal trauma in infancy and childhood, J. Trauma 8:439, 1968.
153. Thal, A. P., and Wilson, R. F.: A pattern of severe blunt trauma to the region of the pancreas, Surg. Gynecol. Obstet. 119:773, 1964.
154. Thal, E. R., and Shires, G. T.: Peritoneal lavage in blunt abdominal trauma, Am. J. Surg. 125:64, 1973.
155. Thavendran, A.: Selective surgery for abdominal stab wounds, Br. J. Surg. 62:750, 1975.
156. Tostivint, T., *et al.*: Plaidoyer pour la laparoscopie dans les traumatismes abdominaux fermées, J. Chir. (Paris) 102:77, 1971.
157. Touloukian, R. J.: Abdominal trauma in childhood, Surg. Gynecol. Obstet. 127:561, 1968.
158. Trunkey, D. D., Shires, G. T., and McClelland, R.: Management of liver trauma in 811 consecutive patients, Ann. Surg. 179:722, 1974.
159. Ulvestad, L. E.: Repair of laceration of superior mesenteric artery acquired by nonpenetrating injury of the abdomen, Ann. Surg. 140:752, 1954.
160. Upadhyaya, P., Nayak, N. C., and Moitra, S.: Experimental study of splenic trauma in monkeys, J. Pediatr. Surg. 6:767, 1971.
161. Upadhyaya, P., and Simpson, J. S.: Splenic trauma in children, Surg. Gynecol. Obstet. 126:781, 1968.
162. Vallidis, E.: Traumatic haemobilia, Br. J. Surg. 62:234, 1975.
163. Van Wagoner, F. H.: Died in hospital. A three-year study of deaths following trauma, J. Trauma 1:401, 1961.
164. Velcek, F. T., *et al.*: Traumatic death in urban children. Presented at the Annual Meeting, American Academy of Pediatrics, Chicago, October 18, 1976.
165. Villarreal-Rios, A., and Mays, E. T.: Efficacy of clinical evaluation and selective splenic arteriography in splenic trauma, Am. J. Surg. 127:310, 1974.
166. Vital Statistics of the United States, 1974.
167. Vollman, R. W., Keenan, W. J., and Eraklis, A. J.: Post-traumatic chylous ascites in infancy, N. Engl. J. Med. 275:875, 1966.
168. Wang, C. C., and Robbins, L. L.: Roentgenologic diagnosis of ruptured spleen, N. Engl. J. Med. 254:445, 1956.
169. Wangensteen, O.: *Cancer of Esophagus and Stomach* (New York: American Cancer Society, Inc., 1951).
170. Warren, K. W., and Wagner, R. B.: Long-term results of nonpenetrating pancreatic trauma, Lahey Clin. Bull. 16:218, 1967.
171. Waugh, G. E.: Traumatic rupture of the common bile duct in a boy six years old, Br. J. Surg. 3:685, 1916.
172. Welch, C. S., *et al.*: Is conservative care of minor splenic injury feasible? (Forum), Mod. Med. 41:96, 1973.
173. Welch, K. J.: Traumatic pancreatitis in childhood, Newton-Wellesley Med. Bull. 11:22, 1959.
174. Welch, Kenneth J.: Right hepatic lobectomy for blunt trauma with adjunct hypothermia (nonpenetrating abdominal injuries in children). Presented at the Annual Meeting, American Association for the Surgery of Trauma, San Diego, Calif., October 5, 1960.
175. Welch, Kenneth J.: Abdominal and Thoracic Injuries, in Mustard, W. T., *et al.* (eds.), *Pediatric Surgery* (2d ed.; Chicago: Year Book Medical Publishers, Inc. 1969), Vol. 1, pp. 708–731.
176. White, P. H., and Benfield, J. R.: Amylase in the management of pancreatic trauma, Arch. Surg. 105:158, 1972.
177. Widmann, W. D., and Laubscher, F. A.: Splenosis: A disease or a beneficial condition? Arch. Surg. 102:152, 1971.
178. Yellin, A. E.: Pancreatoduodenectomy for combined pancreatoduodenal injuries, Arch. Surg. 110:1177, 1975.
179. Yellin, A. E., Vecchione, T. R., and Donovan, A. J.: Distal pancreatectomy for pancreatic trauma, Am. J. Surg. 124:135, 1972.
180. Żachary, R. B., and Emery, J. L.: Abdominal splenosis following rupture of the spleen in a boy aged 10 years, Br. J. Surg. 46:415, 1959.

14 Lyle J. Micheli

Musculoskeletal Injuries

THE BASIC PRINCIPLES OF orthopedic trauma management in children will be outlined, particularly as related to the coordination of management of the multiply injured child. The details of attaining and maintaining reduction of specific fractures are to be found in recent texts dealing with fractures in children.[2, 10, 11, 16]

The Clinical Setting: Epidemiology of Injury

The patterns of trauma in general, and trauma to children in particular, have cultural and social determinants that make it imperative that the physician, surgeon or public safety officer who is concerned with the management and, in particular, with the prevention of trauma have a complete understanding of the clinical setting of injury. Such injuries as sideswipe injury of the elbow, wringer injury of the arm and cart spoke fracture dislocation of the ankle are seen rarely now, and in their place are seen such injuries as Little League elbow, power lawn mower injuries and seat belt fractures of the spine.

Owing to advances in the prevention and treatment of congenital, metabolic and infectious disease in children, trauma has increased in importance as a cause of concern for the pediatric physician. Trauma now is the leading cause of death in children, and an increasing proportion of pediatric morbidity is due to trauma.

A recent trend in pediatric trauma has been the increasing number of children sustaining injury from motorized vehicles, including automobiles, snowmobiles, trail bikes, drivable power lawn mowers, etc., with a resultant increase in severity of injury and the need for a comprehensive multidisciplinary evaluation of the injured child.

Another trend is the increasing participation of children in organized competitive athletics rather than free play activities. Factors in this trend include an increased emphasis on athletic excellence at an early age, limited facilities for spontaneous recreation and well-meaning but misguided parental enthusiasm. There now is evidence that this increase in organized competitive athletics has increased the incidence of serious injury in this age group.[8]

Both of these trends present us with the opportunity of decreasing the incidence and severity of childhood injuries if studies of the epidemiology and mechanism of injury in these settings are carried out and then acted on. This is particularly true of organized sports injuries. Athletic competition is by its very nature a structured activity in which the rate or severity of injury can be directly affected by changes in the rules of the game, techniques of coaching and officiating and alteration in the design of protective or competitive equipment.

The relative incidence and severity of neonatal fractures and birth trauma appear to be decreasing, doubtless reflecting increased awareness and improved obstetric techniques.[5] Recently there has been an increased awareness, and perhaps increased incidence, of injuries to children from direct abuse or negligence, frequently dubbed "The Battered Child Syndrome," or trauma X. The combination of multiple fractures at varied stages of healing, subdural hematoma, failure to thrive and skin bruising usually are diagnostic.[14]

Types of Extremity Injuries in Children

Just as with adults, extremity trauma in children can run the full gamut from simple contusion of soft tissue and muscle, or strain of the musculotendinous units, through sprain of the ligamentous supports of the joints, dislocation of the articulating bones of a joint or fracture of the long bone of the extremity, with possible associated major neurologic or vascular damage. The pattern of injuries seen in children who have sustained extremity injuries differs from that seen in adults. The type of injury sustained by a child from a given trauma depends on the relative age and stage of development of the child at the time of injury. As an example, extremity injuries in the neonatal infant often result in a separation of the largely cartilaginous end of the long bone from the shaft of the bone rather than joint injury or fracture of the shaft because an infant's ligaments are stronger than adjacent bone and epiphyseal plate. These injuries can present problems in initial diagnosis because of the absence of radiographic abnormalities despite extensive swelling, deformity and lack of the use of the extremity. On occasion, the instillation of contrast material such as Renografin 60 into the joint as an arthrogram has been helpful to assess alignment of the joint. Usually, however, simple traction to align the extremity without deformity has been satisfactory. Subsequent follow-up reveals the early and rapid appearance of extensive bony callus, with early clinical stabilization of the injury. In the older child, extremity trauma frequently will result in fractures of the shaft of the long bone, and joint injury or dislocation is relatively rare. Finally, in the preadolescent or adolescent child, and particularly the child who has toughened his bones and ligamentous structures by athletic training, extremity injuries frequently result in fractures through the epiphyseal plate or growth plate near the end of the long bones rather than in joint injuries or shaft fractures, and a high index of suspicion must be maintained in order to detect these injuries.

Epiphyseal plate, or growth plate, fractures are, of course, peculiar to the child. The growth plate consists of a somewhat irregular cartilaginous disk located near either end of the long bones between the epiphysis and metaphysis of the bone and is responsible for the longitudinal growth of the bone (Fig. 14–1). Its microanatomy consists of multiple columns of cartilage cells in various stages of transformation from immature cells on the one end to degenerated rem-

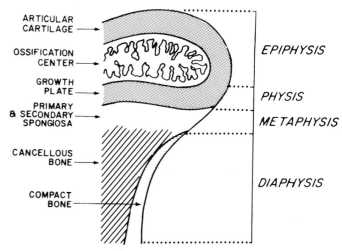

Fig. 14–1.—Growth plate.

nants of cells at the other end of the column, which form the latticework for the new bone formation taking place in the shaft. This rather intricate structure is less resistant to deforming force applied to the extremity than either the ligaments of the joints or the bony cortex in the shafts of the long bones, and mechanical disruption of the child's bone frequently occurs through the substance of the growth plate itself. In the event that portions of the germinal cell layer of the plate are destroyed by the injury, or that the subsequent alignment of the fractured growth plate fragments is such that columns of healing bone form across portions of the plate, subsequent growth of the bone may be affected. Loss of limb length, angular deformity or joint incongruity are the frequent sequelae of growth plate injury.[1] It is this concern for the potential complications of growth plate fracture in the child that has caused many medical observers to question the advisability of participation in heavy contact sports before growth has been completed.

The potential for problems following epiphyseal fracture depends on both the extent of growth plate damage and the specific growth plate involved. As an example of the latter, fractures involving the growth plate of the proximal humerus rarely result in subsequent growth or joint complication whereas fractures of the distal femoral growth plate have a high incidence of subsequent problems. In 1963, Salter and Harris[12] classified epiphyseal injuries into 5 types, with the relative potential for growth plate damage and future growth problems increasing from type 1 to type 5. This classification is the one used most frequently today to describe and classify growth plate injuries (Fig. 14–2).

Type 1. The fracture line extends transversely across the entire growth plate, probably through the layer of calcified cartilage cells, and nowhere passes across the germinal cells of the plate.

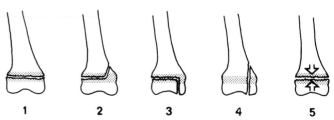

Fig. 14–2.—The Salter-Harris classification of epiphyseal fractures.

Type 2. The fracture line passes partly along the growth plate transversely but then passes into the metaphysis longitudinally and includes a metaphyseal fragment of bone that is attached to the remaining intact growth plate.

Type 3. The fracture line passes transversely across a portion of the growth plate and then passes longitudinally across the proliferating cell layer of the growth plate and epiphysis into the joint. Anatomic reduction and internal fixation are required, since this is an articular fracture. Growth plate injury is seen relatively frequently.

Type 4. The fracture line passes longitudinally across the growth plate from the metaphysis to epiphysis, with the potential for longitudinal bony bridging and joint incongruity unless exact anatomic realignment is attained and held.

Type 5. This epiphyseal injury is diagnosed retrospectively when growth in a portion or all of a given growth plate fails to occur following injury. This injury is believed to be due to an excessive compression force being applied across the growth plate, with resultant death in the germinal cell layer of the plate.

Certain other fractures are seen in children with relative frequency. Pathologic fractures are defined as fractures that occur through bone of abnormal composition. Any fracture following trivial injury must be suspect. A number of conditions in children can cause generalized or localized alteration of bone structure and relative weakening of the bone. Osteogenesis imperfecta is a congenital disease of altered collagen structure in which there is relative weakness of bone and connective tissue. Multiple fractures, sometimes in utero, are seen following minimal trauma. These fractures are best managed by techniques that minimize immobilization and restore motion rapidly. Internal fixation with intramedullary rods of these deformed and fractured bones rather than external plaster immobilization has allowed early motion and ambulation, with an over-all decrease in the incidence of fractures and duration of disability in these children.[15]

Cystic lesions of the long bone, due to such processes as unicameral bone cyst, eosinophilic granuloma, cartilaginous tumors, etc., can be a site of fracture of the long bones. Attention to bony detail at the site of all fractures is necessary, and consultation with the possibility of biopsy should be sought in any questionable lesion.

Special Considerations: Injuries in Children

The rate of healing of injured tissue in children is accelerated, with the most rapid rate of healing seen in the neonate, and a progressive decrease in this capacity noted thereafter, until, in the older teen-ager, the healing rate following injury is similar to that seen in the adult. Nonunion is relatively rare in children's fractures, and, when seen, usually is the result of attempted open reduction.

In addition, dramatic realignment of fracture fragments often is seen in children because of the remodeling of bony architecture possible in the child. This remodeling is due to both the growth plate, which tends to lay down new bone in line with the axis of the limb as a whole, and direct remodeling of bony architecture at the site of the deformity itself, with bone deposition on the concavity of the deformity and bone resorption in the convexity (Fig. 14–3).

It follows that the capacity for remodeling will be greatest in younger children with at least 2 more years of growth remaining and in fractures near the ends of long bones, in close proximity to the growth plate. In addition, the greatest remodeling occurs in deformities in the plane of motion of the joint nearest to the fracture. Remodeling is relatively less effective in correcting angulation out of the plane of motion of the joint, particularly near the midshaft region of the long bones, and, of course, will never connect rotational malalignment or displacement of the joint surfaces in an intra-articular fracture. Exact realignment of fracture fragments, in addition to being unnecessary in certain situations because of this capacity for remodeling, may be contraindicated in others. It has been shown that in fractures of the shaft of the femur, the bony healing causes stimulation of the rate of growth of the femoral plates, with 1 cm or more of permanent leg length increase possible in the young child. An overlap of fracture fragments of 1 cm has been recommended in these fractures.[7]

In children, permanent joint stiffness due to immobilization alone is seen rarely whereas joint stiffness following extended plaster immobilization is a real concern in the management of adult fractures.

For these reasons, open reduction and internal fixation are required less frequently to attain a satisfactory result in children's fractures. Manipulation to attain reduction, and external immobilization or traction to maintain reduction, even for prolonged periods, generally are sufficient to manage children's fractures. Open reduction is required to attain realignment of intra-articular fractures or to reduce and fix certain other fractures, such as displaced fractures of the femoral neck, where the potential for remodeling is minimal and there is a hazard of avascular necrosis if early exact realignment and fixation are not attained.

An exact understanding of the conditions under which

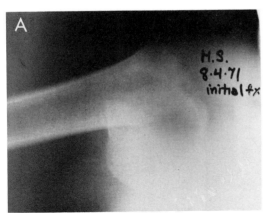
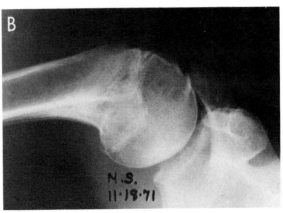

Fig. 14–3.—Remodeling in childhood fractures. **A,** initial alignment of fracture of the proximal humerus in a 12-year-old child. No reduction performed. **B,** alignment 3 months later, with remodeling evident.

remodeling will be effective in correcting deformity is necessary in order to manage children's fractures, and a vague impression that remodeling "probably" will make right a malaligned fracture in a child is never sufficient reason to avoid proper manipulative reduction or even open reduction and fixation, if necessary.[10]

In recent years, disproportionate emphasis has been placed on the capacity for remodeling of children's fractures, with the result that too often malaligned fractures have been accepted without proper reduction or immobilization and without subsequent improvement by remodeling.

Injuries of Special Concern

It is beyond the scope of this chapter systematically to discuss children's fractures, and the reader is referred to textbooks of children's fractures for further reference.[2, 10, 16] I will discuss a number of trauma situations in which the injuries sustained are seen frequently by pediatric surgeons in the course of managing the multiply injured patient or when called on to deal with the complications of orthopedic injuries or procedures.

Initial management of extremity injuries in the multiply injured child is straightforward and relatively simple, but, unfortunately, errors frequently occur at this stage of management. The neurovascular status of the extremity and whether open injuries of the bones or joints are present must be determined immediately. A tiny cut from within the skin outward caused by the end of a fracture fragment can have serious results if unrecognized and the fracture site becomes infected. On at least two occasions we have seen gas gangrene with subsequent loss of an extremity result from an unappreciated open fracture.

Absent extremity pulses require thorough assessment to determine whether they reflect generalized hypovolemia or an extremity injury. It must be remembered that dislocations of the shoulder, elbow, hip or knee may cause serious vascular injury but be inapparent radiographically if they have undergone reduction spontaneously or in the course of manipulation while the patient is en route to the hospital. Ultrasonography using the Doppler technique has proved to be useful in certain cases in which peripheral pulses were not palpable initially.

Having completed the initial assessment, proper splinting of each potentially injured extremity is carried out before sending the child for a radiograph or while further evaluation of the neurologic, cardiothoracic or abdominal status is being carried out. The newer pneumatic splints provide excellent immobilization of most arm, knee and lower leg injuries. In addition, swelling is reduced while the low pressure splint is in place. In injuries about the elbow and in severely displaced forearm fractures, pneumatic splints should be used only if their relative straightening effect on the extremity will not cause excessive pain or increase the potential for neurovascular injury. If there is doubt, it is better to splint the extremity in the position of deformity until consultation is obtained. Rapid splinting of a deformed arm can be carried out with a longitudinal splint of 6–8 layers of 3″ or 4″ plaster of Paris padded with webril or sheet wadding and held in place by loosely applied elastic bandages. In the conscious child who is able to sit, simple immobilization generally is sufficient for injuries of the shoulder or upper arm.

Hip and thigh injuries, including proximal fractures of the femur, often cannot be immobilized properly using a pneumatic splint. A Thomas splint or a Keller-Blake splint with half ring is required to immobilize the extremity and provide stabilizing traction.

Open fracture and joint injuries in children are a subject of special concern because of the increased incidence of these injuries in recent years and the serious consequences attendant on inappropriate treatment. They require immediate attention if proper cleansing of the wound is to be attained and infection avoided.

Initial management should include washing the surrounding skin and wound margins with sterile saline or Betadine soap to remove gross contaminants and then covering the exposed wound and tissue with Betadine-soaked sponges and sterile gauze prior to splinting. As soon as the patient's general condition permits, and preferably within 6 hours of injury, proper cleansing of the wound and alignment of the fracture should be carried out in a sterile environment with appropriate anesthesia. Multiple cultures of the wound are obtained. An initial culture of the uncleansed wound is sent for aerobic and anaerobic bacterial culture. The wound then is alternately lavaged with normal saline and Betadine solution. We prefer an external saline irrigation setup. After gross clot and debris have been removed, nonviable subcutaneous tissue, fascia and muscle are debrided by sharp dissection. The initial debridement should remove all obviously nonviable tissue, but tissue of questionable viability should be preserved until a second debridement 24 hours later, if necessary. The Water Pic system can be useful if there are multiple small fragments or road debris embedded in the wound. Debridement is done without tourniquet to facilitate the differentiation of viable from nonviable tissue. An elastic Esmarch bandage is available to apply proximal to the debridement site if uncontrolled or excessive bleeding occurs in the process of debridement. Bone fragments that are contaminated or have lost soft tissue attachments are removed from the wound, but longer fragments, which are essential to maintain stability, may be left in place initially if they are free from contamination and in a viable soft tissue bed. Following initial debridement and lavage, a second set of cultures is obtained and intravenous antibiotic treatment is begun. At present, we prefer cephalothin or a combination of oxacillin and gentamicin, depending on the extent of contamination. Intravenous antibiotics are continued for at least 48 hours, or until final wound closure. The results of initial culture may dictate a change of antibiotics in 48 hours.

Only after wound cleansing and debridement have been performed are attempts made to realign the fracture. If the fracture is stable following reduction, simple plaster immobilization, with an appropriate window cut in the plaster to facilitate wound care, may be all that is required. In fractures of the femur or humerus, postoperative immobilization with skeletal traction through the tibia or olecranon often is satisfactory.

In injuries where there is extensive soft tissue loss, particularly those involving circumferential wound care, or in cases where the injured child is uncooperative or agitated, several newer apparatus have been used effectively to maintain proper alignment and stabilization of the extremity while facilitating wound care, including complete immersion of the extremity in a Hubbard tank or whirlpool baths. Presently, we are using two systems in this fashion: The Wagner apparatus, primarily designed as an instrument for leg lengthening, and the Hoffman apparatus, both of which provide external skeletal fixation using transcutaneous pins placed above and below the fracture site and connected by carefully engineered external frames that provide three-dimensional stabilization and have the capacity for subsequent alteration of fragment position or alignment in a measured fashion (Fig. 14–4).

These external fixation devices provide sufficient stability to maintain extremity alignment despite segmental bone loss in an extremity, and can be used to provide stabilization across a joint such as the elbow when extensive comminution is present.

Closure of deep fascia is unnecessary following fracture debridement and is contraindicated in the lower leg or forearm, to avoid the possibility of fascial swelling, compression and neurovascular compromise. Wound closure in open fractures is unnecessary and offers no clear advantages in most cases, particularly in view of the serious and even life-threatening complications of primary wound closure. We do prefer soft tissue coverage over tendons and ligaments, as they have poor tolerance for direct exposure to air or dressings. Pedicle flaps are used to attain skin coverage over them and the wound is opened in another site.

No wound should be closed at any stage of care if the margins do not come together easily and without tension. Forced closure almost invariably is disastrous, particularly in the forearm, lower leg or foot. Better to have to deal with the possibility of a delayed split-thickness skin graft or flap coverage of a skin defect rather than take the risk of wound slough, neurovascular compromise, deep infection or gas gangrene. This is particularly important in degloving or partial avulsion of an extremity, where portions of skin and subcutaneous tissue have been separated from underlying fascia. Attempts to "tack" these margins back into place almost invariably result in further skin loss.

Open injuries of joints require opening, lavage and debridement. Gas in the initial radiography may be the only indication of an unsuspected puncture wound. Careful inspection of the open joint must be carried out at the time of debridement to detect foreign bodies that are not evident radiographically. On at least two occasions we have discovered unexpected fragments of wood or plastic in such joints. If adequate sharp debridement of the wound edge is possible, the wound margins are closed and the drainage of the joint carried out for a period of 48 hours using Penrose or Memovac drainage, along with systematic antibiotics and appropriate immobilization.

Injuries about the elbow in children are a cause of special concern because of the frequent difficulty in primary treatment of these injuries and the serious complications that can occur in the course of treatment.

In particular, supracondylar fractures of the elbow are a major concern. These are the most frequent fractures about the elbow. The fracture line generally lies immediately proximal to the condyle and passes through the olecranon fossa. Usually there is posterior and medial displacement of the distal fragment. It is imperative to have a child with this injury anesthetized and the fracture reduced as rapidly as possible, for the development of swelling about the elbow prior to reduction is doubly detrimental—not only does it render it difficult to flex the elbow beyond 90 degrees, essential to both attain and maintain reduction, but it also increases the possibility of subsequent neurologic and vascular complications.

Initial assessment of neurologic and vascular status is essential, as the incidence of traumatic neuropathy of radial, ulnar or median nerves at the time of initial evaluation is high (8–20% in reported series). Initial vascular compromise can be seen but, in addition, initial detection of radial and ulnar pulses and subsequent loss in the course of management is an important sign of impending ischemia (Fig. 14–5).

Vascular compromise of the arm following elbow fracture is one of the most feared complications in the management of children's fractures. The absence of the radial pulse alone does not indicate ischemia, but the loss of a pre-existent pulse along with pain in the hand, pallor of fingers or paralysis of the extremity and intrinsic muscles of the hand are definite signs of impending ischemia. Pain elicited on passive extension of the fingers is a further confirmatory finding.

In the event of impending ischemia, the first step is to remove constricting bandages and extend the elbow to the point at which the radial pulse returns or the hand develops adequate circulation. Proper management of the fracture at this point generally will require the use of traction to maintain alignment of the fracture. Either skin traction of the Dunlap type or skeletal traction with a pin through the olecranon is used. We prefer olecranon skeletal traction with the arm overhead, as it leaves the elbow area free from all constricting dressings and the arm elevated (Fig. 14–6).

If signs of impending ischemia, including progressive loss of active and passive extension of the fingers, hypesthesia

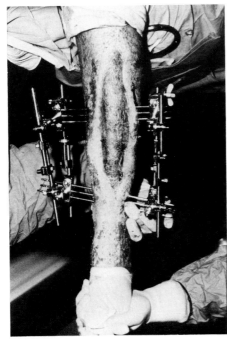

Fig. 14–4.—Hoffman apparatus used to immobilize a lower leg with septic nonunion of the tibia and fibula.

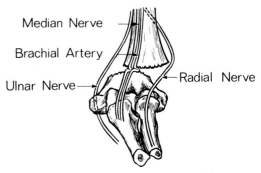

Fig. 14–5.—Supracondylar fracture of the elbow. This most commonly results in posterior and medial displacement of the distal fragment, with possible injury of the brachial artery and median nerve by the distal end of the proximal fragment, and stretching of the radial and ulnar nerves.

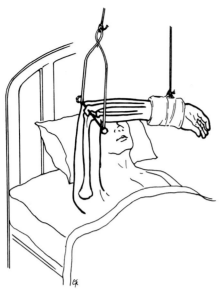

Fig. 14–6.—Overhead olecranon skeletal traction used to manage elbow fractures in children.

and pallor, persist beyond 1 hour despite these steps, surgical exploration and decompression of the fascial compartments and muscles of the forearm should be undertaken.[3] After complete fasciotomy and epimysiotomy of the forearm muscles from above the elbow to below the wrist have been carried out, the brachial artery must be inspected in the area of the fracture. Evidence of arterial spasm frequently is present. Stripping of the adventitia, lidocaine drip and mechanical distention generally are adequate to restore flow. If the vessel has been divided or lacerated, the area of injury should be resected and a vein graft inserted. After the artery has been dealt with, the fracture is reduced and fixed with two Kirschner wires pinned proximally across the fracture site at the level of the condyles (Fig. 14–7).

Arteriography must not be used as the sole indication for decompressing a forearm with impending ischemia, since swelling and necrosis within the fascial compartments of the forearm may progress unchecked following a period of ischemia despite the subsequent restoration of blood flow at the elbow. Cases of progressive ischemia of the forearm in the presence of a normal arteriogram have been reported. The decision to decompress the forearm must be based on clinical evidence of progressive ischemia and not on arteriography. Time must not be lost waiting for arteriography.[6]

As a general rule, it is best to avoid the use of enclosed long arm casts in the management of fracture about the elbow. The swelling associated with elbow injuries can be significant and a patient with an enclosed circumferential cast is subject to the possibility of excessive pain, if not neurovascular compromise, if the cast is not split. It generally is safer to use a combination of splints with circumferential wrappings above and below the elbow. After several days, when the swelling has begun to subside, a circumferential cast can be used if required to maintain position.

Extremity injuries and orthopedic procedures about the hip or knee also carry with them the possibility of neurovascular compromise or injury. Sciatic nerve palsy, particularly of the peroneal portion, is seen after traumatic hip dislocations.[4] Instrumentations and pinnings about the hip carry the possibility of both intrapelvic and extremity vascular injury. We have seen injury of the external iliac vein following pin transfixion of the femoral head and acetabulum.

The superior gluteal artery can be injured in the process of obtaining a posterior iliac bone graft. It may well be necessary to obtain intrapelvic exposure of the vessel as it retracts

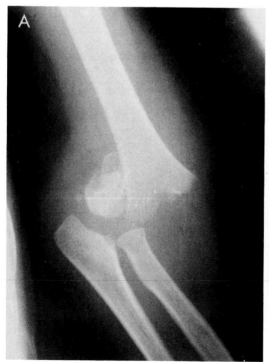

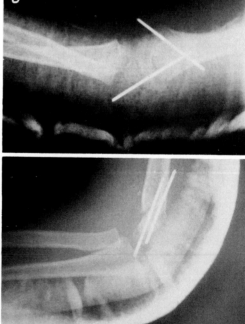

Fig. 14–7.—Supracondylar fracture of the elbow. **A,** the fracture with posterosuperior displacement of the distal fragment. The neurovascular structures are at risk from the sharp end of the shaft. **B,** the fracture re- duced, pinned and the elbow maintained in flexion. Pulse and sensation must be monitored frequently.

inside the sciatic notch. The route of choice is the retroperitoneal inguinal approach to the internal iliac artery.

Femoral fractures and femoral procedures such as osteotomy and plating can be complicated by injuries to the superficial femoral artery. It is imperative to use a technique of immobilization that permits assessment of the neurovascular status of the child after injury, and routine neurovascular check should be a part of the nursing routine following femoral fracture or instrumentation. It is worth noting that femoral fracture alone can result in blood loss to a degree to induce hypovolemic shock in a child. In addition to proper splinting, an intravenous line should be in place as part of this initial management of a child with suspected fracture of the femur. Direct injury to a portion of its major arterial trunk in association with fracture dislocation may result in ischemia of the lower extremity and require emergency assessment and repair. In addition, the lower extremity is subject to secondary neurovascular injury, usually involving muscle and nerves in one or more of the fascial compartments of the lower extremity, with injury the result of increased swelling and pressure within the closed fascial compartment. The anterior compartment, containing the major dorsiflexors of the foot and the nerves to the dorsum of the foot, has been involved most frequently.

Ischemic contracture of the lower limb has been seen following femoral fractures and, in particular, with Bryant's traction treatment of femoral fractures. With Bryant's traction, skin traction straps are applied to both lower extremities and overhead traction is applied with the hips in a position of 90° flexion and the knees in full extension. Several factors appear to be responsible for the development of lower leg ischemia in this situation, including the positioning of the knees in full extension and the application of potentially constrictive circumferential wrappings around the lower extremity. In addition, use of this technique in children weighing over 25 pounds or older than 2 years appears to have increased the risk of ischemic complications. The development of ischemia in this situation has never been demonstrated to be due to major arterial injury or constriction. In addition, a number of cases have been reported in which the nonfractured extremity developed ischemia while in this traction, thus further implicating the technique itself.[9] As in the management of this problem in the upper extremity, all constrictive bandages should be removed and the limb placed in a relaxed position. If signs of ischemic and muscular neurologic dysfunction persist, early decompression of the involved compartment must be carried out. Arteriography may demonstrate the need for major artery exploration in addition to fascial compartment decompression, but, as in the forearm, the decision to decompress must be based on assessment of the neurovascular status of the extremity and not dictated by arteriographic findings.

Injuries about the knee in the child and adolescent, particularly when the result of major trauma, frequently are misdiagnosed and undertreated. Injuries at the knee may result in fracture through the growth plate, with the ligamentous structures of the knee remaining intact (Fig. 14–8). Careful clinical assessment and attention to radiographic detail of the growth plate generally are sufficient to make the diagnosis of epiphyseal injury. In a significant number of cases, however, serious ligamentous injuries can occur without associated fracture. By the time the child is seen in the hospital Emergency Room, swelling about the knee, and joint effusion, make clinical assessment difficult, and the presence of effusion and swelling actually may impart a false clinical stability to the knee. Initial radiographs generally are unre-

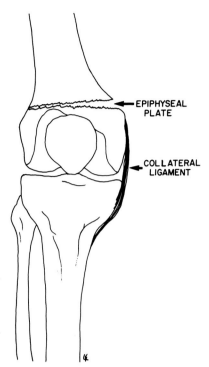

Fig. 14–8.—Injury to the knee in the child may result in fracture through the growth plate rather than ligamentous disruption.

markable, and the injured child all too often is splinted and given crutches, with subsequent evaluation 1–2 weeks following injury. Unfortunately, the best results following ligamentous disruption about the knee are obtained by immediate repair of the damaged ligamentous structures. Attempts to correct the instability of the knee by late reconstruction procedures are less successful and significantly more complicated.

The major difficulty in providing proper care to a child with a significant ligamentous injury of the knee is that of initial detection. Clinical evaluation is difficult if more than 1 hour has passed since injury, and plain radiographs generally are not helpful. Careful clinical history often is vital. A severe twisting injury induced by significant extrinsic force, accompanied by a "pop" in the knee and a sensation of the knee tearing or coming apart, is suggestive. Frequently there is a sensation of instability of the knee immediately after injury and the patient describes his knee as wobbly and tending to give way when he attempts to put weight on the extremity.

In the patient suspected of having a significant ligamentous injury of the knee, two further examinations can be carried out separately or in combination. Using sterile techniques, aspiration of the knee can be performed, followed by instillation of 10–15 ml of 1% lidocaine and 30–40 ml of Renografin 60. This usually provides adequate anesthesia of the knee joint to relieve protective muscle spasm. A stress radiograph then can be obtained in an attempt to demonstrate ligamentous instability. In addition, extravasation of contrast material through sites of ligamentous disruption on AP and lateral radiographs can be seen if the knee is compressed with an elastic wrap.[17] If this local anesthesia is not adequate to relieve protective muscle spasm, and significant suspicion of major ligamentous injury exists, the patient should be examined under general anesthesia and immediate operative repair carried out if ligamentous instability is demonstrated.

REFERENCES

1. Aitken, A. P.: Fractures of the epiphyses, Clin. Orthop. 41:19, 1965.
2. Blount, W. P.: *Fractures in Children* (Baltimore: The Williams & Wilkins Company, 1955).
3. Eaton, R. G., and Green, W. T.: Epimysiotomy and fasciotomy in the treatment of Volkmann's ischemic contractures, Orthop. Clin. North Am. 3:175, 1972.
4. Funk, F. J.: Traumatic dislocation of the hip in children. Factors influencing prognosis and treatment, J. Bone Joint Surg. 44-A: 1135, 1962.
5. Gresham, E. L.: Birth trauma, Pediatr. Clin. North Am. 22:317, 1975.
6. Griffin, P. P.: Supracondylar fractures of the humerus: Treatment and complications, Pediatr. Clin. North Am. 22:477, 1975.
7. Griffin, P. P., Anderson, M., and Green, W. T.: Fractures of the shaft of the femur, Orthop. Clin. North Am. 3:213, 1972.
8. Micheli, L. J.: The Young Athlete, in *Sports Medicine and Phys-iology* (Philadelphia: W. B. Saunders Company, in press), Chap. 18.
9. Nicholson, J. T., Foster, R. M., and Heath, R. D.: Bryant's traction: A provocative cause of circulatory complications, JAMA 157:415, 1955.
10. Rang, M.: *Children's Fractures* (Philadelphia and Toronto: J. B. Lippincott Company, 1974).
11. Rockwood, C. A., and Green, D. P.: *Fractures* (Philadelphia and Toronto: J. B. Lippincott Company, 1974).
12. Salter, R. B., and Harris, W. R.: Injuries involving the epiphyseal plate, J. Bone Joint Surg. 45-A:587, 1963.
13. Shanard, W. J.: *Pediatric Orthopaedics and Fractures* (Philadelphia: F. A. Davis Company, 1971).
14. Smith, C.: The battered child, N. Engl. J. Med. 299:322, 1973.
15. Sofield, H. A., and Millar, E. A.: Fragmentation, realignment, and intramedullary rod fixation of deformities of the long bones of children: A ten-year appraisal, J. Bone Joint Surg. 41-A:1371, 1959.
16. Tachdjian, M.: *Pediatric Orthopaedics* (Philadelphia: W. B. Saunders Company, 1972).
17. Wang, J. B., and Marshall, J. L.: Acute ligamentous injuries of the knee. Single contrast arthrography—a diagnostic aid, J. Trauma 15(5):431, 1975.

15 William J. Pitts

Snakebite

A BITE FROM A VENOMOUS SNAKE is an uncommon injury of children in the United States. It can range from a difficult, diagnostic dilemma to one of the most challenging emergencies encountered.

Snakebite: Facts and Figures

An estimated 8000 bites by venomous snakes occur each year in the United States.[1] Sixty per cent to 65% of these are minor,[2] but in the remainder the venom load will be substantial enough to pose a serious threat to life or limb.

Parrish[2] reported 6678 venomous bites treated in the United States during 1959. More than half of these cases occurred in people below 20 years of age, with the greatest incidence in the 10–19 year age bracket. Ninety-six per cent of bites involved a limb, the lower extremity most frequently. McCollough[3] observed that in Florida 15% of the traumatic amputations in children were a consequence of venomous snakebite! Parrish[4] reported a mortality of 0.21% among treated patients, with 40% of the deaths occurring in the less than 20 year age group, 20% below the age of 5 years.

Table 15–1 gives the geographic distribution of Parrish's 6678 bites. Venomous bites are rare in New England, relatively infrequent among northern border states but progressively increase in frequency in the southern half of the country. The states with the highest incidence of snakebite fatality, in order of decreasing frequency, are Arizona, Georgia, Florida, Alabama, South Carolina and Texas.[4]

Snakes: Their Bites and Their Venoms

THE SNAKES.—Two of the world's five families of venomous snakes occur in the United States. Those of greatest significance belong to the family *Crotalidae* and include species of rattlesnakes (genus *Crotalus* and *Sistrurus*) and several species of cottonmouth and copperhead of the genus *Agkistrodon*. Two species of coral snake are the only North American representatives of the second family, the *Elapidae*.

More than 99% of the venomous bites sustained in the United States are inflicted by members of the family *Crotalidae*, the remainder from the eastern coral snake and from imported species in zoos, private collections and in research laboratories.[2]

All members of the family *Crotalidae* have paired facial pits, vertically elliptical pupils (in distinction to the round pupils of most nonvenomous species) and have noncleft ventral plates, or scutes, extending from the anal plate caudad along the ventral surface of the tail. These features serve to differentiate the cottonmouth from nonvenomous water snakes, with which it is confused.

The eastern coral snake is encircled by bands of red, yellow and black. Although occasionally confused with the scarlet king snake and other nonvenomous species of similar coloration, the coral always can be differentiated by the simple verse, "If red touches yellow, can kill a fellow!" A coral snake's snout is black, it has no pits, it has round pupils, it has cleft ventral caudal scutes and its tiny delicate fixed anterior fangs often are obscured by mucosal folds.

For the average feeding strike, the snake rations its venom to 10–25% of that available. If thoroughly aroused, frightened or injured, the snake may resort to multiple strikes or to a bite-and-squeeze type of envenomation, with expenditure of 75% or more of its venom capacity. Children, with their reduced body mass, have more severe reactions than do adults. They are more likely to receive multiple strikes than

TABLE 15–1.–VENOMOUS SNAKEBITES IN THE UNITED STATES
(Annual Incidence°)

Alabama	208	Massachusetts	2	Rhode Island	0.3
Arizona	102	Michigan	58	(One every 3 years)	
Arkansas	307	Minnesota	3	South Carolina	184
California	221	Mississippi	236	South Dakota	31
Colorado	41	Missouri	234	Tennessee	79
Connecticut	4	Montana	38	Texas	1408
Delaware	8	Nebraska	46	Utah	20
Florida	350	Nevada	7	Vermont	0.3
Georgia	530	New Hampshire	1	(One every 3 years)	
Idaho	10	New Jersey	25	Virginia	217
Illinois	35	New Mexico	71	Washington	25
Indiana	45	New York	37	West Virginia	210
Iowa	9	North Carolina	856	Wisconsin	15
Kansas	115	North Dakota	5	Wyoming	21
Kentucky	143	Ohio	45	District of	
Louisiana	334	Oklahoma	206	Columbia	5
Maine	0	Oregon	14		
Maryland	42	Pennsylvania	74	TOTAL	6677.6

°Suggested annual incidence based on data 1958 and 1959.[2]

the adult, who is able to escape more rapidly, and the venom dose therefore is greater.

THE VENOM.—Snake venom is a protein-rich mixture containing many enzymes, polypeptide toxins and other substances.[8] The composition varies considerably among species, producing a wide spectrum of effects—some proteolytic, others coagulant and still others hemolytic, hemorrhagic or neurotoxic.[7] Bradykinin, histamine and serotonin may also be released from the tissues by the venom enzymes, adding to the tissue damage.[12] Bradykinin, released by L-arginine esterase, is believed to produce the intense local pain of crotalid venom destruction and produce immediate transient hypotension and also nausea, vomiting and increased perspiration.[9] Phospholipase-A converts serum lecithin to the lysolecithin,[8] which may produce acute renal failure secondary to massive hemolysis. Other enzymes and toxins, with considerable variation among different families and species, produce the wide spectrum of local and systemic effects often seen.[10-13]

Clinical Manifestations

CROTALID ENVENOMATION.—Burning pain and progressively advancing edema and ecchymosis in the soft tissues surrounding the fang punctures are typical and appear rapidly after envenomation. The extent of the reaction depends on the amount of venom injected. In certain circumstances, however, particularly following envenomation by the eastern diamondback and the Mojave rattlesnake, neuromuscular effects may predominate in the early period, with muscle fasciculations, dysphonia, respiratory difficulty and profound weakness or partial motor paralysis.

Nausea and vomiting are common symptoms, as are increased perspiration, scalp and perioral numbness and tingling of the fingers. Loss of consciousness, convulsions and repeated vomiting may occur in children.

In cases of mild envenomation, edema and ecchymosis progress slowly, extending only a few inches (Fig. 15–1) when maximally developed in 12–24 hours.[16] More rapid advancement following more potent envenomation may produce enough swelling of the extremity to compromise distal circulation and tissue perfusion, which may lead to superficial necrosis and intracompartmental muscle ischemia and fibrotic contracture or frank gangrene.

Huge volumes of fluid may accumulate within the swelling extremity, with hypovolemia, hypotension, shock and cardiac arrest. Marked reduction of a previously elevated hematocrit may indicate extensive hemolysis. Defibrination of the blood may also occur, with consequent autoanticoagulation and multifocal spontaneous hemorrhage, which may be life-threatening.

In 1955, Wood, Hoback and Green[14] offered a system of grading to assist the therapist in identifying the degree of severity of a case of envenomation based on the extent of the local reaction correlated with the presence and intensity of systemic symptoms. Their classification is summarized in Table 15–2 with the addition of Grade 0[15] and Grade IV.[18] Antivenin doses are based on this grading system. Antivenin dosage often must be increased by 50% in the management of small children. The intravenous route of administration is now considered standard.

Russell[1] reported no deaths in 550 cases managed by prompt intravenous antivenin therapy. Defibrination, spontaneous hemorrhages and severe hemolysis were totally prevented by adequate, early doses of antivenin.[19] No amputations were performed and fasciotomies were not necessary if antivenin was used early and *in adequate dose.*[1] Serum sickness was observed with increased frequency as larger doses of antivenin were used but this responded to standard treatment.[19]

ELAPID (CORAL SNAKE) ENVENOMATION.—Minimal swelling and discomfort may be the only objective findings when the patient presents for evaluation following this type of bite. The patient may remain asymptomatic for up to 7 or more hours postenvenomation, followed by subtle neurologic changes, which progress rapidly to bulbar paralysis, respiratory arrest and death. If life support measures are successful, total motor paralysis supervenes, which lasts for several days. Clearance of neurologic symptoms reverses in the order of development.

Therefore, the greatest danger of coral snake envenomation is failure to recognize its lethal potential because of the paucity of early objective findings.[6]

Ancillary Measures and Alternative Approaches

THE TOURNIQUET.—Compression of subcutaneous venous and lymphatic afferent channels has been found to be

TABLE 15-2

					"Standard"[d] TREATMENT
	CROTALID ENVENOMATION SYNDROME CLASSIFICATION OF SEVERITY				
		LOCAL TISSUE CHANGES		SYSTEMIC CHANGES	ANTIVENIN DOSAGE SCHEDULE
GRADE	FANG MARKS	Extent of Edema in Inches— Within 12 Hrs		Nausea, Vomiting, BP ↓ Pulse ↑ Resp. ↓ Convulsions, Numbness	No. of Ampules, All Intravenous
0[b]	Present	0		0	0
I[a]	Present	1–5		0	Usually None
II	Present	6–12		Mild	2–4
III	Present	12+		Moderate	5+
IV[c]	Present	Extensive and rapidly advancing		Severe	10–20–30+

[a]Modified from Wood *et al.* [14]
[b]Added by Parrish.[15]
[c]Added by McCollough and Gennaro.[18]
[d]See text from Van Mierop.[11]

of definite value as a first aid measure in moderate and severe crotalid envenomations, particularly when treatment is delayed. Loss of tagged venom from envenomated extremities of dogs was reduced from 20% to 9% within a 2-hour period by simple tourniquet compression of more proximal tissues.[20]

INCISION AND SUCTION.—In 1927, Jackson[17] demonstrated the effectiveness of suction through cruciate incisions in experimental envenomation. One-quarter-inch linear incisions now are preferred—one through each fang puncture. McCollough and Gennaro[18] demonstrated that more than 50% of venom can be recovered if suction is begun within 3 minutes of envenomation. Routine incision and suction is not advised in bites of lesser virulence or in those of greater virulence if professional care can be obtained promptly.

EXCISION—SUPPLEMENTING ANTIVENIN.—In 1955, Parrish[21] demonstrated that 7 cm diameter circular excision 30 and 60 minutes postinjection of 6 MLD rattlesnake wounds in dogs resulted in the survival of two-thirds of the animals. Snyder[20] successfully performed excision in 23 patients in conjunction with regional intra-arterial administration of antivenin; no soft tissue loss occurred from the bite and only 1 patient had serum sickness. Skin grafts were needed in several patients.

Excision of envenomated tissue is of definite value for the extremely seriously bitten child and for the strongly antivenin-sensitive adult. Excision in bites involving hands and fingers—particularly in mild to moderate envenomation—requires considerable individualization.

Treatment Recommendations

First Aid Measures

1. Transport the bitten individual to the nearest source of competent professional care.
2. A tourniquet to restrict lymphatic and venous drainage should be applied well above the bite and left in place until the patient is hospitalized. If tourniquet readjustment is needed, a second tourniquet should be placed above the first before removing it.
3. Incision and suction if necessary in moderate or severe bites should be performed *immediately* or not at all.

4. The use of ice or refrigerant packs applied to the bite wound may be dangerously injurious to envenomated tissue and is not recommended under ordinary circumstances.
5. Antivenin should not be given as a first aid measure unless personnel are equipped to manage allergic complications.
6. The bitten person should be kept N.P.O. en route.
7. Positive identification of the snake is helpful.

Definitive Care

1. No therapy is indicated without confirmed envenomation.
2. The tourniquet is left in place until antivenin therapy is begun.
3. A history of the patient's general health, presence of allergy and details of the envenomation is obtained if possible.
4. An intravenous line is established. Blood is obtained for:

   a) *Routine hemogram.*
   b) *Coagulation profile.*
   c) *Serum creatine phosphokinase (CPK) level.* (This enzyme, rapidly elevated in response to skeletal muscle and cardiac muscle damage, may be important in the detection of subfascial envenomation.[12])
   d) *Type and crossmatch.* Hemolysis interferes with crossmatching.

5. Antivenin is administered intravenously after appropriate sensitivity testing, with epinephrine (1:1000) immediately available for control of unexpected allergic reaction.

The total dose of antivenin given is of critical importance. Whereas dose ranges as suggested in Table 15-2 are generally adequate, the therapist must be alert to the possibility of *undergrading* the envenomation in the initial evaluation and to the fact that the actual antivenin need may be greater than that initially estimated. The delivery of a total dose completely sufficient to accomplish total venom neutralization is the clear goal of such therapy. Adequacy of treatment is assessed by lasting cessation of pain, control of advancing edema, and improvement in vital signs and the patient's sense of well being. Also evident will be measurable correction of derangements in the clotting mechanism and systemic functions.

In certain cases, surgical decompression of tightly edematous tissue will be necessary for efficient antivenin delivery to the spreading venom inoculum at the bite site.

6. A central venous line and an indwelling urinary catheter may be needed in severe envenomations.

7. Serial measurements of the circumference of the bitten extremity are obtained.

8. Tetanus prophylaxis is administered if necessary.

9. The circulatory status of the bitten extremity must be watched carefully; excessive tension in fingers or hand is managed by incisions placed along preferred lines.

10. Fasciotomy, if indicated, should be done through single or multiple transverse skin and subcutaneous tissue incisions.

REFERENCES

1. Russell, F. E.: Snake venom poisoning in the United States. Experiences with 550 cases, JAMA 233:341, 1975.
2. Parrish, H. M.: Incidence of treated snakebites in the United States, Public Health Rep. 81:269, 1966.
3. McCollough, N. C.: The juvenile amputee. Preliminary report of the problem in Florida, J. Fla. Med. Assoc. 46:302, 1959.
4. Parrish, H. M.: Analysis of 460 fatalities from venomous animals in the United States, Am. J. Med. Sci. 245:129, 1963.
5. Wingert, W., and Wainschel, J.: Diagnosis and management of envenomation by poisonous snakes, South. Med. J. 68:1015, 1975.
6. Parrish, H. M., and Khan, M. S.: Bites by coral snakes: Report of 11 representative cases, Am. J. Med. Sci. 253:561, 1967.
7. Russell, F. E.: Pharmacology of animal venoms, Clin. Pharmacol. Ther. 8:849, 1967.
8. Minton, S. A., Jr.: Venom Diseases (Springfield, Ill.: Charles C Thomas, Publisher, 1974).
9. Brown, J. H.: Toxicology and Pharmacology of Venoms from Poisonous Snakes (Springfield, Ill.: Charles C Thomas, Publisher, 1973).
10. Jiminez-Porras, J. M.: Biochemistry of snake venoms, Clin. Toxicol. 3:389, 1970.
11. Van Mierop, L. H. S.: Poisonous snakebite—a review. 1. Snakes and their venoms. 2. Symptomology and treatment, J. Fla. Med. Assoc. 63:191, 1976.
12. Gennaro, J. F., Jr.: Personal communication. (Information based on studies by Szabo, P., and Gennaro, J. F., Jr. and reported at International Symposium on Toxicology, Costa Rica, August, 1976.)
13. Markland, F. S., and Pirkle, H.: Characterization of a thrombin-like enzyme from Crotalus adamanteus (eastern diamondback rattlesnake), Toxicon 14:412, 1976.
14. Wood, J. T., et al.: Treatment of snake venom poisoning with ACTH and cortisone, Va. Med. Mon. 82:130, 1955.
15. Parrish, H. M.: Poisonous snakebites resulting in lack of venom poisoning, Va. Med. Mon. 86:396, 1959.
15a. Gingrich, W. C., and Hohenadel, J. C.: Standardization of Polyvalent Antivenin, in Buckley, E. E., and Porges, N. (eds.), Venoms (Washington, D. C.: American Association for the Advancement of Science, 1956), Pub. No. 44, pp. 381–385.
16. Parrish, H. M., et al.: Snakebite—a pediatric problem, Clin. Pediatr. 4:237, 1965.
17. Jackson, D.: First aid treatment for snakebite, Tex. St. J. Med. 23:198, 1927.
18. McCollough, N. C., and Gennaro, J. F., Jr.: Evolution of venomous snakebite in the southern United States from parallel clinical and laboratory investigations. Development of treatment, J. Fla. Med. Assoc. 49:966, 1963.
19. Wainschel, J.: Personal communication, February, 1977.
20. Snyder, C. C., et al.: A definitive study of snakebite, J. Fla. Med. Assoc. 55:330, 1968.
21. Parrish, H. M.: Early excision and suction of snakebite wounds in dogs, N. C. Med. J. 16:93, 1955.
22. Antivenin (Handbook) (New York: Wyeth Laboratories, Division of American Home Products Corporation, Copyright 1961, revised 1963 and 1968), pp. 35–38.

16 R. Marshall Pitts
Spider Bites

HISTORY.—Although more deaths are reported from stings of the Hymenoptera, especially the honeybee, than any other venomous creatures, including snakes, in the United States,[24] certain arthropods—scorpions, tarantulas and black widow spiders—are more infamous in the history of humankind than the Hymenoptera. Scorpions, the oldest land animal, were the first to come out of water onto land in the Silurian epoch, long before insects emerged. They are the most renowned poisonous arthropod in fable, folklore and astrology.[6] Tarantulas famous from the spider panic of the seventeenth century in Italy, in which they were thought to cause a frenzied "dance of death,"[33] are frightening in size and appearance but relatively harmless to humans. Black widow spiders, probably the most universally *feared* "insect" from ancient times, deserve their bad reputation for their decidedly unpleasant and sometimes dangerous bite.[5]

Macchiavello[19] first associated the "gangrenous spot" of Chile with the bite of the brown spider, Loxosceles laeta, in 1937. This did not receive much scientific recognition in the United States until 1957, when Atkins[3] connected "necrotic arachnidism" with the bite of a brown spider of the same species in the United States, Loxosceles reclusa. In 20 years, the Loxosceles reclusa has achieved notoriety as possibly a more dangerous spider than the black widow.

Insects and Arthropods

Of 302 deaths from insects and arthropods recorded in the United States from 1950 to 1959, Hymenoptera (bees, wasps, yellowjackets, hornets and ants), accounted for 229 (76%), scorpions 8 (3%) and spiders 65 (21%).[24] Severe reactions and fatalities due to stings of Hymenoptera usually are anaphylactic in type.[22] The stings of scorpions found in the United States are painful but not dangerous, with the exception of the "lethal scorpion" of the Southwest, Centruroides sculpturatus. This scorpion injects a neurotoxin with a strychnine-like action,[6] which may lead to severe convulsions and death, especially in children. An antivenin is available.*[30]

Of about 50 species of spiders in the United States impli-

* Poisonous Animal Research Laboratory, Arizona State University, Tempe, Arizona.

cated in bites of humans, only 2 are significantly venomous.[27] These spiders, commonly known as the black widow and the brown recluse are about the same size, and both are important in pediatrics because death from spider venom almost always is confined to the very young or the debilitated.[28] The bites of the black widow and the brown recluse spiders may have surgical implications.

Spider Characteristics

The scientific names for the black widow and brown recluse provide insight into the lore and character of these arthropods. The scientific designation of the black widow, *Latrodectus mactans*, means "murderer-killer." The spider is called "widow" because the smaller male sometimes is eaten by his hungry mate. The distinctive mature female has a black body with a round, bulbous, shiny abdomen containing a red hourglass marking on its underside (Fig. 16–1). The warmer climate areas of the world are her habitat. The black widow spider typically is found in the outdoor privy, under the toilet seat, attracted by the moisture and the flies.[5]

The scientific designation for the common brown spider, *Loxosceles reclusa*, "the secluded one," appropriately indicates its shy, nonaggressive nature. Both male and female are venomous and about the same size. The brown recluse has a tan to brown body approximately ½ inch long with a leg span of about 2 inches. A distinctive dark, violin-shaped marking appears on top of the spider's cephalothorax, which provides easy identification and accounts for the nickname "fiddle-back" spider (Fig. 16–2). This venomous spider is found most commonly in the south central United States. The brown spider is a hunter that forages for food at night. He is likely to hide out in the daytime in packing crates, old clothes, bedclothes and other dark, undisturbed places.[9] Seventy-five per cent of bite victims are in bed, or dressing, when bitten.[18] Modern society has diminished the black widow menace with indoor plumbing.[5] Conversely, improved transportation and central heating are increasing the brown spider's threat by spreading his habitat.[15]

Spider Venom

Black widow spider venom is a neurotoxin that produces little reaction at the site of the bite but promptly leads to the clinical syndrome of painful muscle cramps, abdominal pain and profuse sweating.[16] Other signs and symptoms, such as fever, hypertension, drowsiness, delirium, constricted pupils and excessive salivation, may be present. The most prominent sign is the agonizing abdominal pain and rigidity, which suggests other diseases, such as perforated peptic ulcer, renal colic, acute pancreatitis, acute appendicitis, enteritis, food poisoning and tetanus.[12] Usually the severe symptoms gradually subside over a period of 2–8 days.[5] Most of the deaths reported from spider bites have been due to the black widow.[24]

The bite of the brown recluse spider has been described as a "bite with a delayed fuse." The venom is a cytotoxin and

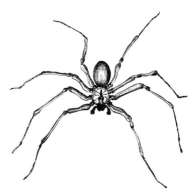

Fig. 16–2.—Brown recluse spider—actual size. Note "fiddle" shape on cephalothorax.

hemolysin.[20] The victim may feel little pain initially, but local pain, vesication and erythema appear in 2–8 hours (Fig. 16–3). Systemic symptoms, notably fever, malaise and vomiting, may appear in 12–24 hours; these findings may be particularly severe in children.[11, 31] Deep local necrosis of skin and subcutaneous tissue may follow in 2–5 days. Undoubtedly, most bites are milder than those with necrosis and so go unreported.[8] In one series, 31 of 336 bites had severe necrosis.[11] Rarely, necrosis spreads widely in an irregular, star-shaped pattern.[13] Local excision with primary closure, or skin grafting, may be necessary.

The principal systemic effects of *Loxosceles* venom appear to be rapid hemolysis and thrombocytopenia.[10] Hemolysis usually develops within 24 hours and is more common and more severe in children.[11] Fulminating systemic viscerocutaneous loxoscelism is characterized by general symptoms, such as fever, malaise and vomiting, followed by hemolytic anemia, hemoglobinuria and diffuse intravascular coagulation. Death may result. Severe local and systemic loxoscelism rarely coexist.[2]

Treatment

BLACK WIDOW BITES.—The treatment of black widow bites is directed at symptomatic relief, and the use of the specific antivenin. There is no effective first aid treatment

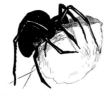

Fig. 16–1.—Black widow spider—actual size—protecting egg sac.

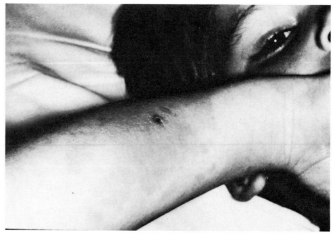

Fig. 16–3.—Brown spider bite on arm of 6-year-old boy. Note necrotic spot and surrounding erythema. Child was febrile and nauseated.

for spider bites.[26] The black widow victim should be hospitalized and promptly treated with antivenin (Latrodectus mactans—MSD[21]) for early relief from symptoms. Antivenin should be administered intravenously in severe cases, and to all children less than 12 years of age. Precautions with the antivenin should be taken, as with any product prepared with horse serum.[21] The child should receive the entire contents of the restored antivenin vial. Symptoms usually subside in 1–3 hours, but a second dose of antivenin may be necessary.

Calcium gluconate USP, administered intravenously, is standard treatment for muscle cramping but is not as effective as methocarbomol NF (Robaxin), IV.[27] The dosage of calcium gluconate is 500 mg/kg/24 hours or 12 gm/M[2]/24 hours in divided doses. It may be given orally or intravenously.[29] The dosage of Robaxin is 60 mg/kg/24 hours or 2 gm/M[2]/24 hours divided into 4 doses (IV) by slow push or continuous drip.[29]

Narcotics should not be used in children with black widow bites because of the danger of a synergism with the black widow venom, which can lead to respiratory paralysis.[30] Small amounts of sedatives may be required for extreme restlessness. In severely ill children, positive-pressure breathing and careful monitoring in an intensive care unit may become necessary.

Atropine is effective for rapid symptomatic relief from black widow symptoms, and may be more readily available than antivenin.[14]

BROWN RECLUSE BITES.—Most brown spider bites, including small necrotic spots, may be left untreated.[2] Treatment of more severe bites is controversial. Most authors recommend early surgical excision of necrotic spots greater than 1 cm. This excision should include all devitalized fat and fascia.[4] Secondary closure, with skin grafting after 3–5 days, is the usual treatment, although primary closure sometimes is possible. Auer and Hershey[4] reported satisfactory results in all patients in whom excision was carried out within 10 days from the bite.

Whether local injection of steroids around a severe local lesion can lessen the severity of the lesion is questionable.[8, 17] This approach is considered important by some authors,[11] who caution that massive doses must be administered within 24 hours of the bite.[1, 10, 13] Eighty mg of triamcinolone suspension is recommended—20 mg into each quadrant around the bite.[2]

Steroids should not be withheld from children with systemic disease. Early coagulation studies are important to detect thrombocytopenia and hemolysis.[2, 32] Steroids must be administered early and in massive amounts.[2, 9, 10] In cases of severe hemolysis, exchange transfusion has been used with dramatic effect.[23, 25] More investigation is necessary to define better therapy for the brown spider bite.[7]

An antivenin is available for the *Loxosceles laeta* species of South America, but commercial production of an antivenin for the *Loxosceles* species of the United States has not been achieved.

Good housekeeping practices and liberal use of insecticides undoubtedly are important prophylaxis against brown spider bites, but care in shaking out seldom-used clothing and airing material taken from storage may be better.[2]

REFERENCES

1. Anderson, P. C.: Treatment of severe loxoscelism, Mo. Med. 68:609, 1971.
2. Anderson, P. C.: What's new in loxoscelism?, Mo. Med. 70:711, 1973.
3. Atkins, J. A., *et al.*: Probable cause of necrotic spider bite in the Midwest, Science 126:73, 1957.
4. Auer, A. F., and Hershey, F. B.: Surgery for necrotic bites of the brown spider, Arch. Surg. 108:612, 1974.
5. Baerg, W. J.: The black widow and five other venomous spiders in the United States, Ark. Agr. Exp. Sta. Bull., p. 608, 1959.
6. Baerg, W. J.: Scorpions: Biology and effects of their venom, Ark. Agr. Exp. Sta. Bull., p. 649, 1961.
7. Berger, R. S.: A critical look at therapy for the brown recluse spider bite, Arch. Dermatol. 107:293, 1973.
8. Berger, R. S.: The unremarkable brown recluse spider bite, JAMA 225:1109, 1973.
9. Butz, W. C.: Envenomation by the brown recluse spider (Aranae, Scytodidae) and related species. A public health problem in the United States, Clin. Toxicol. 4:515, 1971.
10. Dillaha, C. J., *et al.*: North American loxoscelism. Necrotic bite of the brown recluse spider, JAMA 188:33, 1964.
11. Fardon, D. W., *et al.*: The treatment of brown spider bite, Plast. Reconstr. Surg. 40:482, 1967.
12. Frazier, C. A.: *Insect Allergy* (St. Louis: Warren H. Green, Inc., 1969).
13. Frazier, C. A.: Spider Bites (Black Widow and Brown Recluse) and Scorpion Stings, in Conn, H. (ed.), *Current Therapy 1976* (Philadelphia: W. B. Saunders Company, 1976), p. 871.
14. Gotlieb, A.: Atropine for spider bite, Harefuah 68:223, 1965.
15. Hite, J. M.: Biology of the brown recluse spider, Ark. Agr. Exp. Sta. Bull., p. 711, 1966.
16. James, J. A., *et al.*: Reactions following suspected spider bite, Am. J. Dis. Child. 102:141, 1961.
17. Jansen, G. T., *et al.*: The brown recluse spider bite: Controlled evaluation of treatment using the white rabbit as an animal model, South. Med. J. 64:1194, 1971.
18. Lessenden, C. M., and Zimmer, L. K.: Brown spider bites, J. Kans. Med. Soc. 61:379, 1960.
19. Macchiavello, A.: La Loxsceles laeta causa del arachnoidismo cutaneo, o mancha gangrenosa, de Chile, Rev. Chil. Hist. Nat. 41:11, 1937.
20. Majeski, J. A., and Durst, G. G.: Necrotic arachnidism, South. Med. J. 69:887, 1976.
21. Merck Sharp and Dohme package insert for antivenin (Latrodectus mactans), AHFS Category 80:04, 6145208, April, 1972.
22. Mueller, A. L.: Further experiences with severe allergic reactions to insect stings, N. Engl. J. Med. 26:374, 1959.
23. Nicholson, J. F., and Nicholson, B. H.: Hemolytic anemia from brown spider bite, J. Okla. State Med. Assoc. 55:234, 1962.
24. Parrish, H. M.: Analysis of 460 fatalities from venomous animals in the United States, Am. J. Med. Sci. 245:129, 1963.
25. Riley, H. D.: Brown spider bite with severe hemolytic phenomena, J. Okla. State Med. Assoc. 57:218, 1964.
26. Russell, F. E.: Bites of Spiders and Other Arthropods, in Conn, H. (ed.), *Current Therapy 1970* (Philadelphia: W. B. Saunders Company, 1970), p. 878.
27. Russell, F. E.: Venomous Animal Injuries, in *Current Problems in Pediatrics* (Chicago: Year Book Medical Publishers, Inc., July, 1973).
28. Schmaus, J. W.: Bites of Spiders and Other Arthropods, in Conn, H. (ed.), *Current Therapy 1970* (Philadelphia: W. B. Saunders Company, 1970), p. 803.
29. Shirkey, H. C.: Table of Drugs, in *Pediatric Therapy* (St. Louis: The C. V. Mosby Company, 1975).
30. Stahnke, H. L.: How to get stung by a scorpion, Desert Magazine, August, 1960.
31. Subcommittee on Accidental Poisoning, AAP: Treatment of brown recluse spider bites. Newsletter supplement, April 15, 1970.
32. Vorse, H., *et al.*: Disseminated intravascular coagulopathy following fatal brown spider bite (necrotic arachnidism), J. Pediatr. 80:1035, 1972.
33. Whitcomb, W. H., and Weems, H. V.: The tarantula, Fla. Dept. Agr. and Consumer Serv. Entomology Circular 169, 1976.

17 AURELIO C. USON / JOHN LATTIMER

Genitourinary Tract Injuries

MORE CHILDREN die as a result of traumatic injuries each year than from the next three leading causes of death combined. Injuries to the genitourinary system comprise 2.4–7.0% of all traumatic lesions and, lately, they seem to occur in clinical practice with increasing frequency.[75]

Trauma to the genitourinary organs can be direct, as from a bullet or a knife, or indirect, as from a sudden jerk or whip-like force generated during a fall or when the body is thrown suddenly against an immobile hard object, as in an automobile crash. Furthermore, injuries can be closed, without disruption of the body wall, or open (or penetrating) with a perforation through the soft tissues. About 80% of the penetrating injuries damage intraperitoneal organs or other deep structures. There are also spontaneous or non-traumatic types of genitourinary injuries. In these instances, there frequently is a predisposing cause or pathologic condition that greatly increases the chances of "spontaneous" rupture or laceration. Large silent hydronephroses, ectopically placed kidneys and greatly distended, thin-walled bladders are examples. On the other hand, there have been instances in which children have been involved in accidents of great violence, yet miraculously escaped any injury. By and large, the greatest number of severe genitourinary injuries in children result from traffic accidents, provoked trauma (the battered child) and accidental falls, kicks or blows that occur at play or during competitive athletics. Still another type of genitourinary injury is iatrogenic, such as can occur during urethral instrumentation with metal sounds or cystoscopes or during endoscopic or open surgery. Occasionally, the kidney or ureter is perforated during retrograde pyelography or during the replacement of a nephrostomy tube (Fig. 17–1), particularly if a catheter is passed with a stylet.[8]

Despite severe and multiple injuries of the genitourinary tract or other parts of the body, children tend to recover much better than do adults. For instance, we have seen children who were severely injured, with multiple fractures and kidneys dislocated into the pleural or peritoneal cavities, who appeared to be only moderately ill and recovered promptly following nephrectomy and adequate treatment of their other injuries (see Fig. 17–6).

Other things being equal, the results of therapy for trauma to the genitourinary tract depend on: (1) the time interval between injury and treatment; (2) the type and severity of injury; (3) the structures, organ(s) and system(s) involved; (4) the presence of shock, peritonitis or coma; (5) the understanding of the problem, coupled with available diagnostic and therapeutic facilities; and (6) the collaboration of trained personnel during the preoperative evaluation and postoperative care and control. The results of therapy for severe trauma to the genitourinary organs have improved steadily as a consequence of increased knowledge and familiarity with this problem, coupled with refined diagnostic devices, therapeutic techniques and hospital facilities. Prevention of motor vehicle accidents, introduction of safer vehicles, better supervision of children and proper use of diagnostic and therapeutic tools no doubt would further decrease the number of accidents and genitourinary trauma in children.

Kidney Injuries

In 1966, Smith et al.[66] reported an incidence of 1 case of renal injury in every 860 pediatric admissions. According to these authors, renal injuries occur about 3 times more frequently during the second decade of life than during the first and affect boys 3 times as often as they do girls.

The kidneys are more vulnerable to injury in infants and children than in adults because of the less protected position of these organs during childhood. At this age, the kidneys lie mainly within the abdomen, their perirenal fibrous fatty envelopes are poorly developed and the kidney substance is fragile. There is also an increased morbidity after kidney injuries in children because of the closer relationship of the kidney to the peritoneum, the more delicate structure of the intra-abdominal organs, the disproportion between size and force of trauma relative to the size and strength of the anatomic structures, plus the inability of small children to complain or to protect themselves. Despite this increased vulnerability of the kidney to injury, children usually recover better than adults because of the greater capacity of their tis-

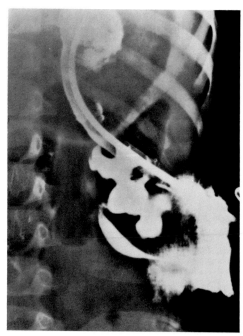

Fig. 17–1.—Penetrating injury caused by nephrostomy tube mounted on a stylet during an attempt to replace the tube. Hemorrhage and extravasation made nephrectomy necessary.

sues to recover spontaneously, their lesser incidence of concomitant diseases and their good general reserve.

ETIOLOGY.—Most renal injuries in children are of the closed variety and are produced by an indirect type of blunt trauma. Only occasionally does a bullet or knife injure the kidney directly. With the latter type of renal wound, other serious injuries in the peritoneal cavity or elsewhere in the body almost always are present. Trauma of sufficient force to fracture the lower ribs or the transverse processes of the thoracolumbar vertebrae usually injures the kidney also. In fact, a fragment of a fractured vertebra or a segment of the eleventh or twelfth rib can injure the underlying kidney.

Pre-existing renal abnormalities such as horseshoe kidney, ectopic kidney, renal cysts, renal tumors (nephroblastomas) and particularly hydronephrosis make the kidney vulnerable to trauma of a degree that might not be sufficient to damage an otherwise normal kidney. Children known to have urinary tract abnormalities should avoid contact and competitive sports until such abnormalities have been corrected.

Associated Injuries

According to Morse et al.,[49] as many as 40% of the pediatric renal injuries are accompanied by cerebral, spinal cord, bony, pulmonary and intraperitoneal (visceral, mesenteric and vascular) injuries as well as damage to other organs of the genitourinary system. Furthermore, about 25% of the children with left renal injury may also have a rupture of the spleen.

SYMPTOMS AND SIGNS.—Hematuria, pain, tenderness and abdominal rigidity usually are present with renal injury. Their degree of severity depends on the type of trauma, extent and severity of the renal lesion and any concomitant injuries, plus the general condition of the child.

If there is a perirenal hematoma or urinary extravasation, an abdominal mass sometimes can be palpated under a fairly rigid and tender abdominal wall. Paralytic ileus may indicate the presence of a retroperitoneal or intraperitoneal hemorrhage or urinary extravasation.

Hematuria with thread-like clots usually is pathognomic of renal injury.[21] Occasionally the bladder is distended with clots, the child is unable to void and anuria occurs as a result of the increased intravesical pressure.

Shock, in varying degrees, is a common feature in severely traumatized children with extensive kidney injuries. Shock may be produced by the initial physical impact on the splanchnic, celiac and other important neuroplexuses, but in kidney injuries it often is due to hypovolemia as a result of massive retro- or intraperitoneal bleeding.

It is, of course, essential to diagnose the condition and treat the traumatized child, regardless of the type of genitourinary tract injury, before the state of shock becomes irreversible.

Fever may be present because of absorption of blood, and its occurrence does not necessarily indicate sepsis. Urinalysis may disclose microhematuria, leukocyturia and mild proteinuria. Anemia and a decreased hematocrit value reflect blood loss; increased serum creatinine concentration may reflect diminished renal function as a direct result of injury or indirectly from underperfusion; and significant leukocytosis may reflect visceral injury, with relative lymphocytosis being more indicative of splenic injury.

PATHOLOGY.—The pathologic types of renal injuries (Fig. 17–2) have been classically divided as: (1) injuries of the kidney appendages—perirenal fat, ureter, renal vascular pedicle, (2) injuries of the kidney proper and (3) combinations of the two.

In the first group, the most important injury is that involving the main renal artery or vein. In these cases, massive bleeding occurs, producing perirenal hematomas, often with communication into the pleural or peritoneal cavity. The kidney, dislocated from its vascular pedicle, becomes necrotic even without intrinsic parenchymal lacerations.

Injuries of the kidney proper can be subdivided into (a) simple cortical contusions of kidney without deep parenchymal damage and with integrity of the true renal capsule; (b) deep lacerations of the kidney substance with concomitant rupture of the fibrous capsule or a calix, or both capsule and calices; (c) superficial lacerations of the renal cortex with associated tears of the fibrous capsule; (d) rupture of the pelvis; (e) the "shattered" kidney.

In general, the pathologic findings following renal trauma depend on the type and severity of the kidney injuries, degree of vascular damage, presence or absence of infection and the time interval between trauma and diagnosis. Renal infarction, infection, calcification, perirenal cyst formation (with or without hypertension) may be seen as late sequelae in some of these children.

With extensive rupture of the renal pelvis, urinary extravasation develops, with subsequent encapsulation, infection or reabsorption (in mild cases).

DIAGNOSIS.—With our present knowledge regarding genitourinary trauma and the refined laboratory and radiologic techniques now available, an accurate diagnosis can be made promptly in most children with renal injuries.

In children with multiple traumatic lesions, the team approach for correct diagnosis and adequate management is recommended. During the process of diagnosis, the following points are important: (1) the type of trauma; (2) the type and severity of symptoms and signs present; (3) realization that shock may occur quite suddenly, even as the child waits for x-ray study, for example; and (4) prompt blood count, urinalysis and plain radiographs of the chest and abdomen. The urologist should be concerned with establishing, as quickly as possible, an accurate diagnosis of the type, extent and complications of the renal injury. The status of the contralateral kidney and the remaining parts of the genitourinary tract and the over-all condition of the child should be evaluated also. The physician does well to be aware always of possible concomitant injuries and the possibility of massive secondary bleeding even in children with milder renal trauma.

Whenever possible, an infusion intravenous urogram with tomography should be obtained without delay. This study can be performed if the systolic blood pressure is above 70 mm Hg and if the radial pulse is palpable.

A plain film of the abdomen may reveal obliteration of the renal silhouette and psoas shadow, scoliosis with the concavity toward the injured side, free subdiaphragmatic air, urinary ascites, penetrating fragments of foreign bodies and bony fractures (ribs, transverse processes of thoracolumbar vertebrae, pelvic bones, etc). The urographic findings vary greatly according to the causation, pathologic type and severity of the injury. Usually the renal segment that has been injured may excrete the contrast medium poorly after a delay or not at all. Pooling of the extravasated contrast medium may appear within a parenchymal tear, alongside the neck of an intrarenal calix or just underneath the fibrous capsule.

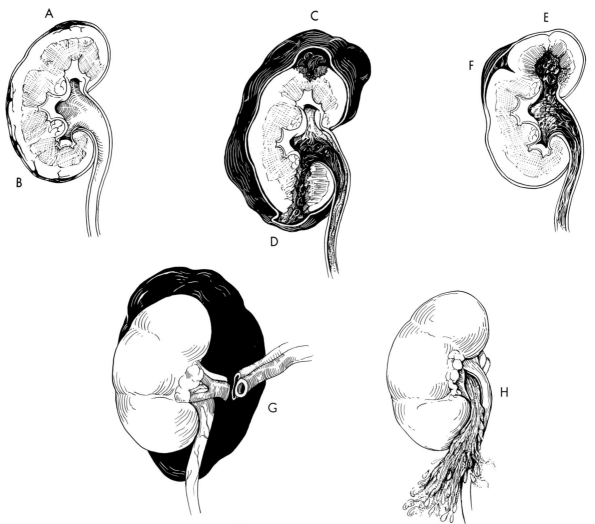

Fig. 17–2.—Pathologic types of renal injury. **A,** simple small, single laceration; capsule intact. **B,** multiple superficial lacerations with possible fragmentation of renal cortex; capsule intact. **C,** extensive laceration of renal parenchyma and adjacent fibrous capsule but without gross penetration into the renal pelvis; perirenal bleeding with hematoma formation is usual. **D,** same as **C,** but with laceration into the pelvis; here, gross hemorrhage into the collecting renal system is also present. **E,** laceration of parenchyma with penetration into the calix and profuse bleeding into the pelvis. **F,** deep laceration of renal parenchyma with subcapsular hematoma. **G,** complete severance of renal vascular pedicle with massive perirenal, retroperitoneal or intraperitoneal bleeding. This is an unusual type that may kill the child by exsanguination, although at times bleeding stops as a result of tamponade and arterial spasm. Recovery usually is good after nephrectomy and ligation of the renal pedicle. **H,** rupture of renal pelvis, seen in rare instances of renal trauma; hydronephrosis may be an important underlying factor. Urinary extravasation with perirenal collecting and infection may develop, requiring incision and drainage of the extravasated area, suture of the pelvic rent and temporary nephrostomy.

Extravasation around the kidney (parenchyma and/or pelvis) is proof of parenchymal or pyelocaliceal rupture. Absence of renal visualization usually suggests severe injury, with fragmentation and/or infarction of the renal substance. The pelvis, ureter and bladder may show filling defects due to the presence of blood clots.

Retrograde ureteropyelography rarely is necessary to delineate the site and extent of the renal injury. A normal retrograde pyelogram of a kidney that has shown nonvisualization of the contrast medium by infusion urography should suggest renal artery division or the thrombosis seen in patients injured by high-voltage electricity.

Transfemoral arteriography is a safe and valuable procedure for exact delineation of the extent and severity of the underlying pathologic anatomy of the renal parenchymal vasculature and other coexistent intra-abdominal injuries. Displacement of the intraparenchymal arteries as a result of hematoma, extravasation and/or segmental renal infarction,

stretching with outward displacement of the capsular artery over a perirenal hematoma, intraparenchymal renal extravasation due to rupture of interlobar and/or arcuate arteries, vascular narrowings or "amputations" due to spasm, periarterial compression and/or thrombosis, usually are visualized on selective angiographic studies of injured kidneys.

Renal scan using ([197]Hg) chlormerodrin or (^{99m}Tc) DTPA is a safe and simple method of studying the integrity of the renal parenchyma. A scan suggestive of a major kidney injury should be confirmed by selective renal angiography.

Nephrosonography may determine the presence of a nonvisualized kidney or monitor the magnitude of extravasation of blood or urine. In traumatized children who are brought in with shock, peritonitis or coma, these life-threatening situations take precedence, but once the child recovers sufficiently, a correct diagnosis of the underlying kidney injury should be established without delay, followed by a well-outlined plan of treatment.

TREATMENT.—The therapeutic complexities posed by children with renal injuries can be quite puzzling. The treatment hinges mainly on the type, extent and severity of the renal injury as well as the nature of the overall clinical situation in each particular case. For these reasons, only general guidelines can be suggested.

An orderly and thorough (multidisciplinary) diagnostic approach is a prerequisite for adequate decision making regarding therapeutic priorities.

Maintenance of lifesaving functions and control of serious complications should be the primary objectives. Attention to cope with any derangement in respiratory and cardiocirculatory functions by providing an adequate airway, control of hemorrhage, restoration of blood volume and prevention of shock and/or infection is mandatory. Surgical repair of the major visceral perforations, including kidney, ureter or bladder, as well as important cerebrospinal and vascular injuries is next in priority.

About 40% of patients with renal injuries have other injuries in the urinary tract or elsewhere. The liver and spleen frequently are involved.

The management of blunt renal trauma has been a controversial topic. The disagreement between proponents of expectant management and the advocates of immediate surgery has not produced any conclusive evidence as to which approach is associated with the best salvage of kidney function and fewest and least severe complications.

In blunt renal trauma, as a general rule, it pays to be as conservative as possible regardless of the severity of the presenting clinical picture. We agree with Peters and Bright's flow sheet for the management of blunt renal injuries (Fig. 17–3).

In cases of "major" renal injuries such as the comminuted kidney and avulsion of the renal pedicle, or in the multiple injury patient, surgical intervention usually is carried out at the earliest possible moment. Nephrectomy should not be done without evidence of a healthy contralateral kidney unless there is no other way to save life and plans for transplantation are set in motion.

Operative exploration is demanded when the child shows symptoms and signs of impending shock (falling blood pressure, increased pulse rate, perspiration, drop in hemoglobin and hematocrit) that cannot be prevented by the usual conservative measures such as bed rest, administration of plasma expanders, blood and angiotonic agents, fluid and electrolyte replacement and sedation. Operation is also indicated in children whose bladders become distended with clots that cannot be drawn out by bladder irrigation through a urethral catheter or by spontaneous voiding, or when there is evidence of a ruptured spleen or liver or of a bowel perforation. Finally, operation may be needed at some later date in children who fail to recover completely due to such complicating factors as perirenal hematoma, extravasated urine, recurrent severe kidney bleeding, large renal infarction, a painful, partly calcified retroperitoneal mass, cyst or abscess, an expanding aneurysm or the finding of a contracted kidney with hypertension.

With open injuries of the kidney, it should be remem-

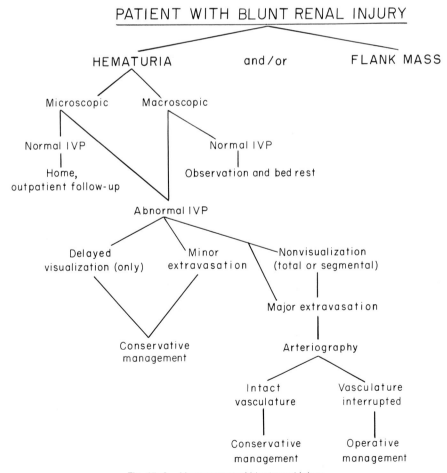

Fig. **17–3.**—Management of blunt renal injury.

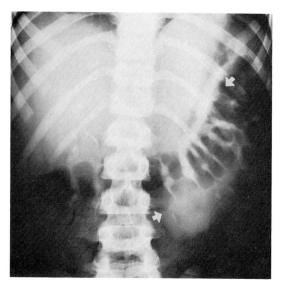

Fig. 17–4.—Renal injury. Enlargement of left kidney shadow with nephrogram *(arrows)* during intravenous pyelography. This kidney, with a small laceration causing extravasation of blood around it, recovered spontaneously and completely.

bered that some of these children may also require tetanus antitoxin.

From the practical standpoint, the management of a child with renal injury may fall in one of the following categories.

1. Children with slight or moderate degrees of renal injury, and without evidence of extra-urologic injuries. In this group nonoperative management is the treatment of choice (Figs. 17–4 and 17–5). The child should be placed on bed rest at least until the hematuria has ceased. He should receive antibiotics to prevent infection, analgesics and tranquilizers for sedation and good hydration. Intravenous administration of mannitol, particularly if there is bilateral renal trauma or extensive muscle trauma with minimal kidney involvement, can be added to the therapeutic regimen. Peritoneal dialysis or hemodialysis may also be necessary.

2. Children with *C* and *D* renal injuries (Fig. 17–2) should also, in principle, be treated conservatively, but as the clinical picture develops, under close vigilance and control, a good proportion of these children will require operative treatment. Whenever there is a suspicion of a concomitant intraperitoneal injury, it is wise to have a bowel expert and a vascular surgeon on the team to be ready to cope adequately with any problem that may be encountered. Maximal preservation of viable renal substance is the desideratum, although, at times, it is quite difficult to predict or to achieve.

3. Children with *H* renal injuries (Fig. 17–2) should be operated on without delay. Such renal injuries usually are associated with a large and tense perirenal hematoma as well as other intraperitoneal visceral injuries of variable severity and complexity. Nephrectomy usually is the treatment of choice, but, again, only after careful appraisal of the functional status of the contralateral kidney, adequate control of the major sources of bleeding, removal of the hematoma and thorough inspection and palpation of the injured kidney.

Traumatic injury of the renal artery occurs about 2 cm from its origin, mostly in the left renal artery, and is associated with intimal disruption. Levine and Hessl[40] have reported successful revascularization, after removal of the thrombus and repair of the intimal laceration, as late as 18 hours after the injury.

According to Javadpour *et al.*[31] and Morse *et al.*,[49] about 70–80% of children with renal trauma may be managed conservatively whereas the remaining 20–30% require surgical intervention and, of these, 5–7% undergo nephrectomy.

OPERATIVE TECHNIQUE.—Certain technical details in the surgical management of renal injuries need emphasis. One must secure control of the renal pedicle before Gerota's fascia with its enclosed and tense hematoma is entered. The exposure of both renal pedicles and control of further hemorrhage from the injured kidney are best achieved through a transperitoneal midline incision from xiphoid to pubis. This approach permits the repair or removal of the injured kidney, a thorough exploration of all intra-abdominal organs and the management of other visceral injuries encountered at operation. Early renal pedicle exposure with adequate control of the renal blood flow has considerably reduced the incidence of nephrectomy, often performed in haste for pro-

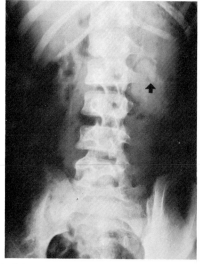
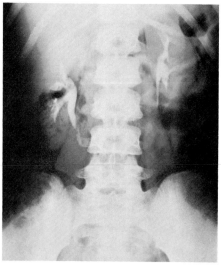

Fig. 17–5.—Renal injury. *Left,* intravenous pyelogram showing extravasation from the lower calix of the left kidney *(arrow)* following a blow to this area. There was blood in the urine. *Right,* a year later, after conservative treatment, the kidney secretes contrast medium normally and the lower calices are sharply defined, although more medial than usual.

fuse and uncontrollable bleeding. A bleeding kidney may have its vascular pedicle controlled and the kidney corpus wrapped in crushed ice until aortic, caval, splenic or other major bleeding is controlled. Renal arcuate arteries are individually ligated with 4-0 chromic catgut figure-of-8 sutures. Collecting system lacerations are repaired with running sutures of 4-0 or 5-0 chromic catgut. The denuded renal parenchyma is covered with previously reflected renal capsule, omental fat or any fatty tissue from the lumbar region. Once the renal injury has been repaired and the kidney repositioned, a portion of retroperitoneal fat is interposed between the lower renal pole and adjacent ureter in order to prevent any ureteral kink or secondary adhesions and ureteropelvic obstruction. Any collection (sanguineous, serohematic or urinary) is cultured and the renal fossa drained through the flank.

COMPLICATIONS.—Early complications of renal trauma include: secondary hemorrhage, urinary extravasation (urinomas), urinary ascites, shock, abscess formation and renal failure. They are likely to occur in the "conservatively" managed patient with major renal trauma. Delayed complications or sequelae are less common and their true incidence is not known, because of lack of any large prospective long-term studies. They include hypertension, stone formation, pararenal pseudohydronephrosis, renal pseudocysts with or without calcifications, segmental caliectasis, arteriovenous fistula, renal atrophy, urothorax and renointestinal fistulas. Obviously, the treatment of the delayed complications must be highly individualized. Harmful complications require correction whereas minor ones are best left undisturbed and evaluated periodically.

Ureteral Injuries

ETIOLOGY.—The ureter rarely is injured by blunt or penetrating trauma. Mertz et al.[46] reported ureteral injuries in 4% of children who sustained some form of renal trauma. The ureter may be compromised in blunt trauma by sudden hyperextension of the dorsolumbar spine or upward displacement of the kidney. Gunshot wounds occasionally may just "bruise" the ureteral wall or may partially or completely transect it. Iatrogenic ureteral injuries in children are seen much more rarely than in adults. Occasionally, a ureter may be cut during the removal of a large retroperitoneal tumor such as sympathicoblastoma or the ureter be perforated by a ureteral catheter. Again, a "pathologic" ureter (megaureter, retrocaval ureter, duplicated ureter, etc.) is far more vulnerable to injury than a normal one. Ureteral damage from high-energy radiation can result in fibrosis, with subsequent obstruction and hydroureteronephrosis.

DIAGNOSIS.—Not infrequently, patients with ureteral injuries remain asymptomatic or their urologic complaints are overshadowed by those of other injuries; they return some time later with malaise, fever, flank tenderness, abdominal distention, anuria, flank mass or urinary fistula. Infusion intravenous urogram with delayed pictures and ureteral tomography and, particularly, retrograde ureterography will confirm the diagnosis (Fig. 17–6). Here again, a broad-spectrum antibiotic should be mixed with the contrast medium. Ureterograms can be made with the ureteral catheter or with a plug-type catheter obstructing the lower end of the ureter through which contrast medium is injected. If the ureter has been ligated accidentally, the late dissolution of the suture may result in a urinary fistula at the suture site or in relief of the stricture.[28] Usually, however, the ureter will be obstructed and necrosis will occur at the site of the obstructing suture, with subsequent fistula formation.[61] Anuria following extensive abdominal operations always should suggest the possibility of bilateral occlusion of the ureters. Injuries to the ureter may drain into the peritoneal cavity, filling it with a mixture of blood and urine as in the case of renal injuries.

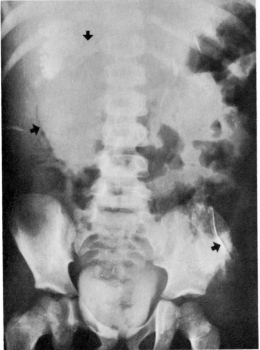
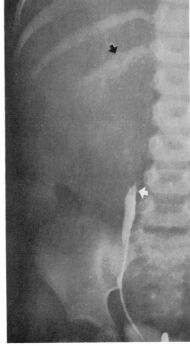

Fig. 17–6.—Ureteral trauma. X-rays of a 3½-year-old girl who was run over by a truck, sustaining fractures of the left iliac crest *(arrow)*, right twelfth rib *(arrow)* and rupture of ureter *(white arrow)*. There is large urinary extravasation below the right kidney with hydronephrosis *(arrow, left)*. The diaphragm was ruptured and the right side of the chest was full of urine. Nephrectomy with repair and drainage resulted in good recovery.

DIFFERENTIAL DIAGNOSIS.—Wound disruption often will cause a copious exudate that may be confused with urine. An increasing retroperitoneal extravasation of urine may cause symptoms and signs simulating peritonitis; and oliguria or anuria may raise the suspicion of kidney damage. Giving the patient a few tablets of methylene blue by mouth may clarify whether the wound drainage is urinary, and retrograde or intravenous pyelograms usually will show any injury to the ureter. Fistulas from ureter or bladder into the vagina are not as common in children as they are in adults, aside from the congenital circumstance of ectopic ureteral opening into the vagina or urethra.

TREATMENT.—The ureter should be repaired over a splint or T-tube as quickly as possible. If there is reason to suspect that the tissues will be friable or fragile or that infection will impair healing, an interval of 3–4 months should be permitted before the plastic repair is done. In these cases, the urine should be temporarily diverted above the injury. Minor injuries to the ureter usually will heal spontaneously with chemotherapy despite urinary extravasation. It is necessary to be sure that a ureteral catheter will pass freely up and down the ureter before conservative treatment can be advised. It is beneficial to leave a large-size ureteral catheter in the kidney pelvis for 4–5 days to permit the ureteral wound to seal over. Such catheters, however, usually fall out spontaneously and quickly. If the injury is discovered early, it may be repaired over a T-tube or splinting catheter with nephrostomy tube in place. If the lower end of the ureter is necrotic or cannot be made to reach the bladder, a full-thickness bladder flap can be rolled up into a tube to reach the lower end of the ureter (see Chap. 115). If the ureter will reach the bladder easily, it can be tunneled through the wall of the bladder obliquely for a distance of 2 or 3 cm to provide a valve-like connection (see Chap. 115). Such a tunneling operation must be done with great care because of the small size of the child's bladder. Anastomosis of the ureter to the bowel is to be discouraged in children in view of the poor long-term results. If the ureter will not reach the bladder, a segment of small intestine may also be used to splice out the length of the ureter.

Transureteroureterostomy and renal autotransplantation may also be attempted in selected cases. It should be emphasized that a ureter that has been "bruised" by a bullet or bony fragments may slough days or weeks later, and that a ureter lacerated or transected by a bullet has sustained more damage than actually can be seen at the time of emergency exploration. As a rule, both ends are refreshed for 1 cm beyond the edges of the visible damage before any form of anastomosis is undertaken.

Any attempt at proper leakproof and successful ureteral repair must include adequate preservation of blood supply, a tension-free suture line, proper alignment of both ureteral ends, "fat-padded" anastomosis and good drainage.

POSTOPERATIVE COURSE.—Most ureteral anastomoses do well postoperatively. Intravenous pyelograms and calibration of the site of anastomosis with cystoscopic catheters are desirable at intervals of 3–4 months for at least a year. This is done to be sure that the anastomosis remains patent. Occasionally fibrosis takes place around the ureter as a result of the extravasation of urine. If concomitant injuries to other organs overshadow the ureteral injury, insertion of a temporary nephrostomy tube is desirable and a ureteral splinting catheter may be run down the ureter at the time of implantation of the nephrostomy tube. The site of the extravasation can be drained through the flank at the time of nephrostomy. Broad-spectrum antibiotics usually are not indicated while the patient is having ureteral "splints" and urethral catheters. At this time, adequate suppressive therapy is recommended. Antibiotics should be used when all urinary tubes have been removed, starting the night before and according to the urine culture report and susceptibility test.

COMPLICATIONS.—Persistent urosepsis, stricture formation, fistulization and urolithiasis are the more common complications. They should be dealt with accordingly. However, removal of an infected, hydronephrotic, poorly

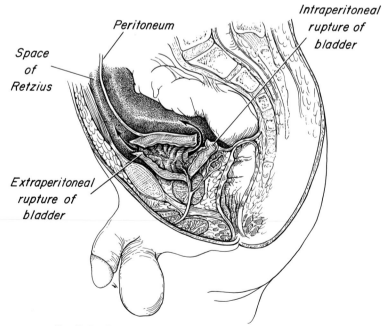

Fig. 17–7.—Bladder rupture, extraperitoneal and intraperitoneal.

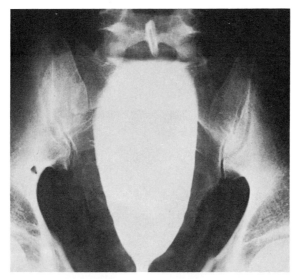

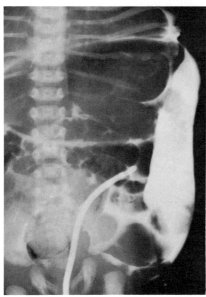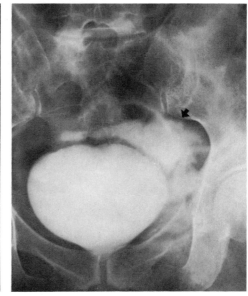

Fig. 17–8 (top).—Cystogram showing the bladder compressed from side to side, with apex elevated above the pubis and top flattened by peritoneal reflection. This is characteristic of a bladder compressed by perivesical hematoma or extravasation, as seen with fractures of the bony pelvis (near left acetabulum) or with extravasation from extraperitoneal rupture of bladder or urethra.

Fig. 17–9 (bottom, left).—With intraperitoneal rupture of the bladder, con-

trast medium from cystography may flow out freely to fill the peritoneal cavity, as in this child with a paper-thin bladder that ruptured spontaneously. There also was deficiency of the abdominal musculature.

Fig. 17–10 (bottom, right).—Intraperitoneal extravasation of contrast medium *(arrow)* following a blow on the full bladder in accident that also fractured the left upper pubic ramus.

functioning kidney, as a result of such complications, may be a better choice than another futile attempt at ureteral repair.

Bladder Injuries

The location of the bladder during infancy and childhood is abdominal rather than pelvic. Thus, it is covered largely by peritoneum and presents a greater risk of being damaged by generalized abdominal trauma. According to Mertz *et al.*,[46] bladder injuries are found concomitantly in about 3% of children with renal injuries.

ETIOLOGY.—Trauma to the bladder can be blunt or penetrating. Blows on the abdomen may cause rupture of the full bladder, with urinary extravasation, either extraperitoneally, when the rupture involves the bladder neck or lower half of the bladder, or intraperitoneally if the rupture takes place in the dome (Figs. 17–7 and 17–8).

Blunt trauma (falls, blows, kicks, crushing, etc.) severe enough to cause fractures of the pelvic bones is likely to produce bladder injury. The injury usually is caused by a sudden increase in intravesical pressure and/or by extrinsic compression or tearing by sharp bony spiculae. Penetrating wounds of the bladder (high-velocity missiles, stab wounds, falls on sharp objects, picket fences or bedposts) have been reported with wounds of entry in the lower abdomen, rectum or vagina.

Iatrogenic vesical injuries, usually in the form of a single perforation, do occur occasionally in the course of endoscopic manipulations and pelvic or inguinal operations (pelvic tumors, herniated bladders in infants). Spontaneous bladder rupture has been seen in children with bladder outlet obstruction and hugely distended, thin-walled bladder (prune bellies, hypotonic neurogenic bladders).

DIAGNOSTIC MEASURES.—Although the history of a blow on the abdomen or trauma to the pelvis will help with older children, younger children often are unable to give an accurate account of what happened, and a search for bruises, abrasions or ecchymoses must be made. There is a tendency to spasm of the abdominal muscles, with either intraperitoneal or extraperitoneal extravasations, but usually the spasm is not of the same hard consistency as with peritonitis unless the urine is infected. With intraperitoneal ruptures, the child does not void[62] and the abdomen becomes progressively distended, particularly after a day or two. Signs and symptoms of septic peritoneal irritation then may appear. A fluid wave can be elicited, and lateral films of the abdomen will show the intestines floating on the extravasated urine. Catheterization may produce large amounts of urine, particularly if the rent in the bladder wall is of large dimension. Cystograms with fairly large amounts of contrast medium (100–200 ml) mixed with an antibiotic will reveal the perforation. If large amounts of fluid are not used, plugs of omentum may prevent the laceration from opening up at the time of cystography. Retroperitoneal rupture may be followed by a surprising amount of soft induration around the bladder base, which can be felt on rectal examination. As this extravasation of blood and/or urine increases, it will compress the bladder from the sides until, on a cystogram, the bladder shadow becomes a long, narrow oval extending from the prostate area upward to the peritoneal reflection, where the shadow is flattened across the top (Fig. 17–8). The area of extravasation may show a ground-glass appearance. Cystograms usually are effective in indicating the diagnosis and often will show the entire peritoneal cavity (Fig. 17–9). The dilution of the contrast material sometimes makes it less clear than expected, and it should be kept in mind that only a faint shadow of the peritoneal cavity may be visible (Fig. 17–10). There may be a denser collection in the cul-de-sac. Cystoscopic examination may show a plug of omentum in the rent, which will have the characteristic refractile granular appearance of fat when seen through the cystoscope. At times, a spontaneous rupture of the urinary bladder may occur and is likely to produce a misleading clinical picture of low-grade peritonitis. Infusion excretory urography with tomography to check on the integrity of the upper urinary tracts as well as retrograde urethrography to exclude concomitant urethral injury are indicated.

TREATMENT.—Although a small extraperitoneal tear or laceration may be treated conservatively by urethral catheter drainage for 7–10 days, the majority of cases will require surgical exploration through a suprapubic midline incision. Shock and continued hemorrhage must be treated first, but operation almost always is necessary to evacuate the extravasation and to repair the rent. Extraperitoneal rents are not easily detected in some cases, but intraperitoneal rents are easily found when the bladder is opened. The peritoneum should also be opened and drained of urine. An intraperitoneal rent should be repaired both on the peritoneal surface and on the bladder surface, with rows of interrupted catgut sutures, using 00 plain catgut on the inside of the bladder and 00 chromic catgut on the outside of the bladder. Silk should not be used where it could be exposed to urine. A small cystostomy tube of the sump type (Freyer or Marion) is the safest, although Malecot catheters are used by some for suprapubic drainage during healing. It may be removed after 5 days and an indwelling urethral catheter used thereafter. Early surgical treatment combined with chemotherapy is eminently satisfactory in treating these injuries. If peritonitis and/or perivesical phlegmon is permitted to develop before operation is performed, the results are less predictable and lethal sepsis may result. If the patient is in precarious condition as a result of a bullet wound, exsanguinating hemorrhage, multiple fractures or other complicating factors, a sump-type drain should be placed quickly in the bladder, the vesical rent closed very superficially, the extravasation widely drained, the patient permitted to revive and definitive operation performed at some later date.

Intensive supportive treatment and postoperative chemotherapy are required.

Widely accepted principles for the management of a ruptured bladder include: (1) debridement of damaged tissue, (2) layered closure of the vesical defect with absorbable suture material, (3) drainage of the perivesical space, (4) urinary diversion, via a suprapubic catheter in most instances, and (5) prophylactic use of broad-spectrum antibiotics.

COMPLICATIONS.—Urosepsis, abscess formation, delayed hematuria, vesical calculi, periureteral fibrosis, vesicocutaneous fistulae, etc. may be encountered.

Urethral Injuries

Injuries to the posterior urethra in boys and girls frequently are the result of pelvic fractures produced by car accidents, falls, blows, etc.[37] This portion of the urethra is solidly fixed by the urogenital diaphragm in the pubic arch, so that any displacement of the pubic bones is likely to tear or avulse the underlying urethral segment. Posterior urethral injuries produced by instrumentation at the time of cystoscopy, catheterization or sounding are seen occasionally.

Anterior urethral injuries as a result of blunt trauma most frequently are caused by the straddle type of injury. The bulbar urethral segment in boys and the juxtameatal portion of the urethra in girls are those usually affected.

DIAGNOSIS.—Posterior urethral injury should be suspected when the child presents with a pelvic fracture and

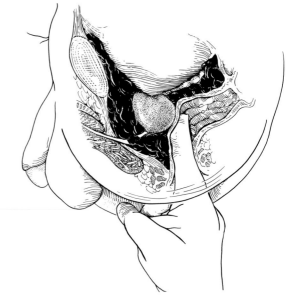

Fig. 17–11.—Complete rupture of posterior urethra. Rectal digital examination discloses a tender, boggy mass in the place occupied by the prostate, which sometimes is palpable, but in a higher position, and movable.

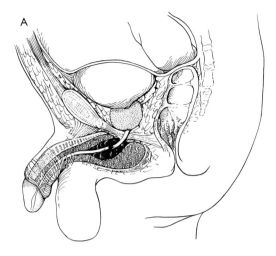

Fig. 17–12.—**A,** rupture of bulbar urethra with periurethral bleeding and hematoma formation. **B,** rupture of urethra and corpora cavernosa with large / hematoma formation extending under Colles' fascia and involving the lower abdominal wall, penis, scrotum and perineum.

urinary retention or is voiding with difficulty and passing blood per urethram. A distended bladder and a soft, fluctuant pelvic mass usually are palpable by rectal digital examination[11] (Fig. 17–11). Even when the bony fragments have again resumed their normal position, it must be assumed that at the moment of fracture there was some displacement and the urethra may have been traumatized. This is also true if one of the sacroiliac joints has been dislocated by the trauma. Usually, the extravasation of blood and urine is upward into the periprostatic and perivesical space, producing an x-ray deformity similar to that seen with extraperitoneal rupture of the bladder (Fig. 17–8). If trauma is very severe, blood and urine may leak downward and appear in the scrotum or layers of the perineum (Fig. 17–12). Infection is somewhat more likely to occur in this area because the urethra may contain organisms, even in children. Drainage and urinary diversion, therefore, are also important for this injury.[16]

After urethral laceration, a drop or two of blood usually appears at the meatus, unassociated with urination. If the patient attempts to urinate, a swelling may appear in the perineum or scrotum and urine may fail to appear at the meatus. Leakage into the periurethral tissues may occur even though most of the urine does come through the penis, in the case of small lacerations of the urethra. Suprapubic bulging and tenderness may be present on palpation, due both to the extravasation and to any fractures of the pelvis. A plain film of the abdomen should be taken to see whether there is any ground-glass appearance of the tissues in the pelvis to suggest extravasation. Catheterization should be attempted with a Foley catheter of appropriate size. If it will pass into the bladder, enough isotonic contrast medium to fill the normal child's bladder, mixed with antibiotic, should be instilled. If the catheter will not pass, contrast medium should be instilled into the urethra for the purpose of getting a urethrogram to locate the exact site of the injury and its extent,

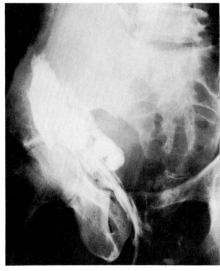

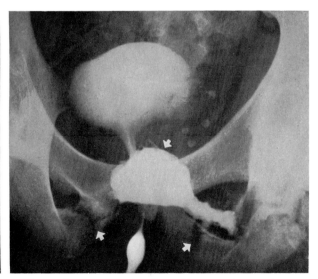

Fig. 17–13 (left).—Extravasation of contrast medium upward around the bladder from a rupture of the posterior urethra by an instrument that created a false passage up under the bladder.
Fig. 17–14 (right).—Contrast medium from a urethrogram leaking out into / a large pocket where the urethra was cut across *(upper arrow)* by a bullet that fractured both pubic bones *(lower arrows)*. Note that the contrast medium is running out into the fracture site through the tract caused by the bullet.

as described above. Fistulous tracts may be seen leading toward the fracture sites or perforating injuries (Fig. 17–14). Complications may occur in the form of late hemorrhage, abscess, urethral stricture at the injury site and, later, sexual impotence.

TREATMENT.—If a urethral catheter that is appropriate for the size of the child's urethra can be passed into the bladder, this, plus chemotherapy and the drainage of any obvious extravasation, usually will be sufficient. Such a catheter should

be left in place for 21–30 days. If a catheter or sound will not pass, the urethra must be exposed and both ends of the urethra approximated either by traction on a Foley catheter (if one can be introduced) or by suture of the laceration. Immediate surgical procedures usually are difficult, as they are complicated by massive hemorrhage, the presence of extravasated urine and pronounced edema of the tissues. As a consequence, most cases are treated by cystostomy and the passage of sounds or catheters down from above or in both directions simultaneously, until the tips of the two in-

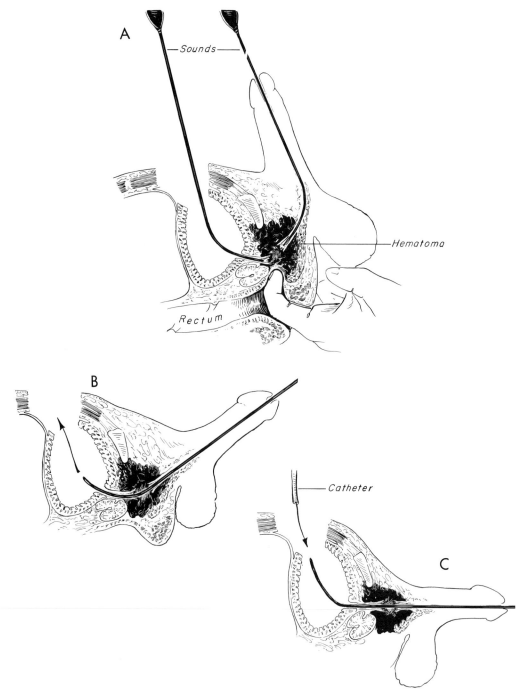

Fig. 17–15.—Method for treating complete transection of the bulbous urethra by passage of sounds in through both ends of the urethra toward the site of injury. **A–C,** the tips of the two sounds usually can be clicked together in the perineal hematoma and the lower one guided to the upper one so that it can be brought up through the proximal portion of the urethra into the bladder. *(Continued.)*

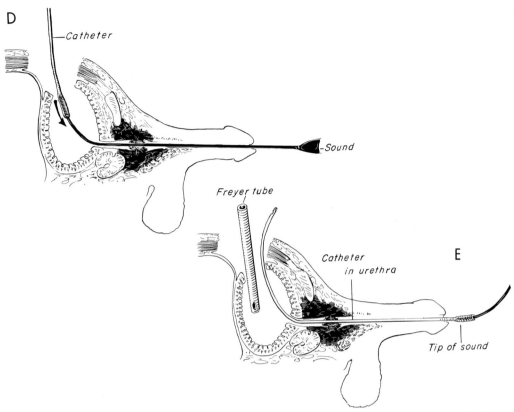

Fig. 17–15 (cont.).–D and **E,** a small catheter can be pressed tightly over the tip of the sound, then drawn antegrade through the urethra and the injured area, to act as a splint around which the torn urethra can heal in continuity. Special instruments have been devised to make this maneuver easier, but they usually are not necessary.

struments can be brought together and one guided up through by the other. A catheter then is threaded down through the injury site and left as a splint (Fig. 17–15). If a Foley catheter can be introduced from below, the bulb can be inflated within the bladder so that gentle traction can be exerted on the bladder neck to pull it downward to join the severed lower end of the urethra. The traction should be left on approximately 3 days, after which it can be released and the catheter now used as a splint. Drains should be placed at the site of the extravasation and left in place for 5–7 days. The area of extravasation and hematoma should be thoroughly impregnated with antibacterial agents such as dilute neomycin-bacitracin solution. The splinting catheter should be left in the urethra for 3–4 weeks if there is some assurance that the urethral ends have been brought close together. When there is doubt as to the accurate approximation of urethral stumps, the catheter should be left in for 6 weeks. Chemotherapy according to the specific sensitivity of the organisms recovered from culture is advisable during the early stages of convalescence. After the drains are out and the patient is afebrile, the chemotherapy can be withdrawn until the day when the catheter is removed. At that time, it should be resumed with a broad-spectrum antibacterial agent and, thereafter, monthly urine cultures should be done until the urine remains sterile.

All patients who have had severe urethral trauma will tend to develop strictures of the urethra to some degree at the site of the scar or repair (Fig. 17–16). Thus, periodic dilations of the urethra must be carried out with great faithfulness in the weeks or months after the indwelling catheter is removed. Intensive treatment to rid the patient of chronic urinary infection is essential after the catheter is removed. According to Malek,[2] early urinary diversion and urethral realignment has yielded better results than urinary diversion and later repair of the urethral stricture. Scar tissue may impair the function of the urethral sphincter and impotence may also be a complication. Severe strictures may follow and possibly may require subsequent urethroplasty of the Johanson,[32] Lapides,[39] Turner-Warwick[71] or Waterhouse[74] type. Slight extravasation during transurethral resection of the bladder neck in children does not usually require cystostomy and can be treated with an indwelling urethral catheter and adequate chemotherapy unless fever, abdominal distention and paralytic ileus occur.

COMPLICATIONS.—The sequelae of posterior urethral injuries, especially in boys, may be quite severe, indeed the beginning of a lifelong tragedy.[42] Urethral strictures, periurethral fibrosis, urinary incontinence, penile erectile impotence and infertility may appear regardless of the type and timing of the surgical technique used. Parents must be informed and forewarned of these complications, lest they later blame them on the surgeon.

Injuries to the Penis

The skin, fascial coverings and corpora of the penis in infants and children may be injured by a variety of causes. For instance, penoscrotal injuries in the newborn inflicted during breech delivery have been reported by Nielson *et al.*[51]

Children will occasionally insert the penis through a metal washer or ring, or mothers may tie a string, thread or hair around the penis in an attempt to improve urinary con-

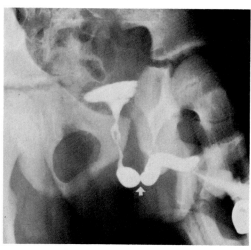

Fig. 17–16.—Strictures such as that shown by the arrow usually occur at the site of injuries to the urethra and must be dilated persistently until they stay open permanently.

trol. Subsequent edema of the foreskin may make it difficult to find the constricting band and to differentiate it from paraphimosis. The tight portion of the foreskin should be slit dorsally to relieve the obstruction, and in the course of doing so any obstructing band usually will be found. Occasionally, the glans penis may be amputated during circumcision or overvigorous attempts to relieve the chordee accompanying hypospadias. In these cases, little can be done other than to relieve the stenosis of the meatus that may follow and to attempt to reconstruct a structure resembling a new foreskin from the skin of the shaft of the penis. This will conceal the loss of the glans. In these cases, it sometimes is desirable to give gonadotropic hormone at the rate of 500 units every other day for 6 weeks to children over 5 years of age. This will cause the penis to enlarge greatly and will make plastic revision of the penis easier. It may also enlarge any remnant of glans to some degree. At puberty, the structure will enlarge considerably more.

Avulsion of the skin of the penis may occur if it is caught in moving machinery, such as a washing machine.[3, 24, 25] Profuse bleeding may occur, requiring evacuation of hematomas. The penis may be tunneled under the skin of the thigh until the skin has "taken." The penis then may be released and the skin used to cover the denuded shaft. Occasionally, the shifting of skin from other sites may be necessary to increase the length or size of the phallus. If the corpora or the urethra is lacerated, the remnants should be meticulously sutured and washed with antibacterial solutions.

Since the blood supply to this area is good, healing may follow even severe trauma.

Mild contusions can be treated by local application of an ice bag, by bed rest and occasionally by temporary urethral drainage. When the foreskin has been caught in the zipper of the child's pants, the zipper is to be cut away from the pants and one proceeds immediately with circumcision. Penile fracture and dislocation should be reduced with evacuation of extravasation, repair of the lacerated corpora and provision of temporary drainage of the bladder via an indwelling urethral catheter.[26]

Partially or completely amputated penises have been successfully reanastomosed at various levels and following periods of ischemia up to 6 hours.

Complications of penile injury include urethral stricture,

ventral chordee, penile shortening, gangrene and sexual impotence.

Scrotal Injuries

Avulsion of the skin of the scrotum may occur if the child's genitalia are caught in machinery.[68] In this case, the testes, if unharmed, may be inserted into pouches under the skin of the thighs and this skin raised at a later date to make a new scrotum. If any remnant of the scrotal skin remains, it may be possible to stretch it into a fairly good scrotum at some later date. Here again, the administration of gonadotropic hormones at the rate of 500 units every other day for 6 weeks will cause a distinct increase in the size of the scrotal sac, the skin of which then may be useful for making a new scrotum.

Injuries to the Testes

The testes and their appendages usually are spared from serious injury because they are highly mobile structures within the scrotal sac.

ETIOLOGY.—Blunt trauma to the testes may result from falling astride a solid object, kicks, blows or pinching. Testicular rupture usually is caused by a severe direct blow that traps the testes against the pubis or the thighs. The resultant hematocele contains, at times, fragments of the testicular substance.

DIAGNOSIS AND TREATMENT.—Testicular injury usually is accompanied by severe nausea, testicular pain and epigastric discomfort. Vomiting may also be present. A large, tender scrotal mass usually is present. The testes and adnexa may be visible through an avulsed scrotum. The possibility of underlying testicular tumor, torsion of the spermatic cord, epididymitis, etc. must be borne in mind. Bed rest with an icebag over the traumatized part is indicated if the injury has just occurred, but after the first 12 hours, warmth usually is more comfortable and more effective in reducing the swelling. Laceration of the testes may cause hematocele, which may require evacuation if painful. Lacerations usually will stop bleeding spontaneously. Most of the blood vessels of the testis run immediately under the surface of the tunica albuginea, and suture ligatures applied to the margins of the laceration should include the vessels just beneath the surface of the tunica albuginea near the bleeding point. Thus, the bleeding can be stopped with a minimal disturbance of the remaining testicular tissue. If a testis is partly removed by the injury, the remainder of the testis should be left undisturbed whenever possible, since there is some hope that it may survive. Cold compresses applied to the area may reduce the metabolism of the tissue sufficiently to permit the remaining testis to survive. If the tunica albuginea can be sutured together over the broken end of the testis, this may help it to seal off and resume at least some endocrine function. If the testis continues to slough, it always can be removed later.

Because of the activity of the cremaster reflex in children, the testes may be·pulled up into the inguinal canals at the time of injury and become fixed there because of the formation of scar tissue in the adjacent areas. Operation may be required to get the testes back into the scrotum or into a newly constructed scrotum. Even an atrophic remnant of testis may have endocrine function and is worth preserving. Undescended testes and testes ectopically placed are vulnerable to local injury or to spontaneous torsion with subsequent infarction.

REFERENCES

1. Alyea, E. P.: Upper urinary tract injury, Urologists' Correspondence Club Letter, Nov. 9, 1949.
2. Aschner, P. W.: Accidental injury to ureters and bladder in pelvic surgery, J. Urol. 69:774, 1953.
3. Baxter, H., et al.: Complete avulsion of skin of penis and scrotum; surgical, endocrinologic and psychologic treatment, Plast. Reconstr. Surg. 4:508, 1949.
4. Bonner, C. D., et al.: Local injections of hydrocortisone as a new and effective treatment for strictures of the urethra and meatus, N. Engl. J. Med. 253:130, 1955.
5. Boone, T. B., Jr.: Traumatic lesions of the urogenital tract, Tex. J. Med. 55:749, 1959.
6. Brown, W. E., and Sutherland, C. G.: The repair of ureteral injuries: Experimental studies, clinical application, and review of the literature, Am. J. Obstet. Gynecol. 77:862, 1959.
7. Bunton, G. L.: Intraperitoneal rupture of the bladder in a child, Postgrad. Med. J. 28:117, 1952.
8. Burghele, T.: Traumatic lesions of the urinary tract secondary to urologic investigations, Rumanian Med. Rev. 9:41, 1965.
9. Campbell, M. F.: Urogenital Injuries, in Urology (2d ed.; Philadelphia: W. B. Saunders Company, 1963), Vol. III, Chap. 43.
10. Carlton, C. E., and Scott, R.: Penetrating renal injuries: An analysis of 100 cases, J. Urol. 84:599, 1960.
11. Constantian, H. M., and Felton, L. M.: Separation of the urethra from the bladder due to fracture of the pelvis, J. Urol. 68:823, 1952.
12. Cullen, T. H.: Avulsion of the skin of the penis and scrotum, Br. J. Urol. 38:99, 1966.
13. Culp, D. A., et al.: Experiences with the Johanson-Denis Brown technique of urethroplasty, J. Urol. 77:446, 1957.
14. Da Motta-Pacheco, A. A.: Orquiepididimite traumatica, Rev. Paul. Med. 41:335, 1952.
15. De la Pena, A., et al.: Cistoperineoplastia tubular intraesfinteriana en el hombre, Cir. Ginecol. Urol. 11:467, 1957.
16. Deweerd, J. H.: Management of injuries to the bladder, urethra and genitalia, Surg. Clin. North Am. 39:973, 1959.
17. Edmondson, H. T., et al.: Pneumoperitoneum: A rare sign of urinary bladder rupture, Am. Surg. 30:721, 1964.
18. Fish, G. W.: Complete evulsion of the urinary bladder, Urologists' Correspondence Club Letter, June 27, 1961.
19. Fontaine, R., et al.: Selective angiography in blunt trauma to kidney, J. Chir. 91:31, 1966.
20. Forbes, K. A.: Appendico-vesical fistula, Ann. Surg. 160:801, 1964.
21. Forsythe, W. E., and Persky, L.: Comparison of ureteral and renal injuries, Am. J. Surg. 97:558, 1959.
22. Fraley, E. E., and Halverstadt, D. B.: Unsuspected Wilms' tumor: Dangers in the conservative therapy of renal trauma, N. Engl. J. Med. 275:373, 1966.
23. Gausa Raspall, P., and Gausa Rull, P.: Traumatismos del pene, Ann. Inst. Corachan 16:92, 1964.
24. Gelb, J., et al.: Total reconstruction of the penis. A review of the literature and report of a case. Plast. Reconstr. Surg. 24:62, 1959.
25. Goodwin, W. E., and Thelen, H. M.: Plastic reconstruction of penile skin: Implantation of the penis into the scrotum, JAMA 144:384, 1950.
26. Gross, M., Arnold, T. L., and Waterhouse, K.: Fracture of the penis: Rationale of surgical management, J. Urol. 106:708, 1971.
27. Harrow, B. R.: Strangulation of penis by a hidden thread, JAMA 199:135, 1967.
28. Hinman, F., Jr.: Recovery of renal function after ureteral deligation, AMA Arch. Surg. 78:518, 1959.
29. Hodges, C. V., et al.: Renal trauma: A study of 71 cases, J. Urol. 66:627, 1951.
30. Irvine, R. O. H.: Renal failure after trauma, N. Z. Med. J. 64:321, 1965.
31. Javadpour, N., Guinan, P., and Bush, I. M.: Renal trauma in children, Surg. Gynecol. Obstet. 136:237, 1973.
32. Johanson, B.: Reconstruction of the male urethra in strictures, Acta Chir. Scand. (supp.) 176:5, 1953.
33. Joubert, J. N.: Injuries to the urethra, S. Afr. J. Med. Sci. 32:919, 1958.
34. Kaiser, T. F.: Immediate management of injuries of the lower urinary tract, Hosp. Med. 3(No. 2):53, 1967.
35. Kaiser, T. F., and Farrow, F. C.: Injury of the bladder and prostatomembranous urethra associated with fracture of the bony pelvis, Surg. Gynecol. Obstet. 120:99, 1965.
36. Kenyon, H. R., and Hyman, R. M.: Total autoemasculation. Report of three cases, JAMA 151:207, 1953.
37. Kisner, C. D.: Injuries of the urethra, with special reference to those occurring in fractures of the pelvis, S. Afr. J. Med. Sci. 32:1105, 1958.
38. Knappenberger, S. T., et al.: Complete avulsion of the renal pedicle by non-penetrating trauma, with survival, J. Urol. 89:316, 1963.
39. Lapides, J.: Simplified modification of Johanson urethroplasty for strictures of deep bulbous urethra, J. Urol. 82:115, 1959.
40. Levine, E. F., and Hessl, J. M.: Renal artery occlusion following blunt abdominal trauma, J. Urol. 112:553, 1974.
41. Lipshutz, H.: Ureteral injuries during abdominal and pelvic surgery: T-tube splinting in ureteroneocystostomy, J. Urol. 81:728, 1959.
42. Malek, R. S.: Genito-Urinary Trauma, in Kelalis, P. P., King, L. R., and Belman, A. M. (eds.), Clinical Pediatric Urology (Philadelphia: W. B. Saunders Company, 1976).
43. McCrea, L. E.: Rupture of the testicle, J. Urol. 66:270, 1951.
44. McKay, H. W., et al.: Management of the injured kidney, JAMA 141:575, 1949.
45. Mertz, H. O.: Injury of the kidney in children, J. Urol. 69:39, 1953.
46. Mertz, J. H., Wishard, W. N., Jr., Nourse, M. H., et al.: Injury of the kidney in children, JAMA 183:730, 1963.
47. Moir, J. C.: Vesicovaginal fistula caused by wedge resection of bladder neck, Br. J. Surg. 53:102, 1966.
48. Morgan, A.: Traumatic dislocation of the testis, Br. J. Surg. 52:669, 1965.
49. Morse, T. S., Smith, J. P., Howard, W. H. R., et al.: Kidney injuries in children, J. Urol. 98:539, 1967.
50. Nation, E. F., and Massey, D.: Renal trauma: Experience with 258 cases, J. Urol. 89:775, 1963.
51. Nielson, H. K., Ferris, D. O., and Logan, G. B.: Injury of the penis, scrotum and buttocks of the newborn resulting in gangrene, Am. J. Dis. Child. 75:85, 1948.
52. Ormond, J. K., and Fairey, P. W.: Urethral rupture at apex of the prostate, JAMA 149:15, 1952.
53. Parkhurst, E., and Landsteiner, E. K.: Management of renal trauma, Surg. Gynecol. Obstet. 105:393, 1957.
54. Peltier, L.: Complications of pelvic fractures, Hosp. Med., p. 88, April, 1967.
55. Persky, L., and Joelson, J. J.: Spontaneous rupture of renal pelvis secondary to a small ureteral calculus, J. Urol. 72:141, 1954.
56. Powers, J. H., et al.: The traumatic rupture of the posterior urethra, N. Y. J. Med. 32:1188, 1932.
57. Prather, G. C., and Kaiser, T. F.: The bladder in fracture of bony pelvis: Significance of the "tear-drop bladder" as shown by cystogram, J. Urol. 63:1019, 1950.
58. Reid, R. E., and Herman, J. R.: Rupture of the bladder and urethra: Diagnosis and treatment, N. Y. J. Med. 65:2685, 1965.
59. Reisman, D. D., et al.: Early deligation of the ureter, J. Urol. 78:363, 1957.
60. Rieser, C.: Diagnostic evaluation of suspected genitourinary tract injury, JAMA 199:124, 1967.
61. Rieser, C., and Edmond, N.: Diagnosis of bladder rupture, J. Urol. 90:53, 1963.
62. Rexford, W. K.: Rupture of the bladder and acute retention of urine, Am. J. Surg. 46:641, 1939.
63. Robbins, J. J.: Injuries of the testicle, J. Ky. Med. Assoc. 69:747, 1961.
64. Sargent, J. C., and Marquardt, C. R.: Renal injuries, J. Urol. 63:1, 1950.
65. Selikowitz, S.: Aspects of genitourinary trauma, Cook County Hosp. & Hektoen Inst. Med. Res., Chicago.
66. Smith, M. J. V., Seidel, R. F., and Bonacarti, A. F.: Accident trauma to the kidneys in children, J. Urol. 96:845, 1966.
67. Staubitz, W. J., et al.: Management of ureteral injuries, JAMA 171:1296, 1959.
68. Sutton, L. E.: Reconstruction following complete avulsion of the skin of the penis and scrotum: Report of a case, N. Y. J. Med. 43:2279, 1943.
69. Thompson, I. M., et al.: The acute abdomen of unrecognized bladder rupture, Arch. Surg. 90:371, 1965.
70. Todd, A. A. D.: Genitourinary complications of blunt pelvic trauma, Can. J. Surg. 7:43, 1964.
71. Turner-Warwick, R. T.: The management of traumatic urethral strictures and injuries, Br. J. Surg. 60:775, 1973.
72. Villanueva, A.: Invagination technique for urethral reconstruction, Arch. Pathol. 70:253, 1955.
73. Wasko, R., and Goldstein, A. G.: Traumatic rupture of the testicle, J. Urol. 95:721, 1966.
74. Waterhouse, K., Abrahams, J. I., Gruber, H., et al.: Transpubic approach to lower urinary tract, J. Urol. 109:486, 1973.
75. Waterhouse, K., and Gross, M.: Trauma to the genito-urinary

tract: Five year experience with 251 cases, J. Urol. 101:241, 1969.

76. Watkins, J. P., *et al.:* Traumatic severance of renal pedicle without death, J. Urol. 98:167, 1967.

77. Winstead, G. A.: Infarct of the testicle: Report of three cases, J.

Urol. 69:830, 1953.

78. Wishard, W. N., Jr.: Surgical injuries of the ureter and bladder, J. Urol. 73:1009, 1955.

79. Zufall, R.: Traumatic avulsion of the upper ureter, J. Urol. 85: 246, 1961.

18 J. Donald McQueen

Trauma to the Central Nervous System

HISTORY.—Trephining ranks as one of the earliest of surgical procedures, well documented by the existence of a large number of perforated prehistoric skulls. The supply is particularly great in Peru, but specimens have been found in numerous parts of the world. Many authorities believe that trauma constituted one of the common indications.[7, 8, 11, 21]

The other lines of evidence for early craniectomies come from the depictions of pre-Inca Peruvian ceramics and from the Hippocratic writings, which emphasize the need for prophylactic trephining and also for craniectomies for certain skull fractures. The indications do not match those of current practice.[10] Celsus (A.D. 34) and his contemporaries advocated removal of depressed bone.[4] Much later, Rhazes directed attention to the compression of the brain in contradistinction to emphasis on the state of the overlying bone.[21]

Comparatively little was added during the Middle Ages, the Renaissance and through the time of the Napoleonic wars. Most trauma surgery was performed in the military sphere and major interest was directed to open wounds with depressed and penetrating bone. Exceptional surgeons such as Percival Pott and Charles Bell recognized the significance of progressive stupor and trephined the intact skull for intracranial blood collections. These procedures must have been performed very infrequently, and Godlee, for example, recorded the performance of only 1 craniectomy in the University College Hospital, London, in 1857.[20]

The decade of enlightenment for neurosurgery came between 1860 and 1870. This emphasis excludes the obvious importance of the advances in anesthesia, which came before, and the introduction of diagnostic studies, which came later, but it stresses the relatively short period when enormous advances were made in three pertinent areas. Development of accurate knowledge of cerebral localization was marked by Broca's 1861 paper on the mapping of motor speech in the second and third left frontal convolutions.[2] Hughlings Jackson's detailed scrutiny of clinical seizure activity was inaugurated by a paper in the same year and he soon was able to localize the motor cortex and other areas on the basis of clinical phenomena.[12-14] Fritsch and Hitzig utilized direct electrical stimulation in 1870 to demonstrate and map the motor cortex of the dog.[6] The second important advance was antisepsis, with the appearance of Lister's fundamental work in 1867.[18] The third significant area is less obvious—appreciation of certain signs of intracranial hypertension and brain compression. The major effort was made by Leyden, who, in 1866, described in detail many of the effects of extradural balloon compression in the dog.[17] These included slowing of the cardiac rate, respiratory irregularities and dilatation of the pupil. He mentioned pressor responses 35 years before Cushing's report.

These developments appeared to have little impact on practice at the time of the Franco-Prussian War in 1870.[8] However, Macewen was able to diagnose a frontal lobe abscess and to localize and operate on a dural tumor and a subdural hematoma in this next decade, guided by the neurologic changes. He thus relied on more than that mental faculty described by Jefferson as a "surgeon's instinct" and inaugurated the modern neurosurgical era.[15] The exact time of this change was 1876—the year of Macewen's first case. It is of note that a significant part of his early work in this field was directed to the care of trauma cases.[16] Three of the 7 patients in his early series harbored intracranial hematomas and were seen prior to the times of Godlee's celebrated glioma resection.

Caveness[3] recently has discussed the incidence of acute head injuries in the United States for the year 1974. He notes a total of 8 million head injuries (or 13.7% of all trauma) and 1.9 million serious injuries (or 3.2% of total trauma). The latter category includes: concussion, skull fracture, intracranial hemorrhage, cerebral laceration and other intracranial injury. Childhood head injury victims constitute a very significant proportion of this number of nearly 2 million. Many of the clinical and pathologic aspects are shared with the adult group; however, dissimilarities are prominent. Three of the most striking distinguishing features are: the special circumstance of birth injury, the amazing resiliency of the young brain and the common absence of alcoholism as a potentiating factor. It is convenient to subdivide pediatric head trauma into three periods: later childhood, at birth and during infancy.

Management in the Emergency Room

Primary attention always is given to maintenance of a free airway. This may simply require positioning of the tongue or jaw, although tracheal intubations (or rarely tracheostomies) are needed with more serious injuries. Bronchial secretions often accumulate and occasionally pulmonary edema is found. The mouth, pharynx and tracheobronchial tree are, accordingly, suctioned assiduously. Vomiting and aspiration of gastric contents are common, and a nasogastric tube is to be passed and the stomach emptied.

The second consideration is hypovolemic shock. Signs of shock point to associated injuries and are not due to head injury, with the exception of terminal or near-terminal states in brainstem lesions, extensive scalp injuries with great external hemorrhage and perhaps the extradural hematoma of infancy. Associated injuries occur in about one third of serious head trauma cases, and such lesions as retroperitoneal hematomas and ruptured spleens are not rare. They may be difficult to diagnose in the unconscious patient. The control of hemorrhage, such as that from a ruptured spleen, will be given priority over neurosurgical procedures, although, in rare instances, trephine openings may be placed at the time of laparotomy.

An intravenous line is placed immediately for the administration of 5% dextrose or Ringer's lactate solution and blood is replaced as required. Inappropriate ADH secretion may occur with head injury as with other trauma, and may lead to dilutional hyponatremia and water intoxication, especially when large amounts of fluids are given because of associated injuries. Most of these complications can be prevented with care, and blood samples should be withdrawn for electrolyte determinations promptly and repeatedly. A fluid balance chart should be initiated for the careful recording of intake and output.

A special effort should be made in the Emergency Room to obtain a detailed account of the injury from witnesses. Knowledge of the prior status of the patient is as important as, for instance, the existence of a seizure disorder. Similarly, knowledge of the sequence of events after the accident is of great significance. Progressive deterioration in the state of consciousness is a strong inducement to operative intervention. The presence or absence of a lucid interval should be ascertained, although this is less common in the presence of an extradural hematoma in childhood than in later life. These points are fundamental in patient management and are stressed because the search for pertinent information in the Emergency Room commonly is deficient.

The physical examination should be carried out quickly. The points to be stressed in the neurologic component are evaluations of: (1) the state of consciousness, (2) vital signs, (3) pupillary size and reactivity, (4) lateralizing motor changes and (5) other evidence of altered brainstem function.

A change in the state of awareness is the pre-eminent sign. It seldom is misleading, although patients with mass lesions may improve temporarily as the brain accommodates to the pressure from a hematoma or during the relaxation phase of a cerebrospinal fluid pressure wave. It is important to document clearly the level of responsiveness and to avoid the unqualified use of such a term as coma. With severe injuries, it is also essential to start a coma chart and to carefully document the effect of verbal and painful stimuli, the presence of spontaneous motion and other pertinent data, noted below.

Alterations in the vital signs are of special importance. Bradycardia is one indication of intracranial hypertension that will prominently influence the neurosurgeon. However, physiologic slowing of the pulse should be considered, and contusions at the base of the brain will also induce this change in the absence of a mass lesion. The systemic blood pressure will tend to rise. Respiratory changes are varied and are incompletely understood. The Cheyne-Stokes respiratory pattern points to a deep hemispheral or diencephalic lesion and possibly to transtentorial herniation. It is also found with posterior fossa lesions. Slow and labored breathing appears with herniation from above and with direct pressure below the tentorium. Ataxic respiration occurs with lesions of the posterior fossa and neurogenic hyperventilation accompanies tegmental disturbances. All indicate a state that demands immediate action.

Dilatation of a pupil and an impaired response to light point to uncal herniation and an excellent chance for a mass, such as a large hematoma. Local trauma and pre-existing disease must be considered. The pupillary change usually will match the site of the lesion; however, false localization is found in 15–20% of cases.

Motor responses are important in many ways. One of the most obvious is the opportunity to establish lateralizing findings. These may be detected by analyzing spontaneous movement or by the response to pain. Hemiparesis is a valuable lateralization sign, although an expanding lesion may be on the same side as the motor loss if the brainstem is displaced so that contralateral motor fibers are compressed at the unyielding tentorial edge.

Other tests for brainstem function, of limited use in the Emergency Room setting, are carried out in certain instances and particularly at those times when one is concerned with the presence of an irreversible lesion. The stimulus for the oculocephalic reflex or doll's head phenomenon is rapid head turning; the normal response is a contraversive conjugate deviation. Caloric stimulation is applied with ice water irrigation of the external auditory canal in the presence of an intact tympanic membrane. Nystagmus is normally induced with the rapid component to the opposite side. The slow phase is manifested by sustained deviation to the side of syringing. Its retention is a hopeful prognostic sign in the unconscious patient. The corneal reflexes are among the last responses to disappear with progression.

The scalp is carefully examined for signs of local injury and may have to be shaved. Open wounds are meticulously examined and cerebrospinal fluid leaks looked for.

Three general courses of action are available after the initial examination and treatment. In desperate situations, because of deep unresponsiveness and the other changes noted above, one may go directly to the Operating Room in search of an intracranial hematoma. This decision is made reluctantly and only when the situation warrants the risk of abandoning standard diagnostic tests. It usually is wise to obtain skull films on the way to the Operating Room.

In the second group of children, major concern exists regarding the presence of a surgical lesion, and the data at hand indicate that time is available for a definitive diagnostic study. Skull and cervical spine films are made, followed by either arteriography or CT (computerized tomography) scanning. The latter technique is becoming increasingly popular for the demonstration of intracranial blood deposits, edema and other lesions. Head immobilization has been a major problem with the restless child. However, recent advances permit a scanning time of less than 10 seconds, which increases the likelihood of successful examination.

Several CT scans are shown in Figures 18–1 to 18–8. An external hematoma is shown in Figure 18–1 and bilateral subdural hygromas are indicated in Figure 18–2. These are examples of conditions in which the selection of a site for a bur hole or craniectomy is facilitated by the scan. Depressed fractures are shown in Figure 18–3, a brilliant demonstration of the site of a deep bony spicule. Figure 18–4 illustrates a large area of contused brain with hematoma and

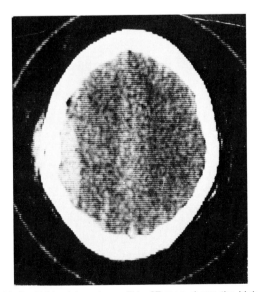

Fig. 18–1.—Epidural hematoma. This CT scan shows the high-density lesion to the left.

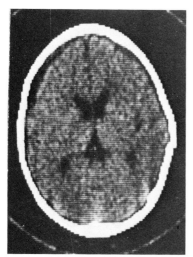

Fig. 18–2.—Subdural hygromas. This CT scan shows the bifrontal low-density collections in a 6-year-old child with acute trauma.

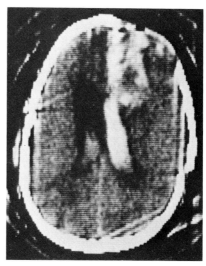

Fig. 18–4.—Intracerebral hematoma. This CT scan shows the high-density blood in the right frontal region with an extension into the ventricular system.

points to the need for a frontal lobectomy and the insertion of an intraventricular drain. Another hematoma is illustrated in Figure 18–5. The findings in Figure 18–6 point to a totally different benefit. Focal edema (with no hematoma formation) is shown in a case in which operative intervention was correctly avoided. Figure 18–7 illustrates a comparable situation with brain swelling. Occipital lobe infarction, one of the most devastating effects of intracranial hypertension, is demonstrated in Figure 18–8, a scan that was obtained in a case of acute trauma.

Arteriograms are necessary in many instances, performed either in lieu of a CT scan or sometimes as a complementary study, as in the instance of an inadequately visualized, isodense subdural hematoma.

The third and major group of injured children are those admitted for observation under conditions in which immediate action is not necessary. Alterations in the state of consciousness then may be followed more adequately to permit a rational approach to therapy. Similarly, motor losses may be analyzed repeatedly and the opportunity exists, for exam-

ple, to observe recovery after a contusion. Such diagnostic studies as echoencephalography are ideal for this group, and further tests will be performed as indicated.

An outline for management in the Accident Room is given in Table 18–1. This is presented to indicate the 3 groups and not to give absolute indications for procedures. Clearly, all patients with pupillary dilatation do not require arteriographic studies or CT scans, and all patients with a deteriorating neurologic status do not go directly to the Operating Room.

Operative Management

Intracranial hematomas are evacuated through trephinations, craniectomies or via a craniotomy. In recent years, two major changes have occurred in the selection of operative procedures. It is possible, with the use of the diagnostic studies noted above, to restrict the number of bur hole

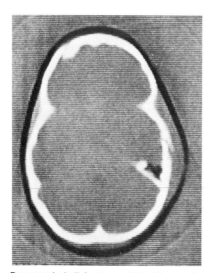

Fig. 18–3.—Depressed skull fractures. This CT scan depicts depressed bone in the right parietal and left frontal regions. It is particularly helpful in recognizing the site of deep bony spicules.

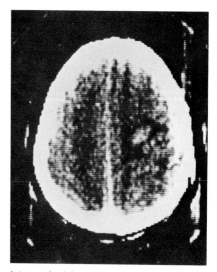

Fig. 18–5.—Intracerebral hematoma and edema in a 14-year-old child with acute trauma. The hematoma is marked by the high-density area in the right central region. It is surrounded by a low-density area of edema.

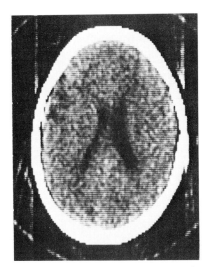

Fig. 18−6.−Brain edema. Focal edema is shown by the low-density lesion to the left. The left lateral ventricle is also narrow.

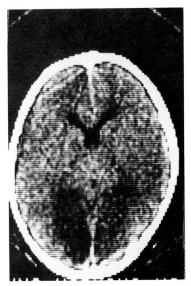

Fig. 18−8.−Infarction of occipital lobes after head trauma in a 6-year-old child. These are shown by the low-density areas posteriorly and follow transtentorial herniation with compression of posterior cerebral arteries.

placements and to avoid the use of 6 sites, so often necessary in the past. The second change is the wider use of craniotomies as compared with trephinations. This permits the more adequate removal of such clotted blood deposits as are found in acute and subacute subdural hematomas.

The extradural hematoma is a relatively rare lesion and accounts for only 2% of childhood head injury admissions.[19] Most extradural hematomas are found in the temporal region in association with a linear fracture and a torn middle meningeal artery. These collections are approached through a vertical or curvilinear temporal incision through the temporalis muscle, which is used later to cover the bony defect. Trephinations are made with the Smith perforator or a McKenzie perforator and a bur, and are rapidly expanded to craniectomies the size of a silver dollar or larger. The mass of black clot is readily apparent as the bone is perforated; it is quickly aspirated after the bony opening has been rongeured to adequate size. The meningeal vessel is cauterized

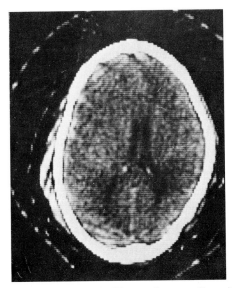

Fig. 18−7.−Brain swelling. This CT scan shows swelling with a shift of the thinned ventricles from left to right. Note the high-density subgaleal hematoma in the left parietal region.

at the site of the tear and extensively along its course. It often is necessary to follow the artery to the base, and to plug the foramen spinosum with a small piece of cottonoid. Other areas then are cauterized because of the secondary oozing that occurs as the hematoma separates dura mater from bone. Extradural hematomas also form, less commonly, after venous sinus tears. In the posterior fossa they are rare, but should be considered when a linear fracture is shown to traverse a major venous sinus in that area. The overall surgical results are excellent. However, the fact that only 70% of cases in the Boston series were categorized as normal in final status emphasizes the need for prompt diagnosis and treatment.

The subdural hematoma of infancy is a special case and is discussed subsequently. The chronic form of subdural hematoma is uncommon in later childhood; however, the acute forms occur as at other ages. A craniotomy flap often is useful because of the presence of clotted blood. Other subdural collections may be managed differently. Hygromas such as those depicted in Figure 18−2 may be easily evacuated through bifrontal trephine openings or small twist-drill holes. Intracerebral hematomas may also be evacuated with varied approaches. The striking lesion depicted in Figure 18−4 consists of a mixture of blood and destroyed brain and requires a generous approach through a craniotomy flap. Small craniectomies may be used in other instances.

Brain swelling is shown in Figure 18−7. In severe form, the brain herniates through the tentorial notch to produce a clinical picture identical to that found with a large mass lesion. The pertinent features include drastic alterations in the state of consciousness, third nerve palsies and long tract signs. Massive decompressions may be considered when this state is advanced and refractory to other forms of treatment. These procedures are performed by turning down and removing large bone flaps and opening the dura mater, unilaterally when the process is predominantly on one side or bifrontally when it is generalized. This technique is utilized very rarely in practice and it is better, in most instances, to rely on the use of controlled respiration.[9] For this, mild hyperventilation is maintained via the retained endotracheal

TABLE 18-1.—MANAGEMENT OF MAJOR ACUTE HEAD INJURY
IN THE ACCIDENT ROOM

GROUP	INDICATIONS	DISPOSITION	DIAGNOSTIC STUDIES
1	Rapid neurologic deterioration Failure of vital signs Compound head injury	Operation	X-ray skull
2	Depressed state of consciousness Dilated and unreactive pupil Bradycardia Neurogenic hypertension Lateralizing motor changes	Neuroradiology	CT scan or arteriogram
3	Improving neurologic status Minor changes in items in group 2	Observation	X-ray skull C spine Echoencephalogram

tube and PA_{CO_2} values are held in the range of 25–30 torr. Intermittent curarization often is required. Positive end-pressure respiration is useful for associated respiratory problems; however, Aidinis *et al.*[1] recently have presented experimental data that point to untoward effects in patients with head injury.

An extradural pressure sensor is quite helpful in these cases and permits the long-term monitoring of intracranial pressures. The device is inserted through a bur hole placed as an independent procedure or alternatively in conjunction with a craniotomy when swelling coexists with a mass, such as with an acute subdural hematoma.

Prompt explorations are carried out for compound injuries. The wound is carefully examined in the Emergency Room and a special effort is made to obtain adequate skull films with tangential views. A CT scan often is of great help (Fig. 18–3). At the time of exploration, the bony edges are rongeured to provide a small craniectomy, a debridement is carried out to remove all foreign material and the wound is liberally irrigated. Great care is required in those instances in which dural rents have occurred. Devitalized brain and blood clots are removed with suction and a determined effort is made to find any pieces of bone or foreign body, since retention may lead to the establishment of epileptogenic foci or to abscess formation. Dural defects are closed with pericranial tissue. A cranioplasty usually is carried out at a later time.

For closed depressed fractures, an early exploration is indicated if the depression is pronounced or if there is concern regarding dural penetration. Conversely, minimal depressions may be dismissed without an operative procedure. A large intermediate group is treated semielectively within the first 24 hours. A skin flap is turned over the involved area and the depressed bone elevated in any of a variety of ways. Often, an adjacent bur hole is placed and a dissector is introduced to pry out the bone. Alternatively, a small hole may be nibbled in the margin of intact bone and the fragments elevated directly with a rongeur. The bony defect is filled with bone chips in some instances; primary or secondary cranioplasties are fashioned with methyl methacrylate in others.

Medical Support

Glucocorticoids are given commonly and almost routinely with severe head injuries, and particularly in life-threatening situations. Obviously, they may be withheld in the presence of such complications as acute gastric bleeding. Dexamethasone is a popular choice and is given with an initial dosage of 10 mg and a continuing dosage of 4 mg q6h for the older child. This dose may be augmented to much higher levels as a heroic measure, although the efficacy is not established. Antacids are given via a nasogastric tube in all instances.

Serum electrolyte concentrations are obtained frequently and fluids are restricted during the first few days because of the tendency to water retention, manifested as a dilutional hyponatremia. Refractory states will require the use of intravenous mannitol infusions. Parenteral hypertonic saline may be needed with extreme changes.

Hypertonic mannitol is administered as a 20% solution in a dosage of 1–3 gm/kg. It is given rapidly and is preferred over urea because of its nonpenetrating characteristics. The administration of mannitol results in a shift of water out of normal brain and, accordingly, it may be needed under desperate conditions in the Emergency Room prior to exploratory trephinations. However, such brain shrinkage may permit expansion of an intracranial hematoma, and mannitol, therefore, should be used with great caution until the results of arteriography or CT scanning are available. Later, it may be used intermittently for a temporary effect; for example, when high CSF pressure waves are detected with extradural sensors or when clinical concomitants appear.

General hypothermia is a useful measure and many patients with major head injury are placed on cooling blankets. Rectal temperatures may be lowered to approximately 90° F to limit metabolic activity significantly in the damaged brain. Unfortunately, it usually is an impracticable form of management because of shivering and the need for repeated curarization. Therefore, this technique is used in most instances only to combat hyperthermia and to hold rectal temperatures at or slightly below the normal range.

Continued vigilance regarding respiratory function is of the utmost importance. The need for attention to PA_{CO_2} levels has been noted. The monitoring of PA_{O_2} levels and the use of humidified oxygen are similarly emphasized. Anticonvulsants are uncommonly required in the Emergency Room for head injury. The over-all effect of injury in the acute phase is one of depression and only about 5% of trauma cases will manifest seizure activity initially. Diazepam is the drug of choice and should be given intravenously when needed. The incidence of convulsions increases rapidly in the following days and weeks and the prophylactic use of diphenylhydantoin should be considered when there is gross brain damage.

Antibiotics are given for compound injuries, specifically including the basal skull fracture with sustained cerebrospinal fluid otorrhea. A penicillin preparation is used commonly and is continued for 7–10 days after cessation of the flow. There is wide divergence of opinion on the choice and timing of the drugs.

Injury at Birth and during Infancy

Such changes as temporal lobe damage and bleeding into the subarachnoid space induced at birth may take a good deal of the neurosurgeon's attention days, weeks or years later. However, most of the immediate problems in the perinatal period are not amenable to neurosurgical intervention. Much of the damage follows antenatal and perinatal anoxia rather than mechanical injury.[5] Bleeding occurs most commonly into the subdural space. These hematomas are acute and are to be distinguished from the more chronic form. They often follow tears of the tentorium cerebelli or the falx cerebri with major venous sinus involvement. The subdural space sometimes is needle aspirated in the lateral margin of the fontanelle, and the lateral ventricle occasionally is tapped for blood. Treatable extradural, subdural and temporal lobe hematomas occur in the perinatal period and these should be kept in mind, although they are quite rare in comparison with the devastating bleeds into the subdural space.

The ping-pong ball depressed fracture and the cephalhematoma are two of the well-known lesions of the newborn. The depressed fractures are easily reduced through a small adjacent bony opening. This may be performed a day or two after birth with local anesthesia. The cephalhematoma occurs in association with about 2% of deliveries and consists of a subperiosteal collection, usually unilateral and parietal. The blood infiltrates the tissues. Aspiration is not effective and invites infection.

The subdural hematoma represents a relatively common problem in infancy and these cases account for many of the head injury admissions of the Boston series.[19] Seventeen per cent were in this category and almost all were found in infancy. They also represent the second most common cause of abnormal head enlargement. These collections resemble the chronic subdural hematomas of the adult, but significant dissimilarities are found. Bilateral collections are more frequent in the pediatric group and are present in about 80% of cases. The fluid also tends to be more serous, at least at the time of definitive operation, and often is in the form of an effusion. The infant may present either with excessive irritability or with drowsiness; other presenting symptoms include seizures and failure to thrive. Enlargement of the head occurs preferentially in the coronal plane and produces a box-like configuration, unlike the hydrocephalic contour. The fontanelle usually is tense and retinal hemorrhages are common. Transillumination is a useful technique, particularly for the young infant. The diagnosis, however, is best made with a subdural tap, arteriogram or CT scan. The initial treatment consists of repeated tapping of the subdural space with a 20-gauge needle at the extreme lateral margin of the anterior fontanelle. The head is carefully immobilized by an assistant because of the potential harm from needling. The skin is manually displaced at the point of insertion in order to obviate later overlapping of the puncture holes through skin and dura mater and resultant leakage. The needle is passed through the dura in a direction at a right angle to the skull and the fluid is allowed to drip slowly until a total of about 25 ml is obtained. Many collections are treated successfully with repeated taps. These commonly are performed bilaterally. The use of other techniques is demanded if these collections persist beyond 7–10 days despite daily evacuations. In the past, osteoplastic craniotomies frequently were performed to permit the wide removal of subdural membranes. These procedures are used currently and are particularly helpful when the membranes are very thick. However, there is a growing tendency to substitute a shunting procedure, particularly for the infant harboring a large effusion. It is advisable to shunt the fluid to the vascular compartment when the protein content is high and to use either this procedure or diversion to the peritoneal space when it is low. The over-all results are good, with satisfactory results in 75% of cases.

The battered or abused child is of particular concern to the neurosurgeon, since a significant amount of damage is inflicted on the head. The inadequacy of the history is notorious and, therefore, special diagnostic effort is demanded. A meticulous examination for cutaneous injury is performed and varied and multiple lesions commonly are found. Funduscopic examination may give evidence of recent head trauma and point to the diagnosis of a subdural hematoma. A roentgenographic skeletal survey typically shows multiple fractures of various ages. Linear skull fractures are common and are found in half of the cases with subdural hematomas. Spinal trauma occurs infrequently but should be kept in mind. One of the most appalling injuries recorded on our service was that of an infant who probably was hyperextended with such force as to disrupt the spinal column, producing a permanent paraplegia.

The extradural hematoma of infancy represents a special injury because of the fact that hypovolemic shock may appear from the intracranial blood loss. In the adult, the presence of systemic hypotension points to an associated injury or to brainstem involvement. In the infant or young child, the head is disproportionately large and the brain is able to adapt to large hematomas. Hence, these clots may reach such a size as to provoke hypotension. The clinical picture is that of a combination of drowsiness with signs of shock, including pallor, tachycardia and eventually hypotension. This combination constitutes one of the most unequivocal states for emergency action in neurosurgical practice.

The leptomeningeal cyst induced by trauma is another specific and rare lesion of infancy or young childhood. At this age, the dura mater is adherent to bone at the suture lines and may be torn as the skull is fractured linearly. This permits the egress of cerebrospinal fluid and cyst formation. The cyst tends to progress and to erode the bone edges, producing the "growing fracture of childhood." The operative management often is a formidable problem and is directed at removal of all cystic components and scar plus repair of the dura mater, and sometimes a cranioplasty.

Spinal cord injuries are extremely rare in infants and children and account for only 0.5% of major trauma to the central nervous system. They occur most commonly after breech extractions but are also noted in older children after diving or automobile accidents or falls. The battered child may also appear with this injury.

Special care is required in the interpretation of the lateral cervical spine film of the infant, since the normal degree of laxity may permit enough movement to simulate a dislocation.

Most of the injuries in both age groups involve the cervical region. Alignment usually is normal in the infant and sandbag support is sufficient for immobilization. If traction is needed, it may be applied through steel wires traversing adjacent bur holes in both parietal regions.

Fracture-dislocations are the rule in the older child, although normal alignment is found in about 15% of cases. Skull tongs are applied in the Accident Room and 5–10 pounds of traction applied initially. This weight may be increased to 15–20 pounds if required for reduction.

A decompressive laminectomy will be performed if there is roentgenographic evidence of bony impingement on the cord or if the clinical status worsens. Conversely, laminectomy may be rejected if there is immediate and total loss of power below the level of the injury or if the neurologic status improves. The decision concerning decompression often is difficult and frequently it is made after a positive contrast myelogram is performed. There is a growing tendency against the performance of laminectomies for major spinal cord injuries aside from the penetrating spinal injury, in which prompt debridement and decompression are mandatory.

REFERENCES

1. Aidinis, S. J., Lafferty, J., and Shapiro, H. M.: Intracranial responses to PEEP, Anesthesiology 45:275, 1976.
2. Broca, P.: Nouvelle observation d' amplémie produite par une lesion de la moitié postérieure des deuxième et troisième circonvolutions frontales, Bull. Mem. Soc. Anat. Paris S-2:398, 1861.
3. Caveness, W. F.: Epilepsy, a product of trauma in our time, Epilepsia 17:207, 1976.
4. Celsus, A. C.: *De Medicina.* Translated by Spencer, W. G. (Cambridge, Mass.: Harvard University Press, 1935–1938).
5. Courville, C. B.: *Birth and Brain Damage* (Pasadena, Calif.: M. F. Courville, 1971).
6. Fritsch, G., and Hitzig, E.: Über die elektrische Erregbarkeit des Grosshirns, Arch. Anat. Physiol. 37:300, 1870.
7. Grana, F., Rocca, E. D., and Grana, R. L.: *Las Trepanaciones Craneanas en el Peru en la Epoca Pre-Hispanica* (Lima: Imprenta Santa Maria, 1954).
8. Gurdjian, E. S., and Webster, J. E.: *Head Injuries, Mechanisms, Diagnosis and Management* (Boston: Little, Brown and Company, 1958).
9. Hayes, G. J., and Slocum, H. C.: Achievement of optimal brain relaxation by hyperventilation techniques of anesthesia, J. Neurosurg. 19:65, 1962.
10. Hippocrates: On Injuries of the Head, in *The Genuine Works of Hippocrates.* Translated by Adams, F. (London: The Sydenham Society, 1849).
11. Horrax, G.: *Neurosurgery: An Historical Sketch* (Springfield, Ill.: Charles C. Thomas, Publisher, 1952).
12. Jackson, J. H.: Cases of epilepsy associated with syphilis, Med. Times Gaz. 1:648, 1861.
13. Jackson, J. H.: Clinical remarks on cases of temporary loss of speech and power of expression (epileptic aphemia?, aphrasia?, aphasia?) and on epilepsies, Med. Times Gaz. 1:442, 1866.
14. Jackson, J. H.: Clinical remarks on the occasional occurrence of subjective sensations of smell in patients who are liable to epileptiform seizures or who have symptoms of mental derangement and in others, Lancet 1:659, 1866.
15. Jefferson, G.: Sir William Macewen's Contribution to Neurosurgery and Its Sequels, in *The Selected Papers of Sir Geoffrey Jefferson* (Springfield, Ill.: Charles C Thomas, Publisher, 1960).
16. Jennett, B.: Sir William Macewen: 1848–1924. Pioneer Scottish neurosurgeon, Surg. Neurol. 5:57, 1976.
17. Leyden, E.: Beiträge und Untersuchungen zur Physiologie und Pathologie des Gehirns, Virchow's Arch. 37:517, 1866.
18. Lister, J.: On the antiseptic principle in the practice of surgery, Lancet 2:353, 1867.
19. Matson, D. D.: *Neurosurgery of Infancy and Childhood* (Springfield, Ill.: Charles C Thomas, Publisher, 1969).
20. Rowbotham, G. F.: *Acute Injuries of the Head* (Baltimore: The Williams & Wilkins Company, 1964).
21. Walker, A. E. (ed.): *A History of Neurological Surgery* (Baltimore: The Williams & Wilkins Company, 1951).

19 Richard G. Eaton
Management of Acute Hand Injuries

OPTIMAL MANAGEMENT of an acutely injured hand begins with an accurate anatomic diagnosis. Only when the injured parts have been clearly identified can a rational plan for repair and reconstruction be established. This axiom is particularly true in dealing with an injury that may involve multiple tissue systems, such as the motor or sensory nerves or tendons in the hand of a child. The ease and accuracy of evaluation vary inversely with age, the child under 3 years providing a particular challenge to the examiner's diagnostic expertise. By considering the injury topographically, the not-infrequent sequelae of missed diagnosis in childhood will be minimized. Fortunately, the child's freedom from disabling adhesions and painful neuromata, and his capacity for vigorous nerve regeneration and rapid fracture healing, compensate somewhat for the often unavoidable inadequacies of physical examination following acute trauma.[5]

Evaluation of the Injured Hand

The child rarely is able to provide an accurate description of his injury. Parents or adults infrequently witness the event, hence their history often is secondhand and of uncertain reliability. Diagnosis depends almost completely on the physical examination. The first step in evaluating the injury is to gain the confidence of the usually terrified young patient. Occasionally, in the hysterical child, a short-acting intramuscular sedative will permit the otherwise impossible examination of a complex injury.

SENSATION.—In the usually inarticulate child, evaluation of sensibility can be the most difficult determination. It must be done *prior to* any portion of the examination that might cause pain. Absence of a normal sweat beading in the tangential beam of a penlight would suggest nerve deficit. Light stroking of each finger may indicate anhidrosis and loss of sympathetic tone and thus confirm injury to a peripheral nerve trunk. *Never use a pin.* Pain inflicted at this point in the examination may destroy all rapport with the patient. Under 5 years of age, an objective response to blunt two-point testing is not possible; however, in the school-age child, patient application of the usual paper clip or blunt forceps, requesting a one- or two-point response, may provide fairly accurate evaluation of peripheral nerve defects (Fig. 19–1). In forearm or wrist lacerations, immersing the hand in warm water or soap solution for as little as 10 minutes often will produce wrinkling in the normally innervated areas whereas the denervated fingers remain smooth, providing a topographic impression of peripheral nerve trunk injury.[3, 16]

MOTOR.—A tentative diagnosis of most injuries can be made by careful analysis of the resting attitude of the hand and the site of laceration. This diagnosis then is confirmed through systematically ruling out the damage to all topographically related structures. Absence of, or a deficit in, the normal position of rest or lack of tone at a single joint would suggest a tendon division or proximal muscle paralysis (Fig. 19–2). Shortening, angulation or rotation of the digit due to a displaced fracture often is not obvious in the pudgy hand of a young child; however, with experience, even such subtle deformities can be readily appreciated. With the hand in supination (palm up), external rotation of the thumb or lack of the palmar cupping provided by thenar muscle tone would suggest a median nerve injury and loss of the abductor brevis or opponens pollicis muscle tone.

In the unconscious or totally uncooperative patient, flexor muscle and tendon continuity can be tested by squeezing the distal third of the volar forearm (Fig. 19–3). Such a maneuver should produce involuntary mass flexion of all digits. Lack of motion of any digit would suggest musculotendinous disruption. Localized pressure over the distal flexor carpiradialis tendon will produce the same reflex flexion of the thumb. For additional confirmation, *passive* wrist flexion and extension, utilizing the tenodesis effect of flexor and extensor muscle tone, often will bring out defects in tendon continuity (Fig. 19–4).

In some suspected tendon injuries, when the diagnosis still is uncertain, and once sensibility has been satisfactorily evaluated, a gently administered local anesthetic wrist block

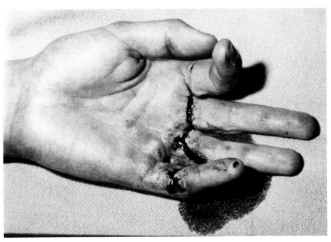

Fig. 19–2.—The resting attitude of the injured hand. In this patient, it suggests division of the profundus and superficialis tendons to the middle and ring fingers and division of the flexor profundus tendon to the fifth finger. Compare these to the resting position of the interphalangeal joints in the normal index finger.

will enable the child to perform pain-free active flexion and extension of otherwise pain-splinted fingers. By observing defects in active motion, suspected tendon, musculoskeletal and nerve injuries can be confirmed.

Occasionally, circumstances preclude a satisfactory initial

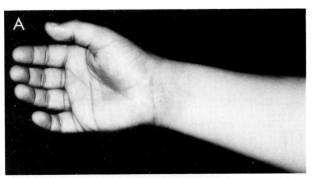

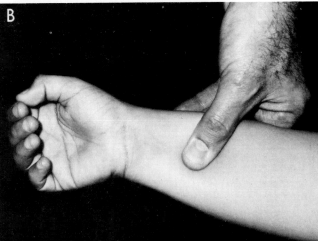

Fig. 19–3.—Test for musculotendinous continuity. **A,** the position of rest or physiologic balance. **B,** local pressure over the distal third of the finger flexor muscle group produces involuntary mass flexion of the fingers. With distal lacerations, lack of flexion at any digit in such testing would indicate disruption of musculotendinous continuity.

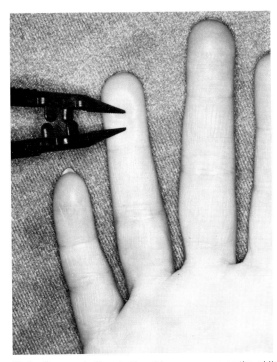

Fig. 19–1.—Sensory testing. In the older, more cooperative child, light application of *blunt* forceps, for a one- or two-point response, often will confirm nerve injury.

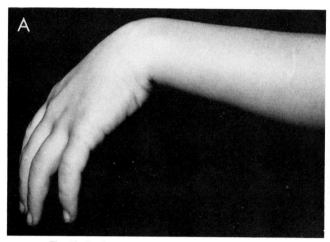
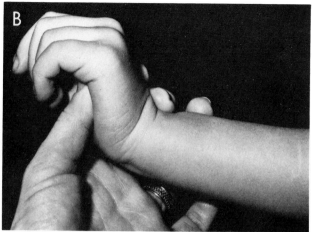

Fig. 19–4.—Passive tenodesis test. Applicable to the infant, the unconscious child and effective even under general anesthesia. In the presence of intact flexor tendons, the maneuver produces flexion of the fingers.

evaluation. In such cases, the skin can be closed under local wrist block anesthesia and the hand immobilized for 3–5 days. Under such a regimen there is a rapid loss of wound sensitivity, permitting a more meaningful examination in 5 days. At this time, while end-to-end repair still is accomplished easily, a delayed primary tendon or nerve repair can be done under elective general anesthesia.

X-RAY.—All but the most trivial hand injuries should receive roentgenographic evaluation. Since the exact nature of the trauma often is obscure, significant skeletal injury may not be appreciated. In the child with open epiphyses, comparable views of both hands are imperative. Fingers must be evaluated by both PA and lateral roentgenograms of the *individual finger* instead of the usual PA and oblique views of the *hand.* A thin, flexible paper cassette or dental film is useful in obtaining the true lateral views of children's digits.

Treatment

With an anatomic diagnosis established, specific treatment can begin. Immediate repair is ideal as long as anesthesia does not involve increased risk. Emergency general anesthesia techniques are *not* justified, since, with adequate wound cleansing, temporary immobilization and antibiotics, the same surgical result can be obtained when the repair is done 6–12 hours later, under optimal circumstances. A surprising number of injuries that do not require more than 30 minutes of tourniquet time can be repaired with local or regional anesthesia under moderate sedation. Every effort should be made to minimize the psychic trauma of the injury and its required treatment.

Skin and Subcutaneous Tissue

FINGERTIP AMPUTATIONS.—Steel doors, bicycle chains and lawn mowers nip off an alarmingly large number of children's fingertips. Fortunately, many are incomplete amputations, a small bridge of skin remaining intact. With gentle handling, a minimum of sutures and dependable immobilization, these incomplete amputations, even when significantly crushed, usually will survive in children. Complete transections through the distal phalanx rarely survive when reattached. However, some skilled in microsurgery have reported successful reimplantation of digits amputated

through the middle phalanx in children as young as 3 years of age.[11]

In children under 12 years suffering a transection *through* the distal phalanx, even a skin graft is not required. Grafts in this area frequently become thickened and corrugated, producing a painful, fissuring verrucous-like plaque that often requires subsequent excision and secondary grafting (Fig. 19–5). The preferred treatment for fingertip amputations in children under 12 years of age, with a defect less than 1.0 cm in diameter, is to reduce the cross-sectional area and prevent eversion of the skin edges by means of a subcuticular, absorbable pursestring suture. If any bone remains exposed, it should be conservatively resected to lie within the soft tissue. The remaining defect is dressed with nonadherent fine mesh gauze and carefully immobilized. The wound is redressed in a similar fashion at 5-day intervals until epithelialized, much like a skin graft donor site. Rapid epithelialization occurs and, with subsequent maturation and contracture, the defect shrinks to at least 50% of its original

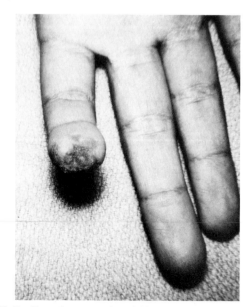

Fig. 19–5.—Fingertip amputation. Initially resurfaced with a medium split-thickness skin graft, recurring painful fissures in the dry, thickened graft required excision and direct closure.

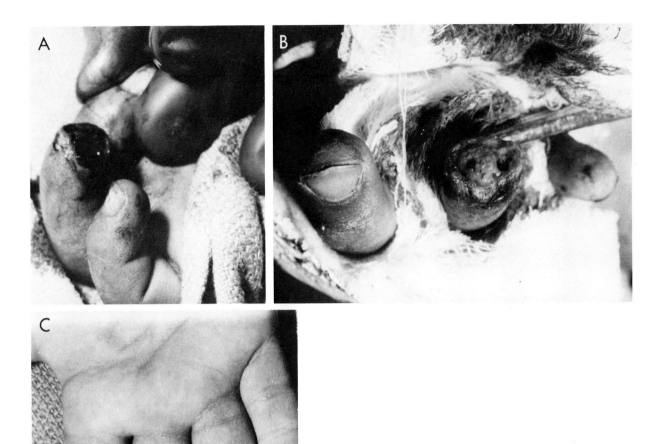

Fig. 19–6.—Open amputationplasty. **A,** clean transection through distal phalanx at base of the nail, approximately 1.0 cm in diameter. **B,** 5 days postsubcuticular pursestring suture and conservative resection of exposed bone. **C,** follow-up after 1 year. The defect has contracted, drawing supple, well-innervated skin over the stump.

size, creating a remarkably well-rounded nontender stump (Fig. 19–6).

FINGERNAIL INJURIES.—Nail plate and matrix injuries likewise are quite common. Partial nail plate avulsion is a superficial injury requiring only a trimming of the detached portion of the nail. Reinserting the superficially dislocated root of the nail into its former subeponychial pocket should be avoided, since this may seal a potential abscess cavity. Conservative trimming of the detached portion of the nail will suffice.

In all nail injuries, two potentially serious problems must be considered. The first involves laceration or displacement of the matrix. Untreated lacerations of the nail matrix, particularly the germinal matrix, may result in permanent deformity of nail growth. Matrix lacerations and displacement must be ruled out, even if this requires removal of the nail plate. Meticulous repair of nail matrix lacerations with 6-0 and 7-0 absorbable sutures minimizes scar in this sheet of germinating tissue and will ensure optimal regeneration of the nail.

A second serious problem is the possibility of unrecognized damage to the subjacent epiphyses. Nail matrix actually is specialized periosteum, the proximal germinal matrix margin lying just distal to the cartilaginous epiphyseal plate. PA and lateral roentgenograms of the injured area as well as the contralateral digit are required for proper evaluation. Traumatic distortion of the distal nail sufficient to dislocate the nail plate from its eponychial cul-de-sac occasionally will cause fracture through the cartilaginous plate. Matrix may become interposed and normal healing cannot occur (Fig. 19–7). Should closed manipulation not produce a per-

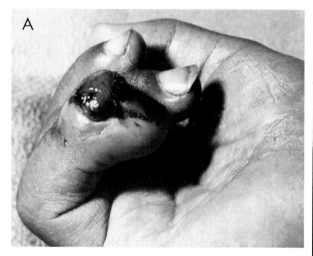
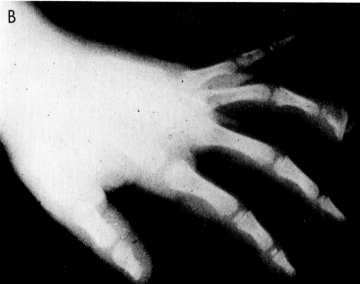

Fig. 19–7. – Infant with displaced open epiphyseal fracture and granuloma formation. **A,** tentatively diagnosed as a sarcoma until history of trauma 3 weeks earlier was obtained. **B,** radiograph of displacement. Following re- moval of interposed nail matrix and granulations, excellent metaphyseal-epiphyseal contact was restored and healing occurred without deformity.

fect reduction, open reduction, removing interposed matrix, may be required.

UNTIDY WOUNDS. – Complex laceration-avulsion wounds such as produced by fireworks, dynamite caps and home-made bombs occasionally create very serious, untidy wounds. With the remarkable regenerative power of the child, most complex wounds heal quite well. Conservative debridement is the rule, giving marginally viable tissue the benefit of the doubt.

Tendon Injury

Flexor Tendon Injury

Recognition and accurate diagnosis are particularly critical for the injured tendon. With isolated flexor tendon lacerations, the lack of flexor tone at one or more joints distal to the laceration is pathognomonic of complete transection (see Evaluation). Because of the child's lesser tendency to disabling adhesion, direct primary repair of lacerated tendons in "no man's land" is much less controversial than in adults. In recent years, experienced hand surgeons are reporting satisfactory results following repair of both profundus and superficialis tendons within the fibrous digital sheath, even in adults. *It must be emphasized, however, that the quality of the repair is directly related to the surgeon's experience with tendon surgery.*[1, 2, 6, 8, 13, 18]

DIGIT. – Primary repair within the digital sheath should be considered only when an experienced surgeon is available, even if this means delaying primary repair as long as 10 – 14 days. The profundus tendon has the highest priority for repair, the superficialis being repaired only in the most favorable circumstances. A skillfully performed elective (late) tendon graft will also yield satisfactory, often superior, results and should be included in the initial considera- tion.[2, 8, 10]

PALM. – In the palm, where combined nerve and tendon injuries are the rule, primary repair yields far superior re- sults. When lacerated in the palm, the superficialis tendons may retract proximally into the wrist and require a separate wrist incision to facilitate atraumatic retrieval and passage of the proximal stump back through the carpal canal. The prox- imal end of the profundus tendon usually is restrained by an intact lumbrical and can be located invaginated within its proximal muscle belly. Both profundus and superficialis tendons can be successfully sutured in the palm as long as the juncture does not encroach on the proximal pulley of the flexor tendon sheath when the finger is in full extension. Meticulous, atraumatic technique using 5-0 and 6-0 wire or monofilament synthetic suture yields most favorable results.

WRIST. – In wrist lacerations, the finger flexor tendons and nerves should be repaired as a primary procedure. When both superficialis and profundus tendons to the same finger are divided in the carpal canal, maximal postoperative ten- don excursion is better ensured if only one, the profundus, is repaired.[14] Lacerated *wrist* flexor tendons need not be re- paired, since immobilization in slight wrist flexion provides satisfactory approximation of the ends, which quickly bridge with scar within their well-defined paratenon sleeves. Per- fect continuity without a restraining wrist flexion contrac- ture is the rule.

TENDON GRAFTING. – The timing of a flexor tendon graft is important, since the unoccupied pulley system tends to collapse progressively with time. Grafting within 3 months of the injury is most desirable. In late tendon grafting, or whenever the critical pulleys at the metacarpal head and midphalanx levels are not satisfactory, a two-stage pro- cedure may be required.[9] At the first stage, the pulleys are reconstructed over an inert flexible tendon implant. At a second procedure 6 – 8 weeks later, the implant is replaced with a free tendon graft, exposing only the proximal and dis- tal ends of the implant tract.

Despite the seemingly improved prognosis for primary repair of divided tendons within the flexor sheath of chil- dren, one recurring fallacy must be noted. For the inexperi- enced surgeon to "give it a try" (primary repair) assuming that if it fails, a tendon graft always can be done later, is a philosophy that has led to the devastation of countless fingers and hands. It is a philosophy condemned by the *experienced* tendon surgeon, who all too often is called on to salvage a stiff, immobile finger with extensive tendon-to-tendon or tendon-to-bone adhesions, an obliterated flexor pulley system and secondarily contracted joints. The prognosis for such a finger, even with the best surgical care, is much inferior to that following an elective tendon graft.[6] To avoid such disasters, primary tendon repairs within the flexor digital sheath should be undertaken only by the experienced tendon surgeon.

Extensor Tendon Injury

MALLET FINGER.—Rupture of the extensor tendon insertion from the base of the distal phalanx, when not complicated by intra-articular or epiphyseal fracture, has an excellent prognosis in children. The distal joint should be securely immobilized in full extension for 5 weeks. A tape-padded paper clip or half-inch aluminum splint is applied to the skin and the entire hand and arm securely immobilized in plaster. Older, more reliable children may not require such a restrictive dressing; however, unless the distal joint immobilization is undisturbed for a full 5 weeks, the result may be compromised.

CENTRAL EXTENSOR MECHANISM INJURIES.—Interruption of the central slip of the digital extensor mechanism, whether by sharp laceration or dehiscence following blunt trauma, is manifested as a loss of extension of the middle phalanx. Since this injury represents only a partial interruption at the center of the triangular extensor aponeurosis, simple splinting of the finger in full extension will relax the tension in the area of injury, resulting in almost anatomic reapproximation. The defect usually will heal itself with minimal impairment of function. Direct suture of clean lacerations may be considered, but carries the risk that additionally traumatized tendon will become adherent to the underlying joint capsule and periosteum, resulting in restricted excursion of this complex extensor mechanism.

Nerve Injury

Nerve injury must be ruled out in *any* laceration or crush injury that overlies a major nerve trunk or one of the peripheral branches (see Evaluation). The best time for nerve repair in the palm and forearm is within 24 hours of the injury, preferably in conjunction with tendon or muscle repair. Early exploration is particularly important should there be any doubt of injury, since it is only in the freshly cut state that a partially divided nerve can be anatomically repaired. Fibrin, edema and scar formation rapidly obscure axonal architecture, making satisfactory later repair almost impossible. Even microsurgical dissection of neuromata in continuity poses a significant hazard to the intact fascicles.

Rules regarding laceration of digital nerves are less rigid. Division of *both* digital nerves demands early repair, since such an injury renders the entire digit anesthetic. Exploration of isolated radial or ulnar digital nerve injuries is optional, since the nerve may have suffered only neuropraxia, and furthermore, the finger is only partially anesthetic and *late* repair of these purely sensory nerves yields equally satisfactory results. Should the nerve not be repaired primarily, however, the parents must be advised that a disruption may be present and subsequent examination and treatment arranged.

Magnification, whether by 2× to 4.5× loupes or through an operating microscope, is a great asset in the accurate reapproximation of divided nerves. Use of delicate microsurgical instruments and 8-0 to 10-0 nylon suture material ensure a meticulous technique and minimal postoperative fibrosis.

In discussing nerve injuries, Wakefield[18] states: "There is nothing in the surgery of trauma, apart from the technical skill and experience of the surgeon, that has such a profound effect on prognosis as the age of the patient." McEwan,[15] comparing a single surgical team's results with nerve repairs in children and adults, noted that 66% of the children regained 5 mm or better two-point discrimination compared with only 15% of adults.

Skeletal Injuries

Significant skeletal injuries of the hand are less frequent in the child. Shorter phalangeal length, resilient cartilage and thick periosteum as well as less exposure to complex machinery would seem to account for this difference. In children under 3 years, fractures are predominantly due to crush injuries, which create longitudinal fracture lines (Fig. 19–8). In this age group, the phalanx is predominantly a centrally ossified cartilage model of the adult bone. Displacement usually is minimal, healing rapid and remodeling quite dependable. Minimal immobilization is required.

The majority of children's hand fractures occur toward the end of the growth period, between ages 11 and 16. During this period, under the influence of increasing growth hormone, there is rapid longitudinal growth. The cartilaginous epiphyseal growth site is wider and more vulnerable to shearing or lateral stress.[7] Athletic activities also begin to peak during this period and epiphyseal fractures are much more frequent. The Salter-Harris classification of epiphyseal fractures is helpful in understanding the fracture pathomechanics as well as establishing the prognosis for growth[17] (see Chap. 14). Minimal displaced epiphyseal fractures often are not recognized until comparison with the roentgenograms of the normal contralateral digit. Dislocations are quite uncommon in the child, as adjacent epiphyseal cartilage plates usually fracture before the tensile strength of the ligament is exceeded.

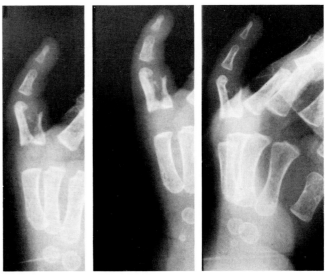

Fig. 19–8.—Longitudinal fracture in an 8-month-old infant. Such fractures usually are caused by crush injuries.

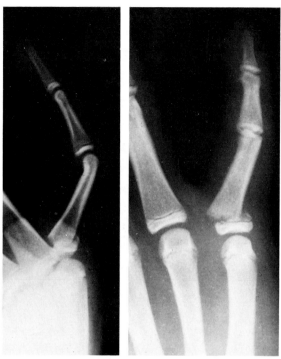

Fig. 19–9.—Radiograph of Salter-Harris type II fracture of the fifth finger. The finger rests in a cocked-back, ulnar deviated position. Such a deformity demands accurate realignment and immobilization in flexion.

Two-thirds of all children's hand fractures involve the thumb (34%) and the fifth ray (30%). More than half (55%) of all fractures involve the proximal phalanx. The most frequent fracture is the epiphyseal fracture of the fifth finger, proximal phalanx[4] (Fig. 19–9). The finger typically rests in a moderately hyperextended ulnar angulated position. Roentgenographic deformity of greater than 20 degrees dorsal angulation, and any lateral angulation or rotation, must be corrected. A simple reduction maneuver consists of firm longitudinal traction as the fifth finger is hyperflexed and angulated toward the distal pole of the carpal scaphoid. Following reduction, the proximal phalanx is immobilized in a secure plaster gauntlet in 50 degrees metacarpophalangeal flexion for 3 weeks. The interphalangeal joints may be left free.

Leonard and Dubravcik,[12] analyzing a series of children's hand fractures, observed that 75% were minimally displaced and required only external immobilization, 15% needed reduction and external immobilization and only 10%, predominantly displaced articular and condylar fractures, required open reduction. In young children, the cast is best extended above the flexed elbow to ensure continuity of immobilization.

REFERENCES

1. Bell, J. L., Mason, M. L., Koch, S. L., and Stromberg, W. B.: Injuries of the flexor tendons of the hand in children, J. Bone Joint Surg. 40-A:1220, 1958.
2. Bora, F. W.: Profundus tendon grafting with unimpaired sublimis function in children, Clin. Orthop. 71:118, 1970.
3. Bunke, J. H., Jr.: Digital nerve repair, Surg. Clin. North Am. 52:1267, 1972.
4. Eaton, D. H.: Personal communication.
5. Eaton, R. G.: Hand problems in children, Pediatr. Clin. North Am. 14:643, 1967.
6. Eaton, R. G., and Littler, J. W.: Flexor Tendon Grafting, in Goldwyn, R. M. (ed.), *The Unfavorable Result in Plastic Surgery* (Boston: Little, Brown and Company, 1972).
7. Harris, R. W.: The endocrine basis for slipping of the upper femoral epiphyses, J. Bone Joint Surg. 32-B:5, 1950.
8. Herndon, J. H.: Tendon injuries in children, Orthop. Clin. North Am. 7:717, 1976.
9. Hunter, J., and Salisbury, R.: Use of gliding artificial implants to produce tendon sheaths. Techniques and results in children, Plast. Reconstr. Surg. 45:564, 1970.
10. Kelly, A. P.: Primary tendon repair, J. Bone Joint Surg. 41-A:581, 1959.
11. Kleinert, H. E.: Personal communication.
12. Leonard, M. H., and Dubravcik, P.: Management of fractured fingers in the child, Clin. Orthop. 73:160, 1970.
13. Lindsey, W. K., and MacDougall, E.P.: Direct digital flexor tendon repair, Plast. Reconstr. Surg. 26:613, 1970.
14. Littler, J. W.: Principles of Reconstructive Surgery of the Hand, in Converse, J. M. (ed.), *Reconstructive Plastic Surgery* (Philadelphia: W. B. Saunders Company, 1964), p. 1669.
15. McEwan, L. E.: Median and ulnar nerve injuries, Aust. N. Z. J. Surg. 32:89, 1962.
16. O'Rian, S.: New and simple test of nerve function in the hand, Br. Med. J. 3:615, 1973.
17. Salter, R. B., and Harris, W. R.: Injuries involving the epiphyseal plate, J. Bone Joint Surg. 45-A:587, 1963.
18. Wakefield, A. R.: Hand injuries in children, J. Bone Joint Surg. 46-A:1226, 1964.

20 James A. O'Neill, Jr.

Burns

ACCIDENTAL INJURY is the main cause of death in children between the ages of 1 and 15 years. Motor vehicle-related injuries rank first in importance, followed by burn injuries and drowning. Approximately one-third of the 300,000 individuals hospitalized and the 8000 who die from burn injuries in the United States each year are children.[11]

The overwhelming majority of burn injuries in childhood occur in the child's home environment as the result of an accident. The obvious inference is that somewhere between 80% and 90% of such injuries are potentially preventable. The pattern of injury appears to be related to age and sex. In the children under 3 years, contact with hot liquids resulting in scald burns is by far the most common cause of both minor and major burns injuries. Boys are injured in this fashion more than twice as often as girls, since males appear to be more active and inquisitive than females in this age group. Most scald burns result when a young child pulls a pot of boiling water or coffee off a stove over his head, chest and arms. Occasionally, a small child will manage to turn the hot water tap on in a bathtub and scald himself, or be carelessly or deliberately placed in a bathtub full of scalding water by an adult. Although scald injuries ordinarily have been considered to result in only partial-thickness skin destruction, we have found that a number of very young children may sustain full-thickness injury because of the thinness of their skin.

Flame burn injuries are seen most commonly in children over the age of 3 years and there is no sex predilection. Even though children's sleepwear now is reasonably protective because of governmental restrictions in manufacture, flammable fabrics still are involved about 60% of the time. Matches, space heaters, outdoor fires ignited with gasoline and stoves are the most common factors related to flame injury. Flame burns ordinarily are full-thickness and constitute most of the major burns and the majority of the fatal burns.

Care of Minor Burns

Minor burn injuries may be classifed as partial-thickness, involving no more than 15% of body surface, or full-thickness, involving no greater than 2% of body surface. Generally, these are the patients who will not require intravenous fluids for their care. More strict criteria must be applied to those children who are under a year of age and to those who have burns involving the face, hands, feet or perineum. Principles of care relate to the problems involved with the injury itself and the practicalities of office management and instructions that parents can be expected to carry out.

Scald injuries resulting from contact with hot liquids, and occasional flash fire burns, are responsible for the overwhelming majority of minor burn injuries. Parents may be instructed to apply ice packs or towels soaked in ice water to minor partial-thickness burns as a temporary first aid measure to alleviate pain. Definitive wound care is in order after that.

The main problems associated with minor partial-thickness injuries are pain, superficial infection, bothersome wound drainage and prolonged convalescence. Closed dressing care, open therapy with the use of topical antibacterial agents or a combination of these two methods satisfy the needs of patients with minor burns. Whether open or closed treatment is used, it generally is preferable to leave blisters intact in patients with minor burns, since such individuals are much more comfortable under these circumstances, and the burns may even heal somewhat faster than if the blisters are unroofed. Minor burns will become colonized by surface bacteria, but the quantities of organisms ordinarily are insufficient to produce invasive burn wound sepsis or conversion of partial-thickness to full-thickness injury. Such superficial infections usually do cause an increase in pain and a delay in wound healing.

The traditional method of care of minor burns involves the use of occlusive dressings as outlined by Harvey Allen in the early 1940s.[5] After thorough cleansing of the wound, a dressing is applied beginning with nonadherent petrolatum gauze followed by bulky gauze dressings covered with roller gauze and stockinet. This method is particularly useful on extremities. Published descriptions of this form of therapy indicate that dressings should be changed every 3 days or so. However, our experience indicates that occasional bothersome superficial infection will occur if dressings are not changed on alternate days or sometimes every day. The closed method is particularly useful in children, who tend to rub or scratch areas of burn, but the method is difficult to use for burns on certain areas of the trunk or around the head and neck. Open therapy is the better option in such cases.

Although serious or invasive infection is not a primary consideration with minor second degree burns, superficial infections are common, and this has led us to use open therapy with application of topical antibacterial creams, as is done with inpatients. Following cleansing of the burn with sterile saline in the physician's office or the Emergency Room, either silver sulfadiazine or gentamicin cream is applied twice daily, with twice daily cleansing in warm water at home. These children ordinarily are quite comfortable and healing usually is complete within 10–14 days. Office follow-up every 5–7 days usually is sufficient, and secondary infection is essentially eliminated, since these topical agents tend to control the staphylococci and streptococci that ordinarily colonize these wounds.

Oral antibiotics generally are not indicated except in those children who have known streptococcal infection in the pharynx or those treated by the closed method, who develop erythema and tenderness around the periphery of the burn wound, indicating infection.

Patients with small full-thickness burns may be treated through the phase of eschar separation by either of the above-mentioned modes of therapy on an outpatient basis. They then may be admitted to the hospital for skin grafting.

Care of Major Burns

Children with burns in excess of 15% of body surface are best treated in the hospital, and intravenous fluid therapy usually is required. The same consideration would apply to infants with smaller burns, those with full-thickness injuries in excess of 5% of body surface or when the face, hands, feet or perineum are involved. Those with severe injuries in excess of 30% of body surface are best managed in a specialized burn care facility.

Special Physiologic Considerations

The principles of burn care related to children are essentially those applied to adults except for quantitative differences. Infants and children under the age of 2 years represent a departure from the latter statement.

Perhaps the most important feature of the young child in comparison with the adult is the great disparity in surface area as related to body weight. From a metabolic point of view, surface area may be mathematically related to water turnover, caloric expenditure and numerous other metabolic parameters (see Chap. 3). For this reason, the burned child has a much greater evaporative water loss relative to weight than does an adult. By the age of puberty, the surface area to body weight ratio of the child becomes approximately the same as that of the adult.

Because of the relatively greater surface area of the infant and child, and because of the thinner skin and subcutaneous tissue, young subjects tend to lose body heat to a greater degree than do adults. A further difference exists in the infant under 6 months, in whom temperature regulation is partially by means of nonshivering thermogenesis, a metabolic process in which stores of brown fat are catabolized under the influence of catecholamines.[16] This process requires the expenditure of large amounts of oxygen, so prolonged hypothermic episodes in young infants may result in excessive lactate production and acidosis. For these reasons, external heating devices are extremely useful in order to maintain ambient temperatures at a high enough level to diminish the temperature gradient between the patient and the environment and thus minimize heat loss from the patient.

A further consideration relates to gas exchange and pulmonary function. Pulmonary ventilation and perfusion ordinarily are quite efficient by 1 month of age but there is a limit to how much work of breathing a very small child can do. Pulmonary compensation for the high basal metabolic needs of infants and small children, and the added increase in metabolic demands related to thermal injury, is limited and may be easily exceeded. If there is superimposition of either inhalation injury or upper airway obstruction due to edema, early institution of ventilatory assistance may be required.

Renal function is another age-related consideration. As a result of the imbalance in the maturation of glomerular and tubular function, the glomerular filtration rate in the infant does not reach adult levels until approximately 9–12 months of age.[17] Prior to this time, the small subject has only about one-half the osmolar concentrating capacity of the adult so that water loads are handled inefficiently. Free water clearance is time-dependent and can be shown to diminish as water loading continues.[56] It is for this reason that stressed infants are likely to retain a large portion of a water load administered as part of a fluid resuscitation regimen.[15] The more the stress the more evident this phenomenon becomes. Fortunately, excessive water retention usually is not a major problem because of the tendency for evaporation of water from the burn wound.

Cardiovascular function ordinarily is up to the increased demands of the child unless there is underlying heart disease. However, it may be more difficult to estimate the adequacy of cardiac output in children than in older individuals, since those under the age of 1 year tend to have a labile peripheral circulation due to an increased tendency to severe vasoconstriction, especially with hypothermia.

Initial Evaluation

A quick glance at a burned patient (Fig. 20–1) by an experienced individual ordinarily is all that is required to categorize the severity of injury. It is important to know when, where and how the burn occurred and the nature of the burning agent. If one determines that there is a strong possibility that smoke inhalation occurred, one may be more aggressive with airway management. In addition to knowing the circumstances of injury, it is vital to obtain information about the child in terms of whether there is a past history of disease, whether the child has been fully immunized, whether he is on medication and whether there has been a recent infection of any sort. If the nature and distribution of the burn cannot be explained on the basis of the history offered, one must be alert to the possibility of child abuse. In a recent review of child abuse cases at Vanderbilt Medical Center, burns represented one of the most frequent forms of deliberate injury sustained by abused children.[38]

Burn injury is unique in that the extent of injury may be mathematically described in terms of total surface area burned. The full extent of injury is also proportional to the depth of injury, but this factor ordinarily is not considered when estimating the need for fluid replacement. The so-called rule of nines is an accurate method for the estimation

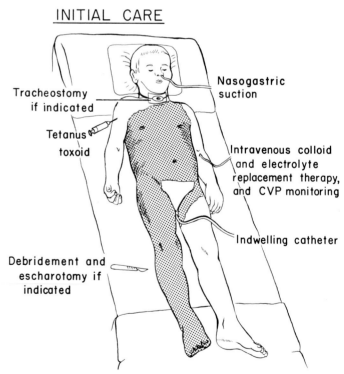

INITIAL CARE

Tracheostomy if indicated

Tetanus toxoid

Debridement and escharotomy if indicated

Nasogastric suction

Intravenous colloid and electrolyte replacement therapy, and CVP monitoring

Indwelling catheter

Fig. 20–1.—Immediate considerations in the care of the severely burned child.

of surface area in individuals over the age of 10 years.[5] The Lund and Browder chart and various modifications of that were developed for use in children under this age in order to consider the relatively greater surface area of the head and somewhat lesser surface area of the lower extremities in infants and young children[30] (Fig. 20–2). It is easier to evaluate the full extent of injury once a major burn has been cleansed with warm water and debridement performed. The patient's weight must be determined as soon as possible on admission before large volumes of intravenous fluid are given. This is important not only in terms of initial estimation of fluid requirements but also in terms of providing a standard of weight to be related to later water balance and nutritional management.

Although physical examination usually is sufficient in terms of providing adequate information for judging the seriousness of injury, special consideration must be given to electrical and chemical injuries, in which extensive tissue damage may be present with few external signs.[21] One may also underestimate the depth of immersion burns in infants.

Treatment

Airway Management

As with any other injury, immediate evaluation of the adequacy of the patient's airway is of prime concern. Those who were burned in an enclosed space or who have hoarseness, persistent coughing or facial burns must be observed for signs of inhalation injury. A chest x-ray should be obtained on admission, primarily for purposes of comparison, since physical and x-ray findings indicative of significant pulmonary injury may not become evident for 24 hours or even longer.[1] The most common form of respiratory difficulty seen in the young age group is upper airway obstruction from edema of the head and neck, glottic and supraglottic

BURN ESTIMATE AND DIAGRAM
AGE vs. AREA

Area	Birth 1 yr.	1-4 yr.	5-9 yr.	10-14 yr.	15 yr.	Adult	2°	3°	Total
Head	19	17	13	11	9	7			
Neck	2	2	2	2	2	2			
Ant. Trunk	13	13	13	13	13	13			
Post. Trunk	13	13	13	13	13	13			
R. Buttock	2½	2½	2½	2½	2½	2½			
L. Buttock	2½	2½	2½	2½	2½	2½			
Genitalia	1	1	1	1	1	1			
R.U. Arm	4	4	4	4	4	4			
L.U. Arm	4	4	4	4	4	4			
R.L. Arm	3	3	3	3	3	3			
L.L. Arm	3	3	3	3	3	3			
R. Hand	2½	2½	2½	2½	2½	2½			
L. Hand	2½	2½	2½	2½	2½	2½			
R. Thigh	5½	6½	8	8½	9	9½			
L. Thigh	5½	6½	8	8½	9	9½			
R. Leg	5	5	5½	6	6½	7			
L. Leg	5	5	5½	6	6½	7			
R. Foot	3½	3½	3½	3½	3½	3½			
L. Foot	3½	3½	3½	3½	3½	3½			
						TOTAL			

Fig. 20–2.—Calculation of surface area of a burn. This modification of the Brooke Army Hospital chart is a useful tool for accurate determination of surface area burned, depending on the age of the patient.

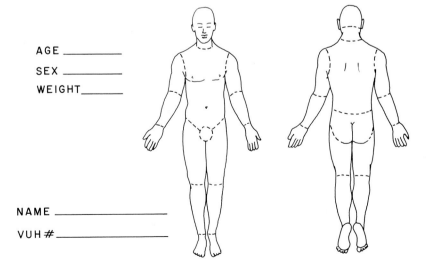

AGE _____

SEX _____

WEIGHT_____

NAME _____

VUH # _____

areas. Immediate nasal or orotracheal intubation is indicated in those patients who have significant respiratory distress on admission or in whom there is any possibility of later compromise of the airway by edema (Fig. 20–3). If one delays institution of nasotracheal intubation, severe swelling may make insertion of a tube impossible. Tracheostomy is reserved for those who require intubation longer than a few days, when airway management is difficult because of profuse secretions or when prolonged ventilatory assistance is required. Tracheostomy is associated with a higher incidence of tracheal and pulmonary complications, so it should be used only when necessary. Regardless of whether nasotracheal intubation or tracheostomy is used, these airways must be managed with extreme care from the standpoint of aseptic technique for suctioning and in the care of humidification equipment. Those patients who are suspected of having sustained inhalation injury must be observed carefully clinically and with daily chest x-rays for up to 5 days, since the characteristic pulmonary findings indicative of this type of damage may take that long to become manifest. The most helpful diagnostic and therapeutic tool in the management of patients who have inhalation injury is the serial determination of arterial blood pH, PCO_2 and PO_2. Significant hypoxemia may be managed initially by nasotracheal intubation and spontaneous breathing with or without continuous positive airway pressure. Those who develop progressive hypoxemia or significant lactic acidosis are best managed by means of controlled ventilatory assistance. Bronchoscopy may be required in those who develop problems with secretions that cannot be evacuated by airway suctioning and which result in atelectasis.

Nasogastric Drainage

Children who have burns in excess of 20% of body surface or those with associated injuries may have marked tachypnea associated with acute gastric dilatation and vomiting. A nasogastric tube should be passed early in order to avoid gastric distention, vomiting and possible aspiration of gastric contents. Ileus associated with early circulatory problems in small children may also be alleviated by nasogastric drainage. Ordinarily, this no longer is a problem after 48 hours have passed. A nasogastric tube is an important feature of the management of those patients who must be transported from one facility to another.

Fluid Therapy

Children with burns greater than 15% of body surface usually are best treated with intravenous fluids. A secure intra-

venous catheter should be placed, via a cutdown or percutaneously, with strict aseptic precautions and sterile dressings to avoid serious infectious complications. Catheters should be placed in unburned sites. Although percutaneous, subclavicular subclavian catheters are useful for the administration of fluids and the measurement of central venous pressure, their use is associated with a higher incidence of pneumothorax in children under the age of 6 years except in experienced hands. It is our preference to use a dressing incorporating povidone-iodine ointment as a further measure to avoid infectious complications, particularly suppurative thrombophlebitis.

Those individuals with burns of greater than 20% of body surface should have a urinary catheter inserted in order to monitor urinary flow. Foley balloon catheters should not be used in infant and preschool males because of potential stricture formation at the level of the membranous urethra. A small straight catheter or feeding tube generally is better in these subjects. After the third postburn day, catheters usually are not required for monitoring purposes and should be removed.

Burn injury is unique in the sense that the magnitude of injury may be partially estimated when one knows the extent of surface area involved. Evans, Artz and Reiss and others have developed formulas designed to estimate the amount of fluids required by burn-injured patients.[18, 50] The Evans, the modified Brooke and the Parkland fluid formulas may be used to estimate fluid requirements in children, but the Parkland regimen is the most practical method and the only one based primarily on physiologic observations (Table 20–1). Ringer's lactate is the best intravenous fluid to use initially in all patients.[7] Ringer's lactate in 5% glucose sometimes is useful in small infants, but it should not be used in the many patients who demonstrate a hyperglycemic response to injury.[3] This may be especially marked in the first 48 hours following burn, and insulin is required in occasional instances. Baxter's studies have demonstrated that the administration of colloid provides no benefit during the first 24 hours following injury.[7] The studies by Pruitt and coworkers[47] have confirmed this observation, demonstrating that plasma volume expansion during the first 24 hours following burn is dependent on the rate of fluid administration rather than the type of fluid administered, whether crystalloid or colloid. Baxter and Shires[10] have shown that the majority of plasma and extracellular fluid losses occur within the first 12 hours following burn and that the loss diminishes rapidly to almost zero for an additional 12 hours. Thus, the majority of fluid and sodium replacement must be given during the first 12 hours, trailing off after that for another 12 hours. In keeping with this line of reasoning, after the first 18–24 hours following burn, it may be preferable to change from Ringer's lactate to ½ normal saline in 5% glucose be-

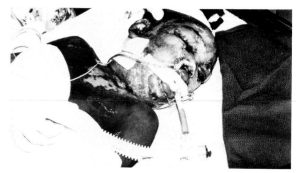

Fig. 20–3.—Orotracheal intubation. Many patients with laryngeal edema or head and neck swelling may have upper airway obstruction relieved with an endotracheal or nasotracheal tube alone. Delay may make intubation impossible. Tracheostomy is performed for those requiring prolonged intubation.

TABLE 20–1.—ESTIMATION OF FLUID
NEEDS IN THE FIRST 48 HOURS
(Parkland Formula)

First 24 hours	
Ringer's lactate	4 ml/kg/% burn
Second 24 hours	
D_5 ½ normal saline	½–¾ first day's needs
5% albumin	As indicated
Guidelines for First 48 Hours	
Urine volume	Peripheral circulation
Vital signs	Hematocrit, electrolytes
Sensorium	Central venous pressure

cause of the infant's tendency to retain sodium and water after that time. Since albumin cannot be shown to exert any beneficial effect during the first 24 hours following burn, it is our preference not to administer any during this interval. However, it can be shown to expand plasma volume after 24 hours, and Birke and his group[12] have demonstrated that burns of moderate size result in albumin losses equal to twice the total plasma pool during the first 4 days. Hence, any albumin administered probably is best given after 24 hours following injury.

By far the most important principle to note is that all fluid formulas are simply methods of estimating fluid requirements. It is the individual response to fluid therapy that determines the rate at which fluids should be administered. The most helpful clinical guide to fluid replacement is urinary output. During the first 48 hours following burn, adequate urine flow is approximately 1 ml/kg/hr or 750 ml/m²/24 hr. This is approximately 10–20 ml/hr in children up to the age of 2 years, 20–30 ml/hr in those 2–5 years of age and 30–50 ml/hr in those older than this. Individual hourly output may vary considerably, but the average should approximate the above-mentioned values. Although urinary output is a good guide, it certainly is not absolute, since significant physiologic derangements may exist despite apparently adequate urine flow.[41] Urine specific gravity may be a helpful guide at first but is increased when there is significant glucose, protein, mannitol or topical antibacterial breakdown product present. It is particularly important to judge the adequacy of cardiac output. In serious burns, cardiac output may diminish as much as 50% from resting values even before plasma volume drops.[8] As resuscitation continues, cardiac output usually rises to levels 3 or 4 times normal.[33] It is impractical to measure cardiac output in most patients but estimation is possible and is based on careful clinical assessment of the adequacy of peripheral circulation, maintenance of vital signs near normal levels, a normal blood pH and a clear sensorium. Serial measurement of central venous pressure may be helpful, and venous pressure is best maintained in the range of 3–6 cm of water. After 24 hours, capillary integrity appears to be renewed and reabsorption of fluid begins. After 48 hours postburn, reabsorption of fluids lost from the capillary bed ordinarily results in diuresis unless tubular necrosis has occurred early. The fact that capillary losses do not continue after the first 18–24 hours is also the reason that colloid administered during this interval appears to provide a sustained improvement in cardiac output and plasma volume. It does not appear to be necessary to give repeated infusions of colloid after the first 48 hours, from the standpoint of volume support. The essential features of early resuscitation then would primarily be emphasis on administration of the bulk of sodium-containing crystalloid during the first 12 hours based on closely followed clinical criteria and administration of colloid only after the first 24 hours, when capillary integrity should have been re-established.

By the time 48 hours have passed, fluid loss no longer is of the type due to transcapillary leakage but to vaporization of water from the wound surface.[58] Studies by Moncrief and Mason[34] indicate that evaporative water loss is the main consideration after 48 hours and that the losses are 85% free water. Calculations based on vaporizational heat loss as well as direct measurements of evaporative water loss indicate that infants and young children lose somewhere in the vicinity of 1–2 ml/kg/% burn/24 hr in addition to their usual daily maintenance requirements of fluids and electrolytes (Table 20–2). These losses continue until the burn wound is either

TABLE 20–2.—ESTIMATION OF FLUID NEEDS AFTER 48 HOURS

Evaporative loss	
D₅ 0.2 normal saline	1–2 ml/kg/% burn/24 hr
Daily maintenance	
D₅ normal saline	According to size
Potassium	As indicated
Guidelines after 48 Hours	
Body weight	
Serum sodium, potassium, osmolality	

epithelialized or covered with grafts. By 48 hours, the initial ileus usually seen with large injuries has passed and it then is possible to initiate oral or tube feedings. It is in the best interest of the patient to remove the intravenous catheter as soon as possible, but it must be kept in mind that oral fluid requirements generally are slightly greater than intravenous requirements. Frequent milk feedings are extremely valuable in children as a method of providing both calories and sufficient fluids to cover evaporative water losses. Ordinarily, tube feedings are required for the management of the infant or very young child with a large burn injury. Tube feeding formulas must provide no more than one-half to two-thirds of a calorie per milliliter of feeding if hyperosmolality is to be avoided in individuals with large evaporative water losses. In addition to following the serum sodium and osmolality as a guide to the adequacy of water replacement during the phase of evaporative water loss, daily measurement of body weight is essential. Infants and children with extensive burns usually gain as much as 20% of their basal weight during the first 48 hours of fluid resuscitation. In most situations, this is gradually lost over the subsequent 5–7 days. By this time, basal weight should have been achieved again and one then aims to maintain this at a steady level.

Although the serum sodium may be easily maintained either with intravenous therapy with 0.2 normal saline in 5% glucose or with most oral diets, the same is not necessarily true of the serum potassium. During the phase of diuresis, which lasts 5–7 days, a great deal of potassium ordinarily is lost via the kidneys. Occasionally, this may result in serious or even lethal arrhythmias, especially in patients who are on assisted ventilation or those receiving digitalis. Serial determinations of serum potassium usually serve as an adequate guide to replacement.

Although blood was emphasized as being the ideal form of early colloid replacement when the Evans formula[18] was described, this no longer is believed to be true. Volume losses during the capillary phase of fluid resuscitation are primarily plasma, and immediate red cell hemolysis rarely exceeds 10%.[33] It is generally accepted that blood should not be administered in the first 48 hours postburn unless associated injuries have resulted in blood loss or there has been a severe pre-existing anemia. Hemolysis becomes manifest after 48 hours and packed red cells then may be administered as indicated. It is our preference to keep the hematocrit above 35 volumes per cent, since it will fall precipitously in most children with large injuries due to the fact that the life span of much of the red cell mass usually is diminished under these circumstances.[6] Although the red cell destruction that occurs acutely may not be sufficient to require immediate blood replacement, impressive hemoglobinuria may occur in some individuals with large, deep injuries. Administration of small doses of mannitol and increasing the rate of fluid infusion ordinarily are sufficient to clear severe hemoglobinuria in a matter of 3 or 4 hours.

Nutrition and Metabolism (Table 20-3)

The metabolic response to severe thermal injury is characterized by hypermetabolism. Early studies suggested that this hypermetabolism was the result of vaporizational heat loss, which is known to be an energy-consuming process.[58] However, studies by Zawacki et al.[60] suggested that the degree of hypermetabolism noted in severely burn-injured individuals was independent of vaporizational heat loss for the most part. Mention already has been made of the requirement for marked increases in cardiac output seen in the postburn period, and these increases are proportional to oxygen consumption. Wilmore and co-workers[57] have reported studies that indicate that the severe hypermetabolism seen in patients with extensive burns is related to increased sympathetic activity, catecholamines, insulin and glucagon being the mediators of this response. Despite the fact that this marked hypermetabolic response to injury continues until the patient's wound is covered, it is possible to increase protein and calorie intake to a level that will meet these increased needs. In the past, severe malnutrition seen in patients with extensive injuries was known to be associated with delayed wound epithelialization and diminished graft acceptance. Recently, it has been shown that patients with large injuries and marked malnutrition have a higher incidence of sepsis and diminished neutrophil function.[25] We have previously noted that children with burns in excess of 40% of body surface who lost as much as 20% of their basal weight had a high incidence of sepsis and death. It has been our recent observation as well as that of others that patients who can be maintained in positive nitrogen balance with good weight stabilization have a lesser incidence of sepsis and improved survival.

The increased calorie and nitrogen requirements in these subjects must be met by one of two methods, since there is no practical way at present to diminish these needs. Certainly it is possible to utilize intravenous parenteral nutrition either totally as a temporary measure or as a supplement on a long-term basis, but the incidence of infectious complications related to the intravenous catheter is something that must be considered seriously. By far the most satisfactory method of meeting the patient's nutritional needs is via the gastrointestinal tract. We find that tube feedings are required in addition to oral feedings in the vast majority of children with large burn injuries. The smallest tube possible should be utilized in order to minimize the problem of esophagitis and gastroesophageal reflux, and patients should be maintained in a slightly elevated position. Vomiting or diarrhea may temporarily complicate patient management with tube feedings, and, in these instances, a variety of elemental diets may be used to advantage. One should aim to provide these children with approximately 100 calories and 3 gm of protein equivalent per kilogram of body weight daily so that basal weight may be maintained.

TABLE 20-3.—METABOLIC NEEDS
IN BURNED CHILDREN

Water	Maintenance plus 1–2 ml/kg/% burn/24 hr
Electrolytes	1.5 mEq/kg/24 hr of sodium and potassium
Calories	At least 80 cal/kg/24 hr
Protein	20 gm/m²/24 hr of nitrogen or 125 gm/m²/24 hr of protein
Blood	Keep hematocrit over 35%
Weight	Beware of weight loss exceeding 15% of preburn weight

Lowrey[29] and others have reported the occasional occurrence of hypertension in burned children, which seems to be associated with prolonged catecholamine and renin excretion. This complication has been infrequent and transient for the most part in our patients.

Wound Care

As soon as provisions have been made for airway management and establishment of a secure route for fluid administration, debridement is performed. Cleansing should be performed gently with warm water or saline, preferably in a Hubbard hydrotherapy tank. Loose tissue and hair should be removed and we prefer to unroof blisters in patients with extensive burn injuries. Soaps containing hexachlorophene should be used sparingly or not at all in burn-injured children, since such subjects are prone to develop seizures from excessive absorption. General anesthesia is not required and intravenous sedation with small doses of morphine or meperidine hydrochloride is sufficient. Burned extremities should be elevated as much as possible in order to minimize accumulation of edema.

Escharotomy (Fig. 20-4)

The administration of large volumes of fluid for resuscitation necessarily results in the accumulation of extensive amounts of edema. When circumferential full-thickness burns are present on the extremities or the trunk, vascular compromise of the fingers or toes or respiratory embarrassment may occur from progressive augmentation of edema. Although elevation of the involved extremities may alleviate the effects of edema to some extent, escharotomy may be required. Moylan and co-workers[36] have suggested the use of the Doppler ultrasonic flowmeter to indicate whether critical reduction in blood flow to the hands or feet has occurred. We have used this routinely and have found it to be extremely valuable. The escharotomy technique described by Pruitt and associates[44] involves an incision through es-

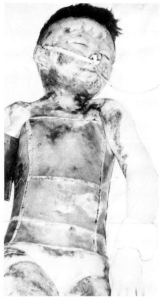

Fig. 20-4.—Escharotomy. To relieve severe constriction and interference with breathing from a circumferential full-thickness burn of the trunk, as in this child, or in a full-thickness circumferential burn of an extremity, threatening its circulation, incision is carried through the eschar into the fat.

char alone on the lateral and medial aspects of the extremity throughout the area of burn. Deeper incisions, particularly fasciotomy, are not required, except perhaps in certain electrical injuries. If escharotomy is going to be required, it ordinarily will be needed within the first 12–24 hours.

Topical Antibacterial Therapy

Fatal burn wound infection has been recognized for more than 100 years, and the concept of topical therapy was recognized even then. Rabin and co-workers[48] reported in 1961 that *Pseudomonas aeruginosa* is the principal bacterial organism associated with lethal burn wound infection, although organisms in almost endless variety are involved in burn wound colonization. Teplitz[53] has described the pathologic features of burn wound sepsis, and experimental models have been developed for the purpose of testing topical antibacterial agents. It appears that bacterial invasion takes at least 4 days to become established in adults, but this may occur in 48 hours in young children, probably because of their thinner skin. The 0.5% silver nitrate soaks applied through bulky dressings, used with great benefit in the past, have been largely replaced by topical creams, easier to use and not requiring dressings.[35] Silver nitrate soaks are quite effective against Pseudomonas organisms and a variety of others as well. In 1965, Lindberg, *et al.*[28] reported the use of 10% mafenide hydrochloride cream. It was effective against Pseudomonas organisms but caused pain and an acidosis related to carbonic anhydrase inhibition. The 10% mafenide acetate cream in current use tends to minimize the problem of acidosis and has proved to be effective in diminishing mortality from burn wound sepsis in children with burns of less than 70% of body surface.[45] This would appear to be the best drug for patients with extensive burns involving thick eschar, since mafenide penetrates eschar to a greater degree than other topical agents. However, mafenide cream application is associated with severe pain in the child with significant areas of partial-thickness burn, and 1% silver sulfadiazine cream is a better choice under these circumstances. Fox and associates[19] have shown that silver sulfadiazine is effective against Pseudomonas without producing pain or significant metabolic toxicity. Approximately 8–10% of individuals treated with mafenide or silver sulfadiazine develop sensitivity rashes. The majority of these will respond to diphenhydramine hydrochloride, but occasionally it will be necessary to discontinue the topical agent. Under these circumstances, silver nitrate soaks are useful. Despite the effectiveness of the various topical antibacterial agents, invasive burn wound sepsis still occurs, particularly in patients with large burn injuries. Before the advent of topical therapy, burn wound sepsis was diagnosed primarily on the basis of the clinical appearance of the patient and his wound. Since the advent of topical therapy, it has been recognized that invasive burn wound sepsis may be present even though the classically described wound findings are absent. For this reason, most workers recommend that representative burn wound biopsies and quantitative cultures be performed weekly or more often in patients with burns greater than 40%.[9, 46] Levels of bacteria greater than 10^4 organisms per gram of tissue indicate impending burn wound sepsis, and a change in therapy is in order. Counts in excess of 10^5 organisms per gram of tissue are diagnostic of invasive sepsis. Massive parenteral antibiotic therapy, changes in topical therapy and subeschar infusion of antibiotics are approaches sometimes useful under these circumstances.[9] Burn wound biopsies may also indicate the presence of opportunistic invasion by other organisms, such as *Providencia stuartii*, *Serratia marcescens*, candida, phycomycetes, herpesvirus and others.

Systemic Antibiotic Therapy

During the 1940s, streptococcal cellulitis was a frequent early complication of burn injury and, on this account, intravenous penicillin was recommended to be given on a prophylactic basis for the first 3–5 days postburn.[27] This was prior to the use of effective topical therapy, and since the latter has been introduced, the incidence of streptococcal infection has fallen. Recent studies by Larkin and Moylan[23] seriously question the value of prophylactic penicillin therapy and suggest that the use of early prophylactic penicillin may be harmful from the standpoint of sensitivity and the establishment of resistant flora. It is recommended that systemic antimicrobial agents should be administered on the basis of information gained from bacteriologic cultures. It is worthwhile to obtain weekly wound surface cultures and, as indicated, quantitative cultures from burn wound biopsies, so that appropriate systemic antibiotics may be administered to patients whose infection escapes from control by topical antibacterial therapy. Routine bacteriologic surveillance of other sources of infection is vital to management and includes monitoring of urine, blood, intravenous catheters, pulmonary secretions and any other possible source or site of infection. Prophylactic penicillin is indicated where autografting is being performed. Liedberg *et al.*[27] have reported studies demonstrating that the presence of group A beta-hemolytic streptococcus within the burn wound is associated with rapid loss of autograft.

Other Aspects of Infection Control

Tetanus immunization was given routinely in the past to all patients with burn injuries. Current information would indicate that antibody response is adequate in those who have been immunized within the prior 7–10 years. We administer tetanus toxoid to those who have not been immunized for 5 years and to those who have associated tetanus-prone soft tissue injuries. Children who have not been previously immunized to tetanus should receive tetanus toxoid and tetanus immune globulin.

Arturson and associates[4] have shown that immunoglobulin G levels are depressed in seriously burned patients for at least a month following burn. For this reason, they and others have recommended that gamma globulin be administered during this phase. There are no controlled studies of its value.[4, 51] Alexander and co-workers[2] and O'Neill and his group[40] have reported studies indicating that early immunization with heptavalent Pseudomonas antigen is a worthwhile protective measure in terms of preventing sepsis, but the method still is experimental. Numerous other immunologic deficits have been reported throughout the immunologic arc, such as defects in opsonization, chemotaxis and neutrophil function.[25, 55] Under these circumstances, administration of fresh-frozen plasma may be helpful.

Continuing Care and Coverage of the Burn Wound

The key to control of infection and to patient survival is expeditious closure of the burn wound. With adequate topical antibacterial therapy, partial-thickness areas of the burn wound usually heal within 2–4 weeks, depending on the size and depth of the injury. Full-thickness eschar ordinarily separates spontaneously by 3–4 weeks, but this process may be accelerated by daily careful debridement of the necrotic tissue as it softens and separates during this interval. This probably is best performed while the patient is being cleansed and given physical therapy in a hydrotherapy tank each day. Depending on the amount of eschar removed, one may continue to use topical therapy on the entire wound or cover the debrided areas with biologic dressings while using topical therapy on the remaining eschar. The vast majority of patients are best treated in this fashion. McMillan[32] has described the procedure of early excision and grafting without the use of topical therapy in certain children with limited areas of burn. Burke and co-workers[14] have carried this approach to its radical extreme in a daring experimental study in a few massively burned children in whom early staged excision of their wounds was performed in association with allograft coverage under immunosuppressive therapy. To date, the validity of the latter approach for patients with massive injuries has not been confirmed by other workers. Janzekovic[22] has reported impressive results with partial tangential excision and grafting of extensive areas of predominantly deep partial-thickness burn. Other approaches to early eschar removal include laser excision and application of enzymatic agents.[26] Unfortunately, results with enzymes designed to hasten eschar separation have been disappointing, since an increased incidence of sepsis has been noted with their use when large areas of burn have been treated early.[20]

Physiologic Dressings

As soon as most of the eschar has been removed from full-thickness injuries, and healthy granulations are present, preparations should be made for autografting. Experience would indicate that complete acceptance of autograft is not ordinarily achieved immediately following eschar debridement and that an additional phase of wound care is desirable. Zaroff and co-workers[59] demonstrated the value of repeated applications of allograft to full-thickness burn wounds in preparation for autografting. Since allograft may be difficult to obtain, others have reported the use of porcine xenografts and certain prosthetic materials in the same fashion[13, 37] (Fig. 20–5). Physiologic dressings decrease the loss of protein, red cells, water and heat. They limit bacterial growth and thereby protect and improve the character of granulation tissue and also enhance the rate of healing of partial-thickness burns. Patients are more comfortable with their wounds covered and are better able to move injured extremities. Such coverage is also helpful to patients who have limited donor sites and are being carried through successive phases of autografting. Ordinarily, physiologic dressings are changed daily at first and then every 3–5 days until they become firmly adherent. At this point, autografting usually is successful. Firm acceptance of a physiologic dressing by the burn wound would appear to be a reliable test of the wound's readiness for definitive closure; this may be the most important contribution of this method to patient care.

Autografting

Complete coverage of all areas of full-thickness burn should be accomplished in one stage if possible, but if the wound is too extensive, or if all areas are not ready for grafting, autografts should be applied to priority areas first, such as the head and neck, hands, feet and areas around joints. Strip grafts are the best form of wound coverage, since scarring is minimized when the entire wound can be covered

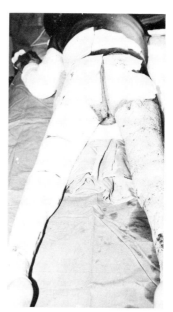

Fig. 20–5. — Prosthetic coverage of clean burn wounds. This child has both pigskin and the artificial prosthetic Epigard. Autografting is not likely to be successful immediately after removal of the eschar, and when the dressing becomes firmly adherent, the wound is ready for removal of the covering and grafting.

with skin. However, expansion mesh grafts are preferable when donor areas are limited.[52] The mesh graft technique is also extremely useful in patients with full-thickness burns in which there are multiple scattered epithelial islands. It generally is preferable to apply strip grafts to the wound without sutures and to leave them open with the patient appropriately restrained. Under these circumstances, the strip grafts may be examined frequently and areas of suppuration or seroma formation drained or unroofed as indicated. Grafts to circumferential burns of the extremities are best covered with firmly applied bulky dressings. Forty-eight hours following autografting with strip grafts, daily treatments in the Hubbard hydrotherapy tank are resumed so that dressings may be changed, grafts debrided and physical therapy attended to. On the other hand, mesh grafts, which usually are applied with a 3 to 1 expansion ratio, require coverage with fine mesh gauze and a bulky gauze dressing moistened at frequent intervals. After 72 hours, these patients once again are returned to hydrotherapy. In those occasional instances in which suppuration and loss of mesh graft occurs, the wounds ordinarily will clean up following a few days of application of fine mesh gauze impregnated with topical antibacterial cream and daily cleansing in the Hubbard tank.

The donor site is an important consideration. A child's skin is thin. Skin may be obtained from donor sites repeatedly, every 2–4 weeks, depending on the rate of donor site healing. We prefer to cover donor sites with a single thickness of fine mesh gauze, which is allowed to separate spontaneously as the donor area re-epithelializes. In those very rare instances in which donor sites become infected, topical antibacterial therapy usually is effective.

Although the physical therapist's contribution to patient care is important throughout all phases of treatment, it is particularly important during and following the phase of wound coverage. Appropriate use of splints, traction and active movement is essential to an optimal functional result. Larson et al.[24] recently have recommended the use of compressive wraps or garments for 6–12 months in order to prevent and treat hypertrophic scar formation[24] (Fig. 20–6). In our experience, the use of this method has substantially reduced the number of reconstructive procedures required by patients with extensive burns compared to prior experience without the use of compressive dressings.

Complications Associated with Burn Injury

The most common cause of death in burn patients is pneumonia. Although many of these pneumonias are related to invasive wound infection, the majority are airborne.[1] Appropriate antibiotic therapy, vigorous pulmonary toilet and intensive ventilatory support are the mainstays of treatment. It must be remembered that some cases are iatrogenic, caused by inadequate sterile technique in the management of artificial airways and inhalation equipment.

Another form of iatrogenic and potentially lethal infection is suppurative thrombophlebitis,[42] seen primarily in burn-injured patients who require intravenous catheters. Characteristically, several days following removal of an intravenous catheter, patients may develop sepsis with no obvious cause. Under these circumstances, old cutdown incisions should be opened and the course of the possibly involved vein gently milked in the direction of the incision. If pus appears within the incision or if there is obvious redness and swelling along the course of the vein, the area should be explored and all of the involved vein excised. The usual organisms involved are *Staphylococcus aureus* and a variety of gram-negative bacteria. Less aggressive therapy than excision of the vein usually is unsuccessful.

Gastrointestinal problems rank high on the list of complications of burn injury. The most common of these is gastroduodenal ulceration—Curling's ulcer. The incidence is higher, lethality greater and serious bleeding and perforation more common in children than in older individuals. In an environment where there is diminished renewal of protective gastric mucus, relative gastric hyperacidity may po-

tentiate mucosal ulceration and lead to serious bleeding or perforation.[39] Endoscopic evaluation of seriously burned patients indicates that mucosal congestion and some degree of ulceration occur in essentially every seriously burned patient. The use of frequent milk feedings, maintenance of optimal nutrition and possibly administration of vitamin A have been associated with a marked reduction in the number of children who have required operation because of the complications related to Curling's ulcer.[31, 49] When massive bleeding does occur, it usually is seen between the fifth and tenth postburn days. It may be treated initially with blood transfusions, nasogastric drainage, iced saline gastric lavage and other supportive measures. The decision to resort to operation should be based on the same criteria used for any patient with serious acute gastrointestinal hemorrhage. When operation has been required, vagotomy, antrectomy and excision of the ulcer, if possible, has been the most successful method of approach in our hands.[43]

Although reference has been made above to a number of complications and others of a more obscure nature have not been discussed, attention must be paid to psychologic considerations. Children who have extensive burns characteristically regress to earlier stages of development. Additionally, they may develop extreme hostility toward their parents and others involved in their care. Self-destructive behavior such as bruxing of teeth and dislodgment of healed skin grafts may require administration of sedatives and appropriate restraint devices. Administration of small doses of drugs such as diazepam may be helpful, but care must be exercised with any drug excreted via the liver, since hepatic dysfunction is a common long-term problem in patients with large injuries. During periods of extreme disorders of behavior, the situation may require a great deal of understanding and support on the part of all members of the burn team for the patient and his family. A cheerful environment, availability of toys and television and a humane approach to painful procedures are helpful. Fortunately, all of these undesirable psychologic changes seem to gradually revert to normal as children recover. We have been gratified to note on long-term follow-up that the vast majority of these children have few or no apparent emotional scars, but a great deal of effort has been expended to achieve this result.

Results

Morbidity and mortality figures have declined over the past 10 years as a result of improvements in fluid therapy and respiratory care, better bacteriologic control with topical agents and physiologic wound dressings, more expeditious wound coverage, better nutrition, centralization of care and a number of other advances. These improvements have been even more remarkable in children than in adults. Bruck and co-workers[13a] at the U. S. Army Institute of Surgical Research reported that topical antibacterial therapy resulted in a change of the LD_{50} burn from approximately 35% of body surface to 65% in a group of 412 children. These figures have been reproduced and even surpassed in a number of centers.[31a] At present, the average burn size in hospitalized patients at our institution is around 30%, although the range is from 10% to 95% of body surface. The over-all mortality is approximately 10% and the LD_{50} burn is around 70%. There has been no mortality in burns under 30% of body surface. The burn in excess of 70% of body surface is a significant challenge and still associated with a disappointingly high mortality. In our hands, these results appear to be the same throughout the 0–14 year age group.

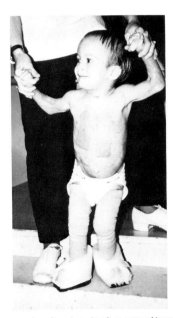

Fig. 20–6.—Compression dressings in after-care of burns. Constant physical therapy is vital to a good functional result. Compression dressings as shown here prevent hypertrophic scarring and promote better function. Note the special shoes constructed to protect this child's feet, which suffered loss of all skin and toes.

Morbidity patterns have changed a great deal in our experience, but the trend is also in a favorable direction. Burn wound sepsis is causing fewer deaths in our patients than before the time of effective topical agents, but it still is a problem in patients with burns in excess of 60%. Also, Pseudomonas is less often the offender than previously and new opportunists are emerging.

Prior to the time frequent milk feedings were given early postburn, severe manifestations of Curling's ulcer occurred in 10% of patients and associated mortality was at least 50%. Since the advent of frequent milk feedings 6 years ago, we have not had to operate on a single child for gastrointestinal bleeding, and none have died on this account.

Improved techniques of physical therapy and compression dressings following grafting have reduced the morbidity related to scar hypertrophy and contracture enough to represent a significant contribution to care. Still more needs to be accomplished in this regard.

The length of hospital stay has also diminished. Patients who are treated for partial-thickness burns that do not require grafting generally are hospitalized for from 5 to 14 days, depending on the size and depth of the injury. Patients who need grafting have required from 2 weeks to 4 months of hospitalization, depending on the extent of the injury, how many grafting procedures are required and how much early rehabilitative work is needed.

As more information comes to light and more is understood about the pathophysiology of injury, further improvements in morbidity and mortality can be expected.

REFERENCES

1. Achauer, B. M., *et al.:* Pulmonary complications of burns: The major threat to the burn patient, Ann. Surg. 177:311, 1973.
2. Alexander, J. W.: Immunologic Considerations and the Role of Vaccination in Burn Injury, in Polk, H. C., and Stone, H. H. (eds.), *Contemporary Burn Management* (Boston: Little, Brown and Company, 1971), p. 177.
3. Allison, S. P., Hinton, P., and Chamberlain, M. J.: Intravenous glucose-tolerance, insulin, and free-fatty-acid levels in burned patients, Lancet 2:1113, 1968.
4. Arturson, G., *et al.:* Changes in immunoglobulin levels in severely burned patients, Lancet 1:546, 1969.
5. Artz, C. P., and Moncrief, J. A.: *The Treatment of Burns* (2d ed.: Philadelphia: W. B. Saunders Company, 1969).
6. Baar, S., and Arrowsmith, D. J.: Thermal damage to red cells, J. Clin. Pathol. 23:572, 1970.
7. Baxter, C. R.: Crystalloid Resuscitation of Burn Shock, in Polk, H. C., and Stone, H. H. (eds.), *Contemporary Burn Management* (Boston: Little, Brown and Company, 1971), p. 7.
8. Baxter, C. R., Cook, W. A., and Shires, G. T.: Serum myocardial depressant factor of burn shock, Surg. Forum 17:1, 1966.
9. Baxter, C. R., Curreri, P. W., and Marvin, J. A.: The control of burn wound sepsis by the use of quantitative bacteriologic studies and subeschar clysis with antibiotics, Surg. Clin. North Am. 53:1509, 1973.
10. Baxter, C. R., and Shires, G. T.: Physiological response to crystalloid resuscitation of severe burns, Ann. N. Y. Acad. Sci. 150:874, 1968.
11. Berman, W., *et al.:* Childhood burn injuries and deaths, Pediatrics 51:1069, 1973.
12. Birke, G., *et al.:* Studies on burns. IX. The distribution and losses through the wound of ^{131}I-albumin measured by whole-body counting, Acta Chir. Scand. 134:27, 1968.
13. Bromberg, B. E., Song, I. C., and Mohn, M. P.: The use of pigskin as a temporary biological dressing, Plast. Reconstr. Surg. 36:80, 1965.
13a. Bruck, H. M., Asch, M. J., and Pruitt, B. A.: Burns in children: A 10-year experience with 412 patients, J. Trauma 10:658, 1970.
14. Burke, J. F., *et al.:* Immunosuppression and temporary skin transplantation in the treatment of massive third degree burns, Ann. Surg. 182:183, 1975.
15. Cameron, J. S., and Miller-Jones, C. M. H.: Renal function and renal failure in badly burned children, Br. J. Surg. 54:132, 1967.
16. Dawkins, M. J. R., and Scopes, J. W.: Nonshivering thermogenesis and brown adipose tissue in the human newborn infant, Nature 206:201, 1965.
17. Edelmann, C. M., and Spitzer, A.: The maturing kidney, J. Pediatr. 75:509, 1969.
18. Evans, E. I., *et al.:* Fluid and electrolyte requirements in severe burns, Ann. Surg. 135:804, 1952.
19. Fox, C. L., Roppole, B. W., and Stanford, W.: Control of Pseudomonas infection in burns by silver sulfadiazine, Surg. Gynecol. Obstet. 128:1021, 1969.
20. Hummel, R. P., *et al.:* The continuing problem of sepsis following enzymatic debridement of burns, J. Trauma 14:572, 1974.
21. Hunt, J. L., *et al.:* The pathophysiology of acute electrical injuries, J. Trauma 16:335, 1976.
22. Janzekovic, Z.: The burn wound from the surgical point of view, J. Trauma 15:42, 1975.
23. Larkin, J. M., and Moylan, J. A.: The role of prophylactic antibiotics in burn care, Am. Surg. 42:247, 1976.
24. Larson, D. L., *et al.:* Techniques of decreasing scar formation and contractures in the burned patient, J. Trauma 11:807, 1971.
25. Lennard, E. S., *et al.:* An immunologic and nutritional evaluation of burn neutrophil function, J. Surg. Res. 16:286, 1974.
26. Levine, N., *et al.:* Use of carbon dioxide laser for debridement of third degree burns, Ann. Surg. 179:246, 1974.
27. Liedberg, N. C., *et al.:* Infections in burns. II. The pathogenicity of streptococci, Surg. Gynecol. Obstet. 98:693, 1954.
28. Lindberg, R. B., *et al.:* The successful control of burn wound sepsis, J. Trauma 5:601, 1965.
29. Lowrey, G. H.: Hypertension in children with burns, J. Trauma 7:140, 1967.
30. Lund, C. C., and Browder, N. C.: The estimation of areas of burns, Surg. Gynecol. Obstet. 79:352, 1944.
31. McAlhany, J. C., Czaja, A. J., and Pruitt, B. A.: Antacid control of complications from acute gastroduodenal disease after burns, J. Trauma 16:645, 1976.
31a. McCoy, J. A., Micks, D. W., and Lynch, J. B.: Discriminant function probability model for predicting survival in burned patients, JAMA 203:644, 1968.
32. McMillan, B. G.: Indications for early excision, Surg. Clin. North Am. 50:1337, 1970.
33. Moncrief, J. A.: Burns, N. Engl. J. Med. 288:444, 1973.
34. Moncrief, J. A., and Mason, A. D.: Evaporative water loss in the burned patient, J. Trauma 4:180, 1964.
35. Moyer, C. A., *et al.:* Treatment of large human burns with 0.5% silver nitrate solution, Arch. Surg. 90:812, 1965.
36. Moylan, J. A., Inge, W. W., and Pruitt, B. A.: Circulatory changes following circumferential extremity burns evaluated by ultrasonic flowmeter: An analysis of 60 thermally injured limbs, J. Trauma 11:763, 1971.
37. O'Neill, J. A.: Comparison of xenograft and prosthesis for burn wound care, J. Pediatr. Surg. 8:705, 1973.
38. O'Neill, J. A., *et al.:* Patterns of injury in the battered child syndrome, J. Trauma 13:332, 1976.
39. O'Neill, J. A., *et al.:* Studies in the pathogenesis of Curling's ulcer, J. Trauma 7:275, 1967.
40. O'Neill, J. A., Nance, F. C., and Fisher, M. W.: Heptavalent Pseudomonas vaccination in seriously burned children, J. Pediatr. Surg. 6:548, 1971.
41. O'Neill, J. A., Pruitt, B. A., and Moncrief, J. A.: Studies of Renal Function during the Early Postburn Period, in Artz, C. P. (ed.), *Research in Burns* (Bern: Hans Huber, 1971), p. 95.
42. O'Neill, J. A., Pruitt, B. A., and Moncrief, J. A.: Suppurative thrombophlebitis, a lethal complication of intravenous therapy, J. Trauma 8:256, 1968.
43. O'Neill, J. A., Pruitt, B. A., and Moncrief, J. A.: Surgical treatment of Curling's ulcer, Surg. Gynecol. Obstet. 126:40, 1968.
44. Pruitt, B. A., Dowling, J. A., and Moncrief, J. A.: Escharotomy in early burn care, Arch. Surg. 96:502, 1968.
45. Pruitt, B. A., *et al.:* Successful control of burn wound sepsis, JAMA 203:1054, 1968.
46. Pruitt, B. A., and Foley, F. D.: The use of biopsies in burn patient care, Surgery 73:887, 1973.
47. Pruitt, B. A., Mason, A. D., and Moncrief, J. A.: Hemodynamic changes in the early postburn patient: The influence of fluid administration and of a vasodilator (hydralazine), J. Trauma 11:36, 1971.
48. Rabin, E. R., *et al.:* Fatal Pseudomonas infection in burned patients: A clinical, bacteriologic and anatomic study, N. Engl. J. Med. 265:1225, 1961.
49. Rai, K., and Courtemanche, A. D.: Vitamin A assay in burned patients, J. Trauma 15:419, 1975.

50. Reiss, E., *et al.*: Fluid and electrolyte balance in burns, JAMA 152:1309, 1953.
51. Stone, H. H., *et al.*: Evaluation of gamma globulin for prophylaxis against burn sepsis, Surgery 58:810, 1965.
52. Tanner, J. C., Vandeput, J., and Olley, J. F.: The mesh skin graft, Plast. Reconstr. Surg. 34:287, 1964.
53. Teplitz, C.: Pathogenesis of Pseudomonas vasculitis and septic lesions, Arch. Pathol. 80:297, 1965.
54. Teplitz, C., *et al.*: Pathology of low tracheostomy in children, Am. J. Clin. Pathol. 42:58, 1964.
55. Warden, G. D., Mason, A. D., and Pruitt, B. A.: Evaluation of leukocyte chemotaxis in vitro in thermally injured patients, J. Clin. Invest. 54:1001, 1974.
56. Wilkinson, A. W.: Some aspects of renal function in the newly born, J. Pediatr. Surg. 8:103, 1973.
57. Wilmore, D. W., *et al.*: Catecholamines: Mediator of the hypermetabolic response to thermal injury, Ann. Surg. 180:653, 1974.
58. Wilson, J. S., and Moncrief, J. A.: Vapor pressure of normal and burned skin, Ann. Surg. 162:130, 1965.
59. Zaroff, L. I., *et al.*: Multiple uses of viable cutaneous homografts in the burned patient, Surgery 59:368, 1966.
60. Zawacki, B. E., *et al.*: Does increased evaporative water loss cause hypermetabolism in burned patients?, Ann. Surg. 171:236, 1970.

21 Paul V. Woolley, Jr. / Jack H. Hertzler / Joseph O. Reed

The Battered Child

INTEMPERATE VIOLENCE directed against the immature has been an element of varying importance in all cultures and has never been foreign to our own. Recognition of the extent and varied manifestations of the malady has come as a shock to the community over the past 25 years, so that current interest transcends professional boundaries to involve medicine, the law, sociology and the several behavioral sciences.

In the past, it has been difficult to estimate with precision the frequency with which wanton injury is visited on infants and young children, since earlier data were accumulated in patterns skewed toward the interest and experience of individual observers.[2, 10] It was to correct this imbalance that Kempe and his colleagues[5] introduced the term battered-child syndrome to cover the gamut of physical, emotional and nutritional abuses recognized by the alert physician. This change in orientation has resulted in a deluge of lay and medical literature that gives an impression of a sizable increase in abuse, but we have not been able to document this at our institution, where careful records have been monitored for more than two decades and attention given to changes in definition, in reporting and in awareness. We can all agree that the problem is not diminishing, as witnessed by the fact that we alone recorded roughly 300 instances in 1976.

The Background of Child Abuse

Man lives in a world of violence, cruelty and disorganized behavior, to much of which he becomes inured without a very deep understanding of motivations. Child abuse is a facet of the over-all problem and one would not expect to find easily elicited and universally common denominators. Actually, we are working in an unusually difficult zone of comprehension, since we have no concise definition of child abuse, rarely a competent complainant and frequently no witnesses. Certain patterns are quite clear and others assume sufficient form for valid consideration while well-constituted multidisciplinary groups the country over continue to study the problem.

The vast majority of injuries are inflicted by persons having natural, legal or de facto control of the victim; e.g., parents, other adult relatives and paramours, guardians and baby-sitters. Sibs are, in our experience, decidedly in the minority and, when implicated, frequently are acting out the pattern of a generally disturbed ménage. When only one person is deemed abusive, it may be either male or female, more commonly female in most studies. In many homes, battering seems almost a conspiracy or, at the least, a permissive attitude characterizes the nonviolent partner.

It is clear that homes in which battering occurs are not set apart by economic status, intellectual or educational level or social heritage of the occupants. Each exerts a quantitative influence but none is a determinant. The impression that abuse is entirely an urban disease of ignorance and poverty or that it is limited to one racial group is largely a figment of methods for ascertainment, reporting and investigation.

In our state of incomplete knowledge, we still look on physical trauma in infancy and childhood as arising under a spectrum of environmental and interhuman situations. Probably simplest on the scale is what might be termed a generally unprotective environment. Here, active aggression is not as important as is a more subtle element—the failure in the positive responsibility of parents to provide for their children a safe and secure home. Many cannot do this because of factors such as low intelligence, alcoholism or an incomplete family unit with an excessive load thrown on the survivor. These factors are compounded by inadequate equipment, slovenly housekeeping and the general defeatism of poverty. Victims of such situations might be regarded as "passively battered." A step above this environment in the spectrum might incorporate mental inadequacy, with the attending lack of self control and poor judgment where an element of aggressive behavior would be present.[9]

Homes in which poverty and lack of education or intelligence are not major problems are being studied in increasing number, with almost as many conclusions as there are investigators.[6] Young age of parents, frequently with an accompanying lack of close or wholesome ties to family and community, is a common factor in our material. Many observers are impressed by the number of parents who were themselves rigidly or sternly dealt with during childhood or were deprived of a close and dear person during the formative years. Everyday terms, such as "angry personality," "easily frustrated," "in a period of unusual stress," "heavy drinker" and the like, appear recurrently. Overt psychosis is encountered rarely in the reports from most investigators.

Currently, a number of studies are concerned with defining attitudes and patterns that might characterize the actual or potential batterer and these, if successful, might allow a prophylactic approach to some dangerous situations.

The victim himself must form part of the background for abuse. In many instances, a single child is selected from several to bear the brunt of violence while the remainder are spared. We have seen one of twins severely handled while the mate is spared. We do not believe that this whipping-boy situation is as prevalent as it appeared to be earlier, since when abusive households are studied over longer periods we find recurring violence toward new members and an unusual incidence of "accidents." More than 80% of seriously battered children have been under 3 years of age. It is self-evident that when ease of frustration is a major factor in abuse, some children will prove more frustrating or abrasive than others. "Irritable," "poor sleeper," "stubborn," "hard to train" are terms frequently used in characterizing injured children whereas several we have seen are known from earlier admissions because of eczema, cerebral palsy, vomiting or chronic diarrhea.

Lesions Associated with Physical Abuse

Inflicted injuries run roughly the same gamut of tissue and organ damage as do those purely accidental. In general, most infants survive the first year or two of life without major mishap, and when an accident does occur, all damage can be explained by a single vector of force. With active aggression,

on the other hand, injuries tend to be repetitive and cumulative and the lesions resulting from a single episode frequently do not conform to a uniform vector. To illustrate, an infant is examined after the mother supposedly fell down 6 steps while carrying the baby. We would not be surprised to find a fracture through the midportion of the femur and a linear fracture of the skull. However, we would be most alarmed to find a fractured skull plus small metaphyseal disruptions at each knee, since the latter usually come from torsion, not from a fall. It would also be disturbing to find the fresh skull fracture but to notice callus around the break in the femur!

Skeletal Injuries

These can be of any type, but attention is called to the frequency with which metaphyseal injuries are present. These are caused by such torsions as might arise from violent shaking or twisting and most commonly are seen around the knee. They are explained anatomically by the firm attachment through Sharpey's fibers of the periosteum to the cartilage of long bones in contrast to the loose arrangement along the diaphyses. These fractures vary in appearance from small triangular chips (Fig. 21-1, *A*) to more linear fragments termed "bucket handles" (Fig. 21-1, *B*). They are accompanied clinically by pain and periarticular swelling. Associated ecchymoses are infrequent. Calcification along the adjoining shaft, from which the periosteum has been stripped or elevated, usually appears within 7-10 days and thereafter healing is quite rapid, so that within 2-4 months the injury appears as cortical thickening, which, in turn, gradually remodels, with complete healing (Fig 21-1, *C*). Discovery of one area of metaphyseal damage should automatically suggest a search for similar lesions elsewhere as well as a complete survey to rule out other evidence of battering. It was this classic pattern that earlier suggested an

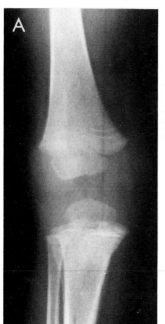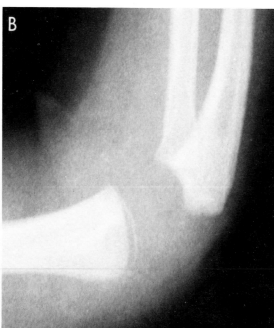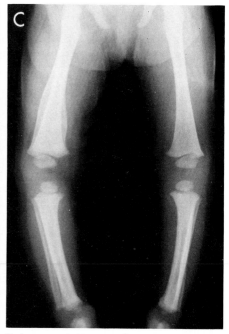

Fig. 21-1.—Metaphyseal fractures from torsion or shaking injuries. **A,** oblique fracture of the tibia, laterally through the epiphysis, producing a characteristic triangular fragment and marked swelling of soft tissue of knee and thigh. The 22-month-old girl had multiple other injuries (see Figs. 21-3, **A** and 21-4), reputedly inflicted by mother's "boyfriend." **B,** "bucket handle" linear, transverse fracture of humerus. This 7-week-old infant was said to have "had a fall"—an unlikely cause of this injury. **C,** healing metaphyseal fracture. A large calcified subperiosteal hematoma with healing metaphyseal fracture of right femur. Note also "greenstick" fracture of left distal tibia. The child was 7 months of age and was admitted with recent fracture of the left radius.

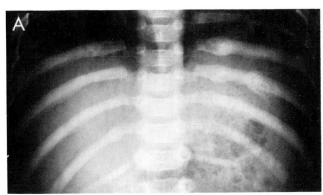

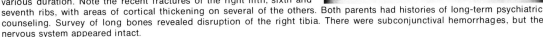

Fig. 21-2.—Rib fractures. These occur rarely from accidents but are relatively frequent in battering. **A,** a 4-month-old admitted initially because of poor weight gain. Skeletal survey revealed multiple fractures of ribs and an area of calcification in the region of the pancreas. There also were healed fractures of the left humerus and radial diaphyses, plus assorted bruises. **B,** a 10-week-old baby with multiple rib fractures of various duration. Note the recent fractures of the right fifth, sixth and seventh ribs, with areas of cortical thickening on several of the others. Both parents had histories of long-term psychiatric counseling. Survey of long bones revealed disruption of the right tibia. There were subconjunctival hemorrhages, but the nervous system appeared intact.

increased metaphyseal fragility and led to confusion between traumatic changes and scurvy, a condition in which all bones are evenly involved by the underlying deficiency.

We are impressed by the rarity with which fractured ribs are encountered following accidents as compared with the relative frequency in battering. Probably distortion by compression leads to this deformity rather than a direct blow or fall, such as would commonly occur accidentally (Fig. 21-2). Skull fractures (Fig. 21-3) vary in form and extent and tend to be linear or stellate rather than depressed. Rarely are they accompanied by contusions and the majority probably result from angulation of cranial bones rather than from a direct blow. The usual lack of correlation between radiologic evidence of fracture and the presence or extent of underlying damage is exhibited. Only about half of the subdural hematomas or brain contusion in our material were accompanied by visible fracture of the skull (Fig. 21-3, *B*).

We carried out, at the time of our initial interest in trauma to the skeleton (Figs. 21-4 and 21-5), an extensive survey

of bone pathology seen in infancy and came to the conclusion that rarely must a serious differential diagnosis be entertained.[10] This view, in general, still is current, provided that good-quality films of the entire skeleton are available and the interpreter has had reasonable experience with radiography in small children. Baker and Berdon[1] have studied and illustrated a variety of generalized and local skeletal lesions that predispose to fracture.

Injuries to the Nervous System

These rank next to skeletal lesions in frequency and account for the major part of serious permanent disability. They occur separately or in conjunction with other lesions of battering. Acute or chronic subdural hematoma (Fig. 21-3, *B*) is the form most commonly encountered, frequently the obvious anatomic expression of brain injury or the residuum of earlier brain contusion.

Recently, much interest has centered about the ocular in-

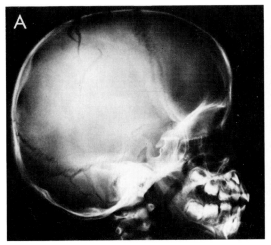

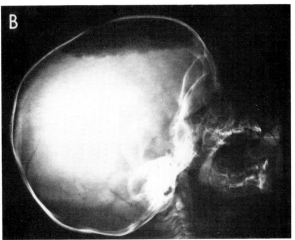

Fig. 21-3.—Skull fracture. **A,** skull of a 20-month-old showing biparietal fractures with widened sutures, indicating elevated intracranial pressure. This is the same infant shown in Figures 21-1, **A** and 21-4. **B,** parietal skull fracture with elevated intracranial pressure. Air outlines a dilated subdural space and the bubbly appearance of remaining fluid indicates its high protein content. A subdural-peritoneal shunt was performed and the patient currently functions at a surprisingly good level.

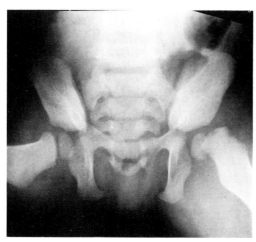

Fig. 21–4.—Epiphyseal separation. Posterior and medial separation of right capital femoral epiphysis in the patient shown in Figures 21–1, **A** and 21–3, **A.**

juries found in battered and abused children.[4, 7] Most common have been lesions characterized by bleeding into the various compartments, especially into the retina. A group of 58 children, of whom 26 had been battered and the remainder had sustained comparable head trauma through other forms of violence, have been examined here with the rather startling finding that 16 of the 17 with retinal hemorrhage were from the battered group and only 1 among those with head injury from other sources.[3] Although the cause of this discrepancy is not currently clear, it certainly indicates that children with head injury plus retinal hemorrhage deserve careful environmental scrutiny as well as inspection for other tissue injuries.

Cutaneous and Soft Tissue Injury

This is common at all ages and often is the only evidence of battering in older children. It usually is seen as bruises or hematomas. Frequently these occur in interpretable patterns when an object such as a belt or a hairbrush has been used. Five children in whom skeletal defects were found had been referred initially for study of purpura secondary to coagulation defects and in none had trauma received serious consideration. Burns are also encountered and it is wise to consider abuse whenever the thermal injury does not fit well with the proffered explanation. Small circumscribed burns frequently are from lighted cigarettes.

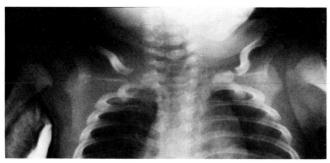

Fig. 21–5.—Injuries probably produced by jerking or shaking child by the arms. Bilateral fractures of the clavicles with separation of the ossification center of the left humeral head. The cast on the right arm is for immobilization of undisplaced fracture through the humeral diaphysis.

The external genitalia rarely have been the focal point for injury in the generally battered child but may, of course, be involved along with other soft tissue structures.

Intra-abdominal Injuries

Intra-abdominal injuries from battering are more common than we once believed, since more than 30 such children have been admitted in recent years. Of these, 24 required laparotomy and all recovered. A history of trauma was obtained initially for 75% of these children but rarely was the true circumstance confessed. Nevertheless, one-half were admitted with the correct diagnosis. The most common complaints for the group were vomiting and distention and the most frequent physical findings were distention and absence of bowel sounds.

An average of 5 specific anatomic injuries were defined in each patient, damage to bowel and solid viscera occurring with roughly equal frequency and lesions to peritoneum or mesentery next in order. This emphasizes the need for thorough preparation to manage a complex variety of disruptions as well as the necessity for gentle, careful but complete examination of all organs and all quadrants of the abdomen.

It is obvious that the possibility of blunt trauma must be given prime consideration among diagnoses whenever physical findings and laboratory or radiologic data do not conform to the more common clinically recognizable pediatric surgical conditions of the abdomen.

Recognition of Physical Abuse

There is no sine qua non for physical abuse. The thought that adults, especially parents, are capable of serious physical brutality to infants is foreign to most physicians and so repulsive that many, consciously or unconsciously, deny the possibility in an individual patient. This is especially evident when there is close parent-physician rapport or if the family is identified as being of the same economic or cultural group as the examiner—a colleague, for instance. Such attitudes explain many of the vagaries in reporting.

This taboo, with wider recognition of the problem, is breaking down—a most salutary trend that can only benefit patient, parent and physician through early detection. Rarely are episodes of battering isolated, and repetition is the rule. Better to be wholesomely suspicious than to run the risk of a truly regrettable later incident.

The following short rules have been helpful to us.

1. Be skeptical when evaluating the volunteered explanation for any injury. Recall the formula we learned in high school physics, $F = MA$ (force = mass × acceleration), and decide if the midthigh of a healthy 6-month-old baby (weighing 14 lb) is likely to fracture transversely by being accelerated through the 15 inches separating a couch from a carpeted floor—or if a fracture of the skull would result under the same circumstances.

2. When one injury is evident, look for others; metaphyseal disruption especially should call for a complete survey, including radiograms of all bones plus the skull, careful examination of the abdomen and demonstration of an intact nervous system with absence of retinal hemorrhage.

3. Regard more than one accident resulting in definite tissue injury during the first 18 months of life as rare in a well-regulated household.

4. Remember that battering encompasses more than tissue damage and appraise the over-all growth and nutritional status of the injured infant. Does he appear to be well cared for? Are his weight and height acceptable for his age?

5. Include some medical background in your histories, especially as it relates to the material included earlier on abusive households.

6. Are the reactions of parents to child and of child to parents appropriate to the situation that has led to their visit? Are the parents as protective and solicitous as those whose child might be seen because of an acute abdomen or following a car accident? How do the parents interreact with each other and does either make an effort to talk to you privately? Do neighbors or relatives attempt to communicate with you?

7. Consider the fact that parents have sought your assistance as implied consent to more than immediate care of injury. Utilize the help of colleagues and other health professions (social service, psychologists, etc.) when indicated.

8. Be realistic and do not talk about vague states such as "purpura," "mild osteogenesis imperfecta" or "subclinical scurvy." Each can be proved or disproved scientifically.

Treatment and Prophylaxis of Battering

Therapy for inflicted injuries does not differ from that of similar anatomic deviations acquired accidentally. The primary aim of the physician is to see that no further abuse befalls either the patient or other members of the household, and the best rule we can give in this respect is: *Never relinquish control of a maltreated child until he can be turned over to some other responsible person or agency.* This frequently necessitates appeal to court or to law enforcement departments, but that certainly is justified in view of the repetitive nature of violence and the high mortality among patients released to the same environment in which the initial trouble appeared.

The ultimate disposition of battered children can be made only after careful study of the individual milieu. Rarely is the physician equipped by training, emotional structure or time to undertake such investigations. These are better conducted by individuals with a good background in social work and familiarity with patterns of child abuse. They frequently are available on the hospital staff, and recently personnel in various courts, the women's division of the police and child protective agencies have been trained for these activities. Investigation must be conducted with a purely nonpunitive outlook, since the punishment for offenses is the responsibility of constituted courts and the physician's ends are met when his patient is ensured a protective environment.

It is obvious, working with a spectrum of situations, that solutions will cover a broad range of possibilities, and currently these are being evaluated in a number of centers. Sometimes material assistance and moral support for those in whom frustration and immaturity are evident suffice. In others, a close and constant tie to a person skilled in interhuman relations has helped. Some situations benefit from psychiatric approaches at various levels of sophistication and, in a residue, the household is so disturbed that long-term removal of the victim by court action is necessary. Even this is not a cure-all; several of the children in our series were battered in foster homes after having been removed from the natural household because of abuse or neglect.

Increased awareness by the community of the seriousness of the child abuse problem has resulted in legislative acts in almost all states, and the individual physician should be familiar with the rules in his specific area. These are essentially quite similar to those governing the reporting of dangerous communicable diseases. They make mandatory the notification of suspected child abuse to a designated agency by physicians, hospitals and certain other persons or agencies. These acts in many areas are of great help to physicians and deserve our support. Most provide immunity for the reporter who acts in good faith and, conversely, regard as a misdemeanor failure to submit a report when it is indicated. Usually reports are filed and tabulated in a central repository, which also is a boon to the physician in permitting detection of parents with a propensity to visit a different office or emergency facility with each episode of trauma. The broad base of eligible reporters permits the physician to shift the onus for reporting to others (a hospital, for instance) when he enjoys a professional or social relationship with the involved family or for other reasons is reluctant to act. It is obvious that no amount of legislation can help unless supported by an enlightened concern on the part of the community, the courts and the medical profession. At present, attitudes vary from an extreme of complete permissiveness or avoidance to one of unconstructive vindictiveness.

Another area of statutes with which the physician should be familiar concerns the right or duty of courts responsible for child welfare.[8] Here, again, there is great variation in interpretation and practice. We have been fortunate in working with courts whose concept of the law charges parents to provide for their children a safe and wholesome home. The occurrence of physical injury is de facto evidence that this is not being accomplished, and thus it becomes the prerogative of the court to assume a variable degree of jurisdiction. With this philosophy, it is not necessary to name a specific offender or to initiate criminal action to obtain our aim, which is, again, a protective and wholesome environment for the child.

REFERENCES

1. Baker, D. W., and Berdon, W. E.: Special trauma problems in children, Radiol. Clin. North Am. 4:289, 1966.
2. Caffey, J.: Multiple fractures in long bones of infants suffering from chronic subdural hematomas, Am. J. Roentgenol. 56:163, 1946.
3. Eisenbrey, A. B.: Unpublished data.
4. Harcourt, B., and Hopkins, D.: Ophthalmic manifestations of the battered-baby syndrome, Br. Med. J. 3:398, 1971.
5. Kempe, C. H., *et al.*: Battered-child syndrome, J.A.M.A. 181:17, 1961.
6. Lystad, M. H.: Violence at home—a review, Am. J. Orthopsychiatry 45:328, 1975.
7. Mushin, A. S.: Ocular damage in the battered-baby syndrome, Br. Med. J. 3:402, 1971.
8. Paulsen, M. G.: The legal framework for child protection, Columbia Law Rev. 66, 1966. (Reprints of this work have been prepared by the Children's Bureau, Department of Health, Education, and Welfare, Washington, D. C.)
9. Smith, S. N., Hanson, R., and Noble, S.: Social aspects of the battered baby syndrome, Br. J. Psychiatry 125:568, 1974.
10. Woolley, P. V., Jr., and Evans, W. A., Jr.: Significance of skeletal lesions in infants resembling those of traumatic origin, JAMA 158:539, 1955.

22 PETER K. KOTTMEIER

Birth Trauma

THE TERM BIRTH INJURY often has been used as synonymous with avoidable injury caused by negligence, an inaccurate implication in the vast majority of complications occurring at birth. For the purpose of this chapter the discussion of surgical aspects of "birth trauma or injury" will include perinatal complications that may become apparent at birth or within the first few days of life.[29] They can be spontaneous or induced and occasionally related to metabolic changes, such as hypoxia. Perinatal complications related to metabolic changes alone or late manifestations such as gastrointestinal perforations, which usually occur after several days of life, will not be included.

Sir Francis Bacon's (1561–1626) statement, "It is as natural to die as to be born and to a little infant, one is as painful as the other," has been supported by numerous medical reports through the past century. Probably the oldest known case of birth trauma was described by Wells,[67] who found a congenital epiphyseal humeral fracture and hemiplegia in a 25-year-old man who died approximately 330–350 years A.D. Detailed autopsy and clinical studies relating birth trauma to fetal presentation and type of delivery appeared in the early nineteenth century.[31, 50, 59]

A review of the medical literature on birth trauma in the nineteenth century and the first half of the twentieth century shows that despite advances in perinatal care and the increased use of cesarean section, the over-all incidence of birth trauma and the order of frequency in which it occurs have changed very little. We recorded an incidence of 0.7% (Table 22–1). Recent diagnostic advances, such as sonography, amniocentesis and intrauterine fetal radiologic studies, can lead to an early diagnosis of potential risks and thereby to avoidance of serious birth trauma under certain circumstances. The prenatal diagnosis of a fetal intra-abdominal mass (Fig. 22–1), which could have led to a potential disaster if the pregnancy were allowed to progress to a spontaneous vaginal delivery, presents one of the promising developments in the care of high-risk infants.[64]

Infants at Risk

The infant's size at birth is related to the variety of birth trauma likely. The large infant appears especially vulnerable to fractures,[4, 6] nerve injuries[21] and visceral injuries, such as to liver, spleen and adrenal.[2, 52] Tank *et al.*[61] emphasized that birth trauma in full-term infants is twice as common as in premature infants. Premature infants, on the other hand, although less susceptible to skeletal trauma, are more likely to sustain visceral or CNS injury.[12] Respiratory complications, such as pneumothorax, also occur more often in premature infants, especially those with "RDS."[13] Coagulation defects in newborns have been reported as contributing factors in liver, splenic and adrenal rupture.[24, 38, 55] Asphyxia and visceral congestion have also been found to be frequently associated with hepatic and adrenal hemorrhage.[36] Pre-existing congenital lesions, such as hydronephrotic kidneys or urinary tract obstructions, are known to be causative factors of urinary ascites.[47] Fetal presentation and type of delivery are closely related to birth trauma. In 1891, Spencer[59] reported head injuries "to occur more often with forceps delivery than with breech presentation, and more often with breech than head presentation." In view of the infrequent use of forceps, breech delivery now is one of the leading causes of major birth trauma, including major CNS, spinal cord, nerve, skeletal and visceral complications. Both the position of the fetus and the assistance required to deliver the infant can lead to major complications.[61] Although certain fetal presentations or disproportion of fetus and maternal pelvis can be expected to contribute to birth trauma, almost all forms of birth trauma can occur in spontaneous, full-term and apparently uncomplicated deliveries.

Head and Neck Trauma*

Peripheral Nerves

Facial Nerve Trauma

Facial nerve paralysis can be caused by either peripheral or central nerve trauma. Central facial nerve trauma leads to a spastic paralysis, peripheral trauma to a flaccid paralysis.[37] All but 2 of 21 infants in Rubin's review[49] were delivered by forceps. Paine[42] found, however, that in most cases the pressure of the infant's face against the pelvis, especially the sa-

*See Chapter 23.

TABLE 22–1.—INCIDENCE OF BIRTH TRAUMA, 1965–1974,
DOWNSTATE MEDICAL CENTER, SUNY
(Total No. Deliveries: 59,963; No. Birth Trauma: 437 [0.7% of All Deliveries])

TYPE OF BIRTH TRAUMA	NO.	% OF DELIVERIES	% OF BIRTH TRAUMA
Peripheral nerve	167	0.27	38.2
Pneumothorax	120	0.20	27
Fracture	69	0.11	16.1
Intracranial hemorrhage	40	0.06	9.1
Other	41	0.06	9.3

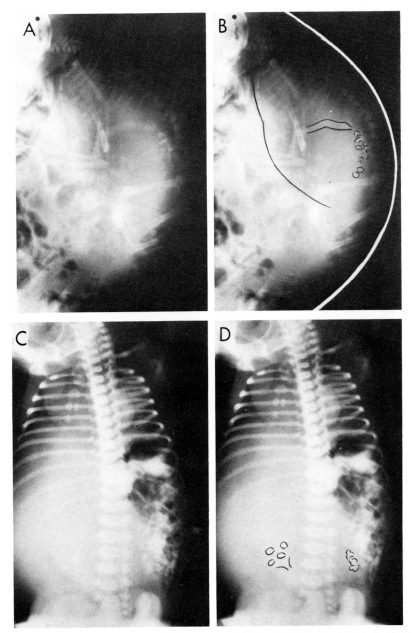

Fig. 22–1.—Fetal intra-abdominal mass antepartum discovery. A 19-year-old primigravida presented during the 36th week of gestation with hydramnios. Sonography demonstrated a single fetus in the vertex position with a cystic intra-abdominal mass. Radiographs obtained 18 hours after instillation of 30 ml of diatrizoate into the amniotic sac show the fetal colon displaced posteriorly. Both kidneys appear normal. **A** and **B**, radiographs are printed upside down to display the fetus right side up. Transverse colon and kidneys are retouched in **B**. **C** and **D**, radiographs of the infant taken immediately after delivery. A large intra-abdominal mass is seen with displacement of the intestine (kidneys retouched in **D**). A large right ovarian cyst was removed immediately after cesarean section. (**A** and **B** reproduced, with permission, from Valenti, **C.**, et al., Am. J. Obstet. Gynecol. 123:216, 1975.)

cral prominence, is responsible for the facial nerve injury. The differentiation between central and peripheral damage can be of therapeutic significance. Compression of the middle third of the facial nerve can occur within the undeveloped mastoid process without radiographic evidence of fracture but require operative decompression.[42]

Although most infants with facial nerve paralysis show complete recovery at 1 year of age, persistent deficits were found after 1 year in 15–35%.[35, 49] A satisfactory result can be expected if at least beginning recovery is noted within 3 weeks.

Brachial Plexus Trauma

Infants with brachial trauma often are large and labor is difficult, with frequent shoulder dystocia or breech presentation.[15, 21, 65] The dominant involvement of the right plexus has been related to the more common LOA presentation, which leaves the right shoulder impinged against the pubic arch.[15] Differentiation between separation of the humeral epiphysis and brachial plexus paralysis can be difficult. Fracture of the humeral epiphysis leads to swelling of the shoulder and pain on motion. In the Erb-Duchenne upper brachial plexus injury there is lack of shoulder motion, but without pain, and there is retention of muscle function of the hand. The arm appears adducted and the forearm cannot be supinated. The hand usually is in a "waiter's tip position," with winging of the scapula.

In the Klumpke type of lower brachial plexus palsy, sensory deficits usually are present, in contrast to the Erb paralysis. Ipsilateral Horner's syndrome, due to damaged sympathetic fibers of the first thoracic root, can accompany the Klumpke brachial paralysis. Phrenic nerve trauma and diaphragmatic elevation are found in approximately 5% of patients with Erb-Duchenne paralysis.[21] Electromyography not only serves as a diagnostic tool to determine the extent and site of the injury but also as a baseline for prognostic evaluation. In Gordon *et al.*'s review,[21] only 9% showed impairment at 12 months of age. Others[15] found residual damage in more than 50% of all children, including delay in bone growth. Treatment includes eletrotherapy, splinting and continuous exercise.

Phrenic Nerve Paralysis

Traumatic paralysis of the phrenic nerve leads to an upward displacement and lack of motion of the involved diaphragm. A history of difficulty during delivery, especially with breech presentation, is common. The elevation of the diaphragm leads to compression of the ipsilateral lung and occasionally also interferes with the function of the contralateral lung. Paralysis of the left diaphragm can also lead to gastrointestinal symptoms with esophageal reflux.[7] Phrenic nerve paralysis may be difficult to differentiate from congenital diaphragmatic eventration or diaphragmatic hernia. Electric phrenic nerve stimulation has been used to differentiate paralysis from eventration. In our own experience, paradoxic motion can be present in either. Unless significant respiratory or gastrointestinal symptoms exist, delay in operative treatment and evaluation of returning function is justified. In infants with respiratory difficulties or significant gastrointestinal reflux, prompt operative intervention is indicated to repair a hernia or imbricate an eventration.

Torticollis

The "tumor" in the sternocleidomastoid muscle, leading to the characteristic head inclination seen in torticollis or "wryneck," was first described by Dieffenbacher in 1830 and its relationship to trauma pointed out by Strohmeyer in 1838.[51] Numerous articles since that time have either supported or disputed possible causes for the localized fibrosis of the sternomastoid muscle: ischemia, vascular necrosis, arterial or venous thrombosis and/or hemorrhage. Sanerkin and Edwards'[51] microscopic findings, with additional vascular injection studies, appear to confirm earlier reports that the traumatic disruption of muscle fibers, rather than hemorrhage, is primarily responsible for the development of the fibrous "tumor" and shortening of the muscle. Spontaneous recovery, even in children with facial distortion, was reported by Schmidt in 1890 and Spencer[58] in 1893, suggesting that operative intervention rarely is indicated. After a flurry of operative interventions within the past 2 decades, partly based on electromyographic studies, the present trend has been return to the nonoperative intervention practiced in the nineteeth century. Passive and active exercise should be encouraged, although in most infants recovery will be spontaneous. (See Chap. 38.)

Fractures

Most long bone fractures are seen in infants with breech presentation.[43] Clavicular fractures occur most often in large infants with vertex presentation and shoulder dystocia.[4, 44] Traumatic birth fractures, especially of long bones, or dislocations, must be differentiated from pathologic fractures in osteogenesis imperfecta or defects such as tibial pseudarthrosis.

Clavicular Fracture

Fracture of the clavicle, the most common fracture in the newborn, usually occurs in the middle third as greenstick type and occasionally is associated with a brachial plexus injury. Treatment rarely is indicated, unless marked displacement has occurred, when a figure-of-eight bandage can be applied. Healing takes place within a few weeks. Callus is radiographically present by the fourth or fifth day. Union is rapid. Complete remolding almost always takes place.

Humerus

The fracture, transverse or spiral, most often involves the middle third of the shaft. The pull of the deltoid muscle leads to an anterior angulation of the proximal fragment.[6] Temporary disappearance of the radial pulse is seen occasionally, yet vascular compromise is exceedingly rare. Humeral fracture and Erb's paralysis can occur simultaneously, one potentially masking the other. Therapy consists of strapping the arm to the chest. Complete healing takes place within 3 weeks.

Femur

Femoral fractures usually occur in the middle third, transverse and complete. The proximal fragment is abducted and flexed by the psoas muscle, placing it at a right angle to the distal fragment. Treatment consists of Bryant's traction for 3 weeks. Late results of femoral fractures are uniformly excellent, an example of Preston Wade's facetious remark: "In children it is only necessary to have both fragments in the same extremity to remold malunion."[54]

Epiphyseal Separation

Epiphyseal fractures, in order of frequency, can involve the distal femoral, upper and lower humeral and the proximal femoral epiphysis. Epiphyseal displacement usually is associated with a fracture of the metaphysis.[33]

HUMERUS.—Pain on passive motion and a palpable and sometimes visible deformity of the proximal end of the humerus indicate an epiphyseal fracture. Radiographs can show calcium deposits, especially when periosteal stripping has occurred. If the nucleus is visible, it is displaced laterally in relation to the shaft of the humerus. After healing takes place, the fractured epiphysis usually appears first on radiographs and is larger than the one on the uninjured side.[23] As in all doubtful epiphyseal dislocations, an arthrogram, with either air or contrast material, can establish a reliable radiographic diagnosis. Although remodeling of a residual displacement usually is rapid and complete,[6, 23] inadequate reduction of epiphyseal fractures can lead to irreparable deformities.[30] The treatment of both upper and lower humeral epiphyseal fractures consists of gentle remodeling and sling immobilization in 90° flexion.

FEMORAL EPIPHYSIS.—Mortens and Christensen[39] and Lindseth and Rosene[34] reported more than 50 proximal femoral epiphyseal fractures in the newborn. The term "pseudodislocation" of the hip has been used to describe epiphyseal fractures,[23] but it refers only to the displacement of the epiphysis and what clinically may appear to be dislocation. There are no proved cases of true "traumatic dislocation of the hip" in the newborn. The clinical differential diagnosis rests between a proximal femoral fracture and a "congenital" hip dislocation. Although a suggestive clinical history, such as breech delivery with an audible snap, may be present, the diagnosis often is difficult.

Clinical findings consist of flexion and abduction of the thigh, with external rotation. Shortening of the injured extremity usually is apparent and the child will avoid movement of the extremity.[34] If the diagnosis cannot be made with certainty, an arthrogram should be performed. An attempt to test the mobility of a partially separated epiphysis can be disastrous, changing a partial into a total epiphyseal separation. The treatment of both upper and lower epiphyseal fractures consists of Bryant's traction for several weeks.

Dislocation

Although various dislocations, including olecranon and mandible, have been reported, most represent only sporadic occurrences. Dislocation of the knee, however, has been documented in several hundred infants.[60] Dislocation of the knee has been divided into two causes. The first is mechanical, most commonly due to manipulation during delivery. The second consists of either a primary mesenchymal defect, usually leading to multiple defects, or a traumatic developmental malposition in utero. The dislocation of knees, with hyperextension, may be the cause rather than the result of breech presentation, preventing a cephalic presentation. Depending on the severity of the tibial displacement, three groups have been identified: (1) congenital genu recurvatum: hyperextension of the knee with intact femoral-tibial articulation; (2) subluxation: some displacement, but the disruption of the knee joint is not complete; (3) dislocation: complete disruption of the femoral-tibial articulation.

In the last there is anterior displacement of the tibia. The hamstring muscles are dislocated anteriorly, acting, therefore, as extensors rather than flexors. The affected knee is hyperextended and the femoral condyles are palpable in the popliteal fossa. In infants with mechanical dislocation, conservative therapy usually is successful when instituted promptly. The tibia is flexed and the dislocation reduced. The knee then is flexed to the fullest extent compatible with maintenance of circulation and sensation. The anterior mold is applied and after 1 week further flexion is obtained in repeated intervals until 90–125° flexion can be maintained. Radiographic proof of reduction is necessary to rule out recurrent dislocation while in flexion. After complete reduction, with attainment of full mobility, a brace is applied until ligamentous stability is present. In children with multiple deformities or dislocations, the final result is less promising, and operative intervention may be necessary.[60]

Respiratory Distress*

Pneumothorax

Pneumothorax has been reported to be more common in the newborn period than at any other time of life.[13] First

---

*See Chapter 46.

reported by Ruge in 1878, it is predominantly seen in prematures under 2500 gm of birth weight. It frequently is associated with a history of meconium or blood aspiration. Uneven pulmonary inflation, with airway pressures ranging from 40 cm to 100 cm of water during the first few breaths, is assumed to be greatly responsible for the formation of the pneumothorax. The elevated transpulmonary pressure can lead to rupture of air along perivascular planes into the mediastinum and then into the pleural space. The incidence of pneumothorax is particularly high in infants with interstitial emphysema or RDS and those with ventilatory assistance.[28]

Depending on the degree of pneumothorax, the infant's symptoms may be minimal and the pneumothorax found accidentally on radiographs. With increasing pneumothorax, the clinical findings range from irritability and tachypnea to cyanosis. A small unilateral pneumothorax usually does not require treatment, but careful observation for increase or bilateral occurrence is warranted. In patients with significant clinical symptoms or radiographically increasing or bilateral pneumothorax, a small catheter should be inserted through one of the upper anterior intercostal spaces and connected to underwater drainage.

Tension Pneumothorax

In contrast to the simple pneumothorax, where respiratory insufficiency usually develops slowly, both tension pneumothorax and tension pneumomediastinum can represent acute and threatening emergencies (Fig. 22–2). The clinical signs consist of cardiopulmonary collapse and cyanosis with shift of the mediastinum to the contralateral side with tension pneumothorax. Although x-rays usually are necessary to identify the extent of a simple pneumothorax, in infants with tension pneumothorax the therapy—immediate aspiration

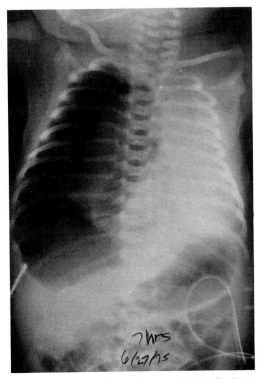

Fig. 22–2.—Tension pneumothorax at 7 hours of age, following respiratory distress after birth. The radiograph demonstrates a right-sided tension pneumothorax with mediastinal shift to the left; the left lung is compressed.

followed by the insertion of a thoracostomy tube— may have to precede radiographic confirmation in view of the rapidly deteriorating condition of the infant.

Although tension pneumomediastinum may not have the immediate deleterious effect of the tension pneumothorax, it can also severely interfere with cardiac return and pulmonary function. In one of our infants, with a jugular catheter in place, a tension pneumomediastinum developed coincidentally and the central venous pressure rose to 23 cm of water. After substernal drainage, the central venous pressure dropped almost immediately to 5 cm of water, with simultaneous clinical improvement of the infant.

Pharyngeal Perforation*

In 1876, Ruge[50] reported a pharyngeal injury in a newborn following a breech delivery, presumably due to the force of the obstetrician's finger. His report was followed a century later by Girdany *et al.*,[19] who reported 2 infants with pharyngeal perforations presenting with clinical symptoms of salivation. Presenting symptoms usually have consisted of dysphagia mimicking esophageal atresia, duplication or pseudodiverticulum. Two infants seen in our institution were suspected to have had traumatic intubations leading to pharyngeal perforation. One presented with a large posterior mediastinal collection, connected to the pharynx (Fig. 22–3). The other developed a small posterior pharyngeal diverticulum, which closed spontaneously. Since the extent of the pharyngeal perforation and the formation of the "diverticu-

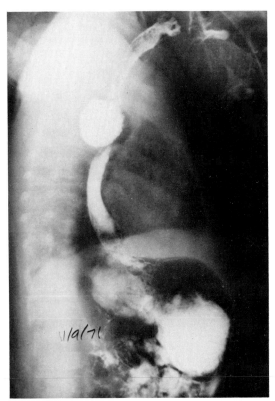

Fig. 22–3.—Pharyngomediastinal fistula with contrast material collecting in the posterior mediastinum. The infant had been intubated after birth. He later developed dysphagia. At operation, what appeared to be a traumatic pharyngomediastinal fistula was found, with fibrosis and inflammatory reaction and without any epithelial lining or structures compatible with congenital enterogenous cysts or duplication.

*See Chapter 43F.

lum" varies considerably, variable symptoms can be expected, based on the extent and location of the lesion.

Tracheobronchial Perforation

Accidental perforation of the trachea during intubation has been reported by Serlin and Daily.[53] A recent report by Anderson and Chandra[3] described accidental perforation of the pulmonary parenchyma in 3 infants on four occasions during aspiration. In an experimental study, they found that customarily used suction catheters can be advanced without major force, most readily through both the lower and the right middle lobe bronchi into the pleural space. It is more than likely that the same mechanism, unrecognized before, may be responsible for a much larger number of infants with pneumothorax, who had required frequent pulmonary toilet. Anderson and Chandra present a chart for maximal safe length of tube for endotracheal suction by body weight.

Hydropneumothorax

ESOPHAGEAL PERFORATION.—Several reports describing esophageal perforation in the newborn stress that esophageal perforation may occur spontaneously, without prior instrumentation.[14, 63, 68] Although no definite cause has been established, most authors assume that the increased intraesophageal pressure during delivery leads to a spontaneous perforation of the esophagus filled with amniotic fluid.

Aaronson *et al.*[1] reviewed 30 infants with a rupture of the esophagus during the first 48 hours of life. The predominant symptoms (in half of the infants) consisted of rapidly developing respiratory distress and regurgitation of bloody material. In 80%, the perforation occurred on the right side, with the development of a tension hydropneumothorax. The perforation occurred most often in the midesophagus, next most commonly in the lower esophageal segment. A sudden respiratory collapse accompanied by a right-sided hydropneumothorax is almost pathognomonic for esophageal perforation in the newborn. Prompt thoracocentesis, followed by thoracotomy and repair of the perforation, is necessary.

Chylothorax*

Recent reviews of chylothorax in infancy by Tischer,[62] Brodman *et al.*[10] and Bensoussan *et al.*[5] discussed the findings of chylothorax in more than 30 infants. The clinical symptomatology appears uniform: the spontaneous development of a hydrothorax, usually right, without an appreciable history of birth trauma. The findings are related to the chylous pleural effusion, with moderate respiratory insufficiency and occasional lymphocytopenia. Infection was reported in only 1 patient, after repeat aspiration.[5] Only 3 of 34 infants had a febrile course. In 6 of 60 patients, the chylothorax was bilateral. The cause of the chylous effusion in the newborn is not known. Only a few cases with apparent malformations of the thoracic duct have been reported.[8, 46, 62] Although the hypothesis that leakage of lymph is secondary to a congenital weakness of the thoracic duct has been advanced by several authors,[8, 46, 48, 62] it is difficult to understand why simple drainage should be adequate in the majority of cases.

Aspiration of the hydrothorax at birth usually reveals serosanguineous fluid. Only after formula feeding has been started does the effusion assume the typical turbid character of chyle, with fat present.

In the majority of infants, operative intervention is unnec-

*See Chapter 46.

essary. Although the use of medium-chain triglycerides appears to diminish the fat content in the chyle, a significant reduction of chylous flow apparently can be achieved only by placing the gastrointestinal tract completely at rest.[9] Hyperalimentation then can be used to carry the patient through the short period (usually not more than a few weeks) required to allow spontaneous resorption of the chylothorax. The initial treatment consists of pleural aspiration followed by the insertion of a thoracostomy tube, if necessary. Only if drainage persists for a prolonged period does operative intervention appear to be justified.

Abdominal Distention

Hemoperitoneum has remained one of the most serious complications of birth trauma since the early reports in the nineteenth century, when hepatic, splenic and adrenal hemorrhage were well recognized as causes of hemoperitoneum, shock and death. In vivo diagnosis and operative salvage have been reported only since 1934.[38] The liver is the organ most likely to be injured during the birth process.[20, 26, 38, 45]

Hepatic Hemorrhage

Both premature and large infants are at risk, especially with difficult or prolonged labor. Breech presentation and manipulation has been looked on as the most common cause of hepatic trauma. However, hepatic hemorrhage can present in all infants, regardless of size and the type of delivery. Two mechanisms are thought to cause hepatic trauma: (1) thoracic compression, which pushes the liver out of the hollow of the diaphragm, pulling the hepatic ligaments, with subsequent tear of the liver parenchyma at the site of their insertion; (2) direct pressure on the liver, leading to subcapsular hemorrhage or rupture.

Congestion, hypoxia or coagulation defects may contribute to the susceptibility of the liver to hemorrhage.

Subcapsular hematomas are more common than primary rupture of the liver. Infants with subcapsular hemorrhage usually are asymptomatic at birth; only occasionally can the hematoma be felt on palpation. Although the infant's hematocrit may drop slightly, major changes usually do not occur for approximately 48 hours, when the capsule ruptures and free bleeding ensues. Vascular collapse, abdominal distention and a rapid drop of the hematocrit follow. A bluish cast of either abdomen or umbilicus, Cullen's sign, may be one of the most obvious signs of a hemoperitoneum in infancy. With a patent processus vaginalis, scrotal hematoma can suggest intraperitoneal bleeding. In patients with primary rupture, major bleeding takes place immediately, explaining the high percentage of fetal deaths with massive liver rupture.

Abdominal radiographs may present a "floating intestine," indicating free intraperitoneal fluid. In patients with subcapsular hemorrhage or delayed rupture, a radiographic diagnosis can be obtained through an umbilical venogram.[32] Sonography may be helpful in differentiating a solid hepatic tumor from an unruptured cystic subcapsular hematoma. Abdominal paracentesis represents the fastest way to obtain a diagnosis of hemoperitoneum. Regardless of the site of bleeding, immediate operative intervention is indicated.

In view of the marked blood loss (the average reported loss was between 200 and 350 ml[11, 38]), adequate transfusion and control of coagulation problems should be initiated, followed by prompt exploration. Fear has been expressed that liver lacerations are difficult to control at operation in infants,[11] but liver repair, including major resections, can be accomplished with no more difficulty in infants than in older children.

Spleen

Although splenic ruptures in the newborn occur less often than hepatic, more than 40 cases have been reported.[26] In several reports, the infants involved were reported to be above average[27, 52] weight but the removed spleen was of normal size. In other reports, both infants and spleens were within normal limits.[41, 55]

Pre-existing pathology, such as a pseudocyst or associated coagulation defects, has been cited.[24, 27, 55] The mechanism of splenic rupture is assumed to be similar to that of rupture of the liver: a tear of the ligamentous attachment to the spleen, especially the lienorenal ligament. Difficult deliveries, shoulder dystocia, association with fracture of the clavicle, Erb's paralysis and association with liver hemorrhage have been reported.[22, 27, 57]

Unlike the bleeding with a hepatic subcapsular hematoma, splenic bleeding is prompt and the average blood loss ranges from 200 to 600 ml.[52] Sudden pallor, hypotension, abdominal distention and occasionally a bluish cast of the umbilicus or the abdominal wall can appear. Diagnostic work-up and therapy are identical in all infants with suspected hemoperitoneum: abdominal paracentesis, transfusion, control of coagulation problems and operative intervention.

Confronted with a lacerated spleen, the surgeon's choice in the past was simple: splenectomy. Although Eraklis *et al.*[17] in 1967 thought that fatal septicemia after splenectomy occurred only in infants with associated hematologic diseases, their assumption no longer is accepted (see Chap. 13).

Myers[40] in 1962 and Smith[56] in 1964 advocated postsplenectomy penicillin coverage as prophylaxis for the fatal meningococcal or pneumococcal infection that has been reported after splenectomy. One of our infants with a central necrosis of the stomach and splenic rupture at birth survived uneventfully for almost 2 years after a staged gastrectomy and splenectomy and died within 24 hours from a sudden fatal septicemia without associated hematologic diseases. He was not on prophylactic penicillin coverage.

The repair of lacerated spleens presently is being pursued by various medical centers. Although there still may be a question as to whether a splenic repair is justified, prophylactic penicillin coverage, in our opinion, is not open to question.

Adrenal Hemorrhage

As in other facets of birth trauma, Spencer[59] deserves credit for the first comprehensive description of adrenal hemorrhage, followed in 1901 by Hamill,[25] who discussed an infant with adrenal hemorrhage, following a spontaneous delivery, in 1892 at St. Christopher's Hospital in Philadelphia. His review of minor and major adrenal hemorrhage and its relationship to abnormal and normal delivery still is valid.

In more recent reports,[12, 45] the previous findings have been confirmed. Adrenal hemorrhages occur most commonly on the right adrenal (78%) and bilaterally in approximately 8%. The anatomic position of the right adrenal is assumed to be responsible for its frequent involvement.

1. The right adrenal is more likely to be exposed to me-

chanical compression, located as it is between liver and vertebra.

2. It is sensitive to intracaval pressure changes, since it drains directly into the vena cava. Difficult deliveries, episodes of hypoxia and coagulation defects are common associated factors in infants with adrenal hemorrhage.

Adrenal hemorrhage can manifest itself in two major ways:

1. Hemorrhage, especially in the newborn.

2. Adrenal insufficiency, which usually develops after birth.

Signs of intracapsular, retroperitoneal or intraperitoneal hemorrhage usually occur between birth and the fourth day of life. Depending on the degree of hemorrhage and its localization, signs and symptoms range from limited blood loss with slight intestinal ileus to massive intraperitoneal bleeding. Minor intracapsular bleeding usually requires no therapy. It may present later as calcification of the adrenal, reported by Wagner[66] as the "rim sign" occurring as early as the twelfth day of life. With limited retroperitoneal hemorrhage, transfusion and close observation may suffice. In infants with massive retroperitoneal or intraperitoneal hemorrhage, abdominal exploration is warranted. The operative procedure consists of evacuation of the adrenal hematoma, ligation of bleeders or adrenalectomy. Although unilateral adrenalectomy is well tolerated, hydrocortisone coverage may be necessary. In view of the potentially increased risk of infection due to decreased adrenal function, antibiotic coverage is advisable. Extensive adrenal hemorrhage, especially if bilateral, may lead to early signs of adrenal insufficiency: electrolyte and fluid imbalance, convulsions, collapse and infection. Appropriate fluid and electrolyte replacement, antibiotics and hydrocortisone are required.

Radiographic examination may be essential to differentiate between adrenal hemorrhage and other lesions, such as adrenal neuroblastoma. The "rim" calcification, seen in adrenal hemorrhage, differs from the diffuse calcification in neuroblastoma. Right adrenal hemorrhage can also lead to inferior vena cava occlusion, as shown in 1 of our infants (Fig. 22–4), which is less likely to occur with neuroblastoma. Sonography can be helpful in differentiating a solid suprarenal tumor from a cystic lesion, such as adrenal hemorrhage.

We have had 3 patients with adrenal hemorrhage. The first 2 were operated on and recovered uneventfully. The third patient, with a confined bilateral adrenal hemorrhage demonstrated by x-ray, was observed closely and by 13 days of age the flank masses had disappeared and urography revealed a normal renal axis.

Kidney

Rupture of the kidney as a cause of hemoperitoneum in the newborn has been reported in only 4 cases.[16, 18, 47] Three of these kidneys were normal, and in 2 patients associated hepatic or splenic hemorrhage was found. The fourth kidney was found to be hydronephrotic and rupture occurred during a spontaneous delivery.

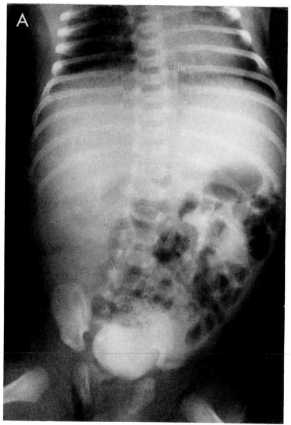 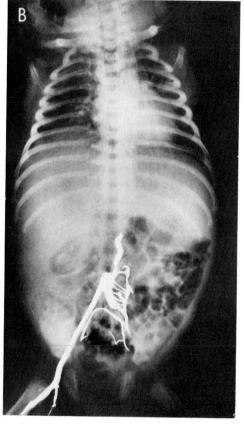

Fig. 22–4.—Adrenal hemorrhage. Radiographs of an infant with sudden abdominal distention, right flank mass and fall in hematocrit. **A,** urogram with a normal left kidney. The right kidney is not functioning. **B,** retouched venogram with caval obstruction and obvious collaterals, suggestive of caval compression by a right adrenal hemorrhage. At operation, a large right adrenal hematoma was evacuated and bleeders ligated. The infant recovered uneventfully and had normal bilateral renal function. (Reproduced, with permission, from Gross, M., *et al.,* J. Pediatr. Surg. 2:308, 1967.)

REFERENCES

1. Aaronson, I. A., Cwyes, S., and Louw, J. H.: Spontaneous esophageal rupture in the newborn, J. Pediatr. Surg. 10:459, 1975.
2. Abramson, A. M. (ed.): *Resuscitation of the Newborn Infant* (St. Louis: The C. V. Mosby Company, 1973).
3. Anderson, K. D., and Chandra, R.: Pneumothorax secondary to perforation of sequential bronchi by suction catheters, J. Pediatr. Surg. 11:687, 1976.
4. Bauer, O., Weidenbach, A., and Thieme, R.: Die knochernen Geburtsverletzungen des Neugeborenen, Munch. Med. Wochenschr. 1092:998, 1967.
5. Bensoussan, A. L., Braun, P., and Guttman, F. M.: Bilateral spontaneous chylothorax of the newborn, Arch. Surg. 110:1243, 1975.
6. Bianco, A. J., Schlein, A. P., Kruss, R. L., and Johnson, E. W.: Birth fractures, Minn. Med. 55:471, 1972.
7. Bishop, H. C., and Koop, C. E.: Acquired eventration of the diaphragm in infancy, Pediatrics 22:1088, 1958.
8. Boles, E. T., and Izant, R. J.: Spontaneous chylothorax in the neonatal period, Am. J. Surg. 99:870, 1960.
9. Brodman, R. F.: Chylothorax of the newborn, Arch. Surg. 111:499, 1976.
10. Brodman, R. F., Zavelson, T. M., and Schiebler, G. L.: Treatment of congenital chylothorax, J. Pediatr. 86:516, 1974.
11. Brown, J. J. M.: Hepatic haemorrhage in the newborn, Arch. Dis. Child. 32:480, 1957.
12. Brown, S. J., Dunbar, J. S., and MacEwan, D. W.: The radiologic features of acute massive adrenal haemorrhage, J. Assoc. Can. Radiol. 13:100, 1962.
13. Chernick, V., and Avery, M. E.: Spontaneous alveolar rupture at birth, Pediatrics 32:816, 1963.
14. Chunn, V. D., and Geppert, L. J.: Spontaneous rupture of the esophagus in the newborn, J. Pediatr. 60:404, 1962.
15. Eng, G. D.: Brachial plexus palsy in newborn infants, Pediatrics 48:18, 1971.
16. Eraklis, A. J.: Abdominal injury related to the trauma of birth, Pediatrics 39:421, 1967.
17. Eraklis, A. J., Kevy, S. V., Diamond, L. K., and Gross, R. E.: Hazard of overwhelming infection after splenectomy in childhood, N. Engl. J. Med. 276:1225, 1967.
18. Geley, von L., and Hartl, H.: Massive Parenchymblutungen beim Neugeborenen, Munch. Med. Wochenschr. 111:2206, 1969.
19. Girdany, B. R., Sieber, W. K., and Osman, M. Z.: Traumatic pseudodiverticulum of the pharynx in newborn infants, N. Engl. J. Med. 280:237, 1969.
20. Goodman, J. M.: Liver trauma in the newborn: A case report, J. Trauma 14:427, 1974.
21. Gordon, M., Rich, H., Deitschberger, J., and Green, M.: The immediate and long-term outcome of obstetric birth trauma, Am. J. Obstet. Gynecol. 117:51, 1973.
22. Gruenwald, P.: Rupture of liver and spleen in the newborn infant, J. Pediatr. 33:195, 1948.
23. Haliburton, R. A., Barber, J. R., and Fraser, R. L.: Pseudodislocation: An unusual birth injury, Can. J. Surg. 10:455, 1967.
24. Halvorsen, J. F.: Rupture of the normal spleen occurring as a birth injury, Acta Obstet. Gynecol. Scand. 50:95, 1971.
25. Hamill, S. McC.: Hemorrhage into the suprarenal capsule in stillborn children and infants: Report of a case showing rupture of the sac and escape of blood into the perirenal tissues and the peritoneal cavity, Arch. Pediatr. 18:161, 1901.
26. Hasse, W., and Waldschmidt, J.: Das Hämoperitoneum beim Neugeborenen, Chirurg 9:132, 1968.
27. Hottinger, von A., and Gilardi, H.: Geburtstraumatische Ruptur einer normalen Milz, Schweiz. Med. Wochenschr. 88:587, 1958.
28. Howie, V. M., and Weed, A. S.: Spontaneous pneumothorax in the first ten days of life, J. Pediatr. 50:6, 1957.
29. Issel, von E. P.: Vorschlag zur Definition des Geburtstraumas, Zentralbl. Gynaekol. 97:1122, 1975.
30. Jacquemain, B.: Die Bedeutung der geburtstraumatischen Epiphysenlosung am proximalen Femurende, Geburtshilfe Frauenheilkd. 27:690, 1967.
31. Kennedy, E.: Apoplexy of new-born infants, Dublin J. Med. Sci. 10:419, 1836.
32. Keuth, U., Althaus, W., and Feldmann, E. M.: Rontgenologisch dargestellte geburtstraumatische Leberruptur eines Neugeborenen, Monatsschr. Kinderheilkd. 124:38, 1976.
33. Lemperg, R., and Liliequist, B.: Dislocation of the proximal epiphysis of the humerus in newborns, Acta Paediatr. Scand. 59:377, 1970.
34. Lindseth, R. E., and Rosene, H. A.: Traumatic separation of the upper femoral epiphysis in a newborn infant, J. Bone Joint Surg. 53-A:1641, 1971.
35. Lukaszewica, G.: Congenital peripheral paresis of the facial nerve, Ginekol. Pol 35:829, 1964.
36. Lundqvist, B.: Hemorragies intra-thoraciques et intra-abdominales chez le nouveau-né, Acta Gynecol. 9:331, 1929.
37. McHugh, H. E.: Facial paralysis in birth injury and skull fractures, Arch. Otolaryngol. 78:443, 1963.
38. Monson, D. O., and Raffensperger, J. G.: Intraperitoneal hemorrhage secondary to liver laceration in a newborn, J. Pediatr. Surg. 2:464, 1967.
39. Mortens, J., and Christensen, P.: Traumatic separation of the upper femoral epiphysis as an obstetrical lesion, Acta Orthop. Scand. 34:239, 1964.
40. Myers, N. A.: Ruptured spleen: A manifestation of birth injury, Med. J. Aust. 1:809, 1962.
41. O'Neill, E. A., O'Brian, E. R., and Hyun, B. H.: Rupture of the spleen in the newborn infant, JAMA 193:187, 1965.
42. Paine, R. S.: Facial paralysis in children, Pediatrics 19:303, 1957.
43. Panzer, von R.: Geburtsfrakturen, Zentralbl. Gynaekol. 33:1163, 1964.
44. Pockrandt, von H.: Über die Klavikulafraktur bei Neugeborenen nach Spontangeburt, Zentralbl. Gynaekol. 12:407, 1965.
45. Potter, E. L.: Fetal and neonatal deaths, JAMA 15:996, 1940.
46. Randolph, J. G., and Gross, R. E.: Congenital chylothorax, Arch. Surg. 74:405, 1957.
47. Ravich, L., and Schell, N. B.: Rupture of the kidney in the newborn infant, N. Y. State J. Med. 61:2822, 1961.
48. Ravitch, M. M., and Rowe, M. I.: Surgical emergencies in the neonate, Am. J. Obstet. Gynecol. 103:1034, 1969.
49. Rubin, A.: Birth injuries: Incidence, mechanisms, and end results, Obstet. Gynecol. 23:218, 1964.
50. Ruge, C.: Ueber die Verletzungen des Kindes durch die Extraction bei ursprunglicher oder durch Wendung herbeigefuhrter Beckenendelage, nebst kurzer Beleuchtung der Extractionsmethoden, Z. Gebertshilfe Frauenkrank. 1:68, 1876.
51. Sanerkin, N. G., and Edwards, P.: Birth injury to the sternomastoid muscle, J. Bone Joint Surg. 48-B:441, 1966.
52. Schwartz, O., and Cohn, B. D.: Rupture of the normal spleen in the newborn, with survival, Surgery 59:1124, 1966.
53. Serlin, S. P., and Daily, W. J. R.: Tracheal perforation in the neonate: A complication of endotracheal intubation, J. Pediatr. 86:596, 1975.
54. Shaftan, G. W., Kottmeier, P. K., and Klotz, D. H.: *Pediatric Trauma, Quick References to Surgical Emergencies* (Philadelphia and Toronto: J. B. Lippincott Company, 1974), Chap. 37.
55. Sieber, W. K., and Girdany, B. R.: Rupture of the spleen in newborn infants, N. Engl. J. Med. 259:1074, 1958.
56. Smith, C. H.: Indications for splenectomy in the pediatric patient, Am. J. Surg. 107:523, 1964.
57. Sokol, D. M., Tompkins, D., and Izant, R. J.: Rupture of the spleen and liver in the newborn: A report of the first survivor and a review of the literature, J. Pediatr. Surg. 9:227, 1974.
58. Spencer, H. R.: On hematoma of the sterno-mastoid muscle in new born children, J. Pathol. Bacteriol. 1:112, 1893.
59. Spencer, H. R., and Lond, B. S.: On visceral hemorrhages in stillborn children. An analysis of 130 autopsies: Being a contribution to the study of the causation of stillbirth, Obstet. Trans. 33:203, 1891.
60. Stern, M. B.: Congenital dislocation of the knee, Clin. Orthop. 61:261, 1968.
61. Tank, E. S., Davis, R., Holt, J. F., and Morley, G. W.: Mechanisms of trauma during breech delivery, Obstet. Gynecol. 38:761, 1971.
62. Tischer, von W.: Der Chylothorax im ersten Trimenon, Z. Jun. Kinderchir. 5:43, 1967.
63. Tolstedt, G. E., and Tudor, R. B.: Esophageal fistula in a newborn infant, Arch. Surg. 97:780, 1968.
64. Valenti, C., Kassner, E. G., Yermakov, V., and Cromb, E.: Antenatal diagnosis of a fetal ovarian cyst, Am. J. Obstet. Gynecol. 123:216, 1975.
65. Vassalos, E., Prevedourakis, C., and Paraschopoulou, P.: Brachial plexus paralysis in the newborn, Am. J. Obstet. Gynecol. 101:554, 1968.
66. Wagner, A. C.: Bilateral hemorrhagic pseudocysts of the adrenal glands in a newborn, Am. J. Roentgenol. 86:540, 1961.
67. Wells, C.: An early case of birth injury, Dev. Med. Child Neurol. 6:397, 1964.
68. Wiseman, H. J., Celano, E. R., and Hester, F. C.: Spontaneous rupture of the esophagus in a newborn infant, J. Pediatr. 55:207, 1959.

PART III

Head and Neck

PLATE I

A. Congenital Anophthalmia. This infant was born with extensive craniofacial defects, including bilateral anophthalmia, bilateral complete cleft lip and cleft palate. A central nervous system deficit was suspected.

B. Cleft Lip and Palate. An infant boy with a unilateral cleft lip, cleft palate and typical nasal deformity. The defect was repaired at 1 month of age with the use of an inlay flap; particular attention was paid to the correction of the nasal deformity. The associated cleft palate was repaired when the child was 1 year old.

C. Burn Scald. A toddler sustained this injury of the head and neck areas from hot coffee. Because of the proportionately large surface area represented at this age, such a burn is capable of producing shock. Hospitalization and intensive supportive care are necessary. This photograph was taken 48 hours after the scald, when burn fluid sequestration is maximal.

D. Platelet-Trapping Hemangioma. Infant showed no evidence of hemangioma at birth, but 1 month later an uncomplicated lesion appeared in the perioral region. This spread rapidly and, because of platelet trapping, extravasation and infection occurred, resulting in the loss of important features and ultimately in death.

E. Mixed Hemangioma and Lymphangioma of the Parotid and Cervical Region. Frequently, such lesions are occult, deep to the skin layer and invade the parotid gland by direct extension. In this infant, there was a bulky external component. Excision was carried out in two stages, with preservation of the facial nerve.

F. Thyroglossal Cyst. This 2-year-old boy had a classic thyroglossal cyst with a history of sudden enlargement following an upper respiratory infection. The thyroid lobes were normal in size and location. Complete excision of the cyst was performed, including a central block of the hyoid bone. The proximal stalk extended to the base of the tongue at the foramen cecum.

PLATE I

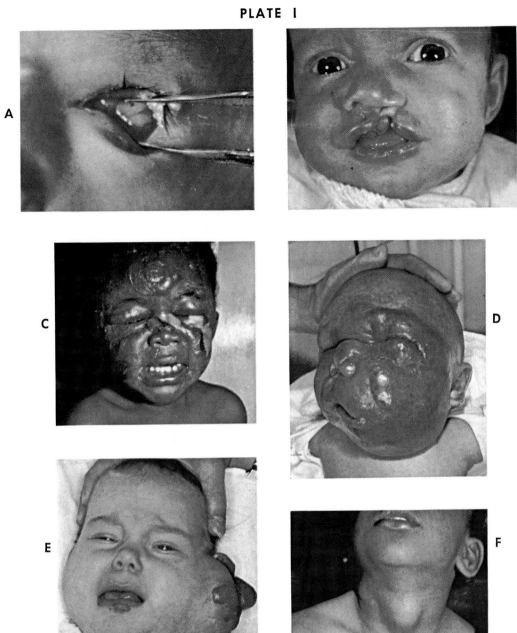

23 J. S. CRAWFORD / ROBERT PASHBY

Eyes and Lids

Injuries

IN YOUNGER CHILDREN, injuries are sporadic and may result from a wide range of causes and in older children, injuries occur from sports. Hockey accounts for an increasing number of injuries. A great deal of interest recently has been aroused in greater protection to the face. Similar protective measures are being taken with the squash player, the football player and with other sports such as fencing.

Wounds to Conjunctiva

Lacerations or other wounds of the conjunctiva in themselves are of little importance. The surgeon must be sure that a conjunctival laceration is not accompanied by a laceration of the sclera. Conjunctival wounds, if small, are left alone and an antibiotic is instilled during the healing. Larger irregular lacerations may be sutured with fine (7-0) gut sutures.

Corneal Injuries

Contusions of the cornea occur frequently and their presence may be verified by the instillation of a drop of 2% fluorescein or the commercially prepared pieces of filter paper impregnated with fluorescein, which are moistened with saline or water and touched to the conjunctiva in the lower fornix. The fluorescein stains the abraded cornea yellow-green. These eyes are quite sensitive because of the exposure of the nerve endings. Treatment consists of instilling an antibiotic ointment and applying a firm eye dressing, tight enough to make sure that the lids are not allowed to move until the cornea is healed. The patch is held in place overnight and the cornea then re-examined with the fluorescein. As long as there is staining, another tight patch is applied, with re-examination the next day.

Small foreign bodies entering the conjunctival sac usually are found on the back of the upper tarsus. As the upper lid moves up and down in the act of blinking, vertical scratches occur on the cornea. The lid must be everted to find these and they then can be removed with a cotton applicator. Foreign bodies embedded in the cornea require the instillation of a local anesthetic and removal with a spud. A small hypodermic needle on the end of a 2-ml syringe is also a very useful instrument for removing these corneal foreign bodies. Retained iron or steel foreign bodies may produce a rust ring in the cornea. Such foreign bodies frequently are easy to remove with gentle curettage.

A direct blow to the eyeball may result in contusion, with the greater damage occurring at the point where the blow is received. A transmitted force may send a wave of pressure through the fluid contents of the eye and produce a contrecoup type of injury to the posterior portion of the globe, resulting in retinal edema, rupture of the choroid or even a rupture of the posterior portion of the sclera. Direct trauma frequently gives rise to injuries of the structures of the anterior segment of the eye, with local damage to the cornea, or even a rupture. There may be a tear in the root of the iris (iridodialysis). There may be splitting of the region of the canal of Schlemm, interfering with the aqueous drainage, occasionally resulting in glaucoma. The lens may be damaged or dislocated. A partial or total cataract may occur.

A severe blow to the eye may cause a wide dilatation of the pupil (traumatic mydriasis) due to a paralysis of accommodation, which results from damage by the pressure wave to the nerves as they pass through the ocular tissue. Ocular hypotony may occur with these injuries due to damage to the ciliary body and the aqueous formation. If the hypotony is marked, papilledema can occur and may last for weeks or months.

Perforating Wounds of the Eye

These vary in size from small puncture wounds to more extensive lacerations. Eyes injured in this manner often are quite sore and painful. If an attempt is made to open the lids, the patient will reflexly squeeze the lids closed. In this case, it is better to put on a clean eye pad and examine the eye under an anesthetic when the appropriate operative repair can be carried out.

If the wound is clean and small and there is no herniation of ocular content, no suturing will be required. Large irregular corneal wounds require direct suturing with fine synthetic sutures (Fig. 23–1) under a microscope because the sutures used are extremely fine (8-0 or 10-0).

If the lens is injured, the full extent of damage may not be determined until some time after the injury. Frequently it is not easy to detect a dislocated lens unless there is a large dislocation. Tears in the lens capsule do not produce immediate opacification of the lens. Instead, the cataract forms slowly and gradually becomes apparent. If the lens becomes swollen, a secondary glaucoma may occur.

Formerly, when a traumatic cataract occurred, the lens was left in place, allowing it to absorb gradually, but, unfortunately, thick secondary membranes frequently resulted. A better end result is obtained if the lens material is aspirated using a 21-gauge needle or, if necessary, an 18-gauge nee-

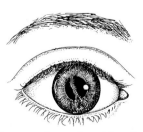

Fig. 23–1.—Irregular corneal wound requiring direct suturing with fine sutures.

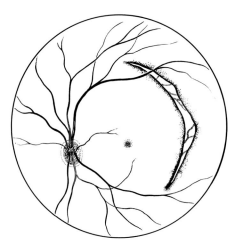

Fig. 23–2.—Rupture of the choroid. This occurred in a child who was struck in the eye with a ball.

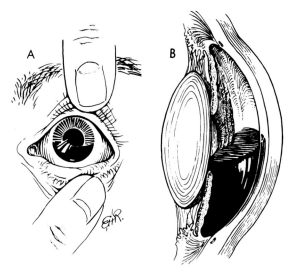

Fig. 23–3.—Hyphema—blood in the anterior chamber.

dle, with the use of a microscope. A contact lens is fitted to the aphakic eye as soon as healing has taken place. This will restore binocular vision and help to prevent development of a secondary strabismus.

Rupture of the Sclera

This may occur either as the result of a severe blow to the eye or as a result of a foreign object passing into the eye. If the sclera is seen to be ruptured, and the break is in the anterior portion of the globe, direct suturing is carried out. If, on the other hand, the eye becomes hypotensive, the child should be given an anesthetic, the conjunctiva incised and the sclera examined to see if a break can be found.

Rupture of the Choroid

A strong blow to the front of the eye may cause a contre-coup injury, and this may be in the form of a rupture of the choroid (Fig. 23–2). This shows up as a yellowish brown streak, occasionally obscured by hemorrhage, which later acquires more sharply defined, heavily pigmented edges. When the rupture affects the macula, vision is reduced, but the rupture may be at other positions on the posterior pole of the eye and not affect sight.

Retinal Tears

A break in the retina may result from trauma to an eye. Detachments occur frequently in patients with retinal tears and are more frequent with patients who have myopia or other retinal degenerative diseases frequently associated with old age.

Treatment of these detachments consists of finding the retinal hole, draining the subretinal fluid and sealing off the hole. The retina is approximated to the choroid by placing a silicone band around the eye. Adhesions between the retina and the choroid are promoted either by applying diathermy to the sclera outside the break or by the use of cryotherapy.

Hyphema

Blood in the anterior chamber (Fig. 23–3) most frequently is caused by blunt trauma but may also occur as a result of a penetrating ocular injury. Hyphema may occur after eye operations or in certain systemic diseases, especially the blood dyscrasias. The prognosis is good with most hyphema patients, and the gross blood clears by the end of 5 days. Secondary hemorrhage is more serious. This occurs because an anterior chamber full of blood blocks the drainage channels (canal of Schlemm). The intraocular pressure of the eye may go up and, in these cases, the hemosiderin in the blood is driven into the corneal stroma and blood staining of the cornea results. Most of the secondary hemorrhages occur on or about the third or fourth day and usually not after the fifth day.

Many of these patients have a sore eye and their parents give them aspirin or various aspirin-containing compounds. Acetylsalicylic acid has an inhibitory effect on platelet aggregation. One normal therapeutic dose of aspirin will prolong the bleeding time and interfere with the platelet aggregation for 5 days or more. For the same reason, it is not wise to give aspirin as a sedative after intraocular operations. Acetamino-

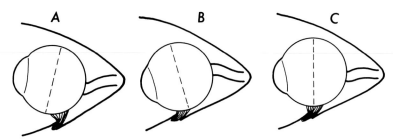

Fig. 23–4.—Blow-out fracture of the orbital floor. **A,** inferior rectus caught posterior to equator. **B,** inferior rectus caught anterior to equator. **C,** inferior rectus caught at equator.

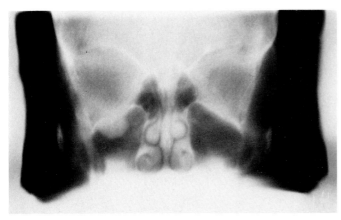

Fig. 23–5.—Fractures of the orbital floor. Tomogram showing the typical "hanging" drop density in the roof of the right antrum.

phen (Tempra) may be used to relieve pain, as it does not have the same effect on the platelets, or codeine if a stronger sedative is required.

Patients with hyphemas should be put to bed with bilateral eye patches. In most cases, the hemorrhage clears quickly and will disappear within 1 or 2 days. If the hemorrhage is slow in absorbing, the binocular eye patches are kept in place for at least 5 days. Studies have shown that bed rest is more important than the binocular patches.

If the intraocular pressure is elevated, for example, to 40 or 50 mm Hg, Diamox may be given to decrease the aqueous formation, and, in some cases, the pressure may be brought down and kept controlled until the hemorrhage is absorbed. If it is impossible to get the intraocular pressure down within 48 hours, irrigation of the blood from the anterior chamber is carried out under general anesthesia. The conjunctiva is incised 3–4 mm from the limbus and the flap of conjunctiva is turned down. The anterior chamber is entered with either a keratome or a Graefe knife, and then, with the use of a curved blunt needle, saline is irrigated into the anterior chamber. Sometimes the irrigation may have to be continued for an hour or an hour and a half before the clot will break up and be irrigated from the eye. The wound in the sclera is closed with 6-0 plain gut suture and another similar suture is placed to close the conjunctival wound. Some surgeons prefer to enter the anterior chamber through the cornea just anterior to the limbus.

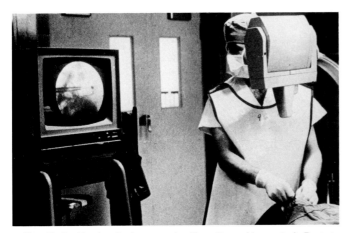

Fig. 23–6.—Foreign body removal with radiographic control. Forceps directed to the site of a foreign body.

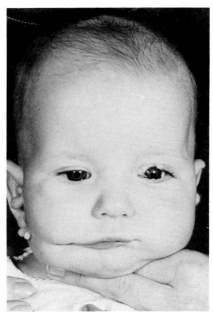

Fig. 23–7.—Coloboma. Multiple congenital anomalies, including coloboma of left upper lid, skin tags about ears and deformity at side of mouth.

Blow-out Fractures of the Floor of the Orbit

These fractures may be limited to the floor of the orbit or they may occur with other fractures of the bones of the middle third of the face associated with fractures extending into the floor of the orbit.

Fractures of the malar-zygomatic complex or crushing injuries of the intraorbital rim may cause a comminution of the orbital floor but are not true blow-out fractures.

A pure blow-out fracture results from a sudden pressure over the rim of the orbit, increasing the intraorbital pressure, and the thin portion of the floor blows out, which may prevent a rupture of the globe. These injuries frequently result from the eye being struck with a ball or a fist.

PHYSICAL EXAMINATION.—These patients are unable to elevate or depress the globe. They have vertical diplopia, decreased sensation over the distribution of the infraorbital nerve. Occasionally there is edema and hemorrhage in the orbit, which may cause proptosis. As this subsides, the patient develops an enophthalmos. The hole in the orbital floor allows the orbital fat, Tenon's capsule and inferior rectus and occasionally the inferior oblique to herniate downward. If the fracture is small, the inferior rectus or inferior oblique may be trapped, limiting the elevation and depression of the globe (Fig. 23–4). Tomograms of the orbital floor usually are needed to demonstrate the fracture (Fig. 23–5).

A traction test using small forceps is carried out by grasping a piece of conjunctiva below the cornea to demonstrate restriction of passive movement of the globe.

TREATMENT.—The present feeling regarding treatment is that time should be allowed for the orbital swelling to subside before the decision is made to repair the hole in the floor of the orbit. Limitation of ocular movement may be due to damage to the extraocular muscle, with hemorrhage, or to nerve damage, and these may gradually recover.

Operation consists of making an incision in the skin at the junction of the lower lid with the cheek. The periosteum is incised and raised from the floor of the orbit. Retractors al-

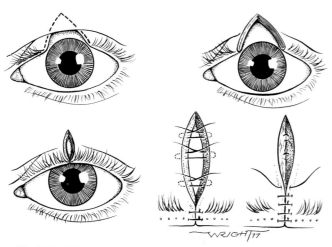

Fig. 23–8.—Primary closure of a coloboma. The edges are freshened, then carefully apposed and sutured in layers.

low examination of the floor of the orbit, and when the hole is located, a thin piece of Teflon or of silicone rubber is placed over the defect in the orbital floor. It may be necessary to wire the Teflon plate to the rim of the orbit.

Foreign Bodies in the Eye and Orbit

Foreign bodies such as BB pellets, shell fragments or chips of metal may strike the eye and end up in the orbit. The diagnosis is made with the help of x-rays and ultrasound. The foreign body may enter the globe and be located anywhere within the eye. Various methods are used by the x-ray department for localizing the position of the foreign bodies.

Removal of a foreign body frequently is quite difficult. If the localization shows that the foreign body is near the front of the eye, and is magnetic, with the aid of a magnet, the foreign body may be drawn into the anterior chamber, a small incision made near the limbus and the foreign body extracted with further use of the giant magnet. If the foreign body is behind the lens and can be moved with the magnet, it should be drawn to the region of the pars plana. Further localization can be carried out with the help of the Berman locator and an incision made through the sclera, the magnet

Fig. 23–9.—Coloboma. Method for partial and total upper lid reconstruction. (Adapted from N. L. Cutler and C. Beard, Am. J. Ophthalmol. 39:1, 1955.)

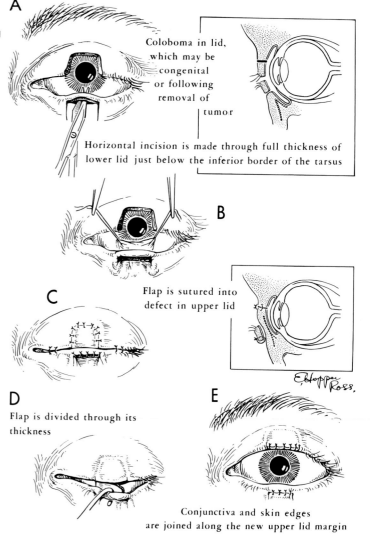

A

Coloboma in lid, which may be congenital or following removal of tumor

Horizontal incision is made through full thickness of lower lid just below the inferior border of the tarsus

B

Flap is sutured into defect in upper lid

C

D

Flap is divided through its thickness

E

Conjunctiva and skin edges are joined along the new upper lid margin

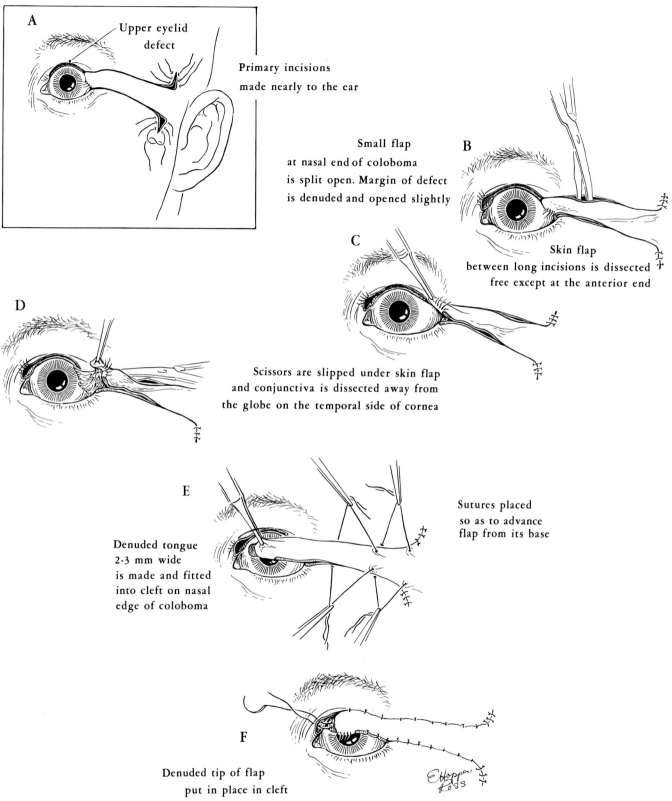

Fig. 23—10.—Coloboma. Wheeler method of repair of congenital coloboma of upper eyelid.

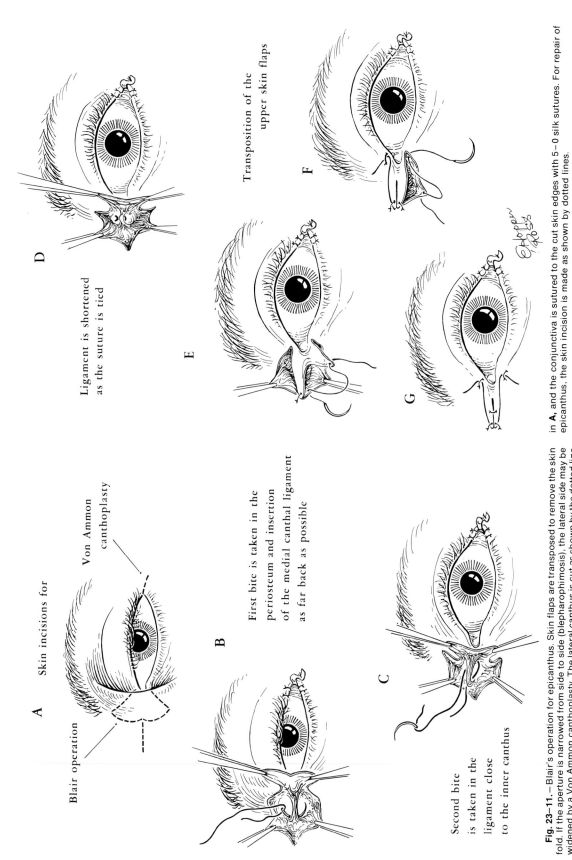

A Skin incisions for

Von Ammon
canthoplasty

Blair operation

B First bite is taken in the
periosteum and insertion
of the medial canthal ligament
as far back as possible

C Second bite
is taken in the
ligament close
to the inner canthus

D Ligament is shortened
as the suture is tied

E

Transposition of the
upper skin flaps

F

G

Fig. 23–11. – Blair's operation for epicanthus. Skin flaps are transposed to remove the skin fold. If the aperture is narrowed from side to side (blepharophimosis), the lateral side may be widened by a Von Ammon canthoplasty. The lateral canthus is cut as shown by the dotted line in **A,** and the conjunctiva is sutured to the cut skin edges with 5–0 silk sutures. For repair of epicanthus, the skin incision is made as shown by dotted lines.

220

tip applied to the lips of the wound and the foreign body extracted.

If the foreign body is nonmagnetic and located either within the orbit or within the eye, the image intensifier is quite useful in the successful removal of these foreign bodies. Unlike the fluoroscope, the x-ray image intensifier is well suited to the operating room, requiring no period of dark adaptation.

In this system, the x-rays are focused on a fluorescent screen mounted against the photocathode, which shows an electronic image on the screen (Fig. 23–6). The screen displays the image on two planes and the system can be rotated 90 degrees to show a third. With the help of a small pair of forceps directed toward the foreign body, the whole maneuver can be watched on the screen and the foreign body located and removed.

Surgery of the Lids

Congenital Abnormalities

COLOBOMA.—This is a defect of the lid margin. The extent of involvement varies and they occur most commonly in the nasal portion of the upper lid (Fig. 23–7). Less frequently, they are found laterally in the lower lid and may be found in the craniofacial dystrophies, such as Treacher Collins syndrome. In large colobomas, the edges are covered with palpebral conjunctiva connecting the lid to the bulbar conjunctiva.

The etiology is uncertain. They may result from arrest of development or from traction by amniotic bands.

Repair of the coloboma depends on the position and extent of the defect. Primary closure, after freshening of the margins of the defect, may be used for colobomas up to approximately 25–30% of the total horizontal lid length (Fig. 23–8) or the Wheeler halving procedure may be indicated.

With a larger defect, 30–50%, a portion of tarsus from the same lid may be rotated to fill the defect. The deep structure defect can be filled by either a mucous membrane graft, a piece of bank sclera or a conjunctival graft from the lower lid. A variation of the Cutler-Beard procedure for upper lid colobomas (Fig. 23–9) and a variation of the Hughes technique for large lower lid colobomas may be used.

Large lower lid defects, 25–50%, are effectively handled by an upper lid tarsoconjunctival advancement flap combined with a split-thickness retroauricular skin graft.

In large defects of the medial side of the upper lid, Wheeler's method of repair (Fig. 23–10) is the method of choice.

EPICANTHUS.—Epicanthus is a circular fold of skin running vertically on the side of the nose, arising in the upper lid and curving down to the lower. It usually disappears with growth of the face and development of the nasal bridge; however, it may persist. It is bilateral, although it may be asymmetric. Congenital ptosis may occur concomitantly. Repair by the Blair operation (Fig. 23–11), Spaeth's technique or the Y-V operation of Verwey (Fig. 23–12) may be used for repair of palpebral epicanthus.

EPICANTHUS INVERSUS.—This condition is similar to epicanthus but the skin fold arises in the lower lid and curves upward to the upper lid (Fig. 23–13). Spaeth's correction is shown in Figure 23–14. The syndrome of epicanthus inversus, blepharophimosis and ptosis frequently is transmitted as a dominant characteristic.

TELECANTHUS.—Telecanthus indicates a wide intercanthal distance with a normal interpupillary distance. It may occur alone or in association with epicanthus and blepharophimosis, and may be unilateral. Repair is made by the Y-V operation or that of Mustardé. In addition, transnasal wiring is used to pull the medial canthus into proper position. These procedures effectively advance the medial canthi by tucking and resecting the medial canthal tendon, and the proper position is held by the wiring (Fig. 23–15). To avoid possible complications of exposed wires in the nasal cavity, strips of fascia lata are tied to the medial canthal tendons and drawn across the bridge of the nose to hold the medial canthi in their new position.

EPIBLEPHARON.—Epiblepharon is a large skin fold hanging down over the margin of the upper lid or, more frequently, occupying a similar position on the lower lid. It usually disappears by the end of the first year. Occasionally, the lashes of the lower lid may turn in and abrade the cornea. This can be corrected by excision of the superfluous skin in the lid fold.

ENTROPION.—Congenital entropion is an inturning of the lid margin, which usually occurs in the lower lid, rarely in the upper. It usually is secondary to epicanthus epiblepha-

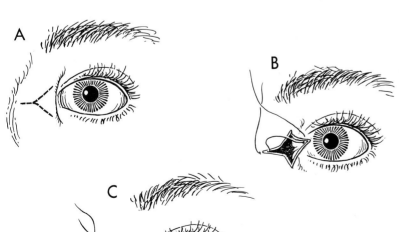

Fig. 23–12.—Epicanthal repair by Y-V operation of Verwey. Skin incision is made as shown in **A** with branches of Y on epicanthal fold. Apex of triangle is fastened medially with one buried Supramid suture, securing the deep side of the apex of the skin triangle to the periosteum as far medially as possible. The surface of the apex of the skin triangle then is sutured to the skin at the end of the nasal incision with silk. Sides then are sutured.

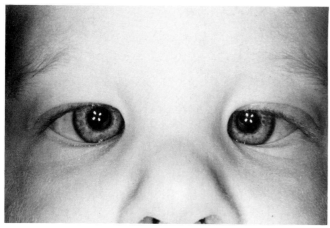

Fig. 23–13.—Epicanthus inversus with ptosis. Skin fold arises in lower lid and extends upward and blends into upper lid.

ron or conditions such as microphthalmos and enophthalmos, in which there is loss of support to the posterior border of the lid. Cicatricial entropion is secondary to any condition causing scarring and shrinkage of the conjunctiva, such as an alkali burn or the Stevens-Johnson syndrome. This may be corrected by a mucous membrane graft. A tarsoconjunctival graft will correct primary congenital entropion caused by absence of the tarsal plate. The treatment of spastic entropion depends on the cause. Taping of the lid to the skin of

the cheek until the inflammation has ceased may suffice or Hill's modification of the Wheeler operation may be required, in which the orbicularis is resected and closure made by suturing the upper edge of the skin incision to the lower border of the tarsus with 3-0 chromic catgut (Fig. 23–16).

ECTROPION.—Congenital ectropion, or outward turning of the lid margin, rarely occurs as a separate entity. More commonly it occurs with congenital ptosis, epicanthus inversus, blepharophimosis, microphthalmos or buphthalmos. Cicatricial ectropion may result from skin diseases or secondary to injuries producing scarring on the skin surface of the lid, such as ichthyosis congenita. Surgical treatment may not be required for minimal ectropion. Ziegler cautery (Fig. 23–17) on the conjunctival surface may correct the problem, and free or pedicle skin grafts or suturing a V incision into a Y may correct cicatricial ectropion. Tarsorrhaphy may also correct the problem.

A wedge resection of tarsus and conjunctiva with apex pointing downward may be required. For a lateral ectropion, Smith's modification of the Kuhnt-Szymanowski procedure is required (Fig. 23–18).

BLEPHAROPTOSIS.—Ptosis of the upper lid indicates a drooping of more than an average amount. The condition may be unilateral or bilateral.

Among the ptosis types, only the following are considered here: (1) Congenital ptosis, (a) with normal superior rectus action; (b) associated with weakness of one or more of the

Fig. 23–14.—Spaeth's correction of epicanthus inversus. **A,** the first incision is along the lower lid margin, 2 mm below the lash line passing through the skin and orbicularis fibers. It is carried upward into the epicanthal fold and then downward. The small piece of skin is removed and, after the tissues are undermined **(B),** the upper margin is moved toward the nose, thus elongating the palpebral fissure and eliminating the epicanthal fold. **C–E** placement of sutures. The suture at **C** is placed first to control the degree of correction. (Adapted from Am. J. Ophthalmol. 41:61, 1956.)

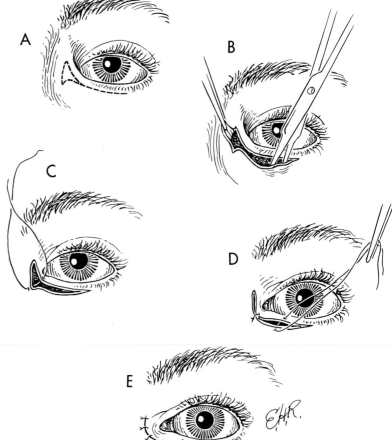

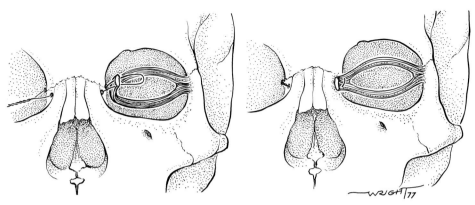

Fig. 23–15.—Transnasal wiring for telecanthus. After disinsertion of the medial canthal tendon, a wire suture is passed through the tendon. An awl is passed through from the region of the opposite medial canthal tendon inser-tion and both ends of the wire suture are drawn through separate holes. The wire is tightened over a bony bridge.

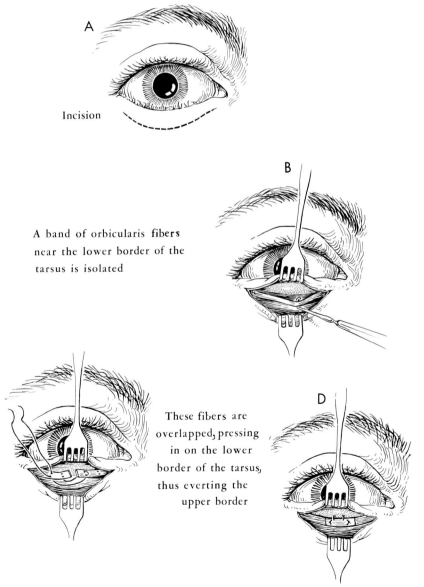

A

Incision

A band of orbicularis **fibers** near the lower border of the tarsus is isolated

B

These fibers are overlapped, pressing in on the lower border of the tarsus, thus everting the upper border

D

Fig. 23–16. — Wheeler repair of spastic entropion (adapted from Bethke).

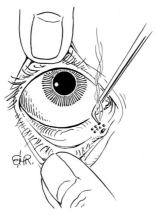

Fig. 23—17.—Ziegler cautery of palpebral conjunctiva to correct eversion of the punctum.

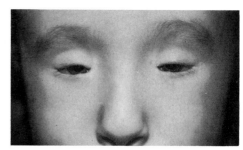

Fig. 23—19.—A child with blepharophimosis and ptosis. The ptosis here is best repaired with fascia lata.

elevator muscles of the eye; (c) associated with the jaw-winking phenomenon of Marcus Gunn; (d) associated with blepharophimosis. (2) Acquired ptosis, (a) local or general disease; (b) neurologic causes; (c) trauma.

The congenital form is most common, most cases being unilateral, with fair to good levator action. About 6% of all cases of congenital ptosis demonstrate the jaw-winking phenomenon of Marcus Gunn, and these are almost all unilateral, but bilateral cases do occur. The affected lid moves upward if the mandible is either depressed or moved to the opposite side. Ptosis associated with blepharophimosis always is bilateral (Fig. 23–19) and occurs in about 3% of cases of congenital ptosis. Only a few of the conditions accounting for acquired ptosis will be mentioned, and only those that occur in children. Acquired ptosis may occur with hemangioma, neurofibromatosis and occasionally after enucleation, usually when there has been no implant in Tenon's

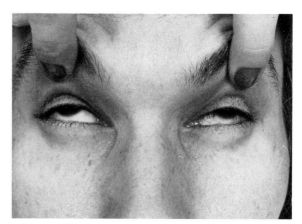

Fig. 23—20.—Bell's phenomenon. Eyes rotate upward and slightly outward when lids are closed. Demonstrated by forcibly elevating lids with examiner's fingers while patient attempts to close lids. Cornea is moved from region of palpebral aperture.

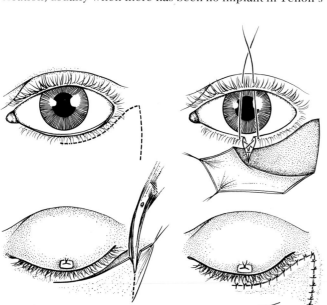

Fig. 23—18.—Smith's modification of the Kuhnt-Szymanowski procedure for lateral ectropion. A skin incision is made and the skin undermined. A full-thickness wedge is resected from the lid and the lid margins are carefully apposed using a suture anchored in the tarsus and brought out through the gray line. The suture then is passed into the gray line of the upper lid and brought out through the skin. The skin of the lower lid is drawn laterally into position and any excess resected before suturing.

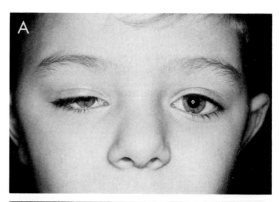

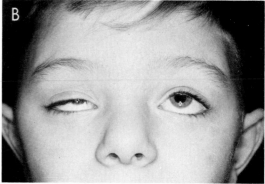

Fig. 23—21.—Lid ptosis with poor levator action.

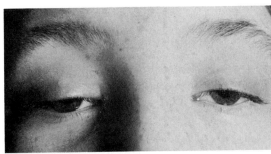

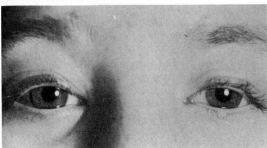

Fig. **23–22.**—A girl aged 9 with bilateral ptosis, with very little levator action.

Fig. **23–23.**—Same girl as in Figure 23–22 after repair with fascia (frontalis suspension).

capsule. Neurologic causes include brain lesions, such as hemorrhage, tumor and trauma. Acquired ptosis may occur with external ophthalmoplegia. Local trauma to the lid may result in ptosis. This may result from cutting the levator muscle or damage to its nerve. Removal of tumors in the lid

has been associated with the onset of ptosis. Removal of lipodermoids at the outer canthal angle has also resulted in ptosis. This may be due to the formation of scar tissue holding the lid down.

Preoperative Examination

The corneal sensation and Bell's phenomenon (Fig. 23–20) should be investigated. The amount of ptosis is determined by measuring the width of the palpebral apertures, noting how much of each cornea is covered by each upper lid. We examine the patient by having him look up and look down, but, most important, in the primary position (Fig. 23–21).

The range of movement of the lid is estimated by measuring the amount of elevation from looking up to looking down. This is done by preventing the frontalis muscle from functioning by holding the forehead with the thumb. The position of the lid fold of the normal lid should be noted so that at the time of operation the fold of the ptosed lid will be placed properly. Photographs of the patient should be taken preoperatively. Full-face photographs are taken with the eyes up, down and in the primary position.

Operative Procedures

(1) Procedure for utilizing the levator muscle. (2) Frontalis suspension operation (Figs. 23–22 and 23–23). (3) Operation using the superior rectus to suspend the lid. (4) Using the corrugator superciliaris muscle.

Operations Using the Levator Muscle

Approach to the levator muscle may be made either through the skin surface or through the conjunctiva. Larger

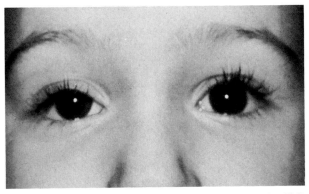

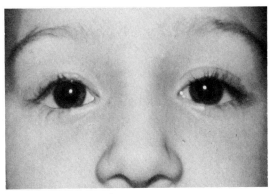

Fig. **23–24.**—Slight ptosis of left upper lid of 8-year-old girl.

Fig. **23–25.**—Same patient as in Figure 23–24 after levator resection through posterior surface of lid.

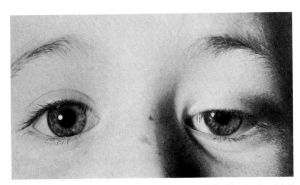

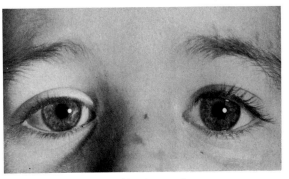

Fig. **23–26.**—A boy aged 4 with ptosis of left upper lid, with good action of levator muscle.

Fig. **23–27.**—Same child as in Figure 23–26 after resection through skin.

degrees of ptosis are treated by the external approach through skin. About 2–3 mm of correction can be obtained by the conjunctival approach, so this method is used in cases of small degrees of ptosis (3–4 mm) (Figs. 23–24 and 23–25). Larger degrees of ptosis are best treated by the external approach through skin (Figs. 23–26 and 23–27).

Operations Using the Frontalis Muscle

Many methods have been used to suspend the lid from the frontalis muscle. At present, autogenous fascia is considered to be the best. Stored fascia that has been treated with cobalt-60 also works quite well, but in 10% of the cases the stored fascia may be absorbed and the ptosis will recur. In the case of the Marcus Gunn syndrome, when the jaw-winking is marked, the levator tendon may be cut to stop the jaw-winking and, later, autogenous fascia used to sling the lid up to the frontalis muscle.

Fasanella-Servat Operation

This operation usually is carried out after age 3½. General anesthesia is mandatory for children and preferable for adults. The lid is everted on a Desmarres retractor and two curved hemostat forceps are placed across the upper border of the tarsus, grasping the conjunctiva, tarsus and levator and Müller's muscles, 3–4 mm behind the everted margin (Fig. 23–28, A).

The hemostats must include sufficient tissue on the nasal and temporal sides of the tarsus so that elevation of the lid will be symmetric. Starting at the temporal side of the tarsus in the region of the lid fold, a 4-0 plain gut suture on a ⅜ of a circle reverse-cutting needle is passed through the lid from the skin side to the conjunctival surface. Using scissors, a cut is made about ½–2 mm above the hemostats for about 5 mm. The suture then is passed deep into the tissue above, including the levator muscle. Moving medially, it is passed into the tarsus deep to the conjunctiva. The tissue above the

hemostats is removed (Fig. 23–28, B) 5 mm at a time and the suture advanced until all the tissue has been cut off. At this point, the suture is pulled tight and then passed back between tarsus and conjunctiva in a lateral direction, superficial to its medial course (Fig. 23–28, C). The result is a double running suture. When the lateral side of the lid is reached, the suture is pulled taut, the needle is passed through to the skin surface close to its point of entry and the ends tied (Fig. 23–28, D). At that time, the retractor is removed and the lid fold checked. If the lid fold does not extend right across the lid, several 4-0 plain gut sutures are passed through the lid and tied on the skin surface. One or two such sutures usually are sufficient. Two modified Frost sutures are placed from the lower lid to the brow, through buttons. After instilling an antibiotic-steroid ointment, they are tied. A tight patch is applied and left in place for 24 hours. During the operation, about 3 mm of the top of the tarsus and 3 mm of levator and Müller's muscle have been removed.

The patient is discharged after the Frost sutures are removed on the second or third day.

Levator Resection Through Skin

Correction of a greater degree of ptosis is possible through a skin incision when the levator action is poor but not absent. The examiner should place his thumb firmly above the eyebrow to stop the frontalis muscle from raising the lid. A millimeter rule is held vertically over the eye and the patient is instructed to look up as far as possible and then look down, also as far as possible. If excursion of the lid is less than 6 mm, the ptosis should be repaired with fascia lata. If there is a 6–7 mm of excursion of the lid, the levator muscle should be approached by a skin incision, since more of the muscle can be isolated and excised in this manner.

TECHNIQUE (FIG. 23–29).—1) Before the levator muscle is resected, one must observe the position of the lid fold on

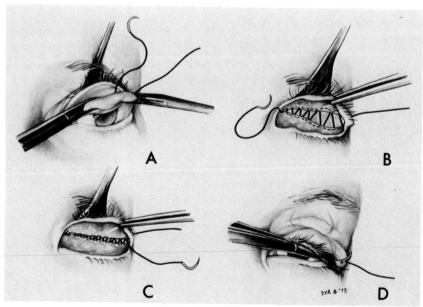

Fig. 23–28.—Fasanella-Servat operation. **A,** the lid is everted on a Desmarres retractor and two curved hemostat forceps are placed across the upper border of the tarsus. A 4-0 plain gut suture is passed through the lid from the skin side of the conjunctival surface but not through it. **B,** the tissue above the hemostats is cut off with scissors; the suture is passed deep into the tarsus and woven across the lid in this manner until it reaches the medial side. It then is pulled taut. **C,** the suture then is passed back, being secured in the deep surface of the conjunctiva on the tarsal side and over to the conjunctiva on the levator side. The suture is woven laterally across the lid superficial to its medial course. **D,** when the lateral side of the lid is reached, the needle is passed through to the skin surface at its point of entry and the suture pulled taut and the ends tied.

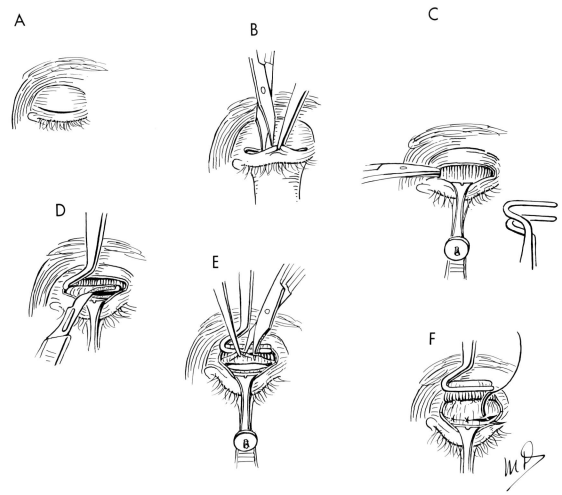

Fig. 23–29.—Repair of ptosis through skin. **A** and **B,** incision through skin and orbicularis oculi; anterior surface of tarsus is exposed. **C,** incisions are made and Berke ptosis clamp is inserted to secure the whole thickness of lid except skin. **D,** tarsus is incised 4 mm from lid border. **E** and **F,** palpebral conjunctiva is dissected off muscle and sutured to tarsus. *(Continued.)*

the normal lid. The distance from the lid border should be measured and the skin incision on the ptotic lid made in a similar position. After the site of the incision has been marked on the ptotic lid, a protective horn plate is placed under the upper lid and the skin and orbicularis muscle are incised the length of the lid. The orbicularis muscle and the skin are dissected and freed from the tarsus down to the edge of the lid. An Erhardt clamp is placed on the tarsus, the lid pulled down and the skin dissected up from the underlying tissues (*A* and *B*).

2) Two buttonhole incisions then are made through the levator and the conjunctiva close to the tarsus, about 25 mm apart. The Berke clamp goes through the incisions to secure the levator muscle. The tarsus is cut across 4 mm from the lid border, and the levator muscle is raised to expose the conjunctival surface (*C* and *D*).

3) An incision is made just below the Berke ptosis clamp (*C*) through the conjunctiva, and the conjunctiva is dissected free from the muscle (*D*). The cut edge of the conjunctiva is resutured to the border of the tarsus with 6-0 plain catgut sutures. This may be done as a continuous suture or as 6 or 7 interrupted sutures (*E* and *F*).

4) The positions of the lateral horn and the check ligaments of the levator now are located by palpation through

the skin of the upper lid while pulling down on the ptosis clamp. These two structures are cut, freeing the levator muscle.

5) The levator muscle is pulled downward and the septum oribtale is cut free from the levator. This is best done just below the orbital rim, where the levator muscle and the orbital septum are separated by a wedge of fat.

6) After that has been done, one may notice the orbital fat to herniate forward. The upper lid then is elevated and the levator muscle pulled down over the lid margin. Four 4-0 double-armed plain catgut sutures are inserted from the deep surface forward through the levator muscle, evenly distributed across the width of the muscle. The sutures are placed in the levator at the level where it crosses the upper border of the tarsus, as a guide to the amount to be resected, which varies between 10 mm and 15 mm. Two ends of each suture are tied (*J*).

7) The distal end of the levator muscle is excised, and then the sutures are passed horizontally into the tarsus and tied (*G*), thus elevating the lid into its new position. Before the sutures shown in *M* are tied, two 3-0 chromic catgut sutures are placed in the lid as shown in Figure 23–29. These chromic sutures hold the lid up at the desired height until all the reaction in the lid has subsided and usually disintegrate

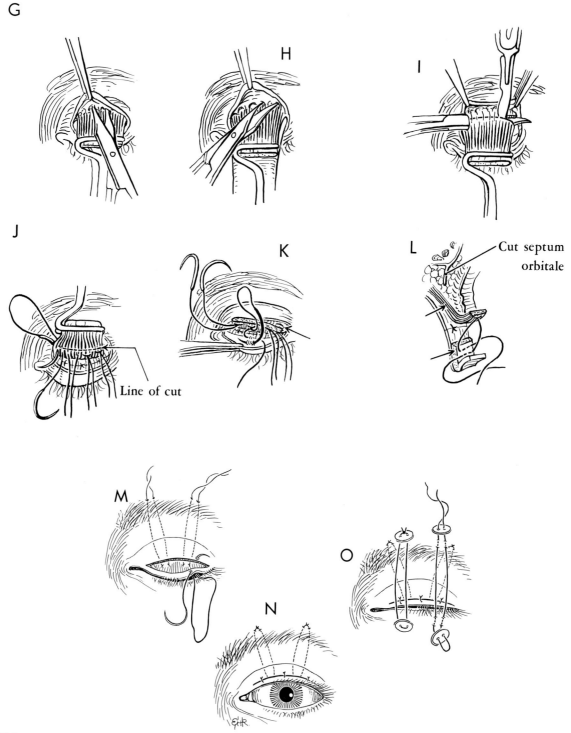

Fig. 23–29 (cont.).—**G** and **H,** superior surface of levator is dissected free. **I,** septum orbitale is incised. Repair of ptosis through skin. **J,** four 4-0 plain catgut sutures through muscle. **K** and **L,** sutures attach shortened levator to tarsus *(arrows)*. **M,** three 4-0 sutures, through tarsus from conjunctival sur-face, form skin fold. **N,** three double-armed 4-0 plain catgut sutures through conjunctival surface. **O,** two modified Frost sutures inserted in lower lid and tied.

in 2 weeks. During the early healing there is a certain amount of swelling in the lid, and this tends to interfere with the results of the levator shortening that was carried out. Since using these sutures, I have been obtaining better re-sults from my levator shortenings.

8) Three other double-armed 4-0 plain catgut sutures then

are placed through the conjunctival surface. One end of the double-armed suture is brought out through the tarsus and the skin below and the other end through the muscle and skin above, thus closing the skin wound and helping to form a good lid fold.

9) Two modified Frost sutures are inserted in the lower

lid and tied *(I)*; then a bandage and adhesive strapping are placed over the eye. The bandage should be left in place for 5 days to help minimize the postoperative swelling.

Repair of Ptosis with Fascia Lata

This operation is used only when there is little or no function in the levator muscle.

PLACING OF THE STRIPS OF FASCIA (FIG. 23–30).— Two pieces of fascia 2 mm wide and 10–12 cm long are used for each ptosed lid. The lid is divided into thirds and skin incisions are made midway between these marks, 2 mm from the lid margin. The incisions in the forehead are made

7 mm above the brow on a line perpendicular to the lid border when the lid is held up with forceps in the desired position. The third incision is made in the forehead midway between the other two incisions and slightly above them *(A)*. The fascia strips are placed in the lid with the help of the Wright fascia needle *(B–D)*. When the needle is passed horizontally between the incisions near the lid border, the needle is passed through the superficial layer of the tarsus. The purpose of using two pieces of fascia in this method is to have the direction of pull at right angles to the new raised position of the lid border. The ends of the fascia are tied in a double knot with a piece of 3-0 chromic catgut tied over the knots *(E)*. An end of each piece of fascia is brought under the

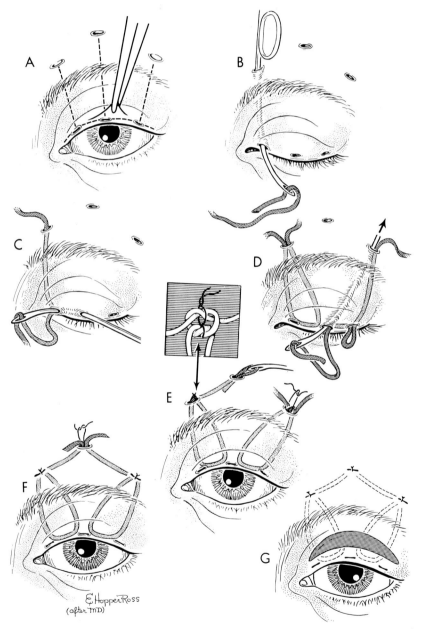

E. Hopper Ross
(after mD)

Fig. 23–30.—Repair of ptosis with fascia lata. **A,** lid is divided into thirds and incisions made in each third, 2 mm above the lash line. Forehead incisions are made 7 mm above the brow on a line perpendicular to the lid border when the lid is held up with forceps in the desired position. The central forehead incision is midway between the other forehead incisions and slightly above them. **B–D,** two fascia strips are placed in each eyelid under the skin and in the orbicularis muscle with a Wright fascia needle. **E,** ends of the fascia are tied in a double knot with a piece of 3-0 chromic catgut tied over the knots. **F,** an end of each piece of fascia is brought under the skin and out through the central forehead incision. **G,** an ellipse of skin is removed in every unilateral case and most bilateral cases.

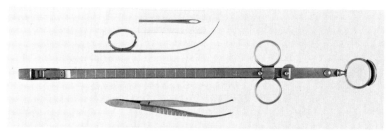

Fig. 23–31.—Wright fascia needle, Crawford fascia stripper and curved forceps for pulling fascia through the end of the stripper.

skin and out through the central forehead incision *(F)*. An ellipse of skin is removed in every unilateral case and most bilateral cases *(G)*. The Wright fascia needle and the Crawford fascia stripper are instruments used for this operation (Fig. 23–31).

Surgical Treatment of Congenital Cataracts and Dislocated Lenses

Until relatively recently, Cordes' conservative approach in the treatment of congenital cataract has had a wide following. He stated, "In view of the inevitable risk, in other words, of anesthetic accident, postoperative infection and surgical complications, congenital cataract surgery should be undertaken only after the most serious consideration." Today, many more congenital cataracts are being removed because anesthetics are better, there are very few postoperative infections and the surgical complications are few.

Assessment of the Cataract

First, precise nature of the lens opacity must be determined. The structure, size and density of the opacity are important. We must determine how much of a visual defect a particular type and size of opacity is causing.

In 1971, Merin and Crawford examined 57 patients with incomplete congenital cataracts to determine the relative effect of type, size and density of the cataract on visual acuity. The densities of the cataract were measured by means of neutral density filters.

The results showed that visual acuity in most patients with unilateral incomplete congenital cataracts was poor, and was about equal to the visual acuity in patients with unilateral complete cataracts (Fig. 23–32). Therefore, both complete and incomplete congenital cataracts should receive the same treatment. Untreated, both groups will develop monocular strabismus and combined strabismic and stimulus-deprivation amblyopia. Surprisingly, the visual acuity bears no relationship to the size of the cataract (Fig. 23–33). The patient with a 5.5-mm cataract would have 20/30 vision or 20/400 vision; poor visual acuity was found in 1 patient with a 6.5-mm cataract and in 1 with a 2.5-mm cataract. The prognosis for the patient with bilateral incomplete cataract, therefore, depends on one factor—the density of the cataract. Optical iridectomy does not improve the prognosis in most cases, particularly when the nuclear opacity is dense.

With the improved surgical methods, the results after operation continue to improve in the bilateral cases, but the visual result in unilateral congenital cataracts continues to be unsatisfactory. Stimulus-deprivation amblyopia, when operation is delayed past 6 months of age, undoubtedly has been a major factor in poor visual results.

In classic studies on stimulus-deprivation amblyopia in cats, Hubel and Wiesel found that kittens that were deprived of visual stimuli in one or both eyes during the first 3 months of life developed profound irreversible amblyopia.

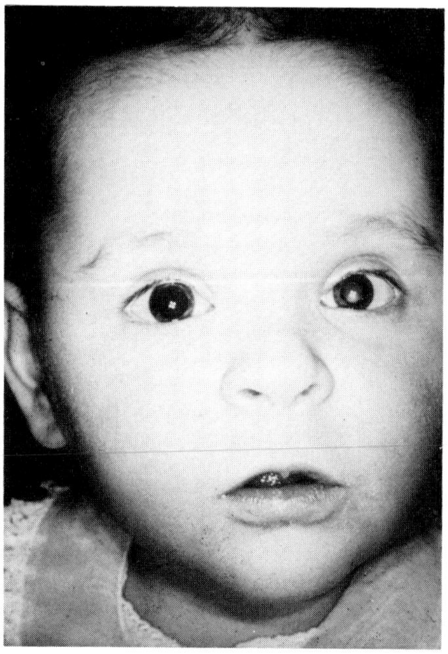

Fig. 23–32.—Unilateral incomplete congenital cataract.

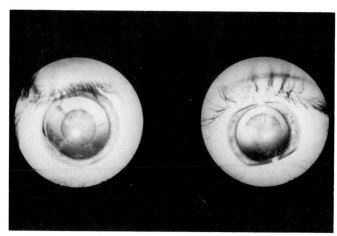

Fig. 23–33.—Bilateral lamellar cataracts in a patient who had an optical iridectomy of the right eye at the age of 6 months. **Right:** cataract size 4.3 mm; visual acuity 20/200. **Left:** cataract size 5.1 mm; visual acuity 20/60. Note that the eye with the larger cataract has the better visual acuity, which bears no relationship to the size of the cataract.

Functional changes occurred in the corticoreceptor fields of the individual retinal units, and histologic degenerative changes took place in the lateral geniculate body. Relative light deprivation resulted in less profound changes in both the cortical fields and the lateral geniculate body. Occlusion therapy in these cases was ineffective. From these investigations and from large-scale clinical experience, we can say that the critical period of visual development in man is in the first 3–4 months of life. Delaying removal of congenital cataract until a child is beyond 4–6 months of age, therefore, may result in stimulus-deprivation amblyopia, nystagmus or strabismus. If a unilateral cataract is allowed to remain longer than 6 months after birth, the blurred image in the affected eye causes an anisometropic amblyopia and an eventual progression to esotropia, which results in strabismic amblyopia. A patient with bilateral lamellar cataracts without a dense nuclear opacity may have clear retinal images, little or no amblyopia and consequently good vision, and in such cases the surgeon may wait until the child is between 4 and 6 years of age to remove the cataract and still obtain a reasonable visual result.

Etiology of Congenital Cataracts

The cause of congenital cataracts can be detected in about two-thirds of the patients. In a study of 386 cases done at The Hospital for Sick Children, Toronto, hereditary cataracts were present in 8.3% of the patients, cataracts associated with systemic disease in 11.9%, cataracts associated with ocular disease in 6% and with convulsions or central nervous system involvement in 22.8%, confirming that infantile cataract is not an isolated disease.

In our experience, the congenital rubella syndrome is the disease that most frequently causes cataracts, (Fig. 23–34), affecting 1 of 5 of our patients. Fifteen of our patients had Down's syndrome and 10 others had congenital cataracts associated with multiple congenital malformations.

The incidence of ocular conditions associated with infantile cataracts shows that persistent hyperplastic primary vitreous is the most common. Aniridia and retrolental fibroplasia are other conditions associated with congenital cataract. In 75 patients with associated central nervous system involvement, 40 had mental retardation and 28 had a history of convulsions. Hypoglycemia was present in 12 of the 75 patients.

Indications for Surgery of Congenital Cataract

Surgery is indicated at 3–6 months of age if the patient has (1) bilateral complete cataracts, (2) unilateral complete cataract or (3) unilateral or bilateral incomplete cataracts in which a dense central opacity exists, allowing for only a poor predicted visual acuity.

If the patient has bilateral complete cataracts, we operate on the first eye at 3–4 months of age, if possible. We wait several weeks until the eye is free from inflammation or any residual effects of the operation and then operate on the second eye. Contact lenses are given if the parents are reliable and cooperative; otherwise, spectacles are prescribed.

If a patient has a unilateral complete cataract, the ophthalmologist must occlude the good eye and provide a contact lens for the eye operated on. Without occlusion and a contact lens, stimulus-deprivation amblyopia is almost certain to develop.

If the patient has bilateral incomplete cataracts in which a dense central opacity exists, and poor visual acuity can be predicted from the cataract density/visual acuity correlation curve, we operate early. Early removal is also indicated for a unilateral incomplete cataract with a dense central opacity if the parents are highly cooperative. If the cataract is associated with ocular or systemic defects, it is better to postpone the operation until the child is older, when a discission and aspiration procedure is done for cosmetic reasons. The above rules also apply to the treatment of rubella cataracts.

Formerly, ophthalmologists were of the opinion that rubella cataracts should not be removed until after 2 years of age. Our present opinion favors early operation. Scheie had reported phthisis bulbi when operation was carried out by a two-stage procedure on rubella cataracts. When a one-stage discission and aspiration technique removes the cataract there usually are no late surgical complications.

The indications for optical iridectomy are controversial. The operation may be indicated if the patient has incomplete cataracts, the fundus can be visualized to some degree and the size of the cataract is less than 4 mm in diameter, or if dilating the patient's pupil results in a pronounced improvement in visual acuity. It may be used as a temporizing operation where there are additional ocular or systemic problems or where the child is grossly retarded. Although it is a benign operative procedure, it probably is not an effective one for many of the cases where it is used.

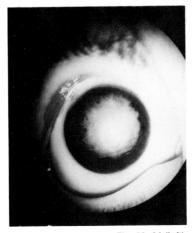 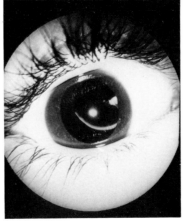

Fig. 23–34 (left). – Rubella cataract.
Fig. 23–35 (right). – Dislocated lens in Marfan's syndrome.

Dislocated Lenses in Children

Marfan's syndrome frequently is accompanied by dislocated lenses (Fig. 23–35). Homocystinuria is a much less frequent cause of dislocated lenses. Many different methods were used to treat these patients. These included intracapsular lens extraction, extracapsular lens extraction by discision alone or facilitated by the Calhoun needle or two Ziegler knives, linear lens extraction and lens discission with aspiration.

The results with discission and aspiration are much improved over the previous methods. Usually a satisfactory result can be obtained with one aspiration whereas with the needling technique alone, repeated procedures were usually necessary.

Surgical Technique for Removal of Congenital Cataracts or Dislocated Lenses

A long beveled tract is made with a Ziegler knife previously dipped in methylene blue. The knife is passed through the cornea into the anterior chamber at the 4 o'clock position temporally. A 25-gauge needle connected to a silicone tube and a 10-ml syringe is passed through the tract until the tip is in the anterior chamber (Fig. 23–36). A limbus-based flap is prepared at the 12 o'clock position and the anterior chamber is entered with the Ziegler knife and the incision widened until it is large enough to admit the

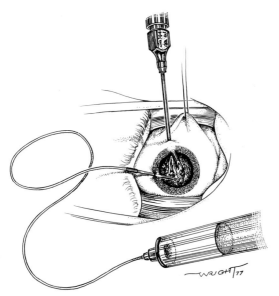

Fig. 23–36.—Aspiration of cataract. A 26-gauge needle (attached by silicone tubing [Dow Chemical Silastic Medical Grade Tubing, Catalog No. 602, 101] to a 10-ml syringe filled with saline) is passed through a slanting Ziegler tract in the lower part of the cornea. The Ziegler knife then is passed through the sclera near the limbus under a conjunctival flap and the cataract "needled." A 21-gauge bent needle (attached to a 2-ml syringe) is introduced through this incision and the cataract aspirated.

end of a 21-gauge irrigating needle (Fig. 23–36). This is attached to a 2-ml syringe filled with saline. The 21-gauge needle is bent with the bevel on top. The needle is inserted into the lens. One-quarter ml of saline is gently pushed into the lens and drawn back into the syringe. Injection of saline and aspiration is repeated, using the needle to break up the lens substance. The other irrigating system maintains continuous flow of saline flushing to keep the anterior chamber full. An operating room microscope is used for the procedure. Occasionally there is a more dense membrane on the surface of the lens, which may need to be removed with a gooseneck forceps. The tip of the 21-gauge needle is used as a dissector to help break up the lens at the time of the aspiration. The incision is closed with one 7-0 chromic catgut suture and the anterior chamber is restored, if necessary, using the irrigating system inserted below. The needle then is removed. It has not been our practice to do a peripheral iridectomy. Atropine ointment is instilled into the eye. In a small percentage of cases there is a formation of a secondary membrane, which may need to be cut. When a rubella cataract is removed, the iris sphincter is cut at 6 and 12 o'clock because it is very difficult to dilate the pupils in these cases.

REFERENCES

1. Converse, J. M., Smith, B., Obear, N. F., *et al.*: Orbital blow-out fractures: A 10 year survey, Plast. Reconstr. Surg. 39:28, 1967.
2. Crawford, J. S., Lewandowski, R. L., and Chan, W.: The effect of aspirin on rebleeding in traumatic hyphema, Am. J. Ophthalmol. 88:543, 1975.
3. Duke-Elder, S.: *System of Ophthalmology*, Vol. XIV, *Injuries*, Parts I and II (London: Henry Kimpton, 1972).
4. International Ophthalmology Clinics, Vol. 14, No. 4, Practical Management of Ocular Injuries, Winter, 1974.
5. Rakusin, W.: Traumatic hyphema, Am. J. Ophthalmol. 74:284, 1972.
6. Beard, C.: *Ptosis* (St. Louis: The C. V. Mosby Company, 1969).
7. Crawford, J. S.: Repair of blepharoptosis with a modification of the Fasanella-Servat operation, Can. J. Ophthalmol. 8:19, 1973.
8. Crawford, J. S.: Repair of ptosis using frontalis muscle and fascia lata, Trans. Am. Acad. Ophthalmol. Otolaryngol. 60:672, 1956.
9. The Ophthalmologic Staff of the Hospital for Sick Children, Toronto: *The Eye in Childhood* (Chicago: Year Book Medical Publishers, Inc., 1967).
10. Harley, R. D.: *Paediatric Ophthalmology* (Philadelphia: W. B. Saunders Company, 1975).
11. The Surgical Staff, The Hospital for Sick Children, Toronto: *Care for the Injured Child* (Baltimore: The Williams & Wilkins Company, 1976).
12. Merin, S., and Crawford, J. S.: Assessment of incomplete congenital cataract, Can. J. Ophthalmol. 7:56, 1972.
13. Merin, S., and Crawford, J. S.: The etiology of congenital cataracts: A survey of 386 cases, Can. J. Ophthalmol. 6:178, 1971.
14. Ryan, S., and von Noorden, G. K.: Further observations on the aspiration technique in cataract surgery, Am. J. Ophthalmol. 71:629, 1971.
15. von Noorden, G. K., Dowling, J. E., and Ferguson, D. C.: Experimental amblyopia in monkeys. Part I: Behavioral studies of stimulus-deprivation amblyopia, Arch. Ophthalmol. 84:206, 1970.
16. Drews, L. C., and Drews, R. C.: Optical iridectomy, Am. J. Ophthalmol. 58:789, 1964.
17. Hindle, N. W., and Crawford, J. S.: Dislocation of the lens in Marfan's syndrome. Its effect and treatment, Can. J. Ophthalmol. 4:128, 1969.

24 Joseph E. Murray / Leonard B. Kaban / John B. Mulliken

Craniofacial Abnormalities

"It is the divine right of man to look human," said Will Mayo. Until recently, there was little hope for the loneliness of patients with facial skeletal malformations who perceived themselves to be less than human, and operations for severe craniofacial deformities consisted essentially of soft tissue rearrangement to create the illusion of correction.[42] In 1949, Sir Harold Gillies was the first successfully to correct the orbital maxillary deficiency in a patient with midface retrusion, by advancement of the facial skeleton.[13] Murray and Swanson[24] performed a similar osteotomy in 1968. Present-day understanding of the anatomy of craniofacial deformities and the techniques for their correction are largely the result of the skill and imagination of one man, Dr. Paul Tessier.[32-39]

Craniofacial deformities may be grouped into two major categories: congenital and acquired. In our clinic, approximately 80% of patients present with congenital malformations of the following major types: (1) craniosynostosis (Crouzon's and Apert's syndromes), (2) orbital hypertelorism, (3) mandibulofacial dysostosis (the Treacher Collins syndrome) and (4) 1st and 2d branchial arch deficiency (hemifacial microsomia). Twenty per cent of our patients present with acquired deformities, consisting of defects secondary to tumors (15%) and trauma (5%).[25]

Congenital Deformities: Anatomy and Clinical Findings

Craniosynostosis with Associated Facial Skeletal Deformity (Crouzon's and Apert's Syndromes)

The estimated incidence of craniosynostosis is 1 per 1000 live births whereas the facial skeleton is affected in only 9–10% of cases.[3, 30] The configuration of the skull deformity in the craniosynostoses depends on the suture or sutures involved. Thus, premature synostosis of the sagittal suture prevents lateral expansion of the calvarium (perpendicular to the fused suture) but permits expansion anteriorly at the coronal suture and posteriorly at the lambdoidal suture. The result is a long, narrow skull (scaphocephaly). Oxycephaly, turricephaly or acrocephaly, all indicating a tall or "tower" skull, would therefore result from premature fusion of the coronal sutures. Other common skull deformities in craniofacial dysostosis include trigonocephaly (metopic synostosis) and plagiocephaly (unilateral coronal synostosis) (Fig. 24–1). Virchow, in 1851, postulated that the skull deformities in craniosynostosis were due to inhibition of growth at the synostosed or fused sutures with compensatory overexpansion of the skull at the open suture lines to accommodate brain growth.[41] For many years it was believed that sutural tissues were the primary growth sites of the skull and that their expansive force pushed the skull bones apart.[20] Included in this doctrine was the belief that the cranial cartilages (condylar, nasal, basal synchondrosal) were also primary growth centers. Recently, however, Moss has established that the sutures are passive areas, allowing cranial expansion, and are not primary regulators of cranial growth.[21, 22] He has also demonstrated that skull growth is determined by growth of the underlying brain, another example of his functional matrix concept. Thus, facial deformities are the result of a disturbance in the complex interaction between the growing facial skeleton and its functional matrix, the expanding brain and overlying soft tissues.

Crouzon, in 1912, first described a group of patients with craniosynostosis and severe midface hypoplasia.[8] A variety of skull types may be seen in Crouzon's syndrome; depending on the cranial suture involved, however, oxycephaly and brachycephaly are the most often observed (Fig. 24–2). The shallow bony orbits produce the characteristic exorbitism and divergent strabismus. The diminished orbital volume is the result of the anterior position of the greater wing of the sphenoid bone, the ballooning of the ethmoid sinuses and the foreshortening of the floor (maxillary hypoplasia) and roof (recession of the frontal bone) of the orbit. During the first 3 years of life, progressive visual loss may occur in patients with Crouzon's syndrome secondary to constriction of the osseous optic canals.[43] Later in childhood, this phenomenon is rare, although the possibility of corneal damage from exposure keratitis always is a threat. Prolapse of the frontal sinus, an inferior position of the cribriform plates and widening of the ethmoid sinuses may produce orbital hypertelorism. Another significant physical finding is the relatively low position of the lateral palpebral ligaments (secondary to hypoplasia of the zygomatic bones), giving an antimongoloid slant to the eyelids.

The maxilla is deficient in three dimensions, producing relative prognathism (the mandible is normal) and the characteristic drooping lower lip. The nose has a typical "parrot's beak" deformity. The narrow, inverted V-shaped maxillary dental arch results in bilateral crossbite. The palate usually has an extremely high vault, but there is a low incidence of bony palatal clefts.[35]

In 1906, Apert described a group of patients with craniosynostosis, midface hypoplasia and peculiar extremity deformities, a syndrome known today by the eponym or as acrocephalosyndactyly.[1] The facial deformities of Apert's syndrome are in many ways similar to those of Crouzon's syndrome. However, there are significant differences between the two groups.[34] Patients with Apert's syndrome more commonly have: (1) isolated involvement of the coronal suture producing oxycephaly (turricephaly, acrocephaly) and a transverse forehead skin furrow, (2) asymmetric exorbitism, (3) more severe lateral canthal dystopia, (4) a significant incidence of clefts of the secondary palate (30% of patients) and (5) anterior open bite (Fig. 24–3). The major distinguishing characteristic of Apert's syndrome is the complex syndactyly of the hands and/or feet, with interphalangeal synostosis, symphalangism and other anomalies producing a "mitten" deformity[18] (Fig. 24–3, D).

233

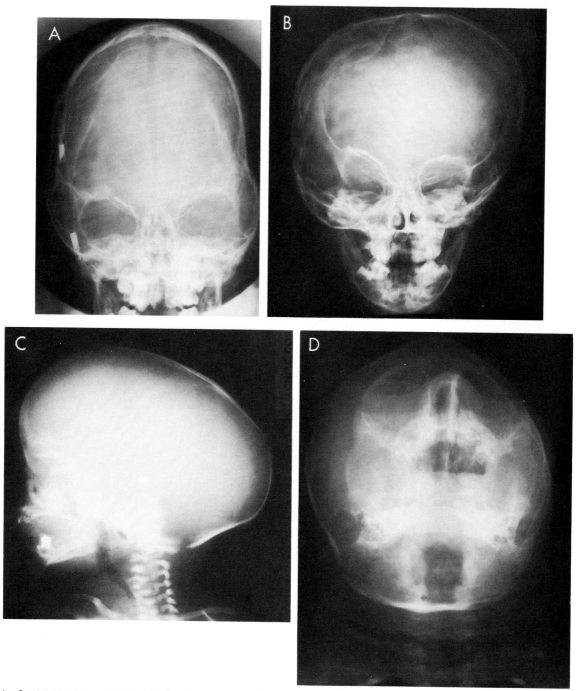

Fig. 24–1.—Cranial dysostosis—characteristic skull shapes. **A,** oxycephaly (turricephaly, acrocephaly)—bilateral coronal synostosis. **B,** plagiocephaly— unilateral coronal synostosis. **C,** scaphocephaly—sagittal synostosis. **D,** trigonocephaly—metopic synostosis.

The genetics of the two syndromes are similar. Crouzon's syndrome is inherited as an autosomal dominant condition, occurring in a frequency of 1 in 10,000 live births; however, 25% of these patients are fresh mutations. Apert's syndrome is less common than Crouzon's syndrome, with an estimated frequency of 1 in 160,000 live births. Apert's syndrome appears to have an autosomal dominant inheritance with low penetrance and there is a higher spontaneous mutation rate than in Crouzon's syndrome.[14]

Orbital Hypertelorism Syndromes

Hypertelorism is a descriptive term denoting an increased distance between the bony orbits. It is a physical finding that may be seen in association with craniosynostosis, craniofacial dysraphism, frontoencephalocele and other facial anomalies, as well as in post-traumatic widening of the nasoethmoidal region. The earlier term "ocular hypertelorism," used by Greig[16] in 1924 to describe 2 patients with

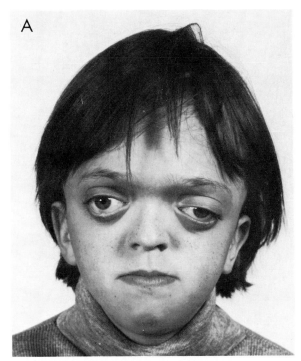

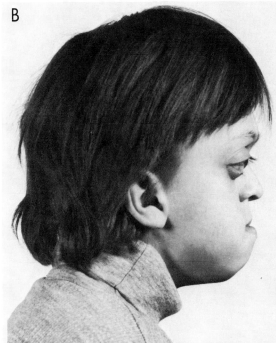

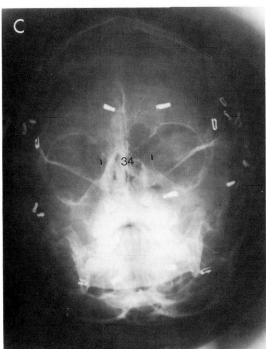

Fig. 24–2.—Crouzon's syndrome. **A** and **B,** an 11-year-old patient illustrates the typical exorbitism, hypoplasia of the maxilla and zygomatic regions and relative prognathism of Crouzon's syndrome. On the PA x-ray **(C),** note the second degree orbital hypertelorism (IOD, 34 mm) and the inferior position of the frontal sinuses and cribriform plates. (On the lateral x-ray, the orbits are shallow and the temporal lobe projects far anteriorly.)

"great breadth between the eyes," is not as useful because soft tissue deformities may give the appearance of hypertelorism without having the true skeletal deformity (Fig. 24–4).

During normal development, the orbital axis converges from 180 degrees during the first 3 months of fetal life to 70 degrees at birth and 65 degrees in the adult. Orbital hypertelorism is the result of any disruption of this narrowing of the orbital axis. For example, a frontoethmoidal encephalocele will, by its physical presence, prevent closure of this angle. However, in most cases, there is no midline mass. Johnston[19] has suggested that median facial malformations resulting in hypertelorism develop because of failure of neural crest cell migration into the developing frontonasal mesoderm.

The principal pathologic anatomy in hypertelorism is widening of the ethmoid sinuses anteriorly, and sometimes inferior displacement of the cribriform plates.[7] The interorbital distance is measured, on the Waters projection, between the medial walls of the orbits, at the junction of the

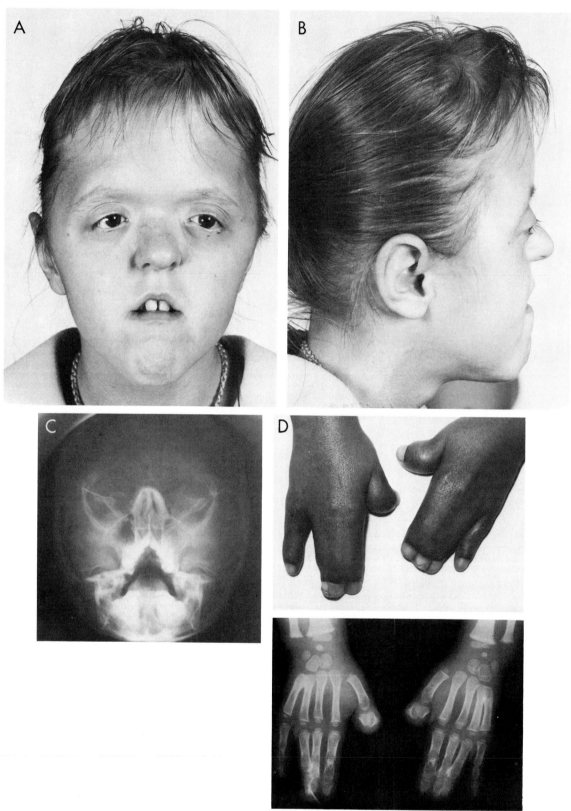

Fig. 24–3.—**A** and **B,** Apert's syndrome in 14-year-old girl. Note the "tower" skull, lateral canthal dystopia, minimal exorbitism and the transverse forehead skin furrow. **(C),** the Waters view x-ray demonstrates the hypoplastic and constricted maxilla as well as the underdeveloped zygomas. In the lateral x-ray, one would see the encroachment of the middle cranial fossa into the shallow orbits, the maxillary deficiency and the characteristic open bite. **D** illustrates the typical hand deformities: acrosynostosis (side to side fusion of distal phalanges), symphalangism, delta phalanx of the thumb, synostosis between 4th and 5th metacarpals.

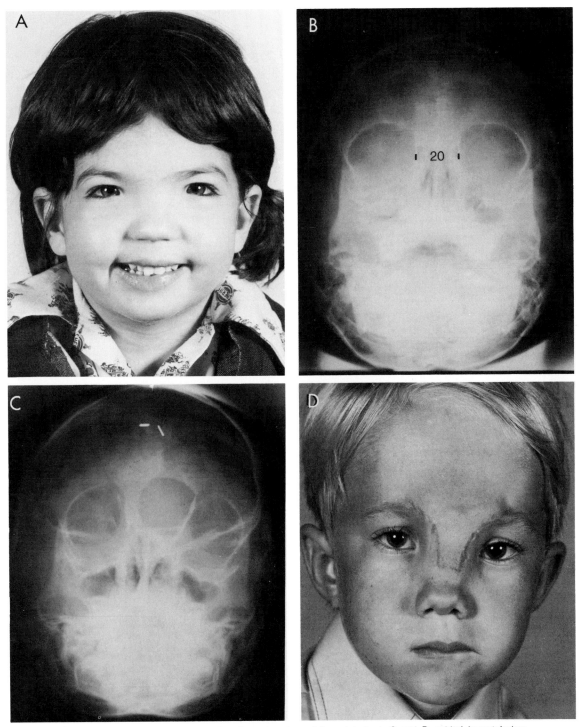

Fig. 24–4.—Hypertelorism. **A** and **B,** telecanthus (pseudohypertelorism). **C** and **D,** orbital hypertelorism secondary to frontoethmoidal encephalocele *(Continued.)*

angular process of the frontal bone with the maxillary and lacrimal bones ("dacryon").[9] The average adult interorbital distance (IOD) is 25 mm in females (achieved by age 13) and 28 mm in males (achieved by age 21).[17] Tessier classifies patients with hypertelorism based on the degree of interorbital widening: first degree, IOD equal to 30–34 mm and second degree, IOD more than 34 mm but with nearly normal orbital shape and orientation. Third degree hypertelorism indi-

cates an IOD equal to or greater than 40 mm; the orbits are lateralized and the cribriform plate usually is prolapsed. It is important to appreciate that despite the orbital divergence, the distance between the optic foramina is not increased (Fig. 24–4, *G*). This anatomic fact allows the movement of the bony orbits medially, to correct the deformity, without compressing the optic nerves.

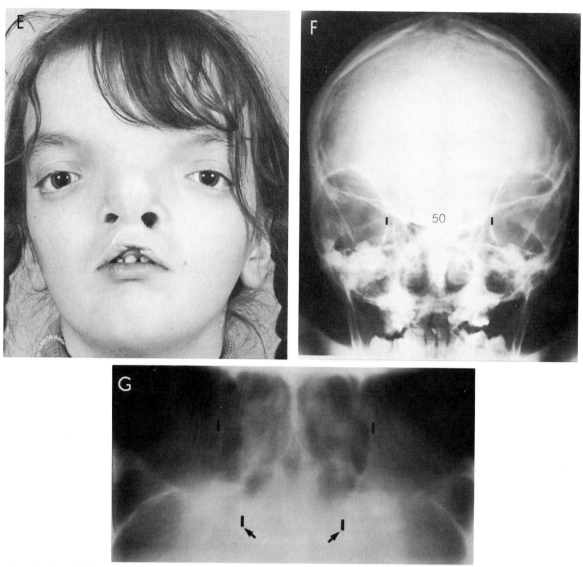

Fig. 24–4 (cont.).—E and **F,** 3d degree orbital hypertelorism. **G,** basal view orbital tomogram of the patient illustrates the widened ethmoid sinuses anteriorly, widened optic axis, yet normal distance between the optic foramina *(arrows).*

Mandibulofacial Dysostosis (the Treacher Collins Syndrome)

This is an easily recognizable facial deformity with a characteristic appearance and occurs in an approximate frequency of 1 in 10,000 live births. It is inherited as an autosomal dominant trait with variable penetrance and expressivity.[14] About 50% of the patients have no conclusive family history of the deformity. This may indicate a high rate of spontaneous mutation or a genetic susceptibility influenced by environmental factors (so-called multifactorial inheritance).

According to Poswillo,[27] the human deformity of the Treacher Collins syndrome may be the result of an insult to the preotic neural crest cells during the first 4–6 weeks of embryogenesis. He has produced a phenocopy of this deformity in rats with vitamin A and has demonstrated focal necrosis of neural crest cells and a deficiency of ectomesenchyme in the 1st and 2d branchial arches.

The clinical features of this syndrome were described by Thomson[40] in 1847, Berry[2] in 1889 and Treacher Collins[5] in 1900. Franceschetti and Klein[12] called this morphogenetic deformity "mandibulofacial dysostosis." The phenotypic expression of this syndrome is variable and produces a wide spectrum of clinical features that are characteristically bilateral and symmetric[31] (Fig. 24–5). There usually is an antimongoloid (downward) cant of the palpebral fissures, frequently a coloboma at the junction of the outer and middle third of the lower eyelids (sometimes the upper) and often absence of eyelashes along the medial one-third of the lower lids. The external ears are malformed and in a low-set position. There usually is a conductive hearing loss in association with the abnormalities of the external and middle ears. The inner ear usually develops normally, perhaps because of its origin from the auditory placode and not from the 1st and 2d branchial arches. Skin tags may be present along a line from the tragus of the ear to the commissure of the mouth, and often there is an extension of temporal hair onto the cheek. The nose is large and beak-like. The zygomatic bones and arches are hypoplastic, or may be present only in vestigial form. The mandibular rami are short, with hypo-

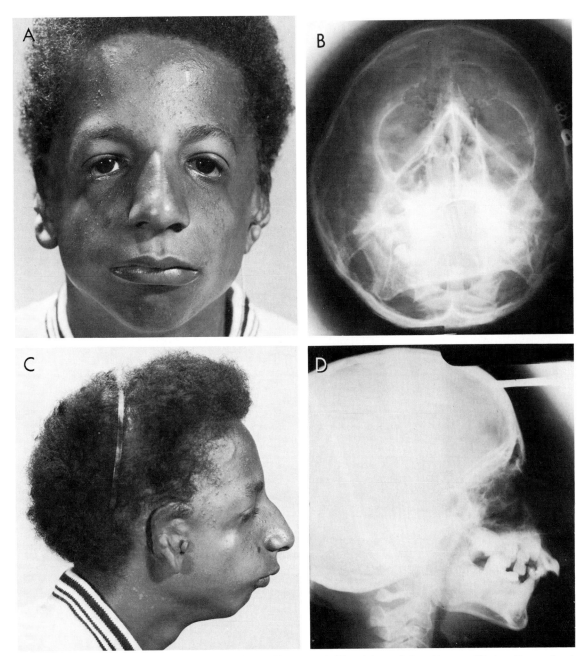

Fig. 24–5.—A 15-year-old patient with Treacher Collins syndrome. The frontal photograph **(A)** and the Waters view x-ray **(B)** reveal the abnormal shape of the orbits and the markedly deficient zygomas. The lateral photo-graph **(C)** and the cephalometric x-ray **(D)** show the nasal and external ear deformities, as well as the mandibular retrusion and concave shape of the inferior border of the mandible.

plastic muscles of mastication, a concave inferior border of the mandible and a retruded chin. The teeth are also hypo-plastic, and malocclusion with open bite may be present. The palate has a high arch, and an overt cleft occurs in 30% of patients.

1st and 2d Branchial Arch Syndrome (Hemifacial Microsomia)

The 1st and 2d branchial arch syndrome has also been called intrauterine facial necrosis, lateral facial dysplasia and hemifacial microsomia.[14] At first glance, the structural deformities are similar to those in the Treacher Collins syn-

drome but there are characteristic differences. The Treacher Collins syndrome is a nearly symmetric bilateral deformity. Hemifacial microsomia is predominantly a unilateral defor-mity, although, in a recent study,[29] 30% of 127 patients had subtle contralateral involvement of the structures of the 1st and 2d branchial arches. Hemifacial microsomia, in contrast to the Treacher Collins syndrome, usually is the result of a spontaneous mutation, with an incidence of 1 in 5642 live births.[15]

Poswillo[26] has presented an animal phenocopy of hemifa-cial microsomia in which drug-induced hemorrhage (from the primitive stapedial artery) causes focal necrosis within the developing upper branchial region. The extent of hematoma formation and embryonic repair determined the degree of distortion of 1st and 2d arch-derived structures. In these studies there was a significant incidence of bilateral, though asymmetric, defects. This animal model offers a possible explanation for the wide spectrum of clinical deformities seen in hemifacial microsomia. In this syndrome, one may find underdevelopment of any or all of the structures of the 1st (zygoma, maxilla, mandible, muscles of mastication, trigeminal nerve, upper part of external ear and parotid gland) and 2d (temporal bone, external and middle ear, facial nerve and muscles of facial expression) branchial arches. Macrostomia often is present in addition to the abnormal upward tilting of the occlusal plane on the affected side. It is thought that the maxillary deformity may be secondary to the influence of the lack of vertical mandibular growth. The mandibular deformity is most severe in the area of the ramus and condyle.

Principles of Surgical Approach

The surgical correction of craniofacial deformities requires the coordination of plastic and oral surgeons, orthodontists, anesthesiologists, neurosurgeons, ophthalmologists, otolaryngologists, radiologists, nurses and social workers.

In the past, operative correction was postponed until the completion of growth. With recent experience and understanding of facial growth, we now operate at an earlier age to facilitate, rather than interfere with, potential growth of the craniofacial skeleton.[10, 25]

Preoperative planning and analysis require clinical photographs, dental models, standard, cephalometric and polytomographic x-rays of the craniofacial skeleton, as well as psychologic, visual and audiometric evaluation. For all pro-

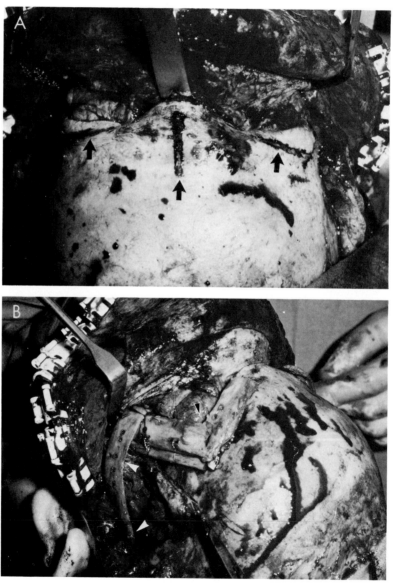

Fig. 24–6.—Intraoperative views of the standard craniofacial dissection in a patient with the Treacher Collins syndrome. **A,** from the head of the operating table. The coronal flap is draped over the face, "V" notched retractor is at the nasofrontal suture. Arrows indicate midline marking and the supra-orbital markings prior to burring. **B,** lateral view. The black arrow on the globe points to rib grafts along the lateral superior orbit. The two white arrows show the zygomatic onlay graft and its relation to the temporal fossa and temporalis muscle.

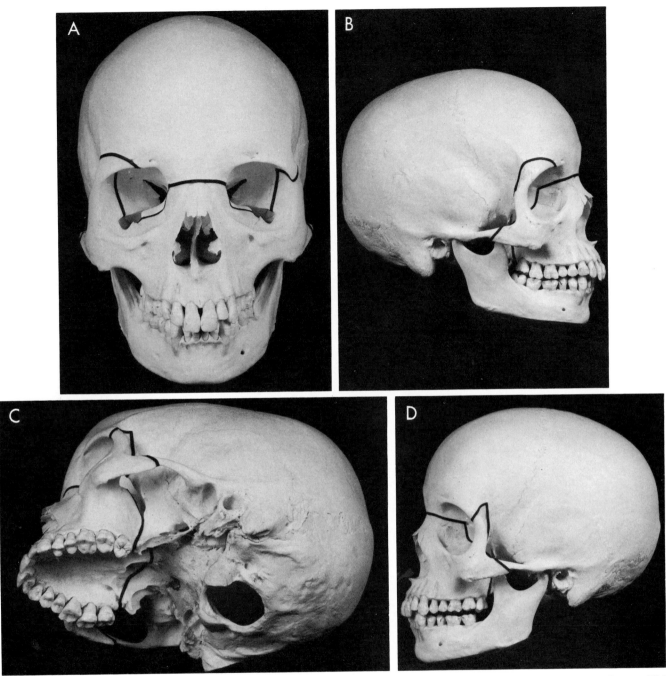

Fig. 24–7.—Le Fort III osteotomy. The four views illustrate osteotomy cuts at the frontonasal, frontoethmoidal, frontozygomatic, frontosphenoid, zygomatic temporal, pterygomaxillary and nasomaxillary suture lines.

A, frontal view. **B,** lateral view; frontozygomatic osteotomy to advance orbital rim. **C,** oblique base view. **D,** lateral view; standard frontozygomatic osteotomy.

cedures, autogenous, costal or iliac bone grafts are obtained as the first step in the operation.

Exposure and Incisions

The operative exposure is similar for midface advancement, correction of orbital hypertelorism and reconstruction of the skeletal deficiency in the Treacher Collins syndrome. A coronal skin incision is made posterior to the hairline and carried down anterior to the tragus of the ears bilaterally.

The facial flap is dissected to the supraorbital rims, a separate periosteal flap is elevated in the frontal region and the temporalis muscle is dissected away from the temporal fossa, to give exposure of the facial skeleton (Fig. 24–6). Conjunctival incisions are made to expose the infraorbital rims, the orbital floors and the anterior walls of the maxilla. For the midface advancement procedure, a third incision is made bilaterally in the maxillary sulcus, for exposure of the pterygomaxillary fissures. In some patients, complete exposure can be obtained through the coronal incision alone.

Osteotomies

Once the soft tissue dissection is complete, the osteotomies may be performed.

LE FORT III OSTEOTOMY.—This is the basic osteotomy for the correction of the midface deficiency in Crouzon's and Apert's syndromes. The osteotomy follows the lines of the Le Fort III fracture or craniofacial disjunction; i.e., frontonasal, nasomaxillary, frontozygomatic, zygomaticosphenoidal and pterygomaxillary junctions are separated. There are several variations in the osteotomies; for example, at the frontozygomatic region and the zygomatic arch region, depending on the underlying skeletal deformity and bone grafting requirements (Fig. 24–7). If the temporal lobes project too far anteriorly, bur holes will provide added exposure and minimize the chance of damage to the dura and brain during the osteotomies.

After the osteotomies are completed, the midface is mobilized and brought forward to a predetermined position in relation to the mandible. It is maintained in this position by wire or elastic fixation of the upper jaw to the lower jaw. Bone grafting of the osteotomy gaps is the next step; finally, split ribs and remaining bone chips are placed as onlay grafts to improve contour deficiencies in the frontal, zygomatic and anterior maxillary regions (Fig. 24–8).

OSTEOTOMIES FOR ORBITAL HYPERTELORISM.—Incisions and exposure are similar to those described for the midface advancement. Next, a frontal craniectomy is done by the neurosurgeon, leaving a rim of intact frontal bone over the supraorbital ridges. The resected frontal bone is

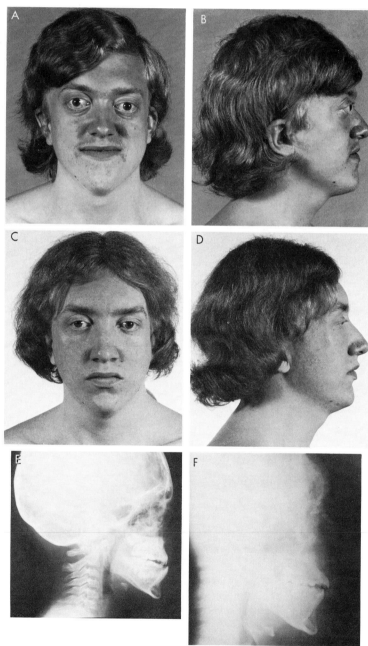

Fig. 24–8.—Crouzon's syndrome. Preoperative and postoperative photographs and cephalometric x-rays following midface advancement. The frontal and lateral views illustrate correction of the exorbitism, elevation of the left orbit and increase in the fullness of the maxilla. (**A** and **B,** preoperative; **C** and **D,** postoperative.) **E** and **F,** the cephalometric x-rays document advancement of the maxilla and correction of the prognathic jaw relationship.

saved, to be replaced later as a graft. With the brain and dura retracted, exposing the floor of the anterior cranial fossa, the fronto-naso-ethmoidal resection is carried out, to narrow the interorbital distance to 20–25 mm. The glabella, nasal bones and a major part of the ethmoid bone and sinuses are removed en bloc. A full-thickness resection of the nasal septum is carried out, and occasionally the turbinates are excised to enlarge the remaining nasal airway (Fig. 24–9).

Osteotomies of the four walls of each orbit are performed posterior to the equator of the globe. Once these osteotomies are completed, the bony orbits remain tethered by two soft tissue pedicles: (1) contents of the optic foramen, the optic canal and the superior orbital fissure and (2) the nasolacrimal ducts. The orbits then are translated medially, rotated into their proper position and vertically repositioned, when necessary. The correction is completed with interpositional

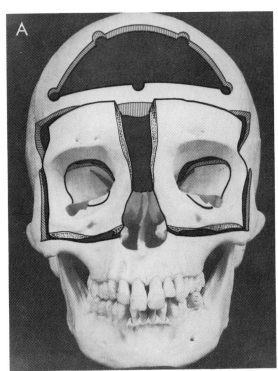
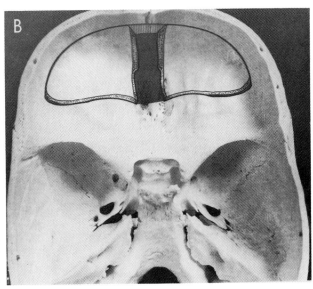
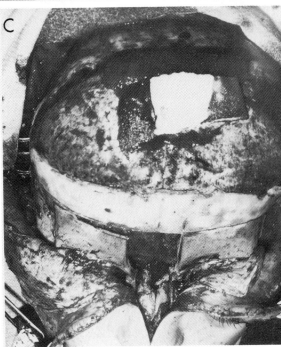
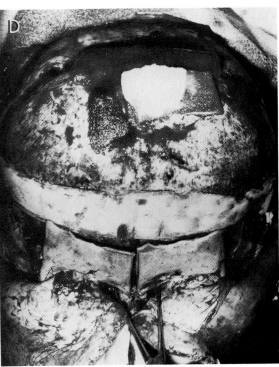

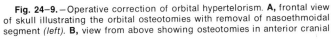

Fig. 24–9.—Operative correction of orbital hypertelorism. **A,** frontal view of skull illustrating the orbital osteotomies with removal of nasoethmoidal segment *(left).* **B,** view from above showing osteotomies in anterior cranial fossa *(right).* Intraoperative views: **C,** during correction of hypertelorism following orbital osteotomies and nasoethmoidal resection *(left)* and **D,** following translocation of the orbits *(right).*

and onlay bone grafts and intraosseous wire fixation. Redundant midline soft tissue is removed and the medial canthi are properly positioned and secured (Fig. 24–10).

Contour Deficiencies (Mandibulofacial Dysostosis)

Individualized surgical correction is required for the wide spectrum of deformities presenting as the Treacher Collins syndrome.

In the past, the eyelid defects were repaired at an early age. Rogers,[28] however, has emphasized that, in many cases, the eyelid surgery should be deferred until the hypoplastic malar regions are augmented.

Two basic approaches to augmentation of the hypoplastic facial skeleton of these patients are undergoing evolution. Some surgeons use alloplastic (silicone) implants over the hypoplastic malar and chin regions in children, augmenting them with larger implants and eventually replacing them

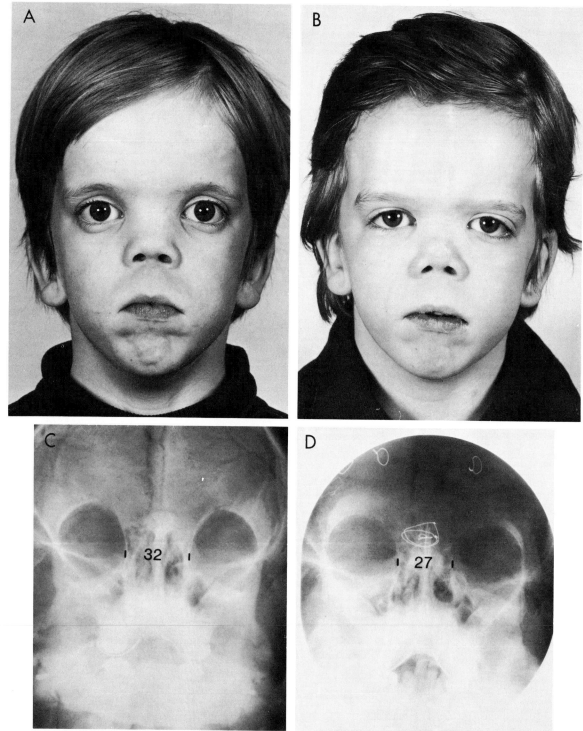

Fig. 24–10.—Hypertelorism. **A,** preoperative and **B,** postoperative photographs and Waters projections of a patient preoperatively **(C)** and following correction **(D)** of 1st-degree hypertelorism (IOD 32 mm to IOD 27 mm).

with bone, if necessary, as the patient grows.[28] Our approach has been to use autogenous bone for correction of the skeletal deficiencies. When the mandibular deformity produces an abnormal occlusion, we prefer to correct this functional problem with mandibular osteotomies in childhood (6–10 years of age), at the same time correcting the contour deficiencies with onlay bone grafts. If the occlusion is normal, we wait until early adolescence and then correct the orbito-malar deficiencies and, if necessary, perform a rhinoplasty and advance the chin point. The orbitomalar regions are approached through the standard coronal incision. Split-rib onlay bone grafts are used to augment the zygomatic arches, the roof, lateral wall and floor of the orbits and the anterior maxilla. The overhanging superior lateral angles of the orbits are burred to create a more normal squared appearance of the orbit (Fig. 24–11).

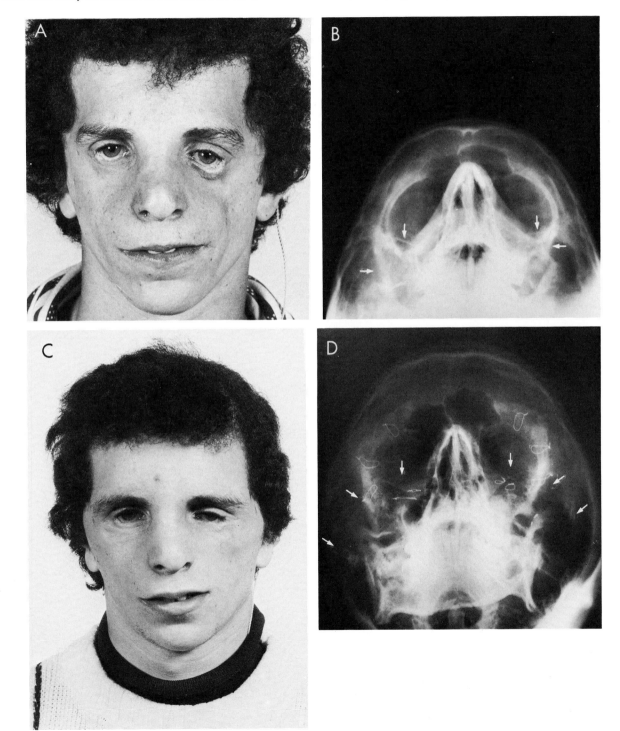

Fig. 24–11.—Treacher Collins syndrome in an 18-year-old patient. The preoperative photograph **(A)** and the Waters view x-ray **(B)** illustrate the deficiency of the malar areas, zygomatic arches and orbital floors *(arrows on the x-ray)*. The postoperative photograph **(C)** and x-ray **(D)** illustrate the change in the orbits achieved by burring the superior lateral orbital rims and by placing onlay bone grafts to the lateral orbit, orbital floor and zygomatic areas *(arrows on the x-ray)*.

Surgical Correction of 1st and 2d Branchial Arch Syndrome (Hemifacial Microsomia)

This is one of the most complex and variable deformities in craniofacial surgery. The affected mandible may be normal in shape but smaller in size (Type I), may have a tempo-romandibular joint with a deformed condyle (Type II) or absence of a temporomandibular joint and no condyle (Type III). Operation varies with the severity of the deformity and the age of the patient. The basic concept of therapy is elongation of the mandible to achieve a horizontal occlusal plane. If operation is performed early, maxillary tilting may not oc-

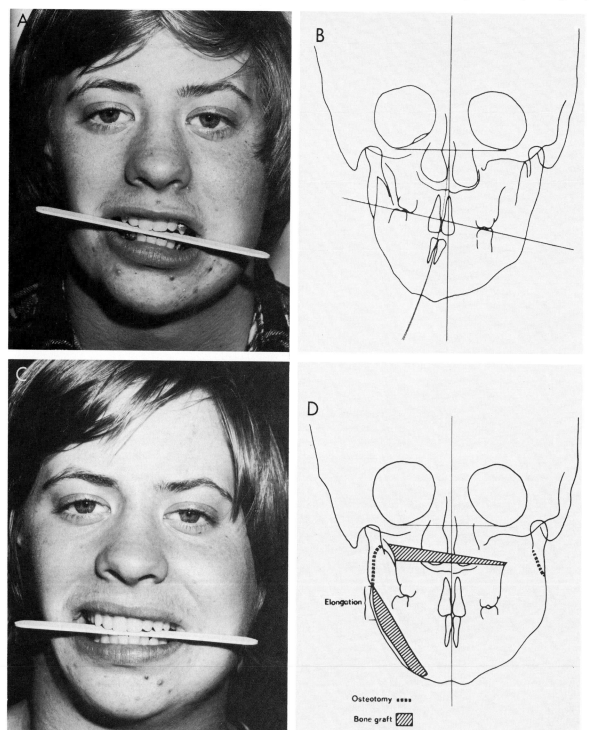

Fig. 24–12.—Hemifacial microsomia. Preoperative and postoperative views of a teen-ager. The preoperative photograph **(A)** and line drawing of the PA x-ray **(B)** demonstrate the tilted occlusal plane, midline shift to the right, hypoplasia of the right mandible and decreased vertical height of the right maxilla and mandible. The postoperative photograph **(C)** and the line drawing of the operation **(D)** illustrate correction of these deformities with a Le Fort I osteotomy to elongate the right maxilla *(shaded area represents the bone-grafted gap),* mandibular osteotomies to elongate the right mandible and onlay bone grafts to improve the contour of the right mandibular body *(shaded area).*

cur. If, however, maxillary development has been impaired and the vertical dimension shortened, correction is accomplished with a Le Fort I osteotomy of the maxilla. In the adult patient with Type II or III deformity, operation is directed toward correction of the temporomandibular joint, the hypoplastic zygomatic arch, the short mandibular ramus and the deficient mandibular contour on the affected side. Facial and dental midlines are restored and the short maxilla and markedly tilted occlusal plane are corrected. The maxilla is lowered on the affected side and bone grafts are placed and fixed in the resultant gap. The maxilla is intruded and fixed on the normal side. This procedure positions the occlusal plane parallel to the interpupillary reference line.

Next, the temporomandibular joint and the ramus of the mandible are exposed via preauricular and submandibular incisions. Onlay bone grafts are used to augment the zygomatic arch and to create a glenoid fossa for the mandibular condyle. The ramus of the mandible is lengthened with an osteotomy or a bone graft to place the new or previously existing condylar head into the glenoid fossa. The body of the mandible may be augmented with split-rib fixation for 6–8 weeks (Fig. 24–12).

In young children with significant deformity, we attempt to elongate the mandible on the affected side with an osteotomy or bone graft. The resulting open bite is maintained with an acrylic splint. Theoretically, this may "release or unlock" the growth potential of the maxilla and allow it to grow downward in a normal fashion. Such treatment may eliminate the maxillary growth deformity in hemifacial microsomia, which we believe is a secondary phenomenon.

Anesthesia and Postoperative Care

The operations described in this chapter involve manipulations of the upper airway and the loss of large volumes of blood (as much as 1–2 blood volume replacements in young children). The airway is maintained by oral or nasoendotracheal tubes wired into position. Only rarely is a tracheostomy required. Blood pressure, fluid and electrolyte balance and blood gases are monitored with intra-arterial and central venous catheters. Large-bore peripheral venous lines are required for blood replacement. A urinary catheter is placed in all patients to monitor urine output and a lumbar cerebrospinal fluid catheter is used when the brain is exposed. Monitoring cerebrospinal fluid pressure with a ventricular "pressure screw" manometer has been described.[11]

The patients remain intubated for 24–28 hours postoperatively in the intensive care unit. Once extubated and ambulatory, they are placed on a high-calorie, high-protein, full liquid diet if they are in intermaxillary fixation or a soft diet if their jaws are not immobilized. Prophylactic antibiotics (penicillin and oxacillin) are started the night prior to operation and maintained for 4 days postoperatively.

Complications

Considering the nature and magnitude of these surgical procedures, the complications to date have been minor and few in number. In our first 106 operations at the Children's Hospital Medical Center, through 1974, there were no deaths or loss of vision.[25] Converse et al.[6] reported 1 death (intraoperative hemorrhage) in 50 patients operated on and Tessier[37] reported 11 deaths in 540 craniofacial operations (2% mortality rate). The major causes of death have been intraoperative hypovolemia and early postoperative cerebral edema.

The most serious intraoperative complications have been related to the upper airway and include obstruction, dislocation or laceration of the endotracheal tube. Pneumothorax, secondary to harvesting of multiple rib grafts, has occurred. Major arterial or venous disruption during the osteotomies may cause acute, life-threatening hypovolemia. Occasionally, we have documented abnormal intraoperative fibrinolysis resulting in a slow, persistent oozing from the entire operative field. On two occasions, this has necessitated terminating the operation. It has been postulated that the manipulation of massive amounts of bone may release fibrinolysins.

Airway obstruction and pneumothorax may also occur in the immediate postoperative period. The possibility of cerebral edema during the first 48 hours postoperatively requires careful monitoring. Early infection within the planes of the soft tissue dissection and related to the bone grafts has been surprisingly infrequent, considering the duration and magnitude of the operations and intraoperative contamination from the nasal and oral cavities.

Late complications include CSF leak (requiring dural repair) and late sepsis with loss of fixation of bone grafts.

A Perspective on Craniofacial Surgery

Thus far, we have discussed only major craniofacial anomalies. Less severe deformities are more common, e.g., mandibular prognathism and maxillary protrusion with or without open bite. These can be corrected with selective osteotomies by standardized techniques, not requiring such extensive soft tissue dissection. For these conditions, the role of orthodontia is critical and must be coordinated with proposals for operation.

Surgical techniques now available allow correction of almost every conceivable deformity of the cranial and facial areas. Practically every anatomic area can be exposed. There is a limitation on time for the soft tissue dissection and blood loss can be extensive, but once osseous exposure is achieved, appropriate osteotomies almost always can be devised.

Limitations in availability of autogenous bone for grafting are more severe in the infant; soft tissues may restrict the distance that osteotomized bones can be translocated, and the canthi may not always remain properly fixed to their sutured sites. Frequently, secondary or tertiary revisions are required to achieve optimal correction. Nevertheless, the major effort to correct the fundamental osseous framework can be surprisingly effective and set the stage for a good result.

Analysis and repair of these major craniofacial defects brings into focus the need for better understanding of facial growth, and slow, steady advances in the study of morphogenesis are accumulating.

The practical question of the proper time for surgical intervention requires controlled experimental work, particularly in primates, in order that clinicians can offer their patients the greatest chance for benefit, with the least chance of morbidity. Recent descriptions of extending the craniectomy for coronal craniosynostosis into the orbit and floor of the frontal fossa are examples of clinical technical advances utilizing these new surgical exposures.

The results of craniofacial surgery, to date, can be documented only with static black and white photographs and radiographic studies. These often do not demonstrate the psychodynamic changes that occur in our patients. The primary motive of the surgeon is to produce a well-rounded human to fulfill his or her full potential in society. Studies in our institution have begun to assess the role of the "body image" concept and its relation to the timing, emotional impact and psychologic adjustment in patients undergoing major alterations in facial anatomy. The psychosocial development of the patients transcends all other considerations.

REFERENCES

1. Apert, E.: De l'acrocéphalosyndactylie, Bull. Soc. Méd. (Paris) 23:1310, 1906.
2. Berry, G. A.: Note on a congenital defect (coloboma) of the lower lid, R. Lond. Ophthalmol. Hosp. Rep. 12:255, 1889.
3. Bertelsen, T. L.: The premature synostosis of the cranial sutures, Acta Ophthalmol. (supp.) 51:47, 1958.
4. Christianson, R. L., and Evans, C. A.: Habilitation of severe craniofacial anomalies, Cleft Palate J. 12:167, 1975.
5. Collins, T. E.: Case with symmetrical congenital notches in the outer part of each lower lid and defective development of the malar bones, Trans. Ophthalmol. Soc. U. K. 20:190, 1900.
6. Converse, J. M., Wood-Smith, D., and McCarthy, J. G.: Report of a series of 50 craniofacial operations, Plast. Reconstr. Surg. 55:283, 1975.
7. Converse, J. M., Wood-Smith, D., McCarthy, J. G., and Coccaro, P. J.: Craniofacial surgery, Clin. Plast. Surg. 1(3):499, 1974.
8. Crouzon, O.: Dysostose cranio-faciale héréditaire, Bull. Soc. Méd. Hôp. (Paris) 33:545, 1912.
9. Currarino, G., and Silverman, F. N.: Orbital hypotelorism, arhinencephaly, and trigonocephaly, Radiology 74:206, 1960.
10. Edgerton, M. T., Jane, J. A., and Berry, F. A.: Craniofacial osteotomies and reconstruction in infants and young children, Plast. Reconstr. Surg. 54:13, 1975.
11. Edgerton, M. T., Jane, J. A., Berry, F. A., and Marshall, K. A.: New surgical concepts resulting from cranio-orbito-facial surgery, Ann. Surg. 182:228, 1975.
12. Franceschetti, A., and Klein, D.: Mandibulofacial dysostosis: A new hereditary syndrome, Acta Ophthalmol. (Kbh) 27:143, 1949.
13. Gillies, H., and Harrison, S. H.: Operative correction by osteotomy by recessed malar maxillary compound in a case of oxycephaly, Br. J. Plast. Surg. 3:123, 1950.
14. Gorlin, R. J., Pindborg, J., and Cohen, M. M.: *Syndromes of the Head and Neck* (2d ed.; New York: McGraw-Hill Book Company, 1976), pp. 220–224.
15. Grabb, W. C.: The first and second branchial arch syndrome, Plast. Reconstr. Surg. 36:485, 1965.
16. Greig, D. M.: Hypertelorism: A hitherto undifferentiated congenital craniofacial deformity, Edinburgh Med. J. 31:560, 1924.
17. Hansman, C. F.: Growth of interorbital distance and skull thickness as observed in roentgenographic measurements, Radiology 86:87, 1966.
18. Hoover, G. H., Flatt, A. E., and Weiss, M. W.: The hand and Apert's syndrome, J. Bone Joint Surg. 52-A:878, 1970.
19. Johnston, M. C.: The neural crest in abnormalities of the face and brain, Birth Defects 11(7):1, 1975.
20. Moss, M. L.: The pathogenesis of premature cranial synostosis in man, Acta Anat. 37:351, 1959.
21. Moss, M. L.: Twenty years of functional cranial analysis, Am. J. Orthod. 61:479, 1972.
22. Moss, M. L.: New studies of cranial growth, Birth Defects 11(7): 283, 1975.
23. Munro, I. R.: Orbito-cranio-facial surgery: The team approach, Plast. Reconstr. Surg. 55:170, 1975.
24. Murray, J. E., and Swanson, L. T.: Mid-face osteotomy and advancement for craniosynostosis, Plast. Reconstr. Surg. 41:299, 1968.
25. Murray, J. E., Swanson, L. T., Strand, R. D., and Hricko, G. M.: Evaluation of craniofacial surgery in the treatment of facial deformities, Ann. Surg. 182:240, 1975.
26. Poswillo, D. E.: The pathogenesis of 1st and 2nd branchial arch syndrome, Oral Surg. 35:302, 1973.
27. Poswillo, D. E.: The pathogenesis of the Treacher Collins syndrome (mandibulofacial dysostosis), Br. J. Oral Surg. 13:1, 1975.
28. Rogers, B.: The surgical treatment of mandibulofacial dysostosis (Berry syndrome; Treacher Collins syndrome; Franceschetti-Zwahlen-Klein syndrome) 3(4):653, 1976.
29. Ross, R. B.: Lateral facial dysplasia, Birth Defects 11(7):51, 1975.
30. Shillito, J., and Matson, D. D.: Craniosynostosis: A review of 519 surgical patients, Pediatrics 41:829, 1968.
31. Stovin, J. J., Lyon, J. A., and Clemmens, R. L.: Mandibulofacial dysostosis, Radiology 74:225, 1960.
32. Tessier, P.: Ostéotomies totales de la face; syndrome de Crouzon; syndrome d'Apert; oxycephalies, scaphocephalies, turricephalies, Ann. Chir. Plast. 12:273, 1967.
33. Tessier, P.: Relationship of craniostenoses to craniofacial dysostoses and to faciostenoses, Plast. Reconstr. Surg. 48:224, 1971.
34. Tessier, P.: The definitive plastic surgical treatment of the severe facial deformities of craniofacial dysostosis, Plast. Reconstr. Surg. 48:419, 1971.
35. Tessier, P.: Orbital hypertelorism. I. Successive surgical attempts, material and methods, causes and mechanisms, Scand. J. Plast. Reconstr. Surg. 6:135, 1972.
36. Tessier, P.: Experiences in the treatment of orbital hypertelorism, Plast. Reconstr. Surg. 53:1, 1974.
37. Tessier, P.: Interview in Contemp. Surg. 8:9, 1976.
38. Tessier, P., Guiot, B., and Derome, P.: Orbital hypertelorism. II. Definitive treatment of orbital hypertelorism by craniofacial or by extracranial osteotomies, Scand. J. Plast. Reconstr. Surg. 7: 39, 1973.
39. Tessier, P., Guiot, G., Rougerie, J., Delbet, J. P., and Pastoriza, J.: Ostéotomies cranio-naso-orbito-faciales hypertélorisme, Ann. Chir. Plast. 12:113, 1967.
40. Thomson, A.: Notice of several cases of malformation of the external ear, together with experiments on the state of hearing in such persons, Month. J. Med. Sci. 7:420, 1847.
41. Virchow, R.: Über den cretinismus, namenthlich in fränhen, und über pathologische schadelformen, Verh. Phys. Med. Ges. Wurzburg 2:241, 1851.
42. Webster, J. P., and Deming, E. G.: Surgical treatment of the bifid nose, Plast. Reconstr. Surg. 6:1, 1950.
43. Wood-Smith, D., Epstein, F., and Morello, D.: Transcranial decompression of the optic nerve in the osseous canal in Crouzon's disease, Clinc. Plast. Surg. 3(4):621, 1976.
44. Zimmerman, A. A., *et al.*: The change in position of the eyeballs during fetal life, Anat. Rec. 59:109, 1934.

25

Ian R. Munro

The Nose

THE MOST PROMINENT AND DISTINCTIVE FEATURE of the human face is the nose. It is subject to trauma, infection, tumors and congenital deformation. Understanding the embryology and anatomy is necessary for diagnosis and treatment.

Embryology

Development of the nose commences during the second intrauterine month and is completed by the end of the third month. The area between the primitive stomadeum and base of the forebrain is called the frontonasal process. On each ventrolateral aspect of this there is an ectodermal thickening called the olfactory (nasal) placode. Elevation of the surrounding ectoderm and thickening of the adjacent mesenchyme converts the placode into an olfactory pit. The lateral margins form the lateral nasal processes. The wide central area becomes the medial nasal process, which is the distal portion of the frontonasal process. The maxillary process grows anteriorly from the dorsal end of the mandibular arch. As this process moves anteriorly, it reaches the lateral nasal process. The ectoderm at the line of fusion becomes buried as a solid cellular rod. Later, this becomes canaliculized to form the nasolacrimal duct. It has a cephalic connection with the conjunctival sac. Caudally, the tube grows downward to open beneath the inferior concha. As the maxillary processes migrate medially, they fuse with the inferior border of the lateral, then the medial nasal process and the frontonasal process until they join in the midline. This converts the olfactory pits into the primitive nasal cavity, with the primitive posterior nares opening into the anterior portion of the stomadeal roof. A transverse furrow develops between the nasal region of the frontonasal process and the frontal region, further defining the nose. The medial nasal process produces two swellings, the globular processes, which initially project anterior to the lateral nasal process and then dorsally and medially to the olfactory pits into the forepart of the stomadeal roof to form the primitive palate. This is continuous above with the short, broad partition of the primitive nasal septum. The tectoseptal extension from each maxillary process extends upward and medially and eventually fuses in the midline at the posterior part of the frontonasal process and the posterior aspect of the primitive nasal septum to form the definitive nasal septum and reaches back as far as Rathke's pouch. A further mesoderm mass from the maxillary process grows medially and inferiorly to form the palatal processes, which eventually fuse with the inferior border of the nasal septum, separating the nose from the mouth.

Elevations appear on the lateral nasal wall to form the superior, middle and inferior conchae.

The ectoderm from the olfactory placode eventually forms the olfactory epithelium in the roof of the nose.

The paranasal sinuses start in late fetal and early postnatal life as diverticula from the lateral nasal walls and invade adjacent bone to form the maxillary, ethmoid, sphenoid and frontal sinuses.

Anatomy

The upper half of the nose is bone. The two nasal bones join the frontal bone superiorly and each other in the midline, where they lie on and are supported by the nasal spine of the frontal bone. Laterally, the nasal bones abut the frontal process of the maxilla, which also forms the lateral part of the upper nose. The nasal septum is formed superiorly by the perpendicular plate of the ethmoid and inferiorly by the vomer, which rests on the nasal crest formed by maxilla and palatine bones. The lower half of the nose is cartilaginous. The quadrilateral septal cartilage supports the framework and joins above with the perpendicular plate of the ethmoid and inferiorly with the vomer. Anteriorly, it rests on the anterior nasal spine of the maxilla. The upper lateral cartilages are triangular and join the septal cartilage in the midline and the nasal bones and frontal process of the maxilla superiorly. The distal half of the nose is formed by the alar cartilages (lower nasal cartilages). The cartilages are U-shaped, with the lateral crura forming the shape of the nostrils and distal end of the nose. Medially, the lateral crura swing downward into the columella to form the medial crura, which lie distal to the septal cartilage and are separated from it by the membranous septum. The lateral crura swing superiorly, as well as laterally, leaving the lateral inferior part of the ala nasi unsupported but filled with fibro-fatty tissue.

Trauma

Because the nose is the most protuberant area of the face, it frequently is injured. If abrasions occur, all foreign material must be removed by scrubbing to prevent tattooing. If dirt is not removed and epithelium heals over it, secondary removal is difficult and produces scarring. Lacerations are treated as elsewhere, with certain modifications. There is little spare skin on the nose, so debridement should be kept to a minimum. Lacerations involving the free alar margins must be realigned precisely to prevent notching, which is difficult to correct secondarily. If the laceration extends to the nasal cavity, the mucous lining of the nose must first be repaired. If the cartilage is divided, it must be repositioned accurately, but sutured only if the free margins do not lie easily in apposition after the mucosa is repaired. The skin must be repaired with 6-0 Nylon sutures, which should be removed in 5 days to prevent stitch marks. Deeper lacerations of the middle or upper nose may involve the nasolacrimal duct, which must be identified and then splinted by a large suture or fine polyethylene tube passed from the lacrimal sac down the duct into the nose and then removed at 2 weeks. Because the blood supply of the nose is extensive, small flaps of skin often may survive if replaced. A trap-door (U-shaped) laceration may heal, with subsequent contracture, causing a heaped-up appearance. Secondary procedures may include revision, Z-plasties, excision and replacement or other plastic maneuvers. Lost skin is best replaced by a free postauricular full-thickness graft for best color match. Lost cartilage, if extensive, must be replaced by nasal, septal or ear cartilage. Loss of part of the alar rim can be replaced by a free composite graft from the ear for defects up to 1 cm. Larger full-thickness losses through the nose may require extensive plastic procedures using adjacent or distal flaps (Fig. 25–1).

Fractures of the nose are common. The nasal septum must be examined for a septal hematoma, which can be either submucosal or subperichondral (Fig. 25–2). This always must be drained through an L-shaped incision at the base of the hematoma. An untreated septal hematoma may result in noninfective lysis of the septal cartilage, with subsequent collapse and distortion of the nose (Fig. 25–3). Sometimes fractures of the bony nasal framework are difficult to diagnose. A history of trauma, combined with nasal bleeding,

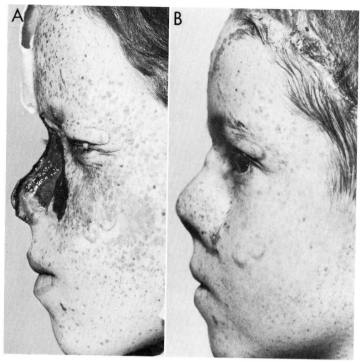

Fig. 25–1. – Loss of a large portion of the nose due to dog bite. **A,** appearance at time of injury. **B,** immediate result after repair by a forehead flap.

ecchymosis and localized tenderness, is the most accurate method of assessment. Radiographs are unreliable in detecting unilateral nasal fractures unless bony displacement is severe. The profile radiograph is reliable only for showing depressed fractures of the dorsum. Inspection and palpation are the best methods of assessing the need for treatment. Soon after the trauma, lateral deviation is visible, or depressed nasal bones can be palpated. If the diagnosis is not certain, reinspection at 3–4 days, when the swelling goes down, may be necessary. Displaced nasal bones can be replaced by closed manipulation for 7–10 days after trauma. The nasal septum must also be repositioned. Light nasal packing for 3 days and an external splint will hold the bones in place. More extensive fractures, or comminution, must be exposed and directly repositioned, if necessary by fine 30-gauge stainless steel direct wiring, using very fine drill

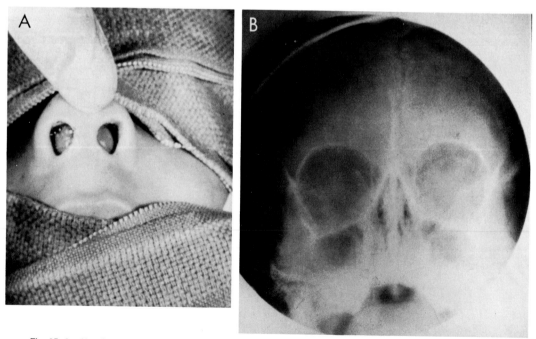

Fig. 25–2. – Nasal septal hematoma. **A,** septum bulges to both sides. **B,** radiograph showing septal hematoma.

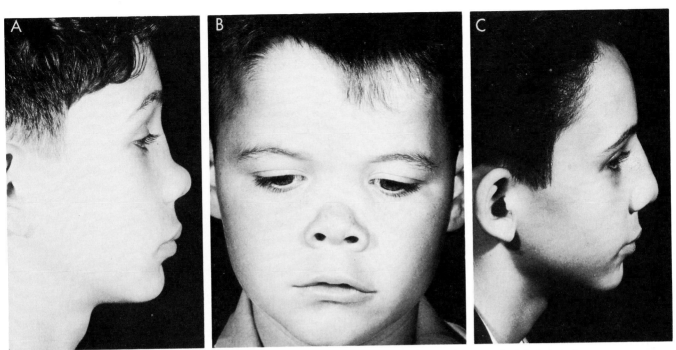

Fig. 25–3.—Septal hematoma, untreated and infected. **A** and **B,** severe nasal collapse from earlier infected nasal septal hematoma. **C,** after reconstruction with an iliac bone graft.

points. Late deformities of the nose occur only when the fractures have not been correctly repositioned and held in place long enough for good healing. Severe injuries to the roof of the nose may fracture the naso-orbital complex. This can cause lateral dislocation of the medial canthal ligaments or posterior displacement of the complex back into the anterior cranial fossa, producing cerebrospinal fluid rhinorrhea. These patients should be referred to large centers with combined teams of neurosurgeons and plastic surgeons. Elevation of the naso-orbital fractures may stop the rhinorrhea. Displaced canthal tendons must be resutured by transnasal wiring. The overlying nasal bones must be wired together directly. This is more reliable than the use of external traction devices or the application of lead plates and trans-

nasal wires. Infections of the nose are dealt with in standard texts on rhinology. Suppurative infections occasionally may cause loss of the columella Fig. 25–4). Plastic reconstruction is carried out secondarily after adequate healing and scar maturation.

Tumors

Swellings of the nose are not uncommon and have great significance for potential difficulty if diagnosed incorrectly preoperatively. They can be classified as follows:

Ectoderm— Epidermoid cysts
— Dermoid cysts or sinuses
— Pigmented nevi — Junctional
            — Compound
            — Intradermal
            — (Giant)
— Calcifying epithelioma of Malherbe
Neurogenic— Meningocele
— Encephalocele
— Glioma
— Neurofibroma
— Chordoma
— Melanoma — Juvenile
            — Malignant
Mesoderm— Lymphangioma
— Lymphedema
— Hemangioma — Capillary — Strawberry nevus / Nevus flammeus / Spider / Telangiectasia
            — Cavernous
— Angioma
— Fibroma
— Lipoma
— Chondroma } Benign or malignant
— Osteoma
— Myoma

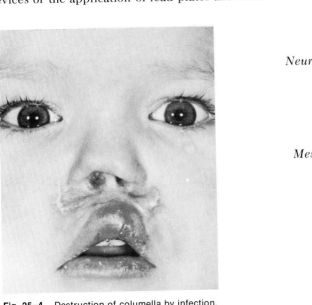

Fig. 25–4.—Destruction of columella by infection.

Mixed—Teratoma
  —Hamartoma
Other Developmental Cysts
—Subalar facial cleft cyst
—Nasoethmoidal facial cleft cyst
—Nasopalatine cyst { Nasal floor
                   { Incisive foramen
—Median anterior maxillary cyst
—Cyst of Jacobson gland

Epidermoid cysts are not common in children. They are lined by squamous epithelium and contain cheesy white keratin. Dermoid cysts are more common and more significant. Usually midline, they lie between the nasal bones or along the nasal septum, widening it. They may have a stalk, running cephalically up the nasal septum, which can reach the base of the anterior fossa. Some dermoid cysts are dumbbell shaped, the stalk passing into the skull, and a second swelling is present inside the skull. The cysts are lined by squamous epithelium with dermal appendages—glands and hair follicles. A sinus tract may open onto the nasal skin anywhere from the tip to the root of the nose and occasionally may be displaced to a more lateral position (Fig. 25–5). Treatment consists of opening the nasal bones as a book flap through a midline incision, then tracing the stalk upward (Fig. 25–6). If it passes into the skull, neurosurgical removal through a craniotomy is mandatory.

Brown pigmented nevi in children usually are junctional but may be compound or intradermal. Treatment is for cosmetic purposes and is best by an elliptical excision. Giant pigmented nevi usually are considered to be those involving 10% of the body surface area; however, even if the area is smaller than this but involves a major area of the face, it is called giant. There is a 10–20% malignancy rate in these after adolescence. Excision of giant nevi is complex and involves a combination of free full-thickness skin grafts and rotation flaps or the use of distant flaps.

The slow development of a painless, flat, hard mass that is adherent to overlying skin but freely mobile beneath usually is due to a calcifying epithelioma of Malherbe. The overly-

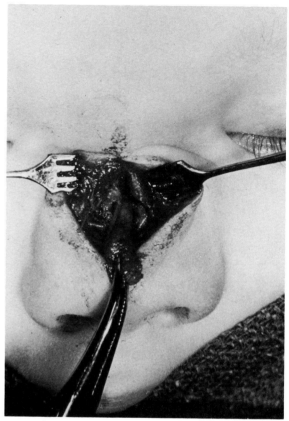

Fig. 25–6.—Dermoid cyst and tract passing into nasal septum—exposed by opening the nasal bones.

ing skin may be thinned and bluish. Progressive growth may cause ulceration of the skin, although occasionally these lesions have undergone slow spontaneous resolution. Simple excision is the best treatment.

NEUROGENIC TUMORS.—During early development there is projection of brain and meninges into the prenasal space between frontal and nasal bones anteriorly and cartilaginous capsule behind. This teat-like projection becomes surrounded by bone—the foramen caecum. If the dural process does not become walled off, a meningocele results. If brain remains in the dura, the lesion is an encephalocele Fig. 25–7). The brain and dural contents may become walled off from the foramen caecum, in which case a nasal glioma remains (Fig. 25–8). These lesions, rare in the Western world, are relatively common in southeast Asia. Suwanwela has classified sincipital encephaloceles into:

A. Frontoethmoidal—(1) Nasofrontal
                    (2) Nasoethmoidal
                    (3) Naso-orbital
B. Interfrontal
C. Craniofacial cleft (Tessier Type 0, 1 or 2)

The tumors are present at birth and often produce orbital hypertelorism, telecanthus and nasal deformity. They are midline or asymmetric, as described in the classification. Meningoceles and encephaloceles are soft, compressible and pulsatile, enlarging on crying. Nasal gliomas are firm and should be differentiated from dermoid cysts and hemangiomas. Openings in the skull can be detected radiographi-

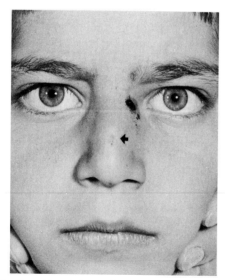

Fig. 25–5.—Dermoid cyst of nose. Arrow shows dimple in midline. Later, a discharging sinus presented, near the right medial canthus, which communicated with the dermoid cyst.

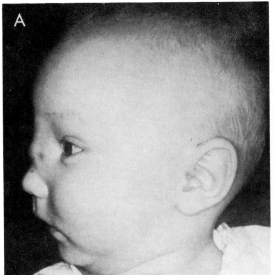

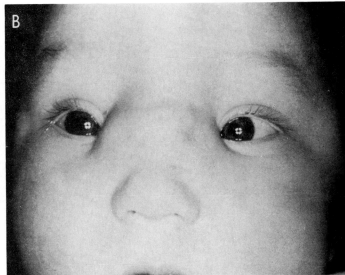

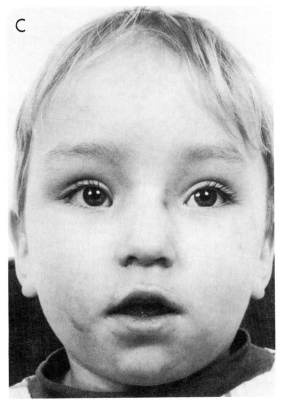

Fig. 25-7.—Nasal encephalocele. **A,** lateral view. **B,** frontal view showing pseudo-orbital hypertelorism. **C,** 2 years after removal of encephalocele and repositioning nasal bones.

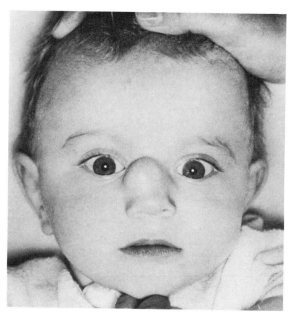

Fig. 25–8.—Nasal glioma.

cally. Air encephalography or computerized transaxial tomography usually will confirm the diagnosis. When a bony cleft is present, with or without an encephalocele, there often is dehiscence of the overlying muscle and replacement by fat. Treatment of a nasal glioma is similar to that of der-

moid cysts—complete excision after splitting the nasal bones. Meningoceles and encephaloceles require complex combined neurosurgical and plastic techniques by a craniofacial team because it often is best to correct the orbital hypertelorism and severe nasal deformity at the same time.

Neurofibromas are not common and usually are associated with neurofibromatosis (see Chap. 135).

Chordomas of the nose are exceptionally rare. They are slow-growing malignant lesions from embryonic remains of the chorda dorsalis. Operation often is ineffective and palliative radiation may be all that is possible.

Melanomas of the nose must be treated as elsewhere in the body. Malignant melanomas are exceptionally rare in children. More common is the rapidly growing juvenile melanoma, which is a benign lesion but difficult to differentiate histologically. It usually presents in early adolescence.

The strawberry nevus always is either absent or extremely small at birth. It starts to enlarge in the first 2 months of life and continues to grow for up to 8 months. These lesions should never be treated surgically or by any other means. They always undergo spontaneous resolution, usually disappearing by age 5 or 6 without leaving any mark on the skin. The excessively large lesions may leave some redundant skin after resolution. This can be excised easily and leaves a smaller scar than would have been achieved by resecting the primary lesions (Fig. 25–9). Rarely, the lesion reacts in a locally malignant fashion as a "field-fire" hemangioma. This grows extremely rapidly. It is subject to hemorrhage and infection, causing local destruction of tissue (Fig. 25–10). High doses of prednisone may stop the relentless growth in some cases.

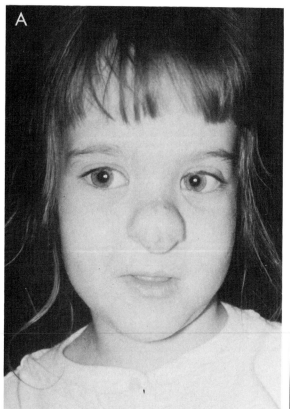
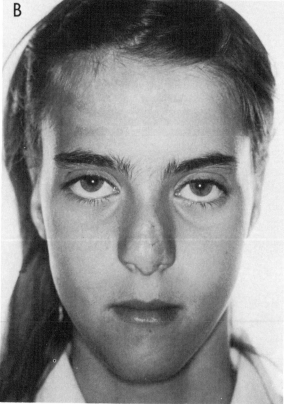

Fig. 25–9.—**A,** strawberry nevus of nose. **B,** same patient 12 years later.
No primary treatment. Patient had very small area of redundant skin excised.

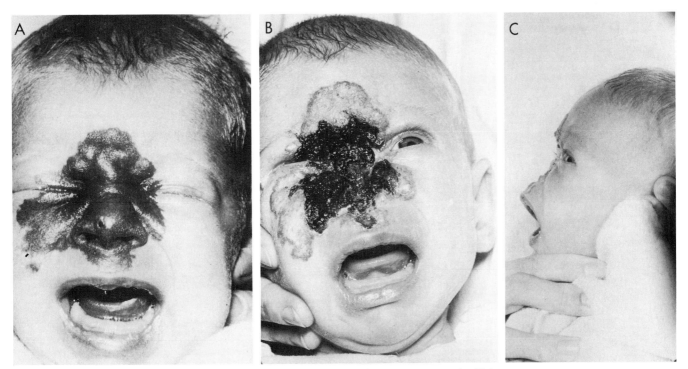

Fig. 25–10.—"Field-fire" hemangioma. **A,** appearance soon after birth. **B** and **C,** same patient 2 months later with destruction of nose.

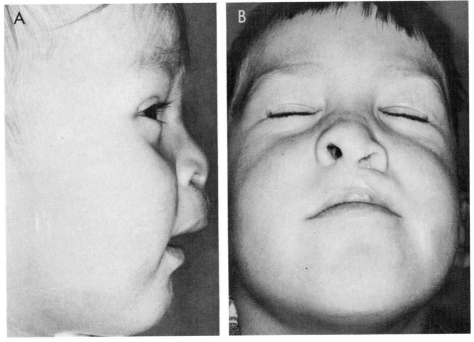

Fig. 25–11.—Nasal deformity associated with cleft lip. **A,** previously repaired bilateral cleft lip showing short columella and splayed nostrils. **B,** previously repaired unilateral cleft lip with typical displacement and flattening of one nostril, deviation of the septum and a short columella on that side.

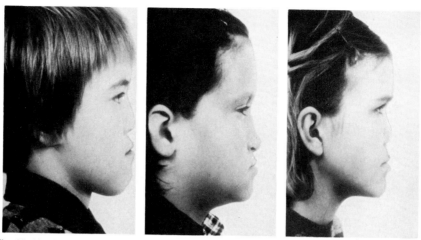

Fig. 25–12.—Maxillonasal hypoplasia (Binder). Three unrelated patients showing typical deformity.

The nevus flammeus (port-wine stain) is the other common hemangioma. This is present at birth, flat and nonexpanding. Surgical tattooing with light-colored pigment superficial to the nevus produces the best cover of this lesion.

Spider nevi and telangiectasia are uncommon in children and may undergo spontaneous resolution. A needlepoint electrocautery to the main vessels can eliminate the smaller lesions.

Cavernous hemangiomas of the nose are uncommon. They are present at birth and do not enlarge. There may be an arteriovenous fistula component. Treatment is delayed until the age of 5 to ensure that there are no signs of spontaneous resolution, such as softening of the mass with the development of gray areas, as occurs in the strawberry nevus. Excision of a cavernous hemangioma is difficult and involves resurfacing the area with free grafts or a forehead pedicle.

Lymphedema is much less common than lymphangioma. The latter presents as a diffuse swelling, usually without skin color change. Present at birth, it may not be obvious for some months. Lymphangioma and lymphedema are both prone to bouts of cellulitis of hematologic origin. Excision of the swelling is difficult because it is diffuse, invading all tissue layers. Residual tissue from incomplete excision has a tendency to enlarge so that often there is little improvement.

All the other benign or malignant mesodermal tumors are rare in children, except the juvenile angiofibroma. This usually presents with epistaxis or nasal obstruction. The tumor must be differentiated from an angiofibrosarcoma, which is extremely malignant and metastasizes early. This tumor is radiosensitive.

Teratomas and hamartomas are also rare. The former can be benign or malignant. Giant teratomas present at birth—epignathus—are massive lesions arising from the base of the skull and passing through the nose into the mouth, causing a cleft palate and immediate postnatal respiratory obstruction. In rare instances, it has been possible to resect these lesions immediately after birth.

Congenital Anomalies

These provide the most interesting plastic surgical nasal problems. The most commonly seen is that associated with a cleft lip (Fig. 25–11). The unilateral cleft lip produces flattening and widening of one alar cartilage and deviation of the nasal septum. The bilateral cleft lip nose has a very short columella, a wide tip and both alar cartilages are splayed laterally (see Chap. 26).

Maxillonasal hypoplasia produces a very characteristic deformity (Fig. 25–12). There is hypoplasia of the entire nose, more severe distally. The nose is unsupported due to absence of the anterior nasal spine. The lower maxilla is hypoplastic, causing a Class III malocclusion. Treatment involves advancing the lower maxilla forward to provide normal occlusion (a Le Fort I osteotomy) and simultaneously advancing the entire nose (an upper Le Fort II os-

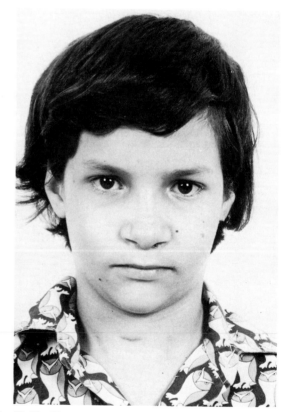

Fig. 25–13.—Maxillonasal hypoplasia three months after correction by combined Le Fort I and Le Fort II maxillary osteotomies, with advancement and iliac bone graft.

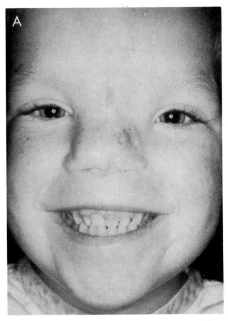
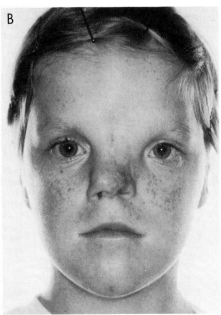
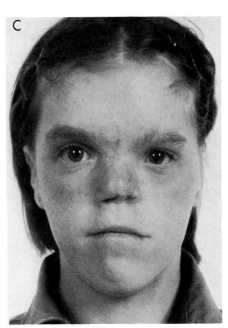

Fig. 25–14.—Incomplete facial cleft involving nose. **A,** patient before operation. **B,** same patient after several years of attempts to correct nasal deformity by soft tissue maneuvers. **C,** same patient after repositioning entire left orbit medially, allowing easy correction of deformity.

teotomy) with an additional bone graft to the dorsum and columella (Fig. 25–13).

Displacements, asymmetries and deficiencies of the nose always have been difficult to correct. Tessier has described a system of facial clefting that explains the pathology of these nasal anomalies and thus helps in providing the correct treatment. He has shown that these patients all have an underlying bone deficiency, incomplete or complete clefting or displacement of the skeleton. This can occur beneath intact skin cover (Fig. 25–14). To provide adequate correction of the external problem, it is necessary first to correct the skeletal problem, either by onlay bone grafts or repositioning the skeleton. Many of the midline or parasagittal bony

clefts causing a wide nose are associated with orbital hypertelorism. It is necessary to reposition both orbits before a good correction of the nose can be achieved.

Coloboma, or notching of one alar rim, is the simplest form of cleft. In most cases there is a displacement of the alar cartilage, often without true deficiency of tissue. This can be corrected by rotation of the displaced rim and advancement of the upper skin (Fig. 25–15). This produces a better nose than the use of small composite grafts of skin fat and cartilage taken from the ear. Larger colobomas may need the use of a forehead flap to bring in enough extra tissue.

Hemi-absence of the nose always is associated with skeletal displacement. Craniofacial correction of the orbital hy-

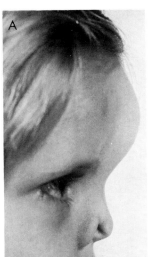
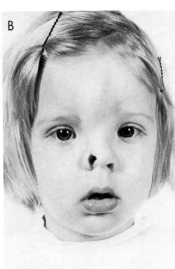
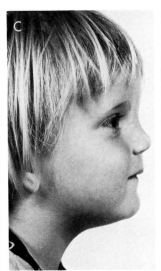
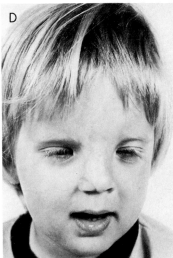

Fig. 25–15.—Unilateral nasal coloboma. **A** and **B,** protuberance of forehead due to lipoma overlying bony depression of forehead (an incomplete facial cleft). **C** and **D,** same patient 6 months after correcting coloboma by rotating alar rim and advancing nasal skin. Lipoma excised and frontalis muscle repositioned through coronal scalp incision.

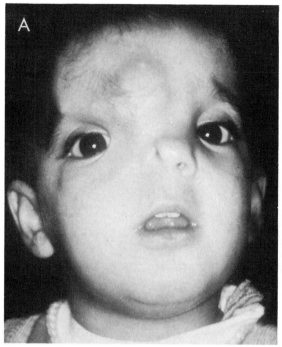

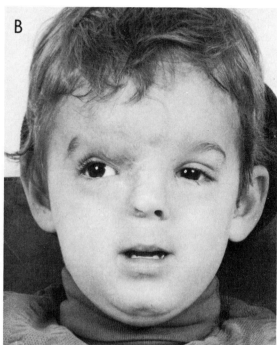

Fig. 25–16.—Hemi-absence of nose, orbital hypertelorism, frontal encephalocele. **A,** before operation. **B,** 2 years after one-stage reconstruction of nose, excision of encephalocele and orbital repositioning.

pertelorism provides enough surplus skin to rebuild the nose from local flaps (Fig. 25–16).

Midline nasal clefts vary from mild (Fig. 25–17) to severe. They often are associated with a median cleft lip. The most significant diagnostic feature of this cleft is the probable association of a degree of holoprosencephaly. This may be associated with severe mental retardation. The majority of patients with nasal clefts, from bifid nose to complete separation, have orbital hypertelorism. Adequate correction of the nose cannot be achieved until this is corrected, even though the nasal elements can be forced together (Fig. 25–18).

Total absence of the nose is extremely rare. Neonates usually have been considered to have obligate nasal breathing. However, infants with complete choanal atresia or absent

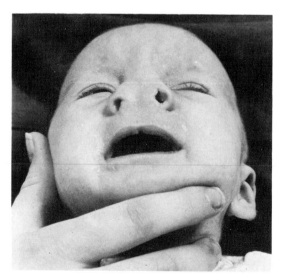

Fig. 25–17.—Partially bifid nose with upper lip notching.

nose can survive. A complete nose can be reconstructed from distant pedicles migrated via a wrist carrier, an inner upper arm flap or a scalp flap (Fig. 25–19).

Another rare anomaly is the lateral nasal proboscis or unilateral tubular nose. One half of the nose is normal and the other half is a tube of skin and subcutaneous tissue attached by a small proximal pedicle and with a dimple at the distal end. The nose can be reconstructed by a succession of operations using just the tube of skin (Fig. 25–20). Some surgeons believe that it is easier to reconstruct in only two operations using a forehead flap.

Oro-orbital facial clefts (Fig. 25–21) are associated with severe rotation and nasal displacement. This often is associated with eye anomalies. Correction combines a variety of advancement and rotation procedures, plus the addition of local flaps.

Choanal atresia is obstruction of one or both nasal cavities. It usually is in the posterior aspect and may consist of mucosal webbing. More commonly there is a solid mass of bone obstructing the nostril. As with total absence of the nose, the child may have difficulty with breathing, especially when suckling. Recurrent bouts of asphyxia or aspiration should lead one to consider the diagnosis of choanal atresia. Passing a fine catheter down the nose confirms such a diagnosis. Correction can be accomplished by forcing a trocar down the nose or using a transpalatal approach to the nose and excising the bone block (see Chap. 29).

Many of the unilateral and bilateral congenital nasal anomalies, as well as some tumors such as encephaloceles, are associated with abnormalities of the nasolacrimal drainage system. If obstruction is suggested by excessive lacrimation, it can be confirmed by inserting radionucleotide substances into the conjunctival sac and following their progress to the level of the obstruction. This is a noninvasive technique and does not require anesthesia in the young infant, as is necessary for dacryocystography.

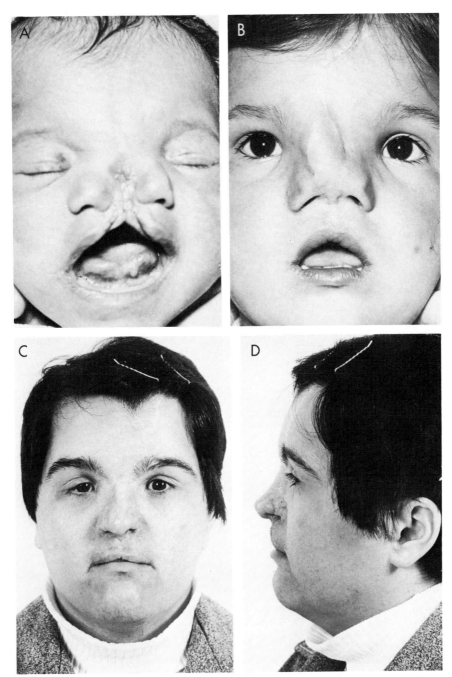

Fig. 25–18.—Completely bifid nose, median cleft lip, orbital hypertelorism. **A,** original appearance, in infancy. **B,** repair of nose and lip by excision of central cleft, forceful approximation of parts and addition of forehead flap. **C** and **D,** 20 years later—correction of intracranial orbital hypertelorism and simultaneous nasal reconstruction.

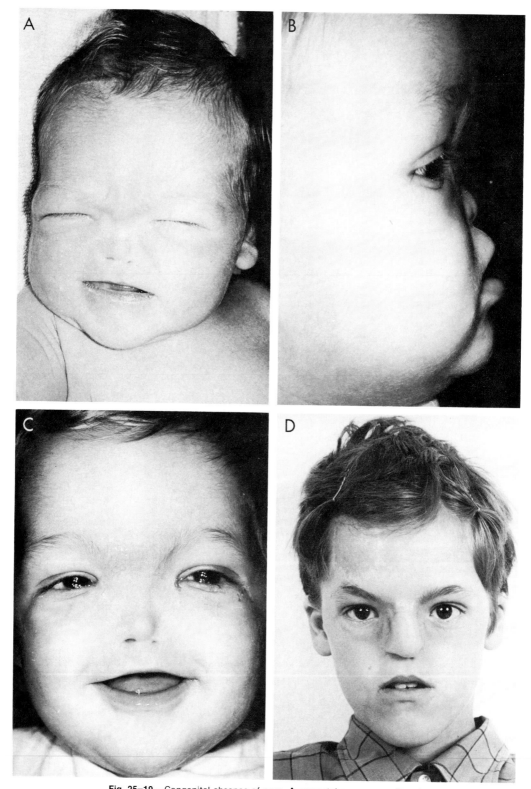

Fig. 25–19.—Congenital absence of nose. **A,** neonatal appearance. **B** and
C, same patient at age 12 months showing absent growth. **D,** same patient with nose reconstructed from forehead.

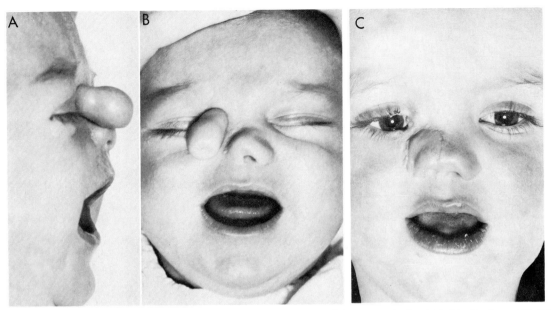

Fig. 25–20.—Lateral nasal proboscis (tubular nose). **A** and **B,** the left side of the nose is normal. The tube of skin and fat (lateral proboscis) hanging from a pedicle, represents the right side. **C**, after repair, using the lateral tubular nose to provide all the needed tissue.

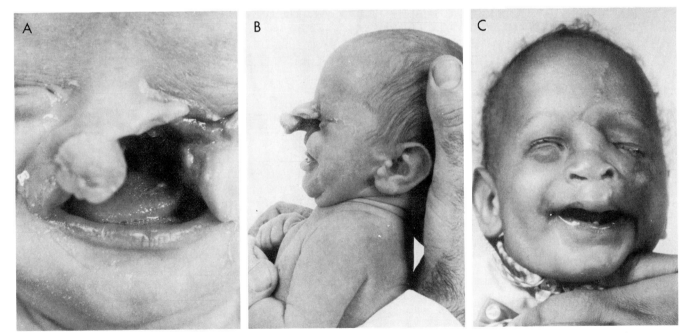

Fig. 25–21.—Complete left oro-ocular facial cleft and right cleft lip. **A** and **B,** this grotesque anomaly, as in this instance, may be associated with ocular anomalies. **C,** 1 year after repair using local flaps and forehead flap.

REFERENCES

1. Baxter, R. J., Johnson, J. D., Goetzman, B. W., and Hackel, A.: Cosmetic nasal deformities complicating prolonged nasotracheal intubation in critically ill newborn infants, Pediatrics 55: 884, 1975.
2. Binder, K. H.: Dysostosis Maxillonasalis ein Arhinencephaler Missbildungskomplex, Dtsch. Zahnaerztl. Z. 17:438, 1962.
3. Boyle, T. M.: The management of nasopharyngeal chordoma by repeated irradiation, J. Laryngol. Otol. 80:533, 1961.
4. Canick, M. L.: Major soft tissue injuries to the nose, Plast. Reconstr. Surg. 32:549, 1962.
5. Erich, J. B.: Nasal duplication, Plast Reconstr. Surg. 29:159, 1962.
6. Fox, J. W., Golden, G. T., and Edgerton, M. T.: Surgical correction of the absent nasal alae of the Johanson-Blizzard syndrome, Plast. Reconstr. Surg. 57:484, 1976.
7. Greeley, P. W., Middleton, A. G., and Curtin, J.: Incidence of malignancy in giant pigmented naevi, Plast. Reconstr. Surg. 36: 26, 1965.
8. Griffith, B. H.: Frontonasal tumors: Their diagnosis and management, Plast. Reconstr. Surg. 57:692, 1976.
9. Kaplan, E. N.: The risk of malignancy in large congenital nevi, Plast. Reconstr. Surg. 53:421, 1974.
10. Kazanjian, V. H.: Treatment of dermoid cysts of nose, Plast. Reconstr. Surg. 21:170, 1958.
11. Kubo, K.: Nasal gliomas, Plast. Reconstr. Surg. 52:47, 1973.
12. Littlewood, A. H. M.: Congenital nasal dermoid cysts and fistulas, Plast. Reconstr. Surg. 27:471, 1961.
13. McGovern, F. H., and Fitz-Hugh, G. S.: Surgical management of congenital choanal atresia, Arch. Otolaryngol. 73:627, 1961.
14. Munro, I. R., Saijo, M., and Mancer, K.: Lymphangioma—a long-term follow-up study, Plast. Reconstr. Surg. 56:642, 1975.
15. Munro, I. R., Saijo, M., and Mancer, K.: Lymphedema—a clinical review and follow-up study, Plast. Reconstr. Surg. 56:513, 1975.
16. Munro, I. R.: Orbito-cranio-facial surgery—the team approach, Plast. Reconstr. Surg. 55:170, 1975.
17. Richardson, G. S., Pinzon, G., Fetterman, G. H., Musgrave, R. M., and Gaisford, J. C.: Calcifying epithelioma of Malherbe, Plast. Reconstr. Surg. 36:263, 1965.
18. Rival, J. M., et al.: Dystose maxillonasale de Binder, J. Genet. Hum. 22:263, 1976.
19. Suwanwela, C., and Suwanwela, N.: A morphological classification of sincipital encephalomeningoceles, J. Neurosurg. 36:201, 1972.
20. Tessier, P.: Anatomical classification of facial, craniofacial and laterofacial clefts, J. Maxillofac. Surg. 4:69, 1976.
21. Thomson, H. G., Birdsell, D. C., and Freiberg, A.: Surgical tattooing—an experimental study, Plast. Reconstr. Surg. 37:482, 1966.
22. Thomson, H. G., Douglas, L., and Munro, I. R.: Surgical tattooing—an experimental study (Part II), Plast. Reconstr. Surg. 39: 291, 1967.

26

W. K. LINDSAY

Cleft Lip

OROFACIAL CLEFTS are the most common of all facial malformations. Cleft lip, with or without cleft palate, is the most common form of orofacial clefting. Most clefts of the lip are associated with dentoalveolar and premaxillary defects anterior to the incisive foramen and frequently are called clefts of the primary palate. Both terms will be used in this chapter.

It is recommended strongly that you read the chapter on cleft palate (Chap. 27) when considering the development and epidemiology of cleft lip.

Normal Lip Development

Facial processes (Fig. 26–1) arise due to migration and later proliferation of neural crest mesenchyme. Coalescence of these facial processes results in the formation of the primary palate or lip, which constitutes the initial separation between the oral and nasal cavities and eventually gives rise to portions of the upper lip and maxilla. First, epithelial invagination cuts off an isthmus of mesenchyme. Next, epithelium surrounds the isthmus and mesenchymal penetration continues to enlarge the isthmus. A small portion of the primary palate forms by an epithelial invagination process. The major portion of the primary palate forms by coalescence of facial processes, apparently through epithelial fusion and mesenchymal consolidation.

Cleft Lip Development

Most clefts of the primary palate or lip appear to result from variable degrees of mesenchyme deficiency in the facial processes that coalesce to form the initial separation between oral and nasal cavities. In some cases, distortion of the processes may be of considerable importance. Defect in, or failure of, the initial epithelial invagination process has been thought by some to cause clefts of the primary palate, but there is little evidence to support this. The majority of studies indicate that a failure of mesenchymal consolidation is the main cause.

Epidemiology

Multiple genetic and, to a lesser extent, multiple environmental factors seem to be involved. Certain clefts result from chromosomal abnormalities, particularly the relatively rare median cleft lip, in which affected individuals rarely survive the first year of life.

Cleft lip is most common in Oriental populations (2/1000), next in Caucasians (1/1000) and least in the American black population (0.4/1000).

Cleft lip is more common in males than in females, but that trend is not so great for isolated cleft lip, being more significant for cleft lip combined with cleft palate.

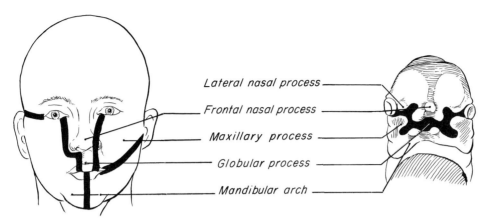

Fig. 26–1.—Facial clefts. *Left,* drawing showing some of the possibilities of facial and lip clefts. *Right,* head of fetus in 7th week. The central nasal processes are separated from the lateral on each side by the lateral nasal grooves, which represent the anterior nares. (Redrawn from Robinson, A. [ed.], *Cunningham's Textbook of Anatomy,* 6th ed.; courtesy of Oxford University Press.)

Associated malformations commonly include hypertelorism and heart, feet and hand anomalies. The incidence of associated malformations is not so great for isolated cleft lip, greater for cleft lip occurring with cleft palate and even greater for isolated cleft palate.

Birth rank, parental age, socioeconomic factors, geographic factors and seasonal variation have been studied in detail, but are not associated with cleft lip epidemiology.

Very few cases of cleft lip are caused by chromosomal aberrations (e.g., trisomy D syndrome with median cleft lip). Another small group result from a more dominant gene (cleft lip associated with mandibular lip pits or van der Woude syndrome), but most cases of cleft lip have a multifactorial etiology. These factors operate by influencing the amount of mesenchyme in those parts of the embryonic facial processes that coalesce to form the primary palate. Any genetic factors predisposing to mesenchymal deficiencies in the developing primary palate could participate in the multifactorial etiology. Environmental components aggravate the deficiency. Very little is known about maternal and external environmental factors in humans.

Risk for Future Siblings

Table 26–1[23] depicts risk figures in a useful way, but a surgeon must realize the problems in taking a meaningful genetic history and should not hesitate to request the expertise of a genetic counselor.

Historical Aspects

It is convenient to classify cleft lip operations by region of lip operated on, even when delving into history.

1. Straight Line Operations

(*a*) Paring the edges of the cleft, followed by straight line closures with figure-of-8 sutures around pins; Paré (1510–1590).[19]

(*b*) Involving the complete length of the lip (Fig. 26–2, *A*); Von Graefe (1825) and Rose (1833)[22]—curved incisions with concavities opposed; Thompson (1912)[27]—a straight incision running obliquely across the lips.

2. Lower One-Third Operations

(*a*) Triangular flap two-limbed incision; Owen (1904)[18]—flap rotated from the medial to the cleft (lateral) side; Mirault (1844),[17] Blair (1926)[1] and Brown and McDowell (1945)[5]—flap rotated from the cleft (lateral) side to the medial side.

(*b*) Triangular flap three-limbed incision (Fig. 26–2, *B*); Simon (1864)[24] and König (1893)[10]—flap rotated from the medial to the cleft side; Tennison (1952),[26] Marks (1953), Brauer (1953), Randall (1958),[20] Cronin (1957), Hagerty (1958) and Skoog (1958)—flap rotated from the cleft (lateral) side to the medial side.

(*c*) Quadrilateral flap (Fig. 26–2, *D*), Hagedorn (1884),[7] Le Mesurier (1935),[11] Axhausen-May (1947, 1955) Brauer (1953), McCash (1957) and Wang (1960)—flap rotated from the cleft side to the medial side.

3. Upper One-Third Flap Operations (Fig. 26–2, C)

Geraldé (circa 1869)—with the cleft representing the diagonal of a Z, the central band of the Z is located on the medial side of the cleft; Millard (1957)[13]—a rotation-advancement technique, similar to a Z-plasty with the central band of the Z on the cleft (lateral) side; Randall (1965)[21]—a temporary lip adhesion operation.

4. Combined Upper and Lower Lip Flaps

Huffman and Lierle (1949)[8] with associate[9] and Skoog (1958)[25]—a series of Z-plasties; Millard (1960)[14] added a small vermilion border flap.

The reader is referred to the text by Millard[16] for the most modern and exhaustive history of this operative procedure.

TABLE 26–1.—PREDICTED RECURRENCE PERCENTAGE

AFFECTED RELATIVES	CLEFT LIP WITH OR WITHOUT CLEFT PALATE	ISOLATED CLEFT LIP
One sibling	4.4	2.5
One parent	3.2	6.8
One parent and one sibling	15.8	14.9

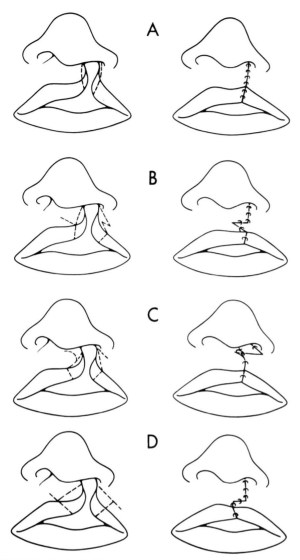

Fig. 26–2.—Basic cleft lip operations, comparative drawings. **A,** straight line operation; **B,** lower one-third triangular flap operation; **C,** upper one-third triangular flap operation; **D,** lower one-third rectangular flap operation.

Neonatal Management

Parents

The surgeon's early concern, on first being asked to see a child with cleft lip, is for the parents. Parents always are upset, and to a much greater degree than is apparent. They always want to know what caused the condition and what they have done wrong, although they may not have the temerity to ask. It often is better to avoid the question of hereditary influences at the time of the first interview, unless it is obvious from the history that heredity was unlikely to have been a significant etiologic factor in their case.

The surgeon then should outline for the parents what can be done for the child, emphasizing the fact that these children can grow up nicely and developing the concept that they should be treated as normal children, without overprotection. In these ways, one can improve acceptance of the child. The prognosis must be appropriately tempered if there are anomalies other than the cleft or if retardation is suspected.

Probably at subsequent visits, the surgeon will be asked

about the risk for future siblings, and he should be prepared to answer questions. Genetic counseling should be arranged if the concern is deep and involved.

Child

It may be possible for the infant with a relatively incomplete isolated cleft lip to be breast-fed. The infants with more severe cleft lip and those with an associated cleft palate almost always require artificial feeding. Feeding problems are related more to the cleft palate than to the cleft lip (see Chap. 27).

Age at Operation

A cleft lip may be repaired immediately after birth or when the baby is showing steady weight gain. The operation can be done quite successfully at any age. A neonatal operation has the advantage of making the baby more acceptable aesthetically to the parents before he goes home. There are two disadvantages. Some associated congenital anomalies may not be obvious in the neonatal period. There always will be residual deformity, if only a scar, after repair of even the most minimal cleft lip, and parents may be disappointed with these residual deformities if they never knew the baby as he was preoperatively.

Most cleft lips are repaired at 6–12 weeks of age. The baby should be showing a steady weight gain and the hemoglobin should be at least 10 gm. These measures favor adequate wound healing and safe anesthesia.

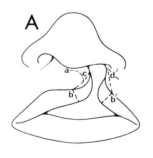
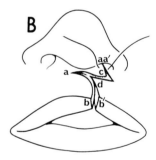
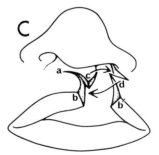
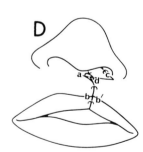

Fig. 26–3.—Upper one-third triangular flap operation. Point *a* is chosen at the midpoint of the base of the columella. It may be moved onto the normal side if necessary for adequate length. Point *b* is the point chosen for the peak of the cupid's bow. The triangular flap *c* is marked out on the normal side of the cleft in its upper portion. The extensive triangular flap *d* is marked out with its short arm commencing under the ala of the cleft side and its long arm running from the floor of the nose to point *b'* on the vermilion border. This point can be moved more laterally if necessary to give adequate lip length. Incisions are made full thickness through the lip. The triangular flap *c* is rotated laterally to the point beneath the ala. The *c* flap may be managed in different ways. The curved line *ab* straightens out by rotation and advancement as *b* and *b'* are approximated. The triangular flap *d* is rotated medially to point *a* beneath the columella.

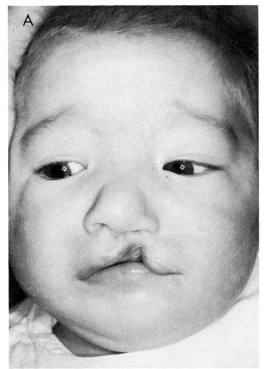

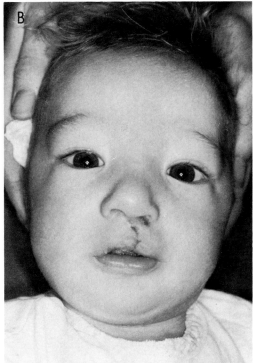

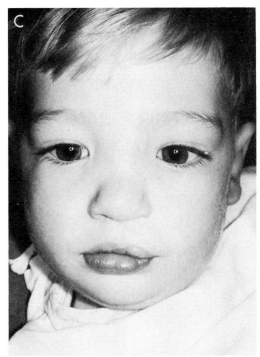

Fig. 26–4.—Upper one-third triangular flap operation. **A,** preoperative incomplete cleft lip; **B,** 6 days postoperative at time of suture removal; **C,** 18 months of age when back in the hospital for palate repair.

Choice of Anesthesia

There still is controversy about the choice of anesthesia. Local infiltration anesthesia combined with epinephrine for hemostasis frequently is used by those performing operations in the neonatal period. Some centers believe that open insufflation general anesthesia is associated with fewer postoperative respiratory complications. Most centers today favor endotracheal anesthesia.

Induction usually is accomplished with intravenous Pen-tothal (Abbott) administered by fine venipuncture. This is followed immediately by a muscle relaxant drug. The child is intubated and maintained on halogen and oxygen throughout the operation.

Neonatal Maxillary Orthopedics

Some centers attempt to reposition the alveolar segments prior to lip surgery[23] by various forms of intraoral and extraoral orthodontic appliances, including adhesive tape pressure and elastic traction.

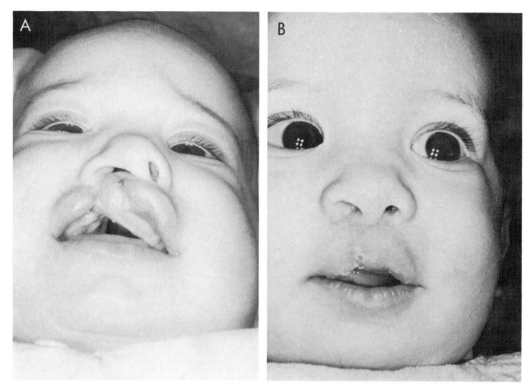

Fig. 26–5.—Upper one-third triangular flap operation. **A,** preoperative complete unilateral cleft lip at 3 months of age; **B,** 7 days postoperative at time of suture removal.

Widely separated alveolar segments in unilateral cleft lip or the projecting premaxillary segment in bilateral cleft lip can be moved best in the first few weeks of life. It is generally agreed that this extra treatment method, for unilateral cases, does make the lip repair easier for the surgeon but that it has no long-term benefit for the patient. Neonatal repositioning is of more value in bilateral cases. The most sophisticated mechanical method of accomplishing this has been described by Georgiade and Latham.[6] The correction that is obtained by neonatal maxillary orthopedics is similar to that which occurs spontaneously in unilateral cases in the few weeks following cleft lip operation. It is quite satisfactory to close the bilateral lip over the untouched premaxilla and await spontaneous repositioning over the next few years.

Lip adhesion or partial straight line closure has been described.[21] Such a partial closure molds the alveoli and makes a complete cleft into an incomplete one. Formal lip repair is performed 6–12 weeks later. It is thought by some that the end result is better after this two-stage procedure.

Surgical attempts to reposition the alveolar segments by osteotomy, before or at the time of the lip operation, are never indicated for unilateral clefts. Some surgeons still osteotomize the prevomerine bone when repairing bilateral complete clefts, but majority opinion indicates that surgical vomerine osteotomy predisposes to later midface retrusion and should be avoided.

The Unilateral Cleft Lip Repair

Upper One-Third Flap Operations (Figs. 26–3–26–5)

This operation[12-16] interrupts the long straight line of repair to a degree, without interfering with the philtral ridge of the lower lip on the cleft side. The operation has been criti-

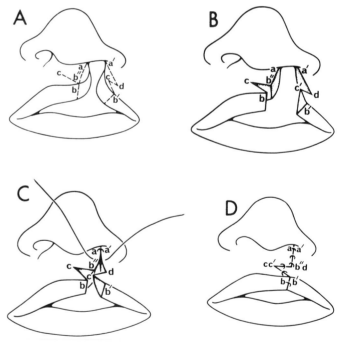

Fig. 26–6.—Lower one-third triangular flap operation. Top points *a* and *a'* are chosen, *a* representing the base of the columella on the normal side and *a'* the level of the ala on the cleft side. Point *b b''* is chosen on the normal side where the peak of the cupid's bow for the cleft side can be visualized. Point *d* is chosen on the cleft side such that *a' d = a b (b'')* and in such a way that *a' d + d b' =* the length of the lip on the uncleft side. A triangle *b' c' d* is marked out. A line *b c* is marked out such that it equals *c' d* or *c' b'*. Note that the peak of the cupid's bow is chosen from the normal side of the cleft in this operation. Full-thickness incisions are made through the lip along those lines. Mucous membrane closure is carried out, followed by closure of the muscle layers and, finally, by closure of the white and red lips approximating *a a', b'' d, c c'* and *b b'.*

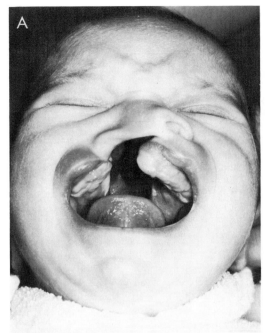

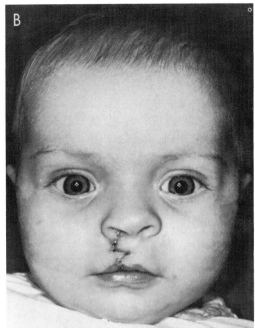

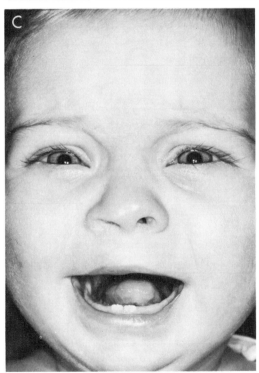

Fig. 26–7.—Lower one-third triangular flap operation. **A,** complete unilateral cleft lip at 3 months of age; **B,** 6 days postoperative at time of suture removal; **C,** 18 months of age when in the hospital for palate repair.

cized for producing a lip that is too tight in its lower one-third because it does not move extra tissue into this region. However, the procedure tends to produce a more natural alar base and nasal floor than do the other operations. The amount of visible scarring is least with this operation. Millard has described this operation in detail.[12-16]

Lower One-Third Flap Operations (Figs, 26–6–26–8)

The flaps may be either triangular[20, 26] or rectangular.[11] They have the advantage of breaking up the straight line so that it does not contact longitudinally and produce the re-

sidual mild cleft lip deformity. They also have the advantage of moving more tissue into the lower one-third of the lip and, in this way, producing a desirable fullness or pout in this area. These operations have the disadvantage of interrupting the philtral groove with a short transverse or oblique line in the lower portion of the lip that may remain quite obvious. They offer less desirable philtral ridge reconstruction on the cleft side and have a tendency to produce lips long on the cleft side unless care is taken with initial measurements and flap design.

This operation has been well described by Tennison[26] and Randall.[20, 21]

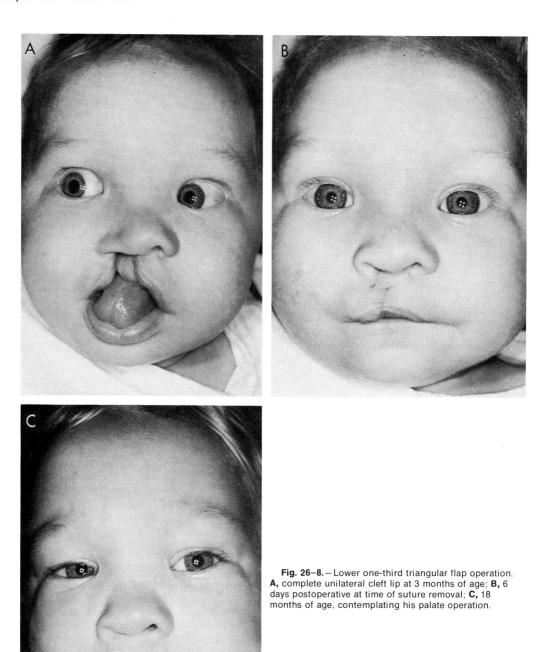

Fig. 26–8. — Lower one-third triangular flap operation. **A,** complete unilateral cleft lip at 3 months of age; **B,** 6 days postoperative at time of suture removal; **C,** 18 months of age, contemplating his palate operation.

Results of Unilateral Cleft Lip Operations

The postoperative result is quite spectacular and parents usually react favorably. Those who do not either have not truly accepted the child or have not been prepared for the limitations of the surgical result.

The results are closely related to the degree of the original deformity. Operations on incomplete cleft lips, even those with a Simonard's membrane, produce better results than do those on complete cleft lips and there are degrees of increasing severity in so-called complete cleft lips. Wide clefts, those with hypoplasia of the marginal tissues, those with a straight or an inverted alar rim and those with gross deviation of the columellar base produce less desirable results after primary lip repair.

Following the lip operation, the incision line is intensely

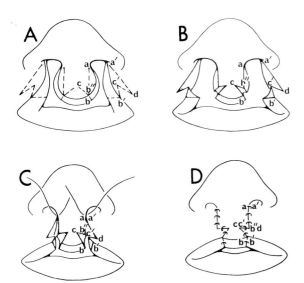

Fig. 26–9.—Repair of bilateral complete cleft lip by lower one-third triangular flap operation. **A,** points *a* and *a'* are chosen as top points at the base of the columella and level of the ala, respectively. Point *b b''* is chosen on the vermilion border of the prolabium. Point *d* is chosen on the lateral segment in such a position that $a'd + db' = 3/8$ inch. Point *b b''* is chosen on the vermilion border of the prolabial segment so that *a, b b'' = a' d*. The triangle *b' c' d* is marked out, and a vertical line is drawn back on the prolabium so that *b c = d c'* or *b' c'*. If point *c* comes at or close to the midline of the prolabium, the operation must be done in two stages. **B,** full-thickness incisions are made. **C,** edges are approximated, and the triangular flap is rotated. **D,** the mucous membrane is closed. The muscle layers are closed. The white lip is closed by suturing *a a', b'' d, c c'* and *b b'*.

red and, during this stage, tends to shorten in the long axis and produce a pull-up deformity. In another few weeks, this shortening decreases as the lip softens and the redness fades. The lip length will return to the approximate level of the original careful measurements the surgeon planned for. It takes 6–12 months for a lip incision scar to resolve proper-

ly. During this period, the alveolar segments are molding together from the force of the repaired lip over them. The anterior portion of the cleft narrows. The projection of the central segment of the alveolus tends to decrease.

The Bilateral Cleft Lip Repair

The surgeon has a greater variety of methods of management and techniques at his disposal for the bilateral cleft lip deformity. Complete cases with severe projection of the premaxilla may require neonatal maxillary orthopedics. A decision will have to be made whether the prolabium will be used for the whole of the center of the lip or only for its upper two-thirds. Will the bilateral cleft be repaired in one or two stages?

Straight Line Operation

This operation (Fig. 26–2, *A*) requires that the prolabium be used for the whole of the center of the lip. It has the advantage of producing the shortest and often least obvious incision lines. The philtral area can be more natural. A lip repaired primarily in this way lends itself well to secondary revisionary procedures. They usually never end up too long. The main disadvantage of this operation is that there is insufficient tissue available for the repair of more severe degrees of bilateral complete cleft lip, so that central one-third "whistle" notch deformities are more prevalent. The reader is referred to the writings of Broadbent,[3, 4] who has modified Manchester's contributions. Direct muscle closure across the premaxilla deep to the prolabium is recommended.

Upper One-Third Triangular Flap Operation

This operation for bilateral cleft lips is not illustrated or described in detail here (see Figs. 26–2, *C* and 26–3). A similar procedure is done on both sides of the bilateral cleft. The prolabium is lengthened by this procedure. Complete

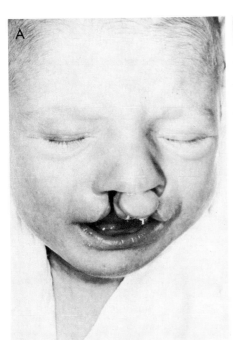

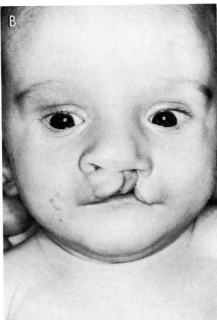

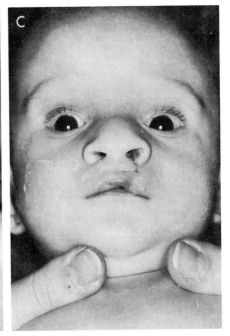

Fig. 26–10.—Lower one-third triangular flap operation. **A,** bilateral complete cleft lip at 3 months of age, preoperative; **B,** 4½ months of age. The right side has been repaired; **C,** 4¾ months of age; the sutures have just been removed from the left side.

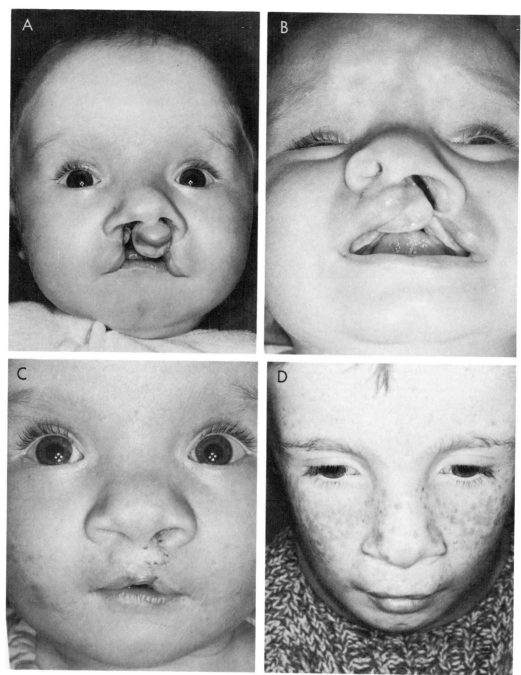

Fig. 26–11.—Lower one-third triangular flap operation. **A,** bilateral complete cleft lip/cleft palate patient; **B,** the right side, the side with the widest cleft, was repaired at 3 months of age; **C,** the left side was repaired at 4½ months of age, shown 1 week later at time of suture removal; **D,** patient at 5 years of age.

bilateral clefts have to be operated on in two stages if this procedure is used.

Lower One-Third Triangular Flap Operation
(Figs. 26–9–26–11)

This operation predicates the use of the prolabium for the whole of the center of the lip. The prolabium is lengthened, so this operation is useful in patients with a small prolabium. If the prolabium is very small, the operation will have to be done in two stages because point *c* (Fig. 26–9) would come

to the midline and the lower portion of the prolabium would have inadequate blood supply.

There is no normal side to measure and match with the cleft side. Therefore, one chooses an arbitrary length of ⅜ inch. Starting measurements longer than this tend to make a long lip whereas shorter measurements produce short lips. The long vertical distances *a b″* and *a′ d* should be ¼ inch and the base of the triangular flaps, *b′ d* ⅛ inch, representing the remainder of the distance to the white line of the lateral segments. The triangular flap *b′ c′ d* may be equilateral or isosceles. The same vertical distance is chosen on the white lip of the prolabium. An incision is marked back into the white lip of the prolabium, which will open up to accommodate the triangular flap. If this incision approaches the midline of the prolabium, the operation must be done in two stages.

Results of Primary Bilateral Cleft Lip Repair

The results with all of the described operations closely parallel the degree of severity and symmetry present preoperatively. The very severe cases, those patients with a small prolabium, a severely projecting premaxilla, wide alveolar gaps and a very short columella, give less desirable results. The markedly asymmetric deformity, complete on one side and incomplete on the other, tends to end up with varying degrees of postoperative asymmetry. The faces of many postoperative bilateral cleft lip patients are unattractive for a variety of reasons. Unattractive features may include medially placed eyebrows, apparent or real hypertelorism, broad nasal bones, wide alae and blunt nasal tips. Faces with combinations of these features may never be considered pretty.

Changes with Time in Bilateral Cleft Lip

Patients vary in the postoperative behavior of their reconstructions. In some, a skimpy prolabium becomes adequate in 2–3 years' time. In many cases, the projecting premaxilla molds into a more attractive position in 2–3 years' time. In others, the face grows out to a slightly molded premaxilla in 5–6 years' time. It is only in the very rare case that a premaxilla will remain grossly projecting after 12 or 13 years. Similarly, a short columella will lengthen absolutely or relatively with time. The possibility of such spontaneous changes should be remembered when discussing and planning revision procedures.

Later Management of Patients with Unilateral Cleft Lip

Almost all patients require specialized orthodontia to improve dentoalveolar and maxillary deformities in the form of crossbites and collapse.[23] This usually is performed in the second dentition. Most patients will require prosthetic replacement of at least 1, and occasionally 2, missing permanent teeth in the line of the cleft. This will take the form of either a removable or a fixed bridge, which cannot be final until growth is complete, at 17–18 years of age.

Revisionary operations may be necessary for the lip and almost always are required for the nose. They may be done at any age if the deformity is gross, but should be deferred until the patient wants them, if the deformity is not severe. Patient self-acceptance is the goal. It must be remembered that there always will be some residual deformity—if only a faint scar.

Common lip revision operations include trimming red lip redundancies and correcting red lip indentations or notches. Spread and hypertrophic scars may be revised by excising in such a way as to narrow scars without lengthening the lip, unless the lip is short.

Operations to improve the position and shape of the nose and nasal orifice frequently are necessary. The alar base may require repositioning and the floor of the nose may need correcting. There always is some slumping of the lower lateral cartilage of the nose in the side of the cleft, which usually requires repositioning by either an internal or external nose operation or by an alar margin excision procedure. Septalethmoid surgery may be necessary to improve the airway.

Major nasal bone and septal surgery is best deferred until growth is complete.

Gross disproportion between the maxilla and mandible may not be correctable by orthodontia. Disproportions due to maxillary collapse or hypoplasia are improved by lower Le Fort osteotomies. Disproportion due to the downward and forward growth of the mandible is improved by mandibular osteotomies.

Later Management of Patients with Bilateral Cleft Lip

The same orthodontic and prosthodontic treatment requirements described for unilateral lips apply to bilateral lips.[23] The methods are different because of the projecting mobile premaxilla and the fact that twice as many permanent teeth usually are absent.

The primary lip repair scar usually is the best because subsequent intervention produces more fibroplasia, but occasionally short lips must be lengthened and long lips shortened, the former being easier. The upper buccal sulcus may require deepening by mucosal advancement or Esser inlay graft. Some primary operations leave red lip or "whistle" notching. Lesser notches are corrected by double local red lip rotation flaps. Grosser deficiencies, particularly when associated with lower lip redundancies, may be improved spectacularly by a cross-lip pedicle flap (Abbé).

The columella usually is short and the nasal tip blunt. Adequate time, up to 6 years, should be allowed to see what spontaneous improvement will come to these relationships and to allow time for the maxillary-premaxillary relationship to improve. The columella can be lengthened by a local rotation flap procedure involving sickle flaps from the vertical lip scar[2] or by rotation of tissue from the floor of the nose. The latter procedure is particularly efficacious if the nasal floor is wide and the alae are widely placed.

Nasal tip blunting causes great concern in young patients. The external midline approach allows approximation of the lower lateral cartilages after incision of fat and skin. The resulting scar is acceptable if the original deformity was severe. Milder tip bluntness can be improved by a paired alar rim rotation flap procedure.[2]

Parental acceptance of the child with cleft lip encourages the patient's self-acceptance, and both are materially assisted by the surgeon, his fellow cleft lip-cleft palate team members and appropriately delivered treatment measures, such as those outlined above.

REFERENCES

1. Blair, V. P., and Brown, J. B.: Mirault's operation for single hare lip, Surg. Gynecol. Obstet. 51:81, 1930.
2. Brauer, R. O.: Lengthening the Columella, in Georgiade, N. G., and Hagerty, R. F. (eds.), *Symposium on Management of Cleft Lip and Palate and Associated Deformities* (St. Louis: The C. V. Mosby Company, 1974), p. 270.
3. Broadbent, T. R., and Woolf, R. M.: Bilateral cleft lip repairs— review of 160 cases and description of present management, Plast. Reconstr. Surg. 50:36, 1972.
4. Broadbent, T. R., and Woolf, R. M.: Bilateral Cleft Lip: One-Stage Primary Repair, in Georgiade, N. G., and Hagerty, R. F. (eds.), *Symposium on Management of Cleft Lip and Palate and Associated Deformities* (St. Louis: The C. V. Mosby Company, 1974), p. 134.
5. Brown, J. B., and McDowell, F.: Simplified design for repairs of single cleft lip, Surg. Gynecol. Obstet. 80:12, 1945.
6. Georgiade, N. G., and Latham, R. A.: Intraoral Traction for Positioning the Premaxilla in the Bilateral Cleft Lip, in Georgiade, N. G., and Hagerty, R. F. (eds.), *Symposium on Management of Cleft Lip and Palate and Associated Deformities* (St. Louis: The C. V. Mosby Company, 1974), p. 123.

7. Hagedorn, M.: Über ein Modifikation des Hasenscharten-operation, Zentralbl. Chir. 11:756, 1884.
8. Huffman, W. C., and Lierle, D. M.: Repair of bilateral cleft lip, Plast. Reconstr. Surg. 4:489, 1949.
9. Jayopathy, B., Huffman, W. C., and Lierle, D. M.: The Z plastic procedure—some mathematical considerations and applications to cleft lip, Plast. Reconstr. Surg. 26:203, 1960.
10. König, F.: *Chirurgie Lehrbuch des Speziellen Chirurgie für Ärzte und Studierende* (4th ed.; Berlin: A. Hirschwald, 1898), Vol. 315.
11. Le Mesurier, A. B.: *Harelips and Their Treatment* (Baltimore: The Williams & Wilkins Company, 1962).
12. Millard, D. R.: Extensions of the rotation-advancement principle for wide unilateral cleft lips, Plast. Reconstr. Surg. 42:535, 1968.
13. Millard, D. R., Jr.: A Primary Camouflage in the Unilateral Hare Lip, in Skoog, T., and Ivy, R. H. (eds.), *Transactions of the International Society of Plastic Surgeons* (Baltimore: The Williams & Wilkins Company, 1957), p. 160.
14. Millard, D. R., Jr.: Complete unilateral clefts of the lip, Plast. Reconstr. Surg. 25:595, 1960.
15. Millard, D. R., Jr., and Pigott, R. W.: Rotation-Advancement in Wide Unilateral Cleft Lips, in Sanenero-Rosseli, G., and Boggio-Robutti, G. (eds.), *Transactions of the Fourth International Congress of Plastic Surgery*, Rome, 1967 (Amsterdam: Excerpta Medica Foundation, 1969), pp. 349–355.
16. Millard, D. R., Jr.: *Cleft Craft. The Evolution of Its Surgery. I. The Unilateral Deformity* (Boston: Little, Brown and Company, 1976).
17. Mirault, G.: Deux lettres sur l'opération du bec-de-lièvre considéré dans ses divers états de simplicité, J. Chir. (Paris) 2:257, 1844.
18. Owen, E.: *Cleft Palate and Hare Lip* (Chicago: W. I. Keerner & Co., 1904).
19. Paré, A.: *Les Oeuvres de M. Ambroise Paré, etc.* (Paris: Masson & Cie, 1575), Livre 17, Chap. 4.
20. Randall, P.: A triangular flap operation for the primary repair of unilateral clefts of the lip, Plast. Reconstr. Surg. 23:331, 1959.
21. Randall, P.: A lip adhesion operation in cleft lip surgery, Plast. Reconstr. Surg. 35:371, 1965.
22. Rose, W.: *Hare Lip and Cleft Palate* (London: Lewis, 1891).
23. Ross, R. B., and Johnston, M. C.: *Cleft Lip and Cleft Palate* (Baltimore: The Williams & Wilkins Company, 1972).
24. Simon, G.: V. V. Bruns Handb. Prakt. Chir. 1:47, 1913.
25. Skoog, T.: Repair of unilateral cleft lip deformity: Maxilla, nose and lip, Scand. J. Plast. Reconstr. Surg. 3:109, 1969.
26. Tennison, C. W.: The repair of the unilateral cleft lip by stencil method, Plast. Reconstr. Surg. 9:115, 1952.
27. Thompson, J. E.: An artistic and mathematically accurate method of repairing the defect in cases of hare lip, Surg. Gynecol. Obstet. 14:498, 1912.

27

W. K. LINDSAY

Cleft Palate

HISTORY.—The condition of cleft palate has been recorded for centuries. The history of its treatment is one of continued improvement. As early as the sixteenth century, these defects were covered or filled with artificial materials, and by the eighteenth century the palate had been closed by suture after cauterization. Throughout the nineteenth century, even before general anesthesia became available in 1869, efforts were directed toward obtaining adequate lateral relaxation to obtain good midline healing. This culminated in 1861 in the work of Von Langenbeck,[43] who used lateral release incisions and hamular infractions, adding to this elevation of full-thickness and mucoperiosteal flaps and attachment of these flaps to the denuded nasal septum. These techniques improved healing.

During the present century, efforts stimulated originally by Veau[42] have been directed toward making the palate as long as possible or the velopharyngeal space as small as possible, and improved speech has resulted. More recently, radical surgery has been criticized for producing excessive dentoalveolar and maxillary deformity.

Geneticists and epidemiologists have done more investigation on this than on any other anomaly.

Dental specialists have worked to improve the aesthetic and functional end results of the cleft palate treatment. Speech therapists have developed effective techniques. The care of the patient with cleft palate has moved into the realm of rehabilitation medicine, where efforts to integrate the work of the medical and paramedical workers have continued to improve the outlook for these patients.

Throughout the years, physical reconstruction has been improved greatly; morbidity and mortality have decreased and become negligible. Speech has improved, but not to the same degree. A significant number of patients with stigmatized speech remain. Surgical controversy in the 1970s centers around a balance between the best speech result and the best facial and dental aesthetic result.

Embryology and Development

The development of the whole palate requires a consideration of two areas: the prepalate (primary or labial palate) and the palate proper (secondary or oral palate).

PREPALATE.—The prepalate is related to the development of the face, lips, premaxilla and upper four incisor teeth, that is, the region anterior to the incisive foramen. Development commences during the 4th week of gestation and is completed by the 7th week. There are both classic and modern theories of embryology for this region.

The classic nineteenth century treatise by His[21] described the normal development as taking place from masses of ectoderm and mesoderm termed processes, three paired lateral and one central. These processes enlarge, grow together and fuse by ectodermal breakdown. Clefts occur when the mechanism of ectodermal breakdown and fusion is halted. This theory now is considered inadequate because it does not explain some of the variables found in this region, such as Simonard's membrane.

The modern twentieth century theory, suggested by Streeter[41] and proved in detail by Stark,[38, 39] describes this general region developing between the primitive oral cavity below and the primitive nasal pits above as a series of mesodermal masses underlying ectoderm in such a way as to form furrows. More specifically, the epithelial anlage of upper lip and premaxilla contains three masses of mesoderm. Each mesoderm mass undergoes a differential surging growth to join the others to form a lip and premaxilla. The process is not one of ectodermal breakdown and classic process fusion. An absence of or a decrease in mass volume of either lateral mesodermal mass volume results in some degree of unilateral or bilateral clefting of the lip and the lateral incisor regions of the alveolus. A similar deficiency in the central of the three mesodermal masses results in the rare clefting of the median lip and central alveolar region.

PALATE PROPER.—The palate proper is related to the development of the hard palate, soft palate, uvula and maxillary teeth—the region posterior to the incisive foramen. Development commences during the 6th week of gestation and is completed by 8½ weeks. The newer concepts of mesodermal penetration do not apply. This region develops bilaterally from the palatal processes or plates of the maxillary bones, which become prominent during the 6th–7th weeks, by which time the prepalate has formed. They extend from the prepalate to the tonsillar pillars and hang vertically beside the tongue. Between the 8th and 9th weeks, the palatal processes commence positional change, from the vertical to the horizontal plane, which progresses in wavelike fashion in a posteroanterior direction under the control of an intrinsic shelf force.[17, 45] For a time, the palatal shelves are kept apart by the tongue, but as the tongue lowers in the floor of the mouth and moves forward, the two palatal plates fuse. Alterations of shelf force produce abnormal degrees of palatal arching. Failure of the tongue to lower produces palatal clefts. The best clinical example of this is found in the Pierre Robin syndrome,[12] in which the combined tongue and palate abnormalities are obvious.

Classification

ANATOMIC CLASSIFICATION.—Davis and Ritchie,[9] Veau[42] and others have described anatomic methods of classification. It is common today to refer to an isolated cleft lip; a cleft lip and cleft palate, unilateral or bilateral, complete or incomplete; and an isolated cleft palate. These methods give little consideration to the alveolus.

EMBRYOLOGIC CLASSIFICATION.—The progress of epidemiologic studies, the need for uniformity of reporting results and the demand for detailed consideration of degree of involvement have led to an embryologic system of classification. The following system of classification is recommended for the future, and the reader should refer to the original papers[2, 40] for details.

Clefts of prepalate (primary palate):
  Cleft lip:
    Unilateral; right, left; extent ⅓, ⅔, 3/3.
    Bilateral; right, left; extent ⅓, ⅔, 3/3.
    Median; extent ⅓, ⅔, 3/3.
    Congenital scars.
  Cleft alveolar process:
    Unilateral; right, left; extent ⅓, ⅔, 3/3.
    Bilateral; right, left; extent ⅓, ⅔, 3/3.
    Median; right, left; extent ⅓, ⅔, 3/3.
    Submucous; right, left, median.
  Cleft lip and alveolar process:
    Any combination of the foregoing types.
    Premaxilla protrusion; slight, moderate, marked, none.
    Premaxilla rotation; right, left, slight, moderate, marked, none.
    Developmental arrestive prepalate; slight, moderate, marked, total.
Clefts of palate (secondary palate):
  Cleft soft palate; extent, palatal shortness, submucous (occult) cleft.
  Cleft hard palate; extent, vomer attachment, submucous (occult) cleft.
  Cleft soft and hard palate.
Clefts of prepalate and palate (cleft primary and secondary palate):

Any combination listed under clefts of prepalate and clefts of palate.
Facial clefts other than prepalatal and palatal:
  Mandibular process clefts—including mandibular lip pits.
  Nasal—ocular clefts.
  Oral—ocular clefts.

OTHER CONDITIONS PRODUCING CLEFT PALATE SPEECH.—These include congenital short palate and submucous (occult) cleft palate, both included in the above classification; congenital suprabulbar paresis[15]; acquired palatopharyngeal paresis, diphtheritic and poliomyelitic; congenital absence of tonsillar pillars; changes following tonsillectomy and adenoidectomy; surgical and traumatic loss of palatal and/or pharyngeal tissue; and mimicry of others.

Applied Anatomy

Operations carried out on a patient with cleft palate are concerned primarily with the anatomy of the hard and soft palates, whereas improvement of speech and total rehabilitation of a patient with cleft palate are concerned, in addition, with the anatomy of the prepalate, the tongue, the nasal pharynx and the oral pharynx.

NORMAL PREPALATE.—The prepalate is covered with mucous membrane continuous with that of the palate proper behind, forming the gingiva in front and densely adherent to the periosteum above. The bone is the premaxilla and composes that portion of the hard palate anterior to the incisive foramen. It thickens in front to form the alveolus, which contains the upper four incisor teeth.

CLEFT PREPALATE.—Prepalatal clefts (Fig. 27–1) usually are associated with vertical lip scars or cleft lips of any degree and may involve alveolar deficiencies varying from a missing lateral incisor tooth in the second dentition to partial or complete clefts of the alveolus unilaterally or bilaterally to complete absence of the premaxilla (the rare condition of median cleft). The only isolated cleft palate with prepalate involvement is that of orofacial digital I syndrome, when atypical alveolar clefting may occur associated with missing teeth and labial-alveolar webs. The premaxilla, in bilateral complete clefts, will be mobile; and often it is protrusive, since it is attached only by the vomerine or the prevomerine[1] bone.

With growth, there will be localized dental disturbance, depending on the severity of the prepalatal cleft, manifested by malformation and rotation of the teeth adjacent to the cleft and frequently by the presence of supernumerary teeth in the deciduous dentition and the absence of teeth in the permanent dentition.[24]

NORMAL PALATE.—The palate proper consists of a hard palate, soft palate and uvula. The hard palate is covered with mucous membrane, which forms rugae on its surface and meets in the midline as a ridge or raphe continuous with the mucous membrane of the prepalate in front and the soft palate behind. The mucous membrane contains mucus-secreting glands. It is continuous laterally with the gingiva of the maxillary teeth.

Normally, the palatine bones are horizontal, with a slight transverse arching. Each is continuous laterally with the maxillary alveolus and superiorly with the vomerine bone in the midline. Posterolaterally, each is separated by a fissure from the pterygoid bone of its side. Each posterior border contains a large and a small foramen for the greater and lesser palatine nerves and vessels.

The soft palate is covered with glandular mucous mem-

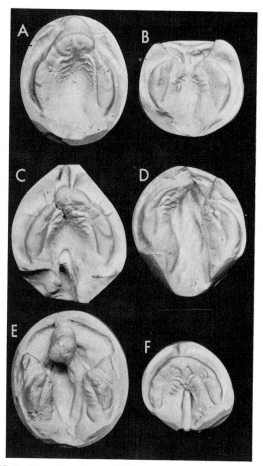

Fig. 27–1.—Examples of types of cleft palate: plaster models from dental impressions under 3 months of age. **A,** cleft of prepalate, left, incomplete. **B,** cleft of prepalate, median, complete. **C,** cleft of prepalate, right, complete, and cleft palate, incomplete. **D,** cleft of prepalate and palate, left, complete. **E,** cleft of prepalate, and palate, bilateral, complete; moderate projection of premaxilla and rotation to right. **F.** cleft of palate involving uvula, soft palate and posterior two-thirds of hard palate proper.

HIGH ARCHED PALATE.—Variation in the transverse arching of the palate is common. Thus, the high arched palate frequently is a normal anatomic variation. But it often is associated with submucous cleft palate, craniostenosis and choanal atresia. It probably is due to failure of the complete positional change of the palatine bones from the vertical to the horizontal plane between the 6th and 7th weeks of gestation.

PREPALATAL-PALATAL CLEFTS.—Such clefts always have some involvement of the uvula and soft palate and almost always have some involvement of the hard palate. The hard palate involvement may be a deficiency of one (unilateral) (Fig. 27–2) or both (bilateral) (Fig. 27–3) palatine bones near the midline. The mucous membrane of the septum and the vomerine will be visible on the uncleft side. A zone in the region of the incisive foramen extending for varying degrees may be intact (incomplete clefts) (Fig. 27–1, *C*). Occasionally, this incomplete involvement consists of a midline posterior hard palate deficiency with the vomerine bone lying free in the midline.

Unilateral prepalatal-palatal clefts, after repair of the lip and again after repair of the palate, may develop a medial shift or collapse of the maxillary or lateral segments, particularly on the cleft side, and a posterior shift or collapse of the anterior or premaxillary segment. The mandible frequently overgrows downward and forward. Associated with this will be dental crowding in the second dentition and decreased vertical growth of the teeth. This complex de-

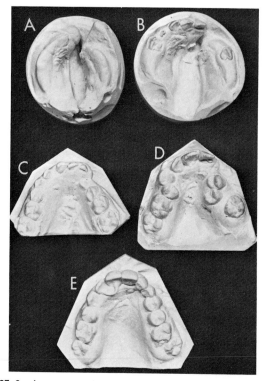

Fig. 27–2.—Appearance of a cleft palate at different ages and after different stages of treatment. **A,** cleft of prepalate, left, complete, unilateral, at 3 months of age immediately before lip surgery. **B,** at 18 months, immediately before palate surgery, showing narrowing of the cleft palate anteriorly. **C,** at 6 years, with palate healed and primary dentition erupted. The model does not show the soft palate repair. **D,** at 11 years, with secondary dentition erupted, to show the dental deformity due to smallness of the maxillae. **E,** 1 year later, following orthodontic repositioning of the maxillae and minor tooth realignment along with prosthetic replacement of the missing left lateral incisor tooth, which should be removable until 18 years of age and then converted to a fixed bridge.

brane on both its oral and nasal surfaces, both being continuous with mucous membrane of the oral and nasal cavities. It is firmly fixed to the posterior border of the hard palate and to the maxillary tuberosities by the palatine aponeurosis. It is suspended from the side walls of the posterior oronasal cavities by the tendons of the tensor palatine muscles curving around the hamulus and by the loose areolar attachment of the levator palatine to the medial pterygoid muscle and its fibrous attachments to the eustachian tubes. It has mobile suspension from the lateral and posterior pharyngeal walls and tongue by the palatopharyngeal and palatoglossal muscles. The bulk of the soft palate is made up of mucous membrane and the paired tensor palatine and levator palatine muscles, which have their broad origins on the base of the skull on the pterygomandibular ligament and the eustachian tubes and which insert into the midline raphe of the soft palate and the palatine aponeurosis.

All muscles except one are native and are supplied by the same nerve—the accessory nerve via the pharyngeal plexus. The tensor palatine muscles are migrant and are supplied by the mandibular (V3) nerve via the otic ganglion.[18] The blood supply is primarily from the posterior palatine arteries.

The uvula is a midline mass of mucous membrane that contains the small uvulis muscle, which appears to have little function and no homologue.

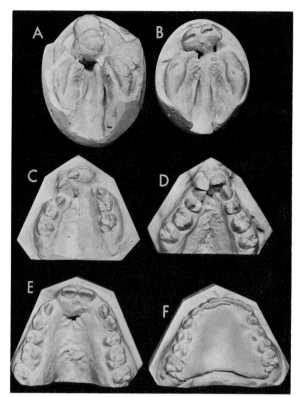

Fig. 27–3.—Appearance of a cleft palate at different ages and after different stages of treatment. **A,** cleft of prepalate and palate, bilateral, complete, with moderate premaxillary projection and mild rotation to right at 3 months of age, immediately before lip repair. **B,** at 18 months, immediately before palate operation, to show medial shifting of the lateral maxillary segments that has occurred. **C,** at 5 years, after eruption of deciduous dentition. The model does not show the soft palate repair. **D,** at 8 years, after eruption of permanent dentition, to show the medial displacement of the maxillary segments and lingual tipping of the incisor tooth. The premaxilla has gradually moved posteriorly without surgical section of the vomerine bone. **E,** at 12 years, following orthodontic repositioning of the maxillary segments and tooth realignment. Note that the residual postalveolar palatal defect has enlarged slightly. **F,** an anterior prosthesis to maintain the new premaxillary and dental positions, supply the two missing lateral incisors and cover the residual anterior oronasal fistula.

formity produces malocclusion, flattening of the upper lip or the whole of the middle third of the face and relative protrusion of the lower lip.

Bilateral prepalatal clefts undergo slightly different dental changes.[24] The premaxilla frequently is protruding at birth. Following lip and then palate repair, the premaxilla gradually recedes and its teeth become tipped lingually. Maxillary collapse proceeds somewhat as in the unilateral case but is modified by the final resting place, size and development of the maxillary "wedge." The deformity will be more or less symmetric.

PALATAL CLEFTS.—Palatal clefts (isolated cleft palate) (Fig. 27–1, *F*) almost always have some involvement of the hard palate in addition to uvular and soft palate involvement. Such involvement may consist of minimal, even submucosal, notching of the posterior border of the hard palate in the midline. Again, there may be midline deficiency of the palatine bones extending anywhere up to the incisive foramen.

Palatal clefts may develop dentoalveolar collapse of the posterior maxillary segments, with crowding of the teeth. Such developments are particularly likely to occur if the cleft and the surgical repair extended well forward into the hard palate and close to the alveolar margins.

Epidemiology

More information is available on the etiology of the cleft lip and cleft palate than for any other congenital anomaly, perhaps because it is common, obvious and produces social disability.

INCIDENCE.—Accurate incidence data for any anomaly are difficult to obtain. A continuing study of a segment of Canada,[6] recording only anomalies reported by physicians at birth and therefore probably low in isolated cleft palate figures, points out that this anomaly, considering cleft lip and cleft palate together, is the third most common, being exceeded only by meningomyelocele and clubfoot. The 1959 figures for this study, using cases per 1000 live births, are: cleft palate, 0.25; cleft lip, 0.34; cleft lip and cleft palate, 0.49; over-all, 1.08 (1:930 live births). An earlier study of the same geographic area[22] reported a similar figure. A United States study[37] supplies the following data on the basis of cases per 1000 live births: cleft palate, 0.79; cleft lip, 0.29; cleft lip and cleft palate, 0.49; over-all, 1.57 (1:640 live births). These are comparable to figures from Denmark.[16] Considering these and other variables, it is reasonable to assume a Caucasian incidence of 1:750 live births. It is generally considered that the black population incidence is lower than these figures and the mongoloid (Japanese) incidence is higher.

ENVIRONMENTAL FACTORS.—Clefts have been produced by severe alteration of certain environmental experimental factors of small animals from susceptible strains at a suitable period of gestation by means of dietary, vitamin and oxygen deprivation, radiation exposure and cortisone administration.[23, 44, 46] This work cannot be applied directly to humans, although there are reports of decreasing the expected incidence of production of this anomaly in mothers who have a known tendency by avoiding deprivation factors.[7, 12]

A number of clinical environmental factors have been studied in 577 consecutive cases.[5, 28] The mean parental ages were compared with a control obtained from the Report of the Registrar General of Canada. No differences from the control were observed for either maternal or paternal age with or without a family history of cleft. No deviations from the expected were found in the analysis of the birth ranks or in correlating birth rank with maternal age. No significant difference was observed when the mean birth weights of infants with cleft palate were compared with the mean birth weights in a large hospital, although the birth weights of the probands were lower than those of their sibs.

With respect to laterality, 43% had left-sided involvement, 24% right-sided involvement and 33% bilateral involvement. The bilateral cases had a greater incidence of both family history and involvement of other members of the family.

The sex distribution is significant. Cleft lip with or without cleft palate is more common in males whereas the isolated cleft palate is common in females. No form of sex-linked inheritance satisfies the ratios, and so it must be concluded that for some unknown reason the male is more susceptible to cleft lip with or without cleft palate and the female to cleft palate alone.

There was a significantly high incidence of severe associated anomalies in both groups, but more so in the isolated cleft palate group. The associated anomalies can be divided into two groups: (1) those occurring in the immediate vicinity:

Pierre Robin syndrome (macroglossia, micrognathia and cleft palate), Klippel-Feil syndrome (short neck, web neck, cervical spine abnormalities, including atlanto-occipital abnormalities),[25] Psaume syndrome[34] or oral-facial-digital syndrome[36] (tongue, floor of mouth, maxillary and mandibular teeth and digital abnormalities); and (2) those occurring elsewhere in the body, particularly congenital heart disease and extremity abnormalities (Ellis-Van Creveld syndrome[15]). This association of a high incidence of congenital abnormalities with cleft palate is suggestive of an over-all disturbance in development.

Studies of the incidence of maternal first trimester disturbances, among which are gestational bleeding, acquired illnesses (rubella, severe nausea, vomiting), operations, accidents and other stresses, have been carried out but have produced no significant data. Similarly, study of social status of the families and previous health of the parents produced insignificant data.

GENETIC FACTORS.—The only established human etiologic factors are genetic. Pioneer work in the field has been reported by Fogh-Andersen.[16]

A study[28] of 750 consecutive cleft cases has shown that approximately 33% of cleft lip patients with or without cleft palate have a history of a similar lesion in the family. Only 25% of isolated cleft palate patients have a similar history.

There is further evidence to suggest that these two groups of lesions are genetically different. A genetic analysis[5] of 413 pedigrees of the above-mentioned series indicates that cleft lip with or without cleft palate is due to at least two pairs of recessive genes if one applies the 40% penetrance observed in cleft twin studies, and that isolated cleft palate is due to a simple dominant gene with greatly reduced penetrance. The most recent suggestion[4] is that cleft lip with or without cleft palate has a multifactorial etiology, involving many genes and environmental factors, and that isolated cleft palate is even more heterogeneous.[35]

Chromosome studies.—An abnormal chromosome pattern has been shown for certain severe types of cleft lip and cleft palate, usually when associated with other anomalies such as microphthalmia.[33] This work has yet to be confirmed by others.

The epidemiologic data that are available suggest an interplay of genetic, environmental and constitutional factors.[17]

Risk for future siblings.—Reliable estimates for counseling parents of affected individuals and the affected individuals themselves are available[5] (Table 27–1). Such counseling is dependent on the ability to take an accurate pedigree and to consider other variables and should be undertaken in consultation with a geneticist.

Treatment

NEONATAL PERIOD.—In a small proportion of cases, usually those in which the patient has associated anomalies such as the Pierre Robin syndrome, a congenital heart defect and mental retardation, there will be respiratory and deglutition problems.

If due to local causes, the respiratory distress manifested by cyanosis and sternal indrawing requires manual or elastic traction repositioning of the tongue and nursing of the baby on the side or face in an assisted environment such as a Croupette. Failure of the baby to improve with such careful positioning requires either tracheostomy or operative forward repositioning of the tongue on the floor of the mouth and the buccal mucosa of the lower lip.[11, 47] Breast feeding is not impossible but usually is contraindicated for both aesthetic and mechanical reasons. The majority of the patients do well with a long, large, soft nipple that has a larger than usual hole in it. Assisted feeding by means of a Brecht feeder may be helpful, but the danger of aspiration must be recognized. A few patients have difficulty in sucking or in swallowing and may require gavage or indwelling plastic tube feedings. The feeding problems do not respond as well to tongue repositioning as do the airway problems. Careful nursing care, requiring great effort and encouragement, is the most important therapeutic factor in the management of neonatal problems, and surgical intervention at this stage rarely is necessary. These infants usually learn to suck, swallow and breathe successfully. The mandible becomes acceptable. Some food will come out the nose until after the palate is repaired.

PRIMARY OPERATION; AGE AT OPERATION.—Consideration must be given to mortality and morbidity, speech results and facial and dental growth and development. Most surgeons agree that it is preferable to have the palate repaired by 2 years of age, before the child has developed many speech abilities and habits. An increasing number of centers operate by 12 months of age, closing just the soft palate or the whole palate, but this has not been shown to improve speech results. Some dental specialists would like to have the operation postponed until 4–7 years of age to decrease the maxillary and alveolar dental deformity, which allegedly is due in part to contracture of the operative scar.

The surgeon has many operations and modifications of operations from which to choose. There are two main groups of operations: those producing adequate lateral mobilization to allow midline closure without tension[29, 43] (Figs. 27–4, 27–7 and 27–10) and those combining these features with complete anterior detachment of the hard

TABLE 27–1.—GENETIC RISKS OF CLEFT

	CLEFT LIP WITH OR WITHOUT CLEFT PALATE (%)	CLEFT PALATE (%)
Frequency in general population (ref. 6)	0.08	0.02
Risk of 2d affected child		
(a) If both parents are normal	3.7	2.5
(b) If 1 parent has cleft similar to patient's	19.4	14.3
Risk of 3d affected child (a and b)	9.0	0.90
Risk of 1st affected child if parent has a cleft	4.04	5.82

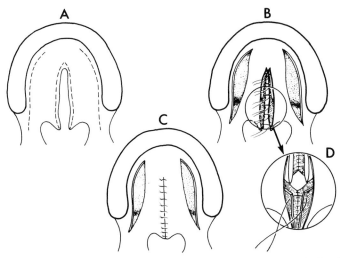

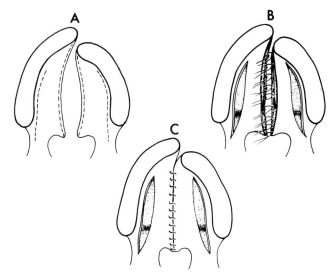

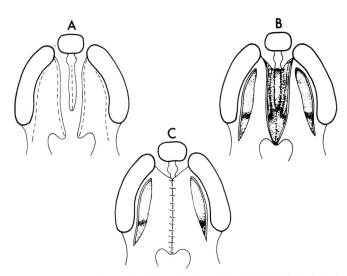

Fig. 27–4.—Von Langenbeck (simple closure) palatoplasty for isolated cleft palate. **A,** the incision lines for the margins of the soft and hard palate and for the soft and hard palate lateral release incisions. **B,** closure of the nasal mucosa. In this case, direct closure leaving the nasal mucosa intact is shown. This is possible only in the narrower and less extensive clefts. Not shown is the fact that the hamuli probably have been infractured, mucoperiosteal flaps have been elevated, leaving the posterior palatine artery intact but freeing it from its foramen, and some tenuous fibers running from the region of the maxillary tuberosity to the vicinity of the posterior palatine artery have been cut. **C,** closure of the oral mucosa. Note that the anterior mucoperiosteum still is intact and there is a bipedicle mucoperiosteal flap on either side. The opportunities for pushback are not as great. The lateral open areas are not as large as with the other operations. **D,** an enlarged drawing of the circled area in **B** to illustrate one of the controversial areas. The nasal mucosa is treated differently by different surgeons. Some transect it and allow some to drop back with the soft palate, leaving the controversial raw nasal area. Some make great efforts to dissect as much mucosa as possible from the nose, leaving the raw area more in the nose than in the nasopharynx. Some utilize an island flap to close the raw area. Some develop Z-plasty flaps of nasal mucosa to gain length and to effect direct closure. Some insert a primary pharyngeal flap. The tensor and levator muscle mass is shown, already dissected away from the posterior nasal spine and the palatine aponeurosis. Some turn the levator back into the posterior soft palate to construct a better sphincter.

and soft palate to allow pushback of the whole palate[10, 42] (Figs. 27–5, 27–6, 27–8, 27–9, 27–11 and 27–12). In cleft lip-cleft palate patients, simple closure palatoplasty produces less dentoalveolar and maxillary deformity than does pushback palatoplasty. The speech results with the two procedures are approximately the same.

There are other worthwhile palate operations, such as closure of the anterior hard palate at the time of lip correction[42] and the use of a bone graft to close the bony defect and prevent maxillary and premaxillary collapse,[30, 32] specific management of the levator muscles by dissection and posterior repositioning[14] and meticulous management of the nasal surface.[8]

SECONDARY OPERATIONS.—Residual oronasal fistulas at, in front of or behind the alveolus may be closed secondarily if they are a cause of foul odors, food impaction or persistent escape of liquids into the nose. This is not recommended routinely because of the possibility of producing dental disabilities, and the region is likely to be reopened if maxillary collapse is to be corrected orthodontically. Later, this region will have to be covered by a small denture carrying the one or two missing teeth, which can be designed to cover the residual prepalatal defect as well. Residual palatal (hard or soft) defects must be closed secondarily.

If the speech result is not acceptable after an adequate

Fig. 27–5.—Von Langenbeck (simple closure) palatoplasty for unilateral complete cleft lip-cleft palate. **A,** the incision lines. **B,** mucoperiosteal flaps have been elevated, although this is not well shown in this diagram. The nasal mucosa is closed. In this anomaly, the nasal nucosa on the noncleft or medial side is continuous with the septum and vomer. More tissue is available to manipulate. It may be dealt with as described in Figure 27–4. The more anterior septovomerine mucosa may be rotated forward for a considerable distance and used to close the alveolar gap in various ways. What one does in this area varies with the original width of the cleft, what was done at the time of lip closure, how much the alveolar gap narrowed after lip closure and how much reopening of the cleft is anticipated by permanent dentition orthodontic expansion. **C,** oral mucosa closure. Note that it is impossible to obtain a two-layer closure of the alveolar portion of the cleft with this operation (see text). Pushback is less. Lateral raw areas are relatively smaller because the mucoperiosteum is not detached anteriorly.

Fig. 27–6.—Von Langenbeck (simple closure) palatoplasty for bilateral complete cleft lip-cleft palate. The configuration of this deformity varies tremendously and line drawings can be misleading. **A,** the incision lines. The inferior border of the vomer is incised and mucous membrane is elevated from both sides of it. **B,** mucoperiosteal flaps are elevated without anterior detachment, keeping the posterior palatine arteries intact. Extensive dissection frequently is necessary in the lateral release incision area for this anomaly. The cleft usually is wide and there usually is considerable hypoplasia. The nasal mucosa is closed. Two suture lines are necessary anteriorly because of the two vomer flaps. **C,** oral mucosa closure. It is impossible to close the anterior portions of the cleft with this operation. However, the amount of palatine bone denuded is less.

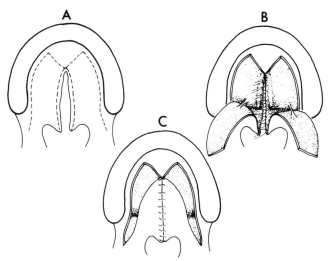

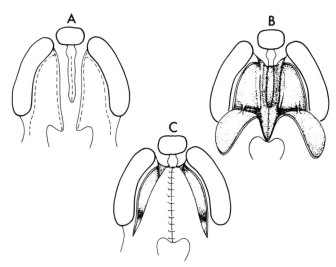

Fig. 27–7.—Two-flap palatoplasty for isolated cleft palate. **A,** the incision lines. Note that the medial and lateral incision lines are joined anteriorly by an oblique line placed to allow V-Y type of closure. **B,** mucoperiosteal flaps are completely elevated based posteriorly and on the posterior palatine arteries. The dissection is otherwise identical to Figure 27–4, *B.* Direct closure of nasal mucosa is shown, but the same variants in management described in Figure 27–4, *D* apply. **C,** the oral mucosa has been closed. The V-Y lengthening principle is used anteriorly to gain over-all palatal length or pushback.

Fig. 27–9.—Two-flap palatoplasty for bilateral cleft of the primary and secondary palate. **A,** the incision lines. The oblique lines joining the medial and lateral incisions must be placed with care if significant V-Y retrodisplacement is to be obtained. **B,** elevation of mucoperiosteal flaps. Closure of mucous membrane. The same variants apply as in Figure 27–4, *D.* **C,** closure of oral mucosa. It will be impossible to obtain complete anterior closure unless the premaxilla has been repositioned by earlier maxillary orthopedics.

trial of speech therapy, and after allowing sufficient time for developmental improvement, velopharyngeal competence should be reassessed by physical examination and speech cephalometry (Fig. 27–13) or cinefluoroscopy. If the soft palate is short but mobile and the pharynx is of normal size, a secondary pushback procedure may be indicated. If the soft palate is short and immobile and the pharynx is either of normal size or larger than normal, a palatopharyngoplasty

(Fig. 27–14) will be indicated. In certain cases, when the palate is both long and mobile but the pharynx is extremely large, pharyngeal augmentation procedures such as the Hynes pharyngoplasty or the insertion of free grafted material beneath the posterior pharyngeal wall[3, 19] may be indicated. Pharyngoplasty, using either the superiorly or inferiorly based flap is the most widely used secondary procedure for velopharyngeal inadequacy and when properly chosen, usually in conjunction with training by a speech pathologist, will give worthwhile improvement to the speech result.

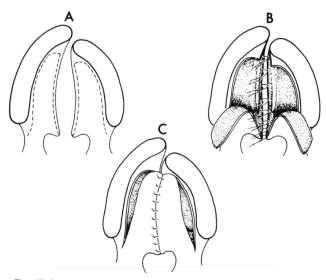

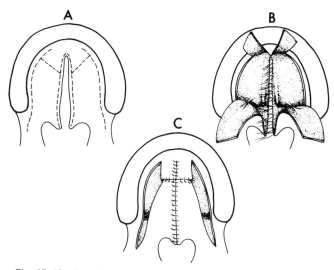

Fig. 27–8.—Two-flap pushback palatoplasty for unilateral complete cleft of the primary and secondary palate. **A,** the incision lines. Note that the medial and lateral incision lines are joined anteriorly by a line placed obliquely in a manner that will allow maximal V-Y retrodisplacement of the mucoperiosteum. **B,** mucoperiosteal flaps have been elevated with posterior palatine arteries intact, but teased out of their foramina. Soft palate lateral release incisions have been made. The hamuli may be infractured. The nasal mucosa is closed with the same variants noted in Figure 27–4, *D* and Figure 27–7, *B* and *C.* **C,** the oral mucosa is closed, using the V-Y shift anteriorly, which shifts not only mucoperiosteum but the whole palate posteriorly.

Fig. 27–10.—Four-flap palatoplasty for isolated cleft palate. This procedure is used by some when the cleft extends forward to the incisive foramen region. **A,** the incision lines. The oblique incision joining the medial and lateral incisions is again made in such a way as to permit V-Y closure and gain length. Care must be taken to retain a base to the anterior two flaps, yet these flaps must be mobile enough to shift them forward. **B,** the four flaps are mobilized and the nasal mucosa is closed directly. The same variants in management of the nasal mucosa apply as described in Figure 27–4, *D.* **C,** oral mucosa closure.

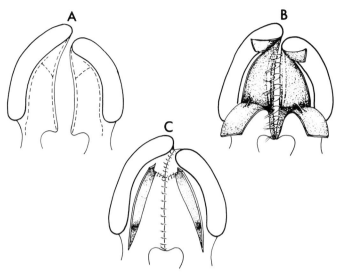

Fig. 27–11.—Four-flap pushback palatoplasty for unilateral complete cleft of the primary and secondary palate. **A,** the incision lines. Anteriorly, these vary considerably with the configuration of the palate. **B,** four mucoperiosteal flaps have been elevated, the two small flaps move medially and anteriorly. The nasal mucosa is closed, with the variants mentioned in Figure 27–7, *B.* **C,** oral mucosa closure. The same variants apply as in Figure 27–4, *D.*

Prosthetic speech appliances may be considered when operation is contraindicated because of poor anesthetic risk.

REHABILITATION.—Successful treatment involves consideration of the following factors: the patient's appearance, including both his external facial and dental configuration, the acceptability of his speech and the success of his rehabilitation, which is a combination of the above as well as his parental and his own mental outlook. The care of other medical and paramedical workers will be required to complete

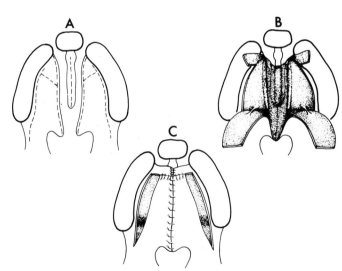

Fig. 27–12.—Four-flap palatoplasty for bilateral complete cleft of primary and secondary palate. **A,** the incision lines. Frequently it is difficult to find very much mucoperiosteum for the anterior two flaps. **B,** dissection of the four mucoperiosteal flaps. Lateral soft palate release dissection, usually involving infracture of hamuli. Closure of nasal mucosa, again utilizing any of the variants noted in Figure 27–4, *D.* **C,** closure of oral mucosa. Again, the premaxilla has not been repositioned and nothing has been done to the alveolar gap region at the time of lip closure, so complete anterior oral closure will be difficult.

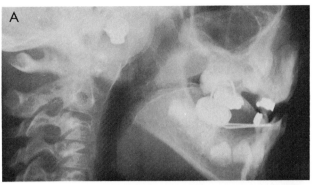

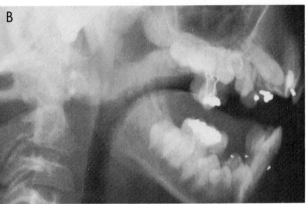

Fig. 27–13.—Speech cephalometric radiograph. The tongue and pharynx may be coated with radiopaque material such as barium paste. The head is held in fixed position by ear markers. Lateral films are taken in the "rest" position, with the patient "blowing" with closed lips and saying "ooh" and "ah." **A,** repaired isolated cleft palate in the rest position, showing a short cleft palate that could not make velopharyngeal closure. **B,** 3½ years later, the same patient in the rest position after pharyngoplasty, showing the soft tissue mass that unites the posterior pharyngeal wall and the soft palate.

the treatment of many patients with cleft palate. Understanding among these people is essential.

Ear, nose and throat.—These children have a higher than usual incidence of otitis media and hearing loss.[5, 13, 31] The early treatment of ear infections is important. The possibility of hearing loss is watched for and the underlying infection treated by the otolaryngologist. The role of the adenoids and tonsils is given serious consideration. Their thoughtless and traumatic removal is contraindicated because of the possibility of enlarging the velopharyngeal space, but carefully done often will benefit these children.

Speech therapy.—The function of speech probably is the most important to others, although not necessarily to the patient. There is no true objective method to measure speech. Subjective methods should be satisfactory, but they are veiled in the personal interests of the examiner, individual opinions as to what constitutes acceptable speech, the surgeon's tendency to think that his own work is satisfactory and the speech therapist's drive to produce "normal speech."

The outstanding problem in the speech of children with cleft palate is nasality (hypernasality or rhinolalia). Some cannot make the necessary closure between soft palate and pharynx to prevent nasal escape on the production of any of the consonants and vowels—with the exception of the nasal consonants m, n and ng. Sometimes a muffled tone rather than nasality is produced, due to depression of the nasal passages, with resultant lack of resonance.

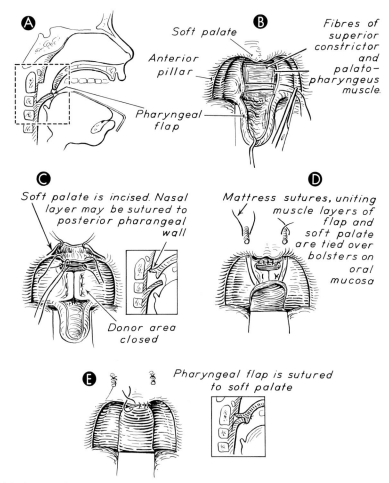

Ⓐ

Soft palate

Anterior pillar

Pharyngeal flap

Ⓑ Fibres of superior constrictor and palato- pharyngeus muscle.

Ⓒ Soft palate is incised. Nasal layer may be sutured to posterior pharangeal wall

Donor area closed

Ⓓ Mattress sutures, uniting muscle layers of flap and soft palate are tied over bolsters on oral mucosa

Ⓔ Pharyngeal flap is sutured to soft palate

Fig. 27–14.—The palatopharyngeal (pharyngoplasty) operation. The procedure for an inferiorly based pharyngeal flap is outlined. For high, very short soft palates the pharyngeal flap should be based superiorly.

The sibilant consonants are the most commonly affected. These involve the sounds, s, z, sh, zh, ch and j or soft g. Different types of lisp may develop—the protrusion, the lateral or the nasal lisp. The explosive consonants p, b, t, d, k and hard g frequently are affected because there is insufficient breath pressure in the mouth to produce them. The articulation of all consonants may be faulty, and then the speech will be unintelligible.[27]

Speech therapy, when indicated, is most valuable between 4 and 8 years of age, although therapists can detect and correct abnormal tendencies in younger children. Advice to parents and demonstration of exercises to build up oral breath pressure are useful in the younger children, to be followed by detailed exercises in the older ones, all followed by tape recordings.

Dental care.—Facial and dental configuration frequently can be made acceptable.[24, 35] This involves the judicious use of orthodontic repositioning of displaced maxillary segments and malaligned teeth, fixed bridge replacement of missing teeth, removable prosthetic replacement of missing teeth when simultaneous coverage of small anterior residual palatal defects is necessary, sacrifice of hypoplastic teeth, construction of more anterior space by procedures such as the Esser inlay graft techniques, the use of a larger anterior prosthesis or, more commonly, Le Fort I type lower maxillary osteotomies in cases with marked maxillary underdevelop-ment and the use of a concomitant mandibular resection when this bone is overdeveloped.

RESULTS OF TREATMENT.—Despite all these measures, a certain proportion of patients are left with inadequate speech. Results are fairly constant in the principal centers, variations probably being due to the lack of a standard, unbiased method of recording results.

The speech results of 612 consecutive cleft palate cases have been assessed by the author, who was not one of the operators. Essentially the same operative procedure was used on all cases (Figs. 27–6, 27–8 and 27–9). The results are summarized in Table 27–2. Avoiding the term "normal," 68.5% of the patients had acceptable speech; 10% had poor speech.

These results have been studied in detail to determine the cause of residual speech defects following palatoplasty. They have been found to be related to many variables, not all of which can be controlled but all of which must be taken into consideration when dealing with the rehabilitation of the patient with cleft palate. These include: the bilateral complete cleft lip-cleft palate patient, a very low intelligence quotient (−80), hearing loss (particularly +20 decibels bilaterally), poor psychosocial family environment, the presence of residual defects in the soft and posterior hard palate and severe dentoalveolar deformities. Secondary pharyngeal

TABLE 27–2.—OVER-ALL SUBJECTIVE SPEECH
RESULTS° OF 612 CONSECUTIVE PATIENTS
WITH CLEFT PALATE

ACCEPTABLE, 68.5%	UNACCEPTABLE, 31.5%
TYPE I, 39.7%	TYPE III, 21.4%
TYPE II, 28.8%	TYPE IV, 10.1%

°Description of speech types:

  I. Normal speech ⎱
  II. Minor articulation defects ⎰   Acceptable
      not stigmatized by cleft palate
  III. Intelligible speech, but
      stigmatized by cleft palate
  IV. Unintelligible speech,   Unacceptable
      stigmatized by cleft
      palate (poor)

flap operations can improve speech results when patients are chosen carefully.[20] The speech pathologist should be involved in the operative selection and the postpharyngoplasty care.

REFERENCES

1. Browne, D.: An orthopedic approach to problems of cleft lip and cleft palate, Trans. Int. Soc. Plast. Surg., 1955.
2. Bull. Am. A. Cleft Palate Rehabilitation: Report of the nomenclature committee of the American Association for Cleft Palate Rehabilitation, 9:39, 1959.
3. Calnan, J. S.: The surgical treatment of nasal speech disorders, Ann. R. Coll. Surg. Engl. 25:119, 1959.
4. Carter, C. O.: Genetics of common disorders, Br. Med. Bull. 25:52, 1969.
5. Cleft Lip and Cleft Palate Research and Treatment Center, The Hospital for Sick Children, Toronto, Canada: Five Year Report.
6. Congenital abnormalities reported on Physician's Notice of Birth Form, Province of Ontario, Department of Health. Courtesy of A. H. Sellers, Director, Division of Medical Statistics.
7. Conway, H.: Effect of supplemental vitamin therapy on the limitation of incidence of cleft lip and cleft palate in humans, Plast. Reconstr. Surg. 22:450, 1958.
8. Cronin, T. D.: Method of preventing raw area in nasal surface of soft palate in pushback surgery, Plast. Reconstr. Surg. 20:474, 1957.
9. Davis, J. S., and Ritchie, H. P.: Classification of congenital clefts of the lip and palate, JAMA 79:1323, 1922.
10. Dorrance, G. N.: The push-back operation in cleft palate surgery, Ann. Surg. 101:445, 1935.
11. Douglas, B.: Treatment of micrognathia associated with obstruction by plastic procedures, Plast. Reconstr. Surg. 1:304, 1946.
12. Douglas, B.: The role of environmental factors in the etiology of so-called congenital malformations, Plast. Reconstr. Surg. 22:94, 1958.
13. Drettner, R.: The nasal airway and hearing in patients with cleft palate, Acta Otolaryngol. 25:131, 1960.
14. Edgerton, M. T., and Dellan, A. L.: Surgical retrodisplacement of the levator veli palatine muscle, Plast. Reconstr. Surg. 47:154, 1971.
15. Ellis, W. B., and Van Creveld, S.: A syndrome characterized by ectodermal dysplasia, polydactyly, chondrodysplasia and congenital morbus cordis, Arch. Dis. Child. 15:65, 1940.
16. Fogh-Andersen, P.: *Inheritance of Harelip and Cleft Palate* (Copenhagen: Arnold Busck, 1942).
17. Fraser, F. C., Walker, B. E., and Trasler, D. G.: Experimental production of congenital cleft palate: Genetic and environmental factors, Pediatrics 19:782, 1957.
18. Grant, J. C. B.: Vessels and Nerves of Soft Palate, in *A Method of Anatomy* (5th ed.: Baltimore: The Williams & Wilkins Company, 1952), p. 748.
19. Hagerty, R. P., and Hill, M. J.: Cartilage pharyngoplasty in cleft palate patients, Surg. Gynecol. Obstet. 112:350, 1961.
20. Hamlen, M.: Speech changes after pharyngeal flap surgery, Plast. Reconstr. Surg. 46:437, 1970.
21. His, W.: Die Entwickelung der menschlichen und thierischer Physiognosen, Arch. Anat. Physiol. Anat., part 384, 1892; Beobachtungen zur Geschichte der Nasen und Gaumen-bildung im meuschlichen Embryo, Abhandl. Math. Phys. Classe Kgl. Sachs. Gesellsch. Wissensch. 27:347, 1901.
22. Hixon, E.: A study of the incidence of cleft lip and cleft palate in Ontario, Can. J. Public Health 42:508, 1951.
23. Ingalls, T. H.: Causes and prevention of developmental defects, JAMA 161:1047, 1956.
24. Johnston, M. C.: Orthodontic treatment for the cleft palate patient, Am. J. Orthod. 44:750, 1958.
25. Klippel, M., and Feil, A.: Un cas d'absence des vertèbres cervicales, Nouv. Inconogr. Salpêtrière 25:223, 1912.
26. Le Mesurier, A. B.: The operative repair of cleft palate, Can. Med. Assoc. J. 33:150, 1935.
27. Lewis, R.: Speech and the cleft palate child, Can. Med. Assoc. J. 71:600, 1954.
28. Lindsay, W. K.: The Hospital for Sick Children, Toronto, Canada. Unpublished data.
29. Lindsay, W. K.: Surgical repair of cleft palate, Clin. Plast. Surg. 2:309, 1975.
30. Lynch, J. B., Lewis, S. R., and Blocker, T. G., Jr.: Maxillary bone grafts in cleft palate patients, Plast. Reconstr. Surg. 37:91, 1966.
31. Masters, F. W., Bingham, H. G., and Robinson, D. W.: Prevention and treatment of hearing loss in the cleft palate child, Plast. Reconstr. Surg. 25:503, 1960.
32. Nordin, K. E.: Bone grafting to alveolar process clefts following treatment of secondary cleft palate deformity, Trans. Int. Soc. Plast. Surg., 1955.
33. Patau, K., *et al.*: Multiple congenital anomalies caused by an extra autosome, Lancet 1:790, 1960.
34. Psaume, J.: A propos des anomalies fasciales associées à la division palatine, Ann. Chir. Plast., Vol. 2, March, 1957.
35. Ross, R. B., and Johnston, M. C.: *Cleft Lip and Palate* (Baltimore: The Williams & Wilkins Company, 1972), p. 62.
36. Ruess, A. L., *et al.*: The oral-facial-digital syndrome: A multiple congenital condition of females with associated chromosomal abnormalities, Pediatrics 29:985, 1962.
37. Shapiro, R. N., *et al.*: The incidence of congenital anomalies discovered in the neonatal period, Am. J. Surg. 96:396, 1958.
38. Stark, R. B.: Pathogenesis of harelip and cleft palate, Plast. Reconstr. Surg. 13:22, 1954.
39. Stark, R. B., and Ehrmann, N. A.: Development of the center of the face with particular reference to surgical correction of bilateral cleft lip, Plast. Reconstr. Surg. 21:177, 1958.
40. Stark, R. B., and Kernahan, D. A.: A classification of cleft lip and cleft palate based upon newer concepts of embryology, Bull. Am. Acad. Cleft Palate Rehabil. 9:45, 1959.
41. Streeter, G. L.: Developmental horizons in human embryos: Age groups XV, XVI, XVII & XVIII, Contrib. Embryol. Carnegie Inst. 32:133, 1948.
42. Veau, V.: *Divisions Palatine* (Paris: Masson & Cie, 1931).
43. Von Langenbeck, B. von L.: Uranoplastic by detaching the mucous periosteal lining of the hard palate, Arch. Klin. Chir. 2:205, 1861.
44. Walker, B. E.: Experimental production of cleft palate in animals, Bull. Am. Acad. Cleft Palate Rehabil. 7:8, 1957.
45. Walker, B. E., and Fraser, F. C.: Closure of the secondary palate in three strains of mice, J. Embryol. Exp. Morphol. 4:176, 1956.
46. Warkany, J.: Etiology of Congenital Malformations, in Levine, S. Z., *et al.* (eds.), *Advances in Pediatrics* (Chicago: Year Book Medical Publishers, Inc., 1947), Vol. 2.
47. Woolf, R. M., Georgiade, N., and Pickrell, K. L.: Micrognathia and associated cleft palate (Pierre Robin syndrome), Plast. Reconstr. Surg. 26:199, 1960.
48. Wynn-Williams, D.: Congenital suprabulbar paresis, Speech Pathol. Ther., p. 18, April, 1928.

28 Milton T. Edgerton

Auricular Deformities

THE ABSENCE OF a major portion of the external ear (microtia) is an uncommon (approximately 1 in every 20,000 live births—Ohmori[13]) congenital deformity in children. Complete absence of the ear (anotia) is exceedingly rare. This chapter will deal with the problems associated with *microtia* and leave for another time the less complex management of lop ear, cryptotia, cup ear and protruding ears. These lesser deformities are not usually associated with stenosis of the external auditory canal and do not require the transplantation of major amounts of tissue.

The human ear is one of the most difficult features in the human body to construct. The complex shape and folding of its surface contour—the firm but flexible specialized cartilaginous framework, the large amount of thin, pink covering skin with little subcutaneous tissue—and the spatial requirements of projection, level and axis have all combined to challenge the ingenuities of generations of plastic surgeons. The solutions are not complete, but great strides have been made in the past decade. It now is reasonable for the parents of a child born with unilateral or bilateral microtia to expect reasonably shaped, sized and positioned ears with ear canal and middle ear reconstruction that, in many instances, will allow the child to go without a hearing aid. In most instances, this reconstruction can be completed by the time the child is of school age.

Etiology

The inheritance of congenital microtia is low and multiple cases in a single family are quite rare. A few of the "thalidomide babies" had microtia in association with other major abnormalities, but environmental teratogenic etiologic factors are poorly defined. Although measles will cause congenital nerve deafness, it is not known to produce microtia of the external ear (Rogers[14]).

Microtia deformity may be limited to the auricle, but in more than 90% of children so afflicted, deformities are found in adjacent anatomic areas that are formed from the first and second branchial arches. When microtia is associated with *unilateral* facial changes, the most common associated deformities are: (1) misplaced ear remnants; (2) abnormally low hairline in mastoid region; (3) cervical sinus tracts; (4) ocular epibulbar dermoids; (5) facial nerve palsies; (6) mandibular hypoplasias; (7) macrostomia. A combination of these defects occurring with microtia on one side of the face is grouped under the syndrome of hemifacial microsomia, or lateral facial dysplasia.

Microtia is bilateral in approximately 15% of the affected children. When other facial deformities are present in patients with bilateral microtia they include most commonly: (1) a low temporal hairline; (2) colobomas and absent eyelashes; (3) hypoplasia of zygomas with antimongoloid slant of eyelid fissures; (4) clefts of bony orbits; (5) micrognathias;

(6) ectopic hair in cheek regions. Varying combinations of these symptoms constitute the syndromes described by Berry and Treacher Collins. They have a high familial tendency.

The external ear is known to form during fetal life from six small "hillocks" that develop from the 1st and 2d branchial arches on either side of the first branchial groove (Fig. 28–1). Between the stages of the 13-mm (38-day-old) and 135-mm embryos, the external ear evolves into almost adult form. The only parts of the adult external ear that eventually form from the mandibular arch are the anterior crus of the helix and the tragus. The hyoid (2d branchial) arch contributes the remainder of the auricle.

Postnatal Ear Growth

Male and female ears are about the same size at birth (Hajnis[9]), but a boy's ear grows faster during the first year of life. Adult male ears average a mean 5 mm longer than girls' ears. At 5 years of age, the average ear is 54 mm long and 33 mm wide. It will grow only 10 mm longer over the remaining life of the patient. This makes it practical for the plastic surgeon to construct an *adult-sized* ear on a 5-year-old child without producing troublesome disproportions.

Use of Prosthetic Ears

Much effort and research have been expended in the attempt to produce artificial ears that will obviate the need for multistaged sophisticated surgical construction from living tissues. To date, these efforts have been complete failures in the treatment of congenital microtia. The new soft vinyls have delicacy and elasticity. They may be colored realistically to match the skin of the opposite normal ear. Repeated use of skin glues frequently causes skin irritation. To reduce this problem, living skin-cartilage "pegs" were constructed in the mastoid region and used as "hangers" for the prosthetic ears. Even so, children will *not* continue to wear even the best prosthetic ears. The problems include: (1) difficulty in blending the edge of the prosthesis with the normal skin; (2) occasional intense embarrassment to the child when the ear gets knocked off at a school recess; (3) problems of getting the ear soiled or having the thin edge break off; (4) considerable expense of regular fabrication and replacement as the prosthesis wears out. Perhaps the greatest hurdle of any maxillofacial prosthesis is (5) the inability of the patient to incorporate a removable and replaceable unit into his concept of his own body image. This inability makes it difficult—or perhaps impossible—to overcome the *personal sense of deformity* by use of an external prosthesis, even when the appearance of the ear is excellent to other persons. The average child would prefer *no* reconstruction to the wearing of an artificial ear.

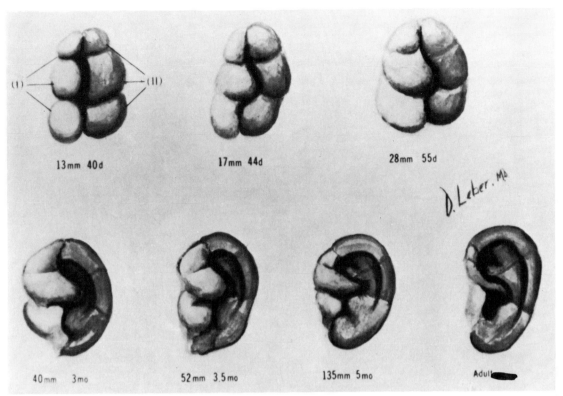

Fig. 28–1.—Embryologic formation of the external ear at the various stages of fetal life (Leber's concept). Note that in the adult ear the only contributions of the first branchial arch would appear to be the root of the superior helix and the tragus.

Choice of Autogenous Costal Cartilage versus Soft Silastic in Ear Construction

For many years, surgeons have tried to use grafts of cartilage to provide a framework in reconstructing the ear. Unfortunately, the hyaline cartilage of a rib lacks the toughness and elasticity of normal ear cartilage. As a result, any frame carved from a rib always lacks the strength, springiness and flexibility of a normal ear.

Dr. V. Blair attempted to overcome the limitations of rib cartilage by harvesting living ear cartilage allografts, donated by mothers for the building of their babies' ears. These ear cartilage grafts gave promising early results but, over a period of several years, the immune responses of the child to the tissue histoincompatibility caused gradual resorption of the cartilage. Surgeons then returned to the use of autogenous cartilage and its problems.

Despite the limitations, Tanzer,[15-17] Fukuda[8] and others[2-5] managed to achieve fine results with costal cartilages by improving carving and splicing techniques. During the 1960s, many plastic surgeons using such methods were, for the first time, able to construct quite acceptable ears for children. Further interest was rekindled in ear reconstruction by early efforts at middle ear reconstruction.[5] Surgeons discovered that skillful middle ear and tympanic membrane reconstruction could be combined with external ear construction to provide useful appearance and acceptable body imagery (Fig. 28–2).

During this same period, a number of surgeons explored the use of various synthetic materials in an attempt to produce an ear framework with qualities superior to carved costal cartilage. In the 1950s, I utilized polyethylene and carved Teflon to produce thin, elastic frames (Fig. 28–2, B). Several patients with these early synthetic frameworks continue to do well after more than 15 years of follow-up (Figs. 28–2, F and 28–7, D and E).

Cronin,[4] Ohmori,[12] Edgerton[5, 6] and others[7, 8] have reported successful use of the soft Silastic (370) ear frame manufactured by the Dow Corning Corporation.

This material is thin, strong, inert, flexible and may have its shape modified in the operating room. The successful results using this method of ear reconstruction are equal or superior to the best results with the costal cartilage technique. Use of a Silastic ear frame also obviates the need for operating on the child's rib cage and a full-sized ear may be constructed at any desired age and with considerable reduction in operating time.

Despite these early promising results, many surgeons found that a high percentage of the implanted Silastic implants became exposed in the postoperative period and had to be removed. It became important to determine what differences accounted for the success of some Silastic implants. As so often is the case in newly developing surgical fields, the answer was found to lie in exacting details of surgical technique.

A summary of the key points in obtaining successful Silastic implants includes the following 10 surgical principles.[6]

1. The design of skin flaps overlying any implant should permit contact with all contours of the implant surface and avoid bridging or dead space.

2. Incisions should be designed so as ultimately to maintain the maximal amount of undisturbed sensation and circulation within the remaining skin overlying the implant.

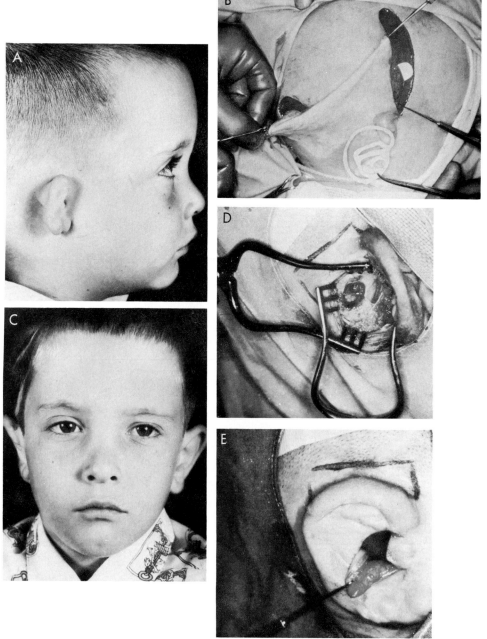

Fig. 28–2.—Unilateral Class II microtia and stenosis of the external auditory canal. **A,** 18-month-old male with characteristic appearance. **B,** external ear reconstruction carried out utilizing a hand-carved, three-ring, Teflon framework for ear support—with scalp hair roll technique to provide covering for the new ear. **C,** at 4 years of age, reconstructed ear has excellent shape, projection and flexibility. **D,** at 5 years of age, reconstruction of the middle ear is undertaken to improve and provide binaural hearing. The reconstructed right ear has been reflected.forward on a pedicle based on the superficial temporal artery. The middle ear has been exposed by removing the cortex of the mastoid bone. A thin skin graft was used to provide a new tympanum. **E,** at the conclusion of middle ear reconstruction, the external ear is returned to its original position with the aid of preoperative dye markings on the side of the head. A pedicle flap from the back surface of the ear is utilized to form a lining for the new external auditory canal. *(Continued.)*

When possible, incision should not cross ridges or high points of the surgical implant. Maximal circulation and cutaneous sensation should be preserved by avoiding encircling incisions of the ear.

3. To prevent wound breakdown and exposure, the surgeon should implant as deeply as possible beneath the skin surface.

4. The wound pocket should be made sufficiently large that the inserted implant will not be compressed on insertion.

5. Hemostasis must be meticulous and, postoperatively, suction drainage will minimize hematoma or seroma.

6. The implant should be well secured to avoid undesired motion. Fixation is best obtained by implant fenestration, by use of flexible, nonabsorbable sutures or by anchorage with fascia.

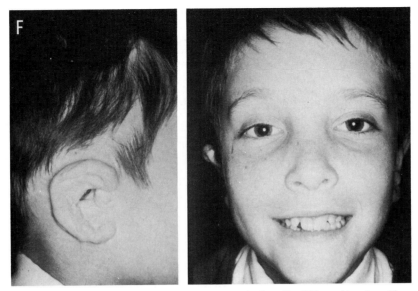

Fig. 28–2 (cont.).—**F,** 2 years later, this boy enjoys the benefits of binaural hearing with only a 20-db hearing loss in the frequencies of conversational voice.

7. Where deep burial of the implant has been impossible, as in the case of the ear, local deep tissue flaps of fascia or periosteum may be primarily interposed between the implant and the overlying skin.

8. The newly constructed ear should be protected postoperatively, but tight pressure dressings over anesthetic skin should be avoided. The active child requires protection for several months until sensation improves. Through-and-through bolster sutures increase the risk of introducing infection and should not be used.

9. When progressive thinning of the skin overlying the implant occurs, an additional surgical stage is needed to

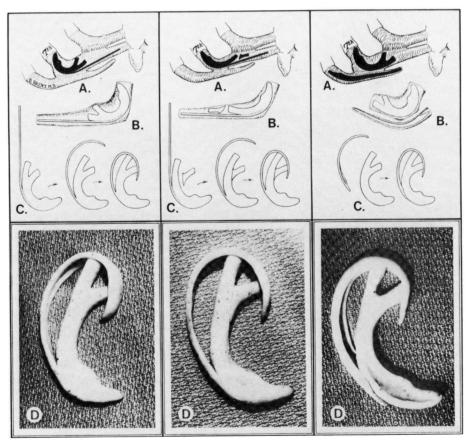

Fig. 28–3.—Brent's method of carving rib cartilage.[2] This shows three methods of fabricating the ear framework using adult size rib cartilage. The two-piece method of construction shown makes it possible to get adequate size ear cartilage even from the ribs of a 4-year-old child.

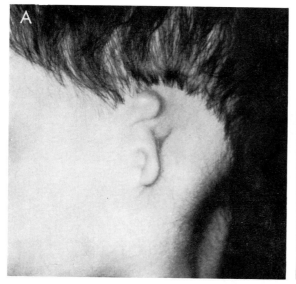

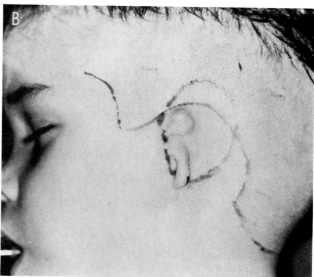

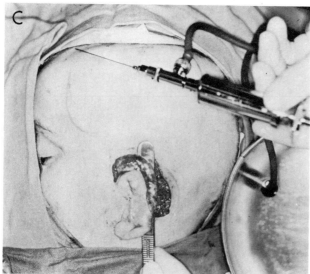

Fig. 28–4. – Class III microtia and atresia. **A,** a 3-year-old child. The right ear is normal. **B,** the hairline has been marked and also an outline to show the desired height of the reconstructed ear. This usually extends 1½–2 cm above the hairline level. **C,** at the first operation, a Silastic frame was inserted through an incision exactly at the hairline and, at that operation, a fan flap from the temporalis fascia and periosteum was reflected downward to cover the upper half of the framework. A color matching skin graft taken from the overlying shaved portion of the scalp then is used to immediately cover that portion of the framework enveloped within the fan flap. A Pipkin syringe is being used to infiltrate the scalp and thus make it easier to remove a skin graft of adequate size. *(Continued.)*

provide augmentation of the tissue overlying the implant. This protection may be provided as "insurance" along with the first-stage elevation of the ear in correction of microtia.

10. In the event of unexpected exposure of Silastic or other synthetic framework, the surgeon should resist the temptation to remove the implant immediately. Experience has shown that many (probably most) such exposed implants may be saved by appropriate use of a salvage flap, as discussed previously.[6]

Using these techniques, I have had to remove only *one* personally inserted Silastic ear frame over the past 10 years. Since 1973 at the University of Virginia, a periosteal fan flap from the temporal region[7] has been utilized *prophylactically* to cover the helix and upper half of the Silastic frame *at the time of initial insertion* of the frame (see Fig. 28–7, *B* and *C*). This prevents later exposure of the Silastic and also allows the surgeon simultaneously to place a color-matched split-thickness skin graft over the elevated helix and its covering fan flap. This fan flap also makes it unnecessary to compress the elastic ear frame against the side of the head in order to bury it in a skin-covered pocket. The evils of internal wound pressure thus are avoided and an additional operative stage is saved for the patient.

Ohmori[13] has further adapted the principle of the fan flap by using it to cover the area of the cavum and canal portions of the Silastic ear frame (where previously he had experienced most of his exposures of frame).

New Cartilage Carving Techniques

In 1974, Brent[2] published a method of ear reconstruction using an expansile framework of autogenous rib cartilage. This ingenious method (Fig. 28–3) uses a thin flexed strip of rib cartilage to create the curving wide outer rim of the helix. The technique makes it practical to obtain an adult-sized cartilage ear frame from the ribs of a 4-year-old child. Even this improved rib cartilage frame lacks the flexibility and lateral projection of the Silastic ear frame.

The Author's Current Approach to Microtia

At the University of Virginia we prefer to see the child with microtia shortly after birth. A careful examination for etiologic agents and associated defects is made. The parents are encouraged to ask questions about the cause of microtia and its correction. They are informed as to the full nature of the deformity and the therapeutic possibilities.

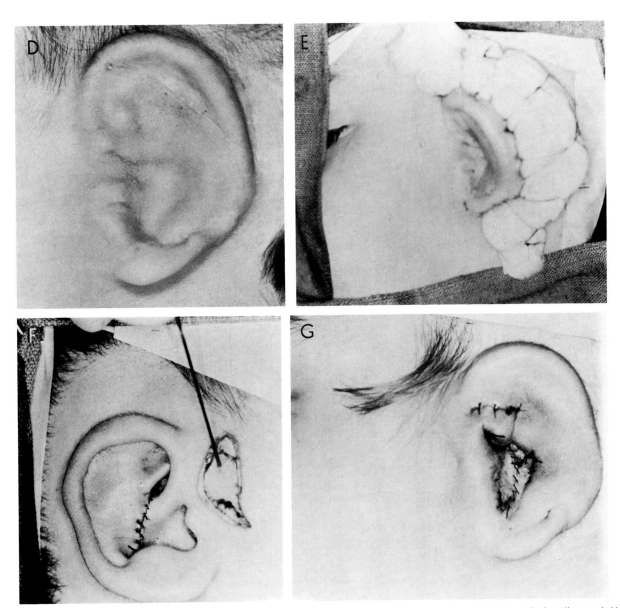

Fig. 28–4 (cont.). – **D,** this one-stage reconstruction of the ear is shown with excellent color match of the skin graft where it may be seen covering the helix and pinna. **E,** further deepening of the sulcus behind the ear may be required at a second operation in some children. Here, this skin graft is being held in position by a tie-on bolus dressing over soft cotton. **F** and **G** illustrate a method of removing a composite graft of cartilage and skin from the cavum of the opposite or normal ear. This graft may be reversed and inserted to produce a canal and cavum of relatively normal appearance in the reconstructed ear. This new canal is easily joined to the middle ear in those children where middle ear reconstruction is deemed advisable.

Baseline tests include photographs of ears and face, cephalometrograms and panorex x-rays, tomograms of the temporal bones, facial nerve testing, impedance audiometry and dental models.

The family is encouraged to believe that a satisfactory basic ear reconstruction can be obtained in two steps. Constructing an external auditory canal will require a third. If indicated, middle ear reconstruction will require a fourth operation. The otologist and audiologist will see the patient on this initial visit.

Beginning at 24–36 months of age, the child with microtia is admitted to the hospital for the first stage of ear construction. The family is given the pros and cons of both the cartilage-framework and the Silastic-frame techniques. With unilateral defects, I usually recommend use of the Silastic frame but clearly warn the family that although the Silastic frame increases the likelihood of getting a better-shaped ear, there is a slightly higher chance of wound complications (10%). If the family is unwilling to accept this risk, we proceed with the autogenous rib cartilage method, using the Brent technique of cartilage fabrication[1] (Fig. 28–3).

Regardless of which framework material is used, the ear lobe remnant is first shifted backward and cephalically, and a periosteal fan flap with an inferior pedicle is elevated in the temporal region (Fig. 28–4). This flap is reflected inferiorly to cover the helix and upper one-third to one-half of the new ear frame. A split-thickness skin graft is taken from a shaved area of the scalp and laid over the periosteum now exposed as a result of reflecting the fan flap over the helix (Fig. 28–4, C).

Stage II may be carried out 3–6 months later when the graft is soft and all edema has subsided. At this step, the posterior surface of the ear is dissected away from the mastoid bone to deepen the posterior sulcus with an additional split-thickness skin graft (Fig. 28–4, *E*).

If the microtia is bilateral, Stages I and II are carried out on both ears in just two stages by operating on both sides at each operation. When *both* external auditory canals are stenosed, the child is fitted with a bone conduction hearing aid at the *initial* visit (in one case at 2 weeks of age).

At present, the otologist on our team (Dr. Robert Jahrsdoerfer) prefers, in cases of bilateral microtia, to reconstruct the more favorable middle ear (as determined by polytomes) at about 4 years of age.[10] By that age, we expect to have already completed reconstruction of the external ears. A joint plastic-otology operation then is performed. The external ear is reflected forward (with its vascular pedicle based on the parotid and superficial temporal artery) (Fig. 28–2, *D*). The middle ear is opened with the aid of a microscope and a thin graft of skin and fascia is used to construct a tympanum. The reflected ear then is returned to its original site and local flaps are used to provide lining for the canal down to the level of the new tympanum. When properly performed in suitable cases, an excellent hearing result may be obtained. At times, a fenestration procedure may be required. The family and patient are cautioned to keep the canal clean and dry, especially after swimming.

The results of middle ear construction have been so encouraging with *bilateral* microtia that we now urge exploration of all *unilateral* cases when the anatomy (as judged by tomography of the temporal bone) appears favorable.

The medical literature suggests that a single good ear and open ear canal is adequate for language development and function. Many otologists advise against middle ear exploration of unilateral cases, citing danger to the facial nerve and postoperative canal hygiene problems as the main deterrents. We have *not* found this to be the case. Several adults with unilateral microtia have given us strong documentation of the values of binaural hearing (Fig. 28–5).

Conclusions

Excellent auricles now may be reconstructed either from carved autogenous rib cartilage or by the use of ear frameworks made from Silastic, Teflon or other suitable synthetic materials. Although poor results often have been obtained with both methods, the good results are convincing evidence that long-term dependable results may be obtained with either approach (Fig. 28–6).

In the hands of most plastic surgeons, ear construction by use of autogenous rib cartilage will be followed by fewer wound complications than occurs with Silastic frame implantation. The elasticity of a compressed and buried silicone rubber framework produces significant pressure on the overlying skin (in contrast to the nonelastic rib cartilage). This "memory" of Silastic causes it to return to its original molded form and will lead to extrusion when the slightest error is made in surgical technique. That same quality of elasticity gives Silastic frame ears a better shape and flexibility than is possible to obtain with carved costal cartilage.

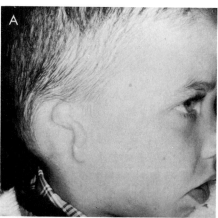

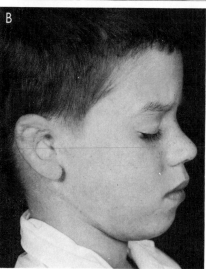

Fig. 28–5.—Right-sided unilateral microtia with some hypoplasia of the ramus of the right mandible and some deficiency of parotid tissue. **A,** at 6 years, before operation. **B** and **C,** result after a three-step reconstruction of the right ear utilizing a cervical skin tube for the additional skin covering for the upper half of the ear. *(Continued.)*

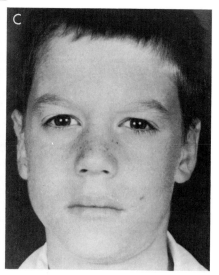

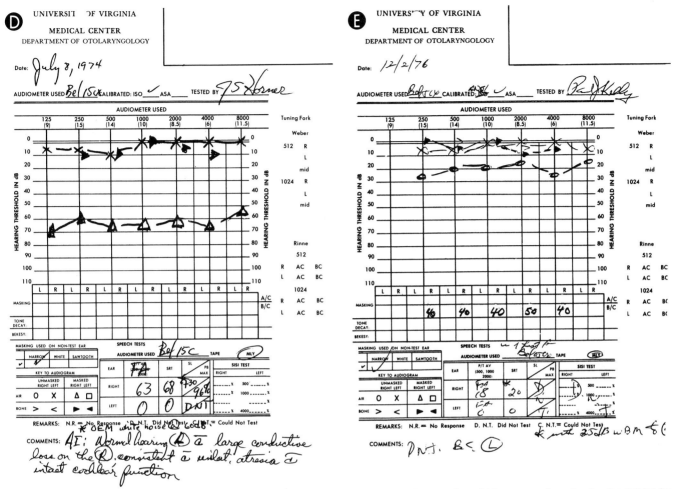

Fig. 28–5 (cont.). – **D,** audiogram on the same patient at 16 years of age, with a marked conductive hearing loss in the right ear. Middle ear reconstruction was performed at that time in a joint plastic and otologic operation.

E, audiogram 2 years after middle ear operation, showing the striking improvement in hearing.

For a time, surgeons believed that the tissues of some individual children would not chemically "tolerate" Silastic, thus leading to extrusion. The author and Dr. C. Bacchetta[6] have been able to show that nearly all children who develop exposure of Silastic may be salvaged by correction of the technical errors that led to the skin breakdown. A true tissue "allergy" to silicone rubber is almost unknown. Clearly, better and more widespread applications of the laws of surgical implants will continue to yield increasingly lower complication rates with each passing year. The routine use of the periosteal fan flap is a new technique that already has reduced the number of complications in our cases.[7]

In Japan, Ohmori[13] and Fukuda[8] already have reported large series of successful ear reconstructions using synthetic ear frameworks (and with only a 10% complication rate). I predict that U. S. surgeons will increasingly turn to the use of synthetic ear frameworks as the number of good results reported continues to increase. If a Silastic frame does not give difficulty during the first 6 months after operation, it is extremely rare for complications to appear later. We now have followed successful synthetic ear framework implants in several children for more than 17 years (Fig. 28–7).

New concepts are emerging in regard to treatment of deafness resulting from the stenosed external auditory canal and deformed middle ear with microtia. The hearing loss almost always is a conductive loss, but in a few instances nerve deafness may coexist and must be detected before operation is undertaken. When canal stenosis is bilateral, most otologists urge the exploration and reconstruction of at least one ear at a very early age. Our own experiences at Virginia would indicate that, in many instances, *even the patient with a unilateral* microtia is a proper candidate for middle ear reconstruction (Figs. 28–2 and 28–5).

Binaural hearing is immensely superior to monaural hearing! We predict that other clinics will increasingly attempt to reconstruct the middle ears of children with unilateral microtia. This will occur naturally as more otologists develop sufficient experience with the difficult anatomic dissections of the deformed temporal bones seen in congenital microtia.

Ear reconstruction still is a difficult challenge for plastic surgeons. The surgeon must have much experience and knowledge if he is to avoid the many pitfalls that await him. Close partnership with a temporal-bone otologist and a pediatric audiologist is essential. If other professionals involved in a craniofacial center are at hand, so much the better.

Some of the most demanding ear construction problems are in children with hemifacial microsomia. In these cases, the microtia is associated with hypoplasia of the mandible and temporomandibular joint, a missing parotid gland, dis-

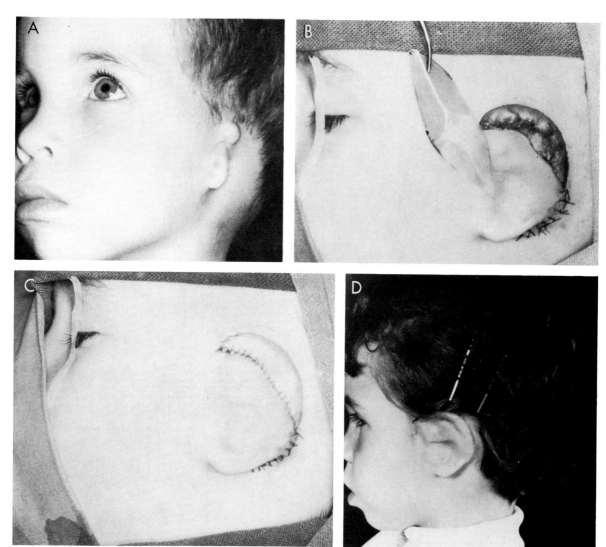

Fig. 28–6.—Four-year-old boy with Class III microtia and stenosis of the left external auditory canal. **A,** appearance before operation. **B** and **C,** at stage one, a Silastic ear framework was inserted through a hairline incision and the ear lobe was rotated downward and backward. At stage two, the framework has been elevated and a periosteal fan flap has been taken from beneath the adjacent scalp region and is folded over the exposed portion of the framework. At this stage, the x-ray film pattern is used to mark out a full-thickness skin graft from the postauricular surface of the opposite ear. This graft is immediately laid over the fan flap, as shown in **C. D,** satisfactory result of this two-stage reconstruction of the external ear. Since this boy is a candidate for middle ear reconstruction, we will defer opening the external auditory canal until his temporal bone growth makes him an ideal candidate for the middle ear procedure.

placed mastoid and small temporal squama, a sometimes paralyzed facial nerve and, in some cases, paper-thin cheek skin. These children need the full services of a craniofacial center.

The reconstruction of the missing ear must, in such cases, be coordinated with the total program of child rehabilitation. Eyelid function, breathing problems or jaw reconstruction may demand attention before one turns to the ear. The small mastoid-parotid complex causes a concavity on the side of the head that may require build-up before starting ear construction. Nevertheless, if the family and child are motivated to undergo the multiple steps required, ear construction should be satisfactory even in children with these complex and multiple deformities.

Only a few years ago a well reconstructed human ear was a rarity. Today there are many reasons for optimism about ear reconstruction. Progress in the use of the miniaturized implantable hearing aids with lifetime batteries soon may further improve the prospects of gaining normal hearing.

REFERENCES

1. Brent, B.: Personal communication, July 28, 1974.
2. Brent, B.: Ear reconstruction with an expansile framework of autogenous rib cartilage, Plast. Reconstr. Surg. 53:619, 1974.
3. Converse, J. M.: On hemifacial microtia. The first and second branchial arch syndrome, Plast. Reconstr. Surg. 51:258, 1973.
4. Cronin, T. D.: Use of a Silastic frame for total and subtotal reconstruction of the external ear: Preliminary report, Plast. Reconstr. Surg. 37:399, 1966.
5. Edgerton, M. T.: Ear reconstruction in children with congenital atresia and stenosis, Plast. Reconstr. Surg. 43:373, 1969.
6. Edgerton, M. T., and Bacchetta, C. A.: Principles in the Use and Salvage of Implants in Ear Reconstruction, in Tanzer, R. C., and Edgerton, M. T. (eds.), *Symposium on Reconstruction of the Auricle* (St. Louis: The C. V. Mosby Company, 1974), p. 58.
7. Fox, J. W., and Edgerton, M. T.: The fan flap: An adjunct to ear reconstruction, Plast. Reconstr. Surg. 58:663, 1976.
8. Fukuda, O.: In Ohmori, S. (ed.), *Plastic Surgery (Keisei-Geka)* (Tokyo: Nanko-do Publishing Co., 1968).
9. Hajnis, K.: *Growth of the External Ear in German Population and Its Use in the Surgery of Congenital Defects* (Prague: Academia, Publishing House of Czechoslovak Academy of Sciences, 1971).

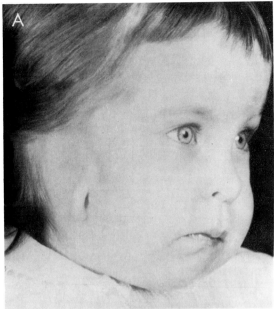

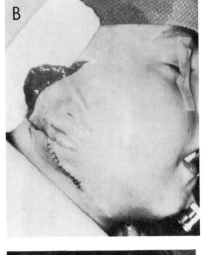

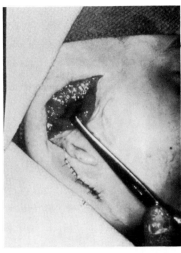

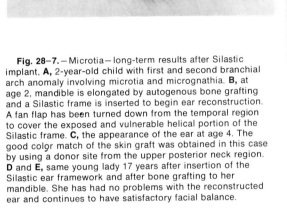

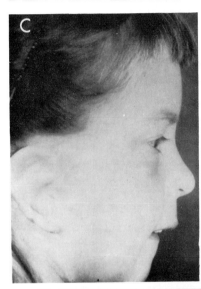

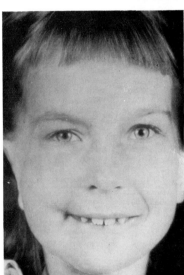

Fig. 28–7.—Microtia—long-term results after Silastic implant, **A,** 2-year-old child with first and second branchial arch anomaly involving microtia and micrognathia. **B,** at age 2, mandible is elongated by autogenous bone grafting and a Silastic frame is inserted to begin ear reconstruction. A fan flap has been turned down from the temporal region to cover the exposed and vulnerable helical portion of the Silastic frame. **C,** the appearance of the ear at age 4. The good color match of the skin graft was obtained in this case by using a donor site from the upper posterior neck region. **D** and **E,** same young lady 17 years after insertion of the Silastic ear framework and after bone grafting to her mandible. She has had no problems with the reconstructed ear and continues to have satisfactory facial balance.

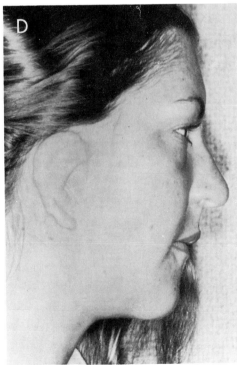

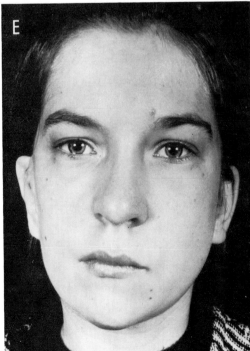

10. Jahrsdoerfer, R. A.: Congenital Ear Atresia, in Tanzer, R. C., and Edgerton, M. T. (eds.), *Symposium on Reconstruction of the Auricle* (St. Louis: The C. V. Mosby Company, 1974), p. 150.
11. Kaseff, L. G.: Investigation of congenital malformations of the ears with tomography, Plast. Reconstr. Surg. 39:282, 1967.
12. Ohmori, S.: Use of Silicone Rubber Frame for the Reconstruction of Microtia Cases, in *Transactions of 5th International Congress of Plastic Reconstructive Surgery* (Sydney, Australia: Butterworths, 1971), p. 467.
13. Ohmori, S.: Congenital deformities of the auricle, Clin. Plast. Surg. 1:3, 1974.
14. Rogers, B. O.: Rare Craniofacial Deformities, in Converse, J. M. (ed.), *Reconstructive Plastic Surgery* (Philadelphia: W. B. Saunders Company, 1964), p. 1213.
15. Tanzer, R. C.: Total reconstruction of the external ear, Plast. Reconstr. Surg. 23:1, 1959.
16. Tanzer, R. C.: Total reconstruction of the auricle: A 10-year report, Plast. Reconstr. Surg. 40:547, 1967.
17. Tanzer, R. C., and Edgerton, M. T. (eds.): *Symposium on Reconstruction of the Auricle* (St. Louis: The C. V. Mosby Company, 1974).

29 F. I. CATLIN

Otolaryngologic Disorders

Surgery of the Tonsils and Adenoids

History

EXCISION of the tonsils was mentioned as early as 1000 B.C. in the Hindu literature.[28] Later ancient medical writers, including Hippocrates, Galen and Celsus,[7] described partial tonsillectomy for chronic infection and for symptoms of airway obstruction. Complete faucial tonsillectomy was performed seldom because of the high incidence of severe or even fatal postoperative hemorrhage. The use of caustics and live cautery was popular in the eighteenth century, but the advent of general anesthesia in the nineteenth century produced a return to the guillotine techniques of excision. Surgical removal of the tonsils and adenoids as performed today is a procedure perfected since 1900 and is estimated to be done over 2 million times a year in the United States.[21]

Evaluation for Surgery of Tonsils and Adenoids

The purpose of the tonsil and adenoid operation is to remove the diseased tissues with minimal anesthetic risk, with least discomfort to the patient, with as little tissue damage as possible and with few, if any, postoperative complications.

Considerable difference of opinion prevails regarding the indications for tonsillectomy and adenoidectomy. Many unfavorable results can be avoided by adequate preliminary evaluation of the patient and observance of the correct indications for operation.

The anatomic relationships of the tonsils and adenoids have certain peculiar aspects that must be considered. Proctor[21] lists four factors of importance: (1) The surfaces of the tonsils and adenoids are exposed to ingested or inhaled foreign material. (2) The tonsil and adenoid crypts are very near adjacent capillaries. (3) A rich lymphatic connection exists between the tonsils, the adenoids and the regional lymph nodes. (4) The tonsils and adenoids are closely related to the oropharynx, esophagus, nasopharynx, eustachian tubal orifices, nasal passages and paranasal sinuses.

The most common childhood diseases of the tonsils and adenoids are acute and chronic infections, secondary extension of microorganisms or toxins into the lymphatics or bloodstream or direct spread of infection to the nose, paranasal sinuses, eustachian tubes, middle ear or lower respiratory tract and enlargement of the tonsils and adenoids, with obstruction of the airways.

A complete and careful history may be the major factor in the decision to operate. Attention should be directed to the incidence and severity of upper respiratory infections, tonsillitis, obstructive symptoms (as from nasal obstruction, mouth breathing and eustachian tube obstruction), otalgia, otorrhea, otitis media, cervical adenitis and bronchitis. Pertinent questions in the history should include general health and hygiene, system review, allergies, operations and injuries, drug and food sensitivity, prior infectious disease, developmental and family history.

The physical examination should include an evaluation of general development and health status, plus a thorough inspection of the neck, cervical glands, ears, nose, nasopharynx, pharynx, hypopharynx, paranasal sinuses, and tests of hearing acuity.

Indications for Operation

INDICATIONS FOR ADENOIDECTOMY. — Adenoidectomy alone is indicated when symptomatic adenoid disease is present without tonsil infection. Acute adenoid infection may cause fever, sinusitis and recurrent otitis media. Adenoid enlargement causes symptoms of obstruction — mouth breathing, snoring, nasal voice, accumulation of nasal secretions and frequent head colds. Blockage of the eustachian tube orifices may produce conductive hearing impairment and/or chronic otitis media.

The child with chronic adenoiditis may present the so-called adenoid facies, with open mouth, high palatal arch and pinched appearance of the middle third of the face. The ears may show signs of middle ear inflammation or infection, with dull, retracted and slightly thickened tympanic membranes and inflammation or fluid in the middle ear.[26] Anterior rhinoscopy shows accumulated secretions. Examination of the nasopharynx may show a large mass of adenoid tissue covered by mucopurulent discharge. The adenoids often fill the nasopharynx, producing signs of obstruction.

In children under 4 years of age, chronic adenoiditis may

occur without chronic infection of the tonsils, and adenoidectomy is the operation of choice, even when one or two attacks of acute tonsillitis have occurred. Removal of both tonsils and adenoids in very young children often stimulates hyperplasia of other lymphoid elements in the oropharynx. Recurrent inflammation of such tissue is difficult to treat and may cause persistent sore throat. In children over 4 years, chronic adenoiditis as a rule is accompanied by chronic tonsillitis, and tonsillectomy with adenoidectomy is necessary.

Several conditions must be differentiated from chronic adenoiditis. Tornwaldt's disease, or infected nasopharyngeal bursa, may produce a chronic nasopharyngeal infection without adenoid hypertrophy. The diagnosis usually is made by examination but, in some patients, only after adenoidectomy.

Retropharyngeal abscess may be confused with a large adenoid mass and should be suspected if a large nasopharyngeal swelling is seen in an acutely ill child who has had a previous adenoidectomy. The abscess is soft and fluctuant, in contrast to lymphoid tissue, and must be examined with *extreme gentleness* in order to avoid rupture, with discharge of the abscess contents into the larynx.

Partial or complete choanal atresia may be confused with obstruction of the posterior nares by adenoids. Passage of a nasal catheter usually will rule out its presence. The posteri-

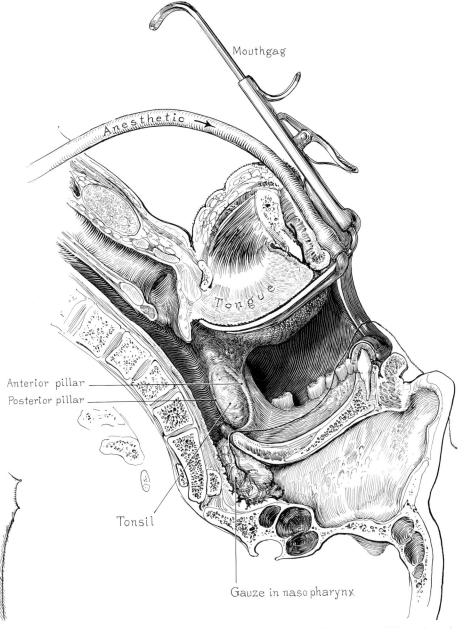

Fig. 29–1. – Tonsillectomy – exposure and packing. The patient is recumbent, the foot of the table slightly elevated. A gauze pack in the nasopharynx prevents saliva, vomitus or blood from entering the nasopharynx. The operator, wearing a headlight, stands at the end of the table. By placing the tongue depressor a little to the right or left of the median line of the tongue, an excellent view of the operative field on that side is obtained. (Figs. 1–5 courtesy of the Department of Art as Applied to Medicine, Johns Hopkins University School of Medicine; from original drawings by Max Brödel for the paper by S. J. Crowe *et al.*[8])

or choanae should be checked for patency during every adenoidectomy.

Adenoid remnants may hypertrophy and require secondary removal. Small amounts of lymphoid tissue about the eustachian tube can produce secondary conductive hearing loss or otitis media. In such instances, the nasopharyngeal strontium-90 applicator technique has been recommended by Boniver and Garson,[5] although the possibility of carcinogenic effects causes many physicians to question use of this form of therapy.[2]

INDICATIONS FOR TONSILLECTOMY.—Whereas chronic adenoid infection may occur alone, chronic tonsillitis in children almost always is associated with chronic adenoiditis. The symptoms of chronic tonsillitis range from frequent recurrent episodes of acute infection to less clearly recognized complaints, such as swelling of the cervical glands or difficulty in swallowing. The chronically infected tonsil may

be enlarged or small, scarred and smooth-surfaced as the result of obliteration of the crypts by infection. The pillars often show capillary injection of their mucosal surfaces. In the course of acute tonsillitis, organisms may break through the tonsil capsule to form a peritonsillar abscess, causing trismus. Most children with chronic tonsillitis exhibit enlarged cervical lymph nodes, especially those at the angle of the mandible.

Indications for the combined operation:
1. Chronic recurrent tonsillitis.
2. Peritonsillar abscess (quinsy).
3. Nasal airway obstruction from hypertrophic adenoids, in association with chronic tonsillitis.
4. Oropharyngeal obstruction. I have personally seen 5 children within the past 4 years with pulmonary hypertension and cor pulmonale secondary to chronic oral and nasal airway obstruction by enlarged tonsils and adenoids.[16]
5. Conductive hearing impairment or recurrent ear

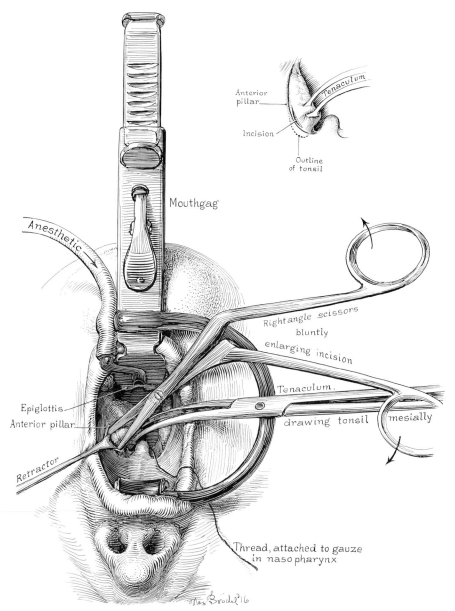

Fig. 29–2.—Tonsillectomy—dissection. The upper pole of the tonsil is gently pulled toward the midline. An incision then is made through the mucous membrane just mesial to the anterior pillar *(inset).* A retractor may be inserted as shown in the large drawing in order to provide better exposure.

infection. Adenoidectomy performed for sensorineural hearing impairment in children who do not have chronic infection is condemned.

6. Nephritis, rheumatic fever, iritis and certain other systemic diseases.[26]

7. Congenital cardiovascular anomalies, which may predispose to bacterial endocarditis.

8. Diphtheria carriers.

9. Recurrent sinusitis, bronchiectasis, asthma and chronic cough are suggested indications with little merit, unless one of the preceding indications is present.

Contraindications to Adenoidectomy and Tonsillectomy

1. Hemophilia and other blood dyscrasias.

2. Disturbances of the bleeding and clotting mechanisms that resist correction.

3. Active pulmonary tuberculosis, uncontrolled diabetes, acute nephritis and active rheumatic fever.

4. General debility.

5. A concurrent epidemic of poliomyelitis in the local community.[1, 9, 11, 22]

6. Acute bacterial illness and the acute exanthemata.

7. Peritonsillar hemangioma.

8. Tumors of the tonsil or nasopharynx, which should be treated either by more extensive operation or by irradiation.

9. Cleft palate. Palatal surgery should precede adenoidectomy and tonsillectomy. Closure of the palate may reduce recurrent eustachian salpingitis and otitis media, or the adenoid tissue may be essential for effective closure of the nasopharynx during deglutition.

10. Congenitally short palate and/or submucous cleft. When palatal closure is incomplete or barely effective, adenoidectomy is contraindicated. In less severe cases, partial adenoidectomy may be considered. Tonsillectomy, if needed, must be performed carefully to reduce secondary scarring.[4]

Preoperative Care

In a survey of 1447 certified otolaryngologists during 1968–1970, Pratt[19] reported 377 fatal cases in 6,175,729 tonsillectomies and adenoidectomies, an incidence of 0.006%. The cause of death was reported to be equally divided into three factors: anesthesia (0.002%), cardiac arrest (0.002%) and postoperative hemorrhage (0.002%).

All candidates for tonsillectomy and adenoidectomy should have a complete history and physical examination as well as adequate laboratory studies, including admission hemogram, prothrombin time, partial thromboplastin time and urinalysis. Foods and liquids should be withheld for 8 hours to avoid vomiting with aspiration. Scopolamine or atropine is given to inhibit respiratory secretions. If the child is likely to be restless or agitated, sedation may be required, using Nembutal, Demerol or Vistaril.

Anesthesia

Tonsillectomy anesthesia is difficult and hazardous; 40% of the deaths studied by the Baltimore Anesthesia Study Commission were associated with difficulties in anesthesia.[21] Student anesthetists, frequently assigned to tonsillectomy and adenoidectomy cases, must be adequately supervised.

Inhalation anesthesia is generally preferred for children. The level of anesthesia should be only sufficiently deep to permit relaxation of the pharyngeal and palatal muscles. Thereafter, the level may be lightened to reduce the likelihood of tracheal aspiration.

Endotracheal intubation should not be an all-or-none practice. The majority of pediatric tonsillectomies can be handled safely without intubation, provided that both surgeon and anesthesiologist safeguard the airway.[9, 12]

Halothane is the anesthetic agent of choice, except in patients with a history of hepatitis.

Operation

Careful adenoid curettage and surgical dissection of the tonsil, adequate hemostasis, gentle handling of tissues and an anesthetic technique that will safeguard the airway are fundamental principles. The use of a properly fitting mouth gag with the patient in the Trendelenburg position will, by elevation of the base of the tongue, maintain an adequate airway and furnish dependent drainage of secretions or blood to the nasopharynx (Figs. 29–1–29–5). Efficient suction must be constantly available—from the start of anesthesia until the patient leaves the operating room.

Adenoidectomy by curettage is best performed prior to

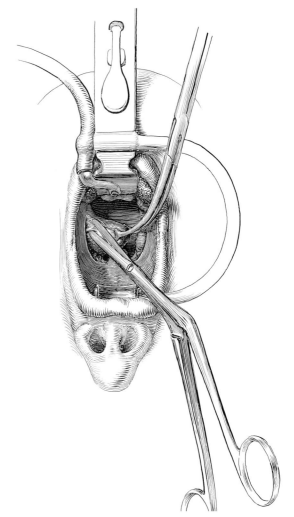

Fig. 29–3.—Tonsillectomy–dissection. The tonsil is removed by a combination of sharp and blunt dissection, made as close as possible to the capsule of the tonsil and carried down to the lower pole, where the tonsil may be severed by scissors or a snare.

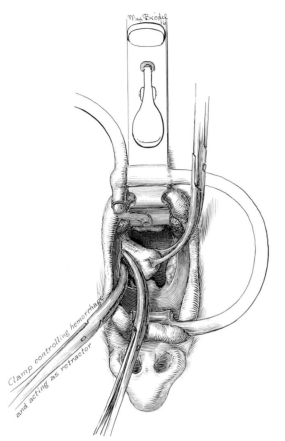

Fig. 29–4. – Tonsillectomy – hemostasis. Every bleeding vessel is clamped as in any surgical operation. This ensures a dry field and lessens the danger of postoperative pulmonary complications.

tonsillectomy so that the nasopharynx can be observed for continuing hemorrhage during the remainder of the operation. Following adenoidectomy, a tagged sponge usually will control bleeding and may remain until the end of the operation.

After operation, the patient is placed in a semiprone position, with the head turned to the side (Fig. 29–6). Hemorrhage occurs in about 1.2–5% of reported cases.[8, 18] Constant nursing attendance, with suction and oxygen nearby, is necessary until the child can handle his own secretions and is in satisfactory condition. The nurse should save all expectorated blood and watch for swallowing of blood, especially in young children. When swallowing movements are observed, when pallor is pronounced or the pulse rate rises, the pharynx should be examined at once.

Pain may be controlled by codeine, acetaminophen or aspirin and seldom is severe beyond the second postoperative day. An ice collar may provide some comfort. Prolonged pain may be an index of secondary complications and deserves investigation.

No nourishment is given orally until the child is able to swallow liquids without danger of aspiration. Parenteral fluids may be necessary,[10] especially in hot weather. Hot, spicy, very acid or rough foods should be avoided for the first 5–7 days. The child's activities should be restricted for the first 2 or 3 days,[15] with a gradual return to normal during the next week. Swimming is not advisable until the tonsil fossae are healed – normally in about 2 weeks.

Complications

Most of the complications following tonsillectomy and adenoidectomy are related to the healing process. The tonsil fossae and adenoid bed become coated with a yellow-white septic membrane that gradually is replaced by granulation tissue in about 1 week, and then by regenerated mucous membrane. Delay in healing may result from diabetes or malnutrition or virulent secondary infection. Any child on steroid therapy is maintained on steroids until healing has occurred.

Severe sore throat postoperatively may result from operative trauma, secondary infection or an impending exanthem. Antibiotics sometimes reduce the soreness by control of the secondary bacterial infection. Earache frequently follows tonsillectomy and adenoidectomy. The ears usually appear normal, in which case the pain is assumed to be of the referred type via Jacobson's nerve to the middle ear. Warm oily ear drops sometimes are beneficial.

Hemorrhage, the most frequent complication of tonsillectomy, occurs early (in the first 24 hours) or late (from the fifth to tenth day). Most early hemorrhage can be avoided by me-

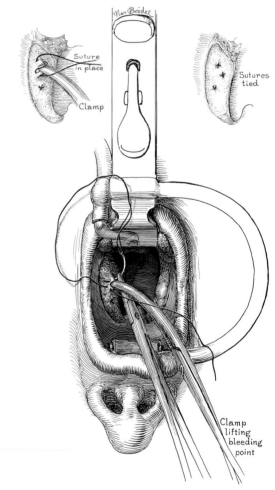

Fig. 29–5. – Tonsillectomy – hemostasis: method of ligating bleeding vessels. Note the small amount of tissue included in the clamp. The sutures are transfixed as superficially as possible and snugly tied. Several operators have found 00 plain catgut to be the best suture material. Because of the possibility of slippage, the ends of the catgut suture should be left somewhat longer than shown in the small illustrations.

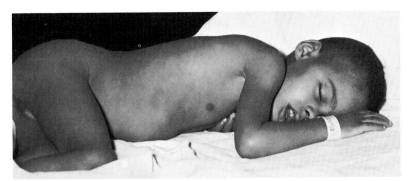

Fig. 29–6.—Tonsillectomy—postanesthesia position. The patient should remain in the semiprone position until fully recovered from the anesthesia. The upper leg and arm may be placed over a pillow to prevent his rolling onto his face. In this position, with head extended, the airway will remain open because the tongue and jaw will fall forward. Secretions and vomitus will tend to run out of the mouth instead of being aspirated. Oxygen, suction and constant nursing care are necessary until the patient is fully awake.

ticulous hemostasis in the tonsil fossae[17] or by the use of a nasopharyngeal pack for adenoid bleeding.

If postoperative bleeding is not controlled after removal of clots from the fossa and the application of gentle pressure with a sponge, the child should promptly be taken to the operating room and anesthetized. The bleeding point then is identified and transfixed. Most patients with postoperative hemorrhage should have blood typing and crossmatching as a precautionary measure.

Late postoperative hemorrhage, usually 7–10 days after operation, results from sloughing of the granulation membrane or tonsil sutures. Parents should be advised to watch for bleeding at this time. The treatment is similar to that for immediate hemorrhage. Procrastination or use of local agents is poor treatment for "tonsil bleeders." Prompt, positive treatment lessens or avoids the possibility of anemia, shock, excessive instrumentation, ingestion of blood and delayed postoperative recovery.

Uncommon complications include lung abscess, cervical emphysema[20] and parapharyngeal abscess.

Follow-up examinations are recommended at 2 weeks, 6 months and 1 year, in order to ascertain the condition of the patient and the value of the operation. Shaikh, Vayda and Feldman[23] report that most tonsillectomy data are of limited value. In 29 reports, only 5 exhibited fair study design; only 10 showed an adequate sample, all were poor in description of illness and treatment and in only 2 was there an adequate follow-up.

Indiscriminate tonsillectomy subjects children to unnecessary risks and discomfort. Tonsillectomy for good indications returns to good health children who previously have been repeatedly or chronically ill.[27]

REFERENCES

1. Anderson, G. W.: Tonsillectomy and poliomyelitis, JAMA 184: 80, 1963.
2. Anon.: Thyroid cancer increase linked to x-ray exposure, Med. News, JAMA 236:2478, 1976.
3. Bateman, G. H., and Kodicek, J.: Primary quinsy tonsillectomy, Ann. Otol. Rhinol. Laryngol. 68:315, 1959.
4. Berner, R. G.: Hazards of adenotonsillectomy in the child with cleft palate, JAMA 181:558, 1962.
5. Boniver, R., and Garson, J.: Beta therapie tubaire par sonde de strontium pour les otites recidivantes, Acta Otorhinolaryngol. Belg. 28:996, 1974.
6. Brain, D. J.: Cryosurgery in benign conditions of the nose and throat, Proc. R. Soc. Med. 67:72, 1974.
7. Celsus: De Medicino, translated by W. G. Spencer (Cambridge, Mass.: Harvard University Press, 1935), Vol. 3, p. 371.
8. Crowe, S. J., et al.: Relation of tonsillar and nasopharyngeal infections to general systemic disorders, Bull. Johns Hopkins Hosp. 28:1, 1917.
9. Davies, D. D.: Anesthetic mortality in tonsillectomy and adenoidectomy, Br. J. Anaesth. 36:110, 1964.
10. Faigel, H.: Tonsillectomy—a bloody mess, Clin. Pediatr. 5:652, 1966.
11. Fischer, A. E., et al.: Poliomyelitic paralysis and tonsillectomy, JAMA 186:873, 1963.
12. Graff, T. D., Holzman, R. S., and Benson, D. W.: Acid-base balance during halothane anesthesia for tonsillectomy, Anesth. Analg. 43:620, 1964.
13. Grahne, B.: Abscess tonsillectomy, Arch. Otolaryngol. 68:332, 1958.
14. Harly, S., and Aastrup, J.: Cryosurgery—principles and applications to tonsillectomy, Acta Radiol. (supp.) (Stockh.) 313:254, 1972.
15. Heasmon, M. A.: How long in hospital? A study in duration of stay for two common conditions, Lancet 2:539, 1964.
16. Luke, M. J.: Chronic nasopharyngeal obstruction as cause of cardiomegaly, cor pulmonale, and pulmonary edema in children, Pediatrics 37:762, 1966.
17. Magielski, J. E.: Electrocautery hemostasis in tonsil and adenoid surgery under Fluothane (halothane) anesthesia: 1,054 cases, Laryngoscope 73:595, 1963.
18. Parkinson, R. H.: Tonsil and Allied Problems (New York: The Macmillan Company, 1951).
19. Pratt, L.: Tonsillectomy and adenoidectomy morbidity and mortality, Trans. Am. Acad. Ophthalmol. Otolaryngol. 74:1146, 1970.
20. Pratt, L. W., Hamberger, H. R., and Moore, V. J.: Mediastinal emphysema complicating tonsillectomy and adenoidectomy, Ann. Otol. Rhinol. Laryngol. 71:158, 1962.
21. Proctor, D. F.: The Tonsils and Adenoids in Children (Springfield, Ill.: Charles C Thomas, Publisher, 1960).
22. Ravenholt, R. T.: Poliomyelitic paralysis and tonsillectomy reconsidered, Am. J. Dis. Child. 103:658, 1962.
23. Shaikh, W., Vayda, E., and Feldman, W.: A systematic review of the literature on evaluation studies of tonsillectomy and adenoidectomy, Pediatrics 57:401, 1976.
24. Volk, B. M., and Brandow, E. C., Jr.: Bilateral tonsillectomy for peritonsillar abscess, Laryngoscope 70:840, 1960.
25. Von Leden, H., and Rand, R. W.: Cryosurgery of the head and neck, Arch. Otolaryngol. 85:93, 1967.
26. White, P. D.: Heart Disease (3d ed.; New York: The Macmillan Company, 1946).
27. Wilson, I. I.: A review of the indications for tonsillectomy, N. Z. Med. J. 61:603, 1962.
28. Wise, T. A.: Review of the History of Medicine (London: J. & A. Churchill, Ltd., 1967), Vol. 2, p. 225.

Surgical Treatment of Hearing Impairment

Operation on the ear is performed for four major purposes: (1) to eradicate progressive disease, (2) to combat life-threatening otic conditions, (3) to modify hearing function and (4) to improve external appearance (see Chap. 28). Surgical procedures designed to modify hearing impairment currently are directed at pathology of the external and middle ear. Those designed to improve hearing by modification of inner ear pathology still are under experimental investigation.

Surgery of Congenital Abnormalities of the Ear

Only certain types of congenital ear anomalies are amenable to operation. In the classification derived from Fraser, four principal types of congenital cochlear disorders are described:[7, 10] (1) the Michel type, characterized by complete failure of development of the internal ear, (2) the Mondini-Alexander type with labyrinthine development arrested after the 6th or 7th month of gestation, (3) the Bing-Siebenmann type, in which a normal bony labyrinth is found in association with maldevelopment of the membranous inner ear, and (4) the Scheibe or cochleosaccular type, in which there is a varying degree of malfunction of the cochlear sensory epithelium. In the last two categories, a limited amount of hearing may exist. Two other categories are described that have malformations other than the inner ear:[5] (5) the Siebenmann type with malformations of the external and middle ear and (6) atresia of the external auditory canal alone.

OPERATIVE INDICATIONS AND CONDITIONS.—As a rule, the condition must be bilateral. The operative hazards, particularly with regard to the facial nerve, are so great that it seldom is justifiable to operate in the unilateral case. Shambaugh[23] and Edgerton (see Chap. 28) believe that unilateral deformities can be benefited enough to justify operation.

Inner ear function should be normal as demonstrated by bone conduction audiometry. Operation should be deferred until the child is old enough to cooperate in audiometry. Brain-stem-evoked-response[12, 25] and cortical-evoked-response audiometry may be of assistance despite the conductive problem. Tomograms always should be taken and should show a normal bony inner ear.

SURGICAL TREATMENT.—Correction of an external auditory canal stenosis or atresia often is successful (see Chap. 28). Further operative procedures will depend on the condition of the middle ear. In the absence of a stapes footplate and round window, the chance for improvement of hearing is poor. The creation of a canal to the inner tympanic wall may permit the use of an ear mold for a hearing aid, provided that inner ear function is adequate (Figs. 29–7–29–11).

Surgery for Infectious Disease

ANATOMIC CONSIDERATIONS.—The primary route for extension of infection to the mastoid cells is by way of the eustachian tube. Early infection may prevent the development of the normal mastoid air-cell structure and result in a sclerotic or infantile mastoid. Various theories of mastoid development have been reviewed by Fowler.[6]

The child is more susceptible to otitis media than is the adult. Nasal secretions are more likely to enter the eustachian tube in the younger child because the infantile eustachian tube is straight, horizontal and relatively patulous, and the tubal orifice lies at the level of the palate and assumes a more superior and posterior position in the nasopharynx only as growth of the face proceeds. In addition, enlargement of the adenoids and adjacent lymphoid tissue in childhood may occlude the eustachian tube, or adenoid infection may, by direct extension, involve the eustachian tube and middle ear.

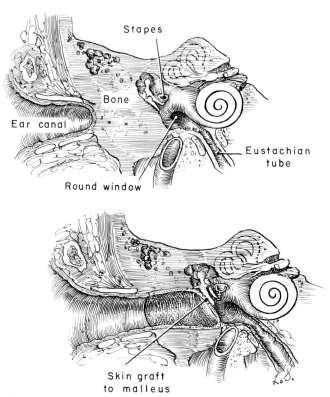

Fig. 29–7.—*Above,* tympanic bony malformation with mobile ossicles. *Below,* repair by skin graft to malleus, (Figs. 7–11 redrawn from Goodhill.[10])

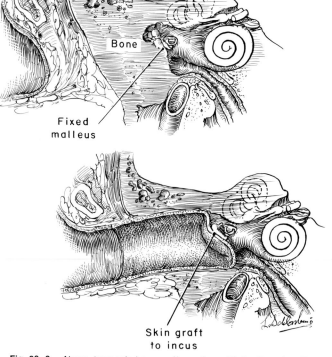

Fig. 29–8.—*Above,* tympanic bony malformation with fixation of malleus. *Below,* repair by skin graft to incus.

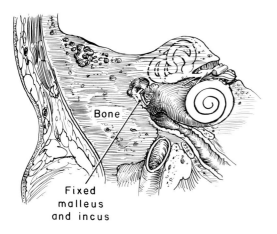

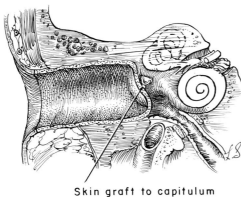

Fig. 29–9.—*Above*, tympanic bony malformation with fixed malleus and incus. *Below*, repair by skin graft to capitulum of the stapes.

SEROUS OTITIS MEDIA.—Chronic serous otitis media is common in children with enlarged tonsils and adenoids and may occur secondary to upper respiratory infection. Allergic factors have been implicated in some cases; air pollution factors have been suggested in others. Occasionally, chronic serous otitis media follows adenoidectomy because of scarring about the eustachian tubal orifice. In children, tumor of the nasopharynx must infrequently be considered in the differential diagnosis.[4]

The *signs* and *symptoms* of serous otitis media include decreased hearing, a sense of fullness and pressure in the affected ear and occasionally tinnitus or pain. Symptoms may be particularly inapparent in young children.

The tympanic membrane usually is slightly retracted and dusky blue, dark red or amber. The audiogram shows a conductive type of hearing impairment. Radiographs of the temporal bone may reveal diffuse clouding in the affected mastoid cells.

The *treatment* of serous otitis media is primarily directed toward removal of underlying causative factors, such as enlarged adenoids; nasal allergy is a factor in about 25% of cases and is managed by antihistamines or desensitization plus nasal decongestants. Every child should be followed to ensure that the otitis has cleared. In persistent cases, myringotomy with aspiration of the middle ear fluids may be necessary, and inflation of the middle ear can be helpful.[16]

If the middle ear fluid obtained during myringotomy is thin and watery, the condition often will improve following aspiration alone. If the fluid is thick and mucoid, recurrence

of fluid is observed commonly. The transtympanic, *pressure-equalizing (P.E.)* tube frequently is used in such instances to permit prolonged aeration of the middle ear cavity for a period of 6–12 months. Complications of P.E. tube use include: middle ear infection, blockage of the tube orifice, persistent perforation of the drum membrane, intrusion of the tube into the middle ear (instead of the usual extrusion into the external auditory canal) and growth of epithelium (cholesteatoma[9]) into the middle ear.[8, 14] The more serious complications are uncommon, and marked improvement of hearing acuity usually is observed following P.E. tube insertion in children of school age.

PURULENT OTITIS MEDIA.—Acute suppurative otitis media is a purulent infection involving the middle ear space and adjacent cells in the mastoid bone. The most common infecting organisms are Pneumococcus, *Hemophilus influenzae* and *Streptococcus pyogenes*.[21] Purulent otitis media usually results from an acute upper respiratory infection.

The *signs* and *symptoms* of acute purulent otitis media are: a sensation of fullness in the ear, decrease of hearing, otalgia and fever. As the infection progresses, pain becomes more severe and tinnitus may appear. The tympanic membrane bulges at first in the pars flaccida, and later the entire membrane is pushed outward with loss of all landmarks except the malleus. In late stages, the membrane may become whitish or yellow and a pulsating discharge may be seen if spontaneous perforation has occurred.

The audiogram or tuning fork tests will show a conductive

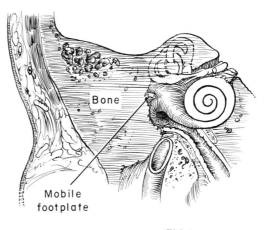

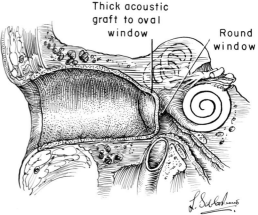

Fig. 29–10.—*Above*, tympanic bony malformations with deformed fixed malleus, incus and crus but with mobile footplate. *Below*, repair by skin graft to oval window, sealing it from the round-window niche.

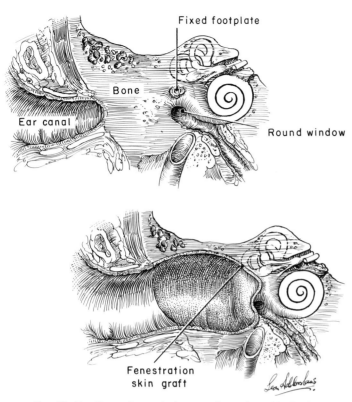

Fig. 29–11.—*Above,* tympanic bony malformation with fixed stapes footplate. *Below,* repair by skin graft to fenestrated horizontal semicircular canal.

hearing impairment and, in general, mastoid radiographs will reveal diffuse clouding of the mastoid air cells, with intact septae.

The *treatment* of acute otitis media depends on the stage of the infection. When signs of middle ear pressure, such as severe pain, are absent and the tympanic membrane is not bulging, antibiotics, nasal decongestants and anodynes, including glycerin-base ear drops, may be sufficient.

When the middle ear infection has progressed to the state of severe pain with bulging of the tympanic membrane, myringotomy, preferably in anteroinferior quadrant, is performed to relieve pressure. The entire thickness of the membrane should be incised and the opening made large enough to permit good drainage. Cultures of the discharge should be taken. If the middle ear already is discharging, the otologist must make certain that the spontaneous opening is adequate for drainage. Aural medication rarely is needed after myringotomy.

Antibiotic therapy must be sufficient to combat the infection adequately and should be continued until the infection is resolved.[19] Mastoiditis should be suspected if otorrhea persists more than 2 weeks.

CHRONIC OTITIS MEDIA.—Many patients with chronic ear disease exhibit perforation of the tympanic membrane with or without aural discharge. When the ear does not respond to topical and systemic therapy, chronic mastoid infection or cholesteatoma in the middle ear or mastoid must be suspected.

Operation for chronic otitis media should be based on the following principles: (1) The chronic disease must be eliminated completely and complications prevented. (2) A closed tympanic cavity must be constructed, properly ventilated through the eustachian tube. (3) At the same time, a system must be created for conduction of acoustic stimuli through the middle ear to the cochlea. The surgical procedure will be modified according to the extent of damage to the middle ear structures. *Tympanoplasty*[28] is contraindicated when complications of the middle ear infection are a danger to life or when there is inadequate function of the inner ear, so that improvement of sound conduction in the middle ear will be without result. Such contraindications include infection of the meninges or lateral sinus, cholesteatoma of the inner ear and severe sensorineural hearing loss. According to the Wullstein[28] classification (Fig. 29–12), Types I, II and III not only furnish protection for the round window but, as far as possible, restore the impedance-matching characteristics of the middle ear structures. Types I and II preserve the attic and ossicular chain, and Type III produces the so-called columellar effect. Types IV and V only provide protection of the round window.

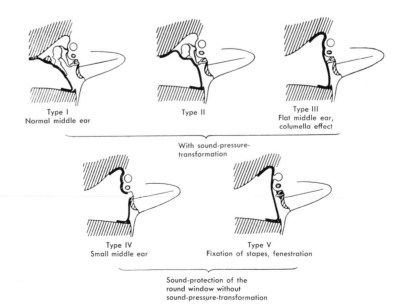

Fig. 29–12.—Conditions offering protection of the various inner ear structures. (Courtesy of H. Wullstein.[28])

TABLE 29 – 1.—LATE RESULTS OF TYMPANOPLASTY°

TYPE OF TYMPANOPLASTY	PREOPERATIVE STATUS OF EAR			
	Discharging Ear		Dry Ear	
	Social Hearing† (SRT 0 – 30 db)	Success‡	Social Hearing† (SRT 0 – 30 db)	Success‡
Type I	73%	83%	83%	92%
Type II	47%	72%	73%	80%
Type III	27%	50%	57%	84%
Type IV	17%	35%	43%	—

° After Tos.[24]
† SRT: Speech reception threshold in decibels.
‡ Success (functional) defined as: social hearing, or air-bone gap, 15 db or improved mean hearing (500 – 2000 Hz), 20 db or obtained speech reception threshold of 30 db or better by speech audiometry.

Successful tympanoplasty with improvement of sensitivity for air-conducted sound most frequently is obtainable when the structures of the middle ear are relatively intact, as in Type I (Fig. 29 – 12). In Type II and more often in Type III, ideal results are fewer and, in Types IV and V, become theoretically impossible. Late results of tympanoplasty reported by Tos,[24] after a postsurgical interval of 2 – 10 years, are summarized in (Table 29 – 1). Note that results are much better for tympanoplasty Types I and II than for Types III and IV; also, that the hearing is better when the preoperative ear is dry. Some of the causes of poor postoperative results cited by Proctor[22] are: (1) graft perforation, (2) frequent presence of sensorineural loss, (3) impaired window function due to increased stiffness from scars, (4) adherence of the tympanic membrane to the promontory, (5) neural loss of more than 10 db, (6) inadequate postoperative eustachian tube function with obliteration of the cavum tympani, (7) graft cholesteatoma, (8) recurrent cholesteatoma, (9) persistence of residual bone infection, (10) nonadherence of the shifted tympanic membrane, (11) progressive necrosis of the stapes and (12) fracture of the stapes. Proctor concluded: "Tympanoplasty is performed to control infection, to prevent recurrent infections and to prevent progression of disease which would result in further hearing loss. The patient should be told that hearing improvement is often minimal and that it may even become worse."

Glasscock[9] followed 90 patients for more than 1 year after an intact canal wall tympanoplasty and noted closure of the air-bone gap within 10 db in 50% and within 20 db in 80%. Glasscock commented that his intact canal wall techniques are not the same as the Wullstein procedures and, therefore, the results cannot be directly compared.

Mastoiditis

Acute mastoiditis generally is a complication of acute otitis media and less commonly results from chronic otitis media. The most frequent causative organisms are Pneumococcus, Hemophilus influenzae, Streptococcus pyogenes and Klebsiella pneumoniae.[21] Two pathologic forms are seen: the coalescent type associated with breakdown of the mastoid air cell walls and the hemorrhagic or thrombophlebitic type, which has been seen more frequently since antibiotics have come into general use.

The frequency of acute mastoiditis has decreased markedly since the introduction of chemotherapeutic agents. Davison[3] noted an incidence of 3% of cases with acute otitis media requiring mastoidectomy in 1954, in contrast to an incidence of 58.9% in 1937. This change is attributed to arrest of the middle ear infection before extension into the mastoid bone has occurred.

The signs and symptoms of acute mastoiditis include otorrhea, pain and tenderness over the mastoid bone, conductive hearing impairment, fever and roentgenographic evidence of cloudiness of the mastoid cells, usually with breakdown of the cellular structure, although this is not always present in fulminating infections. In mild infections, the only symptom may be persistent otorrhea following acute otitis media of 3 weeks' duration, but in more virulent disease, rapid bone destruction with subperiosteal abscess or intracranial complications may appear before otorrhea is present.[1] Bozer[1] and Hoople[13] noted that in many cases of mastoiditis, rupture of the tympanic membrane occurred or myringotomy was performed late in the course of the infection.

Complications of acute mastoiditis arise from spread of the infection to adjacent areas, by direct extension or by a propagating thrombophlebitis. The most common complications are postauricular subperiosteal abscess, preauricular abscess, Bezold abscess in the upper neck, facial paralysis and, occasionally, benign intracranial hypertension. Involvement of the posterior or middle fossa surfaces may produce epidural abscess, meningitis[26] or brain abscess.[18] Extension to the inner ear may produce a serous or suppurative labyrinthitis. Spread to the petrous apex will produce petrositis, often associated with sixth nerve paralysis (Gradenigo's syndrome).[1, 3, 17, 20]

The prognosis for complications of mastoiditis and of acute otitis media has improved since the use of antibiotics. Broydøy and Ellekjaer[2] note a recovery rate of 84% in 1972 for otitic meningitis—a rate comparable to Watson's[25] 84.6% in 1944 (in contrast to 19.6% in 1922). As might be expected, morbidity has increased as death rates decline.[27]

MASTOIDECTOMY.—Simple mastoidectomy is essentially a postauricular incision and drainage procedure (Fig. 29 – 13). The cortex is exposed with a periosteal elevator from the posterior border of the bony external auditory meatus to about 1 cm behind the skin incision. The mastoid cortex and the infected mastoid cells are removed. The antrum is exposed, but the attic space is not entered. A drain is placed in the cavity and brought out through the lower part of the skin incision, which then is closed. Myringotomy is performed if needed. In patients with intracranial complications, exposure of the lateral sinus, middle cranial or posterior cranial fossae may be necessary.

Operations for Ear Trauma

Certain types of aural trauma require surgical intervention. Removal of a foreign body or cerumen impacting the external auditory canal may immediately improve hearing.

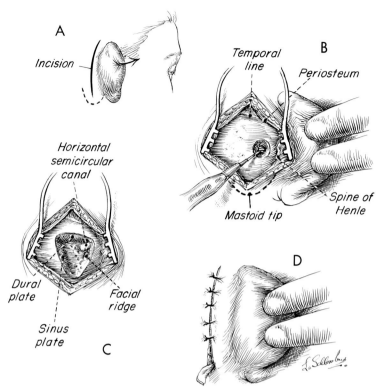

Fig. 29–13.—Simple mastoidectomy. **A,** the usual postauricular incision. **B,** reflection of soft tissue from the mastoid cortex. The spine of Henle on the posterior aspect of the bony external auditory canal represents the approximate level at which excavation of the mastoid bone has begun. **C,** limits of excavation in a simple mastoidectomy: the dural plate of the middle cranial fossa, lateral sinus, facial ridge and horizontal semicircular canal. **D,** closure of the wound. The mastoid cavity has been filled with a drain and a large opening left in the lower part of the incision to provide adequate drainage.

Perforations of the tympanic membrane may follow head trauma. If the perforation is a simple slit, healing usually occurs. A large flap-type rupture may require careful repositioning for satisfactory healing. In some instances, damage to the ossicles may occur without tympanic membrane perforation. If a fracture occurs through the cochlea or if the stapes is driven into the vestibule, vestibular signs may be present: nausea, vomiting and occasionally cerebrospinal fluid drainage through a tympanic membrane perforation or through the eustachian tube into the nose. Facial paralysis may occur in temporal bone fractures, and exploration of the mastoid and repair of the facial nerve are necessary. If a conductive hearing impairment has resulted from trauma and the tympanic membrane is intact, acoustic impedance studies should be undertaken to determine whether or not there is an ossicular disarticulation. Prophylactic antibiotic therapy is indicated in most instances of traumatic injury. In all cases of aural trauma, an otologic examination should be obtained, and audiologic and vestibular function studies as indicated.

Surgery for Tympanosclerosis and Otosclerosis

Otosclerosis is not a disease of very young children. In Guild's[11] series of 1161 routine autopsies, the incidence of otosclerosis in children under 5 was less than 0.6%. In persons over 5 years of age, the incidence was approximately 4%. Occasionally, tympanosclerosis secondary to otitis media is found in children with a conductive hearing impairment that mimics the clinical picture of otosclerosis. After otologic, audiologic and radiologic studies, exploratory tympanotomy may be required.

REFERENCES

1. Bozer, H E.: A study of surgical mastoiditis occurring in children at the Buffalo Children's Hospital during the year 1945 and 1946, N. Y. J. Med. 48:183, 1948.
2. Broydøy, B., and Ellekjaer, E. F.: Otogenic meningitis: A five-year study, J. Laryngol. Otol. 86:871, 1971.
3. Davison, F. W.: Otitis media—then and now, Laryngoscope 65: 142, 1955.
4. Draper, W. L.: Secretory otitis media in children: A study of 540 cases, Trans. Am. Laryngol. Rhinol. Otol. Soc., p. 346, 1964.
5. Dublin, W. B.: *Fundamentals of Sensorineural Auditory Pathology* (Springfield, Ill.: Charles C Thomas, Publisher, 1976).
6. Fowler, E. P., Jr.: *Medicine of the Ear* (2d ed.; Baltimore: The Williams & Wilkins Company, 1948).
7. Fraser, J. F.: Studies in the etiology of congenital deafness (abstract), Clin. Res. 10:212, 1961.
8. Glasgold, A. I.: Cholesteatoma following myringotomy and ventilation tubes, E.E.N.T. Month. 53:274, 1974.
9. Glasscock, M. E.: Ossicular chain reconstruction, Laryngoscope 86:211, 1976.
10. Goodhill, V.: *The Modern Educational Treatment of Deafness* (Manchester, England: Manchester University Press, 1960).
11. Guild, S. R.: Histologic otosclerosis, Ann. Otol. Rhinol. Laryngol. 53:246, 1944.
12. Hecox, K., and Galambos, R.: Brain stem auditory evoked responses in human infants and adults, Arch. Otolaryngol. 99:30, 1974.
13. Hoople, G.: In discussion of Bozer.[1]
14. Hughes, L. A., Warden, F. R., and Hudson, W. R.: Complications of tympanostomy tubes, Arch. Otolaryngol. 100:151, 1974.
15. Jerger, J., and Hayes, D.: The cross-check principle in pediatric audiometry, Arch. Otolaryngol. 102:64, 1976.
16. Kapur, Y. P.: Serous otitis media in children, Arch. Otolaryngol. 79:38, 1964.
17. Korkis, F. B.: Suppurative mastoid surgery yesterday and today, Lancet 2:833, 1954.
18. Kornblut, A. D.: Cerebral abscess—a recurrent otologic problem, Laryngoscope 82:1375, 1971.

19. Lumio, J. S.: Contributions to the knowledge of chronic adhesive otitis, Acta Otolaryngol. (Stockh.) 39:196, 1951.
20. Morse, H. E.: Intracranial complications of chronic mastoiditis, Arch. Otolaryngol. 63:142, 1956.
21. Palva, T., Friedman, I., and Palva, A.: Mastoiditis in children, J. Laryngol. 78:977, 1964.
22. Proctor, B.: What happens in Type III tympanoplasty, Trans. Am. Laryngol. Rhinol. Otol. Soc., p. 396, 1965.
23. Shambaugh, G. S.: *Surgery of the Ear* (2d ed.; Philadelphia: W. B. Saunders Company, 1967), p. 410.
24. Tos, M.: Late results in tympanoplasty, Arch. Otolaryngol. 100: 302, 1974.
25. Watson, D.: Progress in the treatment of mastoid infection and some of its complications, Proc. R. Soc. Med. 41:155, 1948.
26. Whitaker, C. W.: Intracranial complications of ear, nose and throat infections, Laryngoscope 81:1375, 1971.
27. Wright, J., and Grimaldi, P.: Otogenic intracranial infections, J. Laryngol. Otol. 86:1085, 1973.
28. Wullstein, H.: The restoration of the function of the middle ear in chronic otitis media, Ann. Otol. Rhinol. Laryngol. 65:1020, 1956.

Choanal Atresia

Congenital atresia of the posterior nares occurs infrequently. Ersner[5] estimated a bilateral incidence of about 1 per 60,000 persons. The low incidence and resultant unfamiliarity with the symptoms of the anomaly have permitted many cases to escape detection and diagnosis. Recent revival of interest in the correction of this anomaly has resulted in uncovering a substantial number of individuals so afflicted and has improved diagnostic techniques.

The causation of choanal atresia has not been satisfactorily explained. Theories of the mechanisms leading to choanal atresia were reviewed by McKibben[9] and others.[8]

The obstruction consists of a partition attached superiorly to the body of the sphenoid, laterally to the medial pterygoid process, medially to the posterior edge of the vomer and inferiorly to the horizontal plate of the palatine bone (Fig. 29–14). The obstruction may be little more than a membranous septum or may be a solid mass of bone, or bone and cartilage. Each surface is covered with mucous membrane continuous with that of the nasal and nasopharyngeal surfaces. Minute perforations may be present but usually are nonfunctional. The obstructed side is characteristically associated with narrowing of the nasal and nasopharyngeal cavities due to elevation of the palatal arch, a more medial position

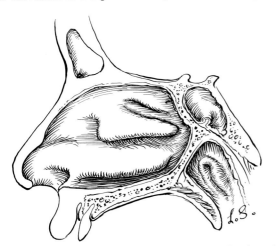

Fig. 29–14.—Choanal atresia. Sagittal section of the head, made just lateral to the vomer, illustrating an extreme form of choanal atresia with dense bony obstruction between the posterior end of the palate and body of the sphenoid. This is the usual site of choanal atresia, but occlusion by membranes or more delicate bony tissue is more common. The obstruction may be unilateral or bilateral.

of the medial pterygoid process and an anterior position of the posterior nasopharyngeal wall. Associated malformations are cited by McKibben.[9]

Symptomatology

INFANTS.—*Cyclic dyspnea.*—Newborn infants ordinarily do not acquire the mechanism of mouth breathing until several days after birth. Dependent as they are on the nasal airway, they may succumb to asphyxia in the presence of bilateral atresia. The term cyclic dyspnea applies to the recurring phases of asphyxia followed by crying, mouth breathing, quiet, then asphyxia again. Feeding usually is impossible in these circumstances.

Dyspnea while suckling.—In some cases, symptoms of suffocation occur only when suckling is attempted, and oral breathing is necessarily impossible. These infants must learn to suck and breathe alternately.

Absence of dyspnea.—An occasional such case has been reported.

OLDER PATIENTS.—The signs and symptoms of complete nasal obstruction are present: mouth breathing, absence of nasal quality to the voice, poor sense of smell and taste and excessive nasal discharge of mucus or tears. Inability to blow the nose is noted, and dryness of the mouth may be annoying.

As a rule, unilateral atresia is unnoticed until later life unless the patent nostril becomes blocked, as in feeding, for example. The symptoms on the obstructed side are nasal obstruction and secretion.

Diagnosis

Whenever an infant has difficulty in breathing and cannot nurse, the differential diagnosis should include choanal atresia, tracheoesophageal fistula, vocal cord paralysis, foreign body, tumors or other obstructive lesions in the nose or nasopharynx. Improved breathing after insertion of an oral airway will suggest the presence of an upper airway obstruction. Many patients show atrophy and underdevelopment of the turbinates, narrowing of the nasal passages and a high arched palate.

Inability to pass a small catheter through the nostrils into the pharynx is strong evidence that the choanae are obstructed. Posterior obstruction of the nasal cavity may be demonstrated by instillation of iodized oil into the nose and roentgenography of the head, with patient supine. In older patients, the obstruction may be seen by anterior and/or posterior rhinoscopy when the accumulated nasal mucus has been removed. In small children, examination under anesthesia may be necessary in order to confirm the nature of the obstruction.

Treatment

The treatment of choanal atresia depends on the severity of symptoms.

Infants with bilateral choanal atresia, who are unable to breathe by mouth, must be provided with an adequate oral airway until mouth breathing has been established or until operative cure has been effected. Constant nursing attendance is necessary to safeguard the airway. Almost all of these infants require feeding by medicine dropper, spoon or stomach tube until they learn to nurse. Operation on the atresia is performed in most of the severe instances within the first few weeks of life. In some infants, bilateral atresia does not cause serious symptoms and may remain unnoticed until later in childhood. As in unilateral atresia, the correction of the anomaly may be performed when convenient.

OPERATIVE REPAIR.—The operative procedure varies according to the age of the patient, the type of occluding tissue and the condition of the nasal structures.[3]

The direct intranasal route for the cure of atresia, the oldest surgical approach, is used today chiefly for the correction of membranous obstructions. The atretic membrane is curetted away and a polyethylene stent inserted between the nose and nasopharynx. The stent remains in place until healing has occurred, on the average in 2–3 months.[11]

The submucous intranasal approach for bony atresia has been used primarily for adults, but with good results reported in some children as young as 2 years.[7] The technique involves incision of the mucosal wall of the inferior nasal septum and floor of the nasal cavity. A tunnel thus is created that is carried back to the bony atresia plate and the mucous membrane overlying the plate elevated in continuity with that of the nasal mucosa. The bony block then is perforated with a chisel and the opening enlarged with rongeurs. The mucosal flap then is returned to its normal position and the mucosa formerly over the bony blocks is incised by flap or cruciate incision, in order to cover exposed bony surfaces. A polyethylene stent is inserted through the nose into the nasopharynx and retained until healing has occurred.

In most infants and small children with bony atresia, the transpalatal approach, first used in the United States by Blair,[2] has been advocated because of the excellent field of view. A palatal flap is created to expose the posterior palatal margin. Owens[10] includes the palatal vessels in the flap in order to preserve the blood supply. Removal of part of the hard palate exposes the obstruction, which is removed by rongeurs or bur. Mucosal flaps from the vomer and anterior and posterior surfaces of the obstruction are used to cover the bony surfaces left exposed by removal of the bony wall. The palatal flap then is returned to its place.

The chief problem in relief from choanal atresia has been postoperative stenosis, which occurs after even slight scar formation because of the narrowness of the nasal passages. Secondary stenosis may be minimized in two ways: (1) enlargement of the posterior choanae by removal of part of the lateral wall of the septum[12] and (2) the use of mucosal flaps to cover exposed bony areas.[4, 10, 11] The use of stents has been subject to debate. In our experience, a properly fitting stent is essential for good postoperative results.

Few large series have been recorded. Johnson[6] listed 2 failures and 9 cures in patients treated by the transpalatine operation. Since few surgeons see this many patients, the need for careful evaluation and handling should be recognized in every choanal atresia that comes to operation regardless of the method of repair selected.

REFERENCES

1. Beinfield, H. H.: Surgical management of complete and incomplete bony atresia of the posterior nares, Trans. Am. Acad. Ophthalmol. Otolaryngol. 60:778, 1956.
2. Blair, V. P.: Congenital atresia or obstruction of air passages, Ann. Otol. Rhinol. Laryngol. 40:1021, 1931.
3. Cherry, J., and Bordley, J. E.: Surgical correction of choanal atresia, Ann. Otol. Rhinol. Laryngol. 75:911, 1966.
4. Dolowitz, D. A., and Holley, E. B.: Congenital choanal atresia, Arch. Otolaryngol. 49:587, 1949.
5. Ersner, M. S.: In discussion of Beinfield.[1]
6. Johnson, S.: Congenital choanal atresia, Acta Otolaryngol. 51:533, 1959.
7. Kazanjian, V. H.: The treatment of congenital atresia of the choanae, Ann. Otol. Rhinol. Laryngol. 51:704, 1942.
8. Lemere, H. B.: Persistent bucconasal membrane in the newborn, JAMA 109:347, 1937.
9. McKibben, B. G.: Congenital atresia of the nasal choanae, Laryngoscope 67:731, 1957.
10. Owens, H.: Observations in treating 7 cases of choanal atresia by the transpalatine approach, Laryngoscope 61:304, 1951.
11. Weseman, C. M.: Management of choanal atresia in the newborn, Laryngoscope 83:1160, 1973.
12. Wright, W. K., Shambaugh, G. E., Jr., and Green, L.: Congenital choanal atresia: A new surgical approach, Ann. Otol. Rhinol. Laryngol. 56:120, 1947.

The Infant Larynx

The common signs of laryngeal disease in early childhood are respiratory obstruction, stridor or abnormal quality of the voice and, less often, aspiration of mucus, food, or both, into the larynx. Stridor may result from extrinsic causes. Only the intrinsic causes of surgical significance will be considered here. Additional information is available in the chapters on tracheostomy (Chap. 39) and endoscopy (Chap. 45). A review of differences between the infant and adult larynx explains why stridor so often is the presenting sign of laryngeal disease in children.

Anatomic Differences

1. SIZE.—The principal anatomic difference between the infant and adult larynx is size (Fig. 29–15). The cross-sectional area of the infant larynx and trachea is relatively smaller than that of the adult when related to total body mass. The greatest narrowing occurs in the subglottic region. Before a diagnosis of congenital stenosis can be established, it is necessary to correlate the size of the infant with the lumen of his larynx. The glottic dimensions in the infant are approximately 7 mm anteroposteriorly by 4 mm across the posterior commissure. The V-shaped glottic airway during inspiration measures about 14 sq mm. It is important to note that edema of 1 mm of the mucosa will reduce the area by 5 sq mm, to about 35% of the original lumen, which will predispose the young child to stridor.

2. CONSISTENCY.—In young children, all laryngeal tissues are softer than in the adult. The cartilages are softer and more pliable and the mucosa is looser and less fibrous. The relatively narrow lumen and the softness and laxity of the

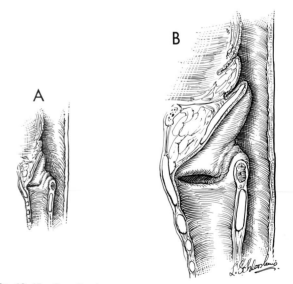

Fig. 29–15.—Growth changes of the larynx. **A,** the 5-week-old infant larynx; **B,** the adult larynx.

TABLE 29-2.—TRACHEAL DIAMETERS FROM
WOOD'S METAL CASTS°

AGE, MO.	NO. OF CASES	TRACHEAL DIAMETER, Mm			
		Abt		Engel	
		Sagittal	Coronal	Sagittal	Coronal
0-1	11	3.6	5.0	5.7	6.0
1-3	35	4.6	6.1	6.5	6.8
3-6	37	5.0	5.8	7.6	7.2
6-12	25	5.6	6.2	7.0	7.8

°After Engel.[3]

infant's larynx are important causes of stridor when the laryngeal tissues are further narrowed by inflammation and edema.

3. POSITION.—The high larynx of the infant descends continuously during development. In the fetus of 5-6 weeks, the larynx is situated opposite the basiocciput, but by the 4th month, the lower border of the cricoid cartilage lies opposite the upper border of the 4th cervical vertebra. At 7 months, the larynx has descended to the middle of the 6th vertebra and is found in this position at term. After birth, further descent occurs until, in adult life, the lower border of the cricoid cartilage lies opposite the lower border of the 6th cervical vertebra and the tip of the epiglottis, which marks the upper border of the larynx, lies opposite the lower border of the 3d cervical vertebra.[9]

According to Wilson,[13] the higher position of the infant's larynx results in a line of entry of air current that is straighter than in the adult and the epiglottis is less overhanging. In later life, when the larynx has descended to its final position, the axes of the pharynx, larynx and trachea meet at a more acute angle. As Wilson noted, not all authors accept this theory, and the effect of position on the production of stridor is subject to question.

4. SHAPE.—The upper end of the larynx and trachea is funnel-shaped in the infant. This shape disappears in the older child and adult female but reappears in a modified form in the adult male, in whom the backward tilt of the cricoid cartilage is replaced by a forward tilt of the thyroid cartilage. The tracheal lumen, however, no longer diminishes as it descends, as in the infant. Measurements by Tucker[12] indicate that the newborn subglottic diameter is 6 mm; narrowness is indicated by a 5 mm diameter and definite stenosis when the diameter is 4 mm or less. There is no uniform agreement as to the relationship of tracheal and laryngeal diameters. Studies by Engel[3] and Bayeaux[2] suggest that the cricoid internal diameter probably is the narrowest portion of the airway, although in the newborn, the tracheal diameter may not be very much larger (Tables 29-2 and 29-3).

The vocal folds are shorter in the infant than in the adult. The epiglottis overhangs the vestibule less than in the adult and is narrower and generally U-shaped. In addition, the

TABLE 29-3.—AIRWAY DIAMETERS FROM ANATOMIC
SECTIONS AND MOULAGE°

AGE, MO.	GLOTTIS, Mm	CRICOID RING, Mm	TRACHEA, Mm
4	23-26	20	22-25
6	26	20	24
8	24	21	24
10	25	22	26
13	25	22	26

°After Bayeaux.[2]

ventricular air sacs of infants are relatively larger in relation to other laryngeal structures than in the adult.

Indications for Laryngeal Surgery

Respiratory obstruction and hoarseness (or abnormal cry) are the two principal indications for laryngoscopy in infants. Other indications include tracheal aspiration and esophageal (or suspected esophageal) obstruction. The reader is referred to the chapters on endoscopy (Chap. 45) and tracheostomy (Chap. 39) for further details.

Causes of Laryngeal Stridor in Infancy

The causes of stridor are intrinsic and extrinsic. Wilson's[13] classification is shown in Tables 29-4 and 29-5. The laryngeal causes of stridor in infancy may be classified under the headings of: congenital anatomic abnormalities; tumors and cysts; inflammatory conditions; neurologic abnormalities; trauma and foreign bodies.

Most intrinsic and some extrinsic conditions that require surgical intervention are diagnosed and treated by endoscopic techniques with or without tracheostomy.

Congenital anatomic abnormalities of the larynx that cause stridor include laryngomalacia, bifid epiglottis, congenital stenosis and cleft larynx.

Laryngomalacia is a benign condition that usually disappears by age 2½ and seldom requires surgical intervention.[1] Tracheostomy has been performed in instances of extreme respiratory obstruction, which is unusual. The symptoms appear at birth or soon after and include attacks of inspiratory stridor (often initiated by an external stimulus), cervical soft tissue retraction and a low-pitched sound that ends, at the cessation of the stridor, with the child exhausted and pale. The attack often is precipitated by placing the child supine. Cyanosis is infrequent and only temporary. The diagnosis is made by direct laryngoscopy. The epiglottis is long and tapering, with its lateral folds rolled posteriorly so as to form a long slit. The aryepiglottic folds are closely apposed and are forced together by any but the slightest inspiratory flow of air. The usual treatment is anticipatory, with gentle handling and positioning of the child plus avoidance of sudden shocks or changes in temperature.

Bifid epiglottis is rare. When laryngeal obstruction is produced by this deformity, tracheostomy and subsequent amputation of the epiglottis have been required.

Congenital *laryngeal webs*, an important cause of stridor in infancy, vary in size from complete laryngeal occlusion, incompatible with life, to a small membranous band across the anterior commissure. Primary symptoms are a poor cry, a weak or aphonic voice and stridor, which may be inspiratory or both inspiratory and expiratory. Feeding problems, dyspnea and cyanosis may also be noted. When the symptoms are mild, the web probably should be left alone. Large webs

TABLE 29–4.—INTRINSIC CAUSES OF LARYNGEAL STRIDOR IN INFANCY°

CONGENITAL ANATOMIC ABNORMALITIES	TUMORS AND CYSTS	INFLAMMATORY CONDITIONS	NEUROLOGIC ABNORMALITIES	TRAUMA	FOREIGN BODY
Laryngomalacia	Papilloma of larynx	Acute laryngitis	Tetany	Birth injury	Vegetable
Bifid epiglottis	Laryngeal cysts	Acute laryngo-tracheo-bronchitis	Neonatal tetany	Post-natal injury	Nonvege-table
Congenital laryngeal stenosis and webs		Diphtheria; postdiph-theritic stenosis	Recurrent nerve paralysis		
Cleft larynx		Exanthema; exanthemata (e.g., measles) and pertussis			
		Tuberculosis			

°After Wilson.[13]

require division, the chief difficulty encountered being re-formation of the web by scar formation. Suspension of a plate between the cords, insertion of a laryngeal stent and tissue grafting to cover the raw surface of the cords[2, 7, 8] have been utilized to prevent this.

Cleft larynx, caused by failure of separation of the larynx and trachea from the esophagus by the 7th or 8th week of gestation, may result in a persistent esophagotrachea. This rare condition was first described in 1792 by Richter.[11] The deformity may vary from a minor deepening of the interary-tenoid cleft in the body of the cricoid cartilage to a wide cleft extending as far as the bifurcation of the trachea (Fig. 29–16). Successful repair of the latter type of deformity has been reported.[10] Tracheoesophageal fistula has been report-ed in association with cleft larynx and may obscure identifi-cation of the cleft. Symptoms include stridor after birth, as-piration after feeding, with cyanosis and subsequent pneu-monia. Clinically, the picture is similar to that of tracheo-esophageal fistula. The larynx is examined and, in the case of small clefts, may be mistakenly interpreted as being normal. If tracheotomy is performed, the child may regurgitate through the tracheostoma. The child fails to thrive, has re-peated respiratory infections and usually dies in early infan-cy from aspiration of food. The diagnosis is best established by direct laryngoscopy. Aspiration may be confirmed by cine-fluorographic studies of the larynx during the act of swal-lowing. Small clefts undoubtedly pass unrecognized; the larger defects require closure of a posterior laryngeal or la-ryngotracheal defect to prevent repeated aspiration pneu-monitis.[5]

Tumors and cysts of the larynx may produce infantile stri-dor. *Papillomas* may be particularly troublesome. The con-dition is not usually seen under 2 years of age. The papillo-mas may be confined to the larynx or may extend above or below the glottic region. Treatment consists of local remov-al, although a variety of therapeutic regimens have been tried in the past, including local use of escharotics, local hormone applications, radiotherapy, antibiotic and steroid therapy and artificial puberty.

Juvenile laryngeal papillomas tend to proliferate about or on the vocal cords, and go into spontaneous remission espe-cially near puberty. In a few instances, the course is aggres-sive, with growth into the trachea requiring tracheotomy for relief from airway obstruction. These have a poorer progno-sis. In general, the less aggressive types should be treated conservatively in an effort to do as little permanent damage as possible while maintaining an airway.

The management of *inflammatory lesions* of the larynx is largely nonoperative except for those instances in which tra-cheostomy is indicated—viz., acute epiglottitis. Laryngo-scopic removal of crusts in diphtheria was advocated by the Jacksons.[6]

TABLE 29–5.—EXTRINSIC CAUSES OF STRIDOR IN INFANCY°

CONGENITAL ANATOMIC ABNORMALITIES	TUMORS AND CYSTS	INFLAMMATORY CONDITIONS	FOREIGN BODY
Dysphagia lusoria (vascular ring)	Hyperplasia of the thymus	Thymic abscess	In the esophagus
Tracheoesophageal fistula	Cystic hygroma	Retro- and parapharyngeal abscess	
Tracheomalacia	Thyroglossal cysts	Mediastinal adenitis, as in mononucleosis	
Congenital goiter			

°After Wilson.[13]

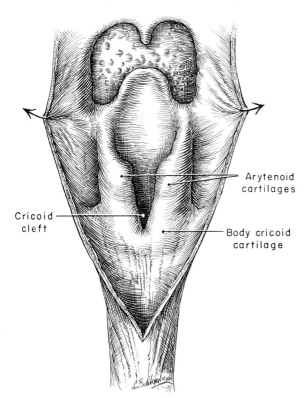

Fig. 29–16.—Laryngeal cleft viewed from behind, the esophagus opened. Newborn larynx with a cleft extending part way through the cricoid cartilage. In extreme cases, the cleft continues between esophagus and trachea, to the level of the tracheal bifurcation.

Arytenoid cartilages

Cricoid cleft

Body cricoid cartilage

vent laryngeal stenosis. A temporary tracheostomy is required while the stent is in place.

Stenosis of the larynx results from infection, intubation[4] and following tracheostomy. The majority of such cases are preventable. Management following the development of stenosis includes excision of the stenotic area, skin grafting and the use of an endolaryngeal stent. The prognosis depends on the site and extent of the stenotic area, the age of the patient plus other individual factors; for instance, the duration of the stenosis and tendency to keloid formation.

Foreign bodies in the larynx may produce stridor or respiratory obstruction. Most vegetable foreign bodies do not lodge in the larynx but cause laryngotracheobronchitis or atelectasis after their passage into the tracheobronchial system. Their management, therefore, includes laryngoscopy and bronchoscopic evaluation and treatment.

REFERENCES

1. Baker, D. C., Jr., and Savetsky, L.: Congenital partial atresia of the larynx, Trans. Am. Laryngol. Rhinol. Otol. Soc., pp. 14–20, 1966.
2. Bayeaux, R.: Tubage du larynx dans le croup, Presse Méd. 1:29, 1897.
3. Engel, S.: *Lung Structure* (Springfield, Ill.: Charles C Thomas, Publisher, 1962).
4. Fearon, B., *et al.*: Airway patterns in children following prolonged endotracheal intubation, Ann. Otol. Rhinol. Laryngol. 75:975, 1966.
5. Harrison, H. S., Fuqua, W. B., and Giffin, R. B., Jr.: Congenital laryngeal cleft: Report of a case, Am. J. Dis. Child. 110:556, 1965.
6. Jackson, C., and Jackson, C. L.: *Bronchoesophagology* (Philadelphia: W. B. Saunders Company, 1951).
7. McHugh, H. E., and Lock, W. E.: Congenital web of the larynx, Laryngoscope 52:43, 1942.
8. McNaught, R. C.: Surgical correction of anterior web of the larynx, Laryngoscope 60:264, 1950.
9. Negus, V. E.: *The Comparative Anatomy and Physiology of the Larynx* (London: William Heinemann Medical Books, Ltd., 1949), p. 175.
10. Pettersson, G.: Inhibited separation of larynx and the upper part of trachea from esophagus in a newborn, Acta Chir. Scand. 110: 250, 1955.
11. Richter, C. F.: Dissertatio medica de infanticidio in artis obstetrica. Thesis for M.D. degree, Leipzig, 1792.
12. Tucker, G.: The infant larynx: Direct laryngoscopic observations, JAMA 99:1899, 1932.
13. Wilson, T. G.: *Diseases of the Ear, Nose and Throat in Children* (2d ed.; New York: Grune & Stratton, Inc., 1962).

Of the neurologic disorders of infancy, *recurrent nerve paralysis* may result from birth injury, infection, maternal disease and surgical injury as well as other causes. When the condition is bilateral, tracheostomy may be required, and the prognosis is poor.

Trauma to the infant larynx includes birth and postnatal injury. As with adult fractures of the larynx, restoration of cartilage position and internal stenting is essential to pre-

30

Kenneth J. Welch / D. S. Trump

The Salivary Glands

SURGICAL LESIONS of the salivary glands are uncommon in infancy and childhood. One may see recurring or suppurative sialadenitis as well as various types of tumors, benign and malignant. Tumors may arise anywhere one might expect salivary gland tissue to be present, including the floor of the mouth, the palate, the submaxillary and parotid regions. Pathologic processes that involve the parotid are important by virtue of frequency of occurrence and the necessity for skillful surgical management.

From 1937 to 1977, 203 children were encountered with surgical lesions of the major salivary glands at the Children's Hospital Medical Center in Boston; 84 patients had neoplasms, 71 had sialadenitis, 41 had sublingual cysts (ranula) and 7 had interesting miscellaneous lesions (Table 30–1). Although most authors have considered neoplasms and sialadenitis separately, it seemed reasonable to combine all surgical lesions of the salivary glands in one chapter because of challenging problems in differential diagnosis and the very important differences in medical and surgical treatment.

Benign Neoplasms

Angioma

From our own survey and other reports (Table 30–2), the most common benign neoplasm affecting the major salivary glands is angioma in one of its several categories.[15, 38, 47, 80] Altogether, 215 cases have been reported. We have encountered 41 patients with hemangioma and 11 with lymphangioma, some having mixed angioma. These tumors present most commonly in female infants at birth or within the first months of life. They usually are confined to the intracapsular portion of the gland with only occasional involvement of the overlying subcutaneous tissue and skin. A surface sentinel lesion may provide the clue to diagnosis, thus eliminating the need for biopsy identification. A review of the literature by Wolfe[83] disclosed that of 48 patients operated on for parotid angioma, 2 died intraoperatively because of the prolonged and difficult procedure, and 12–25% sustained permanent seventh nerve palsy. Kaufman and Stout[45] reported

TABLE 30–1.—SURGICAL LESIONS OF MAJOR
SALIVARY GLANDS (CHILDREN'S HOSPITAL
MEDICAL CENTER, BOSTON, 1937–1977)

Neoplasms		84
Malignant	17	
Benign	67	
Sialadenitis		71
Acute	26	
Chronic	45	
Ranula		41
Miscellaneous		7
TOTAL		203

TABLE 30–2.—BENIGN TUMORS OF THE
MAJOR SALIVARY GLANDS IN CHILDREN
(323 FROM THE LITERATURE TO 1977,*
67 FROM CHILDREN'S HOSPITAL MEDICAL
CENTER, BOSTON, 1937–1977)

Hemangioma	215
Mixed tumor	117
Lymphangioma	23
Lymphoepithelial tumor (Mikulicz's disease)	10
Xanthoma	6
Plexiform neurofibroma	6
Cystadenoma	5
Warthin's tumor	3
Lipoma	3
Neurilemmoma (schwannoma)	2
TOTAL	390

*References: 3, 7, 8, 13–18, 20, 22, 28, 30, 40, 45, 47, 50, 65, 70, 74, 79.

on 3 patients with seventh nerve palsy, and Karlan and Snyder[43] stated that 1 patient in 4 sustained anatomic division. It is apparent that surgical removal of a parotid angioma in infancy provides an uncertain result in terms of ablation and recurrence, plus an unacceptably high risk of producing an expressionless face.

TREATMENT.—Angiomas of the salivary glands may be congenital, but most appear in the first weeks or months of life as a progressive, painless swelling, usually in the region of the parotid gland and only occasionally involving the overlying skin (Fig. 30–1). Provided that there is a cutaneous sentinel lesion over the convexity of the swelling, no biopsy identification is necessary. Group I lesions are spongy, cavernous, moderately cellular and slowly growing. Open rather than needle biopsy is necessary to provide the correct diagnosis and classification from permanent sections. Further treatment is unnecessary and, provided that there is no lymphangioma component, satisfactory involution occurs, with no evidence of the process at age 3–4 years (Fig. 30–2). Group II lesions are firm, microscopically cellular, sometimes called hemangioendothelioma (always benign) and characterized by rapid growth. Biopsy is required; steroids are beneficial (prednisone 1 mg/kg/day). The lesion is observed.

Group III lesions have large arteriovenous communications and grow at an alarming rate. Cardiac overload is common; platelet trapping has been observed. For such patients, we recommend ligation of the external carotid artery, which can be picked up between the branches of the superior thyroid and the lingual arteries. Ligation produces a dramatic decrease in the size of the tumor; involution follows at the customary rate. Prednisone response is variable. On one occasion, surgical excision of such a process has been car-

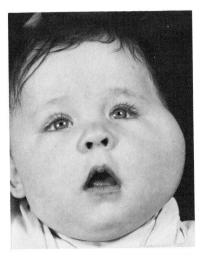

Fig. 30–1.—A 4-month-old girl with rapidly growing cellular hemangioma of the left parotid gland. Treatment consisted of biopsy and observation. There was no residual tumor detectable at age 4 years.

ried out under deep hypothermia with cardiopulmonary bypass (see Chap. 31).

Group IV—In a small group of patients, the hemangioma presents or persists beyond age 5 years. Treatment consists of superficial parotid lobectomy with dissection and preservation of the seventh nerve. Less than 10% of patients require surgical intervention other than biopsy for identification of this usually favorable lesion. Patient observation may be the best policy after tissue diagnosis for most parotid angiomas of infancy and early childhood.

Interstitial irradiation, needle biopsy and injection of sclerosing agents are unwarranted. Permanent injury to one or more of the branches of the facial nerve may occur.

Prior to 1969, the preferred form of treatment for such lesions was biopsy and irradiation or surgical excision with dissection and preservation of the seventh nerve, which was not always possible.[79] Since then, our policy has been to biopsy and observe all such patients presenting in infancy, waiting for involution, which usually occurs. When a sentinel hemangioma provided the diagnosis, no biopsy was performed. Twelve patients were treated by observation; 6 required biopsy. All have involuted satisfactorily. One patient

developed a seventh nerve palsy following biopsy and subsequent rapid growth of the lesion. Prednisone treatment was instituted, with little response and irradiation was considered; fortunately, the process began to involute. The patient did not receive irradiation nor was surgical intervention forced on us. A similar experience has been documented by Williams,[80] who reported 16 children with hemangioma treated operatively with 4 recurrences and 10 patients who were observed following biopsy. The observed patients ranged in age from 1 month to 8 months; all involuted satisfactorily (Fig. 30–2). Twenty patients were female and 6 were male. Four of 10 patients were observed without biopsy because of the presence of a sentinel lesion.

Reports of thyroid malignancy developing many years after therapeutic irradiation of benign lesions of the head and neck make irradiation unacceptable for hemangiomas of infancy and childhood. The ME4 linear accelerator with high collimation tangential to the target will result in significant internal scatter even with lead shielding of the thyroid. At present, there is no known way of avoiding such adverse thyroid stimulation. The subject has been brought into sharp focus recently in the report by Favus *et al.*[26] They reported 1056 patients who received therapeutic irradiation for benign disease in the 1940s and 1950s. Sixteen per cent of patients had palpable nodular thyroid disease. In another 10.7%, abnormal areas were picked up by ^{99m}Tc pertechnetate thyroid imaging. Of patients operated on (71%), cancer was identified in 33% (60 of 182 patients). They consider the problem a major health hazard for at least 35 years in exposed children. The at-risk situation has been known for many years beginning with the report by Duffy and Fitzgerald[23] in 1950, subsequently reported on by Winship,[81] Retetoff *et al.*[60] and Hempelmann.[39] A less pessimistic version of the risk situation appears in a special bulletin of the Massachusetts Medical Society.[76] They conclude that the most commonly encountered lesion is nodularity of the type seen in multinodular goiter rather than neoplasia. Thyroid cancer occurs in approximately 7% of the exposed population. Such patients require annual examination with further investigation if nodularity develops. Risk continues for 35 years. The value of thyroid scanning is controversial because of equivocal findings and additional radiation exposure of a gland already at risk. Equally controversial is the use of thyroid hormone for suppression (0.15–0.20 mg of synthetic thyroxine or 120–180 mg of desiccated thyroid). It is not

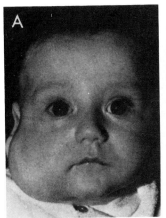
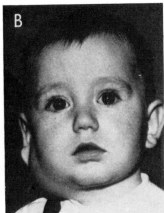
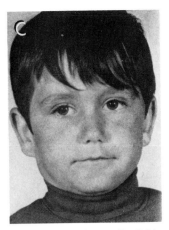

Fig. 30–2.—**A,** parotid hemangioma in a 3-month-old boy. Note the impingement on the ear and the extension into his neck. **B,** the same child at 12 months of age with early sings of involution. **C,** at 6 years of age there is total involution of the parotid hemangioma with slight excess skin, which can be removed later or taken up with additional growth. (From H. B. Williams.[80])

thought to influence in any way radiation-related thyroid carcinoma in man; the risk of thyrotoxicosis after many years of treatment is very real (see Chap. 34).

Lymphangioma

We have encountered 11 patients with primary intracapsular lymphangioma or lymphangioma in a juxtaparotid location with histologic invasion of the gland. A review of the literature shows little interest in this angioma subtype, yet in our experience surgical management has been exceedingly difficult. Chong *et al.*[15] reported 5 cases and Krolls[47] 4; no details are given about surgical treatment. Baum and Perzik[3] encountered 4 patients; 3 had total parotidectomy and 1 died intraoperatively following cardiac arrest. Intracapsular lymphangioma often is a mixed hemangioma in the perinatal period (Fig. 30–3, A). Ultimately, the hemangioma component drops out, followed by persistence or vigorous growth of the lymphangioma component some years later (Fig. 30–3, B). Juxtaparotid lymphangiomas are a separate entity, not to be confused with the bulky hygroma cysticum coli, which involves the major compartments of the neck, infiltrating the floor of the mouth and continuing into the substance of the tongue. Nine patients had lymphangioma restricted to and microscopically invading the parotid gland. All were unilateral.

TREATMENT. *Group I*—Neonates with parotid intracapsular lymphangioma and hemangioma. Treatment consists of biopsy only for histologic identification and sialography (Fig. 30–4) to rule out congenital malignancy. The lesion is observed.

Group II—Neonates with juxtaparotid lymphangioma and histologic invasion of the gland. It is technically impossible to carry out a clean removal of this process without a high risk of seventh nerve palsy. Treatment consists of superficial excision of the lymphangioma in its extraparotid ramifications plus destruction of the deeper intracapsular cysts. This is accomplished by uncapping the cysts and scrubbing the endothelial lining with a mild sclerosing agent under careful direct vision. A useful agent is 0.5% iodine applied with a sterile cotton applicator. These tumors form simultaneously with the major neurovascular supply to the head and neck and are found in and around the ramifications of the seventh, eleventh and twelfth nerves. The seventh nerve trunk measures no more than 0.5 mm in the neonate. While the main trunk of the facial nerve can be identified, the major branches dive into a marsh of multiloculated lymphangioma. It is technically impossible to free them from the tumor. The limited operation may not be the final answer, and recurrences are common but may not be encountered for months or years after the initial subtotal excision.

In summary, we try to remove the bulk of the tumor without sacrificing any structure of functional or cosmetic importance. Repeated small operations usually suffice. One child went 7 years before a recurrence developed. The second operation was relatively simple, with no difficulty in identifying and preserving essential structures.

Group III—Older children with intracapsular lymphangioma or mixed angioma. Surgical excision is carried out electively at age 4, when most of the hemangioma component has dropped out. This may be a primary definitive operation or reoperation following incomplete removal in infancy. This involves total parotidectomy with dissection and preservation of the seventh nerve. Every attempt should be made to clean out the entire process at the time of full dissection. A preoperative parotid sialogram is mandatory (Fig. 30–4). If elements are left behind, reoperation poses a prohibitive risk of seventh nerve damage, since, in addition to residual tumor, there is fibrotic encasement of the nerve and its branches.

Mixed Tumors

Several reports include mixed tumors of the parotid gland in children. They are second only to angiomas in frequency; 117 cases have been reported. Byars *et al.*[9] reported 17 patients evenly distributed from 7 to 18 years of age; 8 were under 14. Howard *et al.*[41] reported on 6 patients; only 1 was operated on before age 14. Chong *et al.*[15] reported 22 mixed tumors in children less than 16 years of age; all involved the parotid. Five had local excision, 4 had subtotal parotidectomy and 12 had conservative parotidectomy with seventh

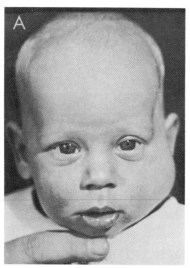
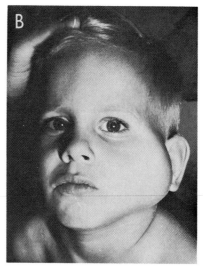

Fig. 30–3.—Mixed angioma (hemangioendothelioma and lymphangioma) of the parotid. **A,** in this 4-month-old boy, the lesion was identified by open biopsy. Irradiation was withheld because of low cellularity and slow growth. **B,** following near "disappearance" of the tumor at age 2 there was sudden regrowth several weeks after an upper respiratory infection. Treatment consisted of total parotidectomy with dissection and preservation of the seventh nerve. The histologic diagnosis was pure lymphangioma. No evidence of recurrence 5 years after operation, and no evidence of facial nerve palsy.

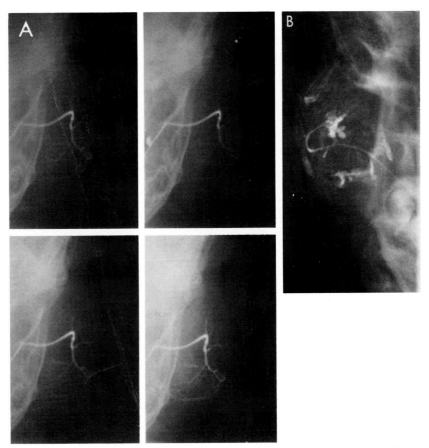

Fig. 30–4.— A, parotid sialograms of a 4-month-old male infant with diffuse parotid hemangioma. The ducts are stretched out by the neoplasm but are otherwise normal. The study does not differentiate hemangioma from other neoplasms; biopsy is required. **B,** parotid lymphangioma, showing displacement of ducts, focal sialectasia and filling defects consistent with multiple spherical, fluid-filled, space-occupying areas of lymphangioma.

nerve dissection. Recurrence was encountered in 3 patients; all were successfully treated by reoperation. Two patients suffered division of the seventh nerve. Baum and Perzik[3] encountered 6 patients, 10–17 years of age. Five were cured by total parotidectomy with no instance of seventh nerve injury; 1 recurred 5 times. Castro[14] reviewed experience with mixed tumors in 19 children. The parotid was involved in 15 patients, the submaxillary gland in 4; 1 was malignant. The treatment carried out is not clear but at least consisted of superficial lobectomy with seventh nerve dissection. Galich[30] encountered 7 patients 17 years and younger with 1 recurrence and 1 seventh nerve palsy. Krolls,[47] reviewing experience at the Armed Forces Institute of Pathology (AFIP), was able to find 55 children with mixed tumors. The parotid was involved in 44 instances, the submaxillary gland in 10. Over-all, treatment was successful; none was malignant. We have encountered 5 patients with mixed tumor of the parotid gland, at variance with other reports; however, we did not include children over age 14. All were satisfactorily treated without recurrence and without seventh nerve damage. Mixed tumor is not uncommon in late adolescence. Nine additional cases have been reported by Foote and Frazell,[28] Grulee[35] and Reiquam.[61]

Miscellaneous Benign Tumors

There are isolated reports of benign tumors corresponding to all of the tissue elements of the salivary glands deriving from fibrous, neural or acinar tissue. Ten patients in this series had miscellaneous benign tumors of the major salivary glands. Three patients had a cystadenoma of the parotid. Two patients had benign lymphoepithelial neoplasm (Mikulicz's disease) and, to date, have not manifested systemic difficulties. The ophthalmologic features of this disease were identified by Sjögren in 1933;[79] keratoconjunctivitis is combined with xerostomia following obliteration of the acinar structure of the lacrimal glands. Grage and Luben[34] reported 6 patients with Mikulicz's disease with multisystem involvement; none were children. In addition, we encountered neurofibroma in 2 children, lipoma in 2 and neurilemmoma (schwannoma) in 1.

Malignant Neoplasms

Seventeen patients ranging in age from 1 day to 4 years had malignancy of a major salivary gland. In 15, the parotid was involved and in 2 the submaxillary gland. There were 10 girls and 7 boys; again, the female preponderance is noted. The lesion was congenital in 2 patients; both are alive and well without recurrence following total conservative parotidectomy with compartmental node dissection (Figs. 30–5 and 30–6). One patient in addition had excision of the mandible. These cases have been reported by Tefft and Vawter.[75, 78] One had adenocarcinoma and the other had duct cell carcinoma. Vawter places these examples of congenital salivary gland malignancy in a special group, which he prefers to call embryoma.

There were 4 undifferentiated sarcomas, 3 adenocarcino-

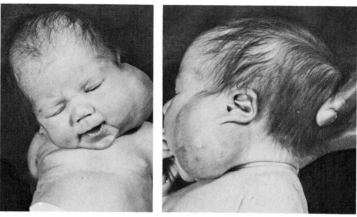

Fig. 30–5.—Congenital duct cell carcinoma in a newborn girl. Treatment consisted of radical parotidectomy and neck dissection. She is well 14 years later.

mas, 2 mucoepidermoid carcinomas, 2 acinic cell carcinomas and 1 example each of undifferentiated carcinoma, malignant mixed tumor, neurofibrosarcoma, adenocystic carcinoma (cylindroma), spindle cell sarcoma and embryonal rhabdomyosarcoma, which appeared to be an intrinsic parotid lesion, although this is debatable. The pathologic classification of 194 neoplasms in children derived from our own experience and review of the literature is listed in Table 30–3.

The most common malignant tumor of the major salivary

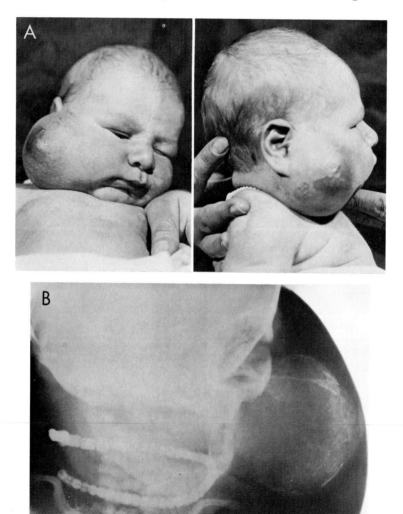

Fig. 30–6.—**A,** congenital adenocarcinoma of the right parotid gland in a newborn boy. **B,** roentgenogram of head and neck showing stippled peripheral calcification.

Treatment consisted of mandibulectomy, radical parotidectomy and neck dissection. He is well 23 years later.

TABLE 30–3.—MALIGNANT NEOPLASMS OF
THE MAJOR SALIVARY GLANDS IN CHILDREN
(177 FROM LITERATURE TO 1977,°
17 FROM CHILDREN'S HOSPITAL MEDICAL
CENTER, BOSTON, 1937–1977)

Mucoepidermoid carcinoma	96
Acinic cell carcinoma	26
Undifferentiated sarcoma	15
Undifferentiated carcinoma	14
Adenocarcinoma	11
Lymphoma	8
Malignant mixed tumor	7
Adenocystic carcinoma (cylindroma)	6
Metastatic	4
Squamous cell carcinoma	3
Neurofibrosarcoma	3
Rhabdomyosarcoma	1
TOTAL	194

°References: 3, 8, 9, 11, 12, 14, 15, 17, 28, 30, 34, 38, 45, 47, 48, 79, 80, 84.

glands in childhood is mucoepidermoid carcinoma, followed in order by undifferentiated carcinoma, undifferentiated sarcoma, adenocarcinoma, adenocystic carcinoma or cylindroma and malignant mixed tumor.[40, 70] These tumors present as rapidly growing, often painful swellings in the region of the parotid or submaxillary gland. There is no clinical feature that permits accurate differentiation from the more cellular benign tumors or from the fulminant form of chronic sialadenitis. For this reason, all patients with a swelling involving a major salivary gland must have sialography and open biopsy for identification. The biopsy specimen should be read in permanent sections; frozen section reports are unreliable.

Both in our series and in the literature there have been many patients without anatomic invasion or interference with the function of the seventh nerve. Normal function of the nerve does not exclude malignancy.

Treatment

Treatment of malignant lesions of the salivary glands varies according to the stage of the disease and the histologic nature of the tumor. Some tumors are small and well confined to the superficial lobe of the parotid gland. These require only conservative parotidectomy with dissection and preservation of the seventh nerve. The poorest prognosis is encountered in patients having undifferentiated or embryonal carcinomas or sarcomas. In our patients, the disease had in all cases spread beyond the limit of resectability when first seen. Consequently, surgical treatment has been limited to biopsy identification and removal of tumor bulk, followed by irradiation and chemotherapy in its various forms. Some tumors were intermediate in their degree of invasiveness and metastasized late or only to regional nodes. For these patients, one must individualize surgical therapy, which can be offered in a number of combinations. If the seventh nerve is involved functionally or is found to be invaded at the time of operation, it must be sacrificed. Further extension of the operation consists of removing the ramus of the mandible and masseter muscle, thus providing access to the pterygoid fossa and lateral pharyngeal wall. Tumors that have moved in this direction usually have a poor prognosis. Mucoepidermoid carcinoma metastasizes frequently to the lymph nodes of the neck and yet only rarely becomes disseminated. For this reason, wide local excision without neck dissection is recommended. If palpable nodes are subsequently identified in the ipsilateral side of the neck, compartmental nodal dissection can be carried out at a second stage, equaling salvage achieved with neck dissection in continuity.

For all but the highly malignant lesions, we favor compartmental node dissection, sparing the sternocleidomastoid muscle and the internal jugular vein. Decision regarding radical surgery depends on the individual merits of the case and on the interpretation of the tumor tissue by a qualified pathologist. It is possible and, on occasion, desirable to do as extensive a resection as possible to provide the greatest chance for survival. In the extreme form, this consists of radical parotidectomy sacrificing the facial nerve, mandibulectomy, dissection of the contents of the pterygoid fossa, removal of the submaxillary gland and radical neck dissection in continuity.

Results

Few details are available about the surgical treatment of the 177 children with salivary gland malignancy encountered in the literature (Table 30–3) except for the recent excellent report by Chong et al.[15] It is even more difficult, except for mucoepidermoid carcinoma and acinic cell carcinoma, to determine the outcome of any form of therapy. In general, the remaining assorted malignancies have in the past had a gloomy outlook, with some recent improvement due to combined triple therapy. With regard to mucoepidermoid carcinoma, 59 children have been operated on.[3, 7, 14, 15, 30, 47, 79] Surgical treatment consists of conservative total parotidectomy with dissection and preservation of the facial nerve. These tumors are slow growing and locally invasive, with little tendency to metastasize. It was necessary to sacrifice the seventh nerve in only 5 patients. One palsy developed after postoperative irradiation—which probably was unnecessary. Compartmental node dissection was done only for clinically palpable nodes. The exact number of neck dissections cannot be determined but regional metastasis did not interfere with longevity. Acinic cell carcinoma was seen in 21 children, all of whom responded satisfactorily to total parotidectomy with no instance of permanent seventh nerve damage.[3, 14, 15, 47, 79] Five patients with malignant mixed tumor survived following conservative parotidectomy, with seventh nerve sacrifice in 1 patient.

In our series (Table 30–4), at the time of writing, 2 patients with congenital parotid malignancy were well 10 and 21 years respectively after operation. A 9-year-old girl with mixed parotid malignancy was well 12 years after wide resection. One girl was well 10 years after parotidectomy with preservation of the seventh nerve for adenocystic carcinoma. Seven of 8 patients encountered since 1967 are alive and well 1–9 years following conservative or radical parotidectomy. In 3, the facial nerve was sacrificed, 1 required extensive resection with mandibulectomy and 2 required compartmental node removal. Irradiation (13 patients) and chemotherapy (6 patients) was used in most (see Table 30–4). Six patients encountered early had highly malignant tumors beyond the limit of resectability and cure when first seen. Treatment consisted of biopsy followed by irradiation and chemotherapy with little or no improvement. All died within a year. We have not encountered a child with primary lymphoma involving a major salivary gland, although this has been reported.[15, 28, 47]

Juxtaparotid Tumors

We call attention to a group of malignant tumors that present as swellings in the region of the parotid gland. Some are

TABLE 30–4.—MALIGNANT LESIONS OF THE MAJOR SALIVARY GLANDS, CHILDREN'S HOSPITAL MEDICAL CENTER, BOSTON, 1945–1977

SEX	AGE	LOCATION		OPERATION	IRRADIATION°	CHEMOTHERAPY	RESULT
M	1 day	Parotid	Adenocarcinoma	RP RN	Yes	No	Well after 14 yr
F	10 days	Parotid	Duct cell carcinoma	RP M	Yes	No	Well after 3 yr
F	6 mo	Submax.	Anaplastic carcinoma	IE	Yes	No	Dead in 7 mo
F	20 mo	Parotid	Mesenchymal sarcoma	B	Yes	Yes	Dead in 8 mo
M	22 mo	Parotid	Mesenchymal sarcoma	B	Yes	Yes	Dead in 6 mo
F	3 yr	Parotid	Adenocarcinoma	B	Yes	Yes	Dead in 6 mo
F	3 9/12	Parotid	Neurofibrosarcoma	RP			Dead in 4 mo
F	9 yr	Parotid	Mixed, recurrent	CP	Yes	No	Well after 5 yr
F	10 yr	Parotid	Adenocystic carcinoma	CP	No	No	Well after 6 mo
M	13 yr.	Parotid	Adenocarcinoma	RP RN	Yes	VAC	Dead in 3 yr
			—————— 1968–1977 ——————				
M	2 4/12	Parotid	Neurofibrosarcoma	CP	No	No	Well after 7 yr
M	5 3/12	Parotid	Embryonal sarcoma	RP	Yes	VAC	Dead in 13 mo
M	8 3/12	Parotid	Undifferentiated sarcoma	RP	Yes	VAC	Alive and well 5 yr
F	10	Parotid	Mucoepidermoid carcinoma	CP	No	No	Alive and well 7 yr
M	13½	Parotid	Mucoepidermoid carcinoma	CP	Yes	No	Alive and well 18 mo
F	14	Parotid	Mixed, recurrent	CP CN	Yes	No	Alive and well 8 yr
F	14 8/12	Submax.	Mucoepidermoid carcinoma	S CN	Yes	No	Alive and well 9 yr

°Orthovoltage before 1967; after 1967, 4 MeV (5000 R).
B = biopsy only; IE = incomplete excision; CP = conservative parotidectomy; RP = radical parotidectomy; CN = conservative node excision; RN = radical neck dissection; M = mandibulectomy; S = total excision submaxillary gland.

nasopharyngeal in origin with a mesenchymal ground substance. The epignathi usually contain tissues of all three germ layers.[24, 69, 84] A third variety is congenital cervicoparotid teratoma[2] (Fig. 30–7).

Cervicoparotid teratoma usually is benign. These present in the neonate and should be excised, including the superficial lobe of the parotid gland, with identification and preservation of the seventh nerve. The lesion is discussed further in Chapter 31.

The diagnosis of juxtaparotid malignancy is aided by sialography. In most cases there is external displacement or compression of the gland, but the duct system is normal (Fig. 30–8). Our patient had an undifferentiated sarcoma of nasopharyngeal origin that involved the parotid gland by contiguity. Subsequently, pulmonary and bony metastases developed.

Secondary tumors are found in the region of the parotid gland, notably metastatic neuroblastoma, retinoblastoma and rhabdomyosarcoma. A discussion of these tumors will be found in Chapter 31.

Ranula

Forty-one patients had sublingual cysts (Figs. 30–9 and 30–10). Some of them were of little clinical importance, appearing as pea-sized swellings to the right or left of the midline in the floor of the mouth adjacent to the frenulum. In a number of patients, the ranula achieved heroic proportions. One neonate had a soft blue cystic subglottic swelling that measured 8.0 × 5.0 cm. This produced airway obstruction and required emergency excision.

TREATMENT.—Errors in management have occurred because of failure to recognize the nature of the process and attempts to excise the cyst completely with a margin of normal tissue. The larger ranulas extend bilaterally or unilaterally from the dental arch to the hypopharynx and under the base of the tongue. An attempt at total excision may result in substantial bleeding and interference with neurogenic apparatus essential to tongue movements and the act of swallowing.

Proper treatment consists of marsupialization of the cyst into the oral cavity.[49] The process may present in a submandibular location (Fig. 30–9) but always should be approached through the oral cavity. This is done under endotracheal general anesthesia with a Dingman double mouth gag and a heavy silk stitch drawing the tongue cephalad after division of the frenulum. The orifice of Wharton's submaxillary duct should be identified with a lacrimal duct probe, and uncapping of the process should be carried out with this

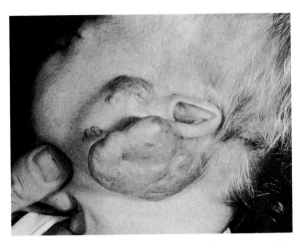

Fig. 30–7.—Congenital teratoma of cervicoparotid area treated by wide, local resection and closure with rotation flaps. The patient was well and free from disease at age 11.

probe in place. On circumscribing the soft blue dome of the cystic process, a large amount of glairy mucoid material is released, revealing the back wall of the cyst. As the uncapping proceeds, the margin of the cyst is anastomosed to the oral mucous membrane with a running interlocking suture of 4-0 chromic catgut. A ranula cavity of any size is obliterated within 2 weeks. Following this procedure, no patient has required reoperation. The submaxillary duct has not been obstructed in the suturing process in this series.

Sialadenitis

Sialadenitis may be encountered as a specific bacterial suppurative infection, a chronic infection without evident etiologic factors or infrequently as granulomatous replacement of the parotid or submaxillary gland.[56, 57, 64] We have encountered 71 children with sialadenitis. Forty-eight patients were males and 23 were females. Male predilection, especially for chronic parotitis, has been noted in other reports.[42, 44]

Acute Sialadenitis

Twenty-six patients had acute sialadenitis. The parotid gland was involved in 18 and the submaxillary in 8. Parotid abscess requiring incision and drainage was encountered in 15. Six patients had incision and drainage of a submaxillary abscess. Acute suppurative parotitis was common in the preantibiotic era and often was the final insult that led to the death of small infants undergoing major surgery for congenital anomalies.

The disease now is most commonly seen in infants, presenting as a painful, red, indurated swelling of the parotid or submaxillary gland. The responsible organism usually can be cultured from the duct orifice. In 16 cases, this was *Staphylococcus aureus*, followed in frequency by streptococcus and d-pneumonococcus. In others, because of the administration of antibiotics before hospitalization, the offending organism was not recovered.

Often, but not always, there is a background of dehydration through vomiting or diarrhea and some constitutional impairment related to concurrent disease. One patient had acute glomerulonephritis. Acute parotitis also occurs in the postoperative period in patients who have undergone multiple surgical procedures. Karlan and Snyder[43] encountered 24 patients with acute sialadenitis. In 2, it was a postoperative complication.

Chronic Sialadenitis

RECURRING PAROTITIS.—This is a well-documented condition in adults,[52, 77] and a number of authors have described the syndrome as it is seen in childhood, with its variations and considerably better prognosis.[2, 27, 42, 44, 52, 64] Katzen and DuPlessis[44] reported on 44 children from South Africa with recurrent parotitis. The condition is rare in blacks. There were 26 males and 18 females. All authors acknowledge that the condition is more common in boys than in girls.

ETIOLOGY.—The cause of chronic sialadenitis is not known. A number of factors have been implicated, but few are applicable in our patients or those in the literature.

Allergy, either as a drug sensitivity (iodide) or food intolerance, has been implicated. There is one report of sialadenitis following periodic treatment of recurring urinary tract infection with sulfisoxazole.[54] Recurring parotitis developed at shorter and shorter intervals after the institution of therapy, and it may be that some drugs are capable of producing distant local tissue sensitization. Opium and other drugs that act on the parotid gland by suppressing secretion may induce parotitis in an indirect way. Many patients had a histo-

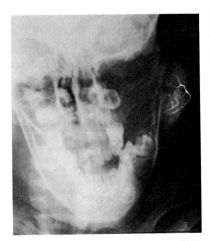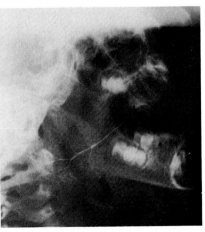

Fig. 30–8.—Undifferentiated sarcoma of nasopharyngeal origin. Sialogram of a patient with a rapidly growing tumor. Note normal duct structure at all levels and lateral displacement of the parotid gland by the underlying tumor.

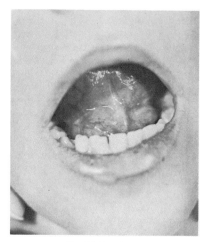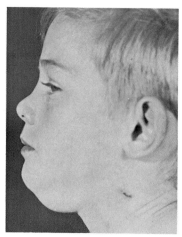

Fig. 30–9.—Ranula. An example with suprahyoid projection. The lesion was treated by unroofing it into the oral cavity.

ry of recent pharyngitis and recurring tonsillitis. Carious teeth were noted in 5 children. A family history was not noted for any of our patients, and no siblings had the disease.[69]

Parotid gland involvement in cystic fibrosis would be a logical entity. The Children's Hospital Cystic Fibrosis Center has under surveillance more than 1200 patients; only 4 developed parotitis. All had sialograms showing minimal ectasia. In all, the parotitis subsided spontaneously and did not recur. Enlarged submaxillary glands are common in patients with cystic fibrosis. They have increased salivary electrolyte values with abnormally high calcium level. Minute calculi could obstruct the drainage apparatus, producing a stagnation background for sialadenitis.

Culture of material expressed from the parotid duct is of little help in this condition, in contrast to acute sialadenitis. Only nonpathogenic organisms are recovered, and these are not consistent.

Inflammatory or congenital stricture of the salivary duct has been implicated, but only 2 patients in 41 had a stenotic duct orifice.

Mumps presents a problem in differential diagnosis with the first attack, but there are several important differences that make it possible to separate the two conditions. Simultaneous bilateral involvement is rare with chronic parotitis. Mumps was mentioned in the records of only 3 patients. An exudate may be obtained from Stensen's duct during a periodic attack of sialadenitis. None is recovered in mumps. The serum amylase content is elevated with mumps and normal with chronic sialadenitis. With mumps there is neutropenia; with sialadenitis there is leukocytosis in the range of 12,000–18,000. In addition to mumps, sarcoidosis, tuberculosis and lymphoma must be excluded.

In some patients, chronic parotitis may represent an autoimmune disorder heralding widespread systemic involvement. Those showing a marked degree of lymphocytic infiltration and islet formation should be observed for the development of systemic disease. There is striking similarity between this variety of chronic parotitis and lymphoid thyroiditis, or Hashimoto's disease.

SYMPTOMS AND SIGNS.—Recurring, painful attacks lasting 1–7 days and aggravated by chewing and swallowing are typical. Physical examination reveals swelling and tenderness limited to the anatomic area of the involved gland without involvement of the overlying skin and subcutaneous tissue. Systemic reactions are variable, but temperature elevation seldom is of more than 1 degree. Examination of the ipsilateral duct orifice at the time of the attack reveals reddening and some pouting. Collected secretions are thick and flocculent, described as snowflake in character. In some cases, the disease is limited to the accessory parotid gland apparatus. This is a small structure centered over Stensen's duct beyond the anterior limits of the true parotid gland. When this alone is involved, it may by local expansion interfere with drainage of the main duct. Between attacks, the gland usually remains somewhat fuller than the uninvolved side and retains local tenderness.

In our series, patients ranged in age from 4 months to 14 years; 4 were infants, 19 were 2–6; 15 were boys; 11 were 6–10 and 8 were 10–14. Eleven children had symptoms from a few weeks to less than 1 year, 21 from 1 to 3 years and 10 from 3 to 6 years. Frequency of attacks varied, but they occurred at least every 3–4 months. The side of involvement seemed to be random. Katzen and DuPlessis[44] reported on 14 patients with right-sided involvement, 12 left and 18 bilateral. Follow-up of our patients revealed that 16 ultimately had bilateral involvement. Most patients start with unilateral attacks, which become bilateral months or years

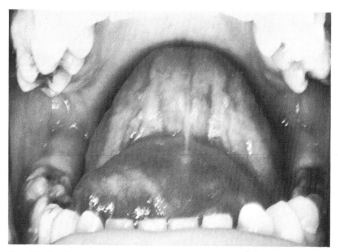

Fig. 30–10.—Large ranula of floor of mouth, lifting the tongue dorsally.

later. Conversely, they rarely suffer simultaneous attacks on the two sides.

DIAGNOSIS.—The diagnosis of chronic sialadenitis rests on the history of the disease, the appearance of a carefully performed sialogram and the histology of the gland determined by open biopsy. At the height of the disease, one sees hyperplasia of duct epithelium and an increased number of mucus-secreting cells. In the periductal tissues there is lymphocytic infiltration, with the formation of some follicles and acinar hypertrophy with fibrosis.

MEDICAL MANAGEMENT.—Treatment of chronic parotitis is in many ways unsatisfactory. Antibiotics commonly are administered at the height of an attack, and the process usually subsides in 3–7 days. However, patients not treated with antibiotics do equally well, with no prolongation of swelling or symptoms. Nonspecific supportive therapy includes attention to oral hygiene, massage of the gland and use of acid sweets and chewing gum. Eleven patients had tonsillectomy; 3 improved and 8 were unimproved. Irradiation for this condition is mentioned only to be condemned. Thirty years ago, 2 patients received 600 R in two doses. Steroids were not used by us or in other reported series in childhood.

Katzen followed up 31 of 44 children by recall or questionnaire. Twenty-one had stopped having attacks, usually at age 11–13, and all by age 15. Most patients are male; therefore, the hormonal surge at puberty would appear to have significance. Of 16 patients in our series still having attacks, 2 have autoimmune disease; 50 others are under 14 years of age. It is hoped that they may go into spontaneous remission at puberty. Karlan and Snyder[43] had good results with nonintervention.

SURGICAL TREATMENT.—The most effective surgical treatment for chronic parotitis is sialolithotomy with removal of one or more opaque calculi identified in a scout film preliminary to sialography. A second procedure of value is the excision of accessory parotid gland apparatus that compresses the midportion of Stensen's duct. If a firm nodule is felt in this location, or if there is evidence of extrinsic compression in the area normally occupied by this tissue, excisional biopsy is indicated, with considerable hope for success. Calibration of Stensen's duct orifice should be routine at the time of sialography, using graded lacrimal dilators, but we encountered stenosis of the duct orifice in only 1 patient. Meatotomy has been recommended and was carried out in 5 patients in one series without significant improvement. Avulsion of the auriculotemporal nerve was performed in 17 patients by Katzen and DuPlessis.[44] Parotitis recurred in 9; in 3, nerve tissue was not found in the pathologic material, and 3 were lost to follow-up. The improvement that occurred in 2 patients was considered fortuitous; both had bilateral disease, and the disease subsided as rapidly on the side not operated on. Ligation of Stensen's duct is thought to be unwise.[21] This is an attempt to produce autoparotidectomy; however, half the patients have suppuration, and in a considerable number an internal fistula develops at some point proximal to the site of ligation.

Total parotidectomy with dissection and preservation of the seventh nerve is reserved for advanced disease. Total parotidectomy was carried out in 7 of 41 patients in our series. In 5, the operation was unilateral and in 2 it was bilateral. In 1 patient, this extensive operation was performed with disease of only a few weeks' duration. The surgeon believed that he was dealing with parotid malignancy, yet there was no preoperative sialogram or biopsy examination. All patients had unremitting disease with advanced sialectasia. Permanent seventh nerve palsy did not occur in any patient.

We believe that parotidectomy for chronic sialadenitis should be reserved for patients with severe, debilitating, recurring attacks, pain, toxicity and total disorganization of the gland.

The surgical procedures carried out in 41 patients with parotid sialadenitis are listed in Table 30–5. The most common procedure was biopsy for identification when sialography was not commonly done or the result was equivocal. The combination of biopsy and irradiation is of historical interest and is mentioned only to be condemned. When calculi were present, sialolithotomy usually was curative. One patient had multiple intraglandular calculi (see Fig. 30–15). Local excision of a small nodule within the substance of the parotid gland without formal parotidectomy was performed in 3 patients. In each case, removal of the process coincided with the abatement of symptoms.

Two patients in the series reported by Katzen and DuPlessis would seem to have been candidates for parotidectomy.[44] One had total disintegration of the gland and a mass compressing the duct suggesting an accessory parotid structure. Another, with disease dating from childhood, and total destruction of the gland, had difficulties in the temporomandibular joint and middle ear, Costen's syndrome. Both appear to be examples of undertreatment.

Of 78 patients reviewed by Maynard,[52] 12 had symptoms dating from puberty and 7 were under the age of 14. In 7, Sjögren's disease and xerostomia developed.

The value of the Gurrey test for parotid function was established by Seward et al.,[68] who studied 86 patients with chronic parotitis. They identified a pathologic condition of the parotid gland consisting of hypersecretion with glandular hypertrophy. Treatment of this condition is bilateral superficial parotid lobectomy. There remains enough hyperfunctioning tissue in the deep lobes to provide oral lubrication.

COMPLICATIONS.—Complications of this disorder are largely iatrogenic. The most serious complication, seventh nerve palsy, may result from parotidectomy, the only definitive therapy for advanced sialadenitis with total destruction of the parotid gland. Complications of parotid gland surgery have been minimal in the entire series, whether performed for sialadenitis or neoplasm. Excluding intentional sacrifice of the seventh nerve in patients with malignancy, only 1 patient is left with any degree of nerve impairment, limited to the mandibular branch. Two patients developed the auriculotemporal syndrome of Frey. This consists of flushing of the side of the face following mastication. It is painless but may

TABLE 30–5.—TREATMENT OF
PAROTID SIALADENITIS

Biopsy only		16
Parotidectomy		7
Bilateral	2	
Unilateral	5	
Sialolithotomy		6
°Irradiation only		5
Local excision		3
Meatotomy		2
°Biopsy and irradiation		2
Total		41

°Prior to 1967.

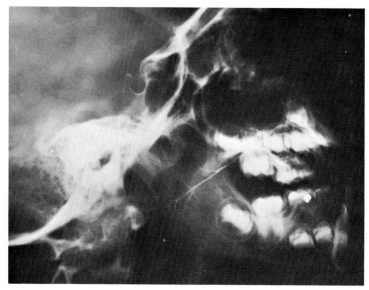

Fig. 30–11.—Unilateral parotitis. Normal sialogram of a 6-year-old boy with contralateral chronic parotitis. There is good definition of main and interlobar ducts, no extravasation into the gland parenchyma and no element of sialectasia.

last for several years after parotidectomy; precise division of the chorda tympani nerve in the floor of the middle ear may be required.

Many adults have decreased to absent salivary output, with distressing dryness, or xerostomia sicca. Meticulous dental care and the application of fluoride may be helpful.

Submaxillary Sialadenitis

Submaxillary sialadenitis occurred in 15 patients. In 4, a calculus was present and in 4 the gland was replaced by granuloma, 1 due to aspergillosis. One child had a foreign body (timothy grass) blocking Wharton's duct, Karlan and Snyder[43] reported 9 cases of submaxillary involvement; 2 were granulomatous. One had a calculus removed and 3 required incision and drainage. Treatment of advanced submaxillary sialadenitis is surgical excision; the gland serves no independent function and presents few anatomic hazards in its removal.

Surgical treatment of our patients consisted of biopsy only in 3 and total excision of the gland in 12, with preservation of the mandibular branch of the facial nerve. One patient developed pseudosarcomatous fasciitis with fusion of the temporomandibular joint (see Chap. 29).

Miscellaneous Lesions

Seven patients had unusual salivary gland lesions. One appeared to have a branchiogenic cyst in the lower third of the neck and below this a draining external fistula.[71] This proved to be an ectopic salivary gland with an external duct. Rothner has reported 3 similar cases.[63] Two patients had aberrant parotid gland tissue; 1 had a leaky palate and 1 had an oncocytoma (oxyphil adenoma) involving the dorsum of

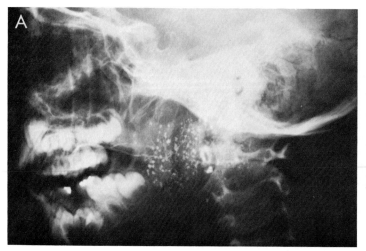
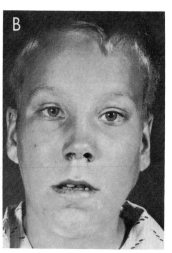

Fig. 30–12.—**A,** sialogram of a patient with a 6-month history of recurring parotid swelling. Note normal duct system and early but diffuse punctate sialectasia. **B,** photograph showing noticeable swelling of left parotid region that remains between attacks which occur every 3–4 months.

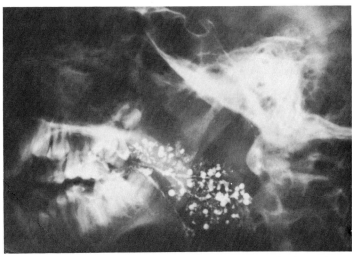

Fig. 30–13.—Chronic parotitis. Sialogram of a patient with advanced saccular sialectasia and widening of interlobar ducts.

the tongue. One had venous thrombosis of the parotid gland. Branchiogenic cysts were encountered within the parotid gland in 2 patients presenting with sialadenitis (see Fig. 30–16).

Sialography

Sialography can be carried out without anesthesia in any child more than 5 years of age. In younger children, a short period of general anesthesia is required.[25] The technique consists of cannulation of Stensen's duct after topical application of Pontocaine and identification of the orifice with a lacrimal duct probe. A blunt lacrimal duct needle attached to a Luer-Lok syringe containing 1 ml of warm Lipiodol is inserted into the duct and 0.5 ml is injected with steady, even pressure. At the same time, the duct is drawn into hyperextension by traction on the cheek. There is moderate discomfort at the time of injection, but this lasts only a few moments. When 0.5 ml has been instilled into the normal duct system, there already is some escape of the medium around the hub of the needle. Further injection results in extravasa-

tion of Lipiodol into the parenchyma of the gland, not only obscuring the fine network of the duct system but ultimately producing a foreign body reaction and compounding difficulties in the already-diseased and fibrotic gland. In one patient, the opaque oil remained in the parotid gland 5 years after sialography. Prominent lymphoid follicles associated with longstanding disease may be evident as filling defects.

There have been no complications resulting from sialography in our experience. The children complain of local tenderness and dull discomfort for 1 or 2 days.

Sialography proved to be 96% correct in differentiating chronic inflammatory disease from neoplasm in a study of 357 patients by Einstein.[25] A normal sialogram is shown in Figure 30–11 and the various grades of architectural disturbance seen in children with sialadenitis are demonstrated in Figures 30–12–30–14. This condition progresses from punctate sialectasis to the saccular form to a widening of the interlobar duct system and, late in the disease, dilation of the major duct system, with progressive disorganization of the gland (Figs. 30–15 and 30–16).

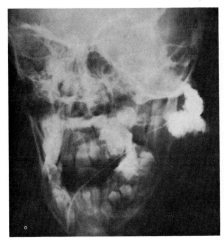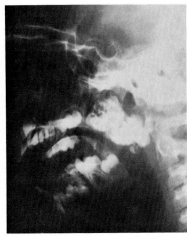

Fig. 30–14.—End stage chronic parotitis. Sialogram showing total disorganization of the parotid gland. The patient had repeated attacks of sialadenitis over a 4-year period, with fever, toxicity, pain and trismus. The disease is unilateral. Total parotidectomy with dissection and preservation of the 7th nerve was performed.

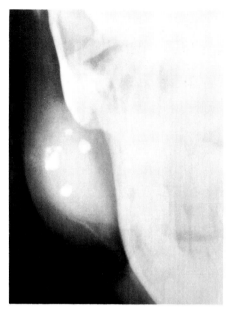

Fig. 30–15.—Sialolithiasis. Multiple minute calculi in the parotid duct of a boy with recurring parotitis and advanced sialectasia.

Most authors recommend biopsy as well as sialography to rule out neoplasia.[14, 47] Scintigraphy has been reported using ^{99m}Tc pertechnetate; most experience is reported in the European literature.[37] Our early experience is inconclusive.

Technique of Parotidectomy

Beahrs has been a constant source of advice and precise techniques for safe and effective parotid gland ablation both for infections and neoplasm.[4-6] Davis made a monumental contribution by dissecting 350 cervicofacial halves to demonstrate the true anatomy of the facial nerve and parotid gland.[19]

When undertaking parotid exploration, the surgeon should be well rested and unhurried and should have refreshed his knowledge of the anatomy and technical details. Endotracheal anesthesia is mandatory. The operative field should be draped with sterile transparent plastic sheeting (Steridrape–3M) to expose the entire side of the face, including the corners of the eye and mouth (Fig. 30–17, A) so that facial twitching may be observed when the nerve is stimulated.

The Y-shaped incision described 50 years ago provides admirable exposure. When the skin flaps are being elevated, it is important to avoid mobilizing the anterior flap as far forward as the anterior border of the parotid gland, for in so doing one may inadvertently transect small branches of the facial nerve as they emerge from the anterior border of the gland (Fig. 30–17, B). With upward traction of the ear lobe and anterior traction of the parotid gland, the dissection is carried along the inferior aspect of the external auditory canal, staying very close to this cartilaginous wall. Many small fibrous septae attach the posterior border of the parotid gland to this structure. As these are cautiously transected, the gland may be reflected anteriorly. As the dissection deepens along the ear canal, the main trunk of the facial nerve as it emerges from the stylomastoid foramen is reached (Fig. 30–17, C). The main trunk of the facial nerve will be found just a little anterior and a little medial to the tip of the mastoid process, which is less developed in infants and young children and assumes a more superficial position. One need not injure the facial nerve if one stays close to the auditory canal while reflecting the parotid gland anteriorly.

The styloid process is not a good landmark on which to rely in identifying the facial nerve. It is absent in approximately 30% of individuals and is extremely small in another 20%. Some authors have recommended identification of the facial nerve by finding its various branches as they emerge from the anterior margin of the parotid gland. This seems less feasible than identification of the nerve as a single trunk, for reasons of both size and variability of peripheral branching.

A nerve stimulator must be available to lend reassurance concerning various septae, which at first appear to be facial nerve. When the nerve finally is exposed, it has an unmistakable appearance, with linear striations. After identification, the nerve trunk can be followed into the posterior aspect of the parotid gland. With strong retraction anterolaterally on the superficial lobe, a plane of cleavage can be developed

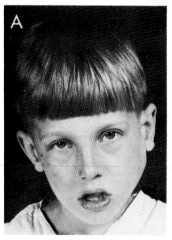
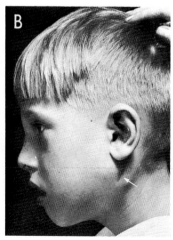

Fig. 30–16.—A, Infected intraparotid branchial cleft cyst in a 10-year-old boy with recurring sialadenitis. He had had attacks for 2 years and grade 3 ectasia. A, frontal view. B, lateral view showing the site of biopsy, which provided the unusual diagnosis. Treatment consisted of superficial parotid lobectomy.

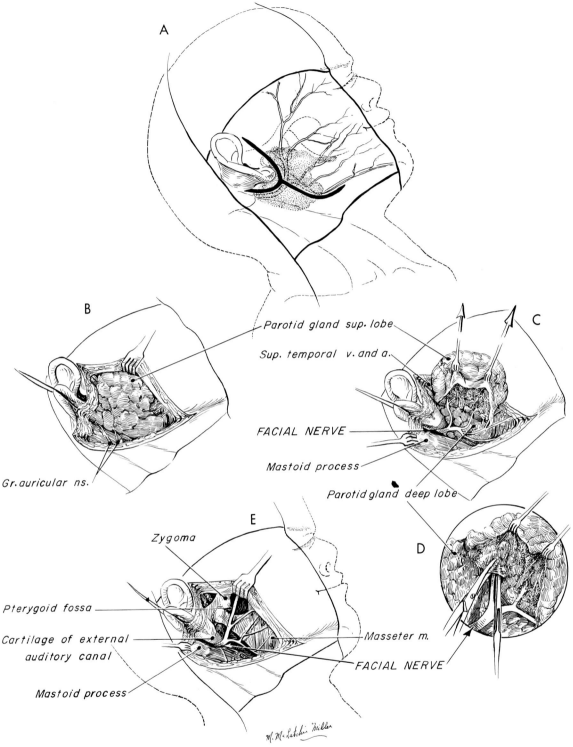

A

B

C

Parotid gland sup. lobe

Sup. temporal v. and a.

FACIAL NERVE

Mastoid process

Gr. auricular ns.

Parotid gland deep lobe

E

D

Zygoma

Pterygoid fossa

Cartilage of external
auditory canal

Masseter m.

FACIAL NERVE

Mastoid process

Fig. 30–17.—Technique of parotidectomy.

between the superficial and deep lobes of the gland. The facial nerve runs in this plane. By alternately spreading and cutting the superficial lobe away from the deep lobe, the various branches can be identified and spared (Fig. 30–17, *D*). Hemostasis must be meticulous, and this portion of the operation must not be hurried. If the lesion is superficial,

it may be removed along with the superficial lobe, leaving the deep lobe undisturbed beneath the facial nerve. If the lesion is deep to the nerve, one can retract the branches of the facial nerve gently, removing the underlying tumor. If the mass seems to be a mixed tumor, it is extremely important not to violate the capsule of the tumor, since these are notoriously prone to seed throughout the operative field and may require reoperation at a later date. If invasion of the facial nerve is apparent, one should suspect carcinoma. However, functional impairment can occur with sialadenitis and with hemorrhage into benign neoplasms.

Facial weakness (20%) may be observed on the side of operation for days or even weeks following extensive mobilization of the nerve, but if one has been gentle in retracting the nerve and no fibers have been severed, complete recovery is the rule.

REFERENCES

1. Arnold, J., *et al.:* 99mTc-pertechnetate thyroid scintigraphy in patients predisposed to thyroid neoplasms by prior radiotherapy to the head and neck, Radiology 115:653, 1975.
2. Bailey, H.: Congenital parotid sialectasis, J. Int. Coll. Surg. 8:109, 1945.
3. Baum, R. K., and Perzik, S. L.: Tumors of the parotid gland in children. Review of 40 cases, Am. Surg. 31:719, 1965.
4. Beahrs, O. H., and Adson, M. A.: Surgical anatomy and technique of parotidectomy, Am. J. Surg. 95:885, 1958.
5. Beahrs, O. H., and Chong, G. C.: Management of the facial nerve in parotid gland surgery, Am. J. Surg. 124:473, 1972.
6. Beahrs, O. H., Devine, K. D., and Wollner, L.: Parotidectomy in the treatment of chronic sialadenitis, Am. J. Surg. 102:760, 1961.
7. Bertelli, A. D., and deFreitas, J. P.: Carcinoma mucoepidermoide da parotida, Rev. Braz. Chir. 54:70, 1967.
8. Bhaskar, S. N., and Lilly, G. E.: Salivary gland tumors in infancy: Report of 27 cases, J. Oral Surg. 21:305, 1963.
9. Byars, L. T., Ackerman, L. V., and Peacock, E.: Tumors of salivary glands in children, Ann. Surg. 146:40, 1957.
10. Byers, R. M., *et al.:* Malignant tumors of the submaxillary gland, Am. J. Surg. 126:458, 1973.
11. Caldwell, R. A.: Case of congenital capillary hemangioma of parotid gland, Br. J. Surg. 39:261, 1951.
12. Campbell, J. S.: Congenital capillary hemangiomas of the parotid gland: A lesion characteristic of infancy, N. Engl. J. Med. 254:56, 1956.
13. Case, J. C.: Carcinoma of parotid gland in youth, Ann. Surg. 111:155, 1940.
14. Castro, E. B.: Tumors of the major salivary glands in children, Cancer 29:312, 1972.
15. Chong, G. C., *et al.:* Management of parotid gland tumors in infants and children, Mayo Clin. Proc. 50:279, 1975.
16. Danziger, H.: Adenoid cystic carcinoma of the submaxillary gland in an 8-month-old infant, Can. Med. Assoc. J. 91:759, 1964.
17. Dargeon, H. W.: *Tumors of Childhood* (New York: Paul B. Hoeber, Inc., 1960), p. 106.
18. Davies, J. N. P., Dodge, O. G., and Burkitt, D. P.: Salivary gland tumors in Uganda, Cancer 17:1310, 1966.
19. Davis, R. A., *et al.:* Surgical anatomy of the facial nerve and parotid gland based on 350 cervicofacial halves, Surg. Gynecol. Obstet. 102:358, 1956.
20. DeLaney, W. E., and Balogh, K.: Carcinoma of the parotid gland associated with Sjögren's syndrome, Cancer 19:853, 1966.
21. Diamant, H.: Ligation of the parotid duct in chronic recurrent parotitis, Acta Otolaryngol. (Stockh.) 49:375, 1958.
22. Dick, A.: Carcinoma in newborn: Report of case, Am. J. Surg. 87:673, 1954.
23. Duffy, B. J., Jr., and Fitzgerald, P. J.: Cancer of the thyroid in children: A report of 28 cases, J. Clin. Endocrinol. 10:1296, 1950.
24. Dummett, C. O., Campbell, T. M., and Giles, J. W.: Epignathoid teratoma, J. Can. Dent. Assoc. 29:788, 1963.
25. Einstein, R. J.: Sialography in the differential diagnosis of parotid masses, Surg. Gynecol. Obstet. 122:1079, 1966.
26. Favus, M. J., *et al.:* Thyroid cancer occurring as a late consequence of head-and-neck irradiation. Evaluation of 1056 patients, N. Engl. J. Med. 294:1019, 1976.
27. Florman, A. L.: Recurrent bacterial parotitis, J. Pediatr. 46:682, 1955.
28. Foote, F. W., and Frazell, E. L.: Tumors of the Major Salivary Glands, in *Atlas of Tumor Pathology,* Sec. 4, Fasc. 11 (Washington, D. C.: U. S. Armed Forces Institute of Pathology), p. 103.
29. Freedman, S. I.: Malignant lymphomas of the major salivary glands, Arch. Otolaryngol. 93:123, 1971.
30. Galich, R.: Salivary gland neoplasms in childhood, Arch. Otolaryngol. 89:878, 1969.
31. Garas, J., *et al.:* Papillary cystadenoma lymphomatosum (Watkin's tumor). Review of 14 operated cases, Panminerva Med. 17:78, 1975.
32. Goldman, R. L., and Perzik, S. L.: Hemangiomas of the parotid in children, Arch. Otolaryngol. 90:605, 1969.
33. Goldman, R. L., and Perzik, S. L.: Infantile hemangioma of parotid gland: Clinicopathological study of 15 cases, Arch. Otolaryngol. 90:605, 1969.
34. Grage, T. B., and Luben, P. H.: Benign lymphoepithelial tumor of salivary glands, Am. J. Surg. 188:495, 1964.
35. Grulee, C. G.: Tumors of parotid in children, Surg. Gynecol. Obstet. 2:31, 1906.
36. Hagler, S., Rosenbloom, P., and Rosenbloom, A.: Carcinoma of the thyroid in children and young adults: Iatrogenic relation to previous irradiations, Pediatrics 38:77, 1966.
37. Haisora, L., *et al.:* Scintigraphy of salivary glands using Tc 99m pertechnetate, Cesk. Stomatol. 73:169, 1973.
38. Hébert, G., Ouimet-Oliva, D., and Ladouceur, J.: Vascular tumors of the salivary glands in children, Am. J. Roentgenol. Radium Ther. Nucl. Med. 123:815, 1975.
39. Hempelmann, L. H., *et al.:* Neoplasms in persons treated with x-rays in infancy: Fourth survey in 20 years, J. Natl. Cancer Inst. 55:519, 1975.
40. Hendrick, J. W.: Mucoepidermoid cancer of the parotid gland in a one year old child, Am. J. Surg. 108:907, 1964.
41. Howard, J. M., *et al.:* Parotid tumors in children, Surg. Gynecol. Obstet. 90:307, 1950.
42. Jones, H. E.: Recurrent parotitis in children, Arch. Dis. Child. 28:182, 1953.
43. Karlan, M. S., and Snyder, W. H., Jr.: Sialadenitis and major salivary gland tumors in children, Calif. Med. 103:178, 1965.
44. Katzen, M., and DuPlessis, D. J.: Recurrent parotitis in children, S. Afr. Med. J. 38:122, 1964.
45. Kaufman, S. L., and Stout, A. P.: Tumors of the major salivary glands in children, Cancer 16:1317, 1963.
46. Kornblut, A. D.: Parotid lymphangioma: Congenital tumor, ORL 35:303, 1973.
47. Krolls, S. O.: Salivary gland lesions in children. A survey of 430 cases, Cancer 30:459, 1972.
48. Lane, S., and Schwarz, A. W.: Infantile hemangioendothelioma of the parotid gland, Am. J. Surg. 96:784, 1958.
49. Mandel, L., and Bauermash, H.: Ranulae, Oral Surg. 10:567, 1957.
50. Marlowe, J. F., and Hora, J. F.: Parotid mucoepidermoid carcinoma in children, Laryngoscope 78:68, 1968.
51. Martinez-Mora, J., Boix-Ochoa, J., and Tresserra, L.: Vascular tumors of the parotid region in children, Surg. Gynecol. Obstet. 133:973, 1971.
52. Maynard, J. D.: Recurrent parotid enlargement, Br. J. Surg. 52:784, 1965.
53. McKnight, H. A.: A malignant parotid tumor in the newborn, Am. J. Surg. 45:128, 1939.
54. Nidus, B. D., Field, M., and Rammelkamp, C. H.: Salivary gland enlargement caused by sulfisoxazole, Ann. Intern. Med. 63:663, 1965.
55. Parsons, R. W.: Heterotopic cervical salivary gland, Plast. Reconstr. Surg. 49:464, 1972.
56. Pearson, R. S. B.: Recurrent swellings of the parotid gland, Arch. Dis. Child. 10:363, 1935.
57. Perzik, J. L.: Diseases of the Salivary Glands, in Gellis, S., and Kagan, B. (eds.), *Pediatric Therapy* (2d ed.; Philadelphia: W. B. Saunders Company, 1966).
58. Rasanen, O.: Sclerosing inflammation of the submaxillary gland, Küttner's tumor, Duodecim 88:646, 1972.
59. Raven, R. W.: Rare tumors of the pharynx and esophagus, Ann. N. Y. Acad. Sci. 114:1061, 1964.
60. Refetoff, S., *et al.:* Continuing occurrence of thyroid carcinoma after irradiation to the neck in infancy and childhood, N. Engl. J. Med. 292:171, 1975.
61. Reiquam, C. W.: Salivary gland tumors in children, Arch. Surg. 84:468, 1952.
62. Rosenthal, S. A., and Teasley, J. L.: Hemangioma of the parotid gland in children, Wis. Med. J. 70:202, 1971.
63. Rothner, A. D.: Aberrant salivary gland fistulas, J. Pediatr. Surg. 5:931, 1973.
64. Royce, S. W.: Recurrent swelling of the parotid gland, Am. J. Dis. Child. 84:468, 1952.
65. Rush, B. F., Jr., Chambers, R. G., and Ravitch, M. M.: Cancer of the head and neck in children, Surgery 53:270, 1963.
66. Scarcella, J. V., Dykes, E. R., and Anderson, R.: Hemangiomas of the parotid gland, Plast. Reconstr. Surg. 36:38, 1965.
67. Schaffer, A. J., and Jacobson, A. W.: Mikulicz syndrome: Report of 10 cases, Am. J. Dis. Child. 34:327, 1927.

68. Seward, H. F. G., Hamilton, D. J., and Paley, D. H.: An investigation of the Currey test for parotid function, Br. J. Surg. 53:190, 1966.
69. Smith, M.: Familial incidence of sialectasis, Br. Med. J. 2:1359, 1953.
70. Snitman, M. F., Thurston, E., and Romanski, A.: Mucoepidermoid tumor of the parotid gland in a 6-year-old child; case report, Surgery 36:966, 1954.
71. Sobieski, E. J.: Branchiogenic cyst within the parotid gland, Arch. Otolaryngol. 32:395, 1965.
72. Soskolne, A., et al.: Minor salivary gland tumors. A survey of 64 cases, J. Oral Surg. 31:528, 1973.
73. Stingle, W. H., et al.: Ectopic salivary gland sinus in the lower neck, Ann. Otol. Rhinol. Laryngol. 83:379, 1974.
74. Sutow, W. W.: Cancer of the head and neck in children, JAMA 190:90, 1964.
75. Tefft, M., Vawter, G., and Neuhauser, E. B.: Unusual facial tumors in the newborn, Am. J. Roentgenol. 95:32, 1965.
76. Thyroid Cancer Following Radiation. Special Bulletin, Massachusetts Medical Society, February 14, 1977.

77. Ulin, A. W., Ehrlich, E. W., and Silk, R. E.: Clinical and surgical considerations of parotid and submaxillary gland disease, Am. J. Surg. 109:731, 1965.
78. Vawter, G. F.: Congenital tumors of the parotid gland, Arch. Pathol. 82:242, 1966.
79. Welch, K. J., and Trump, D. S., in Mustard, W. T., et al. (eds.), Pediatric Surgery (2d ed.; Chicago: Year Book Medical Publishers, Inc., 1969).
80. Williams, H. B.: Hemangiomas of the parotid gland in children, Plast. Reconstr. Surg. 56:29, 1975.
81. Winship, T.: Symposium on thyroid tumors; carcinoma of thyroid in children, Tr. Am. Goiter A. (1951): 364, 1952.
82. Winship, T., and Rosvoll, R. V.: Thyroid carcinoma in childhood: Final report on a 20-year study, Clin. Proc. Child. Hosp. 26:327, 1970.
83. Wolfe, J. J.: Congenital hemangioma of the parotid gland, Plast. Reconstr. Surg. 29:692, 1962.
84. Wowro, N. W., Frederickson, R. W., and Tennant, R.: Hemangioma of the parotid gland in the newborn and in infancy, Cancer 8:595, 1955.

31 K. J. Welch / W. H. Hendren

The Oropharynx and Jaws

A variety of surgical conditions involving the mouth, jaws and pharynx, often presenting as unusual lesions in the newborn, confront the pediatrician. It seemed reasonable to arrange these entities in a single chapter with some unavoidable overlap of common conditions discussed more fully in other chapters. Infections, injuries, anomalies and neoplasms encountered within or adjacent to the oral cavity are discussed. Of interest is the increasing number of autosomal and sex chromosome syndromes associated with the oral anomalies.[26]

Congenital Anomalies of the Lip

Clefts of the Lip

Paracentral cleft of the lip (harelip) is discussed in Chapter 26. Median cleft is far less common, occurring only once in 500 harelip cases. All infants with median cleft have an associated major central nervous system defect.

In 1875, Ahlfeld[2] described a patient with a lateral facial cleft extending up to the ear. Other clefts have been described starting at the mouth and progressing laterally to involve the orbit, zygomatic arch and temporal area. Ballantyne used the term macrostomia and noted the frequent association with deformed ears and preauricular appendages. Lateral facial clefts occur about once in 100 cases of harelip and embryologically represent a failure of fusion of the mandibular and maxillary processes. Lateral cleft lip and paracentral cleft lip or harelip seldom coexist.[10]

In contrast to harelip, a minor degree of lateral facial cleft is not a very striking abnormality, and consequently most of these children are not presented for surgical treatment during the first year of life. They should be operated on between 1 and 3 years of age in order for the postoperative scar to reach its optimal appearance prior to entering school. Usually these clefts are unilateral and the aim surgically is obliteration of the cleft extending from the corner of the mouth into the cheek. It is important to conserve a vermilion flap to line the new, properly located angle of the mouth. The end of this flap is placed as an inlay into the upper surface of the lower lip, thereby avoiding lateral pull on the repaired corner of the mouth as contracture of healing takes place. In other respects, the repair requires careful approximation of the deficient orbicularis muscle and the other components of the cheek. A Logan bow is used postoperatively to prevent direct pull on the suture line. Healing generally is complete in a week, with a uniformly excellent cosmetic result. If there are associated preauricular tabs or accessory ear structures, they should be excised at the same time. The common type of macrostomia is seen in Figure 31–1, A and a dramatic example of bilateral cleft is seen in Figure 31–1, B.

Microstomia

Microstomia is the rarest of all lip anomalies and represents incomplete development of the primitive blastopore. Surgical treatment consists of unilateral or bilateral extension of the diminutive central opening and construction of a vermilion surface by buccal mucosal advancement.[56] Microstomia may also follow loss of perioral tissue secondary to infection, electrical burns or tumors.

Congenital Lip Fistulas

This condition, often inherited, may or may not be associated with cleft lip or palate.[66] The consistent location of the fistulas in the central segment of the lower lip suggests a

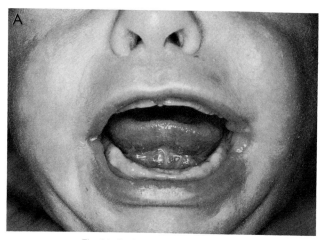
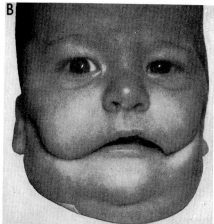

Fig. 31–1.—Lateral facial clefts. **A,** moderate unilateral cleft of the cheek (macrostomia). **B,** extensive bilateral facial clefts extending to temporal areas. (From Blackfield and Wilde.[10])

congenital origin; however, the exact embryologic explanation is lacking. Treatment consists of excision with removal of the two mucous tracts and adjacent glandular tissue. Destruction by electrocoagulation is not recommended. Soricelli *et al.*[59] reported the condition in 6 of 11 members of one family.

Injuries

Burns of the Mouth

Burns of the mouth by caustics still are common because caustic household cleaning compounds are not always put out of the reach of inquisitive toddlers. If there is no evidence of damage to the esophagus in the usual locations at the level of the aortic arch, midesophagus or the esophagogastric junction, they are given a bland diet. Corroded oropharyngeal surfaces are treated by application of sterile mineral oil and usually heal without scarring. The tissue burn already has taken place by the time these children see a physician, and for that reason attempts at local neutralization usually are ineffective. In addition, one does not always know the nature of the compound that produced the burn.

A severe example of burns of the mouth resulting from flames or hot gases and requiring early tracheostomy is shown in Figure 31–2.

ELECTRICAL BURNS.—Electrical burns of all types are being seen with increasing frequency because of the wide use of electric power. They account for 4–7% of all burns, with the highest incidence in Scandinavian countries. Electrical burns of the mouth have been reported sporadically since Pierre[43] called attention to this entity and reported on 11 children in 1961. Thomson *et al.*[64] reported that 43 children were encountered in 20 years at The Hospital for Sick Children, Toronto. Fogh-Anderson and Sorenson[23] reported on 35 children treated in Denmark; 20 were aged 1–2 years, 7 were 2–4 years of age and 5 were under 1 year. We have encountered 8 children with this condition, comprising about 1% of burn admissions. Most cases resulted from biting or sucking the free end of a "live" extension cord. Thus, electrical burns of the mouth occur most frequently in the creeper or toddler, when everything is seen at floor level. The electric cord is a tempting play object, and contact is made at the exposed end or by biting through the insulation. Following completion of the circuit by saliva there are tetanic contractions of the muscles of mastication, causing the jaws to grip the fixture and maintain contact. Unless the child is exceptionally well grounded, electrocution does not occur. There is destruction of tissue beyond the apparent gross limits of the burn, and eventual loss always is far greater than originally estimated. Children with electrical burns of the mouth should be hospitalized for approximately 2 weeks. During this time, the area of gray coagulation necrosis will slough away and alarming hemorrhage from the tongue and lips may occur (Fig. 31–3). Chewing the insensitive tissue may be a factor in starting bleeding. Once the danger of hemorrhage has passed,

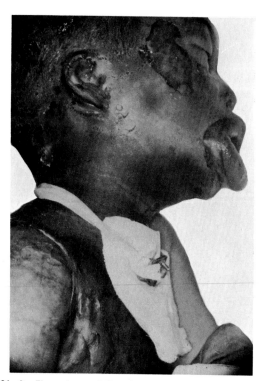

Fig. 31.–2.—Flame burn of the airway and oropharyngeal tissues requiring early tracheostomy. Swelling is maximal at 36 hours.

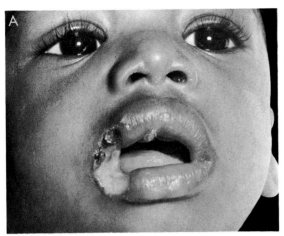

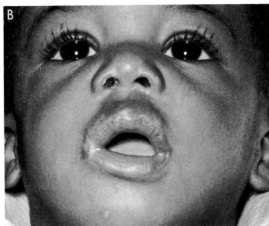

Fig. 31–3.—Electrical burn of the mouth in a 5-month-old child. **A,** immediate appearance. The alveolar ridge and tongue also were involved. Major bleeding occurred on the 7th hospital day. **B,** 6 months later, showing good cosmetic appearance without surgical intervention.

healing occurs rapidly. The temptation is to carry out definitive surgical correction, yet deficiency of lip substance is compensated for by cicatricial closure with surprisingly little deformity. Efforts at plastic reconstruction should be deferred approximately 1 year. At that time, usually very little will be required. The tongue will reshape normally and seldom requires surgical treatment. The lip scar often can be improved, and the only long-range problem is damage to permanent tooth buds in the area of burn. Deep destruction with resulting osteomyelitis of the mandible rarely occurs.

A conservative plastic approach should be adopted. Fogh-Anderson[23] found that 12 children required no surgical treatment whereas 23 had one or more operations. Useful procedures include creation of a sulcus, V-excision of the mature scar, Stein-Estlander-Abbe flap and commissurotomy.

Lacerations

Injuries of the oropharyngeal region are common in childhood, especially in boys. Most are of little consequence, but others may endanger life (Fig. 31–4). Patients with traumatic cleft lip should be hospitalized. Repair must be accurately carried out under endotracheal anesthesia with careful attention to alignment of the vermilion border of the lip. The children should be hospitalized until the lip is completely healed, and the fresh repair should be supported with a Logan bow to prevent disruption or local injury to the suture line.

Lacerations of the cheek in which Stensen's duct may be severed should be repaired by complete external closure and loose internal closure around a rubber slip drain. If the laceration does communicate with the duct, an internal salivary fistula of no consequence will be established.

Major lacerations of the tongue should be sutured because of the frequent occurrence of delayed hemorrhage.

Lacerations of the palate usually occur in active, uncoordinated preschool children, who usually fall with a spoon or stick in the mouth. The object is driven through the palate, producing a traumatic cleft. The injuries vary from simple perforations to complete detachment of the soft palate, often extending into the tonsillar fossa. If the injury is extensive or perforating, the patient should be admitted to the hospital. Because of the proximity of this area to the central nervous system, tetanus prophylaxis is important. The intraoral tissues are exceptionally resistant to infection, and antibiotics have little to offer in most instances. The children should be managed like patients undergoing repair of a congenital cleft palate, by suturing the nasal mucous membrane, then approximating the palatal muscle at the base of the uvula, and finally joining the oral mucous membrane. Chromic catgut is used throughout. Only clear liquids are allowed for 5 days following such a repair, and the arms should be restrained with palate cuffs for approximately 4 weeks.

Braudo[12] reported 4 children who had thrombosis of the internal carotid artery after injury to the soft palate. All patients developed hemiplegia, transient in 3 and permanent in 1. At postmortem examination, 1 was found to have extensive softening of the corresponding hemisphere. These central nervous system difficulties occurred approximately 3 days after injury.

With the earliest detection of neurologic deficit, selective carotid arteriography followed by CAT brain scan could identify the suspected injury to the internal carotid artery at the base of the skull. Combined extracranial and intracranial

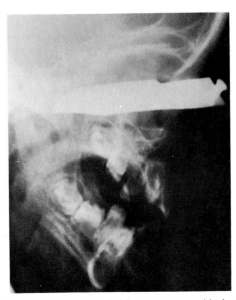

Fig. 31–4.—Knife blade embedded in petrous pyramid of a 1-year-old child. Wound entrance was below the right eye.

exploration might re-establish arterial blood flow to the corresponding hemisphere. Unfortunately, such injuries of the lateral pharyngeal wall usually are considered to be of little consequence and diagnosis is delayed until repair has little to offer.

Hemangioma

Hemangioma may appear as a combined mucous membrane and skin lesion in the region of the oropharynx and is treacherous in this area of rich blood supply. The lesion may be insignificant or absent at birth, first appearing at 1 month of age, and if untreated many progress in several months to massive involvement of the area with secondary infection, ulcerative destruction and loss of important features. Over a long period, these combined capillary and cavernous lesions ultimately involute, but en route to that desirable end, loss of important substance of the lips, nose, eyelids and ears may occur.

Surgical treatment of hemangiomas should be conservative unless the lesion is small or pedunculated and can be removed without sacrifice of important structures (Fig. 31–5). The eventual appearance of most facial hemangiomas is much better than one might originally predict, and operation should be restricted to removal of stromal elements that remain after regression.[30]

The possible extent of such a lesion is shown in Figure 31–6. No hemangioma was present at birth. At 6 weeks of age there were a few surface blotches, and 3 months later there was massive extension of the lesion. It now is well established that bulky hemangiomas occasionally trap platelets, producing thrombocytopenia and secondary bleeding. In this child, the platelet count fell to 20,000 and the head and neck became monstrously deformed because of continued tumor growth and extravasating hemorrhage. Steroids were given. X-ray treatment of the lesion to the limit of skin tolerance (900 R) had no apparent benefit. Platelet infusions also failed to achieve a sustained satisfactory level. The child was hospitalized repeatedly over a 3-year period and ultimately died of exsanguinating hemorrhage after inadvertently driving a fork into his cheek.

Treatment of such a lesion persisting into adult life by wide excision with vascular occlusion using cardiopulmo-

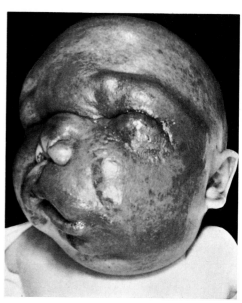

Fig. 31–6.—A platelet-trapping hemangioma, not present at birth but evident at 6 weeks. There were transitory, unsustained platelet rises after prednisone therapy, splenectomy and multiple platelet infusions. Death occurred at 3 years due to exsanguination after a minor local injury.

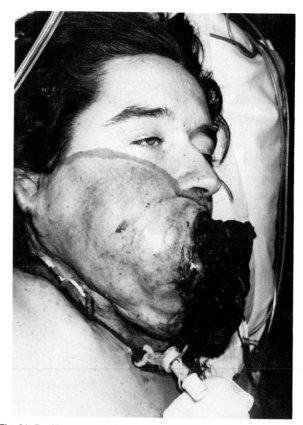

Fig. 31–7.—Massive hemangioma involving the oropharynx and tongue, present from birth, and persistent at age 23. It failed to involute and bled repeatedly, requiring hospitalization and transfusion. Multiple surgical attempts were of no avail and he finally required near-total excision of the process, carried out under total cardiopulmonary bypass with hypothermia. (Courtesy of J. B. Mulliken.)

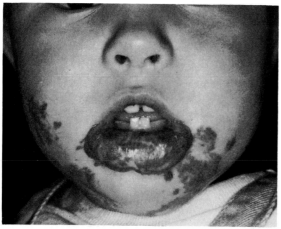

Fig. 31–5.—Hemangioma of lower lip and chin, treated with endoral conservative surgical excision in stages. Thinning of the lip and reconstruction of the vermilion surface was accomplished later by buccal mucous membrane advancement.

nary bypass with deep hypothermia is illustrated in Figure 31–7.

Today, platelet-trapping hemangiomas can be treated by effective methods of platelet transfusion. Fifteen billion platelets can be given in as little as 15 ml of plasma. Under 1 year of age, this results in a normal number of circulating platelets. With this protection, one may wish to excise a hemangioma in which platelet trapping is a threat to life. Diamond has seen 12 such patients, the first recognized some 40 years ago.[18] Good *et al.*[25] reported on this condition, and there are 72 additional cases in the literature.

Lesions of the Jaw

Pierre Robin Syndrome

The Pierre Robin syndrome consists of hypoplasia of the mandible, posterior displacement of the tongue and often an associated cleft palate. Inspiratory obstruction with sternal retraction and failure to thrive are common features (Fig. 31–8). The infant hyperextends the neck to breathe more easily. Attacks of alarming cyanosis are frequent and sudden and can be fatal. Glossoptosis diminishes with growth, and

in most cases embarrassment of respiration and difficulty with feeding improve in 2 or 3 months. Nevertheless, many such infants have died unexpectedly at a time when they seemed to be overcoming their problem.

Tracheostomy should be utilized only as a lifesaving procedure.

A Stamm gastrostomy should be performed in patients who have marked difficulties with feeding. Repeated attempts at oral feeding in the presence of respiratory distress result in aspiration. In an infant, gastrostomy can be accomplished safely under local anesthesia in a few minutes, thereby relieving the nursing staff of many hours of ineffective and dangerous feeding attempts.

Airway obstruction is caused not so much by an oversized tongue as by the hypoplastic mandible and perhaps incomplete development of the intrinsic muscles of the tongue. Micrognathia in itself is an index of immaturity. The jaw steadily lengthens, and at the same time there is marked improvement in the intrinsic operation of the tongue. During this phase of additional local development, surgical procedures have much to offer and indeed may be lifesaving. In 1950, Douglas[19] recommended denuding the undersurface of the tongue and the gingivobuccal sulcus, suturing these

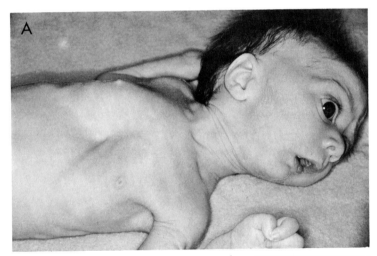

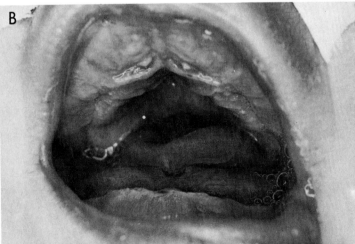

Fig. 31–8.—Pierre Robin syndrome. **A,** 2-month-old infant with micrognathia, glossoptosis and opisthotonic position of the head to improve the airway. **B,** note retrodisplacement of the mandible and tip of the tongue and prominent upper jaw. The associated cleft of the soft palate is thought to be due to abnormal elevation of the tongue during the process of palate closure.

two structures together. He reported 6 patients, with 1 death. In response to a questionnaire, he was able to collect 46 additional instances. Twenty-one were not treated surgically; there were 13 deaths in the untreated group. Twenty-five patients were treated surgically by this method, and there were no deaths. Sometimes the Douglas repair does not hold and the tongue falls back into the throat.

The Douglas repair may be combined with the Duhamel technique, anchoring the base of the tongue forward to the alveolar ridge using no. 1 proline.[20]

We have utilized this method of surgical treatment in 9 patients and all survived.[21] The Duhamel suture must remain in place for approximately 6 weeks; if properly placed, it does not cut through. The procedure is thought not to interfere with the eruption of permanent teeth.

Moderate cases of Pierre Robin syndrome may be managed by feeding the infant in the upright position and subsequently prone positioning with the neck extended by applying traction to a skullcap made of moleskin and stockinet.

A related condition is glossopalatine ankylosis, reported by Spivack and Bennett.[60] The condition is complex and is discussed further under ankyloglossia superior.

Fractures

Fractures of the maxilla and mandible are uncommon in childhood, in marked contrast to the incidence in adults, who usually incur this injury in automobile accidents. Not only are maxillofacial fractures less common in childhood but the child's face is inherently more resilient because of the greater cartilage content.

Diagnosis of a fracture of the *mandible* usually can be made by clinical examination. The fracture is apparent as an irregularity in the mandibular arch with loss of proper dental occlusion, and occasionally with a tear of the oral mucous membrane. The most common site of fracture of the mandible in childhood is the bicuspid area. If there is no significant displacement, no active treatment is necessary. These children have remarkably little discomfort. A liquid or soft diet should be prescribed for about 4 weeks, following which union usually is sufficiently good to permit a full diet. If displacement is present, and if the child has teeth adjacent to the fracture site, interdental wire fixation can be undertaken. External fixation devices are not recommended. If teeth are absent, stabilization of mandibular fragments can be accomplished by open reduction, placing one or two small steel wires very low in the mandibular ramus. As an alternative method of stabilization, one may pass a wire around the symphysis menti and anchor it to the maxilla through a drill hole in the anterior nasal spine. Central bilateral fractures can be supported by a molded splint held in place by wires circumferentially placed around the mandible and the splint.[42] The splint permits the child to open his mouth and it usually is left in place for 4 weeks. These relatively simple techniques avoid the danger of infection and direct injury to tooth buds, which may result from more extensive open reduction methods.

The mandible is fractured next most commonly in the subcondylar region, usually with pain and tenderness in the region of the temporomandibular joint, with considerable trismus and displacement of the lower dental arch. Active treatment of such a fracture seldom is necessary. With subsequent growth, a fracture with considerable angulation may be expected to straighten spontaneously without residual deformity. Very rarely there may be complete separation of the fractured surfaces, with rotation of the proximal frag-

ment, which may require open reduction. In an older child, if the proximal fragment consists of merely the head of the condyle, the simplest management may be to remove the head of the condyle, following which pseudarthrosis occurs, with satisfactory function as a result. Occasionally, interosseous wiring is indicated. A fracture in this area in a small child may result eventually in some degree of facial asymmetry by virtue of interference with the growth center in the mandibular head.

Extensive fractures of the *maxilla* are uncommon in childhood, and when seen should be treated much as they are in older individuals. A depressed malar zygomatic arch may be corrected by simple elevation or occasionally by open reduction with placement of wires for external traction within 72 hours. In older children, after reduction, fixation by wiring the teeth together is a satisfactory method. The primary objective is establishment of good occlusion without injury to permanent tooth buds. Whenever teeth are wired, the patient must be kept under close observation, with wire cutters at hand to be used in the event of distress from vomiting.[55] Gastrostomy is a useful adjunct in some patients.

If open reduction of a maxillary fracture is considered necessary, and this rarely is the case, one must carefully avoid the site of permanent tooth buds. Good healing can be expected in 3–5 weeks with most fractures regardless of their complexity.

Recent experience at Children's Hospital Medical Center, Boston has been documented by Kaban *et al.*,[27a] who reported 122 children treated for facial fractures over a 10-year period.

Tumors of the Jaws

Tumors of the jaws are rare in children, and fortunately benign tumors are predominant, especially those related to dental development. The jaws derive from the first branchial arch and are composed of a mesodermal mass covered with ectoderm. Both tissues can produce a variety of neoplasms. In this area of complex development, inclusions of salivary gland or thyroid tissue may occur.

Jaw tumors usually present as asymptomatic swellings. With growth, they cause irregular displacement and ultimate loss of the overlying teeth, with complicating sepsis. Radiographic and clinical impressions are notably inaccurate, and all lesions must be identified by surgical biopsy. Jaw tumors in children have been classified as follows:[48]

Tumors of dental origin: follicular cysts; dentigerous cysts; ameloblastoma (adamantinoma).

Benign tumors of nondental origin: giant cell; eosinophilic granuloma; fibroma (fibrous dysplasia).

Primary malignant tumors: carcinoma; sarcoma (endosteal fibrosarcoma, osteogenic sarcoma, unclassified).

Metastatic malignant tumors: neuroblastoma; embryonal carcinoma.

BENIGN TUMORS.—Ordinarily, ameloblastoma is a bulky tissue displacing benign tumor, but it may appear in malignant form and has occurred at the age of 5 months. Giant cell tumors should be carefully cleaned out by curettage and cauterization of the tumor cavity. They have a great tendency to recur; therefore, the first operation should be extensive and definitive. Eosinophilic granuloma probably is part of a general metabolic disturbance related to Hand-Schüller-Christian and Letterer-Siwe diseases. It is evident as a swelling of the gums with loosening and bleeding from tooth sockets and ultimate infection. There is no certain method of treatment. Because of the similar histologic and x-ray appearance of jaw fibromas and hyperparathyroidism, calcium, phosphorus and phosphatase blood level determinations are of importance.

Hemangiomas of the mandible and maxilla may present as surgical emergencies. They usually are unsuspected until there is bleeding around a tooth socket either spontaneously or after dental extraction. They are characterized by spurting of arterial blood in large amounts and difficulty with hemostasis by any of the conventional dental techniques. X-ray examination of the jaw reveals the washed-out appearance of bone destruction in the area of the lesion. Ligation of the external carotid artery is of little value. Segmental resection of the maxilla or mandible may be necessary and under some conditions lifesaving. Adjunctive hypothermia has been found useful; and, as with nasopharyngeal angioma, freezing of the lesion with a cryoprobe before surgical resection will reduce blood loss substantially.[17, 62]

Considerable attention has been devoted to a benign lesion of the jaws considered to be a melanotic neuroectodermal tumor of infancy of neural crest origin. In 1 case, this was associated with high urinary excretion of vanillylmandelic acid.[11] Historically, these lesions were considered to be odontogenic and closely related to ameloblastoma. Because of their characteristic pigmentation, they appear to represent a separate entity, also called melanotic progonoma.[29] In most cases, the tumor has become evident before the age of 1 year, predominantly in the maxilla of female patients.[28] Medenis and associates[35] collected 27 cases from the literature, noting the female preponderance and the fact that all patients were under age 6. Conservative resection with curettage to produce bony bleeding appears to be adequate treatment, with infrequent recurrence.

Alveolar margin tumors include epulis (congenital granular cell myoblastoma) (Fig. 31–9) (Cussen[15]) and lymphangiomatous cysts (Levin[31]). Both conditions are treated by local resection. Recurrence is uncommon. Rappaport and Furnas[46] have reported subtotal maxillectomy and mandibulectomy for assorted benign invasive tumors in 13 children, ranging in age from 3 months to 11 years. The conditions treated included tumors of neuroectodermal origin, aneurysmal bone cyst, ameloblastic fibroma, composite odontoma, nasoangiofibroma, hemangioma of bone, giant cell reparative granuloma and osteoblastoma. Patients were followed for an average of 5 years postoperatively with facial and oral photographs, cephalograms and cephalometric analysis, and plaster dental molds were used to document longitudinal and cross-sectional growth patterns. From this considerable experience Rappaport and Furnas conclude that extensive extirpation of facial bones may be performed in children without significantly jeopardizing function or growth. Iliac bone grafts proved highly satisfactory in reconstruction of the mandible without regard to age. Particulate bone was effective in reconstructing large contour defects of the mandible caused by extensive resection of these locally aggressive tumors. Lewin,[32] discussing nonmalignant maxillofacial tumors in children, concluded that reasonably radical resection ensuring complete removal of the tumor offers an excellent chance for permanent cure. In most instances, block resection rather than local excision with curettage will be required. He concluded, as did Rappaport and Furnas, that resection of a skeletal segment involving the facial bones was not more deforming in a child than in an adult and immediate reconstruction can be undertaken. Irradiation has no role in the management of these interesting maxillofacial tumors; operation must be undertaken realistically and aggressively.

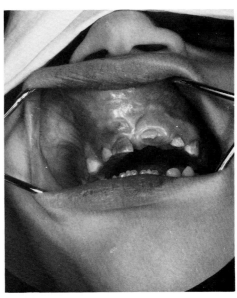

Fig. 31–9.—Epulis (congenital granular cell myoblastoma) involving the maxilla of a 4-year-old boy. The lesion interfered with the eruption of teeth, causing their devitalization. It involved much of the right upper portion of the maxilla, extending into the maxillary antrum. Operation consisted of wide removal and appropriate reconstruction of the maxillary arch.

MALIGNANT TUMORS.—Malignant jaw tumors are rare. Byars[48] reported an endosteal fibrosarcoma in a 3-year-old child. An example of mandibular sarcoma is shown in Figure 31–10.

Osteosarcoma arising in fibrous dysplasia of the facial bones has been reported by Yannopoulos et al.[70] Among the cases reported there were 3 children, ages 6, 8 and 11 years. A review of the literature provided 8 additional cases. Treatment, as with other osteosarcomas of childhood consists of radical local excision followed by irradiation and chemotherapy as methotrexate with citrovorum rescue (see Chap. 8). The possibility of an induced sarcoma following inappropriate irradiation of fibrous dysplasia could not be excluded in 3 cases. Hemangiosarcoma (malignant hemangioendothelioma) of the mandible has been reported in a child by Ghandi et al.[24] Its occurrence in the jaws is particularly rare, only 4 additional cases being reported. Treatment consisted of hemimandibulectomy with suprahyoid neck dissection. The child was entirely well 3 years after operation.

Burkitt's tumor (the African lymphoma).—In 1958, Burkitt[14] described a primitive and at that time unclassified sarcoma arising in multicentric fashion commonly in the jaws of black children in Uganda (Fig. 31–11). He saw 38 patients with the tumor in 7 years, with peak incidence at age 5. The maxilla is involved more often than the mandible, and loosening of molars is the first clinical sign. These tumors grow to huge size, are locally destructive and do not ulcerate. About half metastasize to the abdomen. The regional or distant lymph nodes and spleen are not involved, and there are no changes in peripheral blood. The lesion is essentially osteolytic and is first evident as disappearance of the lamina dura. The obvious relation to neuroblastoma was first considered, but it is a discrete and separate neoplasm. In the relatively small region of Uganda, the tumor attains endemic proportions and is considered the most common malignant tumor of childhood.

The tendency to jaw involvement has a unique age distribution. Below age 3, the jaw tumor has been observed sel-

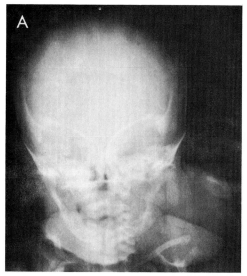
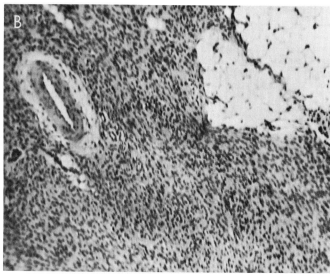

Fig. 31–10.—Sarcoma of the mandible. **A,** roentgenogram of infant with exophytic sarcoma of the mandibular region. These congenital tumors present obstetric difficulties but fortunately are not highly malignant and metastasize late. **B,** photomicrograph of mandibular sarcoma, showing mesenchymal ground substance. These have been classified as embryomas. Although locally invasive, they are resectable when exophytic but seldom when there is invasion of the pterygoid fossa. ×100.

dom. In every child 3 years of age, the jaw tumors have been clinically evident; this incidence diminishes with each year of age, the tumors being seen in only 20% of patients at age 12.[13] Few cases have been seen anywhere in the world beyond age 14. Adatia[1] ably reviewed the literature, focusing attention on the multiracial and world-wide distribution.

Burkitt's tumor is very sensitive to relatively small doses of chemotherapeutic agents, placing it in a favorable category. Burkitt found a significant response to methotrexate in two-thirds of tumors of moderate size and in four-fifths of similar tumors treated with cyclophosphamide (Cytoxan).[13] Of 63 children treated with this agent, 24 had total clinical regression. Regression continued after cessation of therapy. Viral etiology (Epstein-Barr virus) has been implicated, with a favorable tumor-host relationship. Irradiation plays a

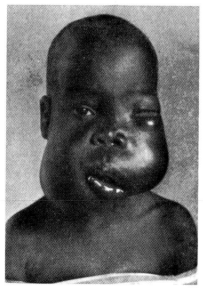

Fig. 31–11.—Burkitt's lymphoma involving the jaws of a 3-year-old boy. Death was due to pulmonary metastasis. (From Burkitt.[14])

minor role; surgical excision, except for identification of the process, seems unwarranted.

A word of caution must be inserted because of the current overdiagnosis of the condition in retrospective review of patients with a probable diagnosis of lymphosarcoma or reticulum cell sarcoma.[40] Reclassification has been based on histologic appearance characterized by proliferation of primitive cells of lymphoreticular tissue and by an abundance of actively phagocytosing histiocytes. Clinical presentation and anatomic tumor distribution similar to that reported in the majority of the African cases has not been required. Several such patients in our institution have blossomed into full-scale lymphatic leukemia. Irradiation and chemotherapy have been of no value at that stage.

Pseudosarcomatous fasciitis.—A perplexing surgical lesion involving the jaws and surrounding mesenchymal tissues initially presenting as a granuloma and later becoming increasingly cellular with a predominance of mesenchymal elements has been called pseudosarcomatous fasciitis.[5] Our patient, a 12-year-old boy, for 5 years had agonizing pain in the distribution of the trigeminal nerve. In addition to stiffening and wasting of the temporomandibular joint became fixed. Some cases have been thought to be due to aspergillosis and were empirically treated with amphotericin B. Because of the histologic nature of the process, prednisone has been administered to toxic levels. Ultimately, because of the unrelieved pain and nutritional difficulties, surgical treatment must be undertaken. This consists of hemifacial resection including the mandible and appropriate resurfacing. This process is radioresistant.[5]

Aggressive fibromatosis of the mandible or palate has been reported by Wilkins *et al.*[68] Four of 6 cases involved children, the youngest age 2. Treatment consists of wide local excision, with rotational flaps or skin grafts. Such lesions are improperly labeled fibrosarcoma and probably all are benign but locally aggressive, invading normal tissues, including bone.

METASTATIC TUMORS.—These may be found in the jaw region or in the glands of the upper neck. Some are occult in the nasopharynx, or the primary site may never be found. Metastatic spread of neuroblastoma to the skull occurs frequently, but the deposits are most common in the calvarium and the retrobulbar tissues. Rarely, first evidence of the tumor may consist of a swelling of the mandible from bony metastasis.

SURGICAL TREATMENT.—Accurate diagnosis of jaw tumors is established by surgical biopsy. Most benign tumors can be adequately treated by wide local excision, occasionally taking a horizontal section of the mandibular ramus. Malignant tumors must be treated by wide local excision with hemimandibulectomy. It is important to maintain the symmetry of the face with proper prosthetic support. Iliac bone grafts for older children are seldom used until facial growth is complete in the second decade.

Infections

Four types of infection with which all surgeons should be familiar are peculiar to the oropharyngeal region.

Ludwig's Angina

This infection is aptly named, angina meaning to strangle or suffocate. The causative organism usually is a streptococcus, although there may be a mixed infection. The most common portal of entry is a carious mandibular molar. Spread through the floor of the mouth is rapid, with involvement of the submaxillary space. In half the patients, Vincent's organisms also are present. A patient with a typical case presents swelling and tenderness of the submaxillary and submandibular regions of the neck, edema of the floor of the mouth and elevation of the tongue (Fig. 31–12). The process may cause complete respiratory obstruction.

Treatment should be started immediately, with large doses of tetracycline and penicillin, to which most patients respond in a gratifying manner. It seldom is necessary to perform tracheostomy or to create large drainage incisions in the submaxillary region, as was formerly done. Pus rarely is encountered early, although at a later stage pus may be found deep between the mylohyoid and geniohyoid muscles or between the geniohyoid and genioglossus muscles. In preantibiotic days, this dreaded infection occasionally spread along fascial planes of the neck into the mediastinum, with fatal outcome.

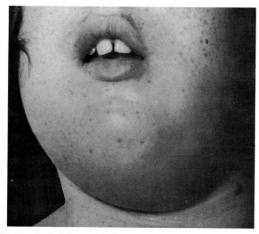

Fig. 31–12.—Ludwig's angina in an 11-year-old girl. Note the brawny edema throughout the submental and submandibular regions. There was elevation of the tongue and mild respiratory embarrassment. The condition responded to antibiotics without need for surgical drainage.

Peritonsillar Abscess

Once a common condition, peritonsillar abscess is seen seldom in this day of early antibiotic treatment of pharyngeal infection. It is extremely rare in small children. Characteristically, there is a history of recent tonsillitis followed by onset of severe pain with unilateral swelling above and medial to the upper pole of the tonsil. Trismus or inability to open the mouth widely is common.

Treatment by prompt surgical drainage is mandatory. Drainage should be carried out under full endotracheal general anesthesia, with the patient positioned in a steep Trendelenburg position to prevent aspiration.

Retropharyngeal Abscess

Retropharyngeal abscess is seen in infants and toddlers but rarely in older children. Symptoms may be those of respiratory obstruction, inability to swallow or stiffness of the neck suggesting a cervical orthopedic problem. Once suspected, diagnosis is best made by palpation of the pharyngeal region, gently sweeping the examining finger across the posterior pharyngeal wall.

Treatment consists of surgical drainage. It is best to drain retropharyngeal abscesses without general anesthesia, because induction of anesthesia may be hazardous when respiratory obstruction is imminent. If the patient is in the Trendelenburg position, well wrapped and with the head well extended, the likelihood of aspiration of pus is minimal.

X-ray examination of both soft tissues and vertebrae of the cervical region is indicated to rule out the presence of an opaque foreign body, which may have been ingested, and to exclude cervical osteomyelitis as the underlying cause.

Noma

Noma is a severe necrotizing infection of mucous membranes that may involve the nose, eyelids, auditory canal or oropharynx. It usually is seen in the first decade of life and nearly always in children with a greatly lowered resistance to infection due to a generalized disorder such as malnutrition, blood dyscrasia, immunosuppression, immune deficiency or exanthematous disease.[61]

No single organism has been uniformly responsible, and culture usually provides evidence of a mixed infection. Vincent's organisms nearly always are present. The infection starts with ulceration of mucous membranes accompanied by a foul odor and progresses rapidly to necrosis and sloughing of tissues. Destruction of much of the face may result (Fig. 31–13).

Treatment consists of massive broad-spectrum antibiotic therapy and vigorous supportive measures directed toward improving the underlying disease state. Necrotic tissue should be debrided.

Tempest[63] has provided a collective review on noma (derived from the Greek "to devour"). It was first described by Tourdes in 1848. Over a 3-year period, Tempest observed more than 300 children suffering from the effects of noma (cancrum oris). This quite fantastic modern-day experience was in Nigeria. Mortality prior to the availability of modern antibiotics ranged from 56% to 88%. In his experience, 95% of cases followed exanthemata, most commonly measles. Severe malnutrition, including kwashiorkor, affected 67% of patients. Prevalence of Vincent's organisms has been ascribed to poor dental care. There was no relationship between noma and sickle cell disease. Only 17 of 250 cases were extraoral in location. Most involved the oropharynx

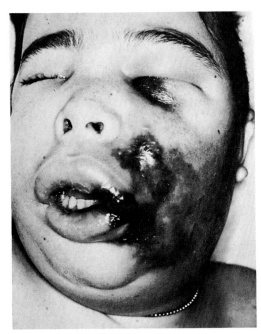

Fig. 31–13.—Noma, or gangrenous stomatitis, destroying a large portion of the left cheek in a 10-year-old child with leukemia.

unilaterally, 66% extending into the maxilla and mandible; 34% of cases were bilateral. Isolated mandibular involvement occurred in 12%. Extensive facial mutilation is graphically portrayed in this report. Much emphasis was placed on reconstruction following loss of important facial features.

Lesions of the Tongue and Oral Cavity

Ankyloglossia Inferior

This condition, called tongue-tie, is common in infancy and often disappears spontaneously or with sucking if the frenum of the tongue is not prominent or is sufficiently thin. In some cases, however, surgery may be necessary to permit normal speech, and operation can be carried out very simply. The handle of a grooved director serves admirably for this purpose. With this instrument, one can elevate the tip of the tongue, permitting the frenum of the tongue to fit between the wing-like projections of the handle. The frenum then is cut transversely to release the tip of the tongue. Bleeding is easily controlled by gentle pressure on a gauze sponge for a minute or two. If surgical release of tongue-tie is deferred until the child is older, general anesthesia is required. The frenulum is divided by electroresection; no sutures are required.

Ankyloglossia Superior

This condition—attachment of the tongue to the roof of the mouth—is a very rare congenital anomaly. It must be recognized at birth, because severe or total respiratory obstruction is inevitable. There is an associated cleft palate corresponding to the synechial margin. Surgical treatment consists of peripheral freeing and suturing of the raw mucous membrane margins of the palate and tongue. Repair of the cleft palate is deferred until the usual age of 12–14 months.[34, 69]

Ankyloglossia superior, glossopalatine ankylosis, has been reported in 33 children by Spivack and Bennett.[60] The condition overlaps with the Pierre Robin syndrome, which is considered by Hanson to be a broad genetic defect demonstrated in 7 of 28 patients (25%).[27] Spivack and Bennett[60] have considerably enlarged on the nature of the disease, pointing out that in the 33 patients studied, fused tongue and palate occurred in 17, micrognathia in 13, macroglossia in 22, cleft palate in 12 and distal anomalies of the extremities in 14. All cases are somewhat different. In severe cases, all four extremities may be involved. In addition, some patients have a median notch involving the lower or upper lip. There may be unilateral or bilateral facial palsy indicating the complexity of the condition and the gross interference with facial bones as well as the petrous portion of the temporal bone. Three patients died without treatment, underlining the extreme urgency of the condition in the neonate lest anoxic brain damage occur because of intermittent respiratory obstruction. Intelligence has been normal in all survivors.

Two unusual infants with congenital fusion of the gums were reported by Snijman and Prinsloo.[57] This fusion was limited to soft tissue synechiae, which were easily divided. The lesion presented in each instance because of inability to feed. The condition may be associated with fibrous ankylosis of the temporomandibular joints. In each instance, the palate was intact; it seemed to have no relationship to glossopalatine ankylosis, although 1 patient did have hemiatrophy of the face and Horner's syndrome.

Cysts

Ranula is a term descriptive of a cyst of the sublingual gland (L., *rana*, frog). It may become very large and interfere with respiration in the newborn. It is fully discussed in Chapter 30.

Cysts of the floor of the mouth are rare except for ranula and lymphangioma in its various forms. Dermoid cysts are uncommon and account for only 2% of head and neck dermoids. These usually are found in the midline deep within the substance of the tongue and, as with dermoids in other locations, often are signaled by the presence of a sinus pore on the surface of the tongue at the junction of the middle and anterior thirds in the midline. Treatment consists of midline longitudinal bivalving of the tongue, tracing the stalk to the dermoid cyst, which is embedded deeply in the geniohyoid muscle. These lesions are approached intraorally, although they may present as a midline swelling of the suprahyoid region.[49]

Schaffer[52a] has encountered 10 neonates with nasopharyngeal dermoid. At times, these were huge and presented at the fauces, obstructing the oral entrance. Treatment of these patients is urgent; suffocation has been reported.

Lingual Thyroid

Thyroid tissue may be situated in the midline of the tongue posteriorly at the site of the foramen caecum, having failed to descend from its embryonic site of origin. Not only may it cause symptoms of dysphagia or respiratory distress but it may be subject to the vagaries of normally placed thyroid tissue. Hyperthyroidism, adenoma and even carcinoma may occur. The lingual thyroid should be totally excised, and although this can be performed transorally, it often is preferable to work through a lateral pharyngotomy or transhyoid approach.[67] In the majority of cases, no other functioning thyroid tissue is present lower in the neck (negative scan), and total surgical excision may be expected to pro-

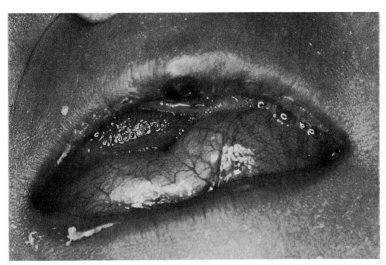

Fig. 31–14.—Cystic hygroma bulging in the floor of the mouth of a 2-day-old infant with a large hygroma encircling the neck. Tracheostomy and feeding gastrostomy were necessary.

duce myxedema. This is not a problem, however, for substitution therapy is both inexpensive and completely satisfactory even in a growing child (see Chap. 34).

Tumors

Several tumors of the tongue and floor of the mouth are characteristic of infancy and childhood.

CYSTIC HYGROMA.—Cystic hygroma of the floor of the mouth often is associated with cystic hygroma involving the neck in a collar-like fashion. Although histologically benign, such a tumor may kill by virtue of distribution throughout the vital structures of the neck. These growths do not respect tissue planes or anatomic compartments. A child with cystic hygroma may have involvement of the floor of the mouth, neck and parotid region bilaterally, and, in addition, the mass may extend caudally into the mediastinum. It is common to see hemangiomatous elements mixed with cystic

hygroma, usually recognizable by a bluish discoloration of the overlying skin. Spontaneous hemorrhage into such a mass is not uncommon. Potts[45] emphasized that operation is never simple. If involvement of the floor of the mouth is extensive, tracheostomy and gastrostomy may be necessary in the first few days of life as a lifesaving procedure (Fig. 31–14). With an extensive hygroma, it is well to limit one's sights to what can be accomplished at a single operation. Thorough cleaning out of a limited area, without injury to such structures as the facial nerve, avoids the necessity for working in that same area subsequently, which is important because reidentification of vital structures may prove difficult. One is never justified in sacrificing important structures, which may be surrounded by hygroma, and should be content with removing as much tumor as possible short of injury to important nerves and vessels. Cysts that cannot be excised safely should be opened. Many infants have been needlessly lost by attempts to excise too much hygroma during one procedure. Although it is tempting, it may prove

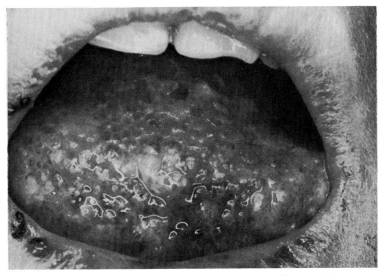

Fig. 31–15.—Diffuse lymphangioma of the tongue of a 10-year-old boy.
Note crusting around the lips, indicating poor oral hygiene.

foolhardy. Similarly, an attempt to clean out one entire side of the face and neck in one operation may force the surgeon to hurry unnecessarily, with resultant permanent injury to an important structure.

LYMPHANGIOMA.—Lymphangioma is the most common cause of macroglossia in infancy.[4] The tumor may be localized to a small area of the tongue or floor of the mouth, or it may involve these areas diffusely. Characteristically, the gross appearance is that of a raised, firm mass in the tongue with a warty-looking surface composed of many tiny cysts, some of which contain lymph and others blood (Fig. 31–15). Recurring attacks of infection, suppurative glossitis, are common and should be treated with antibiotics. Poor oral hygiene is seen frequently, with gingivitis and dental caries. Bleeding into the oral cavity is not uncommon.

Definitive treatment of diffuse lingual lymphangioma may be very difficult. In most instances, surgery is the treatment of choice. Radical extirpation is not necessary, since these lesions are never malignant.[36] One should excise sufficient tumor to reduce the bulk of the mass to a reasonable extent, reshaping the tongue to reduce its size and improve speech. This can be done by resection of the tip of the tongue and bilateral marginal V-shaped wedge resection.[50] Surface vesicles are destroyed by electrocoagulation, followed by re-epithelialization. The size of the tongue may vary from time to time, depending on the degree of lymphatic obstruction and episodes of recurring inflammation. It often is necessary to carry out multiple conservative operative attacks. Several conservative "tailoring procedures" are preferred to widescale definitive excision. Occasionally, one sees a small circumscribed plaque of lymphangioma of the tongue. Surgical excision rids the patient of the annoying mass, intermittent glossitis and considerable worry.

Benign papillomas of the tongue are treated by excision (Fig. 31–16).

Congenital neurofibromatous macroglossia may be seen in childhood, occasionally as a part of generalized neurofibromatosis and in other cases as the only area of involvement.[6] Most cases present with slow-growing hemimacroglossia (see Chap. 135).

Definitive treatment may be impossible due to the diffuse infiltrative nature of plexiform neurofibroma.[47] As in cases of lymphangioma of the tongue, surgical resection is desirable, the goal being to reduce the bulk of the mass and reshape

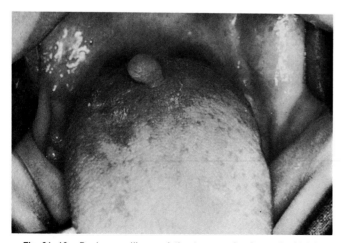

Fig. 31–16.—Benign papilloma of the tongue of a 6-month-old infant, treated by excision.

the tongue in such a manner as to improve function. These lesions are not radiosensitive.

Idiopathic macroglossia occasionally is seen with somatic hemihypertrophy. The condition may be unilateral or bilateral and may be associated with overgrowth of the mandible, one side of the face or the entire body, as reported by Mugnier and Laufer.[37] Shafer[54] prefers the term primary macroglossia. He reported 9 neonates; 7 had omphalocele or umbilical hernia. The reason for the association is not understood (see Chap. 77). Subtotal glossectomy at age 6 months is recommended to prevent prognathism and to ultimately improve speech. Histologic study of resected tongue tissue shows true hypertrophy of muscle cells and increased stromal components with no evidence of neoplasia. Recurrence has not been observed following appropriate surgical treatment.

Lesions of the Nasopharynx

A number of surgical conditions arising in the pharynx and nasal cavities are peculiar to childhood. Pharyngeal cutaneous fistula may present with drainage of saliva from a midline cutaneous opening at the level of the hyoid bone. Surgical treatment consists of pursuit of the sinus tract from the level of the skin opening to the pharynx.[65] Schuring[53] reported a spectacular pharyngeal lesion consisting of a completely formed accessory auricle, the lower half presenting just above the epiglottis, with the balance of the ear embedded in the posterior pharyngeal wall. This may have originated from first branchiogenic cleft apparatus between the mandibular and hyoid arches. Elements usually are retained as the eustachian tube and contribute to the formation of the middle ear. The presence of a completely formed ear in this location more logically relates to the stomadeal plate forming in this bizarre manner.

Nasopharyngeal angiofibroma may be first manifested by a life-threatening bleeding episode both from external loss through the mouth and nares and from flooding of the lungs. Rosen et al.[51] have shown the value of bilateral carotid angiography in demonstrating the major source of arterial supply prior to surgery. Treatment consists of peripheral detachment of the palate on one side and elevation of the mucoperiosteal flap, with care to avoid injury to the contralateral palatine vessels. Palatal tissue is adequately nourished from one side. It may be necessary to remove a portion of the hard palate before attacking the extremely vascular tumor. Use of the cryoprobe has been found to have value, freezing the tumor solid and then cutting it away from its bony attachment. This lesion, except for allergic polyps, is the most common benign tumor of the nasopharynx in childhood but seldom is seen before the age of 7. For this reason, it has been called "juvenile" angiofibroma. Males predominate, with a sex ratio of approximately 4 to 1.[9, 33, 41] Radiation cannot be given in sufficient dosage to destroy the tumor without damaging ossification centers that are important in adolescence when the nasal feature is determined. Both estrogens and androgens have been shown to have an inhibiting effect on the tumor. Estrogens have been given most often in the postoperative period. With adequate removal of the tumor, palatal healing usually is complete and fistulas are uncommon.

Other solid tumors occur in or adjacent to the oropharynx. A dramatic example encountered in the newborn is nasopharyngeal teratoma. These often are pedunculated and protrude from the mouth as a frightening and often ulcerated,

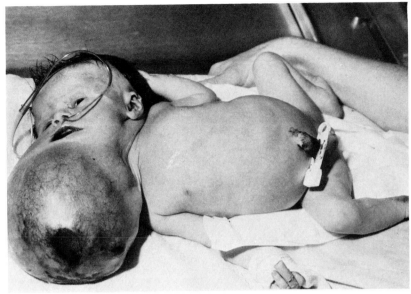

Fig. 31–17.—Cervical teratoma of massive proportions in a newborn. The lesion was successfully removed, preserving all possible skin for adequate restructuring of the mandibular and upper neck regions. Such teratomas generally are mature but have the capability of malignant degeneration in any of the three contributing germ layers. (Courtesy of R. T. Soper.)

orange-sized mass (epignathi). Sollee[58] reported the successful treatment of one of these tumors in a neonate. Fortunately, they are benign. The simultaneous development of the teratoma and the palate interferes with the proper migration of the lateral halves, so the palate may be moderately cleft or absent. Additional cases in the newborn have been reported by Baugh[8] and Ochsner[39] and their colleagues and by Ehrich,[22] who used the colorful term teratoid parasites of the mouth.

Heterotopic brain tissue in the nasopharynx has been reported by Zarem et al.[71] Some 100 cases of extracranial glioma have been reported. We have seen 2 infants with airway obstruction due to a nasopharyngeal mass that ultimately proved to consist of central nervous system tissue, so-called glioma (see Chap. 25). An oncocytoma of the tongue in a 7-year-old patient of Das et al.[16] arose from the dorsum of the tongue at the posterior pharynx and was removed following several episodes of respiratory arrest. The lesion was considered to be a variety of oxyphil adenoma arising from minor salivary glands in the tongue.

Nasopharyngeal carcinoma in children has been reported by Nishiyama et al.[38] Nasopharyngeal malignancy is uncommon and accounted for only 27 of 506 cases as reported by Dargeon.[4] He reported 9 children surgically treated, all below the age of 15 years. The youngest patient was age 7; average age was 12 years. Seven patients died despite surgical extirpation, irradiation and chemotherapy. Two patients were alive 3 and 9 years after treatment. Lymphoepithelioma was the most common histologic type encountered in 6 patients, 2 had transitional cell carcinoma and 1 a poorly differentiated squamous cell carcinoma.

Exophytic cervical teratomas also are seen in the neonate. These may be huge and interfere with breathing or swallowing by raising the floor of the mouth or by local invasion (Fig. 31–17). Platis[44] reported such a case. Of the 71 reported cases, 67 occurred in stillborn fetuses or in newborn infants; 1 was malignant. Of 33 neonates operated on, 21 survived; mortality was 12%. Sixteen were stillborn and 18 died without operation. Three additional cases in the neonate were reported by Ruffolo et al.[52]

REFERENCES

1. Adatia, A. K.: Burkitt's tumour in the jaws, Br. Dent. J. 120:315, 1966.
2. Ahlfeld, F.: Beitrage zur Lehre von den Zwillingen, Arch. Gynäk, 7:210, 1875.
3. Arey, J. B.: Tumors of head and neck, Pediatr. Clin. North Am. 6:2, 1959.
4. Ariel, I. M., and Pack, G. T.: *Cancer and Allied Diseases of Infancy and Childhood* (Boston: Little, Brown and Company, 1960).
5. Arons, M. S., et al.: Hemi-facial resection for rare inflammatory diseases of parotid gland: I. Aspergillosis; II. Pseudosarcomatous fasciitis, Am. Surg. 32:496, 1966.
6. Ayres, W. W., Delaney, A. J., and Backer, M. H.: Congenital neurofibromatous macroglossia associated in some cases with von Recklinghausen's disease: Case report and review of the literature, Cancer 5:721, 1952.
7. Bardwil, J. M.: Sarcomas of the head and neck, Am. J. Surg. 108:476, 1964.
8. Baugh, C. D., and O'Donoghue, R. F.: Teratoma of tonsil causing respiratory obstruction in newborn, Arch. Dis. Child. 30: 396, 1955.
9. Bennett, T. V.: Juvenile angiofibroma of the nasopharynx, Straub Clin. Proc. 32:7, 1966.
10. Blackfield, H. M., and Wilde, N. J.: Lateral facial clefts, Plast. Reconstr. Surg. 6:68, 1950.
11. Borello, E. D., and Gorlan, R. J.: Melanotic neuroectodermal tumor of infancy—a neoplasm of neural crest origin, Cancer 19: 196, 1966.
12. Braudo, M.: Thrombosis of the internal carotid artery in childhood after injury in region of the soft palate, Br. Med. J. 1:665, 1956.
13. Burkitt, D.: The African lymphoma, J. R. Coll. Surg. Edinb. 11: 170, 1966.
14. Burkitt, D.: Sarcoma involving jaws in African children, Br. J. Surg. 46:218, 1958.
15. Cussen, L. J., and MacMahon, R. A.: Congenital granular-cell myoblastoma, J. Pediatr. Surg. 10:249, 1975.
16. Das, S., et. al.: Oncocytoma of tongue in a child, J. Pediatr. Surg. 11:113, 1976.
17. Davies, D.: Cavernous hemangioma of the mandible, Plast. Reconstr. Surg. 33:5, 1964.
18. Diamond, L. K.: Personal communication.

19. Douglas, B.: Further report on treatment of micrognathia with obstruction by plastic procedure: Results based on reports from 21 cities, Plast. Reconstr. Surg. 6:113, 1950.

20. Duhamel, B.: *Chirurgie de Nouveau-né et du Nourisson* (Paris: Masson & Cie, 1953), p. 55.

21. Economopoulos, C.: The value of glossopexy in Pierre Robin syndrome, N. Engl. J. Med. 262:1267, 1960.

22. Ehrich, W. E.: Teratoid parasites of mouth, Am. J. Oral Surg. 31:650, 1945.

23. Fogh-Anderson, P., and Sorenson, B.: Electric mouth burns in children, Acta Chir. Scand. 131:214, 1966.

24. Ghandi, R. K., *et al.*: Hemangiosarcoma (malignant hemangioendothelioma) of the mandible in a child, Oral Surg. 19:359, 1966.

25. Good, T. A., Carnozzo, S. F., and Good, R. A.: Thrombocytopenia and giant hemangioma in infancy, Arch. Dis. Child. 90:260, 1955.

26. Gorlin, R. J., and Redman, R. S.: Chromosomal abnormalities and oral anomalies, Am. J. Surg. 108:370, 1964.

27. Hanson, J. W., and Smith, D. W.: U-shaped palatal defect in the Robin anomalad: Developmental and clinical relevance, J. Pediatr. 87:30, 1975.

27a. Kaban, L. B., Mulliken, J. B., and Murray, J. E.: Facial fractures in children, Plast. Reconstr. Surg. 1:15, 1977.

28. Kerr, D. A., and Weiss, A. W.: Pigmented ameloblastoma of the mandible, Oral Surg. 16:1339, 1963.

29. Körlof, B., and Bergström, R.: Melanotic progonoma of the maxilla, Acta Chir. Scand. 129:292, 1965.

30. Lampe, S., and LaTourette, H. B.: Management of hemangiomas in infants, Pediatr. Clin. North Am. 6:2, 1959.

31. Levin, L. S., Jorgenson, R. J., and Jarvey, B. A.: Lymphangiomas of the alveolar ridges in neonates, Pediatrics 58:881, 1976.

32. Lewin, M. L.: Nonmalignant maxillofacial tumors in children, Plast. Reconstr. Surg. 38:186, 1966.

33. MacComb, W. S.: Juvenile nasopharyngeal fibroma, Am. J. Surg. 106:754, 1963.

34. Marden, P. M.: The syndrome of ankyloglossia superior, Minn. Med. 49:1223, 1966.

35. Medenis, R., Slaughter, D. P., and Barber, T. K.: Melanotic progonoma in childhood, Pediatrics 29:600, 1962.

36. Morfit, H. M.: Lymphangioma of tongue, Arch. Surg. 81:761, 1960.

37. Mugnier, A., and Laufer, J.: Problèmes posés par les macroglossies unilatérales non tumorales du jeune enfant. Actual. Odontostomatol. 79:351, 1967.

38. Nishiyama, R. H., *et al.*: Nasopharyngeal carcinomas in children, Arch. Surg. 94:214, 1967.

39. Ochsner, A., and Ayers, W. B.: Case of epignathus, Surgery 30:560, 1951.

40. O'Conor, G. T., Rappaport, H., and Smith, E. B.: Childhood lymphoma resembling "Burkitt tumor" in the United States, Cancer 18:411, 1965.

41. Osborn, D. A., and Sokolovski, A.: Juvenile nasopharyngeal angiofibroma in a female, Arch. Otolaryngol. 82:629, 1965.

42. Pickett, L. K., and Stark, D. B.: Trauma in and about the mouth in children, Pediatr. Clin. North Am. 3:905, 1956.

43. Pierre, M.: Brulures électriques des lèvres, Ann. Chir. Plast. 6:21, 1961.

44. Platis, J. M.: Teratoma of the neck, Plast. Reconstr. Surg. 34:303, 1964.

45. Potts, W. J.: *The Surgeon and the Child* (Philadelphia: W. B. Saunders Company, 1959).

46. Rappaport, I., and Furnas, D. W.: Tumors of the facial skeleton in children, Am. J. Surg. 130:421, 1975.

47. Rasi, H. B., Herr, B. S., and Sperer, A. V.: Neurofibromatosis of the tongue, Plast. Reconstr. Surg. 35:6, 1965.

48. Richardson, R. J., Robinson, D. W., and Masters, F. W.: Tumors of the mandible in children, Plast. Reconstr. Surg. 23:576, 1959.

49. Rise, E. N.: Dermoid cysts of the tongue and floor of the mouth, Arch. Otolaryngol. 80:12, 1964.

50. Robinson, F.: Lymphangioma of the tongue, Br. J. Plast. Surg. 6:48, 1953.

51. Rosen, L., Hanafee, W., and Nahum, A.: Nasopharyngeal angiofibroma, an angiographic evaluation, Radiology 86:103, 1966.

52. Ruffolo, E. H., Dorr, T. W., and Fletcher, J. C.: Teratomas of the neck: Report of two cases, Radiology 38:223, 1965.

52a. Schaffer, A. J.: Nasopharyngeal Dermoid of the Newborn, in *Diseases of the Newborn* (Philadelphia: W. B. Saunders Company, 1960).

53. Schuring, A. G.: Accessory auricle in the nasopharynx, Laryngoscope 74:111, 1964.

54. Shafer, A. D.: Primary macroglossia, Clin. Pediatr. 7:357, 1968.

55. Sleeper, E. L.: In Cohen, M. (ed.), *Pediatric Dentistry* (St. Louis: The C. V. Mosby Company, 1957).

56. Smith, L. K.: Correction of microstomia, Plast. Reconstr. Surg. 14:302, 1954.

57. Snijman, P. C., and Prinsloo, J. G.: Congenital fusion of the gums, Am. J. Dis. Child. 112:593, 1966.

58. Sollee, A. N., Jr.: Nasopharyngeal teratoma, Arch. Otolaryngol. 82:49, 1965.

59. Soricelli, D. A., Bell, L., and Alexander, W. A.: Congenital fistulas of the lower lip, Oral Surg. 21:511, 1966.

60. Spivack, J., and Bennett, J. E.: Glossopalatine ankylosis, Plast. Reconstr. Surg. 42:129, 1968.

61. Stark, S.: Noma or gangrenous stomatitis, Oral Surg. 9:1076, 1956.

62. Taylor, B. G., and Etheredge, S. N.: Hemangiomas of the mandible and maxilla presenting as surgical emergencies, Am. J. Surg. 108:574, 1964.

63. Tempest, M. N.: Cancrum oris, Br. J. Surg. 53:949, 1966.

64. Thomson, H. G., Juckes, A. W., and Farmer, A. W.: Electric burns of the mouth in children, Plast. Reconstr. Surg. 35:466, 1965.

65. Tscheschmedjiev, J., and Chlebarov, S.: Fistula congenita pharyngocutanea, Dermatol. Wochenschr. 142:764, 1960.

66. Wang, M. K. H., and Macomber, W. B.: Congenital lip sinuses, Plast. Reconstr. Surg. 18:319, 1956.

67. Ward, G. E., Cantrell, J. R., and Allan, W. B.: Surgical treatment of lingual thyroid, Am. Surg. 139:536, 1954.

68. Wilkins, S. A., Jr., *et al.*: Aggressive fibromatosis of the head and neck, Am. J. Surg. 130:412, 1975.

69. Wilson, R. A., Kliman, M. R., and Hardyment, A. F.: Ankyloglossia superior (palato-glossal adhesion in the newborn infant), Pediatrics 31:1051, 1963.

70. Yannopoulos, K., *et al.*: Osteosarcoma arising in fibrous dysplasia of the facial bones. Case report and review of the literature, Am. J. Surg. 107:556, 1964.

71. Zarem, H. A., *et al.*: Heterotopic brain in the nasopharynx and soft palate: Report of two cases, Surgery 61:483, 1967.

Glands of the Neck

ENLARGED CERVICAL LYMPH NODES are by far the most common cause of a neck mass in children. These enlarged nodes usually can be differentiated from other cervical masses, such as cystic hygroma, branchial cleft cyst, thyroglossal duct cyst or dermoid cyst, which generally are spherical, cystic and discrete whereas enlarged lymph nodes are characteristically lobulated, firm and often attached to the surrounding tissues. Cervical lymphadenopathy is due to either infection, hyperplasia or neoplasia (Table 32–1).

The specific lymphatic chain involved in the adenopathy allows the physician to suspect the site of the primary lesion. The skin and subcutaneous tissue of the scalp posterior to the ear drains into the posterior cervical nodes whereas the submaxillary and upper anterior cervical lymphatics drain the buccal cavity, tongue, teeth, gums and pharynx. The

preauricular nodes drain the orbital area and, when enlarged, may be confused with tumor of the parotid gland. Supraclavicular adenopathy may result from drainage of the anterior cervical chain downward or lesions of the mediastinum extending cephalad.

Acute Bacterial Lymphadenitis

The most common cause of sudden lymph node enlargement is acute bacterial lymphadenitis. This process usually is secondary to infections involving the conjunctiva, ear, skin or particularly the oropharynx. The major offending organisms are *Staphylococcus aureus* and *Streptococcus hemolyticus,* group A. Occasionally, gram-negative organisms may be found as the predominant bacteria; with the recent interest in anaerobic cultures, the peptostreptococcus is being isolated more frequently. Cultures from suppurative nodes often are sterile, either because of prior antibiotic therapy or because anaerobic cultures were not done. It is of interest that the most common organism isolated in the early 1940s was the hemolytic streptococcus. Powers and Boisvert[22] reported 79% isolation of hemolytic streptococci in a paper in 1944 and only 17% staphylococci. Scobie[25] demonstrated staphylococci in 67% of cervical lymph node cultures and streptococci in only 7%. Barton and Feigin[4] found that *Staphylococcus aureus* was present in 36% of patients and hemolytic streptococcus in 26% of abscessed glands. This reversal in the bacterial flora undoubtedly is due to the treatment of upper respiratory tract infections with penicillin, which is extremely effective against the streptococcus but not against the numerous penicillin-resistant staphylococci now being encountered.

The diagnosis of acute bacterial lymphadenitis usually is obvious. The condition can be recognized by the sudden onset of a painful cervical swelling 2–3 days after an upper respiratory infection. This is accompanied by fever and gradual reddening of the skin over the affected lymph nodes. Needle aspiration is recommended by some to obtain fluid for culture and sensitivity studies. This often is done even if the lymph node is not fluctuant.

Usually these children are seen first by their pediatrician and placed on antibiotics. Antibiotics are indicated when the patient is febrile and toxic for approximately 1 week. Their long-term use may hinder the resolution of the lymphadenitis. Prolonged use of antibiotics often results in chronic granulomatous lymphadenitis, which neither resolves spontaneously nor suppurates to allow drainage of the mass (Fig. 32–1).

Warm, moist soaks should be used as part of the treatment in order to promote quicker resolution of the problem. If liquefaction of the involved nodes occurs, incision and drainage should be done, but not until the entire mass appears to be fluctuant and broken down. Too early drainage of only a small area of liquefaction often results in subsequent further breakdown of the involved nodes and requires a sec-

TABLE 32–1.—ETIOLOGY OF CERVICAL LYMPHADENOPATHY

INFECTIOUS

1. Bacteria
(a) Gram-positive
    Staphylococcus aureus
    Streptococcus
    Corynebacterium diphtheriae

(b) Gram-negative
    Escherichia coli
    Pseudomonas
    Proteus
    Francisella tularensis

(c) Anaerobic
    Peptostreptococcus

(d) Mycobacteria
    M. tuberculosis
    Atypical

(e) Spirochetes
    Treponema pallidum

2. Fungi
(a) Aspergillus
(b) Cryptococcus
(c) Histoplasma

3. Viruses
(a) Cat-scratch fever
(b) Herpes zoster
(c) Infectious mononucleosis

HYPERPLASIA
1. Nonspecific follicular hyperplasia
2. Giant lymph node hyperplasia (Castleman-Iverson syndrome)
3. Diphenylhydantoin (Dilantin) hyperplasia

NEOPLASIA
1. Primary
    1. Hodgkin's lymphoma
    2. Non-Hodgkin's lymphoma
        (a) Non-Burkitt's lymphosarcoma
        (b) Burkitt's lymphosarcoma
        (c) Reticulum cell sarcoma

2. Secondary
    1. Leukemia
    2. Histiocytosis
    3. Metastatic
        (a) Thyroid
        (b) Neuroblastoma
        (c) Rhabdomyosarcoma

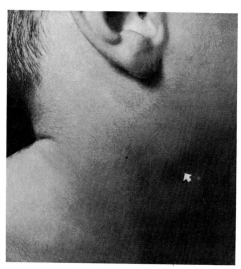

Fig. 32–1.—Chronic lymphoid hyperplasia. An asymptomatic 6-year-old boy with a persistently enlarged lymph node in the right neck for 8 months. Examination of the single node after excision revealed chronic lymphoid hyperplasia that evidently had followed infection of the pharynx. (From A. H. Bill, Jr.[5a])

ondary drainage procedure. Antibiotics should be discontinued shortly after incision and drainage or, as mentioned previously, if after a week to 10 days, the mass is not responding to the antibiotic. The drainage incision always should be placed in Langer's lines and, if possible, beneath the mandible to give a good cosmetic result.

Cervical Tuberculosis

Tuberculosis of the cervical lymph glands has been seen less commonly in the past 10–15 years. Conversely, atypical mycobacterial infections are becoming more frequent. Tuberculous cervical lymphadenitis in children is believed (Lincoln and Gilbert[15] and Kent[12]) to be part of a primary tuberculous infection and not a localized disease process. They found that 5% of all children with tuberculosis developed cervical lymph node involvement, which was confirmed by culture, biopsy and pathologic examination.

These nodes typically are firm, nontender and discrete early in the disease. As the process progresses, they become matted and adhere to the overlying skin. Breakdown of the lymph nodes may occur, with a chronic sinus tract developing (Fig. 32–2). The most characteristic feature of this disease process is the absence of tenderness in the involved areas.

Children with suspected tuberculous lymphadenitis should have the diagnosis confirmed by skin testing with purified protein derivative (PPD) as well as a roentgenogram of the chest. A positive PPD skin test is confirmatory evidence of tuberculous adenitis, and a definitive pathologic diagnosis by node biopsy is not required. However, if the lymphadenopathy is not clinically characteristic or there is a failure of response to treatment, biopsy is necessary to confirm the diagnosis.

The drugs available for the treatment of tuberculosis are streptomycin, para-aminosalicylic acid, isonicotinic acid hydrazide (isoniazid) and, most recently, rifampin. The most generally accepted therapeutic regimen at present is the combined use of isoniazid and rifampin. The new drug rifampin does, on occasion, cause cholestatic jaundice, which

may be compounded in combination with isoniazid. However, this is a rare complication in patients under 20 years of age, so that monthly liver function studies are not recommended in children. This combination of drugs should be continued for an 18-month period, as in any child who either is a positive tuberculin reactor or manifests primary pulmonary tuberculosis.

Surgical intervention plays a limited role in the treatment of tuberculosis. Excisional node biopsy is indicated if the disease cannot be confirmed clinically. A definitive indication for operation involves the child who has incipient rupture of the skin overlying a suppurative tuberculous node or in whom a chronic sinus tract already has developed. In this situation, the lesion may slowly respond to drug therapy alone; however, excision of the involved nodes and sinus tract will result in a more rapid recovery and better cosmetic result. If excision of tuberculous nodes is contemplated, antituberculous drug therapy should be started 3–4 days prior to the operation.

Atypical Mycobacterial Lymphadenitis

Although tuberculous cervical adenitis has decreased in recent years, there now appears to be a definite increase in the incidence of atypical mycobacterial infections. This is due to both our greater familiarity with this entity and the now readily available culture methods.

Pathologically, the atypical mycobacterial infection is indistinguishable by gross and microscopic characteristics from the tubercle bacillus. However, on culture, the atypical mycobacteria can be readily differentiated from the Koch bacillus. Four major groups are recognized. This classification is determined by the pigmentation of the colonies and their response to light.

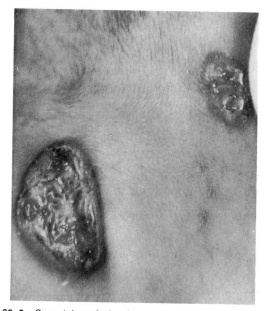

Fig. 32–2.—Open tuberculosis of posterior cervical lymph nodes (ear at right of photo). This 7½-year-old boy had a chronic sore of the scalp behind the right ear, followed by swelling of the right posterior cervical lymph nodes and ultimate breakdown of the nodes. Tuberculin reaction was positive. There was a family history of contact. Treatment in a sanatorium for 7 months with isoniazid and PAS led to healing of the open infection and regression in size of the nodes. After 32 more months of outpatient drug therapy, he was without evidence of disease. (Courtesy of Dr. Helen Marshall, Firland Sanatorium, Seattle.) (From A. H. Bill, Jr.[5a])

TABLE 32–2.—THE CHARACTERISTICS OF ATYPICAL VERSUS
MYCOBACTERIAL INFECTIONS

	TUBERCULOUS INFECTION	ATYPICAL INFECTION
Age	Older	Younger
Geographic location	Urban	Rural
Lymph node involvement	Lower cervical nodes	Upper cervical nodes
Chest roentgenogram	Often positive	Normal
Sedimentation rate	Elevated	Normal
Skin tests		
PPD-S (1st strength)	Positive	Negative
PPD-S (2d strength)	Positive	Weakly positive
PPD-B	Negative	Positive
Cultural characteristic		
Microscopic	Histologically identical	
Culture	Diagnostic	Diagnostic
Response to medications	Good	Poor
Surgical indications	Only for diagnosis or complications of disease	Treatment of choice

Group I.   Photochromogens: colonies become pigmented on exposure to light.

Group II.   Scotochromogens: colonies are pigmented when grown in the dark.

Group III.   Nonchromogens: faintly colored and not influenced by light.

Group IV.   Rapid growers: colonies are present and identifiable after 2 weeks.

Clinically, the atypical mycobacterial lymphadenitis presents in a manner similar to tuberculous lymphadenitis. The upper cervical chains appear to be involved more commonly than other lymphatics. They are nontender and have the appearance of chronicity. The disease entity appears to be most common between the ages of 2 and 8 years. The involved nodes often suppurate and then spontaneously drain, resulting in a chronic sinus tract.

Skin testing is important in differentiating between the atypical and the tuberculous mycobacterial infections (Table 32–2). The double Mantoux test is believed to be of value in that PPD-S (purified protein derivative of mamma-lian tuberculin) usually is negative in the atypical infection and positive in tuberculosis. On the other hand, the PPD-B (prepared from the Battey bacillus, an atypical mycobacteria) often is strongly positive in the atypical mycobacterial lymphadenitis (Fig. 32–3). The tuberculin skin test also tends to be nonreactive in atypical disease and strongly reactive in the tuberculous infections. Chest x-ray always is normal in the atypical disease but may show a pulmonary lesion in tuberculosis.

The importance of differentiating between these two types of infection has been emphasized in the literature[21, 24, 27] on this subject, as the treatment of tuberculous lymphadenitis is mainly drug therapy, reserving operation for the indications described in the preceding section. However, in the atypical mycobacterial infections, it has been demonstrated that antituberculous drug therapy is not generally effective, although a recent report by Mandell and Wright[19] suggests that rifampin may well be useful. Excision of the offending nodes and any sinus tracts, if present, now is regarded as the treatment of choice. It is recommended by some that until the bacterial cultures verify the presence of

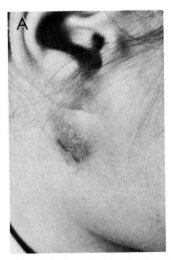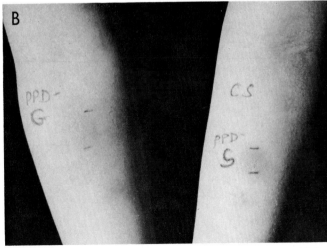

Fig. 32–3.—Atypical acid-fast mycobacterial infection of glands of the neck. **A,** note involved glands at the angle of the jaw, which is typical. The glands were excised, followed by primary healing. A short course of antibiotic therapy was given after removal. **B,** skin tests, which made the diag-nosis. *CS* was cat-scratch antigen (negative); *PPD-S* was intermediate PPD (positive). *PPD-G* was the antigen of one type of atypical acid-fast myco-bacteria; the positive reaction made the diagnosis. (From A. H. Bill, Jr.[5a])

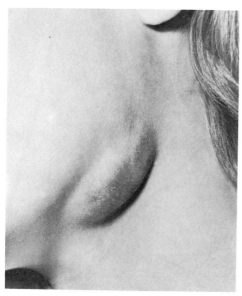

Fig. 32–4.—Cat-scratch fever. This lesion had been present for several months. Cultures of pus withdrawn by needle grew out no organisms. Staining and culture for tubercle bacilli were negative, as were reactions to tuberculin skin tests. Reaction to the skin test for cat-scratch fever was positive. Excision of the lesion resulted in primary healing. (From A. H. Bill, Jr.[5a])

an atypical infection antituberculous therapy should be used. Once the definitive diagnosis had been confirmed, the drugs are discontinued.

Cat-Scratch Fever

Lymphadenitis due to cat-scratch disease appears to be increasing or is at least being diagnosed more frequently.[7a, 20] Except for pyogenic lymphadenitis, it now is the most common cause of cervical node enlargement. These lymph nodes are affected in about 40% of the cases whereas the lymphatics draining the extremities account for the majority of the remaining. The disease is seen mostly in the fall and winter months.

The natural history of cat-scratch fever is that of a small, often insignificant primary lesion appearing as a result of a scratch from a cat, or occasionally a dog or a monkey. Approximately 2–3 weeks later, systemic symptoms of fever, malaise and headache occur, with enlargement of the nodes draining the primary site. The primary lesion itself usually is healed by this time or persists as a small yellow-brown papule. Systemic symptoms may be mild and of short duration or may be severe and persistent. The associated lymphadenitis may resolve spontaneously but may go on to suppuration.

The diagnosis of cat-scratch fever can be suspected from the history of cat scratch but confirmed only by skin test with cat-scratch antigen. The antigen is not available commercially and must be prepared from pus obtained from a suppurative lymph node. Other diagnostic methods being evaluated include serologic testing and in vitro correlation of T-cell mediated immunity.

Treatment is supportive; antibiotics are of no use. If the involved lymph nodes suppurate and become fluctuant, needle aspiration is indicated (Fig. 32–4). Incision and drainage is contraindicated and usually results in a chronic draining sinus. In the face of this complication, excision of the sinus and involved nodes is necessary to eradicate the disease.

Lymphadenopathy Due to Hyperplasia

Nonspecific follicular hyperplasia most often results from previous infection of the upper respiratory tract. Excisional biopsy is indicated when routine diagnostic studies are

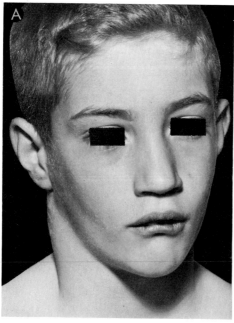
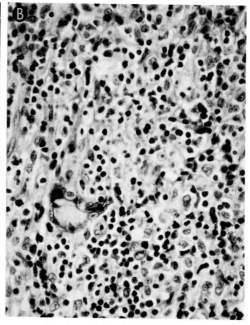

Fig. 32–5.—Hodgkin's disease. **A,** an 11-year-old boy had palpable nodes in the right neck for 2 years, then noticeable increase for 2 months without fever or symptoms. A large mass of lymph nodes was excised en bloc; radical neck dissection was not done. The neck and mediastinum were irradiated. Six years later he showed no evidence of disease. His prognosis for survival approaches 1 out of 3 and becomes better the longer he has no recurrence. **B,** photomicrograph of lymph node, showing giant cell formation and Sternberg-Reed cells. Eosinophils also were present. ×400. (From A. H. Bill, Jr.[5a])

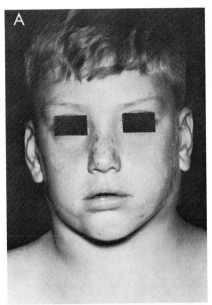 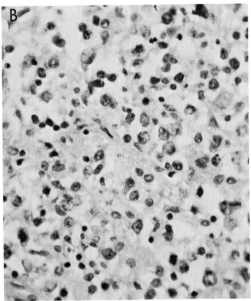

Fig. 32–6.—Reticulum cell sarcoma. **A,** an 8-year-old boy with a 3-month history of increasing swelling of both sides of the neck. When first seen, he also had hepatomegaly and splenomegaly. Biopsy was done. He received irradiation and chemotherapy but died in 2 months of generalized disease. **B,** photomicrograph of lymph nodes from the neck, showing large immature round cells and deposition of reticulum. ×400. (From A. H. Bill, Jr.[5a])

normal and when lymph nodes fail to regress after a reasonable period of observation, usually 6 weeks. Hyperplastic cervical lymphadenopathy also occurs in the Castleman-Iverson syndrome (chronic hypoferrinemia, anemia, growth failure and immunoglobulin abnormalities) or as an allergic response to Dilantin. These two conditions should be kept in mind when evaluating lymphadenopathy so as to prevent an unnecessary operation.

Neoplasia of Cervical Nodes

Leukemia and lymphoma comprise more than 40% of all malignancies in childhood. Leukemia accounts for the majority of the cases. The lymphomas include Hodgkin's disease (Fig. 32–5) and non-Hodgkin's lymphoma[6] (NHL) and are relatively rare. Between 3.5% and 7.7% are NHL, and approximately 30% involve the cervical lymph nodes pri-

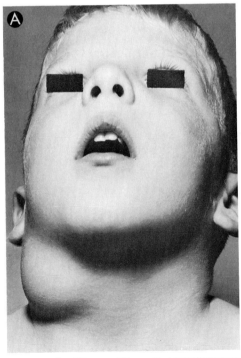 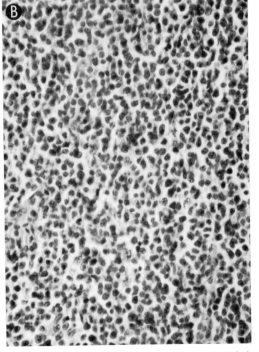

Fig. 32–7.—Lymphosarcoma. **A,** a 4½-year-old boy with gradually increasing swelling of the right side of the neck for 5 months and intermittent unexplained fever. A single greatly enlarged node was found and excised, followed by irradiation of neck and mediastinum. Although he is without evidence of disease 18 months later, the prognosis is doubtful. **B,** photomicrograph of lymph node, showing the large mass of immature cells of the lymphoid series. There was no evidence of leukemia in bone marrow and peripheral blood smears. ×400. (From A. H. Bill, Jr.[5a])

marily:[26] (1) Burkitt's lymphosarcoma,[6a] (2) non-Burkitt's lymphosarcoma (Fig. 32–6) and (3) reticulum cell sarcoma.[13] Hodgkin's lymphoma is discussed elsewhere (see Chap. 33).

NHL occurs 2½ times more frequently in boys than in girls. The peak incidence is between 3 and 12 years of age. Cervical NHL presents as progressive, nonpainful, rubbery lymphadenopathy, usually involving the anterior cervical chain of nodes (Fig. 32–7). Pretreatment work-up in suspected cases should include a complete blood count, a bone marrow aspirate and biopsy, chest x-ray and gallium scan. Excisional biopsy of the involved nodes is necessary to establish the diagnosis.

Until recently, treatment has consisted of surgery and radiotherapy, chemotherapy being reserved for disseminated disease. Radical neck dissection does not appear to improve survival; of 5 children treated by Rosenberg[23] in this manner, 4 succumbed to their disease within 16 months. The Ann Arbor modification of the Rye classification for Hodgkin's disease generally is used for clinical staging of NHL, without the "A" and "B" criteria. The mortality from NHL ranges from 80% to 95% because of the high incidence of leukemic transformation or progression of the disease.

Traggis *et al.*,[26] utilizing surgery, radiotherapy and chemotherapy for all stages of NHL, have reported a 50% survival. Wollner *et al.*[28] recommend aggressive chemotherapy and have shown similar improvement in the survival of children with NHL.

Brecher *et al.*[6] reported cure rates of over 75%, particularly in Stages I, II and III disease; chemotherapy at Roswell Park consisted of vincristine, steroids and methotrexate followed by oral 6-mercaptopurine daily, weekly oral methotrexate and monthly pulses of vincristine, Cytoxan and steroids. Stage IV disease patients in addition are given high-dose methotrexate on three occasions. All patients receive approximately 3000 roentgen units to areas of gross disease.[11a]

Leukemia, the most common cancer in children, may present with cervical adenopathy as the major or only complaint. Routine blood counts should suggest this diagnosis, which may be confirmed by bone marrow examination. Histiocytosis may also present with cervical lymph node enlargement; generally, other clinical manifestations of this disease are present.

Carcinoma of the thyroid may metastasize to the cervical lymph nodes. The primary lesion often is occult. The diagnosis becomes apparent only on excision of the involved nodes.

Neuroblastoma arising in the thorax often spreads to the supraclavicular nodes and may be the first manifestation. On rare occasions, rhabdomyosarcoma metastasizes to the cervical lymph nodes, usually involving the posterior chain.

REFERENCES

1. Altman, R. P., and Margileth, A. M.: Cervical lymphadenopathy from atypical mycobacteria: Diagnosis and surgical treatment, J. Pediatr. Surg. 10:419, 1975.
2. Aur, R. J. A., Hustu, H. O., Simone, J. V., *et al.*: Therapy of localized and regional lymphosarcoma of childhood, Cancer 27:1328, 1971.
3. Bailey, J., Jr., Burgert, E. O., and Dahlin, D. C.: Malignant lymphoma in children, Pediatrics 28:985, 1961.
4. Barton, L. L., and Feigin, R. D.: Childhood cervical lymphadenitis: A reappraisal, J. Pediatr. 84:846, 1974.
5. Belin, R. P., Richardson, J. D., Richardson, D. L., *et al.*: Diagnosis and management of scrofula in children, J. Pediatr. Surg. 9:103, 1974.
5a. Bill, A. H., Jr.: Glands of the Neck, in Mustard, W. T., *et al.* (eds.), *Pediatric Surgery* (2d ed.; Chicago: Year Book Medical Publishers, Inc., 1969), pp. 246–252.
6. Brecher, M. L., Freeman, A. I., Sinks, L. F., *et al.*: Non-Hodgkin's lymphoma in children. (Unpublished data.)
6a. Burkitt, D., and O'Conor, G. T.: Malignant lymphoma in African children, Cancer 14:258, 1961.
7. Carithers, H. A., Carithers, C. M., and Edwards, R. O., Jr.: Cat-scratch disease, JAMA 207:312, 1969.
7a. Debre, R., and Job, J. C.: La maladie des griffes de chat, Acta Paediatr. Scand. (suppl.) 43:1, 1954.
8. Hsu, K. H.: Isoniazid in the prevention and treatment of tuberculosis: A 20-year study of the effectiveness in children, JAMA 229:528, 1974.
9. Jenkin, R. D. T., Sonley, M. J., Stephens, C. A., *et al.*: Primary gastrointestinal tract lymphoma in childhood, Radiology 92:763, 1969.
10. Jones, B., and Klingberg, W. G.: Lymphosarcoma in children: A report of 43 cases and review of the recent literature, J. Pediatr. 63:11, 1963.
11. Jones, B., Kung, F., Nyhan, W. L., *et al.*: Chemotherapy of the leukemic transformation of lymphosarcoma, J. Pediatr. 70:442, 1967.
11a. Kaplan, H. S.: Role of intensive radiotherapy in the management of Hodgkin's disease, Cancer 19:356, 1966.
12. Kent, D. C.: Tuberculous lymphadenitis: Not a localized disease process, Am. J. Med. Sci. 254:866, 1967.
13. Lemerle, M., Gerard-Marchant, R., Sarrazin, D., *et al.*: Lymphosarcoma and reticulum cell sarcoma in children: A retrospective study of 172 cases, Cancer 32:1499, 1973.
14. Lester, W.: Rifampin: A semisynthetic derivative of rifamycin—a prototype for the future, Annu. Rev. Microbiol. 26:85, 1972.
15. Lincoln, E. M., and Gilbert, L. A.: Disease in children due to mycobacteria other than *Mycobacterium tuberculosis,* Am. Rev. Respir. Dis. 105:683, 1972.
16. Lincoln, E. M., and Sewell, E. M.: *Tuberculosis in Children* (New York: McGraw-Hill Book Company, 1963).
17. MacKellar, A.: Diagnosis and management of atypical mycobacterial lymphadenitis in children, J. Pediatr. Surg. 11:85, 1976.
18. Mair, I. W. S., and Elverland, H. H.: Cervical mycobacterial infection, J. Laryngol. Otol. 189:933, 1975.
19. Mandell, F., and Wright, P. F.: Treatment of atypical mycobacterial cervical adenitis with rifampin, Pediatrics 55:39, 1975.
20. Margileth, A. M.: Cat scratch disease: Nonbacterial regional lymphadenitis: A study of 145 patients and a review of the literature, Pediatrics 42:803, 1968.
21. Ord, R. J., and Matz, G. J.: Tuberculous cervical lymphadenitis, Arch. Otolaryngol. 99:327, 1974.
22. Powers, G. F., and Boisvert, P. L.: Age as a factor in streptococcosis, J. Pediatr. 25:481, 1944.
23. Rosenberg, S. A., Diamond, H. D., Dargeon, H. W., *et al.*: Lymphosarcoma in childhood, N. Engl. J. Med. 259:505, 1958.
24. Salyer, K. E., Votteler, T. P., and Dorman, G. W.: Surgical management of cervical adenitis due to atypical mycobacteria in children, JAMA 204:1037, 1968.
25. Scobie, W. G.: Acute suppurative adenitis in children: A review of 964 cases, Scott. Med. J. 14:352, 1969.
26. Traggis, D., Jaffe, N., Vawter, G., *et al.*: Non-Hodgkin lymphoma of the head and neck in childhood, J. Pediatr. 87:933, 1975.
27. Wolinsky, E.: Nontuberculous mycobacterial infactions of man, Med. Clin. North Am. 58:639, 1974.
28. Wollner, N., Burchenal, J. H., Lieberman, P. H., *et al.*: Non-Hodgkin's lymphoma in children: A comparative study of two modalities of therapy, Cancer 37:123, 1976.

33 PHILIP R. EXELBY

Hodgkin's Disease

HODGKIN'S DISEASE is a malignant disease of the lymphatic system characterized by the presence of the Reed-Sternberg cell in the lymphomatous tissue. Although the disease most commonly occurs in young adults, it is seen in children and adolescents and in them presents particular management problems. The modern management of Hodgkin's disease in children has evolved from a better understanding of the clinical spread of the disease, improvements in staging—by clinical, radiologic and surgical techniques—and improvements in radiotherapy and chemotherapy. The surgeon has become increasingly involved in the management of Hodgkin's disease since the introduction of staging laparotomy. Properly carried out, this procedure allows the most precise staging of the disease at this time. There now is considerable experience with staging laparotomy in children, which has contributed to a greater understanding of Hodgkin's disease in them.

A disease characterized by general enlargement of the lymphatics with nodules in the spleen was first described by Malpighi[27] in 1666. In 1832, the pathology was described by Thomas Hodgkin,[17] and 30 years later, Samuel Wilks[50] first used the name Hodgkin's disease. The characteristic cell was described by Dorothy Reed[36] in 1902, although earlier Sternberg[43] and Virchow[48] described a similar cell in Hodgkin's disease. Progress in the treatment of Hodgkin's disease moved slowly until recent years. In 1939, Gilbert[14] noted better radiocurability of the disease when it was limited to one group of lymph nodes rather than multiple groups. In 1950, Peters[31] noted that Hodgkin's disease showed predictable patterns of spread and she later demonstrated[32, 33] the need to radiate nodal areas adjacent to those obviously involved with disease. The first attempts at staging were clinical, including physical examination for evaluation of peripheral nodes, chest x-ray for evaluation of mediastinal nodes and intravenous pyelography for evaluation of para-aortic nodes. The lymphangiogram, introduced in the late 1950s, enabled clinicians to detect disease in the pelvic and retroperitoneal nodes. This technique showed that 30–40% of patients who had demonstrable disease above the diaphragm had unsuspected abdominal disease. In the 1960s, Glatstein,[15] working with Kaplan at Stanford, used exploratory laparotomy as a way of evaluating the lymphangiogram and to determine more accurately other sites of abdominal involvement. A further 15–20% of patients were found to have occult abdominal disease not suspected on clinical or lymphangiographic examination. During this period there were improvements in the histologic classification and methods of treatment in Hodgkin's disease. In 1965, the Rye conference produced a standard staging concept[39] and adopted a modified Lukes and Butler histologic classification.[26] Improvements in radiotherapy technique were described by Kaplan[23, 24] at Stanford (extended field), Johnson at NCI[20-22] (total nodal radiation), Cham, Tefft and D'Angio in New York[3] (involved field radiation), Fuller in Houston[12]

and Jenkin in Toronto.[18, 19] Chemotherapy also developed during this period. Nitrogen mustard had been used as a single agent in the treatment of Hodgkin's disease for many years. This was followed by other agents and later by various multiple drug regimens combining alkylating agents, steroids and Vinca alkaloids. The best known combinations are MOPP (nitrogen mustard, vincristine [Oncovin],[7-9] prednisone and procarbazine), COPP,[25] which substitutes cyclophosphamide for mustard, and ACOPP, which adds adriamycin as a fifth drug.[44, 45] The modern management of children with Hodgkin's disease utilizes all the techniques of diagnosis, staging and combination treatment methods.

Clinical Presentation

The incidence of Hodgkin's disease rises slowly through the childhood years, reaching its peak in young adulthood. The youngest patient seen at Memorial Hospital in New York was 4 years of age, although the disease has been described in younger patients. Boys outnumber girls in a ratio of 3 to 2. Initial presentation usually is painless enlargement of peripheral nodes. At Memorial Hospital, 83% of the children presented with enlargement of the cervical or supraclavicular lymph nodes (Table 33–1). These common sites of presentation in children create difficulty in diagnosis because children so often have enlarged neck nodes associated with respiratory infections, infectious mononucleosis or other childhood diseases. When to biopsy an enlarged neck node in a child may be difficult to decide. Even in the early stages of development of Hodgkin's disease, enlarged lymph nodes may be associated with mild intermittent fever and the whole process may appear to respond to antibiotic therapy. However, the common history is a failure of response to antibiotics and a persistence of enlarged nodes, leading to biopsy. If the biopsy diagnosis is hyperplasia, further observation of the child is necessary and if lymph nodes recur or remain persistently enlarged, a repeat biopsy is necessary and may establish the diagnosis of Hodgkin's disease. Other sites of presentation of Hodgkin's disease in children are rare, the mediastinum being the next most common. Rarer sites include the axillary nodes, inguinal

TABLE 33–1.—CHILDHOOD HODGKIN'S DISEASE (47 CASES). CLINICAL PRESENTATION AND DIAGNOSIS

SITE OF LESION	NO.
Neck node	39 (83%)
Mediastinal mass	4 (8.5%)
Axillary node	1
Inguinal node	1
Parotid mass	1
Cheek mass	1
	47

nodes, bone and lung. Sites such as bone, liver or lung are regarded as manifesting systemic spread of the disease rather than the primary focus, and a careful investigation usually will detect nodal disease. Localized disease below the diaphragm is, in fact, extremely uncommon, and even in those who present with abdominal Hodgkin's disease, cervical and mediastinal nodes usually are involved. The child with Hodgkin's disease may also present with systemic symptoms of fever, sweats, weight loss and malaise. One third of our patients presented with systemic symptoms, most commonly weight loss or fever. Systemic symptoms are seen most commonly in stages III and IV disease.

Staging

Most centers now use the Ann Arbor staging.[2] Stage I is involvement of a single lymph node region or a single extralymphatic organ or site (IE). Stage II is involvement of two or more lymph node regions on the same side of the diaphragm (II) or localized involvement of an extralymphatic organ or site and of one or more lymph node regions on the same side of the diaphragm (IIE). Stage III is involvement of lymph node regions on both sides of the diaphragm (III), which may be accompanied by localized involvement of extralymphatic organ or site (IIIE) or by involvement of the spleen (IIIS) or both (IIISE). Stage IV is a diffuse or disseminated involvement of one or more extralymphatic organs or tissues with or without associated lymph node enlargement. Each stage is divided into A and B categories. A is used for those children without systemic symptoms and B for children with one or more of the following symptoms: (1) unexplained weight loss of more than 10% of the body weight in the prior 6 months, (2) unexplained fever with temperatures above 38° C, (3) night sweats. It is customary to use the letters CS if the staging is clinical and to use the letters PS if the staging is histologic following laparotomy.

Histologic Classification

Following the Rye conference on Hodgkin's disease, the Lukes and Butler histologic classification[26] has been widely used. The four subdivisions in this classification are: lymphocyte predominance (LP), nodular sclerosis (NS), mixed cellularity (MC) and lymphocyte depletion (LD). This classification has proved to be useful, and when combined with pathologic staging has showed an excellent correlation with treatment results. The distribution of histology in our patients is shown in Table 33–2. Nodular sclerosis is by far the most common, followed by mixed cellularity, lymphocyte predominance and lymphocyte depletion. The lymphocyte predominance group is the least malignant and usually is associated with stage I disease. The nodular sclerosis group, which is next in order of malignancy, usually shows isolated cervical nodal disease that may be combined with medias-

TABLE 33–2.—CHILDHOOD HODGKIN'S DISEASE. HISTOLOGY (LUKES-BUTLER CLASSIFICATION)

TYPE	NO.	%
Nodular sclerosis	29	62
Mixed cellularity	10	21
Lymphocyte predominance	7	15
Lymphocyte depletion	1	2
	47	

tinal disease and shows a tendency to involve the spleen and abdominal nodes. The mixed cellularity and lymphocyte depletion groups are increasingly malignant and tend to present in a higher stage and have a more rapid course.[1]

Diagnosis

Definitive diagnosis of Hodgkin's disease depends on histologic examination of a removed lymph node. The biopsy should be adequate and representative of the disease. Unless there are contraindications, cervical lymph node biopsy in a child should also be done under general anesthesia. In addition to the discomfort of the child, "chopping it out in the treatment room" usually results in obtaining inadequate tissue and compromising the diagnosis. The removed tissue must be sent to a competent pathologist, since the diagnosis of Hodgkin's disease in children may be difficult. If, after pathologic examination, doubt exists as to the diagnosis, a repeat biopsy may have to be carried out. We have noted several patients in whom repeat biopsy of cervical lymph nodes showed hyperplasia prior to a definitive diagnosis of Hodgkin's disease.

Investigation of the Child with Biopsy-Proved Hodgkin's Disease

An accurate determination of the extent of disease is essential so that all clinical and occult disease can receive maximal irradiation and normal growing tissue in the child can be spared as much as possible. Failure to irradiate all areas involved with Hodgkin's disease may lead to recurrence and advance in the stage of the disease. Conversely, unnecessary irradiation to the sensitive growing tissue in the child will result in stunting of growth,[34] absorption problems following intestinal irradiation and perhaps the danger of a second primary cancer in the irradiated field years later.[28] It is for these reasons that an exhaustive investigative study is carried out in every child with Hodgkin's disease. This includes clinical, radiologic, laboratory and surgical evaluation.

Clinical Evaluation

A careful history and physical examination should be recorded on all patients. The history should pay attention to the duration of lymph node enlargement, fluctuation of the size of the nodes and a history of associated infections. A detailed summary of the child's growth and weight record is necessary and a record of the systemic symptoms, such as fever, malaise and pruritus. Physical examination should pay special attention to the lymph node regions, including the liver and spleen. Peripheral nodes are easy to evaluate in children, and the size, consistency and fixation of the nodes should be recorded. The size of the spleen and liver often is difficult to evaluate in the child but any enlargement of these organs is notable. A child with a wide costal angle may have a palpable spleen with considerably less enlargement of that organ than a child with a deep costal margin. Even when the spleen is enlarged and palpable, surgical staging has shown that only 50% will be microscopically involved with disease. Liver involvement is equally difficult to determine clinically. It is not uncommon in this disease to see an enlarged liver that on biopsy proves to be normal. Similarly, on rare occasions, nodules may be found in a liver of normal size. However, the accurate recording of peripheral nodal disease and enlargement of liver and spleen is important as a baseline for future evaluation of the progress and treatment.

Radiologic Examination

Routine chest x-ray usually is adequate for evaluation of mediastinal enlargement. In selected cases, mediastinal tomograms may also be necessary to evaluate mediastinal disease and possible spread into the hilar lymph nodes or adjacent lung. The intravenous pyelogram was the only useful abdominal x-ray prior to the lymphangiogram. Despite its limited usefulness, it should be carried out as a baseline study. Deviation of the ureters will be seen only with considerable enlargement of retroperitoneal nodes. Occasionally, massive nodal disease may displace a kidney and, even more rarely, involvement of a kidney by Hodgkin's disease may be demonstrated. An intravenous pyelogram is important in showing the position of the kidneys prior to radiotherapy. *The bilateral pedal lymphangiogram*, introduced in the 1950s, has become the most useful technique in determining involvement of the iliac and retroperitoneal nodes. Para-aortic nodes are common sites of involvement with Hodgkin's disease. Less commonly involved are the common iliac nodes and rarely nodes below that level. It must be remembered, however, that the lymphangiogram demonstrates only those nodes that are in continuity with the flow from the lower extremities and does not show any nodes above the level of the cysterna chyli. The lymphangiogram gives no indication of involvement of celiac axis nodes, porta hepatis nodes or splenic hilar nodes, which may be involved as the only intra-abdominal disease in these children. The lymphangiogram may underestimate the amount of abdominal bulky disease when this extends laterally and cannot be palpated.

COMPUTERIZED TRANSAXIAL TOMOGRAPHY.—This recent development already has proved to be useful in diagnosing abdominal masses in children. It still is in the process of evaluation but may be useful in the determination of celiac axis and gross liver and splenic disease where this cannot be diagnosed by other methods.

SCANS.—Liver-spleen and bone scans are carried out in these children, as well as total body gallium scan. The liver-spleen scan is used for determining size of these organs accurately and in some instances may show nodular involvement. The gallium scan has proved to be one of the most useful tests in detecting foci of Hodgkin's disease in the soft tissues.

Laboratory Studies

Hemoglobin, white cell count, differential, platelet count and sedimentation rate should be recorded. These are essential baseline studies for any child who may get irradiation or chemotherapy. Liver function tests, blood urea, nitrogen and uric acid are carried out routinely. In addition, special biochemical studies, such as serum copper[47] and serum iron, are useful, and, if elevated, may be used in following the course of disease during treatment.

BONE MARROW EXAMINATION.—Bone marrow involvement is rare in children with Hodgkin's disease but biopsy should be carried out as part of the baseline study and now normally is done at the end of the staging laparotomy under general anesthesia.

This initial clinical, radiologic and biochemical evaluation should be carried out as rapidly as possible and the patient prepared for laparotomy. At this stage in evaluation, the clinical and radiologic staging should be noted on the patient's chart for correlation with the staging laparotomy and histologic examination.

Staging Laparotomy with Splenectomy

Considerable experience now is being gathered in both adults and children[11, 15, 16, 37, 38, 46] and, although there are objectors to staging laparotomy in children, it now is carried out routinely in most centers for evaluation of extent of abdominal disease.

Technique (Fig. 33–1)

A paramedian or midline incision is utilized in girls to gain exposure of the upper abdomen for splenectomy and of the pelvis for transposition of the ovaries. A transverse incision provides adequate exposure in boys for splenectomy, liver biopsy and node biopsies as far down as the common iliac nodes. Splenectomy is carried out in all children, taking as long a pedicle as possible in order to remove all the splenic hilar nodes. Accessory spleens are sought and removed, since they may be involved with disease. The splenic pedicle is marked with metal clips for later x-ray identification. The liver is examined and any suspicious areas are biopsied by either wedge excision if the lesions are at the edge of the liver or by needle biopsy. If there is no obvious disease, a sample wedge of at least 1 cm of tissue is taken from both lobes of the liver. Needle biopsy, which was carried out routinely in the beginning of our series, now is done only for suspicious deep nodules. Examination of all the abdominal nodes from the celiac axis down the para-aortic and iliac chain then is carried out and any suspicious nodes are removed and the site marked with metal clips. The lymphangiogram film, which should be present in the operating room, is used to guide the surgeon to any nodes that the radiologist believes are involved. If there are no obviously involved lymph nodes in the abdomen, routine sampling of nodes at different levels is carried out. This includes high and low, left and right para-aortic nodes and common iliac nodes. Again, the node biopsy sites should be marked by

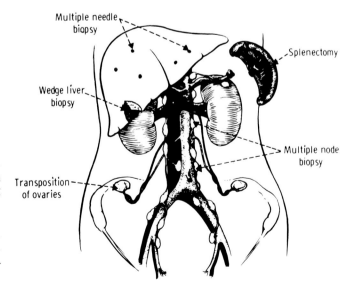

Fig. 33–1.—Evaluation of Hodgkin's disease.

metal clips. A sampling of the celiac axis nodes and porta hepatis nodes is also carried out. Mesenteric nodes are difficult to evaluate, and only grossly enlarged nodes are sampled. In girls, routine transposition of the ovaries is carried out according to the method described by Nahas *et al.*[29] The ovaries are transposed cephalad and laterally and attached to the region of the iliac crest. The position of the ovaries is marked by metal clips to assist the radiotherapist in the design of radiotherapy portals. Prophylactic appendectomy is carried out routinely, since abdominal pain may occur during treatment and the diagnosis of such pain is simplified if the appendix has been removed. Meticulous attention to lymphostasis and closure of the peritoneum at the sites of node biopsy are important to reduce the incidence of adhesions.

Conclusions from Staging Laparotomy

The results of staging laparotomy carried out at different centers are remarkably similar: (1) Approximately 30% of children have the stage of disease changed following laparotomy. Most children have stage increased due to involvement of the spleen, splenic hilar nodes or celiac axis nodes, which may be the only sites of involvement below the diaphragm. (2) Only 50% of palpable spleens show histologic involvement with Hodgkin's disease and 25% of clinically normal spleens show Hodgkin's disease on histologic examination. Clinical and radiologic examination of the spleen and even examination of the spleen at the operating table cannot accurately determine involvement with Hodgkin's disease. We found no correlation between the weight of the spleen and histologic evidence of disease except in very large spleens. Of the 17 histologically positive spleens in our series (Table 33–3), only 8 were palpable on clinical examination and only 7 were enlarged on liver-spleen scan. Even during laparotomy, 6 of the positive spleens appeared completely normal in size and to inspection and palpation. Only by careful histologic sectioning was microscopic disease identified in these 6 spleens. Thirteen had associated nodal involvement, although in 7 it involved only splenic hilar nodes or celiac axis nodes and was not detected by lymphangiogram. (3) Lymph node involvement (Table 33–4) usually can be recognized by the surgeon during laparotomy. Extensive nodal involvement almost always means that the spleen is involved also. In our patients, of whom 14 of 47 had abdominal nodes involved, 9 were diagnosed by lymphangiogram (iliac and para-aortic) and all but 1 had at least one group of positive nodes identified by the surgeon. Two children with positive spleens were thought to have negative nodes but proved to have microscopic involvement of splenic hilar nodes. (4) The liver is involved less frequently than previously thought and always in association with splenic involvement and usually extensive nodal disease. Again, clinical or radiologic enlargement of the liver did not correlate with histologic involvement. (5) The pro-

cedure is relatively safe and complications are uncommon.[41, 49] We have had no major operative complications in the last 40 patients. Fevers often are seen in the first week following a staging laparotomy for Hodgkin's disease, usually are unexplained and resolve without treatment. Late infections attributed to splenectomy have been reported following staging laparotomy.[4, 6, 10, 30, 35] A particularly virulent pneumococcal septicemia has been described by Chilcote *et al.*[5] in these children. All the children who have had splenectomy should receive prophylactic penicillin until they reach adulthood. We have adhered strictly to this policy and have not experienced major infection problems even in children receiving intensive chemotherapy. In common with most other groups, we have had no operative deaths. At present, we believe that staging laparotomy gives the most accurate information of the extent of abdominal Hodgkin's disease and carry out the procedure in all stages I, II and III patients. The information gained is essential to the design of radiotherapy portals and the planning of chemotherapy and outweighs the risks of the procedure, particularly if prophylactic antibiotics are given routinely.

Treatment

Modern treatment of Hodgkin's disease is by irradiation or chemotherapy or a combination of the two modes of treatment.[40, 42] The treatment plan now usually is determined by the pathologic staging and the histologic type of disease.

Radiation Therapy

Various types of radiation therapy have been described in managing Hodgkin's disease in children. Kaplan[24] has been the advocate of extended field irradiation. This is the irradiation of involved node areas and extending to include the next echelon of lymph nodes that appear grossly uninvolved. This is analogous to a cancer operation in which the tumor and surrounding normal tissue are excised to get adequate margins. Johnson[22] has been the advocate of mantle combined with an inverted abdominal Y portal, so-called total nodal irradiation. Results of this treatment have been very impressive, showing that in stages I and II approximately 90% of patients are alive at 5 years. This approach does away with the need for staging laparotomy and relies on clinical and radiologic staging. At our own institution it has been the policy to treat children with involved field irradiation only, based on the extent of disease as determined by clinical, radiologic and laparotomy staging.[3] It is believed that the results are comparable to extended field and total nodal irradiation and spare the child irradiation to growing tissue that is not involved with Hodgkin's disease. If relapse occurs outside the field of irradiation, retrieval is possible by extending the radiation portal at this time. A cooperative study that was set up between various hospitals in the United States and Canada to study the difference between

TABLE 33–3.—STAGING LAPAROTOMY IN CHILDHOOD HODGKIN'S DISEASE— SPLEEN AND LIVER POSITIVE

ORGAN	HISTO (+)	P.E. PAL.	SCAN ↑	SCAN (+)	GROSS ↑	GROSS (+)	LIV (+)	NODES (+)
Spleen	17°	8	7	1$_{GA}$	5	11	3 Spl (+)	13
Liver	3	2	1	1	1	2	3	3

°One case, scan not done.

TABLE 33-4.—STAGING LAPAROTOMY IN CHILDHOOD HODGKIN'S DISEASE—
14 PATIENTS WITH POSITIVE LYMPH NODES

LYMPH NODE	HISTO (+)	GROSS (+)	‡LAG (+)	IVP (+)	IVC (+)	SPL (+)	LIV (+)
Celiac	3°	3	–	–	–	3	–
Splenic	4°	2	–	–	–	4	–
Para-aortic	3	2	3	1	3	2	1
Com. iliac	1†	1	1	1	1	–	–
Diffuse	5	5	5	2	2	5	2
Porta hep.	–	–	–	–	–	–	–
Mesenteric	–	–	–	–	–	–	–

° One patient both celiac and splenic (+).
† Para-aortic node also (+).
‡ 4 false (−), 2 false (+) of all cases.

extended field and involved field irradiation showed no significant difference in survival between the two groups. Further evaluation of these different modalities of treatment must be made. It is obviously desirable to give the child the least amount of irradiation that will cure his disease and to avoid any immediate and late side-effects of treatment.

Chemotherapy

Studies at the National Cancer Institute by DeVita and his colleagues[7-9] resulted in the development of the so-called MOPP regimen, which includes nitrogen mustard, vincristine, prednisone and procarbazine. DeVita used two cycles of nitrogen mustard 6 mg/m² intravenously and vincristine 1.4 mg/m² intravenously on days 1 and 8 of each cycle. Procarbazine is given in a dose of 100 mg/m² by mouth daily throughout each cycle and prednisone 40 mg/m² by mouth each day of cycles 1 and 4. Each cycle is followed by a 2-week rest period. With this regimen there is a remarkable 76% complete response rate in patients with stage IVB disease, with a median duration of response after 6 cycles of MOPP for 36 months. Of those patients achieving complete remission, 70% are alive at 6 years. Similarly good results have been shown by Tan[44] at Memorial Hospital with ACOPP, which is composed of adriamycin, cyclophosphamide, vincristine, prednisone and procarbazine. Adriamycin is given initially 20 mg/m²/day intravenously for 3 doses. After a 2-week rest period, 4 doses of vincristine 1.5–2 mg/m² intravenously are given at weekly intervals. During this 4-week period, procarbazine 50–100 mg and prednisone 1 mg/kg are given daily by mouth. Two weeks after the last dose of vincristine, cyclophosphamide 40 mg/kg is given intravenously as a single dose. After a 3–4-week rest, the cycle is repeated. Treatment is given for 1–2 years, limiting the total cumulative dose of adriamycin to 500 mg/m². The treatment regimen for any particular patient is based on the stage of disease. At our institution, stages I, II and IIIA patients are treated by involved field radiation therapy to a dose of 3500–4000 rads. Stage IIIB patients receive a combination of radiation therapy and chemotherapy. Stage IVA and B patients receive only chemotherapy. Occasionally, in the stage IV patients, radiotherapy may be used for symptomatic disease or disease that may be adjacent to vital structures, such as the trachea. The results of treatment at our institution are similar to those reported from other centers. In stages I, II and III Hodgkin's disease in children, 5-year survival rates of over 80% now are being seen. Even in the advanced stage IV disease, over 60% now can be expected to survive. Hodgkin's disease can, of course, run a chronic course and it is necessary to follow these children for many more years. However, it has been the experience in childhood Hodgkin's disease that there is very little fall-off in survival after the 5-year period.

In the future, as more effective chemotherapeutic agents become available, it may be possible to treat almost all these children by chemotherapy with little or no irradiation. With better diagnostic techniques, it may be that staging laparotomy will become obsolete. At present, however, when modern treatment demands an exact determination of the extent of disease, staging laparotomy remains an important part of the management of these children.

REFERENCES

1. Butler, J. J.: Relationship of histological findings to survival in Hodgkin's disease, Cancer Res. 31:1770, 1971.
2. Carbone, P. P., Kaplan, H. S., Musshoff, K., Smithers, D. W., and Tubiana, M.: Report of the committee on Hodgkin's disease staging classification, Cancer Res. 31:1860, 1971.
3. Cham, W. C., Tan, C. T. C., Martinez, A., Exelby, P. R., Tefft, M., Middleman, P., and D'Angio, G. J.: Involved field radiation therapy for early stage Hodgkin's disease in children, Cancer 37:1625, 1976.
4. Chilcote, R. R., and Baehner, R. L.: The incidence of overwhelming infection in children staged for Hodgkin's disease (abstract), Proc. Am. Soc. Clin. Oncol. 16:224, 1975.
5. Chilcote, R. R., Baehner, R. L., and Hammond, D.: Septicemia and meningitis in children splenectomized for Hodgkin's disease, N. Engl. J. Med. 295:798, 1976.
6. Desser, R. K., and Ultmann, J. E.: Risk of severe infection in patients with Hodgkin's disease or lymphoma after diagnostic laparotomy and splenectomy, Ann. Intern. Med. 77:143, 1972.
7. DeVita, V. T., Canellos, G. P., and Moxley, J. H.: A decade of combination chemotherapy of advanced Hodgkin's disease, Cancer 30:1495, 1972.
8. DeVita, V. T., and Serpick, A. A.: Combination chemotherapy in the treatment of advanced Hodgkin's disease, Proc. Am. Assoc. Cancer Res. 8:13, 1967.
9. DeVita, V. T., Serpick, A. A., and Carbone, P. P.: Combination chemotherapy in the treatment of advanced Hodgkin's disease, Arch. Intern. Med. 73:881, 1970.
10. Eraklis, A. J., Kevy, S. V., Diamond, L. K., and Gross, R. E.: Hazard of overwhelming infection after splenectomy in childhood, N. Engl. J. Med. 276:1225, 1967.
11. Exelby, P. R.: Method of evaluating children with Hodgkin's disease, CA 21:95, 1971.
12. Fuller, L. M., Gamble, J. F., Shullenberger, C. C., et al.: Prognostic factors in localized Hodgkin's disease treated with regional radiation, Radiology 98:641, 1971.
13. Fuller, L. M., Sullivan, M. P., and Butler, J. J.: Results of regional radiotherapy in localized Hodgkin's disease in children, Cancer 32:640, 1973.
14. Gilbert, R.: Radiotherapy in Hodgkin's disease, Am. J. Roentgenol. 41:198, 1939.
15. Glatstein, E., Guernsey, J. M., Rosenberg, S. A., and Kaplan, H. S.: The value of laparotomy and splenectomy in the staging of Hodgkin's disease, Cancer 24:709, 1969.
16. Hays, D. M., Karon, M., Isaacs, H., and Hittle, R. E.: Hodgkin's disease: Technique and results of staging laparotomy in childhood, Arch. Surg. 106:507, 1973.
17. Hodgkin, T.: Some morbid appearances of the absorbent glands and spleen, Trans. Med. Chir. Soc., London 17:68, 1832.

18. Jenkin, R. D. T.: The Management of Malignant Lymphoma in Childhood, in Deeley, T. J. (ed.). *Modern Radiotherapy—Malignant Diseases in Children* (London: Butterworths, 1974), p. 319.
19. Jenkin, R. D. T., Brown, T. C., Petters, M. V., and Sonley, J. J.: Hodgkin's disease in children—a retrospective analysis: 1958–73, Cancer 35:979, 1975.
20. Johnson, R. E.: Updated Hodgkin's disease—curability of localized disease. Total nodal irradiation, JAMA 223:59, 1973.
21. Johnson, R. E., Glover, M. K., and Marshall, S. K.: Results of radiation therapy and implications for the clinical staging of Hodgkin's disease, Cancer Res. 31:1834, 1971.
22. Johnson, R. E., Thomas, L. B., Schneiderman, M., Glenn, D. W., Faw, F., and Hafermann, M. D.: Preliminary experience with total nodal irradiation in Hodgkin's disease, Radiology 104:145, 1972.
23. Kaplan, H. S.: Role of intensive radiotherapy in the management of Hodgkin's disease, Cancer 19:356, 1966.
24. Kaplan, H. S., and Rosenberg, S. A.: Extended field radical radiotherapy in advanced Hodgkin's disease—short-term results of two randomized clinical trials, Cancer Res. 26:1268, 1966.
25. Luce, J. K., Gamble, J. F., Wilson, H. E., Monto, R. W., Isaacs, B. L., Palmer, R. L., Coltman, C. A., Hewlett, J. S., Gehan, E. A., and Frei, E.: Combined cyclophosphamide, vincristine, and prednisone. Therapy of malignant lymphoma, Cancer 28:306, 1971.
26. Lukes, R. J., and Butler, J. J.: The pathology and nomenclature of Hodgkin's disease, Cancer Res. 26:1063, 1966.
27. Malpighi, M.: De viscerum structura, pp. 125–126, 1666.
28. Meadows, A. T., D'Angio, G. J., Evans, A. E., Harris, C., Miller, R. W., and Mike, V.: Oncogenesis and other late effects of cancer treatment in children—report of a single hospital study, Radiology 114:175, 1975.
29. Nahas, W. A., Nisce, L. Z., D'Angio, G. J., and Lewis, J. L., Jr.: Lateral ovarian transposition, Obstet. Gynecol. 38:785, 1971.
30. Nixon, D. W., and Aisenberg, A. C.: Fatal *Hemophilus influenzae* sepsis in asymptomatic splenectomized Hodgkin's disease patients, Ann. Intern. Med. 77:69, 1972.
31. Peters, M. V.: A study of survivals in Hodgkin's disease treated radiologically, Am. J. Roentgenol. 63:299, 1950.
32. Peters, M. V., Brown, T. C., and Rideout, D. F.: Hodgkin's disease—prognostic influence and radiation therapy according to pattern of disease, JAMA 223:53, 1973.
33. Peters, M. V., and Middlemiss, K. C. H.: A study of Hodgkin's disease treated by irradiation, Am. J. Roentgenol. 79:114, 1958.
34. Probert, J. C., and Parker, B. R.: The effects of radiation therapy on bone growth, Radiology 114:155, 1975.
35. Ravry, M., Maldonado, N., Velez-Garcia, E., Montalvo, J., and Santiago, P. J.: Serious infection after splenectomy for the staging of Hodgkin's disease, Ann. Intern. Med. 77:14, 1972.
36. Reed, D. M.: On the pathological changes in Hodgkin's disease with special reference to its relation to tuberculosis, Johns Hopkins Hosp. Rep. 10:133, 1902.
37. Rosenberg, S. A.: A critique of the value of laparotomy and splenectomy in the evaluation of patients with Hodgkin's disease, Cancer Res. 31:1737, 1971.
38. Rosenberg, S. A.: Updated Hodgkin's disease. Place of splenectomy in evaluation and management, JAMA 222:1296, 1972.
39. Rosenberg, S. A.: Report of the committee on staging of Hodgkin's disease, Cancer Res. 26:1310, 1966.
40. Rosenberg, S. A., and Kaplan, H. S.: The management of stages I, II and III Hodgkin's disease with combined radiotherapy and chemotherapy, Cancer 35:55, 1975.
41. Rosenstock, J. C., D'Angio, G. J., and Kiesewetter, W. B.: The incidence of complications following staging laparotomy for Hodgkin's disease in children, Am. J. Roentgenol. 120:531, 1974.
42. Smith, K. L., Johnson, D., Hustu, O., Pratt, C., Fleming, I., and Holton, C.: Concurrent chemotherapy and radiation therapy in the treatment of childhood and adolescent Hodgkin's disease, Cancer 33:38, 1974.
43. Sternberg, C.: Über eine eigenartige unter dem Bilde der pseudo-Leukämie verlaufende Tuberkulose des Lymphatischen apparates, X. Heilk 19:21, 1898.
44. Tan, C., D'Angio, G. J., Exelby, P. R., *et al.*: The changing management of childhood Hodgkin's disease, Cancer 35:808, 1975.
45. Tan, C., Etcubanas, E., Wollner, N., Rosen, G., Gilladoga, A., Showel, J., Murphy, M. L., and Krakoff, I. H.: Adriamycin—an antitumor antibiotic in the treatment of neoplastic diseases, Cancer 32:9, 1973.
46. Tan, C., Exelby, P. R., D'Angio, G. J., Watson, R. C., Etcubanas, E., and Murphy, M. L.: Laparotomy in Staging of Hodgkin's Disease in Children, in *International Congress of Pediatrics, Vienna, 1971.* Proc., Vol. 14, *Malignant Diseases, Radiotherapy and Nuclear Medicine* (Vienna: Wiener Medizinischen Akademia, 1971), pp. 75–80.
47. Tessmer, C. F., Hrgovcic, M., and Jordan, W.: Serum copper in Hodgkin's disease in children, Cancer 31:303, 1973.
48. Virchow, R.: *Die Krankhaften geschwulste*, Vol. 2 (Berlin: A. Hirschwald, 1863), pp. 728–738.
49. Wayne, E. R., Kosloske, A., Holton, C. P., Burrington, J. D., and Hatch, E. I.: Complications of abdominal exploration and splenectomy in staging children with Hodgkin's disease, J. Pediatr. Surg. 10:677, 1975.
50. Wilks, S.: Cases of enlargement of the lymphatic glands and spleen (or Hodgkin's disease), Guys Hosp. Rep. 11:56, 1865.

34

MARK M. RAVITCH

The Thyroid

HISTORY.—Of all the endocrine glands, the thyroid is the one most commonly affected by pathologic changes in size and function both in children and in adults. Thyroid enlargements are obvious and have long been remarked on. Incantations against goiter are found in the Hindu *Atharva-Vedu* dating about 2000 B.C. Shakespeare took note of endemic goiter in *The Tempest:* "Who would believe that there were mountaineers dew-lapped like bulls, whose throats had hanging at them wallets of flesh; or that there were such men whose heads stood in their breasts?"

Renaissance artists often portrayed their women with a full smooth goiter at the throat. Cretins appealed to artistic curiosity. Velásquez left a classic depiction of a goitrous cretin, a dwarf of Philip IV, which hangs in the Prado today. A vivid picture of endemic goiter and cretinism was captured by Felix Platter (1536–1614) in his *Praxeus Medicae,* "and in the Carinthia Valley called Buntzger-

thal, many infants are wont to be afflicted who besides their innate simplemindedness, the head is now and then misformed, the tongue immense and tumid, dumb, a struma often at the throat, they show a deformed appearance and seated in solemn stateliness, staring, and a stick resting between their hands, their bodies twisted variously, their eyes wide apart, they show immoderate laughter and wonder at unknown things."*

The thyroid was described by Galen in his *De Voce* in the second century A.D., but his descriptions of the gland were vague. A much fuller and more accurate account was given by Vesalius in 1543 in Book VI of the *Fabrica.*

---

*Translation by Major, R. H., *Classic Description of Disease* (3d ed.; Springfield, Ill.: Charles C Thomas, Publisher, 1945).

In *Adenographia*, a treatise dealing with the glands of the human body published in 1656, Thomas Wharton gave the gland its present name, from its fancied resemblance to a shield. Wharton made several guesses as to the function of the gland, but the best remembered, and the most often quoted is, "It contributes much to the rotundity and beauty of the neck, filling up the vacant spaces round the larynx and making its protruding parts almost to subside and become smooth, particularly in females, to whom for this reason a larger gland has been assigned, which renders their necks more even and beautiful."

1. Goiter

Goiter means simply an enlargement of the thyroid, whether due to neoplasm, inflammation, colloid accumulation or hyperthyroidism. Most commonly, the term is used to refer to the compensatory enlargement associated with a relative decrease of thyroxine production and increase of colloid, which may arise from a lack of iodine or a number of other defects or deficiencies. The histologic picture in goiters called simple, colloid, endemic, sporadic, congenital, familial, juvenile and pubertal is essentially the same.

PATHOLOGY.—Early in the course of the development of goiter, the gland may show diffuse enlargement and is soft and very vascular. The follicular cells are tall and the interfollicular blood vessels prominent. This very early state of goiter is seen rarely in surgical pathology specimens. At this period, treatment of the deficiency that has resulted in goiter formation will restore the gland to normal. After a time, the changes in the gland become irreversible, and treatment, such as replacement of iodine in a subiodic goiter, results in accumulation of increased amounts of colloid in enlarged follicles, the typical colloid goiter.

If the impairment of thyroxine formation persists, the diffuse enlargement and hyperplasia is replaced by focal areas of hyperfunction scattered through the gland. Microscopically, these areas may be seen as patchy areas of hyperplastic follicles with tall columnar cells, sometimes with the formation of numerous small adenoma-like masses, resulting in a nodular goiter. Often there is considerable fibrosis, and areas of colloid goiter may alternate with areas of hypertrophy and hyperplasia and minute adenomas that often are poorly defined. Foci of intense activity proceed to hemorrhage followed by central necrosis, fibrosis and sometimes calcification. In some instances, the necrotic nodule may be replaced by a single lake of colloid, or new follicles of varying size may grow in it. The multinodular goiter of the older patient is the end result of this cycle of hyperplasia and destruction recurring repeatedly, and usually presents a multiphasic pathologic picture, with different stages of the early and late process being represented in sections throughout the gland.[35]

INCIDENCE.—Goiter is more common in females than in males. The incidence among children varies greatly in endemic and in nonendemic goiter areas. In endemic areas, the highest incidence in all age groups is in girls from 12 to 18 and in boys from 9 to 13.[8, 9, 21] In the endemic areas of the United States, before the use of iodized salt, the thyroid of children commonly became moderately enlarged in early childhood, and by the age of 5, one-fourth of the boys and one-third or more of the girls presented goiters. In a nonendemic area, advanced goiter in childhood, severe enough to require hospital treatment, is relatively infrequent. Wilkins[38] reported that in a 20-year period at the Pediatric Endocrine Clinic of the Johns Hopkins Hospital, 44 children with goiters were treated. Surveys of children in the general population in nonendemic areas reveal an incidence of goi-ter of from 1% to 4%.[8] In 30 years at the Lahey Clinic, 79 children were seen with nontoxic goiters (of whom 22 were proved to have cancer);[1] 58 of the 79 children were girls.

ETIOLOGY.—Compensatory goiter is considered to result from hypertrophy of the thyroid gland in response to a relative lack of thyroxine in the body caused by iodine lack, to goitrogen intake, to stress or to inborn errors of metabolism.[3]

Iodine lack.—The world over, the most common cause of goiter is iodine lack. The normal requirement for the thyroid is $100-200 \mu g$ of iodine per day in the adult, and in childhood and puberty the requirement probably is substantially greater.[24] In a good many parts of the world, the content of soil and water is inadequate to supply the normal needs of the thyroid gland, notoriously in the high mountain regions of the Alps, the Pyrenees, the Himalayas and the Andes. In the United States, before endemic goiter was eradicated by the addition of iodine to table salt as a result of the work of Marine,[20] endemic goiters existed in the Ohio River valley and the Great Lakes region. With the supplementation of iodine intake, the incidence of goiter in children in Ohio fell from 32.3% in 1925 to 4.05% in 1954.[10] When goiter occurs in the presence of adequate iodine intake, other factors must be looked for.

Goitrogens.—A number of naturally occurring substances, as well as some drugs, are known to block the normal formation of thyroid hormone in the gland, resulting in goiter. Such of these goitrogens as pass through the placenta may cause goiter in the fetus. Blizzard's group[4] has demonstrated that thyroxine already is identifiable in the serum of a 78-day-old fetus and that the amount increases in older fetuses in linear relation to gestational age, reaching term levels by 18–20 weeks. Iodine excess, curiously, may act to inhibit thyroxine synthesis and thus provoke TSH (thyroid-stimulating hormone) production and thyroid hyperplasia in both children and adults, and in the fetus.[5, 25] Calcium, fluorine and chloride are other inorganic ions that have been demonstrated to be capable of causing goiter when taken in large amounts. With the exception of calcium, they have not been clinically demonstrated to cause goiter. It is possible that the intake of water with high calcium content in low iodine areas may potentiate iodine lack in the development of goiters.[3, 21]

A number of foods are known to contain goitrogens, among them cabbage, rutabaga, rape seed and soybeans.[31, 36] Infant feeding formulas derived from soybeans have been reported to cause goiter formation.[31]

An increasing number of drugs and other therapeutic agents are known to cause goiter: thiocyanate, potassium perchlorate, sulfonamides, para-aminosalicylic acid, resorcinol, cobalt,[16] arsenic[30] and BAL (British anti-lewisite),[10] all of which appear to be thyroid blocking agents.[3] With the possible exception of para-aminosalicylic acid, most of them are not likely to be given for a long enough period to produce goiters, except possibly in the fetus. The most commonly known goitrogens are the drugs of the thiourea family, in which the thyroid blocking factor is potent and which are therefore used in the treatment of hyperthyroidism. Hyperthyroidism in the mother treated with thiourea drugs may result in goiter in the fetus.

Stress.—Apparently it is possible for the thyroid, while receiving a normal allotment of iodine, to become hyperplastic simply because of excessive demand by the cells for large amounts of thyroxine. This circumstance may occur in children with so-called puberty goiter, a response to the need for extra hormone during this period. Puberty goiter is especially common in girls and may be more frequent and severe where there is a relative deficiency of iodine as well. The increase in size of the thyroid, which occurs during the menstrual period in some women, and the stepwise enlargement of goiters in women during repeated pregnancies probably represent a similar response to demand for increased thyroxine formation.

Inborn errors of metabolism.—This group probably represents the chief cause for sporadic goiter in nonendemic regions (Fig. 34–1). The etiology of these goiters has been elaborated,[32] and active research continues to unravel the responsible types of deficiency in the formation of thyroxine.

At least five principal types of errors of metabolism have been identified, and there probably are many others.[4, 12, 14] The five specifically identified are: (1) Inability to concentrate iodide in the thyroid gland,[11] entirely treatable with Lugol's solution. In any case, goiter is not seen in this group. (2) Ability to concentrate iodide in the thyroid gland but inability to oxidize it to iodine, due to peroxidase enzyme deficiency.[14, 33] (3) Normal production of mono- and diiodotyrosine but inability to convert these substances to thyronines—thought to be due to an iodotyrosine deiodinase defect.[14, 22] Although all the steps through production of thyroglobulin and its breakdown are believed to be normal, iodotyrosine deiodinase is deficient: iodine cannot be retrieved from some of the compounds formed in the metabolic chain, and these compounds are excreted from the body with their iodine, thus creating an iodine deficit.[7, 33, 34] (4) Abnormal release of thyroxine from the thyroid associated with abnormal iodinated polypeptides in the serum.[37] (5) Inborn peripheral resistance to thyroid hormone. In the most striking cases, viz., a syndrome of congenital goiter, deaf mutism, delayed bone maturation, stippled epiphyses and raised levels of circulating thyroid hormone,[26] such patients require as much as 280 micrograms of T_4 to stress thyroidal uptake. Less stubborn resistance to thyroid has been reported,[17] and without deafness and bone changes.

These and other, variant, inborn metabolic defects affecting the thyroid hormone are inherited as simple autosomal recessive traits. The goiter may develop more or less rapidly after birth, or even in childhood or adult life, if at all, presumably depending on the severity of the metabolic error.

Clinical features.—*Congenital goiter.*—The term applies not only to the infant born with goiter but as well to the infant in whom a goiter begins to develop during the first few weeks of life. Congenital goiter (Fig. 34–2), which is very rare in the United States, is common in endemic goiter areas in Europe. According to Aschoff,[2] goiter was present in 50% of all newborn babies in parts of Switzerland as late as 1935, and in Freiberg, Germany, goiter accounted for 10% of the neonatal mortality.

Goiter in the newborn in endemic areas is due mainly to a gross deficiency of maternal iodine intake.[8] In the sporadic goiters of the newborn seen in nonendemic areas, a variety of causes have been observed.[23, 24] Iodine intake by the mother, usually as saturated potassium iodide for asthma or as an expectorant, has led to goiter in the infant.[5, 15] Intake of goitrogens by the mother is an increasing cause of neonatal goiter. Cobalt, thiourea drugs and para-aminosalicylic acid given the mother have all led to goiter in the newborn.[5, 18, 27] It is likely that prolonged intake of any goitrogen that passes the placental barrier will induce goiter in the fetus.

In most instances, no history of maternal goitrogen intake or iodine lack can be elicited. In normal circumstances, maternal thyroxine crosses the placental barrier in small amounts, and the embryo supplies its own thyroxine from

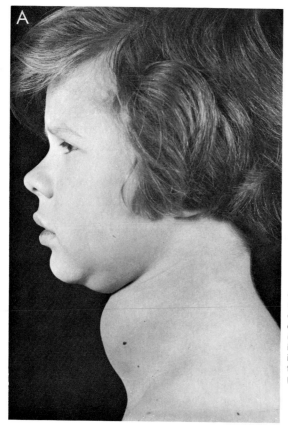

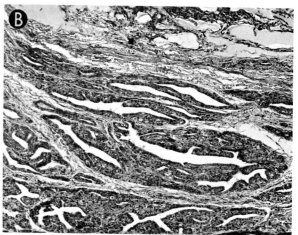

Fig. 34–1.—Sporadic goiter. **A,** this 13-year-old girl had a history of hypothyroidism diagnosed at age 7 months. Goiter was first noted at age 6. She had taken desiccated thyroid sporadically over this period. Analysis of thyroid function suggested an inborn error of metabolism due to inability to couple iodotyrosines. (From Mosier *et al.*[22]) **B,** the variable microscopic picture is illustrated. Empty follicles lined by cuboidal cells with papillary infoldings are seen in the lower part of the section. Thin-walled follicles lined with flattened cells containing quantities of thin, poorly staining colloid are seen in the upper portion.

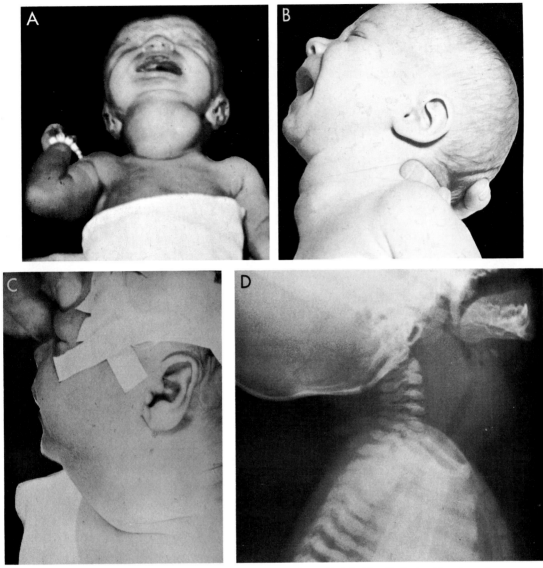

Fig. 34–2.—Congenital goiter: differential diagnosis. **A,** teratoma of thyroid. This infant was born with the huge midline cervical mass causing severe respiratory embarrassment. Diagnosis of congenital goiter was said to have been made and expectant treatment followed. The child died of respiratory obstruction; autopsy revealed teratoma in the position of the thyroid. **B,** hemangioma of neck. A 5-week-old boy, with a swelling present since birth and gradually leading to severe respiratory obstruction. He was admitted in acute distress, with stridor and sternal obstruction. He was intubated without anesthesia, and operation was immediately undertaken for what was thought to be congenital obstructing goiter. An extremely vascular tumor anterior to the thyroid was totally removed; it proved to be a highly cellular hemangioma. Irradiation was given because the tumor seemed to be infiltrating. He was well 12 years later. **C,** congenital obstructing goiter. This infant was referred at 30 hours of age because of increased difficulty in breathing caused by pressure from a large collar-like mass filling the upper neck.

He lay on his left side with the head in extreme hyperextension. The mother had a history of asthma and took saturated potassium iodide, 24 drops a day. An attempt to treat the child by position and oxygen failed, dyspnea persisted and cyanosis developed. He was successfully treated by partial excision of the thyroid. (From Packard et al.[24a]) **D,** congenital obstructing goiter. Lateral roentgenogram of a 2-month-old infant born with a mass in the neck that recently had doubled in size. The mass was large, lobulated, irregular, suggestively cystic, obscured the trachea anteriorly and extended posteriorly to the angle of the mandible. There was marked respiratory difficulty. Subtotal thyroidectomy with removal of the isthmus and portions of the lateral lobes relieved all symptoms. Tumor sections were reported to show a thyroid adenoma of Hürthle cell type. The film shows clearly the large cervical mass and potential airway obstruction from elevation of the base of the tongue and from direct tracheal compression. (Courtesy of Dr. Paul Holinger, Chicago.)

the developing thyroid gland.[6] If a severe error of fetal thyroid metabolism is present, a large goiter may develop in utero. Rarely, a congenital goiter is so large as to cause dystocia at delivery. The head of the fetus cannot flex, and a mental presentation occurs.

Goiter in the newborn due to maternal intake of antithyroid drugs will disappear in 1 or 2 months without treatment. If there is no respiratory obstruction and a valid history of appropriate maternal drug intake is obtained, nothing need

be done. Diagnosis of a congenital goiter due to an inborn error of metabolism is based on the negative maternal history and on specialized tests of thyroid function. In these infants, therapy with desiccated thyroid (120–180 mg daily) is important to shrink the goiter and to avoid the complications of hypothyroidism.

Respiratory obstruction with goiter in the neonate, as with any other cervical tumor, is the surgeon's first concern. Stridor, suprasternal, epigastric and intercostal retraction and

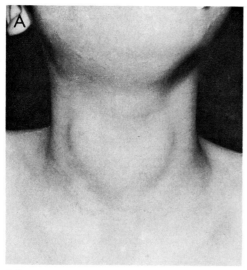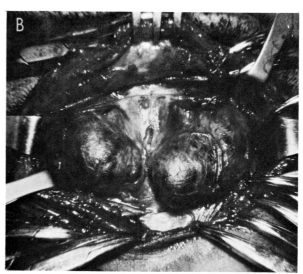

Fig. 34–3.—Colloid goiter. **A,** this 11-year-old girl was euthyroid, but the goiter was nodular and firm, strongly suggesting carcinoma. The mass is clearly visible and symmetric. There were no palpable lymph nodes. **B,** operative view of bilaterally enlarged gland. Size of the mass and its compression by the strap muscles probably caused the feeling of firmness, because, on exposure, the nodules were quite soft. Frozen section showed colloid goiter, so only a little of the prominent portion was removed from each side. Permanent section confirmed the diagnosis, but areas of normal-appearing thyroid acini were found around a bit of attached ribbon muscle. This was considered to represent a benign phenomenon. After thyroid therapy for a year, the gland was much smaller and firmer but still palpably enlarged, although no longer readily visible.

cervical hyperextension characterize the infant with tracheal compression. For some days, an infant with severe respiratory obstruction may appear to compensate for the obstruction, only to grow fatigued and succumb suddenly. Operation should be undertaken if obstruction exists, whether the child "tolerates" it or not. The tracheal intubation probably is the most hazardous moment of the procedure. A formal exposure of the thyroid is undertaken and, at a minimum, the isthmus is resected. As Louw[18] has pointed out, the goiter may completely surround the trachea and it may be necessary to perform a bilateral subtotal thyroidectomy. Schifrin and Hurwitt[28] reported an instance of hypothyroidism developing in a child who had had an extensive thyroidectomy for an enormous obstructing congenital goiter. It is worth remembering, however, that goiter may be the presenting symptom in congenital cretins.[19] Tracheostomy for the child with congenital goiter and respiratory obstruction is difficult until the isthmus has been divided, and after such division may be unnecessary.

Several observations now cast some doubt on the absolute necessity for operation for strangulating neonatal goiter if an intratracheal tube can be maintained in place. Senior and Chernoff,[29] in an infant with an enormous obstructing goiter, born of a mother taking iodine for hyperthyroidism, reduced the gland with desiccated thyroid and extubated the baby successfully after 6 days. Freudenberg,[13] from Kass, successfully treated 3 newborns with obstructing iodine-deficiency goiters and respiratory difficulty with intubation for "a few hours, 3 days and 11 days" and no operation. The goiters receded with the application of 1% iodine-potassium iodide salve to the skin. Most clinics would prefer to use initial intramuscular injections of T₄ followed by oral maintenance doses.[11a]

Juvenile goiter.—An enlargement of the thyroid appearing after the neonatal period and before the onset of puberty requires the exercise of substantial clinical discernment. If the gland is nodular, whether the nodule is single or multiple, soft or hard, in addition to the usual tests of thyroid function, an open biopsy should be performed to rule out the possibility of cancer. If the gland is smoothly and diffusely enlarged and not hard, or if biopsy has shown the nodule or nodules to represent colloid goiter (Fig. 34–3), the treatment is with iodine in endemic areas and with thyroid hormone for children with sporadic goiters presumably due to metabolic thyroid defects. Desiccated thyroid, 120–180 mg daily taken orally, causes suppression of thyroid activity and regression of the goiter through the familiar suppression of the TSH secretion. Several months of therapy may be required to bring about a significant decrease in size of the goiter, and occasionally the ultimate size of the goiter still may be such as to justify a thyroidectomy for cosmetic and symptomatic reasons.

Puberty goiter.—Probably the most common type of goiter encountered in children in nonendemic areas, it is much more common in girls than in boys and usually regresses spontaneously when the period of adolescence is past. As a rule, the goiter is of small to moderate size, diffuse, soft and asymptomatic. If it becomes quite large, desiccated thyroid, 120–180 mg daily orally, will reduce the size of the gland. Operation should not be required and is likely to result in thyroid insufficiency.

REFERENCES

1. Adams, H. D.: Non-toxic nodular goiter and carcinoma of the thyroid in children 15 years of age and younger, S. Clin. North Am. 47:601, 1967.
2. Aschoff, L.: Cited by Clements *et al.*[8]
3. Berson, S. A.: Pathways of iodine metabolism, Am. J. Med. 20: 653, 1956.
4. Blizzard, R. M.: Inherited defects of thyroid hormone synthesis and metabolism, Metabolism 9:232, 1960.
5. Bongiovani, A. M., *et al.*: Sporadic goiter of the newborn, J. Clin. Endocrinol. 16:146, 1956.
6. Carr, E. A., *et al.*: The effect of maternal thyroid function on fetal thyroid function and development, J. Clin. Endocrinol. 19:1, 1959.
7. Chovfoer, J. C., Kassemaar, A. A. H., and Querido, A.: The syndrome of congenital hypothyroidism with defective dehalogenation of iodotyrosines: Further observations and discussion of the pathophysiology, J. Clin. Endocrinol. 20:983, 1960.
8. Clements, F. W., *et al.*: *Endemic Goiter* (Geneva: Health Organization, 1960).

9. Crawford, J. D.: Goiters in childhood, Pediatrics 17:437, 1956.
10. Current, J. V., Hales, I. B., and Dobyns, B. M.: The effect of 2,3-dimercaptopropranol (BAL) on thyroid function, J. Clin. Endocrinol. 20:13, 1960.
11. Federman, D., Robbins, J., and Rall, J. E.: Some observations on cretinism and its treatment, N. Engl. J. Med. 259:610, 1958.
11a. Fisher, D. A.: Comment—on the treatment of congenital goiter, J. Pediatr. 88:527, 1976.
12. Floyd, J. C., et al.: Defective iodination of tyrosine: A cause of nodular goiter?, J. Clin. Endocrinol. 20:881, 1960.
13. Freudenberg, V.: Die Behandlung der Tracheakompression durch Struma congenita, Klin. Paediatr. 186:5, 1974.
14. Gardner, J. U., et al.: Iodine metabolism in goitrous cretins, J. Clin. Endocrinol. 17:638, 1959.
15. Job, J. C., Binet, E., Hénoco, A., and Leroux, J. P.: Goitre néonatal secondaire a l'absorption prolongée d'iodure par la mère. Evaluation du taux sanguin de thyréostimuline hypophysaire (TSH), Presse Med. 79:8, 1971.
16. Kriss, J. P., Carnes, W. H., and Gross, R. T.: Hypothyroidism and thyroid hyperplasia in patients treated with cobalt, JAMA 157:117, 1955.
17. Lamberg, B. A.: Congenital euthyroid goitre and partial peripheral resistance to thyroid hormones, Lancet 2:854, 1973.
18. Louw, J. H.: Congenital goitre, S. Afr. Med. J. 37:976, 1963.
19. Lowrey, G. H., et al.: Early diagnostic criteria of congenital hypothyroidism, Am. J. Dis. Child. 96:131, 1958.
20. Marine, D., and Kimball, O. P.: The prevention of simple goiter in man, J. Lab. Clin. Med. 3:40, 1917.
21. McGavack, T. H.: The Thyroid (St. Louis: The C. V. Mosby Company, 1951).
22. Mosier, H. D., Blizzard, R. M., and Wilkins, L.: Congenital defects in the biosynthesis of thyroid hormone: Report of two cases, Pediatrics 21:248, 1958.
23. Norris, W. J., and Pollock, W. F.: Nodular goiters in children, Am. J. Surg. 90:345, 1955.
24. Oliner, L., et al.: Thyroid function studies in children: Normal values of thyroidal I¹³¹ uptake and PBI¹³¹ levels up to age of 18, J. Clin. Endocrinol. 17:61, 1957.
24a. Packard, G. B., Williams, E. T., and Wheelock, S. E.: Congenital obstructing goiter, Surgery 48:422, 1960.
25. Paris, J., et al.: Iodide goiter, J. Clin. Endocrinol. 20:57, 1960.
26. Refetoff, S., DeGroot, L. J., Benard, B., and DeWind, L. T.: Studies of a sibship with apparent hereditary resistance to the intracellular action of thyroid hormone, Metabolism 21:723, 1972.
27. Riley, I. D., and Sclare, G.: Thyroid disorders in the newborn, Br. Med. J. 1:979, 1957.
28. Schifrin, N., and Hurwitt, E.: Hypothyroidism following thyroidectomy for congenital obstructive goiter, J. Pediatr. 39:597, 1951.
29. Senior, B., and Chernoff, H. L.: Iodide goiter in the newborn, Pediatrics 47:3, 1971.
30. Sharpless, G. R., and Metzger, M.: Arsenic and goiter, J. Nutr. 21:341, 1941.
31. Shepard, T. H., et al.: Soybean goiter: Report of 3 cases, N. Engl. J. Med. 262:1099, 1960.
32. Stanbury, J. B., and Hedge, A. N.: A study of a family of goitrous cretins, J. Clin. Endocrinol. 10:1471, 1950.
33. Stanbury, J. B., Weijer, J. W. A., and Kassenaar, A. S. H.: The metabolism of iodotyrosines: II. The metabolism of mono- and diiodotyrosines in certain patients with familial goiter, J. Clin. Endocrinol. 16:848, 1956.
34. Stanbury, J. B., et al.: The occurrence of mono- and diiodotyrosine in the blood of a patient with congenital goiter, J. Clin. Endocrinol. 15:1216, 1955.
35. Taylor, S.: Physiologic concepts in the genesis and management of nodular goiter, Am. J. Med. 20:698, 1956.
36. Van Wyk, J. J., et al.: The effects of soybean products on thyroid function in humans, Pediatrics 24:752, 1960.
37. Whitelow, M. J., Thomas, S., and Reilly, W. A.: A non-goitrous cretin with a high level of serum PBI and thyroidal I¹³¹ uptake, J. Clin. Endocrinol. 16:983, 1956.
38. Wilkins, L.: Diagnosis and Treatment of Endocrine Disorders in Childhood and Adolescence (2d ed.; Springfield, Ill.: Charles C Thomas, Publisher, 1956).

2. Ectopic Thyroid Tissue

LINGUAL AND SUBLINGUAL THYROID GLANDS.—The thyroid derives embryologically from a midline diverticulum in the ventral wall of the pharynx, first noted about the third week of embryonic life, at a point ultimately marked by the foramen caecum at the base of the tongue.[16] This anlage grows downward as a tubular duct descending in the midline and coming to rest in the familiar location, essentially as a paired organ with a midline connecting bar. Two lateral masses of cells that derive from paired outpouchings of the fourth pharyngeal arch join this midline tissue in its migration but seem not to contribute significantly to the formation of the thyroid gland. If the diverticular character of the tract from the base of the tongue to the region of the thyroid persists, there remains a thyroglossal duct with or without a cyst. Ordinarily, in association with such a patient thyroglossal duct sinus one does not find thyroid tissue (6 of 105 surgical specimens in one series).[19]

Two clinical patterns are associated with maldescent of the thyroid anlage. Lingual thyroid is the result of total failure of migration and presents a solid or cystic mass of varying size at the base of the tongue. If this is large early in childhood or if there is a hemorrhage or cyst formation within it, respiratory obstruction and death may result. More commonly, the patient complains merely of a lump in the throat and, in most instances, is euthyroid. However, Lucot et al.[12] reported 4 children with clinical hypothyroidism and lingual thyroid tissue demonstrable by scintiscan, in the apparent absence of a palpable mass. In essentially all other reports, the presenting sign has been a mass that was digitally palpable and accessible to inspection through the mouth. In some instances, the mass is large enough and its substance sufficiently characteristic to be identifiable as thyroid tissue through the thinned-out pharyngeal mucosa. Niemann et al.[14] report a staggering series of 165 patients with infantile hypothyroidism, of whom 75% were demonstrated to have ectopic thyroid tissue, usually nonpalpable. Strickland et al.,[17] reporting 4 children with median subhyoid ectopic thyroid, point out that all had evidences of hypothyroidism and suggest that the nodules increase in size to the point of clinical prominence in a response, frequently inadequate, to the need for thyroid hormone.

SUBHYOID MEDIAN ECTOPIC THYROID.—This presents as a rubbery midline mass at the level of the hyoid or just below it. Until very recently, these masses more often than not were diagnosed as thyroglossal duct cysts and excised, with belated histologic revelation of their nature and the subsequent development of myxedema in those patients not treated appropriately. The differential diagnosis includes subhyoid median ectopic thyroid, midline cervical dermoid, thyroglossal duct cyst and an occasional enlarged lymph node. In essentially all cases of lingual thyroid and subhyoid median thyroid there is no other normal thyroid tissue, and removal of the ectopic tissue inevitably results in hypothyroidism. As Ward and his group[18] pointed out, this throws great doubt on the significance of the contribution of the lateral thyroid anlagen to the formation of the thyroid gland. If the diagnosis is suspected, it can be confirmed by scintiscan. ¹³¹I, used initially, has been replaced by ¹²⁵I and, more recently, by ⁹⁹ᵐTc pertechnetate isotope, the isotope of choice because of its short half-life—6 hours—low-energy gamma emissions, minimal beta emissions and the ease with which it can be collimated.[1, 10, 15] Scanning establishes the identity of the sublingual or subhyoid mass and, invariably, the absence of normally placed thyroid tissue.

TREATMENT.—The indication for treatment in the case of lingual thyroid is the annoying pharyngeal mass, together with the danger of respiratory obstruction from it. There are a number of reports of cancer developing in a lingual thyroid,[2] most in male patients and all in adults.

Large lingual thyroid masses require excision, and since this is the patient's only thyroid tissue, excision requires lifelong replacement therapy. Excision can be satisfactorily performed through the mouth for the smaller tumors. Ward's lateral pharyngeal approach would seem to be the most satisfactory for the large tumors.[18] If there is no immediate hazard from respiratory obstruction, a trial of thyroid medication may reasonably be undertaken. Lifetime thyroid medication would, in any case, be required, and there is evidence[9, 10] that smaller lingual thyroid masses may become inconspicuous and asymptomatic under effective thyroid replacement medication.

As with any other lesion of the base of the tongue and epiglottis, postoperative edema may threaten the airway and require tracheostomy. The mucous membrane over the sublingual thyroid generally will not be separable from it, and direct closure of the pharyngeal wall and floor of the mouth is required.

The unpleasant cosmetic appearance of subhyoid median ectopic thyroid is the indication for operative treatment. Median cervical ectopic thyroid, whether below or above the hyoid, is most satisfactorily treated by splitting the two halves of the thyroid gland, which retain their lateral arterial supply, so that each half can be placed under its corresponding ribbon muscle, relieving the cosmetic complaint without injuring the gland.[6, 7]

PYRAMIDAL LOBE NODULES.—The pyramidal lobe is the last persistence of the thyroid migration, and adenomas and other nodules may form in it as in any other portion of the thyroid. In such instances, however, one will be able to feel the normal thyroid gland at either side, which is not possible with either the lingual or the subhyoid gland.

LATERAL ABERRANT THYROID.—For some 25 years we have been confident that apparently innocent or papillary-looking thyroid tissue in cervical lymph nodes always represented metastases from a carcinoma of the thyroid, occasionally so small as not to be palpable.[4, 11] The relatively benign nature and long life history of these tumors led earlier clinicians to mistake these lymph nodes, frequently totally replaced by thyroid tissue, for lateral "rests." In the past few years, a number of reports have appeared discarding the term "lateral aberrant thyroid," abandoned a generation ago, but describing "benign metastasizing thyroid follicles," "thyroid follicle inclusions in cervical lymph nodes," "primary thyroid tumors in cervical lymph nodes" and "non-neoplastic thyroid tissue within cervical lymph nodes."[5, 13, 16] The suggestion, as in the former designation of lateral aberrant thyroid, is that this is non-neoplastic and nonmalignant tissue and has no bearing on prognosis or treatment. A study from the M. D. Anderson Hospital seems extraordinarily apropos and would appear to dispose of this argument.[3] Thyroid carcinoma was found unexpectedly in the thyroid gland or lymph nodes at autopsy or in the material removed at operation from 22 patients with squamous cell carcinoma of the head or neck or the lung. Twenty of these had mixed papillary and follicular or pure follicular thyroid carcinoma in the thyroid gland or lymph nodes. Carcinoma was demonstrated in the thyroid glands of 15 of the 22 patients. In the 7 patients in whom no primary thyroid carcinoma was demonstrated, only a portion of the thyroid or none of it had been removed. Carcinoma was discovered in every case in which the whole thyroid gland was available for study, but this often required serial section. Although the primary tumor might be mixed papillary and follicular, the metastases could be either predominantly papillary or predominantly follicular. The conclusion was: "Any thyroid tissue found in a lymph node represents metastatic cancer." The life history of these tumors is so long that no ordinary follow-up study will resolve the question as to whether or not there may be conditions in which non-neoplastic thyroid is found in the neck outside the thyroid gland. Block *et al.*[2] found benign thyroid tissue within the carotid sheath in 2 patients in whom total thyroidectomy had failed to disclose any tumor, although serial sections were not made. What appears to be normal thyroid tissue in the strap muscles of children without any apparent relation to tumors of the thyroid[8] has also been reported.

REFERENCES

1. Aschoff, L.: Cited by Clements *et al.* (reference 8 under Goiter).
2. Block, M. A., *et al.*: Does benign thyroid tissue occur in the lateral part of the neck?, Am. J. Surg. 112:476, 1966.
3. Butler, J. J., *et al.*: Significance of thyroid tissue in lymph nodes associated with carcinoma of the head, neck or lung, Cancer 20:1, 1967.
4. Clay, R. C., and Blackman, S. S., Jr.: Lateral aberrant thyroid: Metastasis to the lymph nodes from primary carcinoma of the thyroid gland, Arch. Surg. 48:223, 1944.
5. Gerard-Marchant, R.: Thyroid follicle inclusions in cervical lymph nodes, Arch. Pathol. 77:633, 1964.
6. Gross, R. W.: *The Surgery of Infancy and Childhood* (Philadelphia: W. B. Saunders Company, 1953), Chap. 66.
7. Haller, J. A., Jr., and Williams, G. R.: Isolated midline thyroid in the thyroglossal duct, Surgery 46:437, 1959.
8. Hazard, J. B., and Smith D. E. (eds.): *The Thyroid* (Baltimore: The Williams & Wilkins Company, 1964), p. 12.
9. Hung, W., *et al.*: Lingual and sublingual thyroid glands in euthyroid children, Pediatrics 38:4, 1966.
10. Katz, A. D., and Zager, W. J.: The lingual thyroid, Arch. Surg. 102:582, 1971.
11. King, W. L. M., and Pemberton, J. de J.: So-called lateral aberrant thyroid tumors, Surg. Gynecol. Obstet. 74:991, 1942.
12. Lucot, H., *et al.*: Quatre cas de thyroïdes linguales chez l'enfant, décelées à l'occasion d'un retard psycho-moteur, J. Radiol. Electrol. Med. Nucl. 46:807, 1965.
13. Nicastri, A. D., Foote, F. W., Jr., and Frazell, E. L.: Benign thyroid inclusions in cervical lymph nodes, JAMA 194:113, 1965.
14. Niemann, N., Pierson, M., Martin, J., and Sapelier, J.: L'ectopie de la thyroïde, cause principale de l'hypothyroïde infantile, Presse Med. 76:659, 1968.
15. Pulito, A. R., and Shaw, A.: Case reports: Median ectopic thyroid gland, J. Pediatr. Surg. 8:73, 1973.
16. Roth, L. M.: Inclusions of non-neoplastic thyroid tissue within cervical lymph nodes, Cancer 18:105, 1965.
17. Strickland, A. L., Macfie, J. A., Van Wyk, J. J., and French, F. S.: Ectopic thyroid glands simulating thyroglossal duct cysts, JAMA 208:2, 307, 1969.
18. Ward, G. E., Cantrell, J. R., and Allan, W. B.: The surgical treatment of lingual thyroid, Ann. Surg. 139:536, 1954.
19. Ward, G. E., Hendricks, J. W., and Chambers, R. G.: Thyroglossal tract abnormalities—cysts and fistulas, Surg. Gynecol. Obstet. 89:727, 1949.

3. Hyperthyroidism

INCIDENCE.—Hyperthyroidism is uncommon in childhood. Bram[5] reported that of 1120 children with goiter, only 128 had hyperthyroidism. He estimated that 2.5% of all cases of hyperthyroidism were found in children. Henoch and Romberg[13] are credited with the first description of hyperthyroidism in a child, a girl of 14, reported in 1851. In 1938, Atkinson[3] was able to collect 208 such cases from the literature. In 1959, Hayles *et al.*[11] reported a total of 253 children treated for hyperthyroidism at the Mayo Clinic between 1908 and 1955, and Saxena, Crawford and Talbot[27] saw 70 cases from 1941 to 1961, accounting for 45% of all goiters seen at the Children's Endocrine and Metabolic Clinic of the Massachusetts General Hospital. In a more recent paper from the Mayo Clinic,[25] of 209 children with goiter, 61 had a diffuse nontoxic goiter, 71 a diffuse toxic goiter and 77 a nodular goiter. Hung,[15] from the Children's Hospital of Washington, in the period 1965 through 1971 saw 77 patients with euthyroid goiters and 68 patients with toxic goiters. The histologic diagnosis in the 77 euthyroid patients was chronic lymphocytic thyroiditis, 43; simple goiter, 28; adenomatous goiter, 4; and hyperplasia of the thyroid, 2.

AGE AND SEX.—Hyperthyroidism may occur at any age in childhood but is increasingly common as adolescence approaches (Fig. 34–4). Congenital hyperthyroidism occurs, presenting a fairly typical picture with exophthalmos, irritability, failure to gain, tachycardia and even heart failure.[10] The usual tests for thyroid hyperfunction are diagnostic, and LATS, secreted by the mother, may be found in the baby's serum. The mothers usually, but not always, are hyperthyroid, the condition is self-limited and may be mild enough to clear up in 2 or 3 months without treatment. The usual antithyroid drugs are used in severe instances.[1, 10, 11, 23, 24] Hyperthyroidism may have its onset in infancy or very early in childhood.[17, 18] About 10% of all reported cases in children occurred between birth and age 5 years, and about two-thirds of all cases in childhood are seen between the ages of 10 and 15.[19] There were only 8 male children among Bram's 128 patients. Other series have reported 2 males out of 50 patients, 36 males out of 253 children.[12, 29]

PATHOLOGY.—The acini show increasing height of the follicle cells with proliferation and hypertrophy of cells leading to an undulating infolding of the epithelium (Fig. 34–5).

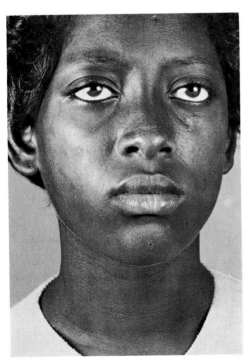

Fig. 34–4.—Hyperthyroidism in a child treated with a thyroid blocking agent. This girl, 14, was first seen with complaint of a mass in the neck, "popping eyes" and sleeplessness for 1 month. The thyroid was symmetrically enlarged. There was mild tremor of the hands. Blood pressure was 125/60, pulse rate 120; PBI was elevated to 13.6 μg/100 ml and ^{131}I uptake to 98% in 3 hours. Given perchlorate, 0.5 gm t.i.d., she became euthyroid in 3 months. Therapy was continued for 24 months, then stopped. She remained euthyroid thereafter. There still is moderate exophthalmos and slight thyroid enlargement. (Courtesy of Dr. R. M. Blizzard, Baltimore.)

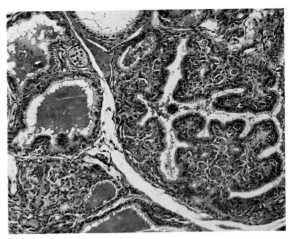

Fig. 34–5.—Hyperthyroidism in a child treated by operation. An 11-year-old boy had a chief complaint of "nervousness" for 3 years. Enlarged thyroid was noted 9 months before admission. BMR was +43 and cholesterol content 155 mg/100 ml. He was given thiouracil for 6 weeks, then Lugol's solution for 2 weeks, followed by subtotal thyroidectomy. He was discharged on the fifth postoperative day. Despite the thiouracil-iodide therapy, the thyroid structure well illustrates the microscopic picture of hyperthyroidism. The follicles are lined with columnar cells and there is papillary infolding of follicular walls. The colloid shows a lacy lining and vacuolization at the junction with follicular cells.

In exophthalmic goiter, the follicular colloid, which normally stains deeply, becomes lighter and vacuolated near the periphery or becomes so conspicuously reduced in quantity that it appears frothy. The proliferation and hypertrophy of the follicular cells lead to striking enlargement of the whole gland. A marked increase of vascularity contributes to the gland's increasing size. Lymphocytes are scattered throughout the thyroid parenchyma and germinal centers may be observed. In some areas of the gland there may be such a dense invasion of lymphocytes that the picture may be confused with struma lymphomatosa. Exophthalmic goiter is an illness that shows cyclic fluctuations, and therefore it is possible to see different degrees of the pathologic picture at different times during the course. Among children, lymphocytic infiltration is found in about 60% of the glands removed.[12] Nodular toxic goiter in a child has been reported in a single instance.[22]

CLINICAL PICTURE.—No more is known of the etiology of hyperthyroidism in children than of that in adults, but notable is the epidemiologic difference, hyperthyroidism in children apparently being found much more commonly in the United States than in Britain and other European countries. The phenomenon of thyrotoxicosis coming on acutely, after severe stress, is common enough in adults, but possibly more common in children. Saxena and his colleagues[27] reported such a close association in one-third of their patients. Six children, for instance, showed evidence of thyrotoxicosis within a few weeks of an automobile accident. Bauer,[4] analyzing 20 instances of hyperthyroidism in children treated at the Children's Hospital, Detroit, found a trigger mechanism in half the cases, varying from acute febrile illness to physical or mental trauma. In familial hyperthyroidism, some cases have their onset in childhood, and even in the neonatal period.[14, 32]

The signs and symptoms of hyperthyroidism in children are those seen in adults but with a varying frequency of some of the manifestations. The most common complaint relates to behavioral disturbances. The child is described as nervous, hyperactive, fidgety, fatigable, irritable, emotionally disturbed, doing badly in school. Appetite is increased. The increase of the size of the thyroid is visible to the parents in at least half the cases. At times, focus on the prominent behavior abnormalities leads to a diagnosis of neurosis or behavioral disorder, and the constant movements occasionally have led to the mistaken diagnosis of chorea. Upward of three-quarters of the children have exophthalmos. A peculiar stare is characteristic and disappears as the hyperthyroidism is controlled, whereas the exophthalmos takes longer to disappear and may persist. Tachycardia and elevated systolic blood pressure are almost invariable. The gland is soft and diffusely enlarged. A bruit over the thyroid commonly is audible. Sweating, weight loss and tremor are seen in about a third of the patients. Actual cardiac failure is uncommon.

DIAGNOSIS. – Occult hyperthyroidism is not a problem in children, and the diagnosis of hyperthyroidism can be made clinically in almost all instances. There have been rapid and sweeping changes in the laboratory diagnosis of thyroid function over the past few years[8a] and the techniques continue to change. The serum T_4 (Murphy-Pattee) or T_4(D) serum T_4 (RIA), serum T_3 and the T_3 resin uptake (RT_3U) are the most commonly utilized. The uptake of ^{131}I finds special uses – infrequently in children, the serum thyroxine-binding globulin (TGB), which affects T_4 and T_3 concentrations, may require measurement in special circumstances. The values of all of these vary from the neonatal period to adult life and, to some degree, from laboratory to laboratory.

TREATMENT. – Thyroidectomy and the administration of thyroid blocking agents are both used at present in the treatment of juvenile hyperthyroidism. Radioactive iodine therapy is too hazardous for use in children, apart from the analogy with thyroid cancer developing after external radiation.[6-8] Sheline, Lindsay and Bell[28] reported the development of adenomas in 2 of 5 children under age 10 who were treated with radioactive iodine. One of these adenomas was classed as a low-grade carcinoma. Several reports have appeared of carcinoma of the thyroid in patients whose hyperthyroidism had been treated some years earlier with ^{131}I.[16] Nevertheless, Saxena and Chapman[26] treated 26 patients under 20 years of age (14 and 15 years) with radioiodine, 100 $\mu g/gm$ of estimated thyroid tissue: 20 had good control of thyrotoxicosis, 2 had poor control and 4 had recurrence. There were 4 instances of permanent hypothyroidism, and in 1 child nodules developed in the gland. In a cautious plea for continued use of ^{131}I therapy, they cite the advantages of simplicity, economy and minimal trauma to the child. By 1970, the group from the Massachusetts General Hospital[9] reported 30 patients treated with radioiodine from 1941 to 1968. In 177 collected cases from the literature, they were aware of 2 cases of cancer reported in patients treated in childhood with radioiodine for thyrotoxicosis. Remission of hyperthyroidism was obtained with a single dose in 25 patients, permanent hypothyroidism developed in 8 patients (26%), recurrence of thyrotoxicosis occurred in a single case 17 years after treatment. Thompson *et al.*[30a] at The University of Michigan, from 1969 to 1976 treated 30 children with ^{131}I, all for special reasons – other severe systemic disease, 5; failure of antithyroid drugs or severe reaction to them, 10; refusal of thyroidectomy, 3; recurrence of thyrotoxicosis in 3 after subtotal thyroidectomy (2 of them operated on "elsewhere"); and after antithyroid therapy, 9. Hypothyroidism had developed in 74% of their patients, and they

believe that "the development of hypothyroidism should be anticipated in virtually all children who receive sufficient ^{131}I to relieve thyrotoxicosis."

The thyroid blocking agents such as propylthiouracil and methimazole can induce a remission but must be taken over a long period to establish permanent remission. The Johns Hopkins group[15a, 31] reported 33 children treated with thyroid blocking agents. Five failed to respond and ultimately came to operation. Nine still were under therapy at the time of the report. Relapses occurred in 7 (21%) and drug reactions in 4 (17%). Nineteen of the children had achieved what appeared to be a permanent remission of their hyperthyroidism and the drug therapy had been discontinued. The average period required to obtain this remission was 28 months. In Bauer's[4] series of 20 patients treated with propylthiouracil or methimazole, 7 had complete or almost complete remission with treatment durations of 3 years, 3¾ years, 6 months, 3½ years, 2⅔ years and 5½ years. Two were operated on primarily and 2 because of drug treatment failure. The others received other drugs with varying effect. The 4 patients operated on had a satisfactory remission and had no relapse after a substantial follow-up; the only complication was mild hypothyroidism in 1. Saxena, Crawford and Talbot,[27] reviewing the reported series of hyperthyroidism in children treated primarily with thiouracils, found a 50% remission rate and a 26% resort to operation. The duration of treatment required was not analyzed, but the individual reports show this to be measured more often in years than in months. In adults, only about half the patients under treatment with thyroid blocking agents obtain permanent remission from hyperthyroidism, and 2–3% of them will develop skin reactions of significant degree.

The Ann Arbor report[30a] includes a total of 71 children treated with propylthiouracil or methimazole. In 4 of the 71, thyrotoxicosis could not be controlled; in 6 of the 71, toxic and allergic symptoms occurred after control was achieved. Their bias had been to use antithyroid drugs only as a preparation for operation, but long-term treatment was undertaken in 20 children in the hope of avoiding operation. All came to operation eventually, 7 for recurrence of thyrotoxicosis, 3 for persistent large goiter, 3 for failure to maintain drug schedule, 4 for emotional or personality problems, 1 for a palpable "cold nodule," 1 for uncontrolled atrial fibrillation and 1 for repeated intrathyroid hemorrhage. This dismal experience reflects the general dissatisfaction with the cure rate and the problems of drug therapy in childhood thyrotoxicosis.

Excision of a large portion of the gland, bilateral subtotal lobectomy, offers the advantage of prompt solution of the patient's problem. In a substantial number of children it is difficult and at times impossible to maintain constant medical supervision for 2, 3 or more years. There is an ever-present risk of discontinuance of drug therapy, with relapse into hyperthyroidism. Proper operative therapy of hyperthyroidism offers a remarkably low incidence of complications. Adequate control of hyperthyroidism in children requires removal of more of the gland than in the adult.

Altman[2] proposes total thyroidectomy, in order to avoid the incidence of recurrence. Of his patients, he had 1 with transient hypocalcemia and 1 who required a temporary tracheostomy. The operative risks seem to us unwarranted, apart from the fact that all the patients require lifelong replacement therapy.

In 95 children with hyperthyroidism treated by subtotal thyroidectomy at the Mayo Clinic between 1934 and 1959 there were no operative deaths and no laryngeal nerve injuries.[12] Permanent hypoparathyroidism developed in 1 patient. Of the 70 patients of Saxena, Crawford and Talbot,[27] 52 underwent subtotal thyroidectomy after appropriate preoperative preparation with blocking agents. In 5 patients (10%), hypoparathyroidism did develop. One child with coincident rheumatic heart disease and severe uncontrolled hyperthyroidism operated on in 1947 in an emergency, died 2 days after operation. There were no instances of recurrent laryngeal palsy, thyroid crisis or malignant exophthalmos. Postoperatively in this series, 35% of the 52 children operated on were hypothyroid, although, with the increase in length of follow-up, the incidence of hypothyroidism decreased. The reverse is true with ^{131}I: the longer the follow-up the higher the incidence of hypothyroidism.

Tank, Bacon and Lowrey,[30] from The University of Michigan, report 64 infants and children seen from 1945 to 1969, of whom they operated on 45. The series included 2 temporary postoperative tracheostomies, 2 permanent but asymptomatic cord paralyses and 2 instances of mild hypoparathyroidism under drug control. This abundance of complications is not explained and is not justifiable. Many surgeons have commented that the decreasing numbers of thyroidectomies performed today limit the training and experience of surgeons, and it may be that thyroidectomy will once more be done by "specialists."[20]

A more recent report[30a] from the same institution for the following 8 years, 1969–1976, lists 41 more children treated operatively at ages of 2–18 years (7 were 10 years of age or less). Thirty-four had bilateral subtotal thyroidectomy, 1 had a total lobectomy on one side and subtotal on the other and 6 had total thyroidectomies. There were no deaths, no recurrent laryngeal nerve injuries, 2 temporary hypocalcemias and 1 recurrence of hyperthyroidism. In the total Ann Arbor experience of 85 children with thyroidectomy in 30 years, only 2 developed recurrent thyrotoxicosis. Hypothyroidism, if it developed, was found in the first year after operation. A more intense evaluation of postoperative hypothyroidism yielded a figure now of 60% as opposed to the 5% of the previous report.[30]

Reports now are appearing of children treated for hyperthyroidism with propranolol.[9, 14, 21] It has been used increasingly in the preoperative treatment of adults.

The Ann Arbor group, who favor subtotal thyroidectomy for thyrotoxicosis in children, now use propranolol along with antithyroid drugs in the preparation for thyroidectomy.

Because of the prolonged treatment necessary to control hyperthyroidism nonoperatively in children, with blocking agents, because of the high relapse and failure rate, because of the unreliability and difficulty of continuous treatment in children, because of the incidence of drug reactions, and because we think that prolonged medical treatment and observation are at least as much of a strain on a child as a brief period of preparation and definitive operation, we continue to favor operative treatment of hyperthyroidism in children. The high incidence of hypoparathyroidism and hypothyroidism after operation in some series is unacceptable and we believe preventable, although possibly at the cost of an occasional recurrence of hyperthyroidism. Ultimately, a nonoperative procedure will prevail, superior to current drugs and operation, but such therapy appears not to be available today.

REFERENCES

1. Adams, D. D., Lord, J. M., and Stevely, H. A. A.: Congenital thyrotoxicosis, Lancet 2:497, 1964.
2. Altman, R. P.: Total thyroidectomy for the treatment of Graves' disease in children, J. Pediatr. Surg. 8:2, 1973.
3. Atkinson, F. R. B.: Exophthalmic goiter in children, Br. J. Child. Dis. 35:165, 1938.
4. Bauer, A. R.: Etiology of juvenile hyperthyroidism, Henry Ford Hosp. Med. Bull., September, 1961.
5. Bram, I.: Exophthalmic goiter in children: Comments based on 128 cases in patients 12 and under, Arch. Pediatr. 54:419, 1937.
6. Clark, D. E.: Association of irradiation with cancer of the thyroid in children and adolescents, JAMA 159:1007, 1955.
7. Doniach, I.: Experimental induction of tumors of the thyroid by radiation, Br. Med. Bull. 14:181, 1958.
8. Duffy, B. J., and Fitzgerald, P. J.: Thyroid cancer in childhood and adolescence: Report on 28 cases, Cancer 3:1018, 1950.
8a. Fisher, D. A.: Advances in the laboratory diagnosis of thyroid disease. Parts I–II, J. Pediatr. 82:1, and 82:187, 1973.
9. Galaburda, M., Rosman, N. P., and Haddow, J. E.: Thyroid storm in an 11-year-old boy managed by propranolol, Pediatrics 53:6, 1974.
10. Gerald, B.: Cardiac failure in infancy secondary to thyrotoxicosis, Radiology 91:50, 1968.
11. Hayles, A. B., et al.: Exophthalmic goiter in children, J. Clin. Endocrinol. 19:138, 1959.
12. Hays, G. C.: Neonatal thyrotoxicosis. Elevated long-acting thyroid stimulator (LATS) in mother and infant, Calif. Med. 110:41, 1969.
13. Henoch, E., and Romberg, M. H.: Cited by Atkinson.[3]
14. Hollingsworth, D. R., Mabry, C. C., and Eckerd, J. M.: Hereditary aspects of Graves' disease in infancy and childhood, J. Pediatr. 81:446, 1972.
15. Hung, W., Chandra, R., August, G. P., and Altman, P. R.: Clinical, laboratory, and histologic observations in euthyroid children and adolescents with goiters, J. Pediatr. 82:10, 1973.
15a. Hung, W., Wilkins, L., and Blizzard, R.: Medical therapy of thyrotoxicosis in children, Pediatrics 30:17, 1962.
16. Karlan, M. S., Pollock, W. F., and Snyder, W. H., Jr.: Carcinoma of the thyroid following treatment of hyperthyroidism with radioactive iodine, (Calif. Med.) 101:196, 1964.
17. Leszynsky, H. E.: Hyperthyroidism in a 3-month-old baby, Pediatrics 47:1069, 1971.
18. Levitsky, L. L., Trias, E., and Grossman, M. S.: Spontaneous thyrotoxicosis in infancy. Report of a case, Pediatrics 46:627, 1970.
19. McClintock, J. C., Frawley, T. F., and Holden, J. P.: Hyperthyroidism in children: Observations in 50 treated cases including an evaluation of endocrine factors, J. Clin. Endocrinol. 16:62, 1956.
20. Parfitt, A. M.: The incidence of hypoparathyroid tetany after thyroid operations. Relationship to age, extent of resection and surgical experience, Med. J. Aust. 1:1103, 1971.
21. Perelman, R., de Gennes, J. L., Devaux, J. P., Pouliot, Ph., and Marie, J.: Maladie de Basedow avec crise thyrotoxique aiguë chez une fillette de 25 mois, Ann. Pediatr. 18:735, 1971.
22. Rosenbloom, A. L., and Pierson, K. K.: Nodular toxic goiter (Plummer's disease) in a child, J. Pediatr. 84:104, 1974.
23. Samuel, S., Gilman, S., Maurer, H. S., and Rosenthal, I. M.: Hyperthyroidism in an infant with McCune-Albright syndrome: Report of a case with myeloid metaplasia, J. Pediatr. 80:275, 1972.
24. Samuel, S., Phildes, R. S., Lewison, M., and Rosenthal, I. M.: Neonatal hyperthyroidism in an infant born of a euthyroid mother, Am. J. Dis. Child. 121:440, 1971.
25. Sanfelippo, P. M., Beahrs, O. H., and Hayles, A. B.: Indications for thyroidectomy in the pediatric patient, Am. J. Surg. 122:472, 1971.
26. Saxena, K. M., and Chapman, E. M.: Proc. 72d Meet., Am. Pediatr. Soc., 1962, abstr. 82.
27. Saxena, K. M., Crawford, J. D., and Talbot, N. B.: Childhood thyrotoxicosis: A long-term perspective, Br. Med. J. 2:1153, 1964.
28. Sheline, G. E., Lindsay, S., and Bell, H. G.: Occurrence of thyroid nodules in children following I^{131} therapy for hyperthyroidism, J. Clin. Endocrinol. 19:127, 1959.
29. Skelton, M. O., and Gans, B.: Congenital thyrotoxicosis, hepatosplenomegaly and jaundice in 2 infants of exophthalmic mothers, Arch. Dis. Child. 30:460, 1955.
30. Tank, E. S., Bacon, G. E., and Lowrey, G. H.: Surgical management of thyrotoxicosis in children, J. Pediatr. Surg. 4:1, 1969.
30a. Thompson, N. W., Dunn, E. L., Freitas, J. E., Sisson, J. C., Coran, A. G., and Nishiyama, R. H.: The surgical treatment of thyrotoxicosis in children and adolescents, J. Pediatr. Surg. 12:6, 1977.

31. Wilkins, L.: *The Diagnosis and Treatment of Endocrine Disorders in Childhood and Adolescence* (3d ed.; Springfield, Ill.: Charles C Thomas, Publisher, 1965).
32. Wilroy, R. S., and Etteldorf, J. N.: Familial hyperthyroidism, including two siblings with neonatal Graves' disease, J. Pediatr. 78:625, 1971.

4. Thyroiditis

Specific thyroiditis is an inflammatory lesion due to an established agent—the organisms of syphilis, tuberculosis or actinomycosis. Until recently, nonspecific thyroiditis has been a wastebasket term applied to inflammatory thyroid lesions without known cause. There is a plethora of synonyms and eponyms—nonsuppurating thyroiditis, granulomatous thyroiditis, Hashimoto's thyroiditis, Riedel's thyroiditis, de Quervain's thyroiditis, giant cell thyroiditis, pseudotuberculous thyroiditis, lymphocytic thyroiditis, struma lymphomatosa. The etiology of some of these conditions is coming to be understood and it is likely that some of these terms will disappear when an etiologic classification can be adopted. For the present, it is useful to continue to use eponyms—de Quervain's,[5] Hashimoto's[10] and Riedel's[20] thyroiditis.

Specific Thyroiditis

Acute bacterial infections of the thyroid gland, uncommon even prior to the days of antibiotics, today are exceedingly rare. Womack[30] pointed out that the thyroid is quite resistant to infection. Injections of pure cultures of staphylococci and streptococci into the superior thyroid artery of dogs rarely induced infection or abscess. When these infections do occur clinically, they appear to be chiefly on the basis of hematogenous seeding of the thyroid following acute upper respiratory infections or, accompanying septicemia, from a focus elsewhere in the body. The most common infecting organism is the staphylococcus, but infections due to *Escherichia coli* and the typhoid bacillus *(Salmonella typhosa)* have also been reported.[12]

The clinical picture in acute infective thyroiditis often is dramatic, with sudden onset of severe pain in the neck, chills, nausea and headache. The rapid swelling of the gland inside its inelastic capsule tends to induce compression of the trachea, with dyspnea and stridor. The gland is extremely tender and stony hard. Pain that radiates to the ear, jaw and face is an early symptom and is almost pathognomonic, occurring in paroxysms and initiated by deglutition. The patient often holds his head acutely flexed. There may be redness of the skin over the area of the gland. The systemic reaction to the infection may be marked to the point of prostration. Necrosis of one or both lobes of the gland, from the increasing pressure within the capsule, has been reported. Suppuration, if undrained, may lead to rupture externally or into the trachea or mediastinum. Symptoms of the milder forms of bacterial thyroiditis and of de Quervain's thyroiditis bear a close resemblance and may be differentiated only by culture and biopsy.

Treatment includes bed rest, hot wet packs to the neck and antibiotics appropriate to the infecting organism. Suppuration is treated by incision.

Nonspecific Thyroiditis

DE QUERVAIN'S THYROIDITIS.—This form of thyroiditis is known also as subacute nonsuppurative thyroiditis, giant cell thyroiditis, granulomatous thyroiditis, acute nonspecific thyroiditis and pseudotuberculous thyroiditis.

Incidence.—The incidence of de Quervain's thyroiditis is difficult to establish. Of 7263 patients undergoing thyroidectomy at the University of California Hospital in a 32-year period, 23 patients had this form of thyroiditis.[16] On the other hand, when a clinical rather than pathologic diagnosis is considered, it appears that the disease is thought to be more frequent than the operative figures suggest. The Hitchcock Clinic in New Hampshire reported seeing 2 or 3 patients with de Quervain's thyroiditis each year.[27] The fact is that in the milder forms of this disease symptoms may be mistaken for pharyngitis[7] and may regress spontaneously. Such patients are not usually hospitalized, and, in the absence of biopsy, definitive diagnosis has been difficult to establish in the past. The disease appears to be most common in the middle years of life, although instances are noted in children from time to time. Females are much more often afflicted than males.

Etiology.—Despite the microscopic evidence of inflammation and the clinical features of inflammation in patients with de Quervain's thyroiditis, culture of thyroid tissue in these patients has revealed no bacterial organisms. A number of observers have suggested that the disease is of viral etiology, citing the fact that often a number of cases may be recognized within a short span of time in a specific area. Eylan and co-workers[6] suggested that de Quervain's thyroiditis is caused by the mumps virus. They observed a large number of cases of subacute thyroiditis in Israel in the course of an epidemic of mumps. Ten of 11 patients examined (only 1 child) had positive complement fixation tests against mumps virus, compared with only 4 of 52 individuals selected at random from the general population. Culture of biopsies of the thyroid gland of 2 of these patients produced a virus that caused encephalitis in hamsters and hemagglutination that was prevented by serum from patients who had had mumps. Hung[14] described a 9-year-old boy with unequivocal mumps and simultaneously a diffusely enlarged, firm and tender thyroid gland. Three years later, the thyroid gland was not palpable, he was undergrown, clinically hypothyroid and laboratory tests substantiated the hypothyroidism.

Pathology.—The thyroid gland usually is not much enlarged but may be adherent to adjacent structures, including the trachea and cervical muscles. The muscles and adhering connective tissues often are edematous. Adherence to adjacent structures often is thought of as chiefly characterizing Riedel's thyroiditis but may occur with de Quervain's thyroiditis as well. In the main, the gland is smooth but occasionally may show bosselations. Various degrees of fibrous replacement of thyroid parenchyma, often with a fibrous trabeculation occur, interlacing in a red vascular parenchyma. Some segments of parenchyma are circumscribed and appear as small colloid-containing nodules generally measuring less than 1 cm in diameter.

Clinical features.—In almost every instance, the patient complains of a sore throat or occasionally of a painful lump in the throat of several days' to several weeks' duration. As a rule, onset of pain is sudden and may be accompanied by chills and fever. At times restricted to one lobe, the pain may migrate from one side of the gland to the other. Pain on swallowing often is referred to the ears. One feels a swollen, tense and tender thyroid gland. Often the diagnosis may be confused with pharyngitis. Some patients present the symptoms of hyperthyroidism. In the early phases of the disease, the PBI level may be considerably elevated, a finding compatible with the symptoms of hyperthyroidism. At the same time, uptake of radioactive iodine by the thyroid will be markedly depressed. This paradox—increased level of thyroid hormone in the serum combined with evidence of depressed function of the thyroid gland—is said to be diagnostic of this form of thyroiditis. Although the PBI level is high, the BEI level has been reported to be low, suggesting that the injured thyroid is producing and spilling into the circulation intermediary products of thyroid hormone metabolism, with depression of thyroxine production.[3, 25, 26]

Treatment and prognosis.—The disease is self-limiting and spontaneous resolution ultimately takes place, although symptoms may persist for several weeks or months. When pain is particularly acute, ACTH and cortisone consistently have led to remission of symptoms. When cortisone is discontinued, the symptoms often recur, so that remission on therapy represents suppression of symptoms. In most instances, the thyroid recovers sufficient function to maintain the patient in a euthyroid state. Most cases of hypothyroidism following de Quervain's thyroiditis have occurred in patients who had subtotal thyroidectomy. Biopsy of the isthmus of the gland may be required to establish the diagnosis. Thyroidectomy is not indicated. In rare instances, the fibrosis and scarring accompanying the disease produce dysphagia, or even dyspnea, which may require subsequent operative therapy.

HASHIMOTO'S THYROIDITIS.—Synonyms of Hashimoto's thyroiditis are struma lymphomatosa, lymphadenoid goiter and lymphocytic thyroiditis (Fig. 34–6).

Incidence.—This is the most common form of thyroiditis in children.[3, 4, 9, 11] In reported series of patients, mostly adults, undergoing thyroidectomy, from 1% to 7% have been operated on for Hashimoto's disease. Almost exclusively a disease of females, the usual age incidence in adults is in the fourth and fifth decades. There are substantial differences between juvenile lymphocytic thyroiditis and adult Hashimoto's disease. The number of cases discovered in children has increased greatly in recent years. The report

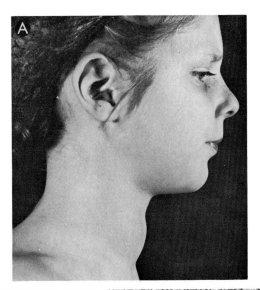

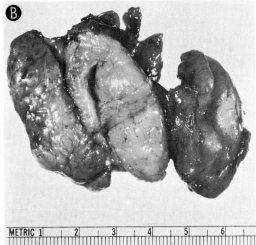

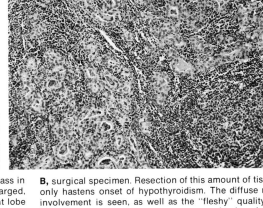

Fig. 34–6.—Hashimoto's thyroiditis. **A,** an 11-year-old girl with a mass in the neck for a year was otherwise asymptomatic. The thyroid was enlarged, measuring 11.5×4.5 cm, and soft and fleshy in consistency. The right lobe was somewhat larger than the left. Blood serum was positive for thyroid antibodies on the guinea pig cutaneous sensitivity test. PBI was elevated and BEI depressed. The 24-hour ^{131}I uptake was low normal at 17%. [131]I scintogram showed equal activity in the two lobes. Clinical diagnosis was Hashimoto's thyroiditis, and operation was elected to confirm the diagnosis. **B,** surgical specimen. Resection of this amount of tissue is unnecessary and only hastens onset of hypothyroidism. The diffuse nature of the glandular involvement is seen, as well as the "fleshy" quality of tissue. Excision of these lesions is temptingly easy because of reduced vascularity and an easily developed plane of dissection. **C,** histologic section showing marked infiltration by lymphocytes. A germinal center is present in the lower portion of the section. Follicles are small. Follicle epithelium is tall and hyperplastic, a feature characteristic of Hashimoto's disease in young patients.

from the Mayo Clinic[8] on the incidence of Hashimoto's thyroiditis found at operation suggests, as others have, that the increase was particularly significant among children. Hung[15] in 7 years found 43 cases in his 77 children with nontoxic goiters. In the same period, Saxena's group[23] saw 70 cases, 45% of all children's goiters.

Etiology.—The finding of circulating antibodies (now at least three) to thyroglobulins by Roitt and Doniach[21] and Witebsky and his colleagues[29] has led to the suggestion that Hashimoto's thyroiditis is due to an autoimmune reaction. Although Witebsky produced the lesions of Hashimoto's disease in the thyroid of rabbits sensitized to a saline extract of rabbit thyroid, passive transfer to monkeys and dogs of antibody-containing serum has not produced thyroid changes in these animals.[21] It is not established that autoimmunity is the cause of thyroid injury rather than the response to it. Nevertheless, the circulating antibodies are found so constantly that the serologic tests for them form an important part of the screening tests for the diagnosis, which ultimately depends on the histologic examination.

Pathology.—The gland is symmetrically enlarged, often to a considerable size. The gland is rubbery, firm or hard, the cut surface lobular, opaque pale pink. The microscopic appearance of the gland varies somewhat, depending on the stage of the disease. Lymphocytic infiltration, often with the development of intrafollicular germinal centers, is a constant finding.[2, 31] Follicles usually are small and colloid is scanty in amount and frequently stains more deeply than usual.[13] Gribetz *et al.*[9] described in 6 patients a variant of this picture, which occurs in younger patients, especially preadolescent and adolescent girls. In the glands of these patients there is hypertrophy of the epithelial cells in addition to the other changes of Hashimoto's thyroiditis. The same changes were observed by Clayton and Johnson[4] in 12 children with Hashimoto's thyroiditis.

Clinical features.—The first symptom noted by the patient always is a swelling of the gland, although occasionally a mild dysphagia calls attention to the condition. There is no history of infection and the gland is not tender. The gland is diffusely and symmetrically enlarged, firm or, in the later stages, hard enough to suggest the woody feel usually associated with Riedel's thyroiditis.

Laboratory data.—The diagnosis is most certainly made by needle or open biopsy of the enlarged gland. The ordinary tests of thyroid function may be suggestive particularly if there is a wide $PBI-T_4$ difference.[22] In 31 of 35 patients from the Children's Hospital of Pittsburgh,[17] the difference was ≥ 2.0 $\mu g\%$. RAI uptake studies have yielded inconsistent results both in uptake and in discharge after perchlorate administration. Tests for antithyroglobin antibody are reported by some to be consistently reliable and by others, less so. The understanding of the significance of the antibodies is further confused by their frequent occurrence in patients with hyperthyroidism.[17]

Treatment and prognosis.—The high frequency of thyroid disease in the families of children with chronic lymphocytic thyroiditis, together with the high incidence in these families of apparently well individuals with significant titers of thyroid antibodies, suggests a genetic background.[19] Winter, Eberlein and Bongiovanni,[28] in an interesting study comparing 18 children with acquired hypothyroidism and 33 euthyroid children with chronic lymphocytic thyroiditis (seen in 7 years), found evidence to suggest that both syndromes were variants of the same disease, based largely on the similar $PBI-BEI$ discrepancy. They consider chronic lymphocytic thyroiditis probably the most common cause of acquired hypothyroidism in childhood.

The majority of patients with Hashimoto's thyroiditis eventually become hypothyroid. Subtotal thyroidectomy only serves to hasten the appearance of the hypothyroid state.[2] The treatment of choice is administration of desiccated thyroid, continued indefinitely, presumably for life. A number of investigators have reported that under this therapy, the thyroid gland returns to normal or near-normal size.[1, 18] Operative intervention is designed to obtain thyroid tissue to confirm the diagnosis, to divide the isthmus as prophylaxis against tracheal compression and to perform subtotal thyroidectomy in the occasional patient whose gland is so large and fibrous that its size is not reduced by desiccated thyroid therapy and in whom symptoms or the cosmetic deformity warrant operation. Skillern *et al.*[24] advocate the use of needle biopsy to confirm the diagnosis.

RIEDEL'S THYROIDITIS (INVASIVE FIBROSING THYROIDITIS, FIBROUS THYROIDITIS, EISENHART STRUMA).—Riedel's thyroiditis is rare in children. The general incidence is said to be about 1 for every 2000 thyroidectomies performed. The disease is encountered commonly in the fourth and fifth decades, Wilkins[27a] found only 5 cases described in children. The thyroid is gradually replaced by extensive fibrosis that involves the thyroid and extends to the surrounding structures, the muscles, trachea and carotid sheath. Grossly, the thyroid appears to be white, avascular and woody, and the ribbon muscles may be involved. The parenchyma is replaced by scar tissue in which giant cells are characteristic.

The chief complaint of these patients is of enlargement of the thyroid gland over a period of 3 months to a year without systemic symptoms or pain.

De Quervain's and Hashimoto's strumas are also associated with some fibrosis and firmness but lack the extreme fibrosis of Riedel's struma. Some authors have emphasized the frequency of dysphagia and dyspnea, presumably due to the heavy fibrous envelopment of the trachea and esophagus, but Woolner *et al.*,[31] who reported the largest series on record (20 cases, none in children), found that although these symptoms do occur from time to time, their frequency is perhaps exaggerated. The entire gland may be involved in about a third of the cases, but in many instances only one lobe or a portion of a lobe is fibrosed.

In patients whose entire gland has been replaced by fibrous tissue, hypothyroidism ensues. But hypothyroidism is not an inevitable sequel of this disease, and many patients may continue to be euthyroid for many years after establishment of the diagnosis. The consistency of the gland in these patients always suggests the possibility of carcinoma. The diagnosis can be made, and carcinoma excluded, only by biopsy.

The present treatment of choice is needle aspiration biopsy or resection of the isthmus of the gland, which provides tissue on which to base the diagnosis and releases the trachea from actual or potential encirclement by the fibrotic thyroid, followed by thyroid replacement therapy.

REFERENCES

1. Astwood, E. B., Cassidy, C. E., and Aurbach, G. D.: Treatment of goiter and thyroid nodules with thyroid, JAMA 174:459, 1960.
2. Blake, K. W., and Sturgeon, C. T.: Struma lymphomatosa, Surg. Gynecol. Obstet. 97:312, 1953.
3. Brown, H., and McGarity, W. C.: Chronic thyroiditis in childhood, JAMA 171:1182, 1959.
4. Clayton, G. W., and Johnson, C. M.: Struma lymphomatosa in children, J. Pediatr. 57:410, 1960.
5. De Quervain, F.: Die akute nichteitrige thyreoiditis, Mitt. Grenzgeb. Med. Chir., supp. 2, p. 1, 1904.
6. Eylan, E., Zumicky, R., and Sheba, C.: Mumps virus and subacute thyroiditis, Lancet 1:1063, 1957.
7. Frid, G., and Wijnbladh, H.: Subacute thyroiditis, struma lym-

phomatosa (Hashimoto's disease) and chronic fibrous invasive goiter (Riedel's disease): A clinical study based on 83 cases, Acta Chir. Scand. 112:170, 1957.

8. Furszyfer, J., Kurland, L. T., Woolner, L. B., Elveback, L. R., and McConahey, W. M.: Hashimoto's thyroiditis in Olmsted County, Minnesota, 1935 through 1967, Mayo Clin. Proc. 45: 586, 1970.

9. Gribetz, D., Talbot, N. B., and Crawford, J. D.: Goiter due to lymphocytic thyroiditis (Hashimoto's struma): Its occurrence in preadolescent and adolescent girls, N. Engl. J. Med. 250:555, 1954.

10. Hashimoto, H.: Zur Kenntniss der lymphomatosen Veränderung der Schildruse (Struma lymphomatosa), Arch. Klin. Chir. 97:219, 1912.

11. Hayles, A. B., et al.: Nodular lesions of the thyroid gland in children, J. Clin. Endocrinol. 16:1580, 1957.

12. Hazard, J. B.: Thyroiditis, Am. J. Clin. Pathol. 25:289, and 25:399, 1955.

13. Heptinstall, R. H., and Eastcott, H. H. G.: Hashimoto's disease, struma lymphomatosa, Br. J. Surg. 41:471, 1954.

14. Hung, W.: Mumps thyroiditis and hypothyroidism, J. Pediatr. 74:611, 1969.

15. Hung, W., Chandra, R., August, G. P., and Altman, P. R.: Clinical, laboratory, and histologic observations in euthyroid children and adolescents with goiters, J. Pediatr. 82:10, 1973.

16. Lindsay, S., and Dailey, M. E.: Granulomatous or giant cell thyroiditis, Surg. Gynecol. Obstet. 98:197, 1954.

17. Loeb, P. B., Drash, A. L., and Kenny, F. M.: Prevalence of low-titer and "negative" antithyroglobulin antibodies in biopsy-proved juvenile Hashimoto's thyroiditis, J. Pediatr. 82:17, 1973.

18. McConahey, W. M., et al.: Effect of desiccated thyroid in lymphocytic (Hashimoto's) thyroiditis, J. Clin. Endocrinol. 19:45, 1959.

19. McConahey, W. M.: Hashimoto's thyroiditis, Med. Clin. North Am. 56:4, 1972.

20. Riedel, B. M. K. L.: Die chronische zur Bildung eisenharter Tumoren führende Entzündung der Schildruse, Verh. Dtsch. Ges. Chir. 25:101, 1896.

21. Roitt, I. M., and Doniach, D.: Human autoimmune thyroiditis: Serological studies, Lancet 2:1027, 1958.

22. Saxena, K. M., and Crawford, J. D.: Juvenile lymphocytic thyroiditis, Pediatrics 30:917, 1962.

23. Saxena, K. M., Crawford, J. D., and Talbot, N. B.: Childhood thyrotoxicosis: A long-term perspective, Br. Med. J. 2:1153, 1964.

24. Skillern, P. G., et al.: Struma lymphomatosa: Primary thyroid failure with compensatory thyroid enlargement, J. Clin. Endocrinol. 16:35, 1956.

25. Steinberg, F. U.: Subacute granulomatous thyroiditis, Ann. Intern. Med. 52:1014, 1960.

26. Towerly, B. T.: A study of idiopathic subacute thyroiditis, J. Clin. Endocrinol. 16:982, 1956.

27. Vanderlinde, R. J., and Milne, J.: Subacute thyroiditis with special emphasis on the problem of early recognition, JAMA 173: 1799, 1960.

27a. Wilkins, L.: The Diagnosis and Treatment of Endocrine Disorders in Childhood and Adolescence (3d ed.; Springfield, Ill.: Charles C Thomas, Publisher, 1965).

28. Winter, J., Eberlein, W. R., and Bongiovanni, A. M.: The relationship of juvenile hypothyroidism to chronic lymphocytic thyroiditis, J. Pediatr. 69:709, 1966.

29. Witebsky, E., et al.: Chronic thyroiditis and autoimmunization, JAMA 164:1439, 1957.

30. Womack, N. A.: Thyroiditis, Surgery 16:770, 1944.

31. Woolner, L. B., McConahey, W., and Beahrs, O. H.: Struma lymphomatosa (Hashimoto's thyroiditis) and related thyroidal disorders, J. Clin. Endocrinol. 19:53, 1959.

5. Cancer of the Thyroid

Cancer of the thyroid, once a medical curiosity in children, has been reported with increasing frequency in recent years. The body over, there are 9 sarcomas for every carcinoma reported in surveys of malignancy in childhood, but carcinoma of the thyroid probably is the most common carcinoma found in children. In the area of the head and neck in children, thyroid cancer is challenged in frequency only by cancer of the nasopharynx.

INCIDENCE, AGE AND SEX.— It is estimated that about 4000 new cases of carcinoma of the thyroid are diagnosed yearly in the United States. About 1 in every 100 of these occurs in a child. Thyroid carcinoma has been reported at every age in childhood but is most common between ages 10 and 14 years. The ratio of females to males is 3 to 1.

PREDISPOSING FACTORS.— Although the etiology of thyroid carcinoma, as of all carcinomas, remains unknown, there appear to be two predisposing factors. The first is goiter, and the evidence for it is chiefly statistical. It is known that the incidence of carcinoma of the thyroid is greater in areas of endemic goiter than in nonendemic areas.[1] Furthermore, since the introduction of iodized salt, the incidence of thyroid carcinoma has tended to decrease from previous levels in endemic areas whereas it has remained unchanged in nonendemic areas.[3]

The second predisposing factor, especially pertinent to children, is exposure of the neck to ionizing radiation during infancy and childhood. This relationship originally was suggested by Duffy and Fitzgerald[5] in 1950. They noted that 3 of 28 children with carcinoma of the thyroid had received prior radiation therapy to the neck. Subsequent studies have repeatedly confirmed this observation.[2] Crile[4] found that 11 of 18 children with thyroid carcinoma had received cervical irradiation. Hayles and co-workers[9] observed that of 59 children with thyroid carcinoma, 30 had had such irradiation. Harness et al.,[7] from Ann Arbor, found that 29 of their 58 children with thyroid carcinoma had received previous ionizing radiation to the head and neck, on the average 9.5 years earlier. All but 2 of the carcinomas were papillary, follicular or mixed; and 2 were medullary with amyloid stroma. There were involved cervical lymph nodes in 88% of the cases and pulmonary metastases in 19%. All their patients underwent total thyroidectomy and subsequently received therapeutic doses of [131]I. Operation included removal of involved nodes or chains. Pellerin et al.[13] had 18 children with cancer of the thyroid, of whom 5 had had previous irradiation 6–14 years earlier. A single child had a medullary carcinoma, with elevated calcitonin, and massive lymph node metastases. In 1951, Horn and Ravdin,[10] reporting from the University of Pennsylvania on 22 patients under age 25 with thyroid cancer, found no note of previous irradiation in the histories. Subsequent specific inquiry yielded the information that at least 50% had, in fact, received thymic irradiation in infancy.[14] Hagler et al.[6] found that of 19 children operated on for thyroid nodules (15 cancers and 4 adenomas), 18 had received therapeutic irradiation 5–17 years earlier.

Most of these children had been irradiated because of supposed thymic enlargement. Simpson and colleagues[15, 16] studied a series of 1722 children treated with x-rays for thymic enlargement from 1926 to 1951; 1400 were traced, of whom 67 were dead of all causes. Seven of these children had leukemia, 6 had thyroid cancer and 4 had developed other cancers. In addition, 9 of the traced children had thyroid adenomas. A control group of 1795 children was also traced. In this group there had been 56 deaths from all causes. None of the children had developed leukemia, none had thyroid cancer and only 1 thyroid adenoma was found. The radiation exposure of the thyroid in some of the instances was estimated to be as low as 50 R. It has been concluded that the thyroid in children is peculiarly susceptible to such x-ray exposure. Certainly, unnecessary irradiation of the necks of children should be avoided.

PATHOLOGY.— The major classifications of carcinoma of the thyroid are papillary, follicular, medullary and anaplastic. Although true papillary and true follicular tumors are seen, many tumors contain both papillary and follicular elements and sometimes are reported as follicular-papillary

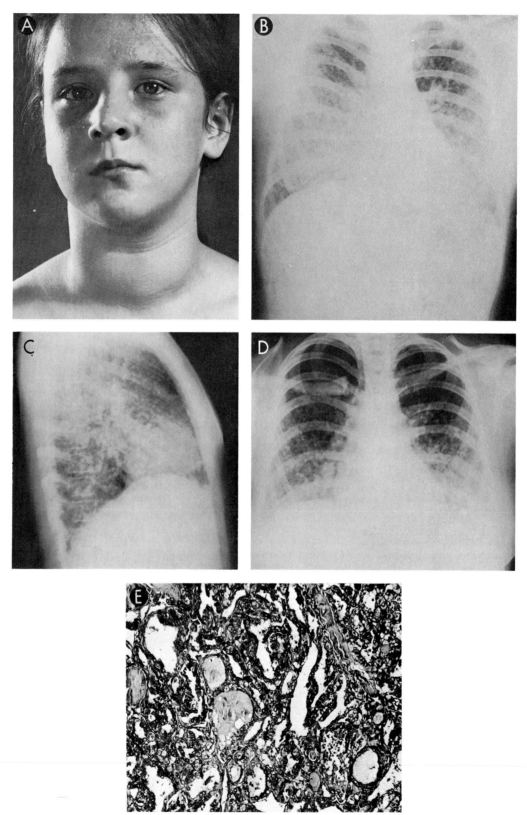

Fig. 34–7. — See legend on facing page.

or papillary-follicular, depending on the predominating type. In an extensive search for both published and unpublished cases of childhood carcinoma of the thyroid in Europe and America, Winship and Chase[19] collected 285 cases (now 800 cases[11]). Of the lesions observed, 85% were papillary or follicular, or contained both elements; 15% of the lesions seen were undifferentiated carcinoma.

CLINICAL FEATURES.—The classic clinical picture in a child with thyroid carcinoma is that of a preadolescent girl who presents with an asymptomatic nodule in one lobe of the thyroid, the existence of which has been known for months or years. Examination frequently reveals enlarged cervical nodes associated with the lesion. Not infrequently, the enlargement of the cervical nodes is the presenting complaint (see p. 354) rather than the lesion in the thyroid itself. The incidence of cervical metastases, when these patients are first seen, has been reported to be as high as 70%, somewhat higher in children than in adults. Usually the involved cervical nodes are movable, smoothly rounded, nontender and discrete. Matting or fixation is uncommon and seen only late in the course of the disease. The lesion of the thyroid gland itself is firm to rock hard and irregular. Occasionally, the gland is diffusely involved, but a mass in one or the other lobe is more characteristic. A nodule in the thyroid of a child is much more likely to be malignant than a nodule in the thyroid of an adult and calls for immediate operative diagnosis. The histories of these patients are marked by repeated delays because of disbelief that a malignancy is possible. If a nodule in the thyroid is found by ^{131}I scintigram to be of functioning tissue, it is less likely to be carcinoma, but the incidence of neoplasms in thyroid nodules in children is so high that operation still must be done. Pulmonary metastases often are present in well-appearing children and do not necessarily contraindicate resection of the primary tumor (Fig. 34–7). Tollefson,[18] from the Memorial Hospital, New York, points out that in his 376 patients with papillary carcinoma, when total thyroidectomy was performed there was an incidence of occult papillary carcinoma of the opposite thyroid lobe of 38%, but that when only a unilateral lobectomy was performed, clinical carcinoma developed in the opposite lobe in only 4.6%.

LABORATORY DATA.—These children almost always are euthyroid. Laboratory studies are of little value in the diagnosis.

TREATMENT.—Although it is agreed that excision is the most effective treatment available for these lesions, controversy prevails concerning the type of excision to be used. Operations advised have included thyroid lobectomy alone for lesions without cervical metastases, total lobectomy on the affected side and subtotal lobectomy on the unaffected side, total thyroidectomy, lobectomy plus prophylactic radical neck dissection on the ipsilateral side and total thyroidectomy plus radical neck dissection. Some have advised the resection of cervical lymph nodes along the jugular

chain on a prophylactic basis whereas others would avoid all prophylactic node operations and would treat cervical nodes when they appear. Even in this instance there is disagreement as to whether a radical neck dissection should be performed or whether only the lymph nodes in the jugular chain and in the bed of the thyroid should be resected. The extremely slow course of this disease makes proper evaluation of the various proposed operative procedures quite difficult.

It is our practice to perform thyroid lobectomy with a modified neck dissection on the side of the lesion. Resection of the sternocleidomastoid is not required, and the jugular vein is spared. Biopsy of the lesion at the time of operation, and a frozen section, may allow this procedure to be carried out in one stage. Thyroid carcinoma often is difficult to establish definitely on frozen section examination, and the dissection may have to be done at a second operation, following confirmation of the diagnosis on examination of the permanent sections. Prophylactic neck dissection is advised, since the incidence of positive nodes found in such sections is well over 50% in adults and may be even higher in children.

Sometimes at operation it is found that total excision is not feasible because of the involvement of vital structures. In such instances, a resection of the greater part of the thyroid gland will facilitate the subsequent effective use of radioactive iodine therapy. The remarkably long survival of children with papillary or mixed papillary-follicular carcinoma, even when all cancer could not be removed, suggests caution in applying operative procedures that require tracheal resection and invite laryngeal palsy or hypoparathyroidism. We have 1 patient alive more than 30 years after incomplete removal of tracheal invasion, and similar cases have been reported.[11, 17]

Follicular tumors are the most likely to take up radioactive iodine, and about 3 of every 4 such tumors will do so. Papillary tumors are much less likely to take up iodine, but about 1 of 4 can be expected to take up some iodine. The very effectiveness of ^{131}I in the case of pulmonary metastases may be the patient's undoing. If the isotope is taken up by metastases widely dispersed through the lung, destruction of the tumor may be followed by pulmonary fibrosis and progressive pulmonary insufficiency. Since a normal thyroid usually will absorb iodine more rapidly than will cancerous tissues, the normal gland first must be eradicated to avoid competition with the carcinoma for the available radioiodine. This is one of the arguments given for total lobectomy on the affected side and all but total lobectomy on the unaffected side at the original operation. However, the inevitable increase in risk of recurrent laryngeal nerve injury and of hypoparathyroidism has made us reluctant to perform near-total thyroidectomy for lesions that are clinically unilobar. There is ample evidence that histologic examination of the apparently uninvolved lobe will show foci of what appear to be papillary carcinoma. However, such lesions rarely, in subsequent years, have manifested themselves clinically as cancer.[18] Since all patients will be permanently on thyroid hormone

Fig. 34–7.—Juvenile thyroid carcinoma with pulmonary metastases and 16-year survival. **A,** the patient, age 11, had had a gradually increasing mass in the neck for 4 years and wheezing respiration on exertion and slight dysphagia for 6 months. She had a history of irradiation to the upper anterior chest at 3 weeks of age for an "enlarged thymus." **B** and **C,** chest films on admission showed extensive bilateral infiltration of lung parenchyma by miliary metastases. On November 6, 1947, most of the thyroid was excised. The carotid arteries were encased by tumor and some malignant tissue was left in these areas. She subsequently received large amounts of radioiodine to a total of 1297 mc between 1948 and 1953. **D,** chest film 2 years later shows

the considerable clearing of miliary infiltration of the lungs following ^{131}I therapy. Apical emphysema is present. The lung lesions picked up ^{131}I avidly, as demonstrated on scintigrams, proving that they were indeed metastatic. The last course of ^{131}I was in 1953. Later, severe pulmonary fibrosis developed, and she died of respiratory insufficiency in 1963. **E,** microscopic details, showing this to be a moderately undifferentiated follicular carcinoma. The tumor cells are seen to produce considerable amounts of colloid, explaining the effectiveness of ^{131}I therapy in this patient. Her course was more characteristic of papillary carcinoma than of carcinoma of this type.

therapy to decrease the TSH stimulus to the gland, total thyroidectomy imposes no special burden in this regard. If the thyroid gland is not excised, its function can be abolished by an initial large dose of [131]I. Residual malignant tissue that does not take up ^{131}I sometimes can be made to do so by the administration of TSH.[12] In those glands that cannot be resected, and will not take up radioiodine, external irradiation may offer some palliative aid.[3] In our own experience and that of others,[11a] the fate of patients treated 15 and 20 years ago suggests that postoperative irradiation for incompletely removed papillary cancers, recently unpopular, is in fact beneficial and should be used.

Undifferentiated carcinoma of the thyroid in children, as in adults, is highly malignant. The survival after diagnosis rarely is more than a year. Papillary or follicular carcinoma of the thyroid is an indolent malignancy. Patients may carry metastatic lesions in the neck for many years before metastases appear elsewhere and may continue to live for a long time with metastases in lungs or bones. The lungs are the most common distant site for metastases, and pulmonary involvement occurs at some time in about 20% of the patients. Because of the slowness of growth and development of this tumor, it is probable that at least a 20-year follow-up must be carried out before the results of treatment can be definitely established. Very few such figures are available. Hayles *et al.*[9] reported that among 9 children followed for 20 years there were 6 survivors, a survival rate of 66.7%. At the end of 30 years, only 1 child of 4 followed was surviving. Available evidence suggests that excess TSH may be a factor in the initiation and growth of thyroid carcinoma. In addition to their primary treatment, all patients with thyroid cancer should receive enough oral thyroid therapy daily to suppress the output of TSH by the pituitary.

REFERENCES

1. Buxton, R. W.: Thyroid disease in childhood, South. Med. J. 50:1175, 1957.
2. Clark, D. E.: Association of irradiation with cancer of the thyroid in children and adolescents, JAMA 159:1007, 1955.
3. Clements, F. W., *et al.*: *Endemic Goiter* (Geneva: World Health Organization, 1960).
4. Crile, G., Jr.: Carcinoma of the thyroid in children, Ann. Surg. 150:959, 1959.
5. Duffy, B. J., and Fitzgerald, P. J.: Thyroid cancer in childhood and adolescence: Report on 28 cases, Cancer 3:1018, 1950.
6. Hagler, S., Rosenblum, P., and Rosenblum, A.: Carcinoma of the thyroid in children and young adults: Iatrogenic relation to previous irradiation, Pediatrics 38:1, 1966.
7. Harness, J. K., Thompson, N. W., and Nishiyama, R. H.: Childhood thyroid carcinoma, Arch. Surg. 102:278, 1971.
8. Hayek, A., Chapman, E. M., and Crawford, J. D.: Long-term results of treatment of thyrotoxicosis in children and adolescents with radioactive iodine, N. Engl. J. Med. 283:949, 1970.
9. Hayles, A. B., *et al.*: Management of the child with thyroidal carcinoma, JAMA 173:21, 1960.
10. Horn, R. C., Jr., and Ravdin, I. S.: Carcinoma of the thyroid gland in youth, J. Clin. Endocrinol. 11:1166, 1951.
11. Klopp, C. T., Rosvoll, R. V., and Winship, T.: Is destructive surgery ever necessary for treatment of thyroid cancer in children?, Ann. Surg. 165:745, 1967.
11a. Lenio, P. T.: External irradiation in treatment of papillary carcinoma of the thyroid, Am. J. Surg. 131:281, 1976.
12. Maloof, F., Vickery, A. L., and Rapp, B.: An evaluation of various factors influencing the treatment of metastatic thyroid carcinoma with I[131], J. Clin. Endocrinol. 16:1, 1956.
13. Pellerin, D., Bertin, P., Vallee, G., and Nezelof, C.: Cancer du corps thyroide chez l'enfant (étude de 18 observations), Ann. Chir. 25:15, and 25:801, 1971.
14. Raventos, A., Horn, R. C., Jr., and Ravdin, I. S.: Carcinoma of the thyroid gland in youth: A second look ten years later, J. Clin. Endocrinol. 22:886, 1962.
15. Simpson, C. L., and Hempelmann, L. H.: The association of tumors and roentgen ray treatment of the thorax in infancy, Cancer 10:42, 1957.
16. Simpson, C. L., Hempelmann, L. H., and Fuller, L. M.: Neoplasm in children treated with x-rays in infancy for thymic enlargement, Radiology 64:840, 1955.
17. Tawes, R. L., and deLorimier, A. A.: Thyroid carcinoma during youth, J. Pediatr. Surg. 3:210, 1968.
18. Tollefson, H. R., Shah, J. P., and Huvos, A. G.: Papillary carcinoma of the thyroid, Am. J. Surg. 124:468, 1972.
19. Winship, T., and Chase, W. W.: Thyroid carcinoma in children, Surg. Gynecol. Obstet. 101:217, 1956.

35   Mark M. Ravitch

The Parathyroids

Hyperparathyroidism

THE CHIEF CONDITION of surgical concern originating in the parathyroid glands in children is primary hyperparathyroidism. Carcinoma of the parathyroid gland has never been reported in childhood.[20]

The first successful removal of a parathyroid adenoma for hyperparathyroidism in an adult was performed by Mandl[17] in 1926. Four years later, Pemberton and Geddie[21] reported successful removal of a parathyroid adenoma from a 14-year-old girl, the first such procedure reported in a child. Wilkins[29] found 10 children with histologically verified primary hyperparathyroidism in the literature between 1930 and 1954. Nolan *et al.*[20] in a review of the literature to 1960,

discovered 22 children in whom primary hyperparathyroidism had been confirmed histologically and added a case of their own. By 1966, the number of reported cases in children had risen to 30.[5] The 1970 report by Bjernulf and others[2] brought the total to 43. By 1975, Mannix,[18] reporting 3 of his own patients and collecting 14 others since Bjernulf's account, put the total at 60 cases of primary hyperparathyroidism in children.

The incidence of functioning parathyroid adenomas in children is equal in the sexes, in contrast to adults, in whom 70% of the lesions occur in women.[8, 30] The youngest reported patient was 3 years of age at the time of diagnosis and had had symptoms for at least a year,[7] but most of the lesions are found in late childhood and early adolescence.

Familial hyperparathyroidism does occur, Macabeo *et al.*,[15] from Lyon, finding a boy of 15 with bony kidney disease relieved by removal of two hyperplastic parathyroids. They studied his family and found 2 of his brothers, 17 and 6 years of age, to have the disease, both chemically and histologically. There have been some 125 cases reported in 37 families, most of the patients being adults. Hyperplasia is more frequent in familial cases than it is in sporadic cases, where adenoma is more common. The relationship between familial hyperparathyroidism and multiple endocrine adenomatosis obviously has been the subject of speculation[13, 27, 28] and is yet unresolved.

PATHOLOGY.—The first detailed descriptions of the pathologic changes in primary hyperparathyroidism were reported by Castleman and Mallory[4] in 1935. Woolner and associates[30] expanded these details with an account of the pathologic examination of specimens from 140 patients with hyperparathyroidism in 1952. Two basic pathologic states of the parathyroids lead to hyperparathyroidism. One is the parathyroid adenoma and the other is primary, *wasserhelle* cell hyperplasia of the parathyroid glands.

In gross appearance, the parathyroid adenoma is yellowish brown, somewhat darker than the normal parathyroid. The cut surface is typically homogeneous, but cysts or areas of hemorrhage may occur. The lesions vary greatly in size. An adenoma as small as 120 mg can give rise to serious systemic symptoms.[30] The most common cell in the parathyroid adenoma is the chief cell, but oxyphilic cells and water-clear cells are also seen.

A striking finding, and one that is distinctive of primary hyperplasia, is the bulk of parathyroid tissue that is found in the neck. All of the parathyroids are involved, and fusion of the upper and lower parathyroids can produce a single irregular mass on either side. On histologic examination, large, clear cells resembling those of hypernephroma with basally oriented nuclei arranged in an alveolar pattern are seen. Primary hyperplasia is easily distinguished from secondary hyperplasia, for the latter condition usually shows a mixture of all cells, with a predominance of chief cells. In infants, the lesion invariably is hyperplasia; in older children, the lesion usually is a single adenoma, except in familial cases.[6]

PHYSIOLOGY.—Parathyroid hormone appears to have two primary sites of action: the mobilization of calcium from bone and the promotion of renal clearance of phosphorus. Some evidence exists that these two functions may be performed by two independent hormones, which may be present in varying concentrations. In any event, in hyperparathyroidism, the osteoporosis of bone, cyst formation, calcinosis, soft tissue calcium deposits, elevated serum calcium and elevated urinary excretion of calcium are all related to the excessive mobilization of calcium from bone. The decreased serum phosphorus and increased urine phosphorus concentrations are a result of increased renal clearance of phosphorus.

The elevated serum calcium also has its own and poorly understood effect on renal function, which results in increased excretion of water, sodium, potassium and chloride, with a lowered urinary specific gravity. Apparently this effect is not a simple osmotic diuresis and cannot be prevented by physiologic amounts of Pituitrin.[25]

CLINICAL FEATURES.—The symptoms of primary hyperparathyroidism are diverse and relatively nonspecific early in the disease. Characteristically, the disease has been present long prior to establishment of the diagnosis. In the 23 children reported by Nolan, Hayles and Woolner,[20] the average duration of symptoms prior to diagnosis was 19.4 months. The general symptoms of hypercalcemia are weakness, lassitude, myasthenia, fatigue, anorexia, constipation, abdominal distention, polyuria and polydipsia. Skeletal changes may result in bone pain or loss of stature. Renal calculi and renal colic occur. Eighteen of their 23 children had renal lithiasis. Alopecia and changes in the fingernails have been noted in a few children.[20] Bone changes have been confused with rickets in some children,[8] and the bone pain has been confused with that from rheumatic fever.[3] In general, symptoms of bone disease are the most frequent form of presentation in childhood (Fig. 35–1), as opposed to the more common presentation with renal disease in adults. However, the presentation varies from hypercalcemic crises[23] presenting a surgical emergency to hyperparathyroidism discovered in a search for the cause of chronic abdominal pain.[9]

Malek and Kelalis,[16] from the Mayo Clinic, found hyperparathyroidism in 6% of children with renal stones, and found renal stones in 6 of their 9 children with hyperparathyroidism (of whom 3 had radiographic evidence of bone disease). One of the children had nephrocalcinosis as well as nephrolithiasis. In all 6 children, the renal function improved after operation, or at least did not deteriorate.

The most dependable roentgenologic evidence of hyperparathyroidism is subperiosteal absorption of bone, which is seen most frequently along the margins of the middle phalanges. The next most frequently observed roentgenologic evidence is the disappearance of the lamina dura of the teeth.

In adults, a varied assortment of associated conditions has been noted accompanying primary hyperparathyroidism. These include hypomagnesemia,[1, 14] pancreatitis[3, 12] and peptic ulcer. Of these, peptic ulcer[26] and hypomagnesemia[14] have also been reported in children. Acute parathyroid crisis in children has been reported at least twice. Reinfrank and Edwards[22] reported a 13-year-old girl with emotional and mental change, drowsiness, generalized weakness, anorexia, abdominal pain and tenderness, BUN of 90 mg and serum calcium of 21.8 mg/ml. At operation, a 6-gm adenoma was removed, with a dramatic response. Stables *et al.*[23] observed an acute intensification of hyperparathyroidism and hypercalcemic crisis in a boy with renal osteodystrophy. Removal of three hyperplastic parathyroids and part of a fourth relieved the symptoms.

Symptomatic hyperparathyroidism has been reported in the neonate in at least 12 instances.[10] As Goldbloom has pointed out, these glands almost always show diffuse, "clear-cell" hypoplasia.[12] In the case report by both Garcia-Bunuel *et al.*[10] and Nguyen *et al.*[19] from the Baltimore City Hospitals, the infant was a "floppy" baby with a high-pitched cry, high arched palate and small rectovaginal fistula. She had the radiologic hallmarks of the disease and multiple healing rib fractures. The serum calcium was 13.4 mg/100 ml. At 15 days, four enlarged, hyperplastic parathyroids were removed. She did well on a high-calcium diet, calcium supplements and administration of dihydrotachysterol (Fig. 35–2).

LABORATORY FINDINGS.—Serum calcium is elevated and serum inorganic phosphorus lowered. In children, normal serum phosphorus levels are a little higher than in adults, being 3.5–4.5 mg/100 ml compared to 3.0–4.0 mg/100 ml.[25] Thus, what would appear to be a low normal value in an adult could be below normal for a child.

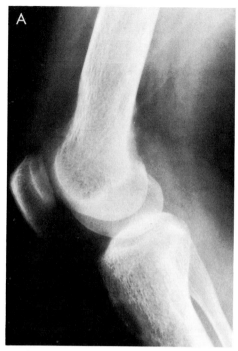
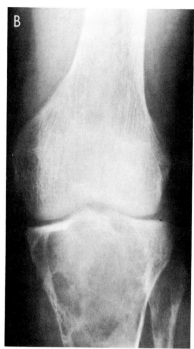
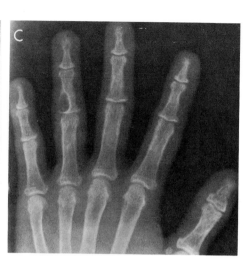

Fig. 35–1. — Osteitis fibrosa cystica in an adolescent. This boy twisted his knee at the age of 16. X-rays at that time showed a lytic lesion of the proximal tibia, which was dismissed as a nonossifying fibroma. The pain recurred 2 years later. **A,** the left knee showed a huge lytic lesion of the entire proximal end of the tibia and smaller rounded lytic lesions in the distal femur. **B,** the opposite knee showed striking subperiosteal resorption of bone in the metaphyses of the femur and the tibia. **C,** the fingers showed a cyst in the middle phalanx of the fourth finger, subperiosteal bone resorption and coarsening of the trabecular architecture. The boy also had lytic lesions in his clavicles. The radiologic findings were diagnostic of hyperparathyroidism. His serum calcium was 13.8 and phosphorus 1.8. A parathyroid adenoma was found and removed at operation. (Courtesy of Dr. A. H. Felman, University of Florida, Gainesville.)

The normal serum calcium level is the same in children as in adults, ranging from 9 to 10.5 mg/100 ml. Even slight elevations above this may be significant. Serum calcium and phosphorus levels may fluctuate widely during the course of hyperparathyroidism, and at times may be normal, so that serial determinations are of importance. Alkaline phosphatase is elevated when skeletal disease is present. Urinary excretion of calcium and phosphate is high and continues to be high, even when the patient is on a low-calcium and/or low-phosphorus diet.

DIFFERENTIAL DIAGNOSIS. — The lesions of bone may be confused with congenital bone cyst, polyostotic fibrous dysplasia, giant cell tumors and osteogenesis imperfecta, but

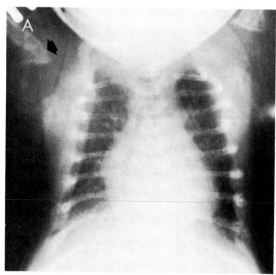
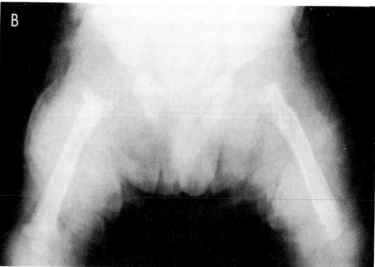

Fig. 35–2. — Neonatal hyperparathyroidism. Newborn girl with hypotonia and a high-pitched cry. Pronounced hypercalcemia (13.9 mg/100 ml) and hypophosphatemia (3.4 mg/100 ml). Roentgenograms show diffuse osteopenia with coarsening of the trabecular architecture and subperiosteal resorption of bone. The changes are greatest in the metaphyses, with pathologic fractures of the right humeral neck *(arrow)* and many ribs. Total parathyroidectomy showed diffuse hypoplasia of all glands, which had a combined weight of 90 mg. Postoperatively, the serum calcium and phosphorus returned to normal and the bones rapidly remineralized. (Courtesy of Nguyen, V. C., *et al.*[19])

the serum calcium is normal in these conditions. Metastatic bone lesions of neuroblastoma or other neoplasms may elevate the serum calcium but serum phosphorus remains normal. Vitamin D intoxication and idiopathic hypercalcemia of infancy are accompanied by an elevated serum calcium content, but, again, the phosphorus level usually is normal and calcium balance studies are normal.

Chronic renal failure, which results in retention of phosphorus and rising serum phosphorus, will stimulate the parathyroid glands to produce secondary *hyperparathyroidism* and can produce an elevation of serum calcium and many of the clinical features seen in primary hyperparathyroidism. Serum phosphorus content is elevated or sometimes normal, but never low in this situation, and this fact provides a clear differential in the diagnosis of secondary and early primary hyperparathyroidism. In the late course of a functioning adenoma, renal calcification and recurrent renal stones may have so damaged the kidneys that serum phosphorus is not cleared adequately and begins to increase. In this instance, differential diagnosis of primary and secondary hyperfunction of the parathyroids may be difficult or impossible on the basis of clinical findings or laboratory tests. Exploration of the neck and biopsy of the parathyroid tissue is the only recourse in this circumstance.

TREATMENT.— The treatment of hyperparathyroidism is excision of the offending tissues. The neck is entered through a transverse cervical incision exposing the thyroid gland. All four parathyroid areas are explored thoroughly in every instance. The finding of one adenoma does not exclude the coexistent presence of one or more other adenomas. Characteristically, in the presence of an adenoma, the remaining parathyroids are small and difficult to identify. If, after a thorough search of the neck, an adenoma has not been found, it is possible that the lesion is in the mediastinum. Mediastinal parathyroid adenomas, reported in adults, have not yet been found in children.

If all parathyroid tissue is found to be hypertrophied, one can presume that the diagnosis is primary *wasserhelle* cell hyperplasia. The treatment in this instance is the excision of all of the hyperplastic tissue except for 0.5 cm³ or so of one gland,[3] an amount adequate to maintain normal calcium and phosphorus metabolism postoperatively. The operation entails little risk, and no deaths in children have been reported from the procedure. Postoperatively, a marked drop of urinary calcium and phosphorus excretion is to be expected. The concentration of serum calcium falls rapidly. Patients with marked bone disease may suffer a transient phase of hypocalcemic tetany.

Following an adequate operation, the prognosis is excellent for long-term survival, provided that renal damage from calcium deposits and stone formation has not become severe in the course of the disease. In a few instances in adults, one or more additional adenomas have manifested themselves a number of years after operation. Local recurrence has also been reported when the capsule of the adenoma was opened and bits of the tumor spilled into the wound.

Secondary hyperparathyroidism occurs in patients with chronic renal failure whose phosphate retention and hyperphosphatemia results in lowered serum calcium with resultant stimulation of parathormone secretion. The general systemic effects, the resultant bone changes and the diffuse deposition of calcium, particularly in the already damaged kidneys, indicate operative correction. Hyperparathyroidism may continue to be a threat even after successful renal transplantation. Of Starzl's 18 patients with renal transplants who underwent parathyroidectomy, 3 were children

and a fourth was 17 years of age.[24] The operation should be the removal of three parathyroids and all but a portion of the fourth. Alternatively, although probably not as safe, all four are removed and portions of one diced and inserted in the sternocleidomastoid muscle — or subcutaneously in the forearm, where they may be observed.[11]

REFERENCES

1. Agna, J. W., and Goldsmith, R. E.: Primary hyperparathyroidism associated with hypomagnesemia, N. Engl. J. Med. 258:222, 1958.
2. Bjernulf, A., Hall, K., Sjogren, I., and Werner, I.: Primary hyperparathyroidism in children, Acta Pediatr. Scand. 59:249, 1970.
3. Bogdonoff, M. D., *et al.*: Hyperparathyroidism, Am. J. Med. 21:583, 1956.
4. Castleman, B., and Mallory, T. B.: The pathology of the parathyroid gland in hyperparathyroidism: A study of 25 cases, Am. J. Pathol. 11:1, 1935.
5. Chaves-Carballo, E., and Hayles, E.: Parathyroid adenoma in children, Am. J. Dis. Child. 112:553, 1966.
6. Corvaglia, E.: L'ipoparatiroidismo cronico idiopatico familiare nell'infanzia, Minerva Pediatr. 25:104, 1973.
7. Crawford, D. J. M., Stefanelli, J., and Alvarez, A. F.: Three unusual cases of hyperparathyroidism, Br. J. Surg. 44:193, 1956.
8. DiGeorge, A. M., and Paschkis, K. E.: Some aspects of tumors of the endocrine glands, Pediatr. Clin. North Am. 6:583, 1959.
9. Frier, B. M., and Marrian, V. J.: Uncomplicated hyperparathyroidism, Arch. Dis. Child. 49:808, 1974.
10. Garcia-Bunuel, R., Kutchemeshgi, A., and Brandes, D.: Hereditary hyperparathyroidism, Arch. Pathol. 97:399, 1974.
11. Geis, W. P., Popotzer, M. M., Corman, J. L., Halgrimson, C. G., Groth, C. G., and Starzl, T. E.: The diagnosis and treatment of hyperparathyroidism after renal homotransplantation, Surg. Gynecol. Obstet. 137:997, 1973.
12. Goldbloom, R. B., Gillis, D. A., and Prasad, M.: Hereditary parathyroid hyperplasia: A surgical emergency of early infancy, Pediatrics 49:514, 1972.
13. Harmon, M.: Parathyroid adenoma in a child: Report of a case presenting as central nervous system disease and complicated by magnesium deficiency, Am. J. Dis. Child. 91:313, 1956.
14. Jackson, C. E.: Hereditary hyperparathyroidism associated with recurrent pancreatitis, Ann. Intern. Med. 49:829, 1957.
15. Macabeo, V., David, L., Frederich, A., and Francois, R.: Hyperparathyroidie familiale: A propos de 3 observations, Pediatrie 30:503, 1975.
16. Malek, R. S., and Kelalis, P.: Urologic manifestations of hyperparathyroidism in childhood, J. Urol. 115:717, 1976.
17. Mandl, F.: Klinisches und experimentelles zur Frage der lokalisierten und generalisierten Osteitis fibrosa, Arch. Klin. Chir. 143:1, 1926.
18. Mannix, H., Jr.: Primary hyperparathyroidism in children, Am. J. Surg. 129:528, 1975.
19. Nguyen, V. C., Sennott, M. W., and Knox, G. S.: Neonatal hyperparathyroidism, Radiology 112:1, 175, 1974.
20. Nolan, R. B., Hayles, A. B., and Woolner, L. B.: Adenoma of the parathyroid glands in children, Am. J. Dis. Child. 99:622, 1960.
21. Pemberton, J. DeJ., and Geddie, K. B.: Hyperparathyroidism, Ann. Surg. 92:202, 1930.
22. Reinfrank, R. F., and Edwards, T. L.: Parathyroid crisis in a child, JAMA 178:468, 1961.
23. Stables, D. P., *et al.*: Parathyroidectomy for hypercalcemic crisis in renal osteodystrophy, Ann. Intern. Med. 61:531, 1964.
24. Starzl, T. E., *et al.*: Renal Homotransplantation — Part II, in *Current Problems in Surgery* (Chicago: Year Book Medical Publishers, Inc., May, 1974).
25. Talbot, N. B., *et al.*: *Functional Endocrinology* (Cambridge, Mass.: Harvard University Press, 1952).
26. Tsumori, H., *et al.*: Juvenile hyperparathyroidism in association with peptic ulcer, J. Clin. Endocrinol. 15:1141, 1955.
27. Wermer, P.: Genetic aspects of adenomatosis of endocrine glands, Am. J. Med. 16:363, 1954.
28. Wermer, P.: Endocrine adenomatosis and peptic ulcer in a large kindred. Inherited multiple tumors and mosaic pleiotropism in man, Am. J. Med. 35:205, 1963.
29. Wilkins, L.: *Diagnosis and Treatment of Endocrine Disorders in Childhood and Adolescence* (2d ed.; Springfield, Ill.: Charles C Thomas, Publisher, 1956).
30. Woolner, L. B., Keating, F. R., and Black, B. M.: Tumors and hyperplasia of the parathyroid glands: A review of the pathologic findings in 140 cases of primary hyperparathyroidism, Cancer 5:1069, 1952.

36 Mark M. Ravitch / Benjamin F. Rush, Jr.

Cystic Hygroma

HISTORY. — The word hygroma stems from the Greek, and directly translated means "a moist or watery tumor." *Dorland's Medical Dictionary* defines hygroma as "a sac, cyst, or bursa, distended with a fluid." If hygroma is given this definition, the term cystic hygroma is redundant. Redundant or not, the term has the advantage of priority and long usage to describe a specific tumor of the lymphatic system occurring predominantly in the cervical region of infants and children. On pathologic grounds, cystic lymphangioma would be more correct, but it is unlikely that the term cystic hygroma will be supplanted.

In 1828, Redenbacker[22] described a cystic hygroma that he termed *ranula congenita*. Adolph Wernher,[29] of Giessen, in a monograph published in 1843, accurately described the gross pathology of the lesion, noted its common location in the neck and its occasional appearance elsewhere in the body, and distinguished it from branchial cleft cysts, tumors of the thyroid and cervical meningocele. Although not certain of its origin, he was sure that it was not due to mechanical factors or to "trespasses of the mother" (Fig. 36–1). He also conferred on the lesion the name cystic hygroma (which had been suggested a year earlier by von Ammon[28]).

In 1872, Koester[13] suggested for the first time the possible derivation of the lesion from the lymphatic system, but a real appreciation of the relation of these tumors to the lymphatics awaited the detailed and meticulous studies by Sabin,[23-26] which she began to report in 1901. Studying pig embryos in Mall's laboratory, she carefully explored the embryology of the lymphatic system. She emphasized the importance of using fresh embryos and remarked that "we are so near the abattoir that the embryos are often brought with the heart still beating."[23]

In 1913, Dowd[7] published from Roosevelt Hospital in New York an account of 4 patients with cystic hygroma. He incorporated in his paper a collective review that had been prepared by C. E. Farr of all cases reported to that date. In addition, he mentioned exchanging ideas and specimens with McClure[15] of Princeton. From the synthesis of thought of the clinician Dowd and the embryologist McClure, it was proposed that cystic hygromas arose from a sequestration of portions of the "lymph sacs," the growth centers of the primitive lymphatic system.[8] In 1938, Goetsch[10] published a classic account of these tumors. His clinical descriptions and studies of the pathology are still quoted in reviews of the subject.

Embryology of the Lymphatics

According to Sabin,[23-26] the lymphatic system arises from the formation of five primitive lymphatics, which she originally called lymph hearts. Sabin stated that these sacs developed from the venous system. Others have proposed that they develop from the coalescence of clefts in the mesenchyme near the veins. In the human embryo of 2 months, the formation of these sacs is complete; they are the paired jugular sacs lateral to the jugular vein, an unpaired retroperitoneal sac at the root of the mesentery and paired posterior sacs in relation to the sciatic veins (Fig. 36–2). Outbuddings from these lymph sacs propagate centrifugally to form the peripheral lymphatic system. The head, neck and arms receive a plexus of lymphatics from the jugular sacs. The hip, back and legs are invaded by lymphatics from the posterior sacs and the mesentery receives its lymphatics from the retroperitoneal sac (Fig. 36–2).

Secondary lymphatic structures developing with or shortly after the development of the primary sacs are the cisterna chyli, the thoracic duct and the subclavian lymph sacs. As demonstrated by their development, these primitive lymphatic sacs possess a considerable potential for growth. It is believed that cystic hygromas develop from portions of these sacs sequestered from the primary sacs during embryonic life. With a few exceptions, cystic hygromas occur in the area of the primitive sacs. By far the most common site of formation of cystic hygroma is in the neck, in the area adjacent to the primitive jugular lymphatic sac — the first of these sacs to form and by far the largest. All sacs are formed by the 8th week.

Natural History

Cystic hygromas occur with equal frequency in males and females, and in black and white children. One of the largest series reported is of 126 cases from Vietnam.[19] They are not common tumors. Anderson[1] reported 20 hygromas among 758 benign tumors seen in a children's hospital in a period of 15 years.

The lesion commonly appears quite early, often being observed at birth. There are reports on record of dystocia at delivery due to the presence of cystic hygromas too large to pass through the birth canal. Fifty percent to 60% of the lesions reported in the literature appeared before the end of the first year of life, and 80–90% appeared before the end of the second year.[5, 11]

Cystic hygromas have been reported to make their appearance in adult life, although rarely. We have seen a cystic hygroma in the neck of a woman of 48. Galofré *et al.*[9] reported on 8 patients past 50; Miller and Taboada's patient was 63.[16]

Often these lesions become manifest rather suddenly and grow quite rapidly. Growth then may stop for a period, to be followed by another episode of enlargement. Gross[11] and others have remarked that a period of enlargement may be preceded by an upper respiratory infection.

Occasionally, cystic hygromas will partially or completely regress spontaneously, either following infection or at times without apparent cause.[19] This is far too uncommon a happenstance to warrant any delay in treatment in the hope that spontaneous regression will occur. Immediate excision is recommended

Pathology

There has been much division of opinion as to whether or not lymphangiomas represent true neoplasms. Lymphangiosarcoma itself is rare, and a sarcoma arising from a previous lymphangioma has, to our knowledge, never been reported.

Nicholson,[18] speaking of angiomas in general, remarked that "angiomata are typical hamartomata, a class of borderline cases between malformations and tumors." Goetsch,[10] in his very careful studies of the pathology of cystic hygroma, pointed out small processes at the fringes of these lesions that he believed represented formation of new tissue by the hygroma. On the other hand, Willis[30] took the view that cystic hygroma represents sequestration of embryonic tissue with no growth potential in the sense that new tissue is formed. He stated: "In my opinion, however, fluid accumulation, the progressive formation of collateral channels and, in some cases, supervening thrombosis and organization, suffice to account for the growth of hygromas. The mingling of lymphatic channels and cysts with the involved tissue is not a proliferative invasive process, but merely a necessary feature of vascular malformation, comparable with that seen in hemangiomas." Certainly, the swellings appear to grow and to involve structures not initially recognized to be affected. This is particularly true of the massive lesions involving the neck and floor of the mouth. Whether this represents progressive invasion or merely accumulation of fluid in previously collapsed spaces is a moot point. Landing and Farber[14] classified lymphangiomas as: (1) lymphangioma simplex—made up of many small lymphatic capillaries; (2) cavernous lymphangioma—made up of larger lymphatic channels and (3) cystic lymphangioma—corresponding to cystic hygroma. They also noted that there is considerable mixing and overlapping, since cavernous lymphangiomas may contain many capillary elements and cystic lymphangiomas may contain both cavernous and capillary elements. They suggest that all these lesions be lumped under the simple term "lymphangioma." The point at which the lesion is too large to be classed as cavernous or too small to be called cystic cannot be defined, and, in our opinion, the position of the lesion in relation to the original lymphatic centers is as important in distinguishing the cystic hygromas as is its microscopic appearance.

Grossly, these lesions are multilobular, multilocular cystic masses composed of many individual cysts that vary from 1 mm to 5 cm or more in diameter. The locules may or may not

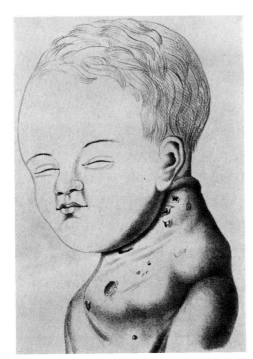

Fig. 36–1.—A neglected, infected and draining cystic hygroma, as illustrated in Wernher's monograph[29] of 1843, the first accurate account of cystic hygroma and its differential diagnosis. The lesion appears to have arisen in the typical location in the posterior triangle of the neck but is so large that most of the neck and a portion of the anterior chest wall are involved. Children with cystic hygroma in Wernher's era usually died when infection occurred; but, in some, infection was followed by sloughing of the cyst lining and spontaneous resolution.

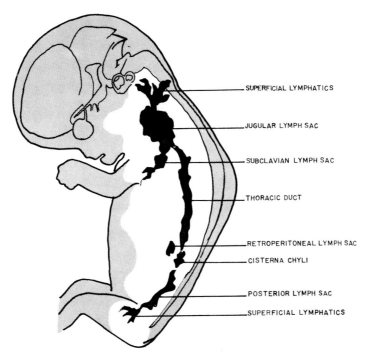

Fig. 36–2.—Lymphatic system in the 30-mm human embryo (about 8 weeks). The major and minor lymphatic sacs are fully developed, and superficial lymphatics are developing from them to spread to the periphery. Prominence of the jugular lymphatic sac in the neck is readily seen. The thoracic duct and cisterna chyli are also present. Sequestration of tissue from any of these structures at this period of development leads to later formation of a cystic hygroma. (After Sabin.[26])

communicate. If there has been no infection, the walls are thin and delicate. The cysts are filled with a serous fluid that may be clear or slightly yellow and occasionally blood stained. The mass often is associated with groups of enlarged lymph glands. The lining of the cyst is a thin pearly or gray, glistening and almost transparent membrane resembling peritoneum or pleura. In the dissection at operation, it usually is found that the mass is less discrete than anticipated, that sheets and tongues of edematous tissue leaking yellow fluid and at times containing small cysts pass in all directions from the periphery, in fascial planes, around and between nerve trunks and vessels. The larger cysts may intercommunicate, and trabeculae often are seen with isolated cords traversing the cystic cavities.

Microscopically, the cyst walls consist of a single layer of flattened endothelium. There may be a moderate amount of fibrous reaction in the surrounding tissue. The cords that pass through some of the cystic cavities actually are muscle fibers, thrombosed blood vessels or bits of fascia, presumably from structures entrapped by the enlarging cysts.

Not infrequently, numerous blood-containing capillaries, sometimes few and small, sometimes many and dilated into cavernous spaces, are seen. These suggest that the defect may not be confined to the lymphatic system but may include the vascular system as well. If vascular elements are prominent, the lesion may be termed a lymphohemangioma.

Clinical Course

Most commonly, the presenting complaint of these patients is of a soft mass in the posterior triangle of the neck (Fig. 36–3). The mass usually can be determined to be fluctuant and lobulated, not attached to the skin and not movable on the deep tissue. It is readily transilluminated, unless the accident of hemorrhage into it makes it tense and firm, as well as rendering it opaque. Three-quarters of the cystic

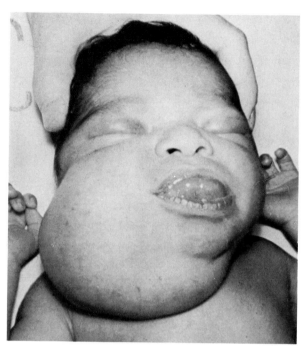

Fig. 36–4.—Massive lymphangioma in a newborn with involvement of the floor of the mouth and elevation of a thickened, probably involved tongue, difficulty in swallowing and breathing. Operation was undertaken within a few days of birth. These represent the most difficult cases operatively. In this instance, all the principal vessels and nerves of the neck were laid out as the lymphangioma was peeled from them. Clusters of thin-walled sacs and strands of whitish tissue went up into the floor of the mouth and far posteriorly, behind the pharynx. Although the carotid artery and the cranial nerves were spared, the omohyoid and digastric muscles and the suprahyoid muscles were in large part excised, and the mandibular branch of the facial nerve was injured. Because of the extensive dissection under the floor of the mouth, a tracheostomy was performed. The immediate outcome was good. The late result is not known.

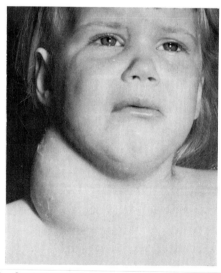

Fig. 36–3.—Cervical cystic hygroma with hemorrhage. A 2½-year-old girl was admitted with a mass in the neck, first noted when she was 15 days old. Originally 2 cm in diameter, the mass gradually increased to 4 cm until 4 days before admission, when she fell and struck the lesion. The mass discolored and rapidly enlarged. The child, previously asymptomatic, developed difficult respirations, especially after exertion, and had to be propped up to sleep. The mass was rather firm but not hard. The clinical impression of cystic hygroma was confirmed at operation, when a large cystic hygroma distended with blood was found. It was adherent to the jugular vein, carotid artery and cutaneous nerves but was fairly well encapsulated, and could be removed intact and in toto.

hygromas seen present in the neck and 20% are observed in the axillary region (Fig. 36–4). The remaining 5% are scattered about the body in the mediastinum, retroperitoneal area, pelvis and groin. The majority of cystic hygromas affecting the neck occur in the posterior triangle, occasionally communicating beneath the clavicle with an axillary hygroma (Fig. 36–5). Some do occur in the anterior triangle and in this location usually appear high in the submandibular region. Often these lesions are associated with intraoral lymphangiomas and are the ones most prone to cause pharyngeal compression and interference with the airway (Figs. 36–4 and 36–6). Cystic hygroma of the parotid region (see Fig. 36–8) may extend from behind the ear almost to the mouth, and from the jaw line to the eye. These are tumors of the parotid region, not of the gland itself, and are chiefly to be distinguished from large hemangiomas of the same tissues.

Two percent or 3% of all cervical hygromas are associated with extensions into the mediastinum that, in some cases, extend to the diaphragm. All patients with cervical cystic hygroma should have a chest film before operation to determine the presence or absence of such mediastinal involvement[6] (Fig. 36–7). Chylothorax and chylopericardium have been complications of cervicomediastinal hygroma.

Except for their visible presence, hygromas usually cause no symptoms. There may be dyspnea and dysphagia and other symptoms indicating compression of the pharynx or structures of the superior thoracic outlet. Rarely, respiratory

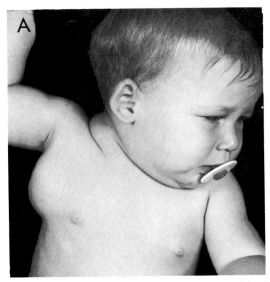

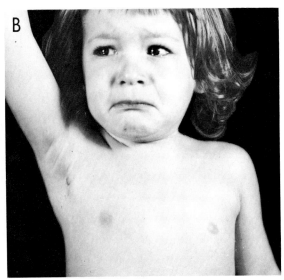

Fig. 36–5.—Cervicoaxillary hygroma recurrent after attempted excision in the neck. **A,** an infant of 9 months immediately before definitive operation, showing the recurrent supraclavicular mass in the posterior cervical triangle and the large communicating axillary hygroma. **B,** 1½ years after operation.

Separate incisions were used, transverse in the neck, and in the line of the axillary crease. The pectoral muscle was not divided. There has been no recurrence, and scars are all but imperceptible.

obstruction has resulted in death of the child before therapy was instituted. Lymphangiomas of the tongue and the floor of the mouth are the most dangerous lesions because of the inherent risk of obstruction to respiration, and are the most difficult to treat[3] (Fig. 36–4).

In the preantibiotic era, infection of these cysts was a much-feared complication. Their location adjacent to the drainage areas from the upper respiratory tract provides an easy path for the ingress of infection, and the lymphatic fluid

contained in the cavities is the culture medium. Incision and drainage of the infected cysts usually resulted in a long and debilitating period of lymphatic fluid drainage from the site of incision, with maceration of the surrounding skin and continued loss of protein. On the other hand, sometimes it eventuated in destruction of the cyst lining by infection, with ultimate cure.

The location and consistency of the lesion usually are so characteristic that differential diagnosis is not difficult. In addition, this is the lesion of the neck most readily transilluminated. Branchial cleft cysts probably represent the most likely diagnostic alternative. Usually they may be differen-

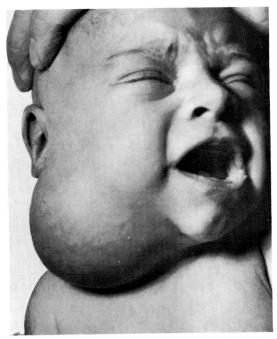

Fig. 36–6.—Cervical cystic hygroma in anterior cervical triangle. Infant at birth had a soft, floppy, cystic mass high in the anterior triangle of the neck, just below the line of the right jaw. In 2½ weeks it had filled rapidly and now, at age 3 weeks, was quite tense. The lesion was excised through a transverse incision; the postoperative course was uneventful.

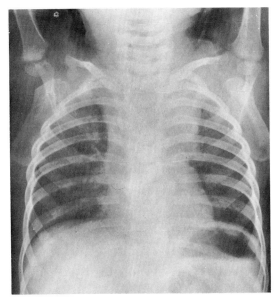

Fig. 36–7.—Lymphangioma of the neck with mediastinal extension. A boy of 4 years had typical cervical lymphhygroma, with radiologic evidence of a mediastinal mass on the same (left) side. The lesion was completely excised in two operations. There was no recurrence. (Courtesy of the Children's Hospital, Detroit.)

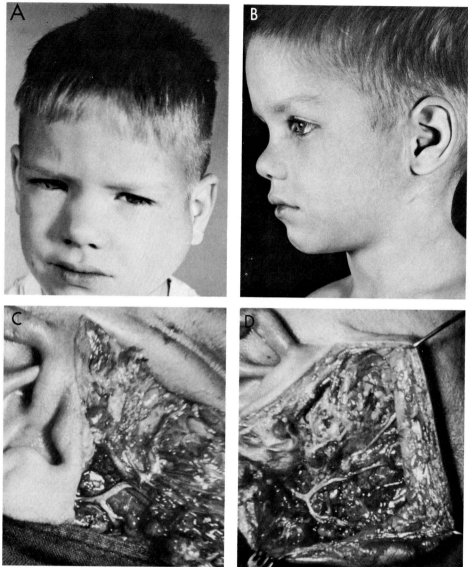

Fig. 36–8. — Parotid lymphangioma. These lesions usually are cystic hygroma, superficial to the parotid gland. **A,** large cystic, transilluminable swelling, anterior to and extending beneath the lobe of the left ear, which had recurred rapidly after attempted excision. There is partial paralysis of the lid. **B,** postoperative result, showing the scarcely perceptible scar. The facial nerve branch, divided at the previous operation, was found and resutured. **C,** operative photograph of similar lesion being excised from over the right parotid.

Traction is being made on the multilocular cyst downward and forward, and the main trunk and two branches of the facial nerve are exposed. **D,** on completion of the procedure, the facial nerve and its divisions lie cleanly exposed over the surface of the parotid gland. Temporary weakness of the corner of the mouth or of the lids may be expected, but one should confidently anticipate avoiding permanent injury to the nerves.

tiated by their preferred location low in the neck along the anterior border of the sternocleidomastoid muscle and by their unilocularity.

Aspiration of a hygroma yields thin, watery fluid that is clear or pale yellow. Aspiration of a branchial cleft cyst yields a thicker fluid. Hamilton Bailey[2] remarked on the constant finding of cholesterol crystals in the aspirate from branchial cleft cysts and believed, as we do, that this is an important distinguishing feature in the diagnosis. Goetsch[10] found that the fluid from cystic hygromas occasionally contained these crystals, although not as frequently.

Deep hemangiomas sometimes may present in the same locations, but they fail to transilluminate, contain blood on aspiration and may be collapsed by constant pressure. Dermoid cysts occur in the neck, may be soft and fluctuant, but

are unilocular, rare in the posterior triangle and not transilluminable. Lipomas occasionally occur in children and may appear to be truly fluctuant, but usually are not transilluminable.

Treatment

Excision is the treatment of choice for these lesions and the only effective treatment available. In an older era, when operation carried great hazards and a mortality of more than 50%,[7, 27] many alternative treatments were attempted, including irradiation, incision and drainage, the injection of sclerosing agents and even the injection of boiling water. None of these proved to be satisfactory.

Because of the hazard of spontaneous infection, of progressive growth leading to substantial disfigurement, with extension into as yet uninvolved areas, and the possibility of dysphagia and suffocation, operative treatment is indicated whenever one of these lesions is encountered. Spontaneous regression is so unlikely as not to be anticipated whereas increase in size is quite likely, so that operation is certain to have to be performed and delay presents no advantages and some risks. Operation should be undertaken just as readily in a newborn as in an older child. The only exception may be the premature infant, in whom operation may await the attainment of normal birth weight.

Cystic hygromas of the neck are best removed through a simple transverse cervical incision under intratracheal anesthesia with a dependable route established for infusion of fluids or blood. Some of the lesions seem fairly well encapsulated and are readily dissected out, but in many instances the lesion, intimately intertwined with the structures of the neck, requires a careful and prolonged dissection to remove the tumor as completely as possible. In some instances, the tumor may closely involve the carotid artery, jugular vein and brachial plexus. Whereas in the removal of other benign cysts it is chiefly the surgeon's pride that suffers if the cyst ruptures, in hygroma, rupture of the cyst may defeat the surgeon. The delicate-walled empty cyst is awkward to handle, the margins difficult to identify.

Axillary hygromas can be approached through incision in the line of the axillary skin crease. It is not necessary or justifiable to divide the pectoralis major. Adequate exposure almost always can be achieved by retraction of the pectoralis.

A special problem occurs if a cervical hygroma extends into the axilla. The infant is draped with that side elevated 15–20 degrees and the arm draped free, the exposed field extending from jaw to nipple and from anterior midline to beyond the posterior axillary line, including the shoulder and upper arm in the field. The cervical portion of the tumor is dissected free, above and to either side, and dissected off the brachial plexus until the hygroma is seen to pass below the clavicle. The axillary portion then is dissected out through a generous axillary incision and dissection extended up toward the clavicle. By alternate traction and dissection, first from above and then from below, the entire specimen is freed and delivered through the passage under the clavicle. A hygroma communicating from the neck into the axilla necessarily has so intimate an attachment to the brachial plexus and the subclavian vessels that a tedious and ticklish dissection is involved.

For a cervical hygroma that extends into the mediastinum, the neck and entire anterior chest are draped out. If the cysts are found in the course of the cervical exploration through a standard transverse incision to extend into the mediastinum beyond reach from above, the incision is carried from its anterior end vertically down the anterior midline and the sternum split so that the cysts may be removed in continuity. The ipsilateral pleura almost certainly will be removed simultaneously. Respiratory embarrassment is an indication for urgent one-stage cervicomediastinal resection and the repeated reports of sudden aggravation of respiratory obstruction counsel operation whenever mediastinal involvement is seen.[12, 17]

Parotid hygromas, so-called, do not involve the gland itself, or no more than its most superficial portion, so that a formal parotidectomy is not required, and there usually is a sharp plane of cleavage between the underside of the hygroma and the superficial surface of the parotid.[20] Incision is made just anterior to the ear as for resection of a parotid tumor (Fig. 36–8, *B*). The facial nerve lies deep to the tumor and should lie bare when the operation is completed (Fig. 36–8, *C* and *D*). The integrity of the nerve must be preserved, but the parents should be warned of the likelihood of temporary paresis after operation.

During dissection of cystic hygromas, particularly those in the neck, any attached structures that suggest lymphatic trunks should be ligated in order to minimize the accumulation of fluid postoperatively. If the hygroma has been very large, a suction catheter always should be placed at the time of operation, both to handle the fluid that may occur in any large wound and specifically to handle any fluid that may have accumulated from transected lymphatic ducts.

Cystic hygroma is not a malignant neoplasm and there is no need to sacrifice normal structures in the course of the operation. This is not to be construed as condoning or encouraging a half-hearted attempt at removal. These tumors can and do recur. Nevertheless, it must be recognized that when sheets of edematous tissue enfold nerves and vessels, complete extirpation is technically impossible. Judging from the pathologic studies by Goetsch,[10] it is likely that even when the surgeon believes that he has removed all of the lesion, some microscopic bits or pseudopods around the peripheral borders of the tumor do remain. In our experience, if all of the macroscopically identifiable tissue is dissected away, recurrence is rare. This reinforces our belief that the lesion is not a neoplasm in the true sense of the word. If, on the other hand, portions of obvious cystic tumor are left behind, the recurrence rate may be as high as 10% or 15%. If some of the tumor must be left, it is important to leave no intact cysts, and all of the cyst wall should be resected in every instance.

The mortality rate for the excision of hygromas should be nil. When very large lesions involving most of the neck or extending into the mediastinum are included in a series, the postoperative mortality is cited at 2–5%.

REFERENCES

1. Anderson, D. H.: Tumors of infancy and childhood, Cancer 4:890, 1951.
2. Bailey, H.: The clinical aspects of branchial cysts, Br. J. Surg. 10:565, 1923.
3. Barrand, K. G., and Freeman, N. V.: Massive infiltrating cystic hygroma of the neck in infancy, Arch. Dis. Child. 48:7, 1973.
4. Bill, A. H., Jr., and Sumner, D. S.: Unified concept of lymphangioma and cystic hygroma, Surg. Gynecol. Obstet. 120:79, 1965.
5. Briggs, J. D., et al.: Cystic and cavernous lymphangioma, West. J. Surg. 61:499, 1953.
6. Childress, M. E., Baker, C. P., and Samson, P. C.: Lymphangioma of the mediastinum: Report of a case with a review of the literature, J. Thorac. Surg. 31:338, 1956.
7. Dowd, C. N.: Hygroma cysticum colli: Its structure and etiology, Ann. Surg. 58:112, 1913.
8. Farr, C. E.: Personal communication.
9. Galofré, M., et al.: Results of surgical treatment of cystic hygroma, Surg. Gynecol. Obstet. 115:319, 1962.
10. Goetsch, E.: Hygroma colli cysticum and hygroma axillare, Arch. Surg. 36:394, 1938.
11. Gross, R. E.: *The Surgery of Infancy and Childhood* (Philadelphia: W. B. Saunders Company, 1953).
12. Kirschner, P. A.: Cervico-mediastinal cystic hygroma: One stage excision in an eight-week-old infant, Surgery 60:1104, 1966.
13. Koester, K.: Ueber Hygroma cysticum colli congenitum, Verh. Phys.-Med. Ges. Wurzb. 3:44, 1872.
14. Landing, B. H., and Farber, S.: Tumors of the Cardiovascular System, in *Atlas of Tumor Pathology* (Washington, D. C.: Armed Forces Institute of Pathology, 1956).
15. McClure, C. F. W., and Silvester, C. F.: A comparative study of the lymphaticovenous communications in adult mammals, Anat. Rec. 3:534, 1909.
16. Miller, J. M., and Taboada, J. C.: Cystic hygroma colli in an adult, Johns Hopkins Med. J. 134:233, 1974.
17. Mills, N. L., and Grosfeld, J. L.: One-stage operation for cervico-

mediastinal cystic hygroma in infancy, J. Thorac. Cardiovasc. Surg. 65:4, 1973.

18. Nicholson, C. W. deP.: *Studies on Tumor Formation* (London: Butterworth & Co., Ltd., 1950).
19. Ninh, T. N., and Ninh, T. X.: Cystic hygroma in children: A report of 126 cases, J. Pediatr. Surg. 9:2, 1974.
20. Noone, R. B., and Brown, H. J.: Cystic hygroma of the parotid gland, Am. J. Surg. 120:404, 1970.
21. Ravitch, M. M.: Radical treatment of massive mixed angiomas (hemolymphangiomas) in infants and children, Ann. Surg. 134:228, 1951.
22. Redenbacker: Dissertation cited by Wernher.[29]
23. Sabin, F. R.: On the origin of the lymphatic system from the veins and the development of the lymph heart and thoracic duct in the pig, Am. J. Anat. 1:367, 1901.

24. Sabin, F. R.: On the development of the superficial lymphatics in the skin of the pig, Am. J. Anat. 3:183, 1904.
25. Sabin, F. R.: The development of the lymphatic nodes in the pig and their relation to the lymph hearts, Am. J. Anat. 4:355, 1905.
26. Sabin, F. R.: The lymphatic system in human embryos with a consideration of the morphology of the system as a whole, Am. J. Anat. 9:43, 1909.
27. Vaughn, A. M.: Cystic hygroma of the neck: Report of case and review of literature, Am. J. Dis. Child. 48:149, 1934.
28. von Ammon: Cited by Wernher.[29]
29. Wernher, A.: *Die angeborenen Kysten-hygrome und die ihnen verwandten Geschwulste in anatomischer, diagnostischer und therapeutischer Beziehung* (Giessen: G. F. Heyer, Vater, 1843).
30. Willis, R. A.: *Pathology of Tumors* (2d ed.; London: Butterworth & Co., Ltd., 1953).

37

ROBERT T. SOPER

Cysts and Sinuses of the Neck

Branchial Remnants

REMNANTS of the embryologic branchial apparatus that persist into postnatal life produce an array of abnormalities in and around the ear and down the lateral aspect of the neck. Of the neck abnormalities of surgical interest in children, branchial remnants are slightly more common than cystic hygromas but are considerably less common than thyroglossal duct remnants.[10] Sinuses, cysts, fistulae and cartilaginous nests are their most common manifestations. The sinuses, fistulae and cartilaginous remnants usually are noted during infancy and young childhood. In contrast, cysts require more time to fill with secretions and produce visible masses, and often are not diagnosed until later childhood or adolescence.

Second branchial remnants are several times more common than derivatives of the first branchial cleft. Remnants of the lower branchial system are rare. Since the branchial apparatus is paired, it is understandable that the remnants are bilateral in 10–15%.[4, 20] Ten percent of patients give a family history of similar branchial remnants in siblings, parents and other relatives.[38] Embryologic patterns eventually dictate the pathologic anatomy. Since surgical removal of these remnants demands regional or local dissection, rather than block excision, knowledge of their developmental anatomy is vital to their safe removal.

Branchial Embryology

During the second to eighth weeks of fetal life, four pairs of well-developed ridges *(branchial arches)* and a poorly defined fifth arch dominate the lateral cervicofacial area of the human embryo (Fig 37–1). The branchial apparatus is first recognized by the tenth day of embryonic life (2.5 mm stage), reaches its apogee of development during the third and fourth gestational weeks, gradually to diminish in size and importance thereafter, disappearing entirely by the fiftieth day of gestation (14 mm stage).

The five pairs of branchial arches are separated by four paired external grooves that are matched by four pharyngeal grooves internally; the four external grooves are known as *branchial clefts* and the four internal grooves are known as *pharyngeal pouches.* The third, fourth and fifth branchial apparatuses are phylogenetically analogous to the respiratory gill apparatus of fishes. Each branchial arch contains mesenchymal tissue, which later develops into cartilage, bone and muscle, as well as blood vessels and nerves. The muscular elements of each arch are supplied by the nerve of that arch. The arches are covered by squamous epithelium (ectoderm) externally and cuboidal epithelium (endoderm) internally. It is helpful to study the contributions of each branchial arch to normal development of the head and neck, in order to understand abnormal development leading to congenital anomalies (Table 37–1).

Throughout normal human development, the branchial clefts and pharyngeal pouches never communicate with each other, remaining separated by a membrane. In contrast, there is free communication in the respiratory gill apparatus of the fish. Only the first pair of grooves and pouches persists as such in the human embryo: external auditory canal (cleft) and eustachian tube (pouch) separated by the tympanic membrane (Fig. 37–2). The second, third and fourth branchial clefts disappear after being buried by overgrowth of the second branchial arch[2, 20] or fusion of different arches[10] during the sixth and seventh weeks of gestation (Fig. 37–1).

In contrast, the endoderm of the second pharyngeal pouch forms the palatine tonsils and the supratonsillar fossa (Fig. 37–2). The third pouch produces the piriform sinus indentation as well as epithelial tissue that ultimately forms the thymus gland and inferior parathyroids. The fourth pharyngeal pouch is bilobed; epithelium from its upper lobe forms the superior parathyroids, which normally come to rest behind the upper pole of the respective thyroid lobes. Thymic descent carries with it parathyroid tissue of third pouch derivation, so that even though it originates higher in the neck, it migrates caudad to fourth pouch parathyroid tissue, ultimately coming to rest behind the lower pole of the lateral thyroid lobes. Epithelium from the lower lobe of the fourth pharyngeal pouch probably contributes the ultimobranchial bodies, which merge with the lateral thyroid lobes; recently they have come into prominence as a likely source of calcitonin (Fig. 37–2).

In the normal course of embryologic events, the first and second branchial arches flourish early to form most of the anatomic structures of the lower face and neck. Three hillocks from each arch cluster around the ostium of the first branchial cleft (the external auditory meatus), ultimately merging to form the external pinna of the ear. The second arch overgrows in a caudad direction to fuse with[10] or cover[2, 20] the lower arches (Fig. 37–1). This buries the epithelial surfaces of the lower clefts, which under normal circumstances atrophy and finally disappear during the sixth or seventh week. Most embryologists believe that abnormal retention of various portions of this buried epithelium produces the majority of branchial sinuses, cysts and fistulas.

shape or contour of the external pinna and malformed malleus and incus, producing congenital deafness. Microtia and aural atresia occur with failure of the first branchial cleft to develop normally. Abnormalities of third, fourth and fifth branchial arches result in abnormalities, cysts and webs of the larynx and aryepiglottic folds.

Lyall and Stahl[20] in 1956, Albers[2] in 1963 and Gray and Skandalakis[10] in 1972 published the most complete and readable summaries of embryologic branchial development and its relationship to lateral cervical cysts, sinuses and fistulas.

Second Branchial Remnants

Remnants of the second branchial cleft and pouch are much more common than those of first branchial origin.[4, 28] Complete fistulas are more common than external sinuses; both of these are more common than branchial cysts, at least during childhood.[4] However, cysts predominate in adults.[20]

By definition, all branchial remnants are truly congenital and are present at birth. Commonly, the tiny external ostium of the fistulas and external sinuses remain unnoticed for some time. Mucoid drainage from the ostium usually is what brings these lesions to the attention of parents; infection due to entrapped bacteria may lead to early detection. Infection is less common in fistulas and external sinuses than in cysts. The cutaneous openings occasionally are marked by skin tabs or bits of cartilage. Often the tract is palpable as a cord-like structure running upward in the neck from the ostium; milking or stripping the tract will provoke a mucoid discharge. The larger fistulas may drain ingested dye or liquids through the ostium (Fig. 37–4).

The external ostium of the second branchial cleft lies along the anterior border of the sternocleidomastoid muscle, generally at the junction of its lower and middle thirds. Because of its embryologic origin, the second cleft tract penetrates platysma and cervical fascia to ascend along the carotid sheath to the level of the hyoid bone. It then turns medially between the branches of the carotid artery, behind the posterior belly of the digastric and stylohyoid muscles and in front of the hypoglossal nerve to end in the tonsillar fossa (Figs. 37–3 and 37–4). External sinuses pursue the same course for variable distances before terminating blindly.

Branchial cysts of second pouch origin usually become clinically evident as gradually enlarging masses that lie deep to the anterior border of the sternocleidomastoid muscle in its upper third (Fig. 37–5). Since it takes time for secretions to accumulate sufficiently to produce a recognizable mass, branchial cysts tend to appear in late childhood, adolescence or young adulthood.[20] Oral bacteria may contaminate those branchial cysts that are associated with a pharyngeal pouch[3, 4, 16, 20] to trigger an infection,[40] which brings the cyst to medical attention. Rarely, branchial cysts are so deep-seated as to bulge into the lateral oropharynx.

About 10% of second branchial cleft remnants are bilateral.[30, 38] There seems to be a familial incidence for fistulas and external sinuses,[20] which has not been reported in branchial cysts. Internal sinuses not associated with cysts are extremely rare (or at least are not often looked for or discovered) but have been reported by Toomey[40] to open onto the posterior tonsillar pillar.

Branchial cysts usually are not difficult to distinguish from cystic hygromas, which are subcutaneous and can be transilluminated. Cysts lie deep to the anterior border of the sternocleidomastoid muscle in its upper third and do not bear the characteristic vascular markings of most hemangiomas (Fig. 37–5). Inflammation of the branchial cyst adds tenderness, erythema and edema to the overlying tissue in approximately 25% of cases.[40] Branchial cysts lie slightly lateral to the jugulodigastric lymph nodes and are not firm or multi-

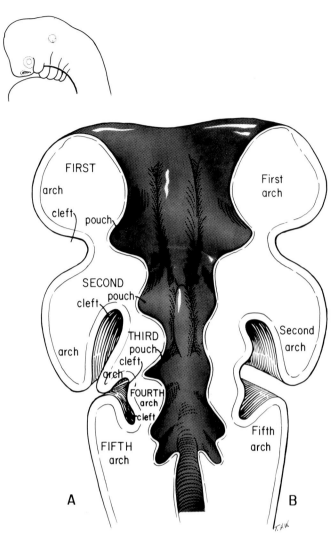

Fig. 37–1.—Coronal view of ventral aspect of fetal pharynx during fifth gestational week. Side **A** represents the more complex changes that occur in the lower branchial apparatus of the human embryo depicted in recent studies[10] whereas side **B** represents the older, more classic view.[2, 20] The inset shows the external view of the fetus and the line of the coronal cut.

Each second and third arch component fuses with its contralateral mate in the anterior midline during their caudad and medial overgrowth and migration. During this fusion process, the right and left anlagen of the hyoid body fuse around the thyroglossal tract (Fig. 37–2). Because of this, removal of the central hyoid body is required when excising thyroglossal tract remnants. Imperfections in midline fusion of the right and left second and third arch ectoderm produce two anterior midline neck defects: the very common dermoid cyst and the very rare midline cervical cleft. A midline cervical cleft likely represents partial failure of the ectodermal derivatives to fuse whereas the dermoid (inclusion) cyst develops when ectodermal cells are entrapped or buried during this fusion process.

Normally, the epithelium-lined lower branchial clefts obliterate and are replaced by mesenchymal structures of the lateral neck. Branchial abnormalities result when portions of buried branchial epithelium fail to obliterate and disappear. These remnants form a cyst if only the midportion of the tract remains. If only the pharyngeal pouch remains, an internal sinus results, which surfaces in the pharynx. An internal sinus (pouch) may be associated with a branchial cyst. If only the outer brachial cleft end of this apparatus is retained, an external sinus is found along the anterior border of the sternocleidomastoid muscle. A fistula results when the membrane ruptures and the entire tract remains patent (Fig. 37–3).

Abnormal development of the first branchial arch results in a host of facial abnormalities, including cleft lip and palate, abnormal

TABLE 37-1.—CONTRIBUTIONS OF BRANCHIAL ARCHES TO NORMAL DEVELOPMENT OF THE HEAD AND NECK

ARCH	ECTODERM Skin	MESODERM Cartilage and Bone	Muscle	Nerve	Artery	ENDODERM Mucous Membrane
#1	Lower face	Meckel's cartilage: malleus, incus, mandible, maxilla	Mastication, floor of mouth, tensor tympani and palati, ant. body digastric	3d division of cranial nerve V	Disappears	Nasopharynx
#2	Lat. and ant. neck	Reickert's cartilage: stapes, styloid process, upper body and lesser cornu of hyoid	Post. belly digastric, facial expression, stapedius	Cranial nerve VII	Disappears	Oropharynx
#3	Small area lat. neck	Lower body and greater cornu of hyoid	Sup. pharyngeal constrictor	Cranial nerve IX	Common carotid	Lower pharynx
#4	None recognized	Thyroid and arytenoid cartilages	Inf. pharyngeal constrictor, cricothyroid m., intrinsic laryngeal m.	Sup. laryngeal branch of cranial nerve X	Lt: aortic arch Rt: subclavian	Hypopharynx
#5	None recognized	Cricoid cartilage	Contributes to intrinsic m. of larynx	Recurrent laryngeal branch of cranial nerve X	Disappears	Hypopharynx

ple. Tuberculous adenitis (scrofula), atypical mycobacterium infections, cat-scratch disease, actinomycosis or other chronic upper cervical lymphadenitis may be confused with a chronically infected branchial remnant. Acid-fast smears and appropriate skin tests, immune titers and cultures should allow correct differential diagnosis.

The lining tissue of both first and second branchial remnants is similar: 90% are lined with squamous epithelium,[40] but ciliated columnar (respiratory) epithelium is also reported.[1, 20] The epithelial lining often is surrounded by muscle fibers. Lymphoid tissue also surrounds the lining and may be abundant enough to develop germinal centers.[1] Inflammatory reaction is in direct proportion to recent infection.

TREATMENT.—The goal of treating all congenital neck sinuses, cysts and fistulas is complete surgical excision undertaken when no inflammation is present. This may be done safely at any age, excluding the neonatal period; in general, the sooner the better. Aspiration of branchial cysts is not recommended, since it generally is not diagnostically helpful and may introduce infection. Contrast injection of fistulas and external sinuses allows a precise "mapping" of the extent of the remnant but is certainly not required for good surgical care (Fig. 37–4, B). Sclerosing solutions are never used.

Recurrence is likely if any part of the epithelium-lined tract is left behind. Since a second operation always is more

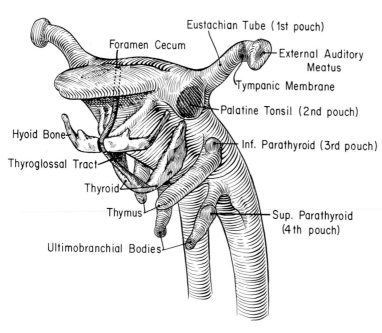

Fig. 37–2.—Three-quarter view of the pharynx during the sixth gestational week showing normal development of the pharyngeal pouches and their contribution to the anatomy of the neck and head.

Eustachian Tube (1st pouch)
Foramen Cecum
External Auditory Meatus
Tympanic Membrane
Palatine Tonsil (2nd pouch)
Hyoid Bone
Thyroglossal Tract
Inf. Parathyroid (3rd pouch)
Thyroid
Thymus
Sup. Parathyroid (4th pouch)
Ultimobranchial Bodies

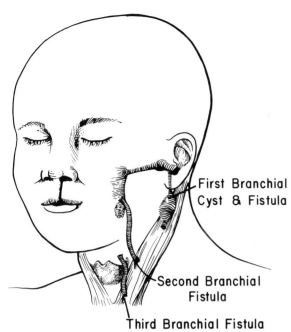

Fig. 37–3.—Diagram of a child with a cleft lip and remnants of the first three branchial systems.

First Branchial Cyst & Fistula

Second Branchial Fistula

Third Branchial Fistula

optimal exposure. The patient's face should be accessible to the anesthesiologist to ensure a safe airway and also for his access to the oral cavity. It helps to have the anesthesiologist insert his finger against the tonsillar fossa to mark the cephalic end of the tract for the surgeon.

External sinuses and fistulas are approached through an elliptical transverse incision around the external ostium, preferably within a skin crease. Dissection is carried down through platysma and then narrowed sharply to the tissue plane immediately surrounding the tract. With upward retraction of the skin and subcutaneous tissues and downward traction on the specimen, the tract is dissected cephalad as high as it is safe to pursue. In the small child and with the ostium located toward the middle of the sternocleidomastoid muscle, the tract can be completely excised safely through one incision.

Fistulas with openings along the lower third of the anterior border of the sternocleidomastoid muscle may require a parallel, higher, so-called stepladder incision for safe and complete removal (Fig. 37–6). Dissection through the lower elliptical incision is carried out as high as exposure allows, at which point a new, higher transverse skin crease incision is made through which the specimen is delivered, and dissection continued as the tract turns medially between the branches of the carotid artery en route to the tonsillar fossa.

Although in earlier years I meticulously identified all the surrounding neck structures, recently I have been content to stay close to the tract during the entire dissection. The wound is drained only if there is current or recent infection. The wound is closed in layers, using inverted knots of an absorbable suture for the platysma. Skin closure is subcuticular. Aerosol spray suffices as the only dressing. Oral fluids are allowed that night and a regular diet the next day. Convalescence is rapid, usually allowing discharge of the patient the day following operation. Recurrences are rare, but happen if a portion of epithelium-lined tract is overlooked.

Branchial cysts are electively excised when they are free from infection. When a cyst abscess has drained (surgically or spontaneously), it is best to wait 3 months for complete

difficult than the first, particularly when dissecting around vital neck structures, complete excision at the first operation is important. Neoplastic degeneration of branchial remnants has not been reported in childhood, but more than 250 cases reported in adults attest to the need for early and complete removal.[5, 14, 16, 21]

Operation is undertaken under general anesthesia with an endotracheal tube and the patient in the supine position; the lower part of the cheek and ear are prepped into the field as well as the entire neck. Slight hyperextension of the neck with the chin turned to the side opposite the lesion provides

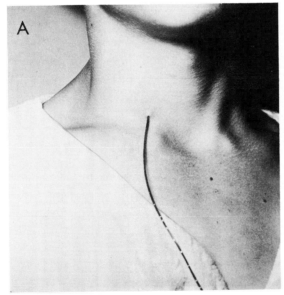
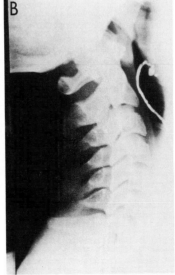

Fig. 37–4.—Fistula of second cleft. **A,** catheter inserted into ostium of second branchial fistula. (From P. P. Rickham, R. T. Soper and U. G. Stauffer, *Synopsis of Pediatric Surgery* [Chicago: Year Book Medical Publishers, Inc., 1975].) **B,** lateral neck radiograph of same patient after injecting contrast dye into the catheter, showing dye puddling in tonsillar fossa.

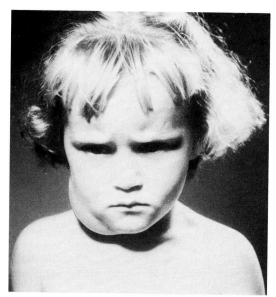

Fig. 37–5.—Right second branchial cyst mass in a child. (From P. P. Rickham, R. T. Soper and U. G. Stauffer, *Synopsis of Pediatric Surgery* [Chicago: Year Book Medical Publishers, Inc., 1975].)

resolution of inflammation before removal. In this instance, an elliptical incision transversely oriented around the drainage scar is necessary whereas in undrained cysts a cosmetically more pleasing skin crease incision is used directly over the mass. Dissection is carried through platysma and the deep fascia. The vertical plane anterior to the sternocleidomastoid muscle is developed and the muscle is retracted laterally. This brings into direct vision the top of the cyst, which then is skirted by sharp and blunt dissection. In the deeper reaches of the dissection, one commonly encounters a tract that pursues a medial direction to terminate in the tonsillar fossa.[16] Pressure by the anesthesiologist's finger on the inside of the tonsillar fossa will make this part of the dissection safer and easier. The end of the tract is suture-li-

gated flush with pharyngeal mucosa. The wound is not drained unless the cyst has been opened or there is unexpected residual inflammation.

Patients with bilateral lesions can have both sides operated on at the same surgical sitting. Appropriate prepping and draping are required for bilateral exposure. The anesthesiologist controls rotation of the head to facilitate dissection first on the one side and then on the other.

Third branchial cleft abnormalities are extremely rare (Fig. 37–3). Theoretically, the external ostium should lie along the anterior border of the clavicular insertion of the sternocleidomastoid muscle. It should track cephalad behind the internal carotid artery into the upper third of the neck, where it turns medially just above the eleventh cranial nerve to the middle third of the neck; it connects with the piriform sinus.[10, 40] We have not encountered this rare anomaly.

Again theoretically, a fourth branchial cleft abnormality should have its ostium low in the neck and travel behind the sternocleidomastoid muscle and either underneath the subclavian artery (on the right side) or underneath the arch of the aorta (on the left side) to reascend in the neck and approach the cervical esophagus.[10, 40] To my knowledge, no such abnormality has been reported.

Anomalies of the First Branchial Cleft

True anomalies of the first branchial cleft are extremely rare. Out of 90 patients with branchial anomalies, Hyndman and Light[12] found only 1 of first branchial origin, Neel and Pemberton[24] reported none out of 319, Rankow and Hanford[28] 3 of 160 and Gross[11] 1 out of 308. Startling exceptions to this customary ratio are the reports by Bill[3] and Bill and Vadheim,[4] who saw 5 patients with first branchial cleft abnormalities during an interval when they treated only 13 patients with second cleft abnormalities.

In 1923, the English embryologist J. E. Frazer predicted that a first branchial cleft anomaly could exist with a tract from the external auditory canal to the skin of the upper lateral neck.[8] Six years later, Hyndman and Light[12] reported

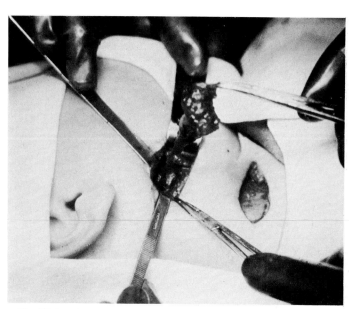

Fig. 37–6.—"Stepladder" incision during removal of right second branchial fistula.

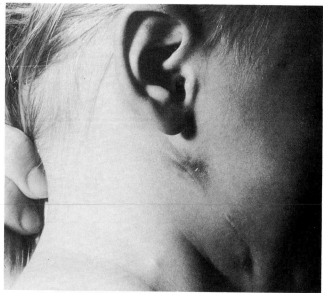

Fig. 37–7.—First branchial remnant, long undiagnosed. Young girl with recurrent infections and abscesses of the upper neck, which ultimately proved to be secondary to a first branchial remnant.

such a patient, and the subsequent years have added other cases. In 1965, Lincoln[18] collected 32 patients with first branchial cleft abnormalities in a review of the literature.

To be excluded from first branchial cleft origin are the relatively common skin tabs and cartilaginous remnants of the ear, as well as preauricular cysts and sinus tracts. Most investigators[10, 13, 20, 27, 33] agree that these minor abnormalities are not of branchial cleft origin but occur simply from abnormal infolding and entrapment of epithelium during merger of the six hillocks (three from the first branchial arch, three from the second branchial arch) that form the external pinna.

There is considerable evidence to support the noncleft origin of *preauricular* cysts and sinuses.[33] The sinuses often are very short and end blindly, never connecting internally to the external auditory canal or eustachian tube; characteristically, they terminate in a strand of tissue that blends with the periosteum of the bony wall of the external auditory canal. Preauricular cysts lie subcutaneously, often are multiple and invade more deeply only if infected. Furthermore, preauricular cysts and sinuses are lined by ectoderm without any hair, in keeping with their origin from the hairless ectoderm forming the external ear. Preauricular cysts may be ignored unless they become infected. After infection has subsided, the external orifice is circumscribed and the short tract, often only 1.0–1.5 cm long, excised—under local anesthesia in older children.

Typically, first branchial cleft cysts present swellings that lie in front of, behind or below the lobe of the external ear or in the submandibular area.[18, 20] External openings of first branchial cleft sinuses lie below the mandible and above the hyoid bone.[3, 18] Recurrent bouts of inflammation and/or spontaneous or surgically aided drainage is the rule, the difficulty often originating in childhood[41, 45] but sometimes not coming to diagnostic clarification or successful surgical treatment until young or middle adulthood[3, 27] (Fig. 37–7). Only one-third of first branchial cleft anomalies have internal openings and are therefore true fistulas;[18] the internal openings involve the external auditory canal, either its bony or membranous portions. Theoretically, this internal connection could be associated with the eustachian tube; Randall and Royster's cases 6 and 7 may be examples.[27] In any event, complete fistulas are understandably associated with drainage from the external auditory canal.

Regardless of whether the abnormality is in the form of a sinus, cyst or fistula, the invariable juxtaposition of the branchial remnant to the parotid gland[17, 45] and facial nerve (seventh cranial)[8] is the most important anatomic feature for the surgeon who is contemplating its excision[18, 19, 27, 33, 41] (Fig. 37–8). Facial nerve anomalies make the dissection more difficult.[17] This operation needs to be carried out after careful consideration of the regional anatomy and with good light and assistance to avoid facial nerve injury. Preoperative "mapping" of the tract with contrast dye and x-rays taken in different planes may aid safe surgical removal.[18]

First branchial cleft sinuses extend medioposteriorly in the neck variable distances, typically in the direction of the external auditory canal, where they terminate blindly (Fig. 37–3). Cysts tend to be located below the pinna or in the submaxillary triangle,[18] although DeBord's second case[6] reports a child with an infected cyst located anterior to the left ear. The first branchial cleft tract can pass superficially or deep to the main facial nerve or bear any variety of relationships to its three main branches, often traveling within the substance of the parotid gland[18, 27, 33, 41] (Fig. 37–8).

Recurrent bouts of infection about and below the pinna

should heighten the likelihood of a branchial remnant in the mind of the surgeon (Fig. 37–7). Cat-scratch disease and other causes of chronic upper cervical lymphadenitis (scrofula, atypical mycobacterium, histoplasmosis, actinomycosis) should be excluded by appropriate skin and blood tests and cultures.

Histologically, first branchial cleft abnormalities are similar to those of second cleft derivation.[18] The tract is lined by stratified squamous epithelium, often with skin appendages such as hair follicles, sweat glands and sebaceous glands. The deeper aspects of the tracts may be surrounded by hyalin cartilage[3, 4] or striated muscle.[27] Acute and chronic inflammation occurs in those with infection. Severe previous infection may completely destroy the epithelial lining.[27]

TREATMENT.—Complete excision is the primary goal in treating all branchial cleft abnormalities. Because first branchial cleft remnants are infected so commonly, antibiotics and warm soaks often are necessary. Abscess formation demands incision and drainage, with appropriate aftercare of the wound. Definitive excision is delayed until all clinical signs of inflammation have disappeared.

Operation must be performed in a regular operating room with adequate equipment (nerve stimulators, probes, etc.) and assistants. We recommend an incision that exposes parotid gland and facial nerve. We use a vertical incision just in front of the ear, curved beneath the lower ear lobule and then carried forward in a curvilinear direction along a skin crease across the upper neck (Fig. 37–8). Naturally occurring external openings are incorporated in an ellipse of the lower sweep of this incision. An external opening that was created by spontaneous or surgical drainage of a cyst abscess often requires a second incision to circumscribe the scar. In any event, an anterior skin flap is developed to expose the superficial lobe of the parotid gland.

The tract then is carefully dissected from below upward. It may be helpful to cannulate and inject the tract with dye to facilitate its dissection, particularly when infection has obscured the path of the tract and complicated its dissection from surrounding structures. As the tract approaches the parotid gland, the root of the facial nerve is identified, preferably from the point where it emerges through the stylomastoid foramen; the faradic nerve stimulator facilitates search for the nerve. The nerve root and its three primary branches are exposed, a step that often requires freeing up the posterior part of the superficial lobe of the parotid gland. Then, and

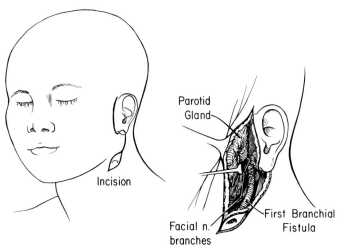

Fig. 37–8.—First branchial fistula—operative removal.

only then, can the relationship of the tract to the nerve or its branches be precisely determined (Fig. 37–8). The tract is freed from the nerve and dissected to its medial extreme, which commonly abuts against (or opens into) the external auditory canal. Occasionally, the tract bifurcates, and both of its branches then must be followed; one will end at or in the external auditory canal and the other may connect harmlessly to an ostium in the ear lobe. The tract is suture-ligated flush with the ear canal, and the specimen is removed. The wound is closed in layers and drained only if inflammatory tissue or pus has been encountered.

As in all other congenital abnormalities, complete excision at the time of the first surgical sitting is desirable. Therefore, patients with first branchial cleft abnormalities should be referred to a surgeon skilled in the embryology and anatomy of this area and capable of extirpating branchial remnants without damage to the facial nerve or other structures in the area.

The postoperative course of these patients usually is uncomplicated, with resumption of feedings the next day. I do not dress the wound unless it has been drained. The drain usually is removed within 48 hours. Mild temporary paresis of the mandibular branch of the facial nerve, which gradually disappears within 6 weeks, is common. A cosmetically pleasing scar results when the tract has been successfully and completely excised.

Midline Neck Masses

Masses that occupy the anterior midline of the neck are fairly common in childhood and usually are of surgical import. The *age* at which they appear often suggests diagnosis. Midline neck masses in the newborn are rare; whereas almost all are benign, they may produce airway problems by distorting and compressing the neonatal trachea. These lesions include cystic hygroma, hemangiomas, teratomas, thyroid hyperplasia and midline ectopic thyroid tissue. From 6 months on, thyroglossal remnants begin to make their appearance as the most common anterior midline neck mass. Excluding goiter, thyroglossal remnants predominate throughout childhood and young adulthood, with dermoid (inclusion) cysts a close second.

Location of the mass often suggests its nature. Thus, a midline submental neck lymph node generally enlarges in response to infection originating near the midline in the floor of the mouth or alveolar ridge. Careful bimanual palpation through the floor of the mouth reveals that the submental mass is not truly solitary or truly midline and is solid rather than cystic; careful inspection of the floor of the mouth often discloses the portal of entry for the infection that triggered the lymphadenitis. Antibiotics and soaks are used in treatment; occasionally, excision is required for differential diagnosis of a submental node that persists.

Dermoid (Inclusion) Cysts

If a midline mass is juxtaposed to hyoid bone, thyroglossal remnants or dermoid (inclusion) cysts are the likely cause. The dermoid cyst is more superficially located than the thyroglossal cyst; it does not move with swallowing or protrusion of the tongue, it often is noted to connect with the underside of the skin and it rarely has any inflammatory trappings. Midline dermoid cysts probably represent entrapment of epithelium of branchial arch origin at the time of embryologic midline fusion. Histologically, they consist of skin epithelium with skin appendages, hair and desquamated epithelial debris that appears cheesy-white. At operation, dermoid cysts lack a deep-seated tract connecting them to hyoid or other neck structures, and their excision is simple and curative.

Midline Cervical Clefts

Although neither producing a mass nor having any embryologic relationship to the thyroglossal apparatus, the very rare midline cervical cleft must be included in any treatise on midline neck abnormalities in children.[11] These curious anomalies present as vertically oriented patches of thinly epithelialized tissue in the low anterior midline of the neck; they measure several centimeters in length and 4–6 mm wide (Fig. 37–9, *A*). They may weep from a raw and reddish surface or have a pale, shiny surface; occasionally they are adorned by skin tabs, short sinuses that end blindly or cartilaginous excrescences.

Midline cervical clefts occur because of imperfect midline

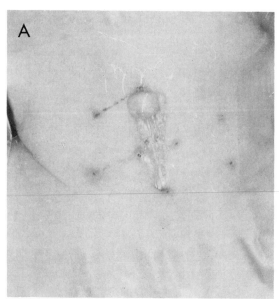
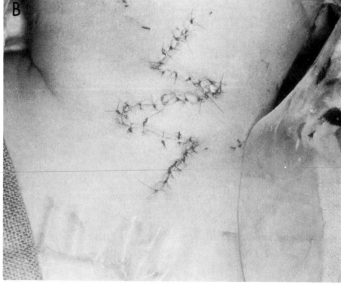

Fig. 37–9.—Midline cervical cleft. **A,** photograph of cleft with skin and cartilaginous excrescence at its upper end. The ink marks were used to fashion **B,** the "Z-plasty" incision that was used to avoid a longitudinal midline scar that might result in a bridling contracture.

fusion of the paired branchial arch tissue during the third and fourth gestational weeks. The abnormality is of cosmetic importance only, and should be removed electively. Excision is easily carried out through an elliptical incision, but at the expense of an unsightly scar that contracts and foreshortens with time. Thus, a series of "Z-plasty" incisions must be used to break up the suture line and leave a functionally and cosmetically pleasing scar (Fig. 37–9, *B*).

Thyroglossal Remnants

Thyroglossal remnants produce midline masses from the base of the tongue to the pyramidal lobe of the thyroid gland. Their most common manifestation is a cyst located at or just below the hyoid bone nearly exactly in the anterior midline of the neck. Second in frequency to cervical adenitis as a cause of neck masses,[13] thyroglossal remnants are 3 times more common than branchial remnants.[10] Undoubtedly they are responsible for the greatest number of *midline* childhood neck masses. Thyroglossal remnants usually are not recognized before the second birthday, and are discovered with increasing frequency throughout later years of childhood. One-third of them are not diagnosed until adulthood.

Embryology of the Thyroglossal Apparatus

Since thyroglossal remnants result from misadventures in the embryologic development of the thyroid gland, both their understanding and principles of treatment are clarified by a review of thyroid embryology.[7, 10, 22, 25, 46] The thyroid gland is the earliest endocrine organ to appear in the pharynx. Its anlage is first recognized toward the end of the second gestational week (2.5 mm stage) as an evagination from the floor of the pharynx between the first and second branchial arches, in the area flanked by the two first pharyngeal pouches and juxtaposed to pericardium. The diverticulum arises from that part of the tongue later marked as the foramen cecum. The thyroglossal tract consists of a column of epithelial cells that canalize to form a lumen.

The tract descends in the anterior midline of the neck following descent of the *septum transversum* and the heart, the head structures of the embryo growing away from it in a cephalad direction. During the sixth week of gestation, the thyroglossal tract is encompassed by fusion of the two halves of the body of the hyoid bone (second and third branchial arch origin), dividing the tract into upper and lower segments (Fig. 37–2). Simultaneously, the thyroglossal tract is buried beneath the second arch epithelium (ectoderm), which fuses superficially in the midline.

During the seventh gestational week, the tip of the thyroglossal tract thickens into recognizable lateral thyroid lobes at the level of the second tracheal ring, which remain connected across the anterior midline by the isthmus. The calcitonin-producing ultimobranchial bodies are contributed to the lateral thyroid lobes by epithelium of the fourth pharyngeal pouch and are the cells incriminated in the rare familial medullary thyroid carcinoma. Normally, all remnants of the thyroglossal tract above the thyroid isthmus disappear during the ninth or tenth gestational week.

Any segment of the thyroglossal tract that does not obliterate results in a midline neck abnormality of some type. The most common and innocent representative is the so-called pyramidal lobe of the thyroid gland, present in about 25%[1] to 50%[10] of people. The pyramidal lobe consists of thyroid tissue that can undergo all the physiologic and pathologic changes of normal thyroid gland (hyperplasia, adenoma, carcinoma). Generally, physical examination distinguishes this tissue as pyramidal lobe, which can be confirmed by thyroid scintiscan. Occasionally, a pyramidal lobe coexists with a thyroglossal cyst.

Ectopic Thyroid Tissue (see also Chap. 34)

An arrest in descent of the thyroid anlage produces ectopic thyroid tissue, which may lie anywhere from the foramen cecum of the tongue to the lower anterior midline of the neck. Ectopic thyroid usually is not associated with normally located thyroid tissue[15, 37] and represents the patient's only source of thyroid hormone. The most common ectopic location of thyroid is at the base of the tongue, more than 300 cases being recorded.[15] Lingual thyroid generally presents a visible and palpable mass at the base of the tongue, which may produce airway problems in the very young if unusually large.[1] Most children simply complain of a "lump in the throat." Since lingual thyroid can undergo all of the physiologic and pathologic changes of normally located thyroid tissue, transoral excision generally is recommended.

The next most common location for ectopic thyroid is in the anterior midline of the neck, just at or below the hyoid bone; at least 18 such patients have been reported.[23, 37] It presents a mass during infancy or childhood that is somewhat cosmetically disfiguring; since ectopic thyroid in this location displays the same physical characteristics as a thyroglossal duct cyst (location, motion with swallowing or protrusion of the tongue, etc.), its differentiation is difficult. If one suspects the true diagnosis preoperatively, thyroid scintiscan will quickly settle the issue; we recommend this if the mass dates back to infancy, as it does in the usual ectopic thyroid. However, thyroid scan should not be considered necessary in the work-up of all children suspected of having a thyroglossal cyst. Gross[11] found only 3 patients with ectopic midline thyroid during a time span in which he saw more than 300 children with thyroglossal abnormalities.

In the past, midline ectopic thyroid has been misdiagnosed at operation as thyroglossal duct cyst and excised. Since the mass generally contains the patient's only thyroid tissue, this renders the patient hypothyroid.[15, 23, 37] Careful inspection of the mass at operation will distinguish ectopic thyroid from thyroglossal cyst; ectopic thyroid is solid, not cystic, and has a deep purple color resembling normal thyroid tissue. Frozen section biopsy confirms its true nature. The surgeon then must explore the lower neck; if a normal thyroid gland is found, the ectopic thyroid is excised with impunity. However, if no normal thyroid tissue is found, two treatment options are open. The thyroid mass can be totally excised, saddling the patient with a lifetime of thyroid replacement. If frozen section reveals adenomas or other thyroid abnormalities, excision is recommended.[15, 23] Alternatively, the mass can be divided vertically in the midline into two halves. Since the blood supply to a midline ectopic thyroid comes in laterally, the vascular pedicle can be mobilized enough to rotate each half of the ectopic thyroid gland laterally underneath the strap muscles, where they remain inconspicuous and still subserve the patient's thyroid requirements.

Thyroglossal Cysts

Thyroglossal cysts are reasonably common; they are 3 times as common as branchial remnants[10] and rank second only to goiter as a cause of anterior neck masses in children.[13] The majority of thyroglossal duct cysts develop in childhood, Sammarco and McKenna[31] reporting 65% of patients less than 20 years of age at diagnosis. The majority make their clinical appearance after the second birthday and fully 50% are clinically apparent by the tenth birthday.[36, 42] Gross' series is restricted to children, two-thirds of whom had symptoms before the sixth birthday.[11] Average age at diagnosis was 4½ years at Childrens Hospital of Los Angeles.[35] In contrast, ectopic midline thyroid produces a midline neck mass from birth onward.

Sex incidence in thyroglossal cysts is about equal,[11, 13, 26, 32, 36] in contrast to most thyroid disorders, in which females predominate. The majority of thyroglossal cysts present simply as asymptomatic masses[11, 13] (Fig. 37–10). However, since thyroglossal cysts retain a connection to

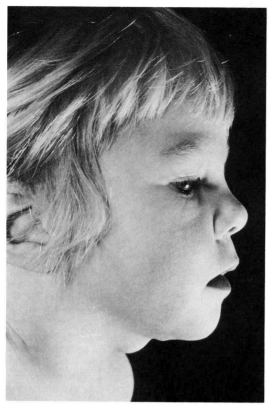

Fig. 37–10.—Thyroglossal duct cyst. Young girl with a midline mass at the hyoid level typical of a thyroglossal cyst.

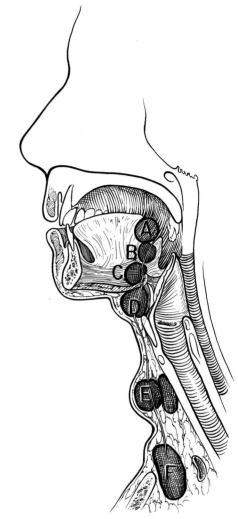

Fig. 37–11.—Thyroglossal cysts—diagram of locations. **A** and **B,** lingual (rare). **C** and **D,** adjacent to hyoid bone (common). **E** and **F,** suprasternal fossa (rare).

the mouth at the foramen cecum, infection by oral bacteria can occur. A cyst that develops an abscess may drain to the outside either spontaneously or by surgical incision. This creates an external draining sinus that periodically seals over only to refester later. The older literature reports that one-third of patients with thyroglossal cyst had external sinuses when first seen,[11, 32] but, in our recent experience, only 5% have drained externally. Thyroglossal cysts never have primary external openings, because the thyroglossal tract embryologically never reaches the surface of the neck. Occasionally, they attach to a pyramidal lobe of thyroid.

Classically, thyroglossal cysts are located in the midline at or just below the hyoid bone (Fig. 37–10). Ward *et al.*[42, 43] reported 105 patients with thyroglossal cysts, of which only 2% were lingual in location; 80% were juxtaposed to the hyoid bone, 25% being submental (just above the hyoid) (Fig. 37–11). Suprahyoid thyroglossal cysts must be distinguished from submental dermoid cysts. A thyroglossal cyst should rise on protrusion of the tongue; a dermoid cyst will not. Only 7% of thyroglossal cysts are suprasternal in location,[42, 43] where they commonly are mistaken for a mass of thyroid origin or a low-lying dermoid (inclusion) cyst. Thyroid scanning will exclude the former whereas the latter is confirmed at operation because it has no cephalad tract; histologic study is the final arbiter.

On physical examination, the thyroglossal cyst mass is smooth, round, elastic and opaque. It is nontender unless infected, when it will also exhibit erythema of the overlying skin. Only about 1% of thyroglossal cysts present lateral to the midline.[32, 35, 39]

Histologic study of the tissue lining thyroglossal cysts generally reveals pseudostratified ciliated columnar respi-

ratory epithelium (60%), with stratified squamous epithelium predominating in the remainder.[1] Occasionally, transitional or cuboidal epithelium is seen.[36] The tissue adjacent to the cysts is fibrous, and upward of 20% harbor recognizable thyroid tissue.[32, 42, 44] Lymphoid tissue is present in about 20% of cases.[1, 44] A thyroglossal cyst that has been chronically inflamed may have its epithelial lining replaced by granulation, inflammatory or fibrous tissue. The tract that connects the thyroglossal cyst to the base of the tongue commonly is lined by mucus-secreting glands,[36, 44] accounting for the mucinous drainage that ensues after spontaneous or surgical drainage of a thyroglossal cyst abscess.

Thyroglossal cysts are treated by complete excision of the cyst and its cephalad tract to the base of the tongue. This goal is best achieved before infection, abscess or drainage occur. We recommend excision when the mass is discovered, unless there are good reasons for delaying operation.

Another reason for early excision of thyroglossal remnants is the occasional malignancy that arises in them. Shepard and Rosenfeld[32] summarized from the world literature 35 cases of carcinoma that arose in thyroglossal remnants. Although the mean age at diagnosis was 55 years, 3 occurred in children during the first decade of life and 3 during the second decade. Twenty-nine were papillary adenocarcinomas of thyroid tissue that was contained within the wall of the thyroglossal remnant and 2 were squamous carcinoma.

Recurrence following excision of an infected or previously drained thyroglossal duct cyst is 1½ times that of an intact cyst.[35] The infected thyroglossal duct cyst is first treated by warm soaks and antibiotics. With actual or impending drainage, incision and drainage is required; excision is delayed until the inflammatory reaction has completely resolved.

A second key issue regarding recurrence centers around removing the midportion of the body of the hyoid bone en bloc with the cyst.[43] Gross[11] had 9 of 27 recur without hyoid bone removal, compared with less than 5% with its removal. The close embryologic association of the hyoid bone to the thyroglossal tract explains the need to resect the central third of the body of the hyoid bone with the thyroglossal cyst (Fig. 37–2), since epithelial tissue commonly is found within the bone or periosteum. Furthermore, since there always is an epithelial connection extending to the base of the tongue, dissection must continue in the midline up to the foramen cecum, where the tract is suture-ligated flush with the tongue mucosa.

Operation is carried out under endotracheal intubation with the patient in the supine position with the head and neck extended. The chin is carefully positioned midline to favor symmetry of the incision.

The transverse incision is carefully made exactly in a skin crease at or just above the palpable cyst. If a sinus is present, it is encompassed by a central ellipse. A vertical incision is never used. A parallel, higher "stepladder" incision is needed only in the rare suprasternal cyst. Aspiration or dye injection into the cyst is not recommended.

The skin incision is carried through platysma and cervical fascia until the cyst wall is exposed. Skin flaps are developed sufficient for careful dissection around the cyst; this dissection is difficult only following recent infection in the cyst. The cyst routinely lies superficial to the sternohyoid muscles and generally is closely attached to the inferoanterior body of the hyoid bone.

When the hyoid bone has been identified and cleared, the scissors are swept under the sternohyoid muscles where they insert into the central body of the hyoid; this insertion is divided, leaving a cuff of muscle attached to bone. The floor of the dissecting field is the tough, distinctive thyro-

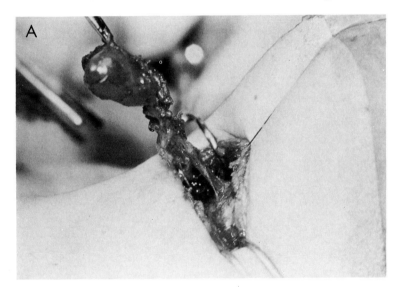

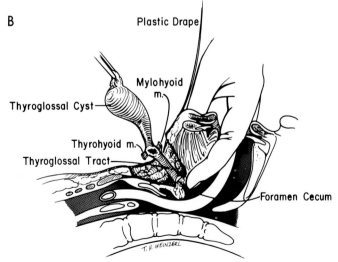

Fig. 37–12.—Thyroglossal duct cyst—specimen and operation. **A,** photograph of removal of thyroglossal cyst, tract and central portion of hyoid bone. **B,** diagram that identifies the surgical specimen seen in the photograph and shows the finger in the mouth to elevate the specimen and mark the foramen cecum for the surgeon.

hyoid membrane. A cuff of mylohyoid muscle is incised above the body of the hyoid bone in a similar manner, thus freeing the central portion of the hyoid bone from its muscular attachments both above and below.

The hyoid bone then is divided so that the central one-third of the body (which is attached to the cyst) is freed; this is done with scalpel or Mayo scissors in the young child and bone cutters in older children. A 1-cm-wide tract of tissue is left attached to the superoposterior border of the freed hyoid bone and this core of tissue is dissected out to the foramen cecum. This is Sistrunk's major contribution to the operation.[34] If one attempts to skeletonize the tract leading from the hyoid bone to the foramen cecum, he may cut across islands of epithelium that protrude as buds from this tract and which, if left behind, lead to postoperative recurrence. Thus, small cuffs of geniohyoid and genioglossus muscles are removed with the tract. This part of the dissection is facilitated by having an assistant elevate the foramen cecum into the dissecting field by finger pressure from inside the mouth. The surgeon then can palpate the finger through the tongue epithelium to pinpoint accurately the upper extent of the dissection (Fig. 37–12).

The tract is suture-ligated with a nonabsorbable suture flush with tongue epithelium and removed. Tongue muscles are loosely reapproximated. Although it is not necessary to coapt the cut edges of hyoid bone, I generally reunite them with a few interrupted nonabsorbable sutures, after which mylohyoid and thyrohyoid muscles are reattached to bone. The wound is drained only if there has been recent infection or if the thyroglossal cyst contents spill into the field. The wound is closed in layers, inverted absorbable sutures being used for the platysma muscle. We close the skin subcuticularly.

Recurrence should be less that 5%,[11, 42] although figures as high as 20% in complicated cases have been reported.[35] Reaccumulation of secretions within a portion of epithelium-lined tract that was left behind is the cause of most recurrences. Recovery usually is prompt, the patient taking oral fluids the night of operation and a full diet the next day. Most patients can safely be discharged from the hospital on the first or second postoperative day. The wounds heal promptly and, if the incision is placed within a skin crease, leave cosmetically pleasing scars.

Low Neck Masses

Special consideration should be given to the infant or child with a cystic mass low in the root of the neck. The majority of these masses are cystic hygromas, 5% of which pass from the neck through the thoracic inlet to involve the upper mediastinum. These are discussed elsewhere (see Chap. 36). Two other possible causes must be considered, both rare: ectopic bronchogenic cyst and ectopic cyst of thymic origin.

Ectopic Bronchogenic Cysts

Most bronchogenic cysts are located in the lung hilum or adjacent to the carina or lower trachea. Rarely, one is found juxtaposed to the lower cervical trachea, in which position it presents as a low neck mass (Fig. 37–13). In this ectopic locale, bronchogenic cysts indent the trachea and generally come to light on investigation of an infant or preschool child with stridor, tracheal deviation or a low-lying neck mass. They characteristically do not connect to the tracheal lumen.

Precise soft tissue radiographs will pinpoint the location of the mass by its tracheal indentation. Operation discloses a unilocular, thin-walled paratracheal cyst that can be dissected cleanly away from the trachea and adjacent great vessels. Diagnosis of the true nature of the cyst generally rests with microscopic demonstration of an inner lining of respiratory epithelium with smooth muscle and occasionally bits of cartilage in its wall.

Ectopic Thymic Cysts

Thymic cysts comprise 5% of mediastinal cysts and tumors.[29] They generally are confined to the upper anterior mediastinum, where they produce respiratory complaints and are discovered on chest radiographs. However, at least 15 neck cysts have been reported[9] that have thymic tissue in their walls, and occasionally mediastinal thymic cysts will enlarge through the thoracic inlet to present a low-lying mass in the root of the neck Fig. 37–14). Understandably, in

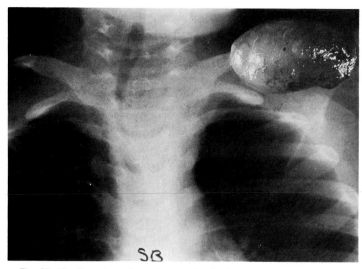

Fig. 37–13.—Bronchogenic cyst presenting in the neck. Radiograph of upper chest and neck showing trachea deviated to the right by a low neck mass that proved to be an ectopic bronchogenic cyst, which is superimposed in the upper right corner of the figure.

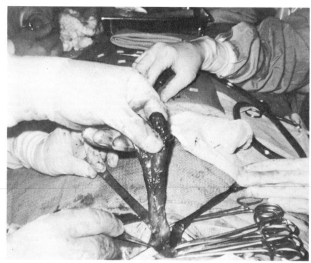

Fig. 37–14.—Cervical thymic cyst. Left-sided neck cyst, which proved to be an ectopic thymic cyst, being dissected from the anterior mediastinum through a low cervical incision. (Courtesy of Dr. Gary Smith, Burlington, Iowa.)

these ectopic locations they commonly are mistaken for cystic hygromas or branchial cysts. Chest radiographs help diagnose those with mediastinal components: cystic hygroma should pass through the inlet to one side or the other (generally left) whereas the thymic cyst should lie anterior to the trachea; furthermore, the cystic hygroma occupies the superior pleural space and displaces the upper lobe caudad (again generally on the left side) while the main thoracic mass of the thymic cyst occupies the anterior mediastinum. Thymic cysts in the neck are distinguished from branchial cysts only on histologic study; they generally produce a firm, nonmovable and nontender lateral neck mass[10] that lies adjacent to the carotid sheath. Because of their embryologic derivation from the third pharyngeal pouch, thymic neck cysts may have tracts that extend caudad to enter the anterior mediastinum[9] (Fig. 37–14).

The thymic cyst usually can be completely and safely removed via a transverse cervical incision centered over the palpable mass. If those with mediastinal extensions or tracts cannot be safely lifted out of the mediastinum through this incision, it may be necessary to split the upper sternum. The wound is not drained unless the thoracic duct is injured. Chest tubes are necessary only if the pleura is entered. The true nature of the cyst often rests with histologic study revealing thymic tissue in the cyst wall.

REFERENCES

1. Ackerman, L. V., and Rosai, J.: Thyroid Gland, in *Surgical Pathology* (5th ed.; St. Louis: The C. V. Mosby Company, 1974), Chap. 9.
2. Albers, G. D.: Branchial anomalies, JAMA 183:399; 1963.
3. Bill, A. H., Jr.: Branchiogenic Cysts and Sinuses, in Mustard, W. T., *et al.* (eds.), *Pediatric Surgery* (2d ed.; Chicago: Year Book Medical Publishers, Inc., 1969), Chap. 22.
4. Bill, A. H., Jr., and Vadheim, J. L.: Cysts, sinuses and fistulas of the neck arising from the first and second branchial clefts, Ann. Surg. 142:904, 1955.
5. Brauer, R. O.: Congenital Cysts and Tumors of the Neck, in *Reconstructive Plastic Surgery* (Philadelphia and London: W. B. Saunders Company, 1964), Chap. 31.
6. DeBord, R. A.: First branchial cleft sinus, Arch. Surg. 81:228, 1960.
7. Dische, S., and Berg, P. K.: An investigation of the thyroglossal tract using the radioisotope scan, Clin. Radiol. 14:298, 1963.
8. Frazer, J. E., and Bertwistle, A. P.: The nomenclature of disease states caused by certain vestigial structures in the neck, Br. J. Surg. 2:131, 1923.
9. Gaeckle, D. J., Lt., and Gerber, M. L., Capt.: Thymic cyst in the neck, Am. J. Surg. 103:755, 1962.
10. Gray, S. W., and Skandalakis, J. E.: The Pharynx and Its Derivatives, in *Embryology for Surgeons: The Embryological Basis for the Treatment of Congenital Defects* (Philadelphia, London and Toronto: W. B. Saunders, Company, 1972), Chap. 2.
11. Gross, R. E.: *The Surgery of Infancy and Childhood* (Philadelphia and London: W. B. Saunders Company, 1953).
12. Hyndman, O. R., and Light, G.: The branchial apparatus, Arch. Surg. 19:410, 1929.
13. Jaffe, B. F.: Neck Masses and Malignant Tumors of the Head and Neck, in Ferguson, C. F., and Kendig, E. L., Jr. (eds.), *Pediatric Otolaryngology* (Philadelphia, London and Toronto: W. B. Saunders Company, 1972), Chap. 100.
14. Katubig, D., and Damjanov, I.: Branchial cleft carcinoma, Arch. Otolaryngol. 89:750, 1969.
15. Klopp, C. T., and Kirson, S. M.: Therapeutic problems with ectopic non-cancerous follicular thyroid tissue in the neck: 18 case reports according to etiologic factors, Ann. Surg. 163:653, 1966.
16. Lee, K., and Klein, T. R.: Surgery of Cysts and Tumors of the Neck, in *Otolaryngology* (Philadelphia, London and Toronto: W. B. Saunders Company, 1973), Chap. 49.
17. Leonard, J. R., Maran, A. G., and Huffman, W. C.: Branchial cleft cysts in the parotid gland; facial nerve anomaly, Plast. Reconstr. Surg. 41:493, 1968.
18. Lincoln, J. C. R.: Cervico-auricular fistulae, Arch. Dis. Child. 40:218, 1965.
19. Lindsay, W. K.: The Neck, in *Plastic Surgery in Infancy and Childhood* (Philadelphia: W. B. Saunders Company, 1971), Chap. 23.
20. Lyall, D., and Stahl, W. M., Jr.: Lateral cervical cysts, sinuses and fistulas of congenital origin, Surg. Gynecol. Obstet. 102:IAS 417, 1956.
21. Martin, H., Morfit, H. M., and Ehrlich, H.: The case for branchiogenic cancer, Ann. Surg. 132:867, 1950.
22. Meyer, H. W.: Congenital cysts and fistulae of the neck, Ann. Surg. 95:1, 1932.
23. Meyerowitz, B. R., and Buchholz, R. B.: Midline cervical ectopic thyroid tissue, Surgery 65:358, 1969.
24. Neel, H. B., and Pemberton, J. DeJ.: Lateral cervical cysts and fistulae; clinical and pathological study, Surgery 18:267, 1945.
25. Norris, E. H.: The early morphogenesis of the human thyroid gland, Surg. Clin. North Am. 9:1355, 1929.
26. Pemberton, J. DeJ., and Stalker, L. K.: Thyroglossal cysts, sinuses and fistulae, Ann. Surg. 111:950, 1940.
27. Randall, P., and Royster, H. P.: First branchial cleft anomalies, Plast. Reconstr. Surg. 31:497, 1963.
28. Rankow, R. M., and Hanford, J. M.: Congenital anomalies of the first branchial cleft, Surg. Gynecol. Obstet. 96:102, 1953.
29. Ravitch, M. M., and Sabiston, D. C., Jr.: Mediastinal Infections and Tumors, in Mustard, W. T., *et al.* (eds.), *Pediatric Surgery* (2d ed.; Chicago: Year Book Medical Publishers, Inc., 1969), Chap. 29.
30. Rogers, W. M.: Normal and Anomalous Development of the Thyroid, in Werner, S. C., and Ingbar, S. H. (eds.), *The Thyroid* (3d ed.; New York: Harper & Row, 1971), Chap. 22.
31. Sammarco, G. J., and McKenna, J.: Thyroglossal duct cysts in the elderly, Geriatrics 25:98, 1970.
32. Shepard, G. H., and Rosenfeld, L.: Carcinoma of thyroglossal duct remnants, Am. J. Surg. 116:125, 1968.
33. Singer, R.: A new technique for extirpation of preauricular cysts, Am. J. Surg. 111:291, 1966.
34. Sistrunk, W. E.: The surgical treatment of cysts of the thyroglossal tract, Ann. Surg. 71:121, 1920.
35. Snyder, W. H., Jr., and Pollock, W. F.: Thyroglossal Cysts and Midline Clefts, in Mustard, W. T., *et al.* (eds.), *Pediatric Surgery* (2d ed.; Chicago: Year Book Medical Publishers, Inc., 1969), Chap. 22.
36. Stahl, W. M., Jr., and Lyall, D.: Cervical cysts and fistulae of thyroglossal tract origin, Ann. Surg. 139:123, 1954.
37. Strickland, A. L., Macfie, J. A., VanWyk, J. J., and French, F. S.: Ectopic thyroid glands simulating thyroglossal duct cysts, JAMA 208:307, 1969.
38. Swenson, O.: Malformations of the head and neck, in *Pediatric Surgery* (2d ed.; New York: Appleton-Century-Crofts, 1962), Chap. 6.
39. Thompson, C. A., and Smith, J. W.: Thyroglossal duct cyst presenting laterally, JAMA 201:565, 1967.
40. Toomey, J. M.: Cysts and tumors of the pharynx, in *Otolaryngology* (Philadelphia, London and Toronto: W. B. Saunders Company, 1973), Chap. 23.
41. Trail, M. L., Lyons, G. D., Jr., and Creely, J. J., Jr.: Anomalies of the first branchial cleft, South. Med. J. 65:716, 1972.
42. Ward, G. E., Hendrick, J. W., and Chambers, R. G.: Branchiogenic anomalies: Results of 70 cases observed at Johns Hopkins Hospital between 1926 and 1946, West. J. Surg. 57:536, 1949.
43. Ward, G. E., Hendrick, J. W., and Chambers, R. G.: Thyroglossal tract abnormalities, Surg. Gynecol. Obstet. 89:729, 1949.
44. Ward, P. H., Strahan, R. W., Acquerelli, M., and Harris, P. F.: The many faces of cysts of the thyroglossal duct, Trans. Am. Acad. Ophthalmol. Otolaryngol. 74:310, 1970.
45. Weissman, F., and Horwitz, F.: Sinus of the first branchial cleft, Plast. Reconstr. Surg. 31:79, 1963.
46. Wenglowski, R.: Fistulae and cysts of the neck, Arch. Klin. Chir. 98:151, 1912.

38 PETER G. JONES

Torticollis

HISTORY.—Torticollis as a deformity was first mentioned by Plutarch in describing Alexander the Great, but the diagnosis is in doubt.[31] Antyllus may have performed tenotomies in about 350 A.D., but the first authentic division of the sternocleidomastoid was done by Isaac Minnius in Amsterdam about 1641.[36] A sternocleidomastoid tumor was first described by Heusinger[14] in 1826, and torticollis was a subject of interest to Dupuytren[10] and many of the German surgeons of the nineteenth century.[7, 17, 20, 26, 30, 32, 34, 38-40]

There are many causes of torticollis in childhood; for example, cervical hemivertebrae, cervical adenitis, acute fasciitis, abnormal position in utero and imbalance of the ocular muscles, but the most common type of torticollis in pediatric practice is the result of fibrosis in the sternocleidomastoid muscle.

Eight theories have been put forward to explain this condition,[1, 9, 17, 20, 21, 25, 28, 32, 34, 37, 39] but none is completely satisfactory. All one can say is that the condition probably is an idiopathic intrauterine embryopathy,[18] which merely reveals our ignorance.

Pathology

The basic abnormality is endomysial fibrosis, the deposition of collagen and fibroblasts around individual muscle fibers that undergo atrophy. The sarcoplasmic nuclei are compacted to form "muscle giant cells," which appear to be multinucleated although not necessarily large (Fig. 38–1). Macrophages containing hemosiderin are present rarely.

The severity and distribution of the fibrosis differ widely from patient to patient and from one fascicle to another. In some cases (2–3%), it is obviously bilateral, and in an additional number this is suspected but not easily proved.

The remarkably mature fibrous tissue in material from neonates strongly suggests that the disease begins well before birth[8, 9, 18, 24] and probably is the cause, not the result, of obstetric difficulties. The reported incidence of breech delivery varies from series to series,[23] but is about 20%, 7 times the "normal" incidence, which suggests that the fibrosis may affect the position of the fetus in utero and perhaps prevent normal engagement of the head in the maternal pelvis.

In older children there is some additional interfascicular fibrosis, and degenerating muscle fibers can be seen at all ages, probably a form of disuse atrophy produced by limitation of movement by the fibrosis.

Clinical Picture

In a prospective series of 100 infants with sternomastoid fibrosis,[18] 66% had a "tumor" in the muscle. In the other 34% there was fibrosis but no tumor, which would help to explain why only a few of the older children with torticollis have a history of a tumor in the neonatal period (6–20%).

IN INFANTS.—The tumor is a hard, spindle-shaped, painless, discrete swelling 1–3 cm in diameter within the substance of the muscle. It develops some 14–21 days after birth and occurs in about 0.4% of all births, as found in a prospective study.[4] Torticollis is not always present[16]; in the neonate there may be little or no inclination of the head to the side; more often there is pure rotation of the head and face to the side opposite the tumor (Fig. 38–2). The tumor subsequently becomes less discrete and more obviously occupies the whole length of the muscle, which is much thicker than normal.

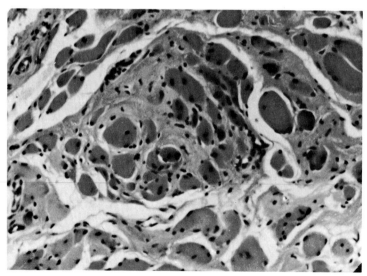

Fig. 38–1.—Specimen from the center of a large persistent sternocleidomastoid tumor in a 9-month-old boy. Note decreased size of muscle fibers undergoing atrophy, some becoming giant cells. The laminae of collagen are thicker than usual.

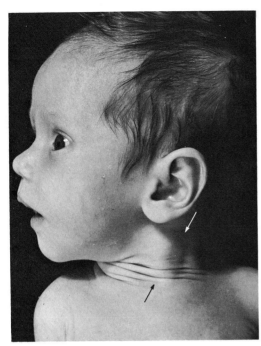

Fig. 38–2.—A tumor affecting both heads of the left sternocleidomastoid of a 3-week-old infant. Note the rotation toward the opposite side and absence of angulation. The tumor is more prominent than usual because of loss of subcutaneous fat associated with pyloric stenosis.

The natural history of the tumor has been determined by a follow-up of 100 infants[18] (Fig. 38–3). In half of them, the muscle became completely normal clinically by the age of 6 months, without any residual fibrosis detectable by synchronous palpation of both muscles. In another 30%, some fibrosis still was palpable at 12 months of age, but not sufficient to cause torticollis.

In a few cases (9%), the tumor persisted throughout the first year of life, or even grew steadily larger, to produce torticollis at the age of 9–15 months.

In infants with fibrosis but no tumor (34%), torticollis was the presenting symptom. The muscle was uniformly fibrous throughout, part or all of it forming a tight band. The outcome and the clinical categories (Fig. 38–4) are much the same as in those with a tumor, although fewer required early operation.

IN OLDER CHILDREN.—Torticollis may develop at any age, and its appearance probably depends on three factors: the severity and the distribution of the fibrosis, and the indi-

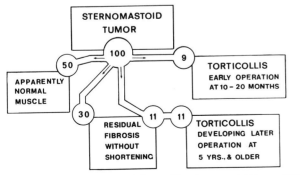

Fig. 38–3.—The outcome in 100 infants with a sternomastoid tumor. These interim figures, obtained when the oldest patient was 12 years old, remained the same after a further 10 years of observation.

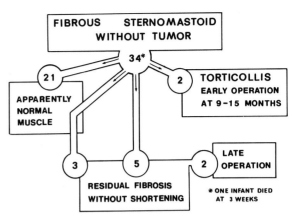

Fig. 38–4.—The outcome in 34 infants with fibrotic muscle but no tumor. One infant died of cerebral birth injuries at 3 weeks of age.

vidual pattern of growth in the particular patient; for example, a sustained spurt in growth at any age may lead to the development of torticollis. In most of the children first seen at 5–10 years of age, fibrous muscular torticollis develops without any known preliminary signs, but in the light of prospective studies it is likely that the latent fibrosis was present and that the fibrosis was congenital, regardless of the age at which the torticollis appeared.

Secondary Effects

Torticollis in early infancy is manifested by rotation of the head toward the opposite side. If this persists for the first 3 months of life and the infant is permitted to lie in this habitual position, the cranium becomes deformed (Fig. 38–5) by gravitational forces that produce a type of craniofacial asymmetry called plagiocephaly (Fig. 38–6). This affects all four quadrants of the cranium, and when the flat frontal area is on the same side as the fibrotic muscle, the plagiocephaly is said to be concordant. In children who have plagiocephaly

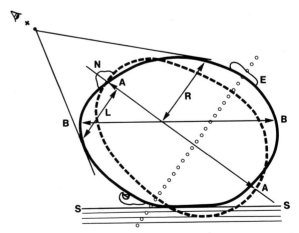

Fig. 38–5.—The development and nature of one isomer of plagiocephaly. The interrupted line indicates the basic symmetric shape of the cranium as seen from the vertex. AA, the normal sagittal axis; SS, the surface on which the head rests, with rotation toward the left. The solid line depicts the plagiocephaly, and BB the new axis of the longest diameter. The right frontal area is flattened; the right ear is situated more posteriorly than the left ear (line of circles), which becomes curled forward during rotation. When viewed from in front at X, the right half of the face (R) appears wider than the left (L). The right sternocleidomastoid was fibrotic and the resulting deformity concordant.

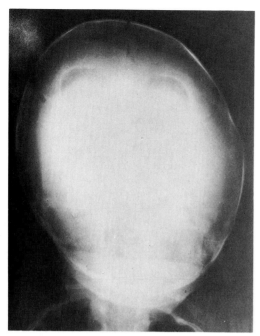

Fig. 38–6.—Radiographic plagiocephaly in child with torticollis—a posteroanterior film taken with head fully flexed and beam directed 30 degrees below the horizontal plane.

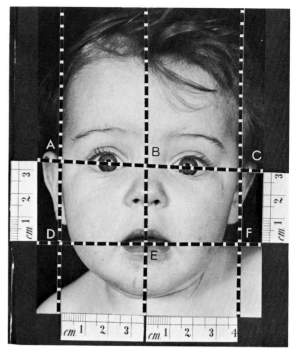

Fig. 38–7.—Assessment of hemihypoplasia on a photograph of a 10-month-old girl with torticollis, showing decreased height and increased width of one half of the face. *ABC,* line drawn through the canthi; *DEF,* line drawn through angles of the mouth; *BE,* the midline. Note that *ABC* and *DEF* are not parallel, *CF* is less than *AD,* and *DE* is less than *EF.*

at birth, it may or may not be concordant with the affected muscle.[18]

Plagiocephaly may be accompanied by an apparent increase of width of one half of the face (Fig. 38–5), which may be confused with hemihypoplasia (see Fig. 38–7) unless it is appreciated that in plagiocephalic asymmetry of the face there is no diminution of the orbitomental distance, but rather a wider half on the flattened side (Fig. 38–5). Having been slowly progressive until the infant is 4–5 months of age, plagiocephaly is halted when the infant can sit up, and slowly returns toward normal in the next 2 years but may never completely disappear.[5]

FACIAL HEMIHYPOPLASIA.—This form of asymmetry occurs with torticollis due to any cause. In infants with marked sternomastoid fibrosis and angulation of the head, it takes about 8 months to develop and the mechanism is unexplained.

Hemihypoplasia (Fig. 38–7) is progressive as long as the torticollis persists, but is halted as soon as the tension in the sternocleidomastoid muscle is relieved by operation. Return toward normal probably continues for as long as there still is active growth in the facial skeleton, up to 18–20 years of age.

ATROPHY OF IPSILATERAL TRAPEZIUS.—This is a constant clinical finding in established torticollis, probably the result of disuse atrophy imposed by the fibrous sternocleidomastoid, and recovers in 2–6 months after operation.

Diagnosis

THE TUMOR.—The clinical signs are virtually diagnostic. Cervical lymphadenopathy, either inflammatory or neoplastic, occasionally may have some resemblance to a tumor but, on palpation, the node or nodes are not in the substance of the muscle.

A primary sarcoma in the sternocleidomastoid could pre-

sent difficulties, but no authentic case has ever been reported.[12]

POSTURAL TORTICOLLIS.—There is a syndrome of congenital asymmetry that includes torticollis[16] and one or more of the following: plagiocephaly, infantile scoliosis and minor asymmetry of the thorax. All are present at birth and steadily improve during the first 6 months. There are no bony abnormalities, no muscular fibrosis and no reduction of the range of passive rotation of the neck despite habitual torticollis. The syndrome probably is a persistence of the position in utero[16]; it improves spontaneously and requires no treatment.

NEUROMUSCULAR INCOORDINATION.—Infants with cerebral palsy, spasticity or athetosis, or normal infants between 4 and 6 months of age with temporary inconsequential delay in coordination, may present an inclination of the head to one side or to the other, or alternating. A careful neurologic examination, the normal texture of the sternocleidomastoid muscles and a full range of passive rotation all point to the correct diagnosis.

OCULAR TORTICOLLIS.—Imbalance of the extrinsic muscles of the eye causes ocular torticollis, which usually does not appear until 6–12 months of age. The sternocleidomastoid muscle is normal, but occasionally fibrosis coexists, in which case it can be exceptionally difficult to apportion the blame correctly. X-rays of the cervical spine are essential to exclude hemivertebrae in infants and dislocation or subluxation in older children.

Management

The natural history of the condition (see Figs. 38–4 and 38–5) shows that in some 80% of affected infants the fibrosis is not sufficient to require operative treatment.

CONSERVATIVE TREATMENT.—The value of passive manipulation has not been proved, although it is widely utilized. It may be beneficial and can do no harm unless the parents are obsessional or overanxious or the patient overreacts. Most mothers become confident and competent enough to place the chin on each acromion six to eight times on four or five occasions each day.

When passive rotation still is limited at the age of 7–8 months, the prognosis must be guarded and careful reviews at intervals of 1 month are necessary. Serial photographs of the face, preferably taken with the head in a cephalostat and under standardized conditions, are most helpful, and serial measurements on them (see Fig. 38–7) provide a more reliable index of progress than memory or clinical impression.

The criterion for operation, regardless of age, is the development of hemihypoplasia. In those with significant torticollis, facial hemihypoplasia invariably is present, although there is not always a linear relationship between the two conditions.

Acquired plagiocephaly, which develops in the first 3 months of life and always is concordant,[18] can be prevented by placing the infant to sleep on each side alternately, avoiding the supine position.

OPERATION.—The muscle can be divided at its upper[21] or lower[31] end or at both sites,[13] but transection in the middle third, through a lateral collar incision, is simplest and provides the best scar.[18] This incision also gives access to the fascia colli, which often is tight and may need to be divided anteriorly as far as the midline and posteriorly to the anterior border of the trapezius.

With the patient supine and a large sandbag under the upper thoracic spine, the head is turned slightly toward the opposite side and double draped so that a complete range of rotation can be effected during the operation without impairing the sterility of the field (Fig. 38–8).

The muscle is dissected at the level where the sternal and clavicular heads converge, some 1–1.5 cm below the exit of the accessory nerve. It then is divided carefully, picking up bleeding points.

The fascia colli then is incised from the anterior border of the trapezius to the anterior midline, although the amount of fibrosis varies from case to case. In severe torticollis, the fascia around the omohyoid muscle and the carotid sheath should also be released.

The head then is fully rotated while a finger palpates the depths of the wound to identify any residual bands requiring division.

The incision is closed with fine sutures to the subcutaneous fascia and a continuous subcuticular polyglycolic stitch to the skin. Two dressings are applied, a small inner layer of gauze and narrow adhesive tape, and a large outer wad of combined dressing or cotton wool, held in place by a wide crepe bandage. The outer dressing holds the head in a slightly overcorrected position and aids hemostasis by obliterating the space, up to 4 cm long, between the cut ends of the muscle.

For 48 hours the patient lies supine without a pillow and with the head held straight between two large sandbags. An alternative method is to nurse the patient on a raised frame with the head hanging over one end so that there is the fullest possible extension of the neck.

On the third day, the outer dressing is removed, the patient sits up and rotation of the head is encouraged by active or passive movements, depending on the age of the patient.[6, 33]

Intensive physiotherapy, including full rotation of the neck in both directions and full extension of the cervical spine, is instituted as soon as possible. The neck-righting reflexes must be re-educated in front of a mirror, a training period lasting at least 3 months.

COMPLICATIONS.—A *hematoma* may develop if hemostasis has been inadequate. It may occur early, in the first 12 hours after operation, or as late as 3–5 days. The wound may need to be opened and the clot evacuated to prevent additional fibrosis during healing.

Disruption of the incision may occur as a result of poor nutrition or overlapping of the skin edges. The wound is closed again with adhesive strips or, if necessary, resutured.

Lack of cooperation is to be expected in patients less than 3 years of age. Older children, too, may fail to achieve complete rotation of the neck by 7–10 days after operation, and if progress is not satisfactory, they can be provided with a light removable wire splint, which can be made in a day or two and so constructed that a slightly overcorrected position of the head is maintained. The splint is removed every 3–4 hours for active exercises.

Experience and Results

A personal series of 78 patients aged 8 months to 19 years has been treated by this method. Complications occurred in 4 children: a hematoma in 2 and the need for a wire splint in the other 2.

The fate of the sternocleidomastoid muscle varied: 38 muscles have partly reunited, 32 have disappeared clinically and in 8 the upper or lower end became attached to part of the fascia colli. Reoperation was necessary in 1 patient.

The scar was temporarily hypertrophic and unsightly in 4 other patients, but this subsided slowly in the following 2 years.

REFERENCES

1. André, N.: *Orthopaedia*, 1743 (facsimile edition; Philadelphia: J. B. Lippincott Company, 1961), p. 96.
2. Armstrong, D., *et al.*: Torticollis: An analysis of 271 cases, Plast. Reconstr. Surg. 35:14, 1965.
3. Brown, J. B., and McDowell, F.: Wry-neck facial distortion prevented by resection of fibrosed sternomastoid muscle in infancy and childhood, Ann. Surg. 131:721, 1950.
4. Coventry, M. B., and Harris, L. E.: Congenital muscular torticollis in infancy, J. Bone Joint Surg. 41-A:815, 1959.
5. Danby, P. M.: Plagiocephaly in some 10-year-old children, Arch. Dis. Child. 37:500, 1962.
6. Dickson, J. A.: The treatment of torticollis, Surg. Clin. North Am. 17:1349, 1937.

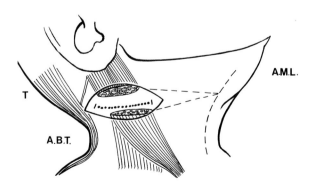

Fig. 38–8.—Operative sketch of division of sternocleidomastoid muscle. The incision (*dotted line*) is placed in a high skin crease at or near the midpoint of the muscle. By use of retraction, the fascia colli is divided as far forward as the anterior midline (*A.M.L.*) and posteriorly as far as the anterior border (*A.B.T.*) of the trapezius (*T*). The accessory nerve lies approximately 1 cm above the line of division.

7. Dieffenbach, J. F.: *Über die Durchschneidung der Sehnen Muskeln* (Berlin: 1841).
8. Dunn, P. M.: Congenital postural deformities: Perinatal associations, Proc. R. Soc. Med. 65:735, 1972.
9. Dunn, P. M.: Congenital sternomastoid torticollis: An intrauterine postural deformity, J. Bone Joint Surg. 55-B:877, 1973.
10. Dupuytren: *Leçons orales de clinique chirurgicale* (Paris: J. B. Bailière et fils, 1839).
11. Golding-Bird, C. H.: Congenital wry-neck (caput obstipum congenitale: torticollis congenitalis), with remarks on facial hemiatrophy, Guy's Hosp. Rep. 162:253, 1890.
12. Gruhn, J., and Hurwitt, E. S.: Fibrous sternomastoid tumor of infancy, Pediatrics 8:522, 1951.
13. Hellstadius, A.: Torticollis congenita, Acta Chir. Scand. 62:586, 1972.
14. Heusinger, K. P.: Berichte von der königlichen anthropanatomischen Anstalt zur Würtzburg, Ber. F. D. Schuljahr 1824/25 (Etlinger, Würtzburg) 4:43, 1826.
15. Holloway, L. W.: Caput obstipum congenitum, South. Med. J. 24:597, 1931.
16. Hulbert, K. P.: Congenital torticollis, J. Bone Joint Surg. 23-B: 50, 1950.
17. Joachimsthal: Cited by Lidge *et al.*[22]
18. Jones, P. G.: *Torticollis in Infancy and Childhood* (Springfield, Ill.: Charles C Thomas, Publisher, 1967).
19. Kiesewetter, W. B., *et al.*: Neonatal torticollis, JAMA 157:1281, 1955.
20. Krogius, A.: Zur Pathogenese des muskularen Schiefhalses, Acta Chir. Scand. 56:497, 1924.
21. Lange, C.: Zur Behandlung des Schiefhalses, Wochenschr. Orthop. Chir. 27:440, 1910.
22. Lidge, R. T., Bechtol, R. C., and Lambert, C. N.: Congenital muscular torticollis: Etiology and pathology, J. Bone Joint Surg. 39-A:1165, 1957.
23. Ling, C. M., and Low, Y. S.: Sternomastoid tumour and muscular torticollis, J. Bone Joint Surg. 55-B:236, 1973.
24. MacDonald, D.: Sternomastoid tumour and muscular torticollis, J. Bone Joint Surg. 51-B:432, 1969.
25. Middleton, D. S.: The pathology of congenital torticollis, Br. J. Surg. 18:188, 1930.
26. Mikulicz, J.: Über die Exstirpation des Kopfnickers beim muskularen Schiefhals neben Bemerkungen zur Pathologie dieses Leidens, Zentralbl. Chir. 1:9, 1895.
27. Moseley, T. M.: Treatment of facial distortion due to wry-neck in infants by complete resection of the sternomastoid muscle, Am. Surg. 28:698, 1962.
28. Nové-Josserand, G., and Viannay, C.: Pathogenie du torticollis congenital, Rev. Orthop. 7:397, 1906.
29. Oribasius: Cited by Lidge *et al.*[22]
30. Petersen, F.: Zur Frage des Kopfnickerhämatoms bei Neugeborenen, Zentralbl. Gynaekol. 10:777, 1886.
31. Plutarch: *Parallel Lives* (Loeb Classical Library) (London: William Heinemann, Ltd., 1958), Vol. 7, p. 230.
32. Schubert, A.: Die Uraschen der angeborenen Schiefhalserkrankung, Dtsch. Z. Chir. 167:32, 1921.
33. Soeur, R.: Treatment of congenital torticollis, J. Bone Joint Surg. 38:35, 1940.
34. Stromeyer, G. F. L.: *Beiträge zur operativen Orthopädik oder Erfahrungen über die subcutane Durchschneidung verkürzter Muskeln und deren Sehnen* (Hannover: Helwig, 1838).
35. Tubby, A. H.: *Deformities* (2d ed.; London: The Macmillan Company, 1912), Vol. 1, p. 56.
36. Tulp, N.: *Observationes Medicae* (Amsterdam: 1671).
37. Van Roonhuyze, H.: *Encyclopedie Méthodique: Partie Chirurgicale* (1670), Vol. 11.
38. Völcker, F.: Das Caput obstipum—eine intrauterine Belästungsdeformität, Beitr. Klin. Chir. 33:1, 1902.
39. Volkmann, R.: Das Sogenannte angeborene Caput Obstipum und die offene Durchschneidung des M. Sternocleidomastoids, Zentralbl. Chir. 12:233, 1885.
40. Witzel, O.: Beiträge zur Kentniss der secundären Veränderung beim muskularen Schiefhals, Dtsch. Z. Chir. 18:534, 1883.

39 EOIN ABERDEEN

Tracheostomy

TRACHEOSTOMY can provide an artificial airway with almost complete safety, but only at the cost of unremitting skilled bedside surveillance for every minute of each 24 hours and by avoidance of operative techniques that have caused major complications. Fatal complications have varied more after tracheostomy than for almost any other operation in surgery (from 0% to over 50%). Obstruction of the tracheostomy tube and distal airways by dried secretions, displacement of the tube and stricture of the trachea are the main lethal complications of tracheostomy reported in the literature for more than two centuries, and implied in the literature for two milleniums. When we surgeons ignore such history, it is our patients who are compelled to repeat the errors of the past.

HISTORY. — Tracheostomy, one of the oldest operations in surgery, has been referred to for more than 2000 years. Many of the early medical writers discussed tracheostomy, although none actually gave a case report. The earliest record is from the Greek physician Asclepiades (b. 124 B.C.),[34] and the operation was commented on by many medical writers during the next 1500 years, some probably only repeating what they had read.[49] The detailed advice given by Antyllus, a physician of the Graeco-Roman period in the second (some say third) century A.D., leaves little doubt that he was guided by hard-won experience, either his own or that of his surgical predecessors.[31] He comments on the advantage of extending the head to bring the trachea forward, the use of a midline skin hook to put tension on the skin, the need to avoid the vessels in the neck, describes how to divide the trachea transversely between the tracheal rings, warns of the danger of dividing the whole trachea and encourages the timid surgeon.

The first actual case reported seems to have been by an Italian surgeon, Brasavolus, who refers to his second successful case in 1546.[49] The great Fabricius of Aquapendente (1537–1619)—who taught anatomy to William Harvey, among others, in Padua—in response stated that not only had he never done the operation but that it was the "scandal of surgery."[30] Other reports appeared from the time of the Renaissance onward during the next three centuries in other parts of Europe, the first British report being by George Martin,[49] who, in 1730, gave an account of a successful tracheostomy on "a young lad" in St. Andrews and referred to two other surgeons in Scotland who were known to have performed successful tracheostomies "within these few years," which implies a more widespread use. The first definitive report on a child was in 1766 by Caron, who treated a 7-year-old boy.[30]

Experimental tracheostomy was demonstrated by Avenzoar, a Moslem physician, who performed a tracheostomy on a goat in 1162 to show his colleagues that the technique, as described, was feasible.[49] The prize for experimental zeal must surely go to Chovell, a young London surgeon, who, in 1733, persuaded a convicted highwayman to allow him to perform a tracheostomy the night before the condemned man's hanging, which must set a grim high-water mark for surgical offers that cannot be refused, even though informed consent may have been somewhat deficient.[34]

The terms "bronchotomy" "laryngotomy" and "pharyngotomy" were used to describe what we now call tracheostomy.[30] "Tracheotomy" was advocated as a term by the eminent Lorenz Heister in 1718 in Germany,[34] but was only slowly accepted into general usage, and the more recent use of the operation is emphasized by the term "tracheostomy." There was an increased use of tracheostomy in the mid-nineteenth century. Montgomery,[52] in 1885, described the technique of tracheostomy care with such precision that he must have had extensive experience, and most of his detailed advice can be followed with advantage today. He concludes by reporting 5 tracheostomies with 4 recoveries and compares this to 7 patients treated without tracheostomy, of whom 6 died. Colles,[21] in 1886, discussed tracheal stenosis after tracheostomy without citing case material but with an authority that could have come only from a large experience, and referred to some recent European reports. O'Dwyer,[55] in 1887, in the second report describing the use of short metal tubes temporarily placed through the larynx for the treatment of croup and diphtheria, recorded the survival of 12 patients among 50 treated with orotracheal tubes, which was an improvement on his results using tracheostomy.

Later important contributions were made by Jackson,[42] who demonstrated that strictures at and below the glottis could be largely avoided by placing the tracheostomy stoma 2 or 3 rings below the cricoid cartilage ("low tracheostomy" rather than "high tracheostomy"). Jackson had also, in 1911, described how a patient could "drown in his own secretion,"[41] but the enormous value of adequately draining or aspirating the respiratory tract was not really appreciated until more than 40 years later.

The early tracheostomy tubes presumably were metal, and the value of a metal cannula to drain a thoracic empyema had been known since Graeco-Roman times. Martin, in his 1730 report,[49] refers to the use of a "pipe" without saying whether this was ceramic or metal, and suggests the value of an inner and outer cannula to make removal of the secretions easier for the patient. The development of metal tubes and of removable inner cannulae (ingeniously constructed, often from silver) progressed until the advent of nonirritant pliable plastic material in the 1950s.[1] A very extensive use of tracheostomy then developed in many centers as the potential safety of the method was demonstrated,[9] but the number of tracheostomies diminished after the mid-1960s as the value of nasotracheal intubation became clear, especially in infants in the first year of life.[3]

Use of Tracheostomy

Many of the advances in pediatric surgery in the past 2 decades have depended on recognizing that respiratory failure played a significant role after a variety of major operations, and on managing that respiratory failure with assisted ventilation. Successful management of the respiratory complications required the development of reliable artificial airways and ventilatory techniques and the use of mechanical ventilators and systems of phased and modulated ventilation (PEEP, CPAP). The underlying surgical conditions included not only those involving the thorax, such as esophageal atresia with tracheoesophageal fistula, congenital diaphragmatic hernia with hypoplasia of the lung, congenital heart disease with congestive heart failure (and/or pulmonary vascular obstructive disease) requiring correction but also conditions not primarily involving the lungs or heart, such as severe burns, major trauma or major sepsis producing shock, prematurity and respiratory distress.

Although tracheostomy has been the method by which surgeons have established an artificial airway for the past 2000 years, the past decade has seen an enormous change as nasotracheal intubation, first reported in 1880 from Edinburgh by Macewen,[3] has been developed to provide a reliable artificial airway without an operation, and this has been of special value in cases requiring short-term ventilatory support. The use of pliable and almost nonirritant plastic material has been even more important for the improvement of nasotracheal tubes than it has been for tracheostomy tubes.

Indications for Tracheostomy

An artificial airway, be it a tracheostomy tube, an orotracheal tube or a nasotracheal tube, is required for one of three basic reasons—to bypass an obstructed upper airway, and so to allow adequate ventilation of lungs, or to drain obstructing secretions from the lower airways and/or to permit assisted ventilation.

The first indication has been used for more than 2000 years; the second has been widely used only over the past 30 years. Upper airway obstructions have been a result of congenital, traumatic, infective or neoplastic lesions of the larynx or pharynx whereas the reasons for draining the respiratory tract may be localized to the lungs or assisted ventilation may be required because of lesions distant from the lungs (which may inactivate the muscles of ventilation and/or the cough reflex, such as head injuries, brain or spinal cord tumors, poliomyelitis, polyneuritis, or some nerve degenerations, or myasthenia gravis).

Indications for Bypass of the Upper Airway

The need to relieve an obstructed upper airway may not always be easy to decide, and the inexperienced observer is wise to provide the artificial airway if in doubt. *Restlessness and a fast pulse rate*, the early warning signs of oxygen deficiency, may not be recognized promptly. The restlessness may be seen as aimless movement of the limbs or the child may thrash about the bed. Vocal noises, if they can be made, usually are meaningless. The older child may repeatedly change position in bed.

Admission to the hospital may cause an ill and frightened child to be even more restless and so increase the oxygen deficit. The comfort of his mother's arms, in a warm and quiet room, may quiet the child and reduce the restlessness. In the environment of a hospital, sedatives, even morphia, have a place, although the danger of using sedatives, instead of a safe airway, to treat the restlessness of oxygen deficiency must be emphasized.[41, 73] Very late there may be cyanosis or diminished consciousness. Severe respiratory obstruction may also be indicated by suprasternal and intercostal retraction and the use of the accessory muscles of respiration. Stridor may become less apparent and deceptively slight in the late stages of obstruction as the volume of each breath becomes diminished. The need for an artificial airway then is so urgent that alternatives to tracheostomy such as orotracheal intubation or, if that is not possible, direct laryngotomy through the cricothyroid membrane may be required.

Laryngotomy has been almost uniformly condemned since Jackson's forcibly expressed criticism in 1921.[42] Brantigan and Grow,[12] however, reported a series of 655 patients having cricothyroidotomy; this series included 12 children, the youngest being 8 months of age. Only one technically related death occurred and no permanent strictures resulted.

Indications for Respiratory Tract Drainage or Assisted Ventilation

The indications for an artificial airway when ventilation becomes inadequate because the lower respiratory tract is occluded by secretions, or because the muscular power to breathe has been diminished or abolished are quite different from those of upper airway obstruction. If surgical help is delayed until the patient has developed hypoxemia, the chances of recovery may be greatly diminished because the lungs may have developed infection and consolidation in addition to atelectasis. If, on the other hand, the need for drainage and assisted ventilation is recognized before the lung has become diseased (and the two nearly always are required together), the patient should never reach the point of severe hypoxemia and need never develop consolidation or bronchopneumonia. The main warning that an artificial airway is required is when coughing becomes ineffective, either because the cough reflex is diminished or because tidal volume is diminished or secretions are increased, especially tenacious and viscous secretions, within the bronchi.

The nature of the primary disease may make the need for an artificial airway and assisted ventilation easily predictable, and assisted ventilation has become part of the postoperative care of many major operations. If there is doubt about the ability to ventilate adequately or to expel the secretions adequately, an artificial airway and mechanical ventilation with good intensive care is wise, but, in nearly all cases after operation, a nasotracheal tube is adequate, and thus is to be preferred. An infant in the first months of life can have a nasotracheal tube in place for weeks, or even months, without serious complications,[4] and even in older children, tracheostomy now is infrequently needed for long-term postoperative ventilatory support.[3]

If the need for an artificial airway is in doubt, lung function, as judged by blood gas levels, may determine the need for mechanical ventilation. The best use of blood gas levels is to make repeated estimations, every 15 or 20 minutes if need be, so that the rate and direction of change can be appreciated, such as an increasing Pa_{CO_2} or a decreasing Pa_{O_2}. The critical level for these blood gases is discussed by Downes and Raphaely in Chapter 2. Tidal volume and physiologic dead space are difficult to measure in the infant and are not used clinically.

Details of Operation

1. Tracheostomy should be performed in an operating room or a suitably equipped intensive care area, with the patient receiving general anesthesia and ventilated through an endotracheal tube. (There is no place now for emergency bedside tracheostomy, because if ventilation is needed with great urgency, the patient should be intubated via the mouth immediately or, if that is not possible, cricothyroidotomy [laryngotomy] should be done rapidly.[12])

2. The head should be fully extended on a narrow wedge placed under the nape of the neck at about the level of the 8th cervical vertebra. The head should be extended so far that the trachea is pulled tight and made to feel subcutaneous,[2] as advised by Antyllus.[31] The patient should be fully draped.

3. Palpation with the nail of the index finger usually will allow the surgeon to count the number of tracheal rings downward from the cricoid ring if the trachea is adequately stretched, and the incision should be placed over the fourth tracheal ring, which usually is just below the lower edge of the thyroid isthmus (the incision is *not* close to the upper sternal edge). The skin is opened with a transverse incision, slightly concave upward, about 12–20 mm in length, depending on the size of the child. The subcutaneous tissue is divided with the electrocautery.

4. Dissection is made in the midline only, strictly in the vertical plane to separate the strap muscles, then through the pretracheal fascia to expose the trachea. If the isthmus of the thyroid obstructs the field, it is easily elevated cephalad with a small retractor. Division of vessels is not usually needed, and division of the thyroid isthmus is required rarely.

5. The trachea is opened by a midline incision through 3 adjacent tracheal rings, usually 3, 4 and 5. A short incision is dangerous, because it results in the tracheal wall being turned into the lumen.[21] No cartilage is excised—ever.[40] The midline vertical incision of the trachea was first suggested by Heister in 1718, and this was an important contribution because a transverse incision between the rings had been used since the second century A.D. on the authority of Antyllus, in the belief that cartilage would not heal. The inherent danger of a transverse incision is discussed later under *Stricture of the trachea.*

6. Complete hemostasis is achieved with the electrocautery, so that no blood drips into the tracheal lumen.

7. The upper end of the incision is held by an assistant using a fine hook—a plastic surgery skin hook being well suited in an infant. The tracheal incision is easily held apart if 3 rings have been completely divided, and a useful instrument for separating the cut edges is a fine nontoothed tissue forceps, placed in the incision with the tips together and allowed to expand open. The regular tracheal dilator such as that designed by Trousseau is much too large for an infant trachea, and actual dilatation of the trachea is never required.

A tracheostomy tube with an external diameter that comfortably fits in the lumen of the trachea is selected. It is surprising how easily an airtight connection can be made between the tracheostomy tube and the wall of the trachea (e.g., OD 5 mm [ID 3.5] diameter tube in a newborn, 5.5 or 6.0 mm OD [ID 3.5–4] at 3–6 months, up to ID 7 mm in older children). Ventilation at pressures of as high as 70 cm H_2O does not require that the tracheostomy tube should fit tightly in the trachea and an inflatable cuff is never required.

Just before the tracheostomy tube is inserted, the anesthesiologist withdraws his orotracheal tube until the tip is lying just above the stoma in the trachea, the tube still through the cords. Now, the tracheostomy tube is inserted. If an adequate tracheal incision has been made, the obliquely cut lower end of the tracheostomy tube is easily introduced. An obturator is needed for the introduction of the tracheostomy tube only if the tracheal incision is too small. The tracheostomy tube is connected by a sterile connector to the ventilator tubing.

After a few breaths, the anesthesiologist inflates his ventilating bag fully, turns the escape valve closed and squeezes the bag with a firm, continuous pressure for about 10 seconds. The surgeon listens for an air leak with his ear placed close to the tracheostomy. If there is an air leak, the tracheostomy tube is removed and a tube one size larger in diameter is placed in the trachea and the check for an air leak repeated. The aim is to place a tube that does not leak at all. A small air leak noted at the time of operation always becomes much larger after some hours. (This is in contrast to placement of a nasotracheal tube when a small amount of air leak is highly desirable, because it guarantees that the tube is not pressing tightly in the region of the cricoid ring.)

9. Aspiration of the tracheal secretions done soon after the initial incision in the trachea may be repeated once the tube is in place.

10. The tube is fixed by a tape tied around the neck (Fig. 39–1). This is an important maneuver and should be done by the surgeon himself. As with the placement of any other tube in the body, the responsibility for accidental displacement belongs solely to the surgeon who inserted the tube. Accidental displacement of the tracheostomy tube can be almost entirely prevented by an adequate technique of tube fixation.

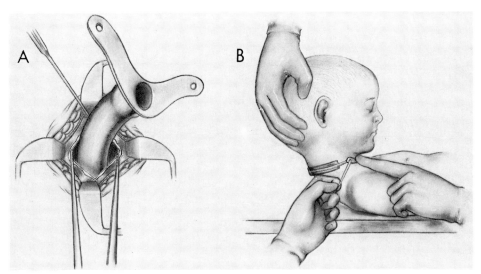

Fig. 39–1.—**A,** the plastic tracheostomy tube is inserted into the trachea, which has been opened by a midline incision through 3 tracheal rings (3, 4 and 5) without excising any cartilage. The transverse skin incision is held open with self-retaining retractors, the tracheal incision is held apart with fine-tipped 6″ tissue forceps and the trachea is stabilized by a plastic surgical skin hook holding the upper angle of the tracheal incision. **B,** fixation of the tube. A tracheostomy tube that fits comfortably but does not allow a gas leak has been inserted into the trachea. The tube is firmly secured by a cotton umbilical tape with the head flexed forward. The skin on the back of the neck is protected by a layer of adherent orthopedic plastic sponge, which is stuck to the tape before it is applied to the patient.

The head should be held flexed forward, because this narrows the diameter of the neck. A good-quality cotton tape, about 8–10 mm wide, is tied first to one wing of the tracheostomy tube flange and placed around the back of the neck and passed through the hole in the wing on the other side and tied with moderate tension on the tape. Any tube that is fixed with adequate tension by tape will tend to have the tape cut into the skin at the back of the neck, and the tape should therefore be padded at the back and the sides of the neck, best done by applying a length of adhesive orthopedic plastic sponge cut to a 12-mm width and a length of 5–6 cm in an infant or longer in an older child. The adhesive sponge is applied to the flattened tape before tying it to the tracheostomy tube, and then, as the tape is tightened, the sponge is positioned between the tape and skin of the patient. When the tape has been tied at both ends, the head is allowed to extend again, and the tension on the tape is checked with a finger.

The tape should not be so tight as to cause venous obstruction nor so loose as will allow the tracheostomy tube to be withdrawn from the wound more than about 1 cm, even if the tube is pulled with firmness. The connection to a ventilator may result in accidental pulling on the tracheostomy tube, but if that has been adequately fixed, accidental displacement should be prevented. The tension on the tape should be checked again by the surgeon 12 hours after operation.

Some surgeons routinely leave a traction suture on each side of the tracheal incision, so that replacement of the tube is made easier should the tube be displaced accidentally. This is a matter of opinion. I have found that the placement of such sutures may make the surgeon less careful about tying the tube into place adequately, and if the tube is displaced accidentally, the sutures may easily pull out if placed between the rings; it could cause necrosis if the suture is placed through the cartilage itself. On balance, I prefer *not* to leave traction sutures in the trachea.

Before taking the child from the operating room, it is wise to irrigate the trachea and bronchi with 1–2 ml of 0.9% saline and to combine this with positioning of the child from one side to the other, also placing the child in head-up and head-down tilt, and accompanying this with vibration of the chest wall and aspiration of the secretion so mobilized.

Postoperative Care

There is almost no field in nursing in which the survival of the patient depends so directly on the skill and devotion of the attending nurse as it does after tracheostomy. Important details are:

1. A special nurse must be available to care for the patient at every hour of the day and night. To cover adequately the 168 hours of each week requires an allotment by the hospital administration of 5 nurses for each tracheostomized patient.

2. Any gas inhaled must be as fully humidified at as near to body temperature as can be achieved.

3. Aspiration is with a sterile catheter:
   a) Whenever secretions are heard obstructing the airway.
   b) When any signs of hypoxemia are observed (the earliest signs are a fast pulse rate and restlessness).

4. Tracheostomy toilet is ordered for intervals as brief as 10 minutes to as long as 2 hours, but rarely longer. The child should be ventilated by hand with 100% oxygen for 2 minutes and then the sterile catheter passed down the tracheostomy, without suction being applied, as far as it will reach and then suction applied and the catheter steadily withdrawn. Rotating the catheter is acceptable, but pushing it up and down is to be avoided. The aspiration should be completed within 10 seconds and the child again ventilated by hand. A specially designed bronchial aspirating catheter with an angled tip facilitates aspiration of the left main bronchus. Otherwise, the left main bronchus is entered in only 10–30% of attempts.[6, 14, 35, 44, 46, 57, 66, 67, 72] Prolonged and strenuous aspiration may cause dysrhythmias, even ventricular fibrillation.[13, 29]

5. Chest physiotherapy is effective for mobilizing secretions and allowing them to be aspirated. Attendants trained

in chest physiotherapy should be available day and night, so that as soon as an area is detected as being underventilated or atelectatic, chest wall vibration and positioning the body both from side to side and head up to head down can be undertaken. Careful auscultation with the stethoscope can detect frequent changes in ventilation and thereby save an excessive number of chest x-rays, although a chest x-ray is advisable whenever a major problem of ventilation seems to have occurred. Mechanical vibration of the chest wall can be more effective than manual vibration, especially in infants.[65]

6. Gastric distention should be watched for, and can be relieved promptly by the passage of a nasogastric tube. Reflux of gastric content is especially undesirable. Aspiration from incoordination of swallowing may be a special problem after tracheostomy, more so than after nasotracheal intubation,[10, 11, 16] but may be especially associated with an inflated cuff.[28]

Since the application of nursing skills is so crucial at this stage, it is the responsibility of the surgeon to see that each nurse is adequately informed of her duties. If tracheostomy is done infrequently, it may be necessary for the surgeon and his resident staff to discuss with each change of nursing staff the essential points of tracheostomy management. This type of intensive care is done well only by those who care intensely, both nurse and surgeon. No nurse should be allowed to be responsible for a patient with tracheostomy if she does not recognize the importance of a rising pulse rate and restlessness and does not appreciate the importance of an adequately saturated ventilatory gas intake and the need for aspiration and careful tracheobronchial toilet. When tracheostomy patients are seen infrequently, it may be difficult for the nursing administration responsible for the allotment of nurses to recognize that 1 nurse per patient requires the allotment of 5 nurses for that patient bed, and it is the duty of the surgeon performing the tracheostomy not only to be sure that the technical details of the operation are performed safely and that the tube is well fixed and the nursing staff adequately instructed but to explain to the administration how closely the risks of lethal complications are related to adequate nursing supervision. If a plastic tracheostomy tube should have to be changed because it is obstructed by secretion there is a need to replace the nurse. However, it is better to instruct the nurse adequately and then neither tube nor nurse will need replacing.

Home care of children with long-term or permanent tracheostomy may become necessary. Fortunately, the respiratory tract becomes able to defend against inspissated secretions after some weeks or months and the patient then can survive safely, breathing ambient air. Effective home care was one of Holinger's important contributions.[38]

Technique of Extubation (Decannulation)

Removing the tracheostomy tube was a dangerous maneuver in the past and a special problem in infants under 1 year of age.[7, 8, 25, 48, 68] The reason for this difficulty was thought to be either a psychologic dependence of the patient on the artificial airway or the development of tracheomalacia in the tracheal cartilages. More recent experience has demonstrated that every child can be successfully extubated at any age, including the early months of life, as long as the trachea is not obstructed. My personal experience is of more than 150 infants having tracheostomy extubation. There were no failures of extubation except in 4 patients with congenital deformity of the larynx, and there were no deaths from extubation. (Tracheal strictures were prevented by avoiding metal

tracheostomy tubes, by avoiding cuffed tubes of all types, by avoiding the excision of any tracheal cartilage or the creation of a flap in the trachea.) Psychologic dependence of the child on the artificial airway never occurred in this experience. The details of the technique of extubation may be important, and those that seemed important in practice are as follows.

1. Extubation should be considered when the patient has been off mechanical ventilation for 2 or 3 days, seems well and is maintaining adequate blood gas levels. If the tracheostomy tube has been in situ for more than 4 weeks, tracheoscopy is performed to exclude a granuloma at the upper margin of the stoma, and to remove it if present.[60]

2. Extubation is performed in the intensive care unit with adequate surveillance and with spare tubes and laryngoscope available.

3. Extubation is made on the morning of a day when the unit is not excessively busy. The child is fasted for 3 hours.

4. A full dose of morphine sulfate (0.2 mg/kg body weight) is given intramuscularly and the child allowed to sleep.

5. The bronchial tree is gently aspirated and the child again allowed to sleep.

6. About 10 minutes later, the tracheostomy tube is gently removed (stolen).

7. The infant is allowed to sleep the next 2 or 3 hours.

8. The neck wound is closed with an adhesive dressing to reduce the air leak.

9. Should respiratory distress develop, the tracheostomy tube is promptly replaced and extubation tried again in a few days.

A preliminary to extubation, when mechanical ventilation has not been needed for 2 or 3 days, is to replace the tracheostomy tube each day with a tube that is progressively one size smaller, until the smallest size (3.5 mm ID) has been in place for a day. This allows the child to breathe around the tube and so to phonate and become accustomed to normal breathing. It also allows the wound to close down around the tube so that the neck wound is small when the tube finally is withdrawn.

Other techniques, described in the past, are better avoided now. One method was progressive occlusion of the lumen of the tube by a series of corks or stoppers so cut as to give graduated obstruction. Such obstruction is unwise if the tracheostomy tube is nearly filling the trachea, and unnecessary if a small tube is in place.

Another technique suggested at intervals over the past 100 years is that of using a fenestrated tube, with a hole in the posterosuperior wall, so as to allow air to pass up through the larynx. This may cause trauma to the posterior wall of the trachea during suctioning and cause granulation tissue to develop. After some personal experience with this method, I agree with Montgomery[52] and Jackson[42] that this method offers extra hazard and no advantage over the small tube extubation method.

In some of the cases in which extubation proved to be difficult at the first attempt, it usually succeeded at the second and sometimes the third attempt. (The *avoidance of tracheal stricture* is essential to guarantee that extubation will be uniformly successful.)

When a tracheostomy tube has been in place for months, or years, and especially if long-term ventilation has been required because of poor pulmonary compliance, extubation may require additional care. The child may be able to breathe spontaneously without ventilatory support for some weeks or months before he can cough well enough to keep the lungs clear of excessive secretions. If the tube is removed too early in these patients, the excessive secretions may prove dangerous several days after a seemingly successful extubation. The answer is to leave a small tracheostomy tube (as small as 2 mm ID) in the trachea for aspiration of the secretions. The tracheostomy does not serve as an airway bypass, and normal nasal humidification is available. Gradually, as the compliance of the lungs improves, the child is able to develop a cough effective enough to remove the secretions from the lungs; this permits the small tube to be removed, but only when the patient has shown an ability to keep the lungs clear, without aspiration, for at least 2 weeks.

Complications of Tracheostomy

It has been the complications of tracheostomy that have made surgeons rightly apprehensive these past 2000 years. In many instances, the complication of the disease, rather than the tracheostomy, led to a fatal outcome. Now that we can recognize the difference, no longer are *any* fatal complications of tracheostomy acceptable in a good intensive care unit.

Infection is the most common complication, and to some degree some infection occurs in every case, but the growth of abnormal bacteria need not necessarily signify cause for concern. If the airways can be kept free from obstruction, and adequate tracheostomy care is given, infection is not likely to be a major problem. However, routine cultures should be taken at least every 3 days.[50] Antibiotics may be useful, more so if instilled into the trachea than if given parenterally,[27, 47] but long-term prophylactic antibiotics usually are inadvisable.

Obstruction by inspissated secretions should be almost totally avoided if the lungs are reasonably normal at the time of tracheostomy. When tracheostomy is required for an airway obstruction as the result of a laryngotracheobronchitis or diphtheria, obstruction by tracheal casts or membranes may occur.

Obstruction of the tracheostomy tube or natural airways by inspissated dried secretions is an ever-present danger with tracheostomy, because tracheostomy not only bypasses the superbly effective natural humidifying apparatus of the nose but also abolishes the aerodynamic explosion with which an effective cough clears mucus plugs so well from the airways. Humidification can be reasonably achieved by well-designed humidifiers, although temperature gradients may deposit water vapor, and so lower humidity when the gas is rewarmed to body temperature. The intratracheal instillation of liquid (usually 0.9% NaCl) will help liquefy secretions that are becoming inspissated, as will extra fluid added by nebulization. Nebulizers, especially ultrasonic nebulizers, must be used with care, as they may add too much water to the lungs, which absorb water rapidly, resulting in water intoxication. Several mucus solvents have been used, but none is reliably effective and nonirritant. Sodium bicarbonate solutions may cause bronchospasm, and the peripheral airways already may be obstructed.[54]

Although natural humidification and natural coughing are superior to the mechanical substitutes, obstruction by secretions need not occur in tracheostomized patients, and in two children's hospitals at least, a large series of patients have been managed with tracheostomy without one patient having obstruction by secretions as a major problem,[3] but both these series had few patients with inflammatory lesions of the upper airways.

Tracheal ulceration or perforation has been reported and may even lead to the erosion of a large artery,[43] carotid or innominate, but this nearly always has been a complication

of rigid tracheostomy tubes. In my own experience it has also occurred with plastic tracheostomy tubes that were cut short, for what at the time seemed good reasons. Since the decision was taken not to cut the tube short, no further case of erosion has occurred in more than 400 infants and children.

Hemorrhage has been a problem at operation,[12a] but rarely is so if the tracheostomy is performed in an operating room with an endotracheal tube for ventilation.

Cannulation of the right main bronchus. If the tracheostomy tube is too long or if the tracheostomy stoma is made too low, cannulation of the right main bronchus can occur quite easily, and if not recognized for some hours, may cause major cardiopulmonary problems. When a tracheostomy tube is inserted, the surgeon should carefully listen to the breath sounds in the left axilla and the right axilla, *with the tracheostomy tube firmly pushed down the trachea.* If the intensity of the breath sounds in the left axilla is equal to that of the right, it may be safely assumed that ventilation of both lungs is adequate and that there is no right main bronchus cannulation. Should the breath sounds in the left axilla be less than on the right, the tracheostomy tube should be withdrawn about 5 mm and auscultation repeated. If withdrawing the tube increases the ventilation of the left lung, it is clear evidence that the right main bronchus is being cannulated, and the answer is *not* to take out the tracheostomy tube and cut it shorter, but, for the reasons given above, simply to place some foam sponge between the patient's skin and the anterior flange of the tracheostomy tube sufficient to position the tube so that both lungs aerate well. This functional method of judging the tube length is safer than interpreting the x-ray appearance and perhaps withdrawing the tube unnecessarily, thereby risking accidental decannulation.

Accidental decannulation was a common problem in the past,[56] but, in my experience, can be almost completely avoided by adequate fixation of the tube.

Granuloma of the trachea can occur, especially in relation to the superior edge of the tracheal stoma.[21, 60] It is to be expected in at least 10% of long-term tracheostomies. Before extubating any child who has had a tracheostomy tube in place for more than 4 weeks, inspection should be made from above with a modern bronchoscope (e.g., Storz). If a granuloma is present, it can be removed quite simply, by first withdrawing the tracheostomy tube and then grasping the granuloma with a skin hook passed through the tracheal stoma, but observed by the endoscopist looking through the bronchoscope. When the obstructing granuloma has been withdrawn into the tracheostomy wound (and this can be easily and best seen through the bronchoscope), it is removed with the electrocautery tip.

Stricture of the trachea. Stricture may develop proximal to the stoma, at the level of the stoma or distal to the stoma.[37]

Tracheal stricture has been the cause of most of the problems of long-term tracheostomy, and has been the reason tracheostomy was so much avoided in patients in the early months of life. My personal experience with tracheostomy in the past 20 years[3] has included almost 1000 children, of whom more than 400 were in the first year of life (300 in the first 3 months). Not one child developed stricture of the trachea. No cartilage was removed from the trachea during tracheostomy. By making an adequate opening (i.e., division of 3 rings), a tracheostomy tube can be inserted comfortably without causing either indentation of the edges of the incision[21] or causing firm pressure on the cut edges sufficient to make the cartilages resorb. If an adequate incision is made, the tube does not compress the tracheal ring just proximal to the stoma, which may be indented by the pressure and cause a particularly troublesome form of stenosis.[7, 48, 64, 68] Subglottic stricture may develop if the stoma is too close to the cords.[42]

Strictures at the level of the stoma are the result of cartilage destruction, either by the surgeon at operation using an excision or tracheal flap technique[40] or using an incision of inadequate length.

The avoidance of rigid (especially metal) tubes is also important in avoiding tracheal ulceration. Any rigid tube must cause unusual pressure areas as the child changes the position of the head whereas a pliable tube will simply reposition itself in the trachea without causing excessive pressure. The response to excessive pressure, especially at the tip of the tracheostomy tube, may be either ulceration, which results in later stricture, or resorption of cartilage, which then is recognized as tracheomalacia.

The avoidance of cuffed tubes is another reason why strictures did not occur in my own experience. Since cuffed tubes were never required, it seems unnecessary to take the risk of stricture that a cuffed tube may offer.[5, 17, 20, 23, 32, 33, 45, 51, 53, 59, 61, 63] Those children requiring high inflation pressures may be better managed with tracheostomy, which thus avoids a cuffed tube, than by nasotracheal intubation, which does require a cuffed tube to control high inflation pressures. An area of pressure from a cuff may denude the underlying epithelium. Experimentally, it has been shown that excision of the mucous membrane is all that is required to produce a stricture.[39] The development of low-pressure (i.e., wide area of contact) cuffs for nasotracheal tubes is important, but it still does not make cuffed tubes acceptable for tracheostomy in children.

Pneumothorax was a problem in the earlier experience with tracheostomy,[62] but has been almost completely avoided since the use of endotracheal intubation, before performing the tracheostomy. This experience has confirmed the theory of Champneys that pneumothorax usually is a sucking injury that occurs only when enough negative pressure is developed in the chest to draw air into the mediastinum, and this requires that the airway be obstructed, when the child can develop a negative pressure of about 40 cm H_2O.[18] Champneys performed some basic experimental studies on stillborn infants in 1882–1883 that demonstrated that pneumothorax never occurred without accompanying mediastinal emphysema, although mediastinal emphysema often was found without pneumothorax.[19] It has been assumed, for many years, that the development of pneumothorax at the time of tracheostomy indicated that the pleura in the neck had been accidentally incised,[24] but any surgeon who has attempted to pass a segment of colon through the apex of the pleural cavity recognizes the anatomic evidence that refutes this explanation. Pneumothorax should be presumed to be evidence of a sucking lesion, which means severe obstruction to air inflow.[58] Mechanical ventilation at high inflation pressures may also cause air leak from the lung. Whatever the cause of pneumothorax, it should be promptly treated with pleural drainage and an underwater seal.

Types of Tracheostomy Tubes

Metal tubes were mentioned in almost all the earlier reports of tracheostomy. The tubes were straight in most descriptions, and a removable inner tube was first suggested by Martin.[49] By the time of Montgomery's report in 1885,[52] double tubes with a removable inner tube were in regular use, and many designs were tried during the next 70 years. At this time, tubes were made of steel or silver, but Colles,[21] in 1886, advised attaching a rubber tube to the end of the metal tube to overcome problems of tracheal erosion from the tip of the metal tube.

Nonirritant plastics greatly improved tracheostomy tubes, as they did nasotracheal tubes and other surgical tubes. The only pliable material that had been widely used up to this time was red rubber, itself a strong tissue irritant.

An effective tracheostomy tube for infants was developed at the Hospital for Sick Children, Great Ormond Street, London, in the late 1950s.[1] The tube design was based on measurements of infants made at autopsy (see also references 15 and 26). The features of the tube were:

1. It was pliable and nonirritant.
2. It was a single tube; that is, there was no removable inner tube.
3. The flange or anterior shield was curved superiorly and laterally in a "Cupid's bow" shape.
4. The outer end of the tube was enlarged to 7 mm ID, so that a 7-mm connector could be inserted without reducing the internal diameter of the air-flow pathway.
5. The tube was curved gradually and was not angled sharply.
6. The lower end of the tube was cut at an angle of about 45° to permit easy introduction into the trachea.
7. There was no cuff on the tube.

These tubes were made in England of polyvinyl chloride[1], sterilized by irradiation, and in the United States a similar tube was made of silicone rubber[36, 69, 70, 71] that could be sterilized by irradiation or heat.

The ideal tracheostomy tube for an infant having mechanical ventilation has not yet been produced. Such a tube should project from the neck shield, to form a male fitting to which the ventilator tubing could be connected as a female fitting and locked in a way that would prevent detachment but yet permit rotation of the tubing, in at least two axes, and also allow easy aspiration by catheter without detaching the tubing.

Metal tubes have served a long and honorable history in tracheostomy, but secretions do adhere to them more readily than to the plastic tubes, and the rigidity of the metal tube makes dangerous pressure points in the trachea much more likely. The metal tracheostomy tube now has an honored place, but it is in the medical museum and not in the human trachea.

Results of Treatment

The deaths of patients having tracheostomy have dominated the attitude of surgeons toward this operation. Tracheostomy should be done only by a surgeon who is aware of the complications that may follow, who is fearful of them and makes *every* effort to avoid them. The fears and apprehensions of the ancient surgeons have been reflected through the ages down to the present day and, even now, some leading practitioners of surgery still avoid tracheostomy whenever possible.

A number of series of tracheostomies in children and infants have been reported.[3, 9, 12a, 36, 38, 56, 73] A simple comparison between different series, to determine whether one technique is superior to another, is of value only if the case material being compared is similar. Not only must the age of the patient and the primary disease be considered but also the climatic conditions at the time (in winter, for instance, air at the freezing point has about one-tenth the water vapor that it will require to be fully saturated at body temperature, and thus the risk of dry tracheostomy is much increased in winter[22]).

An essential part of evaluating any tracheostomy series is to assess the number of deaths that have occurred from complications of the tracheostomy technique. It should be possible to avoid almost completely every fatal complication of tracheostomy. Some series have been reported in infants and children in which all tracheostomy deaths have been avoided.[3] Reference already has been made to 200 consecutive infants at the Hospital for Sick Children, London, and 61 patients at Children's Hospital of Philadelphia without a tracheostomy death.[3] Others[36] have also reported an experience in infants and children without deaths from tracheostomy complications. However, a series can be selected from past reports showing deaths from complications affecting even as much as 50% of patients. There are few operations that emphasize the difference between an "operation" and "surgery." The *operation* of tracheostomy requires certain rules of safe conduct. However, *surgery* includes the organization and supervision of the aftercare, adequate communication with the parents and the child, if old enough, and management of the primary disease that required tracheostomy.

REFERENCES

1. Aberdeen, E.: Tracheostomy and tracheostomy care in infants, Proc. R. Soc. Med. 58:900, 1965.
2. Aberdeen, E.: Tracheostomy in Infants, in Rob, C., and Smith, R. (eds.), *Operative Surgery* (2d ed.; London: Butterworths, 1968).
3. Aberdeen, E., and Downes, J. J.: Artificial airways in children, Surg. Clin. North Am. 54:1155, 1974.
4. Allen, T. H., and Steven, I. M.: Prolonged endotracheal intubation in infants and children, Br. J. Anaesth. 37:566, 1965.
5. Andrews, M. J., and Pearson, F. G.: Incidence and pathogenesis of tracheal injury following cuffed tube tracheostomy with assisted ventilation: Analysis of a two-year prospective study, Ann. Surg. 173:249, 1971.
6. Anthony, J. S., and Sieniewicz, D. J.: Suctioning of the left bronchial tree in critically ill patients, Crit. Care Med. 5:161, 1977.
7. Ardran, G. M., and Caust, L. J.: Delayed decannulation after tracheostomy in infants, J. Laryngol. Otol. 77:555, 1963.
8. Ashcraft, K. W., and Leape, L. L.: The use of a one-way valve to aid in tracheostomy decannulation, J. Thorac. Cardiovasc. Surg. 64:161, 1972.
9. Beatrous, W. P.: Tracheostomy (tracheotomy). Its expanded indications and its present status. Based on an analysis of 1,000 consecutive operations and a review of the recent literature, Laryngoscope 78:3, 1968.
10. Bonanno, P. C.: Swallowing dysfunction after tracheostomy, Ann. Surg. 174:29, 1971.
11. Bone, D. K., Davis, J. L., Zuidema, G. D., and Cameron, J. L.: Aspiration pneumonia, Ann. Thorac. Surg. 18:30, 1974.
12. Brantigan, C. O., and Grow, J. B.: Cricothyroidotomy: Elective use in respiratory problems requiring tracheotomy, J. Thorac. Cardiovasc. Surg. 71:72, 1976.
12a. Bridges, C. P., Ryan, R. F., Longenecker, C. G., and Vincent, R. W.: Tracheostomy in children: A twenty-year study at Charity Hospital in New Orleans, Plast. Reconstr. Surg. 37:117, 1966.
13. Brown, E. B., Jr., and Miller, F.: Ventricular fibrillation following a rapid fall in alveolar carbon dioxide concentration, Am. J. Physiol. 169:56, 1952.
14. Bush, G. H.: Tracheobronchial suction in infants and children, Br. J. Anaesth. 35:322, 1963.
15. Butz, R. O., Jr.: Length and cross-section growth patterns in the human trachea, Pediatrics 42:336, 1968.
16. Cameron, J. L., and Reymonds, J.: Aspiration in patients with tracheostomies, Surg. Gynecol. Obstet. 136:68, 1973.
17. Carroll, R., Hedden, M., and Safar, P.: Intratracheal cuffs: Performance characteristics, Anesthesiology 31:275, 1969.
18. Champneys, F. H.: Artificial respiration in stillborn children. Mediastinal emphysema and pneumothorax in connection with tracheotomy. An experimental inquiry, Med. Chir. Trans. 65:75, 1882.
19. Champneys, F. H.: Addendum: Artificial respiration in stillborn children. (Mediastinal emphysema and pneumothorax in connection with tracheotomy. An experimental inquiry), Med. Chir. Trans. 66:101, 1883.
20. Ching, N. P. H., Ayres, S. M., Spina, R. C., and Nealon, T. F., Jr.: Endotracheal damage during continuous ventilatory support, Ann. Surg. 179:123, 1974.
21. Colles, C. J.: On stenosis of the trachea after tracheotomy for croup and diphtheria, Ann. Surg. 3:499, 1886.
22. Conley, J. J.: Diagnosis and treatment of encrustations in the trachea. Their relation to radical surgery of the head and neck, JAMA 154:829, 1954.
23. Cooper, J. D., and Grillo, H. C.: The evolution of tracheal injury due to ventilatory assistance through cuffed tubes: A pathologic study, Ann. Surg. 169:334, 1969.
24. Dark, J. F.: Tension pneumothorax following tracheotomy, Lancet 1:398, 1952.
25. Diamant, H., Kinman, J., and Okmian, L.: Decannulation in children, Laryngoscope 71:404, 1961.
26. Fearon, B., and Whalen, J. S.: Tracheal dimensions in the living infant (preliminary report), Ann. Otol. 76:964, 1967.
27. Feeley, T. W., du Moulin, G. C., Hedley-Whyte, J., Bushnell, L. S., Gilbert, J. P., and Feingold, D. S.: Aerosol polymyxin and pneumonia in seriously ill patients, N. Engl. J. Med. 293:471, 1975.
28. Feldman, S. A., Deal, C. W., and Urquhart, W.: Disturbance of swallowing after tracheostomy, Lancet 1:954, 1966.
29. Fell, T., and Cheney, F. W.: Prevention of hypoxia during endotracheal suction, Ann. Surg. 174:24, 1971.
30. Goodall, E. W.: The story of tracheotomy, Br. J. Child. Dis. 31:12, 1934.
31. Grant, R. L.: Antyllus, the elusive surgical genius of antiquity: An analysis of his writings, Surgery 50:572, 1961.
32. Grillo, H. C.: The management of tracheal stenosis following assisted respiration, J. Thorac. Cardiovasc. Surg. 57:52, 1969.
33. Grillo, H. C., Cooper, J. D., Geffin, B., and Pontoppidan, H.: A low-pressure cuff for tracheostomy tubes to minimize tracheal injury, J. Thorac. Cardiovasc. Surg. 62:898, 1971.
34. Guthrie, D.: Early records of tracheotomy, Bull. Hist. Med. 15:59, 1944.
35. Haberman, P. B., Green, J. P., Archibald, C., Dunn, D. L., Hurwitz, S. R., Ashburn, W. L., and Moser, K. M.: Determinants of successful selective tracheobronchial suctioning, N. Engl. J. Med. 289:1060, 1973.
36. Haller, J. A., Jr., and Talbert, J. L.: Clinical evaluation of a new Silastic tracheostomy tube for respiratory support of infants and young children, Ann. Surg. 171:915, 1970.
37. Harley, H. R. S.: Laryngotracheal obstruction complicating tracheostomy or endotracheal intubation with assisted respiration: A critical review, Thorax 26:493, 1971.
38. Holinger, P. H., Brown, W. T., and Maurizi, D. G.: Tracheostomy in the newborn, Am. J. Surg. 109:771, 1965.
39. Hughes, R. K.: Resection of the bronchial and the tracheal mucosa, J. Surg. Res. 6:389, 1966.
40. Jackson, B.: Management of the tracheostomy in cases of tetanus neonatorum treated with intermittent positive pressure respiration, J. Laryngol. Otol. 77:541, 1963.
41. Jackson, C.: The drowning of the patient in his own secretion, Laryngoscope 21:1183, 1911.
42. Jackson, C.: High tracheostomy and other errors the chief causes of chronic laryngeal stenosis, Surg. Gynecol. Obstet. 32:392, 1921.
43. Jones, J. W., Reynolds, M., Hewitt, R. L., and Drapanas, T.: Tracheo-innominate artery erosion: Successful surgical management of a devastating complication, Ann. Surg. 184:194, 1976.
44. Jung, R. C., and Gottlieb, L. S.: Comparison of tracheobronchial suction catheters in humans. Visualization by fiberoptic bronchoscopy. Chest 69:179, 1976.
45. Khan, F., and Reddy, N. C.: Enlarging intratracheal tube cuff diameter: A quantitative roentgenographic study of its value in the early prediction of serious tracheal damage, Ann. Thorac. Surg. 24:49, 1977.
46. Kirimli, B., King, J. E., and Pfaeffle, H. H.: Evaluation of tracheobronchial suction techniques, J. Thorac. Cardiovasc. Surg. 59:340, 1970.
47. Klastersky, J., Huysmans, E., Weerts, D., Hensgens, C., and Daneau, D.: Endotracheally administered gentamicin for the prevention of infections of the respiratory tract in patients with tracheostomy: A double-blind study, Chest 65:650, 1974.
48. Lewis, R. S., and Ludman, H.: Decannulation after tracheostomy in infants and young children, J. Laryngol. Otol. 49:435, 1965.

49. Martin, G.: Giving an account of the operation of bronchotome as it was performed at St. Andrews, Philos. Trans. R. Soc. Lond. No. 416, 448, 1730.

50. Matthew, E. B., Holstrom, F. M. G., and Kaspar, R. L.: A simple method for diagnosing pneumonia in intubated or tracheostomized patients, Crit. Care Med. 5:76, 1977.

51. Miller, D. R., and Sethi, G.: Tracheal stenosis following prolonged cuffed intubation: Cause and prevention, Ann. Surg. 171:283, 1970.

52. Montgomery, E. E.: Tracheotomy in croup and diphtheria, Arch. Pediatr. 2:577, 1885.

53. Murphy, D. A., MacLean, L. D., and Dobell, A. R. C.: Tracheal stenosis as a complication of tracheostomy, Ann. Thorac. Surg. 2:44, 1966.

54. Murphy, D. A., and Popkin, J.: Tracheal collapse in tracheostomized infants: Resistance in reference to flow rates in a variety of tracheostomy tubes, J. Pediatr. Surg. 6:314, 1971.

55. O'Dwyer, J.: Fifty cases of croup in private practice treated by intubation of the larynx, with a description of the method and of the dangers incident thereto, Med. Rec. 32:557, 1887.

56. Oliver, P., Richardson, J. R., Clubb, R. W., and Flake, C. G.: Tracheostomy in children, N. Engl. J. Med. 267:631, 1962.

57. Opie, L. H., and Smith, A. C.: Tracheobronchial toilet through a tracheostome, Lancet 1:600, 1959.

58. Padovan, I. F., Dawson, C. A., Henschel, E. O., and Lehman, R. H.: Pathogenesis of mediastinal emphysema and pneumothorax following tracheotomy, Chest 66:553, 1974.

59. Paegle, R. D., Ayres, S. M., and Davis, S.: Rapid tracheal injury by cuffed airways and healing with loss of ciliated epithelium, Arch. Surg. 106:31, 1973.

60. Pearce, D. J., and Walsh, R. S.: Respiratory obstruction due to tracheal granuloma after tracheostomy, Lancet 2:135, 1961.

61. Pearson, F. G., and Andrews, M. J.: Detection and management of tracheal stenosis following cuffed tube tracheostomy, Ann. Thorac. Surg. 12:359, 1971.

62. Rabuzzi, D. D., and Reed, G. F.: Intrathoracic complications following tracheotomy in children, Laryngoscope 81:939, 1971.

63. Rainer, W. G., Sanchez, M., and Lopez, L.: Tracheal stricture secondary to cuffed tracheostomy tubes, Chest 59:115, 1971.

64. Reading, P.: Some post-operative hazards in tracheostomy on infants, J. Laryngol. Otol. 72:785, 1958.

65. Rowe, M. I., Weinberger, M., and Poole, C. A.: An experimental study of the vibrator in postoperative tracheobronchial clearance, J. Pediatr. Surg. 8:735, 1973.

66. Sackner, M. A., Landa, J. F., Greeneltch, N., and Robinson, M. J.: Pathogenesis and prevention of tracheobronchial damage with suction procedures, Chest 64:284, 1973.

67. Scott, A. A., Sandham, G., and Rebuck, A. S.: Selective tracheobronchial aspiration, Thorax 32:346, 1977.

68. Smythe, P. M.: The problem of detubating an infant with a tracheostomy, J. Pediatr. 65:446, 1964.

69. Spooner, T. R.: An evaluation of Silastic tracheostomy tubes, Laryngoscope 81:1132, 1971.

70. Stool, S. E., Campbell, J. R., and Johnson, D. G.: Tracheostomy in children: The use of plastic tubes, J. Pediatr. Surg. 3:402, 1968.

71. Talbert, J. L., and Haller, J. A., Jr.: Improved Silastic tracheostomy tubes for infants and young children, J. Pediatr. Surg. 3:408, 1968.

72. Thiede, W. H., and Banaszak, E. F.: Selective bronchial catheterization, N. Engl. J. Med. 286:526, 1972.

73. Venables, A. W.: Tracheostomy in childhood, Med. J. Aust. 2:141, 1959.

PART IV

The Thorax and Cardiovascular System

PLATE II

A. Congenital Cystic Disease—Left Lower Lobe. Three-and-a-half-year-old child with repeated pulmonary infection. The contrast between the thick-walled scar covering the basal portion of the lobe and the normal upper portion is striking. The diaphragm is at the lower left, just below the lowest of the three white systemic arteries, still undivided, which proceed directly from the aorta to the malformed lobe. These had been demonstrated angiocardiographically. Such systemic arteries may arise from the abdominal aorta and course through the diaphragm. They indicate the congenital nature of cystic disease of the lung and represent a significant operative hazard. There were eight such arteries in all in this patient. Lobectomy was followed by uneventful recovery.

B. Congenital Cystic Disease—Right Lower Lobe. Seven-year-old boy with a lifelong history of repeated severe pulmonary infections, previously diagnosed as bronchiectasis. The entire lobe has been replaced by small and large cysts, lined by a smooth glistening membrane, which histologically showed normal respiratory epithelium. Most of the cysts were filled with a thick glairy mucus, but some also contained air and the roentgenographic films showed multiple fluid levels. Congenital cystic disease causes symptoms usually from repeated infections and occasionally from overdistention of a cyst, particularly in the newborn. Upon diagnosis of the condition, the cyst or lobe should be removed. In this instance, right lower lobectomy was considered curative, for there was no recurrence of symptoms in 14 years.

C. Poland's Syndrome. A 12-year-old girl with absence of the costosternal portions of the pectoralis major, absence of the pectoralis minor, hypoplasia of the skin and subcutaneous fat, underdevelopment of the nipple and breast, and polythelism. In the full expression of the syndrome there is a deformity of the hand, either the mitten hand or ectromelia. The 2d, 3d and 4th or the 3d, 4th and 5th costal cartilages are absent and additional muscles of the thorax may be partially deficient. This girl's hand was normal. She had a deep incurvation of several ribs, successfully treated by multiple osteotomies of the ribs, wedging-out of the incurved segments, and correction of an associated sternal displacement. The result, 10 years later, was gratifying; the chest wall was smoothly rounded, and on it a small breast developed. Nevertheless, she insisted on, and received, a prosthetic mammary implant.

D. Pectus Carinatum, Atypical. Protrusion deformities tend to vary substantially from patient to patient. The depression of the costal cartilages to either side, which is quite conspicuous in this boy, is a fairly constant feature. In him, the sternum is not only prominent, but rotated and there is an extraordinary costochondral prominence on the right. The deformity responded very satisfactorily to staged procedures, involving the resection of the depressed costal cartilages, the excision of chondrosternal prominences and the rotation of the twisted sternum.

E. Pectus Excavatum, Extreme Form. An 11-year-old girl with Marfan's disease. With some hesitation, we have operated upon a number of patients with Marfan's disease and particularly severe deformities. In this child the deformity, observed over several years, had become progressively more embarrassing and disabling. The rotation of the sternum to the right, and the relative underdevelopment of the right breast, so common in pectus excavatum, here are strikingly exaggerated. Patients with essentially a collapse of most of the chest wall on the right may appear not to have pectus excavatum, but probably represent a variant.

F. Ectopia Cordis. This infant, whose naked heart is completely outside of the body cavity, represents the only condition which can truly be called ectopia cordis, as opposed to situations where the heart simply appears to be ectopic, as in children with upper or complete sternal clefts or in children with distal sternal clefts as part of Cantrell's syndrome. In true ectopia cordis, as in this patient, an associated intrinsic cardiac abnormality is usually so severe as to preclude survival, or even the provision of skin covering for the heart.

PLATE II

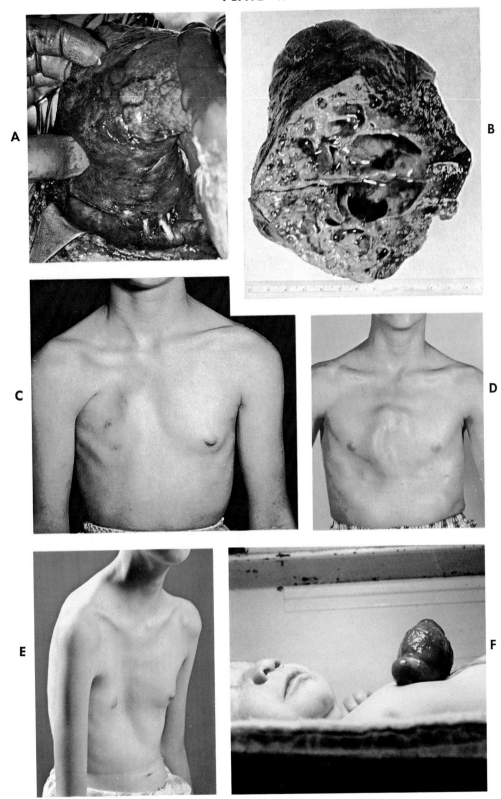

40 Mark M. Ravitch

The Breast

Physiologic Considerations

THE BREAST is a modified sweat gland. At birth there is no difference between the sexes. The tiny nipple is surrounded by an inconspicuous areola and usually no breast tissue is palpable underneath. Microscopically, the area beneath the areola, in which there may be palpable an insignificant nodule, contains rudimentary ducts connecting with the nipple, but no acinar development (Fig. 40–1, A). Within a few days of birth, usually at the end of the first week in the majority of infants, a visible swelling of the breast occurs (Fig. 40–4, A), associated with a secretion of milk or colostrum-like fluid, the "witch's milk" of the laity. It may appear from one breast or both and is equally common in infants of either sex. Histologically, this is reflected by hypertrophy and appearance of acini in the duct system (Fig. 40–1, B) and increased vascularity of the stroma. In one way or another, this response is due to the maternal hormones circulating in the infant. It may be due to the mother's estrogen and prolactin still circulating in the infant, or may be due secondarily to the stimulation of hypophyseal activity by the progressive fall of this blood estrogen concentration within the first week of life.

The enlargement of the breasts frequently is accompanied by visible enlargement of the labia and clitoris and, in an occasional instance, by a bloody vaginal discharge.

These changes regress spontaneously as the inciting factors are removed and endocrinologic balance is restored. Breast enlargement and the other manifestations seldom last more than 2 or 3 weeks.

Congenital Anomalies

CONGENITAL ABSENCE OF BREAST OR NIPPLE.—Amastia or athelism occurs occasionally. While it presages a cosmetic problem in females (it is almost invariably unilateral), its chief significance is its frequent association with underlying defects of the chest wall and pectoral musculature (Poland's syndrome). Trier,[14] reviewing 20 cases of unilateral absence of the breast, 4 of them in males, found in 18 of 20 absence of the corresponding pectoral muscles. He also found 8 cases of bilateral absence of the breast. Bilateral absence of the breast occurs in hereditary anhidrotic ectodermal dysplasia. This is a recessive, sex-linked defect, marked additionally by hypodontia, hypotrichosis, anhidrosis, high brows, saddle nose, thick lips and satyr-like ears.[2] Absence of the pectoralis major, which may also occur independently, is seen with hypoplasia or, more rarely, congenital absence of the breast. Absence of the underlying ribs or costal cartilages is a fairly frequent accompaniment (Fig. 40–2). In such instances there may be total absence of the breast, or merely a decrease in the amount of potential breast tissue so that in females, at puberty, a breast develops

on the affected side but is much smaller than the one on the opposite side.[12]

MULTIPLE NIPPLES OR MULTIPLE BREASTS.—Polythelism or polymastia occurs infrequently (Fig. 40–3). Because of the small size of the normal infant breast and even smaller size of the accessory breasts that occur along the embryonic milk line from the axilla to the normal region of the breast, and then down the trunk, in line with the normal breast, the accessory organs frequently are not noticed until puberty or even until pregnancy causes enlargement of the aberrant breast tissue. In childhood, the accessory breast tissue probably is never sufficiently conspicuous to require treatment.

LATERAL DISPLACEMENT OF THE NIPPLES.—Fleisher[4] has seen 7 infants with bilateral renal hypoplasia, in all of whom the nipples were well lateral to the midclavicular line.

Modifications of Normal Physiologic Changes

Stimulation of the neonatal secreting breast may cause remarkable hypertrophy, which will persist as long as stimulation is continued. The superstition that it is important to remove the witch's milk is responsible for such practice (Fig. 40–4, B).

In girls, the pubertal enlargement of the breasts occurs at a variable period, and at a variable rate, with the onset of puberty, itself variable, anywhere from the age of 9 or 10 to 15 years (Fig. 40–1, D).

In girls at any age before puberty, the breast may respond to the normally present levels of estrogen by moderate hypertrophy. A small mass of breast tissue may be felt beneath the nipple on one or both sides without any striking enlargement of the breasts as such. This mass of breast tissue may remain for a period of time or in some instances may persist until it merges with the pubertal hypertrophy of the breast.

The breast of adolescent boys may vary from a firm discoid, perhaps tender, subareolar nodule to a substantial and conspicuous swelling (Fig. 40–5). The peak incidence is at 14 years, with a spread from 10 to 16. In their large study, Nydick et al.[11] excluded obese boys. The incidence in black boys was lower than in white boys. In the 237 unilateral cases, the right breast was involved twice as often as the left. Probable duration of the mammary enlargement was 2 years There is a positive correlation between size of testes, penis and thyroid and amount of pubic hair and the mammary hypertrophy of puberty. The breast enlargement is transitory (only 7.7% persist for 3 years) and requires neither hormonal nor surgical treatment. Occasional cases of extreme and persistent enlargement may warrant a subcutaneous excision of the breast.

One would expect gynecomastia to be under hormonal control, but only recently have data been presented to sup-

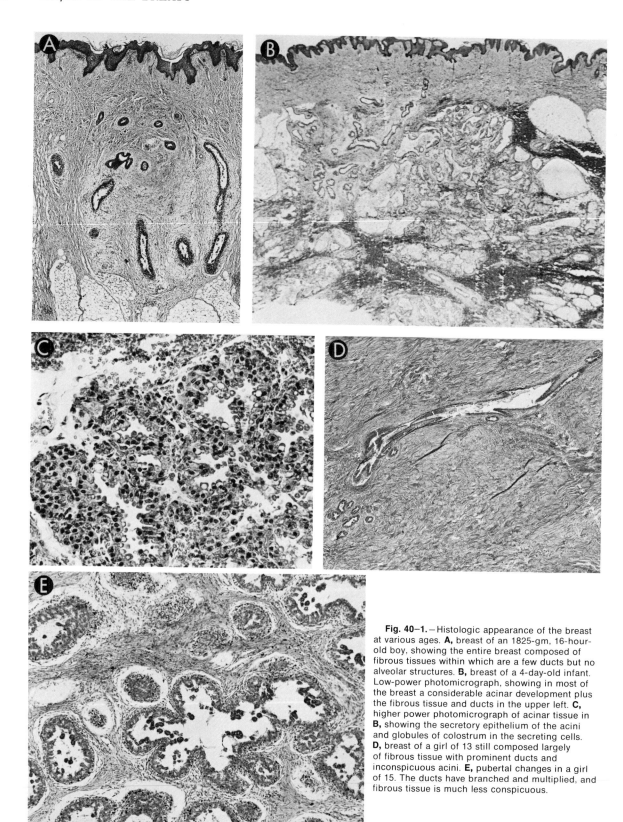

Fig. 40–1.—Histologic appearance of the breast at various ages. **A,** breast of an 1825-gm, 16-hour-old boy, showing the entire breast composed of fibrous tissues within which are a few ducts but no alveolar structures. **B,** breast of a 4-day-old infant. Low-power photomicrograph, showing in most of the breast a considerable acinar development plus the fibrous tissue and ducts in the upper left. **C,** higher power photomicrograph of acinar tissue in **B,** showing the secretory epithelium of the acini and globules of colostrum in the secreting cells. **D,** breast of a girl of 13 still composed largely of fibrous tissue with prominent ducts and inconspicuous acini. **E,** pubertal changes in a girl of 15. The ducts have branched and multiplied, and fibrous tissue is much less conspicuous.

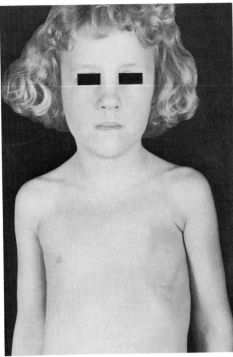

Fig. 40-2.—Congenital absence of the breast (amastia). This child was born without a left breast and nipple, although a faint pigmented area suggests a possible vestige at a point a little lower on the left side than the normal location of a nipple. The conspicuous deformity is due to the frequently associated absence of several ribs and costal cartilages (usually 2d to 4th) and much of the costal portion of the pectoralis major (Poland's syndrome). The thoracic deformity is susceptible of correction.

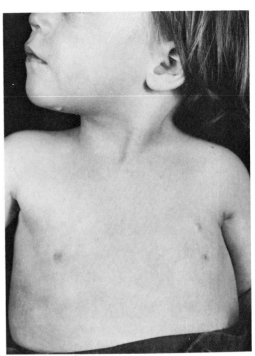

Fig. 40-3.—Polythelism. This child had two well-developed nipples on the left along the course of the embryonic milk line. The supernumerary breast may lactate and, if physically annoying because of proximity to the axilla, or cosmetically disfiguring, may be considered for ultimate removal. This patient had a sacral spina bifida and meningocele.

port this thesis. LaFranchi and others at UCLA[8] suggest, from their data in a study of 16 boys, that "at least in some patients with pubertal gynecomastia, increased levels of serum estradiol or progesterone, or both, and high estradiol/testosterone ratios are causally related to their gynecomastia," finding also that these increased steroid concentrations were transient.

We have seen an instance of unexplained unilateral breast hypertrophy in a small child and there is a report of at least one other.[12, 16]

VIRGINAL HYPERTROPHY OF THE FEMALE BREAST.— This occasionally occurs at puberty and results in the rapid development of enormous mammary glands (Fig. 40-6). These girls present no other evidence of endocrine dysfunction, and the lesion presumably is due to an abnormal local

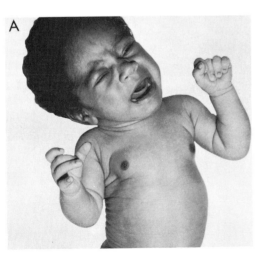 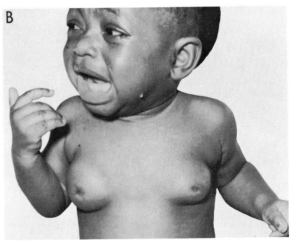

Fig. 40-4.—Neonatal breast hypertrophy. **A,** physiologic hypertrophy in a 12-day-old female with obvious enlargement of the breasts, which secreted "witch's milk." The external genitalia were also conspicuously enlarged. This physiologic phenomenon is due to direct stimulation by still-circulating maternal hormones or possibly to temporary stimulation of the pituitary by sudden reduction of the level of these hormones. **B,** exaggerated hypertrophy in a baby of 8 months whose mother constantly milked the breast to express the witch's milk. The more the breasts responded to the mechanical stimulation the more they were stripped mechanically. The mother could not be persuaded that the condition was self-limited, and manipulation was continued until the child was hospitalized. With application of cold compresses, the breasts soon regressed to normal infantile size.

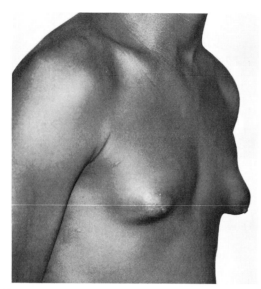

Fig. 40–5. — Pubertal hypertrophy in an adolescent boy. This boy of 11 had normal genital development. Failure of the breasts to diminish in size led to bilateral mastectomy through a subareolar excision. Operation usually is not required.

response of the breasts to physiologic stimulation. The enlargement may be unilateral. The breasts may be so huge as to be cosmetically disfiguring and physically disabling. The condition does not reverse itself and no treatment other than operative removal or a plastic partial excision has been satisfactory.

GYNECOMASTIA. — In occasional adolescent males, one breast or both may hypertrophy to produce a breast that looks and feels remarkably like that of a young woman. This occurs in the absence of any other evidence of endocrine

dysfunction, and such hypertrophy usually persists. The social embarrassment that results justifies subcutaneous excision of the abnormal breasts.

KLINEFELTER'S SYNDROME. — The syndrome of dysgenesis of the seminiferous tubules is associated with small atrophic testes deficient in spermatogenesis and showing hyalinization of the seminiferous tubules. Gynecomastia frequently occurs in these patients.

The fat boy with Fröhlich's syndrome has fatty breasts that seem more a part of his general adiposity than actual gynecomastia.

Precocious Puberty

In girls, various lesions causing physiologic aberrations induce the premature onset of puberty with the usual changes in which the breast takes part, sometimes as the most conspicuous feature.

IDIOPATHIC PRECOCIOUS PUBERTY. — In true idiopathic precocious puberty of unknown etiology, all the physiologic changes of puberty take place. Bilateral breast enlargement generally is the first evidence and is followed by menstruation and the appearance of pubic and axillary hair, and is associated with rapid bone growth and advanced bone age leading to early closure of the epiphyses. Such patients can conceive, as in the famous instance of the 5-year-old Peruvian child reported in the newspapers and commented on by Wilkins.[17]

ALBRIGHT'S SYNDROME (POLYOSTOTIC FIBROUS DYSPLASIA). — In this syndrome, all of the changes associated with puberty may occur in early childhood and are accompanied by the appearance of pathognomonic areas of brownish pigmentation of the skin and diffusely distributed osseous lesions. The basic nature of the endocrine disturbance

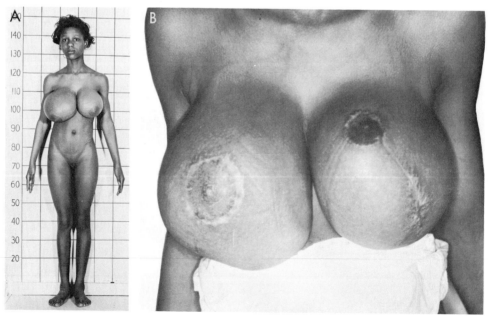

Fig. 40–6. — Virginal hypertrophy of the breast. This girl of 12 for 4 months had noted rapid enlargement of the breasts, more marked on the right, with some pain and tenderness in both. The breasts were engorged and firm and large veins were seen beneath the skin. **A,** the deformity is obvious. She could not wear normal clothing, and operation was undertaken to reduce the size of the breasts. In two stage operations, more than 2500 gm of tissue was removed. The immediate result was quite satisfactory. **B,** in a few months, the breasts began to enlarge again and it was evident that a repeat mammaplasty would be necessary. This is unusual, but ordinarily a reduction mammoplasty for virginal hypertrophy is not performed as early as age 12.

is unidentified. Ovulation does occur, and apparently these patients may grow to maturity.

PRECOCIOUS PUBERTY ASSOCIATED WITH IDENTIFIABLE NEUROENDOCRINE LESIONS. — *Intracranial lesions.* — Various intracranial lesions may manifest themselves by precocious puberty, of which mammary enlargement frequently is the first sign. Midline brain tumors are most characteristically associated with this syndrome, and precocious puberty has been reported with tumors of the pineal body and of the floor of the third ventricle. Most of these tumors are anatomically or pathologically incurable. Inflammatory lesions of the brain — encephalitis, meningitis — have also been held responsible for the appearance of precocious puberty, possibly because of lesions in the same areas of the brain. Neurologic manifestations, such as signs of increased intracranial pressure or of involvement of the hypothalamus — polydipsia, polyuria — are obvious indications in these patients of the cause of the premature enlargement of the breasts.

Ovarian tumors. — A wide variety of ovarian tumors, the most prominent of which is the granulosa cell tumor, may induce premature onset of puberty with accompanying enlargement of the breasts. Chorioepitheliomas, lutein cell tumors and other ovarian tumors can produce essentially the same sequence of events. In the little patient in whom the entire pelvis can be completely explored in the rectal examination, the enlarged ovary provides a ready clue to the cause of the precocious puberty. Removal of the involved ovary brings a rapid reversal of symptoms. The chorioepitheliomas usually are malignant, and the granulosa cell tumors occasionally are malignant.

Adrenal cortical lesions. — The adrenogenital syndrome, whether induced by cortical hyperplasia or by an adrenal cortical tumor, causes early abnormal development of the breasts and genitalia and hirsutism, with or without other cushingoid changes.

Testicular tumors. — Seminomas, chorioepitheliomas and Leydig cell tumors have all been associated with gynecomastia. Treatment is removal of the involved testis.

Liver factors. — Gynecomastia occasionally has been reported in association with juvenile cirrhosis or with severe chronic malnutrition, presumably due to failure of the liver to destroy estrogen, which occurs also in adult male cirrhotics.

Inflammatory Lesions

In the neonate, the engorged breast appears to be particularly susceptible to infection, which presumably enters directly through the ducts in the nipple. Staphylococcic abscesses are not uncommon and are one of the lesions that occur with a staphylococcic outbreak in the nursery. *E. coli* breast abscesses in 2 newborns have been reported by Stetler *et al.*,[13] with the suggestion that the hexachlorophene baths used in the nursery, as an antistaphylococcal measure, allowed the gram-negative organisms to flourish and cause mastitis. In the same decade they reported from Children's Hospital of Philadelphia and Philadelphia General Hospital 38 cases of neonatal mastitis — 27 due to hemolytic staphylococci, 1 to beta-hemolytic streptococci, 1 mixed, 1 no growth and 8 uncultured.

The mild infections in the neonatal breast respond to antibiotics and occasionally to compresses. Evidence of suppuration is an indication for incision. In an occasional instance, a neglected breast abscess results in a widespread phlegmon of the chest wall, with devastating consequences.

Pubertal or prepubertal enlargement of the breast, frequently painful, often is improperly given the title of pubertal mastitis.

Tumors of the Breast

As far as the probabilities are concerned, given a breast mass in a child, the most common cause is pubertal hypertrophy. In the neonate, the mass is most likely to be an abscess. In young girls, a discrete mass within the breast is most likely to be a fibroadenoma. Of 50 patients operated on at Childrens Hospital of Los Angeles,[15] 42 of them girls and 8 of them boys, there were 13 breast abscesses, 9 in neonates, 3 in other infants and 1 in a 6-year-old child. Twenty-nine of the excised masses were fibroadenomas and there was an additional giant fibroadenoma. The youngest patient was 13 years of age and 2 of the patients had not begun to menstruate. Two patients within a year developed new fibroadenomas, which required excision. Less common lesions were chronic cystic mastitis with bloody nipple discharge and intraductal cysts. In the 16-year period under study, no patients were seen with carcinoma of the breast. In 95 patients 12 to 21 years of age who had tumors of the breast removed in a decade at the University of Alabama,[1] 94% of the tumors were fibroadenomas and there were no malignant tumors. A quarter of the patients had multiple tumors. In 90 patients with fibroadenoma, the tumor was multiple in 25%. There were 2 patients with cystic mastitis, 1 with an intraductal papilloma, 1 with a blue-domed cyst and 1 with a lipoma.

BENIGN TUMORS. — Tumors of the breast, either benign or malignant, are uncommon in children. There are occasional reports of cysts of the breast. The most common tumor of the breast in young girls is fibroadenoma, which appears after the onset of puberty. The tumor is benign but in patients of this age group may grow so rapidly and be so large as to suggest, before operation, the possibility that it is malignant. We have seen 2 girls, aged 8 and 10, with bloody nipple discharge due to an intraductal papilloma. Any discrete tumor of the breast should be excised, provided that one makes certain that the lesion is not the much more common pubertal mastitis or hypertrophy, which at times produces a firm little mass suggesting a tumor.

MALIGNANT TUMORS. — Carcinoma of the breast has been reported in a small number of children. Herrmann[7] collected 33 cases of breast carcinoma in patients under 20, but only 12 were aged 12 or less, 1 patient was 13 and 1 was 14. Festenstein,[3] reporting a fatal adenocarcinoma of the breast in a Bantu boy of 14, found reports of carcinoma of the breast in 5 boys aged 6, 12, 12, 13 and 14 years 8 months, and in 5 girls, 2 aged 10, 2 aged 11 and 1 aged 12. The number of reported cases has therefore been the same in the two sexes. Although one is inclined to consider cancer of the breast in young women to be more malignant than the same cancer in older women, it is apparent that cancer of the breast in children is less malignant or at least no more malignant than in adults. Of the 12 patients tabulated by Herrmann,[7] 6 at the time of reporting had no evidence of disease, 1 of them 28 years after radical mastectomy at age 4. The patient mentioned by Haagensen[6] had a tumor from the age of 5 that had been under a physician's observation from the time she was 9 until she was 15, with small growth in that period. The tumor was excised locally after this 10-year history and found to be a fairly characteristic carcinoma infiltrating the fat. The patient was well 11 years later. In Lippitt's 10-year-old girl with a 2-cm lump in her breast, found on routine physical examination, the tumor proved to be a ductal carcinoma involving the areola. She was well 2 years after a simple mastectomy.[9] McDivitt and Stewart[10] make a strong case for the relative benignity of breast cancer in children. Their 7 patients, 3–15 years old, all girls, were free from tumor 2–15 years after operation. The tumor recurred in only 1 of 4 treated by local excision; this child had a second local excision and finally a modified radical mastectomy. None of the children had regional or distant metastases. These authors pointed out some of the distinguishing histologic characteristics of cancer of the breast in children. Cystosarcoma phyllodes has occurred in young girls, and in one instance[5] a 12-year-old premenstrual girl with a lump in the breast of 3 months' duration had a mass 10 × 12.5 × 15 cm, which proved to be a malignant cystosarcoma phyllodes. A year after radical mastectomy the child was well.

Sarcoma.—A handful of cases of sarcoma of the breast in young patients has been reported. Herrmann could find only 3 in patients 12 years of age or under, and all 3 were reported in the last century. Radical mastectomy probably is advisable.

REFERENCES

1. Daniel, W. A., Jr., and Matthews, M. D.: Tumors of the breast in adolescent females, Pediatrics 41:743, 1968.
2. Familusi, J. B., Jaiyesimi, F., Ojo, C. O., and Attah, E. B.: Hereditary anhidrotic ectodermal dysplasia: Studies in a Nigerian family, Arch. Dis. Child. 50:642, 1975.
3. Festenstein, H.: Adenocarcinoma of the breast in a South African Bantu boy aged 14, S. Afr. Med. J. 34:517, 1960.
4. Fleisher, D. S.: Lateral displacement of the nipples, a sign of bilateral renal hypoplasia, J. Pediatr. 69:806, 1966.
5. Gibbs, B. F., Roe, R. D., and Thomas, D. F.: Malignant cystosarcoma phyllodes in a prepubertal female, Ann. Surg. 167:229, 1968.
6. Haagensen, C. D.: *Diseases of the Breast* (Philadelphia: W. B. Saunders Company, 1956).
7. Herrmann, J. H.: Tumors and Other Enlargements of the Breast, in Arial, I. M., and Pack, G. T. (eds.), *Cancer and Allied Diseases of Infancy and Childhood* (Boston: Little, Brown and Company, 1960).
8. LaFranchi, S. H., Parlow, A. F., Lippe, B. M., Coyotupa, J., and Kaplan, S. A.: Pubertal gynecomastia and transient elevation of the serum estradiol level, Am. J. Dis. Child. 129:927, 1975.
9. Lippitt, W. H., Medart, W. S., Jr., and Ramsey, S. N.: Breast cancer in a 10-year-old girl, Surgery 68:395, 1970.
10. McDivitt, R. W., and Stewart, F. W.: Breast carcinoma in children, JAMA 195:388, 1966.
11. Nydick, M., *et al.:* Gynecomastia in adolescent boys, JAMA 178:449, 1961.
12. Ravitch, M. M.: *Congenital Diseases of the Chest Wall and Their Operative Correction* (Philadelphia: W. B. Saunders Company, 1977).
13. Stetler, H., Martin, E., Plotkin, S., and Katz, M.: Neonatal mastitis due to *Escherichia coli,* J. Pediatr. 76:611, 1970.
14. Trier, W. C.: Complete breast absence, Plast. Reconstr. Surg. 36:430, 1965.
15. Turbey, W. J., Buntain, W. L., and Dudgeon, D. L.: Surgical management of pediatric breast masses, Pediatrics 56:736, 1975.
16. Wiedemann, H. R., Harms, D., and Zierott, G.: Linksseitige idiopathische Gynäkomastie bei einem 2¼ jährigen Knaben, Helv. Paediatr. Acta 28:413, 1973.
17. Wilkins, L. A.: *The Diagnosis and Treatment of Endocrine Disorders in Childhood and Adolescence* (3d ed.; Springfield, Ill.: Charles C Thomas, Publisher, 1966).

41 Mark M. Ravitch

The Chest Wall

Congenital Deformities of the Chest Wall

Sternal Clefts

HISTORY.—Clefts of the sternum, which will vary from V-shaped separations exposing the pulsations of the heart to complete separation of the sternal halves with the naked heart outside the pericardium and anterior to the chest wall, always have attracted attention. deTorres[10] in 1740 reported a 1706 case known to him. There are many described in stillborn monsters. As long ago as 1818, Weese's inaugural dissertation systematically discussed the varieties of "Ectopia Cordis"[33] and Breschet's 1826 treatise[4] still is commonly referred to, although the starting point for most current discussions is Greig's 1926 classic.[12]

The literature is plagued with a plethora of case reports describing the varieties of cleft sternum, under various and conflicting terms. It often is not possible, even with assiduous reading, to determine the precise nature of the defect in question. Analysis of the clinical and experimental literature leads to the inevitable conclusion that we are dealing with a continuous spectrum of deformities of the sternum, the heart, the pericardium, the diaphragm and the abdominal wall, which may exist in a variety of combinations, presumably depending on the time, duration and nature of the injury to the fetus. Although the simpler manifestations of "ectopia cordis" generally are seen as isolated defects, the more severe manifestations may be associated with cleft lip, cleft palate, cleft chin, hydrocephalus, exencephalus, craniorachischisis or clubfoot.

From the clinical standpoint there are fundamentally three major groups: (1) Cleft sternum without associated anomalies. The cleft involves the manubrium and a varying extent of the gladiolus, followed by instances in which the sternum is cleft down to the xiphoid, which remains united, whereas in the least common variety the entire sternum is cleft (Figs. 41–1 and 41–2). (2) True ectopia cordis, which is accompanied by varying degrees of cleft sternum, the heart presenting outside the chest wall, usually naked and usually internally malformed (Fig. 41–3). Other major malformations commonly are associated. (3) Cantrell's pentalogy (Fig. 41–4), a syndrome commonly described under the classification of thoracoabdominal or thoracoepigastric ectopia cordis and characterized by a cleft or absence of the distal sternum, a crescentic ventral diaphragmatic defect, a midline ventral abdominal defect or an omphalocele, a defect of the apical pericardium with free communication into the peritoneal cavity, and a cardiac defect, part of which is either a ventricular septal defect or a ventricular aneurysm.

The sternal clefts unassociated with cardiac displacement are readily correctable by appropriate operation, best undertaken in early infancy or the neonatal period. The true ectopia cordis, at this writing, has only once had a successful cutaneous covering of the heart, the patient still awaiting correction of the profound intracardiac anomaly. Patients with the pentalogy syndrome have been operated on in increasing numbers, with correction of both the parietal and cardiac malformations.

Embryology

The basic understanding of the phylogeny and ontogeny of the sternum is essentially that which Hanson[14] presented in 1919. Hanson's opinions, arrived at largely on a comparative anatomic basis, have been reinforced by the experimental work of Fell[11] in the budgerigar, Chen[7] in the mouse and Seno[31] and Pinot[24] in chicks. The sternum develops from an independent blastema in the sixth week, where it is represented by concentrations of mesenchyme in two parallel primordia at some distance from the midline. These paired, longitudinally directed sternal bands converge superiorly and become progressively chondrified, moving toward the midventral line, fusing with each other from cephalad caudally, forming a median cartilaginous plate. The ribs develop independently, from the somites, whereas the sternum derives from the lateral plate mesoderm. The ventrally growing tips of the ribs gradually approximate the sternal bands, and simultaneously the two sternal bands fuse with each other in the midline. Excision of the somites in an embryo will prevent development of the ribs but will not interfere with development and approximation of the sternal bands. Kalter and Warkany[17] described an extraordinary variety of insults to mammalian embryos that can produce cleft sternum.

Subsequently, transverse divisions of the cartilaginous sternum result in the differentiation of segmental sternebrae. These lines of division, or sutures, always occur opposite the ends of each pair of ribs, a further indication that the sternum does not grow from the rib elements, as once was thought. Ossification of the sternebrae is an extremely variable process. The centers of ossification regularly appear in the intercostal levels of the sternum, and may be either single and median or paired. At birth, the sternum is cartilaginous, except for small centers of ossification. Significant sternal marrow spaces are not present until the third year of life and final ossification usually is established by age 14 or 16.

Congenital sternal clefts presumably are the result of the failure of midline fusion of the paired sternal bands. Since fusion occurs first at the cephalic end, one would expect a failure of fusion there to result in the failure of fusion in the entire sternum, yet the cleft of the upper sternum with some fusion of the lower sternum possibly is the most common anomaly of fusion.

Upper Sternal Clefts and Total Cleft Sternum

The most common case reports in patients with cleft sternum are those dealing with a cleft in the superior portion of the sternum, or of all of it except the xiphoid. Although these frequently have been reported under the rubric of ectopia cordis or partial ectopia cordis or cervicothoracic ectopia cordis (because of the absence of the manubrium, the heart appears to be pulsating in the neck) there is in fact no ectopia. The defect varies from a broad U, in which the heart covered only by skin can be seen to pulsate and the defect to bulge with the Valsalva maneuver and collapse paradoxically with inspiration, to a V-shaped cleft of varying breadth, sometimes only 2 or 3 cm, at other times generously wide, and, in either case, sometimes extending to interspace III or IV, sometimes to the xiphoid, where there is a small cartilaginous connection. There commonly is seen a midline cutaneous scar or ridge or red linear discoloration as of a recently healed wound, or skin so thin as to appear in danger of breaking down. This presumably is indicative of a disturbance in, at least, the cutaneous midline fusion. In general,

incomplete or complete clefts of the sternum without ectopia cordis usually have been unassociated with other significant anomalies. The literature is replete with cases of asymptomatic adults with sternal clefts, the most famous being that of Herr Groux of Hamburg, who 100 years ago exhibited himself to hospitals and medical societies around the world.[13] However, the deformity is both alarming and unsightly, and one has an obvious concern for the defenselessness of the heart and great vessels covered only by skin. For these reasons, an increasing number of these patients are coming to operation, almost invariably with success. We have been able to gather 44 patients operated on.[27] The earliest was that of Lannelongue in 1888.[18] The experiences of Maier[19] and of Jewett[16] demonstrate that in the immediate neonatal period direct approximation of the two sternal halves is possible, whether the cleft is complete or incomplete. If the cleft is V-shaped or U-shaped, appropriate notching or transection of the sternal bars or V-shaped wedging of the distal intact portion will be required to permit direct approximation of the sternal halves without buckling. The pericardium usually can be peeled away from the underside of the sternal bars without any difficulty. Within a relatively few weeks, the child may not tolerate the decreased thoracic circumference produced by a direct closure of the sternal halves. With such patients, some variety of the sliding chondrotomy of Sabiston[28] is required (Fig. 41–1). Later in childhood, even this may not be successful. In a 9-year-old patient who did not tolerate direct closure of the sternum after division and approximation of the sternal bands, we used a stainless steel mesh prosthesis, which has given an excellent result for 18 years. Burton,[5] in 1947, used autogenous cartilage grafts to cover the sternal defect. Increasingly in recent years, the patients have been operated on early in infancy, and direct closure of the sternum has been possible with or without sternotomy. Congenital ab-

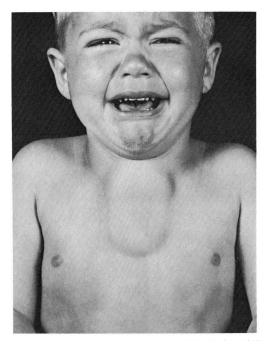

Fig. 41–1.—Upper sternal cleft. Boy of 3 years with a V-shaped cleft in the upper sternum into which the heart bulges, presenting the appearance of cervicothoracic ectopia cordis. Multiple chondrotomies allowed approximation of the sternal edges. Operation in the neonatal period is likely to permit direct closure of such defects without need for chondrotomies or prosthetic materials. (From Sabiston.[28])

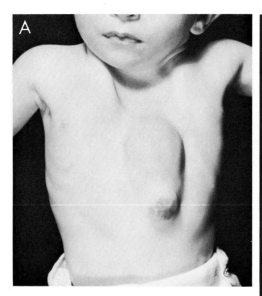

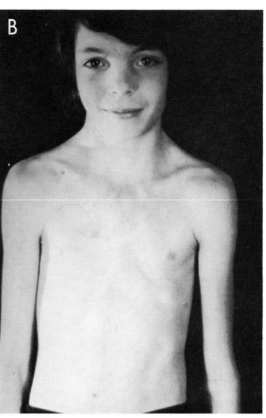

Fig. 41–2.—Complete sternal cleft. **A,** child at 8 months. There is no bony structure between hyoid and pubis. Rib ends are widely separated, and at this time it was thought, even after operation, that there was no sternum, but some years later, lateral roentgenograms showed sternebrae. Note prominence of the heart. Below it, in the pigmented omphalocele-like scar of the umbilicus, the swelling is produced by the liver. The heart was encased in the pericardium, but the pericardium was open to the peritoneal cavity and there was a crescentic diaphragmatic defect. **B,** at age 12. In the first operation, the abdominal portion of the defect was closed by mobilization of local tissues and flaps of the rectus sheath. The edges of the thoracic deformity could not be approximated, so the defect was closed over by a sheet of Teflon felt. A year later, the repair was firm except at the upper end of the Teflon felt, which was lax and, in any case, 2 or 3 cm below the proper upper border of the manubrium. At the second operation, another sheet of Teflon felt was placed above the first and supported by two rib struts taken from the fourth rib on the right. The result has been a sound repair with normal growth of the chest wall and normal expansion of the chest. At the time this photograph was taken there was an area of fluctuation over the graft, which proved to be due to fluid around a corner of the second Teflon graft, which had not "taken." This corner was excised and there has been no further difficulty.

sence of the sternum probably does not occur. We reported it once[26] (Fig. 41–2), mistakenly, in a child who subsequently proved to have a complete cleft of the sternum, and the patient of Asp and Sulamaa[3] probably also was a case of complete cleft of the sternum. In our patient, the associated ventral anterior diaphragmatic defect and omphalocele-like ventral parietal defect suggested a forme fruste of the Cantrell syndrome. That child had no intracardiac defect. In him, at 5 months, the very broad sternal cleft and the time required for closing the abdominal and diaphragmatic defects led to reconstruction of the sternum with Teflon felt, which has given him a good sternum and a firm chest wall for 15 years.[27] Asp and Sulamaa,[3] to avoid the cervical herniation of the lung and unpleasant pulsation in the neck sometimes seen after sternal repair, slid the origins of the sternocleidomastoid muscles medially to meet each other, and Daum[8, 9] extended this to include the insertions of the sternohyoid and sternothyroid muscles as well. Finally, Ingelrans and Debeugny[15] detached and crossed the origins of the sternocleidomastoid muscles, attaching them to the opposite third cartilage on either side, without repairing the superior sternal cleft.

Ectopia Cordis

This appellation properly should be restricted to those instances in which the naked heart is completely outside the chest, either pointing straight forward or commonly touching the chin or ear (Fig. 41–3). We have been able to find 18 operated-on patients with true ectopia cordis of this kind—prethoracic ectopia cordis or ectopia cordis extrathoracica nuda—all unsuccessful but 1.[27] Almost invariably, the heart itself is so seriously malformed that survival would not have occurred had the heart been in its normal position under an intact sternum. Saxena's[29] patient survived initial skin coverage and is awaiting a definitive reconstruction of the cardiac anomaly.

Distal Sternal Cleft (Cantrell's Pentalogy)

In 1958, Cantrell, Haller and Ravitch[6] analyzed the problem of so-called thoracoabdominal ectopia cordis in a paper entitled, "A Syndrome of Congenital Defects Involving the Abdominal Wall, Sternum, Diaphragm, Pericardium and Heart." They presented 5 cases of their own and 15 collected cases of others, separating off a distinct group of patients in whom there was a distal sternal defect, an omphalocele or omphalocele-like parietal abdominal defect, a crescentic anterior diaphragmatic defect, a pericardial defect allowing pericardio-peritoneal communication and an intracardiac defect usually involving a ventricular septal defect, often involving a left ventricular diverticulum (Fig. 41–4). In point of fact, investigation shows that anomalies of this kind can vary widely, and under a variety of titles have been reported in such numbers as to preclude a complete review. The early reports by Ramel[25] in 1778 and O'Bryen[23] in 1837 merit reading for their clarity and their charm. In 1953, Major[20] discussed the condition and reviewed a group of

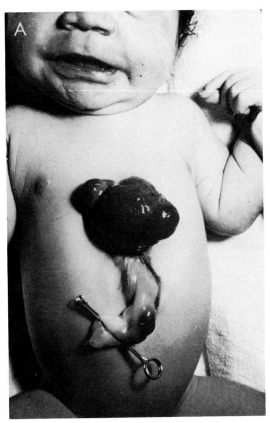

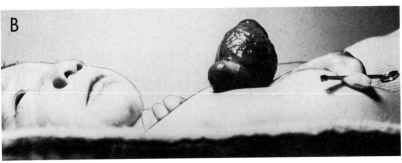

Fig. 41–3.—Newborn infant with true ectopia cordis extrathoracic nuda. The naked heart is exposed to the air through a cleft in the sternum. Such hearts invariably are grossly deformed, frequently with a single ventricle, and thus far only a single child has survived skin coverage and partial replacement within the body. The defect in the sternum may be central, distal, proximal or complete. (Courtesy of Dr. J. A. Knowles.)

cases as, for that matter, had Arnold[2] in 1894. The case of the patient operated on by Scott[30] in 1950 is unique in that "most of the small and large intestines had passed into the pericardial sac." From the standpoint of life, the most serious consideration is the intracardiac defect. Usually this is a ventricular septal defect, but there have also been seen tetralogy of Fallot, cor triloculare with a single ventricle, left ventricular diverticulum, tricuspid atresia and various bizarre anomalies. A ventricular septal defect was at least part of the anomaly in every recorded instance in which there is an adequate description of the heart. An atrial septal defect was present in 53% of the cases; valvular or infundibular pulmonary stenosis occurred in 33%. Of the established cardiac syndromes, only the tetralogy of Fallot was seen with any frequency—20% of the patients—and a left ventricular diverticulum was present in another 20%. More or less remote and unrelated congenital anomalies appear to be rare in most of these patients.

DEVELOPMENT OF THE SPECIFIC DEFECTS.—It has been suggested that the diaphragmatic defect, the pericardial defect and the intracardiac lesions are due to developmental failure of appropriate segments of the mesoderm.

The diaphragmatic defect results from total or partial failure of the transverse septum to develop. When complete, the defect corresponds to that portion of the diaphragm derived from the transverse septum—a ventral defect extending laterally to the region of the pleuroperitoneal folds and dorsally to the point of attachment of the liver and diaphragm. Less extensive defects represent partial rather than total loss of the septum transversum. This anomaly is not related to defects of the foramen of Morgagni.

The pericardial defect involves that portion of the pericardium that normally lies on the diaphragm and which arises from the somatic mesoderm, immediately adjacent to that region of the same layer from which the transverse septum is derived. Defects of this type, of the diaphragm or of the pericardium, without a corresponding defect in the other, would require a highly specific loss of somatic mesoderm and, consequently, are uncommon. It is not surprising, therefore, that coexisting defects of the diaphragm and the diaphragmatic portion of the pericardium are seen in the great majority of the patients under discussion.

The intracardiac lesions result from faulty development of the epimyocardium, which again is derived from the splanchnic mesoderm corresponding to that portion of the somatic mesoderm from which the pericardium is derived. The reason for the predominant occurrence of ventricular septal defects is not clear.

The sternal defect represents not absence of the sternum but failure of fusion of the distal portion. Similarly, the abdominal wall defect constitutes not an absence of normal elements of the ventral abdominal wall but a failure of complete migration of the myotomes, so that differentiation into the various muscle layers occurs at a point abnormally lateral to the midline. The rectus muscles in these patients arise normally from the pubis but diverge as they run cephalad so that they insert into the costal margin at the midclavicular line.

The basic defect in all of these abnormalities could be an absence or deficiency of ventral midline mesenchymal tissue into which the migrating mesodermal structures would normally grow. The time of origin of this syndrome of concatenated defects would have to be prior to, or immediately

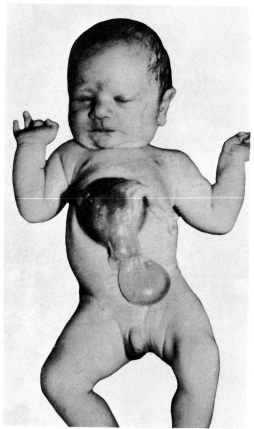

Fig. 41–4.—Distal sternal cleft in pentalogy of defects: sternal cleft, ventral abdominal defect (omphalocele), anterior diaphragmatic defect, pericardial defect, ventricular septal defect (tetralogy of Fallot). The diaphragmatic and midline defects were repaired at once and the cardiac defect left for later repair. (From Cantrell *et al.*[6])

after, the differentiation of the primitive intraembryonic mesoderm into its splanchnic and somatic layers, since derivatives of both of these layers are involved. This would place the time of initiation between the fourteenth and the nineteenth day of embryonic life.

CLINICAL APPROACH.—Apart from the philosophy that has been expressed repeatedly in these pages that congenital anomalies in children are, in general, most satisfactorily treated as soon as they are seen, provided that they are understood and an appropriate operative procedure is available, the children with omphaloceles demand immediate treatment. At the time of correction of the omphalocele, the ventral abdominal defect can be entirely closed, the fissured sternum repaired and the edge of the diaphragmatic defect sutured to the costal arch. In the present state of cardiac surgery, a direct attack on intracardiac anomalies in the neonatal period usually is not feasible. A diverticulum of the left ventricle can, however, readily be excised at the time of the repair.

In children not seen until some years after birth, the nature of the defects, the age of the child and its cardiac status will determine whether the parietal defect and the cardiac defect should be operated on simultaneously, or which should take precedence. In a remarkable instance, Mulder[21] operated on a 15-month-old child, completed the sternal cleft in a median sternotomy, excised a diverticulum of the left ventricle, closed a ventricular septal defect, repaired the

diaphragmatic and abdominal defects and corrected the sternal fissure at the time of closure of the median sternotomy.

From Great Ormond Street, London (1968), Murphy, Aberdeen, Dobbs and Waterston[22] reported the second successful one-stage complete operation in an 11-year-old girl with both a ventricular septal defect and a large left ventricular diverticulum. In this instance, the diverticulum was resected, the ventricular septal defect was patched and the upper part of the parietal defect was closed over with a layer of Marlex mesh.

A third complete one-stage operation was reported from Atlanta, Georgia, in 1973 by Symbas and Ware.[32] The left ventricular diverticulum was amputated and the parietal defects repaired directly.

The manner of repair of the ventral defect will vary with its degree. In defects like those of Mulder's patient, which represent little more than a diastasis recti, the muscles can be readily approximated in the midline. In others, it may be necessary to make relaxation incisions in the rectus sheath or even to turn over flaps of rectus sheath, reinforced by fascia lata. In the small patients, it is possible to close the sternal fissure; in older patients, this has not proved to be possible, and some type of soft tissue or prosthetic repair is required.

REFERENCES

1. Abbott, J.: Absence de sternum chez une femme adulte: Compatibilité de cette anomalie avec la vie et la santé, Gaz. Méd. Paris VII:777, 1852.
2. Arnold, J.: Ueber angeborene Divertikel des Herzens, Virchows Archiv. 137:318, 1894.
3. Asp, K., and Sulamaa, M.: Ectopia cordis, Acta Chir. Scand. 283; 52, 1961.
4. Breschet, G.: Mémoire sur l'ectopie de l'appareil de la circulation, et particulièrement sur celle du coeur, Repertoire Gen. Anat. Physiol. Pathol. Clin. Chir., pp. 1–59, Paris, 1826.
5. Burton, J. F.: Method of correction of ectopia cordis: Two cases, Arch. Surg. 54:79, 1947.
6. Cantrell, J. R., Haller, J. A., and Ravitch, M. M.: A syndrome of congenital defects involving the abdominal wall, sternum, diaphragm, pericardium and heart, Surg. Gynecol. Obstet. 107:602, 1958.
7. Chen, J. M.: Studies on the morphogenesis of the mouse sternum. III. Experiments on the origin of the sternum and its capacity for self differentiation in vitro, J. Anat. 86:387, 1952.
8. Daum, R., and Hecker, W. Ch.: Zur operativen Korrektur der totalen Sternumspalte, Thoraxchirurgie 12:333, 1964.
9. Daum, R., and Heiss, W.: Zur operativen Korrektur angeborener Sternumspalten, Thoraxchirurgie 17–18:432, 1969–1970.
10. deTorres, J. I.: Extract of a Letter from Jos. Ignat. de Torres, M.D. to the Royal Society, containing an extraordinary Case of the Heart of a Child turned upside down, Philos. Trans. London XLI:776, 1740–1741.
11. Fell, H. B.: The origin and developmental mechanics of the avian sternum, Philos. Trans. R. Soc. London 229:407, 1939.
12. Greig, D. M.: Cleft sternum and ectopia cordis, Edinburgh Med. J. 33:480, 1926.
13. Groux, E. A.: Abhandlungen und Notizen uber E. A. Groux's FISSURA STERNI CONGENITA von den berühmtesten Ärzten Europa's (Hamburg: J. E. M. Kohler, 1858).
14. Hanson, R. B.: The ontogeny and phylogeny of the sternum, Am. J. Anat. 26:41, 1919.
15. Ingelrans, P., and Debeugny, P.: Observation de bifidité du sternum associée à une angiomatose trachéale, Ann. Chir. Infant. 6:123, 1965.
16. Jewett, T. C., Jr., Butsch, W. L., and Hug, H. R.: Congenital bifid sternum, Surgery 52:932, 1962.
17. Kalter, H., and Warkany, J.: Experimental production of congenital malformations in mammals by metabolic procedure, Physiol. Rev. 39, Pt. 1, Jan.–July, 1959, pp. 69–115.
18. Lannelongue: De l'ectocardie et de sa cure par l'autoplastie, Ann. Med.-Chir. 4:101, 1888.
19. Maier, H. C., and Bortone, F.: Complete failure of sternal fusion with herniation of pericardium, J. Thorac. Surg. 18:851, 1949.
20. Major, J. W.: Thoracoabdominal ectopia cordis, J. Thorac. Surg. 26:309, 1953.

21. Mulder, D. G., Crittenden, I. H., and Adams, F. H.: Complete repair of a syndrome of congenital defects involving the abdominal wall, sternum, diaphragm, pericardium, and heart: Excision of left ventricular diverticulum, Ann. Surg. 151:113, 1960.
22. Murphy, D. A., Aberdeen, E., Dobbs, R. H., and Waterston, D. J.: The surgical treatment of a syndrome consisting of thoracoabdominal wall, diaphragmatic, pericardial, and ventricular septal defects, and a left ventricular diverticulum, Ann. Thorac. Surg. 6:528, 1968.
23. O'Bryen, J.: A case of partial ectopia cordis and umbilical hernia, Trans. Provincial Med. Surg. Assoc. 6:374, 1837.
24. Pinot, M.: Etude expérimentale de la morphogenèse de la cage thoracique chez l'embryon de Poulet: mécanismes et origine du matériel, J. Embryol. Exp. Morphol. 21:149, 1969.
25. Ramel: Observation de médicine. Sur un coeur situé au dessous du diaphragme, J. Méd. Chir. 49:423, 1778.
26. Ravitch, M. M.: Spectacular problems in surgery. Congenital absence of sternum, Surg. Gynecol. Obstet. 1963.
27. Ravitch, M. M.: *Congenital Deformities of the Chest Wall and Their Operative Correction* (Philadelphia: W. B. Saunders Company, 1977).
28. Sabiston, D. C., Jr.: The surgical management of congenital bifid sternum with partial ectopia cordis, J. Thorac. Surg. 35:118, 1958.
29. Saxena, N. D.: Personal communication, December 18, 1975.
30. Scott, G. W.: Ectopia cordis. Report of a case successfully treated by operation, Guy's Hosp. Rep. 104:55, 1955.
31. Seno, T.: An experimental study on the formation of the body wall in the chick, Acta Anat. 45:60, 1961.
32. Symbas, P. N., and Ware, R. E.: A syndrome of defects of the thoracoabdominal wall, diaphragm, pericardium, and heart, J. Thorac. Cardiovasc. Surg. 65:914, 1973.
33. Weese, C.: Des Cordis Ectopia. Inaugural Dissertation. Vol. I. 50 pages. Starck, Nortlin, 1818.

Depression Deformities

Depression deformities of the sternum—known under such names as pectus excavatum, funnel chest, trichterbrust, schusterbrust and thorax en entonnoir—form the group of deformities that are most commonly treated operatively.

Bauhinus' 1594 case published by Schenck[5] is the earliest written report that has been found. Surgical treatment began with Sauerbruch's first patient, operated on in 1913.[36] Lexer's patient was reported by Hoffmeister in 1927,[16] Sauerbruch's second patient was reported in 1931[37] and in the United States Alexander[3] reported 2 in 1931. The classic review by Ochsner and DeBakey[25] appeared in 1938. The analysis of the clinical problem by A. Lincoln Brown[8] the following year, with a simplified description of the operative technique, initiated the era of modern surgical management.

Pectus excavatum is a deformity of the thorax marked by a sharp posterior curve of the body of the sternum sweeping down from the manubrium, and deepest just before the junction with the xiphoid. The lower costal cartilages bend dorsally to form a depression, the lateral borders of which usually are angled more sharply than the superior and inferior portions of the deformity. Asymmetric deformities are not rare. The concavity usually is somewhat deeper on the right than on the left. Often the sternum is rotated to the right, in extreme cases by 90 degrees, so that what should be the ventral surface of the sternum forms the left side of the deepest portion of the concavity. The right breast in girls occasionally is somewhat less well developed than the left. The deformity may take the form of a broad, relatively shallow deformity that, in an adolescent or a young adult, may measure 17 cm in width, essentially from nipple to nipple, 14 cm or more in length and 3–7 cm in depth. Another type presents as a deep, narrow central pocket and suggests the easy accommodation of a fist or a large ball. These types have been called saucer shaped and cup shaped, respectively. In pectus excavatum in infancy, paradoxic inward motion of the sternum is conspicuous on inspiration, and some degree of deformity persists, even on forced expiration (Fig. 41–5). The deformity usually is present at birth, and progressive.

Infants with this deformity tend to have one of two types of general thoracic configuration. In one, there is a generally well-formed sturdy thorax with a central depression; in the other, the thorax is quite shallow in the anteroposterior diameter even well lateral to the depression. Although the patients with the very broad, shallow-seeming deformities almost invariably have a very shallow chest lateral to the deformities, usually a very long thorax and tend to be asthenic, the deep central defects occur in patients of this type as well as in patients with an otherwise well-formed chest. Pot belly is characteristic of children with pectus excavatum, and Harrison's groove is not rare. As the children grow older, a characteristic habitus develops. The chest is sunken, the abdomen protuberant, the shoulders rounded and the neck slouched forward (Fig. 41–6).

Occurrence

Although it appears that the vast majority of instances are sporadic, a definite familial incidence is seen in other cases (Fig. 41–7) We have operated on many pairs of siblings, on a father and daughter with the same deformity and on 3 children with severe deformity in a family with 2 additional siblings who have had various degrees of somewhat less severe deformity. Sainsbury[35] described a family in which funnel chest was seen in members of 4 successive generations. Occasionally, funnel chest is associated with other skeletal abnormalities. This is particularly true of Marfan's syndrome, the hereditary nature of which is well known. Funnel chest is not rare in association with congenital cardiac malformations. Rickets and scurvy, formerly thought to be causative factors, probably bear no relation to the deformity. Upper airway obstruction early in infancy that persists for a long time, with constant inspiratory retraction of the sternum, ultimately results in a fixed deformity. We have seen this in a child with congenital stenosis of the nares.

Clinical Picture

It is generally stated that pectus excavatum is asymptomatic in infancy and childhood. We have, however, seen 2 infants with severe inspiratory stridor in whom careful study showed no evidence of respiratory obstruction from any of the ordinary mechanisms and in whom the larynx and trachea seemed normal. Both had marked fixed deformity as well as a severe paradoxic sternal retraction. In both, the stridor disappeared immediately after operation, an event that has been noted by others. In a very small number of infants, a history is volunteered before operation of apparent dysphagia or some impediment to the deglutition of food, which is relieved by operation. This is perhaps as difficult to explain mechanically as the relief from stridor in our 2 patients. It is almost a regular event for mothers bringing children in for postoperative examinations to state that the children are eating as they never ate before, in terms of avidity and quantity, and that they are more energetic, more vigorous and more outgoing than ever before. This is true of infants and small children as well as of older youngsters. The first evidences of actual physical difficulty appear in childhood. By radiologic study and by electrocardiography with multiple precordial leads and spatial vector cardiography, the heart usually can be found to be displaced to the left and rotated in a clockwise direction. Presumably as a consequence of the pressure on the heart, and the displacement thus caused, systolic murmurs and cardiac arrhythmias in

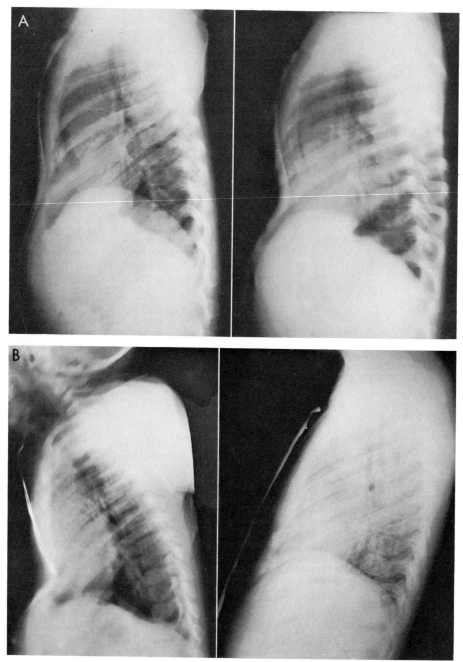

Fig. 41–5.—Pectus excavatum. **A,** C.H., expiration and inspiration showing obvious compression of heart, with the paradoxic inspiratory inward motion of the sternum. **B,** D.P., infant with conspicuous deformity, even in forced expiration during crying. Postoperative roentgenogram shows correction achieved. The lateral views show the depth of the depression but, being essentially sagittal sections, do not indicate the cubic displacement or, of course, the dynamic effects on posture and on heart and lungs.

these children are common. They disappear after operation. Many of the children are thin and asthenic, quiet and do not seem to exercise vigorously. Occasionally, of course, one does see a vigorous, athletic youth with a very deep funnel chest that seems to discommode him not at all, but this is uncommon. More commonly, one is given the story of a child who can hike with his fellows but drops behind on an uphill grade, who can "fool around" a basketball court but not play a game; of a college boy who plays a game or two of tennis but not a set. Exercise tolerance usually is adequate for ordinary activities and moderately reduced for strenuous activities.

Despite a recorded experience extending back now well over half a century, reporting patients invalided by incapacity from exertion and relieved by correction of the severe chest deformity, many continue to contend[15] that although there may be justification for correction of pectus excavatum on cosmetic, psychologic or orthopedic grounds there is no physiologic justification for operation. We have extensively documented elsewhere[32] our own cases of severe cardiorespiratory difficulty in patients with pectus excavatum, relieved by operation. These include a man with two bouts of cardiac failure and fibrillation, a woman with progressive difficulty and incapacity for exercise and tachycardia, pre-

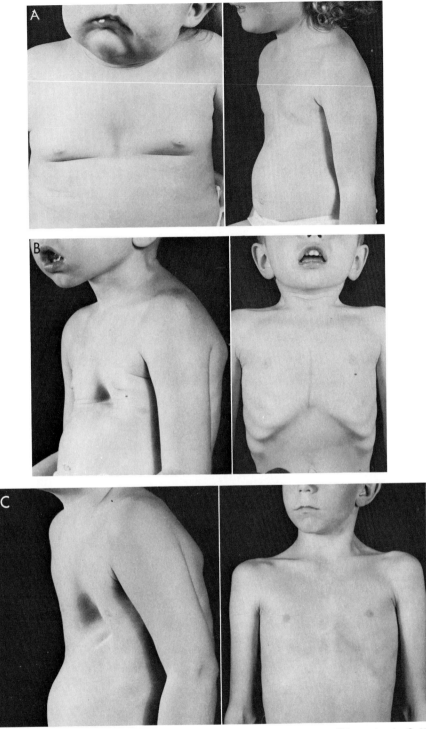

Fig. 41–6.—Pectus excavatum. Types of deformities operated on and results achieved. All left-hand photographs were taken immediately before operation. **A,** L.P., 3½ years since operation. The deformity had been progressing. **B,** J.A., 5 months since operation, showing disappearance of paradoxic sternal motion on deep inspiration—an optimal result. Posture now assumed was impossible previously. **C,** N.J., 7 years after operation. Note erect posture and inconspicuous scar. A slight subcutaneous prominence of the distal end of the sternum and slight depression of the midline beyond the sternum prevent this from being classified as an optimal result. (*Continued.*)

viously treated for 1 year for a presumed hyperthyroidism, and a woman presenting all the signs and symptoms of constrictive pericarditis. A careful reading of the literature from the earliest modern accounts[43] to the most recent[13] uncovers numerous instances of severely symptomatic patients.

There has, for a long time, been a discrepancy between the reported lack of pathologic findings on physiologic investigation on the one hand and, on the other, the very common occurrence of milder symptoms and the occasional occurrence of severe cardiorespiratory symptoms—symptoms of both degrees relieved by operation. The application of appropriate techniques now has demonstrated that the

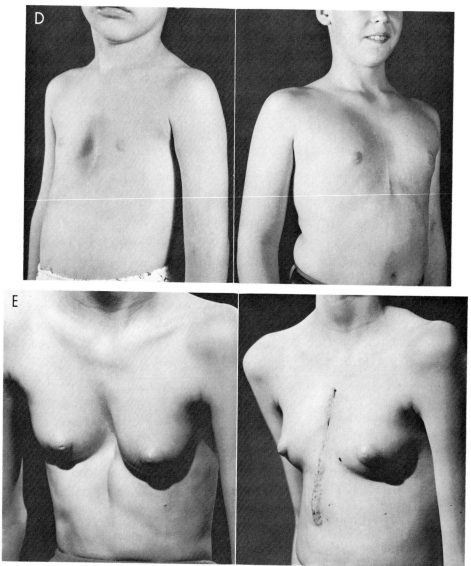

Fig. 41–6 (cont.).—D, G.R., one of two brothers operated on. Before operation, note slumped posture, pot belly and substantial concavity. Satisfactory correction is evident 7 years after operation. **E,** A.B., age 12, with profound pectus excavatum, agenesis of the left lung and disabling shortness of breath. She had given up bicycle riding and had difficulty climbing stairs. There was measured restrictive ventilatory defect. Two years after operation, she has striking return of capacity for exercise, riding her bicycle and climbing stairs with ease. There is substantial return of the ventilatory defect toward normal. Because of the pulmonary abnormality, two Kirschner wires were placed through the sternal marrow, resting on the chest wall; one was removed in 3 and the other in 6 months, with correction well maintained. This is one of the patients whose right breast is smaller than the left.

impairment of respiratory mechanics, the encroachment on the intrathoracic space, the pressure on and the compression, distortion and displacement of the heart do, in fact, produce measurable effects. These studies we have analyzed extensively.[32] The displacement of the heart to the left and its rotation have been abundantly demonstrated by electrocardiography, ordinary roentgenography and angiocardiography. The pancaking of the heart producing a diminished sagittal diameter has been documented and is easily seen in the plain PA film of many children with funnel chest. There is an area of relative lucency on the right side of the heart[11, 29, 34] (Fig. 41–8). Angiography has repeatedly demonstrated compression and deformation of the right ventricle and the right ventricular outflow tract.[1, 17, 32]

The unsophisticated early physiologic studies by us and by others[9] all merely give figures that are, at the most, in the lower normal range. In 1967, Weg *et al.,*[42] in 25 Air Force trainees with pectus excavatum, demonstrated a decrease in the forced expiratory flow and a significant decrease in maximal voluntary ventilation. Significant reports of the range of physiologic dysfunction in patients with pectus excavatum are those from Stockholm[7] and the confirmatory studies by Beiser *et al.*[6] from the National Heart and Lung Institute. Bevegård,[7] in 16 patients ranging from 15 to 63 years of age, pointed out that on transition from rest to exercise in the sitting position, the physical working capacity of his subjects increased significantly less than in normal subjects. The lower physical working capacity is explained by a considerably lower stroke volume during exercise in a sitting position, resulting in a higher pulse rate at a given oxygen uptake. He interpreted this as a result of impaired ventricular filling. The studies from the National Heart and Lung Institute on 6 adults with mild or moderate pectus excavatum, 16 to 44 years of age, tested their response to moderate, upright

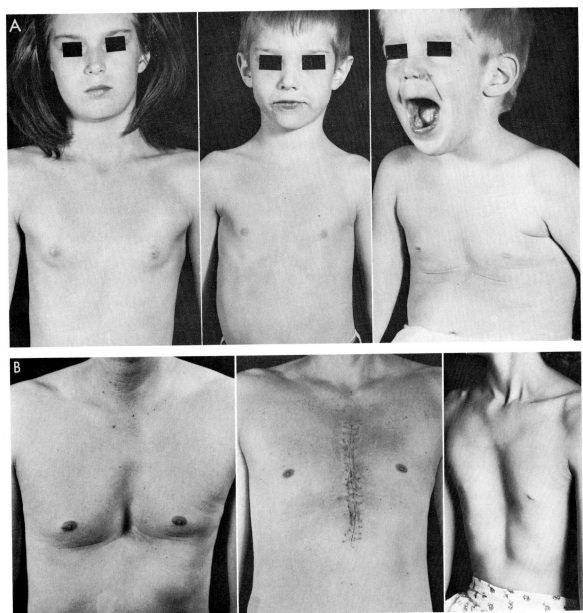

Fig. 41–7.—Pectus excavatum, familial incidence. Most of our cases are not familial, but such incidence is not rare. **A,** B.T. was operated on 9 years earlier at 18 months. Ma.T. was operated on 4 years earlier at 23 months. Mi.T. was operated on shortly after this photograph was taken. Two other siblings had mild deformities, not operated on. **B,** father and daughter. Father was beginning to have some shortness of breath on exertion. Daughter's deformity was still progressing. Both were operated on. Postoperative photograph shows correction of father's deep deformity. Daughter had an equally good result.

treadmill exercise before and after operation. In the supine position at rest, 3 patients had a mild restrictive ventilatory defect. All cardiac catheterization measurements were within normal range. The cardiac output response to moderate supine bicycle exercise was also normal. The response in cardiac output to intense *upright* exercise was below the normal range in 2 patients and at the lower limits of normal in 3. This diminished cardiac output response was due primarily to subnormal increase in stroke volume. Five of the patients had been symptomatic before operation; after operation, 2 of the patients were entirely asymptomatic and 1 who previously had considered himself asymptomatic found himself less fatigued and less short of breath during strenuous activity. Cardiac catheterization data after operation in

the supine position, at rest and during supine bicycle exercise were unchanged, but during intense upright exercise on the treadmill, the cardiac index was increased in each subject on an average of 2.2 liters per minute per square meter, or 38%, without any increase in heart rate at maximal exercise as compared to the preoperative studies. This is attributed to an enhanced stroke volume response. It is worth emphasizing that these significant findings were made in patients who did not have severe deformities. Beiser *et al.*[6] attributed the effects of pectus excavatum on the heart to diminished space in the lower thorax, compressing the heart and interfering with optimal filling of the right atrium and right ventricle, as suggested by us and others before.[40]

The enormous excess functional reserve in the normal

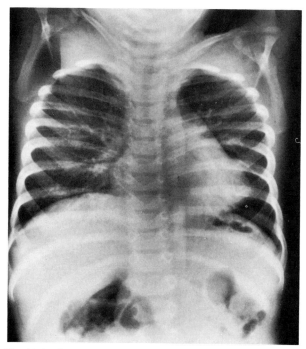

Fig. 41–8.—Pectus excavatum with pancake heart. This roentgenogram shows dramatically the effect of compression of the heart by a deep deformity when the heart does not escape to the left. The large area of relative radiolucency is the result of compression of the heart and a sharp reduction in its AP thickness.[32]

heart probably explains the relative infrequency of recognizable symptoms, particularly in children. Children often are mildly symptomatic, but in the absence of special factors are not severely affected. One of our patients was a 12-year-old girl with severe pectus excavatum as well as agenesis of the left lung (Fig. 41–6, *E*). In her, the combination of these two tolerable physiologic disadvantages produced an intolerable handicap, causing severe symptoms that were dramatically relieved by operative correction of the deformity.

The orthopedic effects of the uncorrected deformity in terms of the slouching, stooped posture are obvious, and the desirability of preventing it is clear, as is the importance of correcting the cardiorespiratory difficulties.

Subject to more argument, perhaps, is the psychologic importance of the cosmetic element of the deformity. It has been a matter of great interest to us that only rarely do parents, or children either, for that matter, present the psychologic effect as a reason for operation. In fact, they usually protest that they want the operation only if it is indicated for "reasons of health." But after operation, attention is centered almost entirely on the visible correction of the deformity and the relief this gives, usually to patient, parent and grandparent. Many children, male and female, come for operation in early adolescence, when they become reluctant to undress before their fellows. The father of one patient with a severe deformity allowed me to feel through his shirt his own extremely severe deformity, telling me that because of it he had never undressed before anyone in his adult life and had never gone swimming in a pool or at the beach. The change in personality of a young adult female after correction of a deep deformity is a striking thing. Shy, introverted, almost depressed individuals seem literally to bloom. How much better to prevent this psychologic maladjustment (Fig. 41–9) than to wait until adult life to correct it.

Indications for Operation

Pectus excavatum causes symptoms in most patients and produces severe symptoms in an occasional one. Operation is recommended (1) to prevent the development of symptoms or to correct those already present, (2) to correct the orthopedic and cosmetic aspects of the deformity and (3) to prevent or correct the psychologic response to the deformity.

Ample experience has demonstrated to us the ease and safety with which the operation can be performed, even in infants, and has convinced us that the younger the patient the easier the operation for both patient and surgeon and the more likely a restitution to a normal thoracic contour. For this reason, operation is advised whenever the patient is seen with a severe defect or a defect that is reliably stated to be progressive. In infants, the persistence of the defect during forced expiration in crying is as significant to us as the depth of the defect on quiet inspiration and the degree of paradoxic motion on forced inspiration. A good many children with relatively minor accentuation of the groove between the pectoral muscles are merely observed. In most such patients, the defect does not advance, but occasionally a mild pectus excavatum deformity deepens strikingly under observation, and operation then is indicated.

The manner of *presentation of operation* to the parents is important. Some parents are incapable of resolving on an elective operation for their children and will not so resolve, despite what may be said. Therefore, it is unfair and unwise to present the case for operation so strongly as to leave them feeling guilty when they make their inevitable decision against operation. It is my custom to state that the deformity usually is progressive and that we are unable to predict in which instances it will be progressive, that mild symptoms are extremely common, that real disability is uncommon and that serious disability is rare. The parents are informed that the risk of operation in infancy is no different from that in later life, that the operation is easier for the small patient and that early operation affords the best chance of restitution to a normal thoracic contour. They are also told that if operation is not performed, it can be undertaken at any time in the future when symptoms become severe, with the full expectation of relief from all symptoms. But the correction of the sternal deformity then will come after the associated abnormal thoracic configuration has been fixed.

Operative Technique

Operation (Fig. 41–10) is undertaken under endotracheal anesthesia. In our earlier operations, transfusion was a regular accompaniment, but with development of the operative technique, we have not, in more than 7 years, transfused any pectus excavatum patients but adults and some large adolescents. Measured blood loss in a small child may be 20–30 ml and in a large teen-ager 100–200 ml. Transfusion is, at times, required postoperatively for anemia, to replace blood that oozed into the mediastinum, principally from the sternal osteotomy. We have never seen operative shock or hypotension and have never had to reoperate for bleeding.

A midline incision from just above the upper border of the defect well down to the epigastrium provides the best exposure with the least difficulty. In small girls we use a transverse submammary incision. This requires more dissection and provides poorer exposure than the midline incision, which is used in all males, in older girls and in younger girls with extensive deformities. Prophylactic postoperative radiotherapy has been recommended, specifically after the

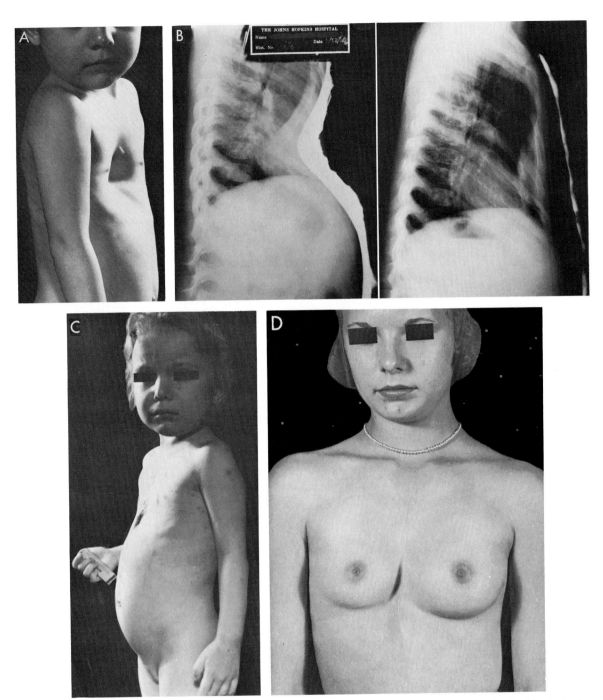

Fig. 41–9.—Pectus excavatum; 12½-year follow-up. **A,** preoperative photograph, showing profound depression and characteristic hunched appearance. **B,** pre- and postoperative roentgenograms, showing extent of the deformity and degree of correction. Contrast is obtained by a midline strip of barium paste squeezed from a tube. **C,** 1 week after operation. **D,** 12½ years after operation. Note the slightly smaller size of the right breast.

operation for pectus excavatum, to prevent the development of keloid.[20] But the incidence of cancer of the thyroid (see Chap. 34) in children treated for enlarged thymus glands with x-ray dosages frequently smaller than would be given to prevent keloid formation has kept us from adopting this measure.

In the vertical incision, skin, fat and the pectoral muscles are reflected in a single flap; in the transverse incision, the skin flaps are developed and then the pectoral muscles stripped back to either side (Fig. 41–10, A). The entire dissection is performed with a fine-needle-tipped electrocautery. If an alert assistant secures the perforating vessels from the internal mammary as they are brought into view by the stripping of the pectorales, the major source of blood loss is avoided. The pectoral muscles are stripped back to expose the deformed cartilages for the entire extent of their deformity. The lower one or two cartilages covered by the rectus muscle are exposed by splitting the muscle. The involved cartilages are removed subperichondrially for the full extent of their deformity (Fig. 41–10, B and C), which may be 5 or

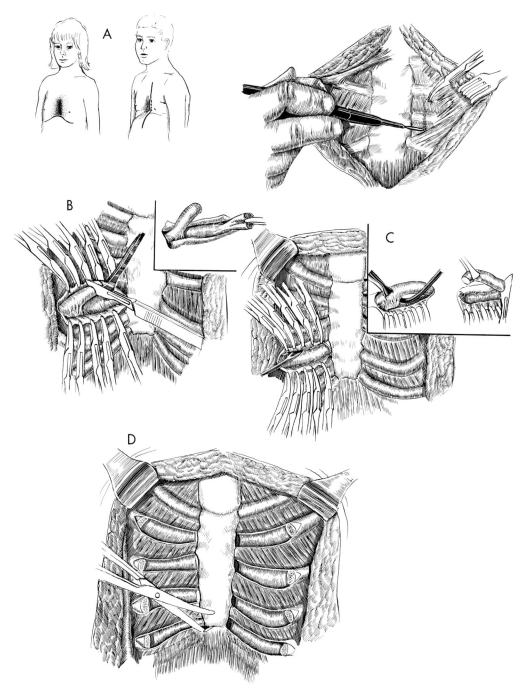

Fig. 41–10.—Operative treatment of pectus excavatum. The slightly bowed, submammary incision is used for little girls; a midline incision for all others. **A,** using the midline incision. After the skin is incised, dissection is carried down to the sternum by electrocautery and the pectoral muscles are dissected back from the sternum and costal cartilages. As the perforating branches of the internal mammary are encountered, they are picked up with a hemostat and coagulated before division. **B** and **C,** the perichondrium is incised longitudinally and a transverse incision made in the perichondrium at either end of the deformed portion of cartilage. If the perichondrial edges are seized with small curved hemostats and dissected away from the car-

tilage with delicate elevators like a Freer or a slender staphylorrhaphy, the cartilage can be either dissected out in one piece, as in **C,** with the right-angle Brophy elevator slipped under it to complete the dissection, or divided in the midportion, as in **B,** and each half stripped out and divided at its end. **D,** all deformed costal cartilages (in this case, four) have been excised the full length of their deformity. In infants, this will all be cartilage. In older children and adults, one will go beyond the costochondral junction of two or three ribs. The xiphoid is shown being divided from the sternum with scissors. A small artery on either side of the xiphoid requires coagulation. (*Continued.*)

6 cm for the lower cartilages and only 2 or 3 cm for the upper cartilages. The fourth, fifth, sixth and seventh cartilages usually are involved, and occasionally the third as well. In the smallest infants, it sometimes is necessary only to resect the fifth, sixth and seventh cartilages to remove all of the de-

formed cartilages. The xiphoid now is divided from the sternum with scissors (Fig. 41–10, *D*), the small artery on either side secured and the right index finger inserted into the mediastinum. In common with most authors, we have not been impressed with the frequency with which we can iden-

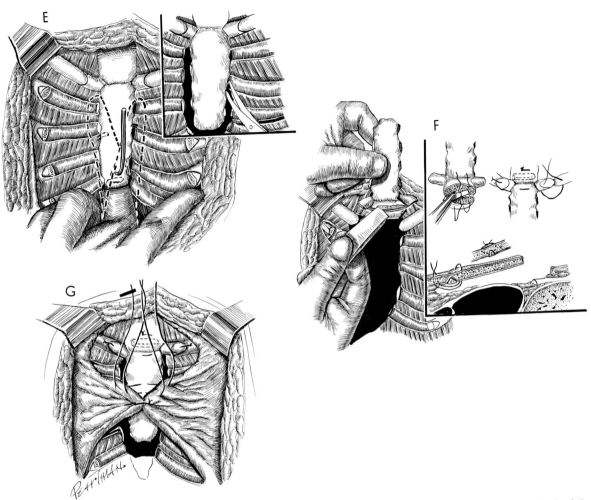

Fig. 41–10 (cont.).–E, the xiphoid having been divided, the sternum is lifted sharply forward with a bone hook, the index finger inserted into the mediastinum, the diaphragmatic attachments, if any, separated and the pleural envelopes displaced back beyond the edge of the sternum on either side. **Inset,** the intercostal bundles are divided from the sternum, with an attempt not to injure the internal mammary vessels. Oblique incisions have been made in the first intact costal cartilage, usually the 2d or 3d. The incision is made from medially and in front to laterally and behind. **F,** the sternum is elevated forward and a wire passed around it in the interspace above the obliquely divided cartilage, to serve as a guide. Care is taken to be certain that the line of the wire is precisely transverse. The posterior cortical lamella is scored with the corner of a sharp osteotome and the sternum fractured forward. **Inset,** a small piece of bone cut from a rib is inserted in the posterior sternal osteotomy and maintained there by silk sutures passed around the osteotomy and either through the bone fragment or around it. The sternum now sits in good corrected or overcorrected position with the medial ends of the obliquely divided cartilage overlapping the lateral ends to which they are sutured with heavy silk. **G,** the sternum is held in overcorrected position by the chock-block bone graft. The obliquely divided costal cartilages are sutured with medial ends overlapping, and now the pectoral muscles are being sutured to each other and to the sternal periosteum in the midline. Care is taken to close the subcutaneous tissue in at least two layers apart from the skin closure. The xiphoid is not reattached, and no muscle covers the space between xiphoid and sternum. The intercostal bundles are not sutured back to the sternum.

tify a tough midline fibrous structure, corresponding to the substernal ligament, thought by some to be a major cause or factor in the deformity.[8] Frequently, the diaphragmatic attachments to the sternum are remarkably light and almost invariably they can be separated with the finger. Very occasionally, a tough strand or two requires cutting. The medial extensions of the pleural envelopes are stripped back with the finger to beyond the sternum on either side, and with the scissors the intercostal bundles are divided from the sternum (Fig. 41–10, E). If care is taken to remain close to the sternum, the internal mammary arteries will not be injured and will be exposed on the underside of the intercostal bundles as this dissection continues. Invariably in older children, and increasingly often in infants, we then transect the first intact cartilage, usually the third or second, close to the sternum. This permits the transverse osteotomy of the ster-

num to be performed one interspace higher than otherwise, and allows for a gratifying overcorrection of the deformity. The cartilage is divided by an oblique incision from in front and medially, to behind and laterally, so that when the sternum is elevated, the medial portion of the cartilage will rest on the lateral (Fig. 41–10, F and G). The sternum is lifted forward, a wire passed around it in the interspace above the divided cartilage and the posterior cortical lamella scored with the corner of an osteotome until the sternum fractures forward (Fig. 41–10, F). The sternum now is isolated like a peninsula, attached at its upper end only by the anterior cortical lamella and its periosteum. A wedge of bone from an exposed rib is pressed into the osteotomy and retained by a heavy silk or synthetic suture through or around it, acting as a chock block (Fig. 41–10, F inset and G). Wire sutures may necrose the soft bone and cut through or may break. The ends of the obliquely transected second or third cartilage now will be found to have a new relationship to each other, the central ends usually being a little cephalad and resting on the lateral ends. This relationship is maintained by through-and-through sutures of silk, providing additional lateral points of fixation of the sternum to the chest wall.

If the sternum is unusually scaphoid, the result of correction of the first angulation at or near the sternomanubrial junction is to bring the tip of the sternum well anterior to the level of the chest wall. In such instances, an anterior transverse osteotomy is performed in the distal portion of the sternum at the approximate beginning of the anterior curve. The distal sternum is bent back and held in this position by inserting another wedge of rib bone into the opened linear osteotomy.

If there is a significant sternal rotation, the sternum is partially transected at the upper end of the twist, forcibly de-rotated and maintained in the corrected position by appropriately placed sutures.[32]

We have not used external fixation since our first two operations, the second of which resulted in a fatal infection, the only death in more than 400 operations. In adults and large teen-agers with extensive rib and cartilage resections and a long sternum exercising great leverage on the repair, in patients referred to us with operative failure and in patients with associated difficulties (the girl with agenesis of one lung, a man with simultaneous resection of emphysematous bullae), we have experimented with additional support of the sternum. A Teflon sling behind the sternum is difficult to make taut. A rib strut is very effective and has been satisfactory in 2 of our patients. For these cases we have, however, settled on one or two Kirschner wires[23] passed through the sternal marrow parallel to the anterior chest wall, the ends curled back on themselves so as not to penetrate the skin. The pectoral muscles cover the wires, which may be removed in 6 months. The ingenious Rehbein splints[33] are more difficult to insert, and the strut bar of steel behind the sternum[2] seems to be a large foreign body. In any case, such fixation rarely is required or used by us.

Injury to the pleura high on the right is not uncommon. The opening usually is left, or sometimes deliberately made, to allow any mediastinal collection to drain into the right pleural cavity for easy absorption. In the deeper deformities, the intercostal bundles, which formerly had an extremely indirect course to the sternum but now are running more directly, are found to be redundant and the excess may be trimmed away and one or two sutures placed to tack the intercostal bundles back to the sternum. If there is the slightest appearance of tension, the sutures are released and the intercostal bundles left unattached. The pectoral muscles are sutured to the sternum and to each other in the midline (Fig. 41–10, *G*) and the skin carefully closed with subcutaneous and cutaneous sutures. As in almost all operations, we avoid dressings. Accumulation of bloody fluid within the mediastinum is not uncommon and requires aspiration, sometimes several times. Rarely, we use catheter suction drainage for 48 hours, but, in general, we prefer to keep the wound closed and to aspirate it as necessary.

Oxygen is not required, but infants who have had an intratracheal tube in place for 1 ½ hours or more breathe moist air for at least 24 hours. No patient has required a tracheostomy. Two patients have received overnight ventilatory assistance—a very large adult and a teen-ager with Marfan's syndrome, who presented with a grotesque recurrence and underwent an extensive operation. Since the xiphoid is not resutured to the sternum, for fear of re-creating the defor-

mity, there is an unprotected rhomboidal area just beyond the tip of the sternum and between it and the xiphoid in which paradoxic motion can be observed for perhaps 1 week. This should be explained to the parents to avoid unnecessary concern. We start antibiotics the night before operation and continue them for 24 hours after operation. The children are allowed feedings and activities as they tolerate them and usually leave the hospital between the seventh and the ninth postoperative day. The parents are asked to see to it that older children avoid rough play for 2 weeks after discharge from the hospital. By the end of the third week, the chest wall is fairly firm and activity may be unrestricted. Adolescents are told to avoid contact sports for 3–6 months. The only complication we have seen after the patient has returned home is the occasional discharge through the incision of a previously unsuspected collection of serosanguineous fluid. The drainage does not persist in such instances and the wound heals spontaneously.

Results

We have operated on more than 400 patients varying in age from 2 months to 40 years. There has been 1 death in the entire group, our second operation—from infection—and we have had 5 other infections. Of children 14 years of age or younger, we have operated on 350. Symptoms always have been relieved, and increased vigor and weight and improved eating habits have been commented on frequently. There has been no frank recurrence of the deformity. In a number of patients, the optimal correction obtained after the operation has been lost. We recommended reoperation in 6 cases. Only 4 patients' families believed that reoperations were necessary, and in these the results have been gratifying. In general, inadequate resection of costal cartilages or a sternal osteotomy not made above the beginning of the downward slope of the sternum seemed to be the explanation of the less-than-optimal results.

Unsightly scars, undue prominence or asymmetry of the sternum occur in some patients. In others, the manubrium itself had been depressed, the entire chest shallow and the satisfactory result, although the best that can be attained, is not a restitution to normal.

Our operation as now performed has resulted from progressive modifications of our original procedure without change of the fundamentals. Nevertheless, mention must be made of the evaluation by Moghissi[24] in 1964 of 58 patients operated on at Southampton by the late E. F. Chin, using Chin's[10] significant modification of the operation we had described in 1949.[30] The evaluation was based entirely on cosmetic results. Twenty-seven chests were rated as normal, 18 as fair (70–90% of normal) and 13 as bad (less than 65% of normal). These figures are so far out of line with our results over a much longer period of observation as to raise a question regarding the general applicability of the observations. The wide interest in surgical correction of pectus excavatum in recent years has resulted in numerous suggestions for operative techniques. Some authors[12, 19] have insisted on the need for external traction for a longer or shorter time, some have used struts of bone,[41, 44] others always secure the chest behind the sternum[26] or through the sternum with a Kirschner wire[23, 28] and some use a heavy metal strut behind the sternum[18, 27] or internal metallic fixation,[33] which may be left or may be removed at a secondary operation. Instead of resecting the cartilages, many authors[1, 14, 22] morcellate the involved cartilages and, on one or another pattern, gridiron the sternum with osteotomies so that when it is pulled into position by external traction or held by a buried strut, the chest wall appears in normal position without the excision of any of its elements. A detailed discussion of the various operative techniques can be found in my monograph.[32]

We have found external traction to be unnecessary in either the more or the less extensive procedures. Morcellation of cartilages and sternum seems to be an unnecessarily large and possibly bloody procedure. The operation described here, which is a modification of that proposed by A. Lincoln Brown in 1939, seems to be the simplest and most effective one.

A word should be said about what has been called the "limited operation," also proposed by Brown. This consists of xiphisternal disarticulation, a freeing of the diaphragmatic attachments to the sternum with the finger and the resection of parts of one or two of the most distal cartilages on both sides. It has been suggested that, in the smallest infants, this will release the sternum from diaphragmatic traction and allow it to regain its normal position. We have experimented with the limited operation on two occasions, and, being dissatisfied with the result achieved in the operating room at the time, proceeded to the formal operation. It has also been our lot to operate on several children on whom the limited operation was said to have been performed and in whom the deformity either persisted or progressed. Even in infants, we doubt that there is a place for the limited operation.

REFERENCES

1. Actis-Dato, A., Gentilli, R. X., and Calderini, P.: I Pectus Excavatum (Torino: Minerva Medica, 1962).
2. Adkins, P. C., and Blades, B.: A stainless steel strut for correction of pectus excavatum, Surg. Gynecol. Obstet. 113:111, 1961.
3. Alexander, J.: Traumatic pectus excavatum, Ann. Surg. 93:489, 1931.
4. Bar, C. G., Zeilhofer, R., and Heckel, K.: Über die Beeinflussung des Herzens und der Atmung durch die Trichterbrust, Dtsch. Med. Wochenschr. 83:282, 1958.
5. Bauhinus, J.: Schenck von Grafenberg, Johannes. Observationum medicarum, rararum, novarum, admirabilium, et monstrosarum, liber secundus. De partibus vitalibus, thorace contentis. Observation 264, p. 516, Freiburg, 1594.
6. Beiser, G. D., Epstein, S. E., Stampfer, M., Goldstein, R. E., Noland, S. P., and Levitsky, S.: Impairment of cardiac function in patients with pectus excavatum, with improvement after operative correction, N. Engl. J. Med. 287:267, 1972.
7. Bevegård, S.: Postural circulatory changes at rest and during exercise in patients with funnel chest with special reference to factors affecting the stroke volume, Acta Med. Scand. 171:695, 1962.
8. Brown, A. L.: Pectus excavatum (funnel chest), J. Thorac. Surg. 9:164, 1939.
9. Brown, A. L., and Cook, O.: Cardiorespiratory studies in pre- and postoperative funnel chest (pectus excavatum), Dis. Chest 20:378, 1951.
10. Chin, E. F.: Surgery of funnel chest and congenital sternal prominence, Br. J. Surg. 44:360, 1957.
11. Edling, N. P. G.: The radiologic appearances of the heart, oesophagus and lung in funnel chest deformity, Acta Radiol. 39:273, 1953.
12. Effler, D. B.: Pectus excavatum: Surgical treatment, Cleve. Clin. Q. 20:353, 1953.
13. Geroulanos, S., Hahnloser, P., and Senning, A.: Trichterbrustkorrektur. Indikation, operatives Vorgehen und Resultate nach einer vereinfachten und modifizierten Methode, Helv. Chir. Acta 41:101, 1974.
14. Gross, R.: Surgery of Infancy and Childhood (Philadelphia: W. B. Saunders Company, 1953).
15. Haller, J. A.: Personal communication, 1970.
16. Hoffmeister, W.: Operation der angeborenen Trichterbrust, Beitr. Klin. Chir. 141:215, 1927.
17. Howard, R.: Funnel chest: Its effect on cardiac function, Arch. Dis. Child. 34:5, 1959.
18. Jensen, N. K., Schmidt, R. W., and Garamella, J. J.: Funnel chest, a new corrective operation, J. Thorac. Cardiovasc. Surg. 43:731, 1962.
19. Lester, C. W.: The surgical treatment of funnel chest, Ann. Surg. 123:1003, 1946.
20. Lindskog, G. E., and Felton, W. L., II: Considerations in the surgical treatment of pectus excavatum, Ann. Surg. 142:654, 1955.
21. Lyons, H. A., Zuhdi, M. N., and Kelly, J. J., Jr.: Pectus excavatum ("funnel breast"), a cause of impaired ventricular distensibility as exhibited by right ventricular pressure pattern, Am. Heart J. 50:921, 1955.
22. Mahoney, E. V., and Emerson, G. L.: Surgical treatment of the congenital funnel chest deformity, Arch. Surg. 67:317, 1953.
23. Mayo, P., and Long, G. A.: Surgical repair of pectus excavatum by pin immobilization, J. Thorac. Cardiovasc. Surg. 44:53, 1962.
24. Moghissi, K.: Long term results of surgical correction of pectus excavatum and sternal prominence, Thorax 19:350, 1964.
25. Ochsner, A., and DeBakey, M.: Chone-chondrosternon, J. Thorac. Surg. 8:469, 1938.
26. Overholt: In discussion of Adkins, P. C., and Gwathmey, O.: Pectus excavatum—an appraisal of surgical treatment, J. Thorac. Surg. 36:714, 1958.
27. Paltia, V., Parkkulainen, V. J., Sulamaa, M., and Wallgren, G. R.: Operative technique in funnel chest. Experience in 81 cases, Acta Chir. Scand. 116:990, 1958/59.
28. Peters, R. P., and Johnson, J.: Stabilization of pectus deformity with wire strut, J. Thorac. Cardiovasc. Surg. 47:814, 1964.
29. Pohl, R.: Trichterbrust und Herzform, Wien. Klin. Wochenschr. 41:1439, 1928.
30. Ravitch, M. M.: The operative treatment of pectus excavatum, Ann. Surg. 129:929, 1949.
31. Ravitch, M. M.: Pectus excavatum and heart failure, Surgery 30:178, 1951.
32. Ravitch, M. M.: Congenital Defects of the Chest Wall and Their Operative Correction (Philadelphia: W. B. Saunders Company, 1977).
33. Rehbein, F., and Wernicke, H. M.: The operative treatment of the funnel chest, Arch. Dis. Child. 32:5, 1957.
34. Rosler, H.: Zur rontgenologischen Beurteilung des Herzgefassibildes bei Thorax deformitäten; [(Kypho)- Skoliose, reine Kyphose, Trichterbrust], Dtsch. Arch. Klin. Med. 164:365, 1929.
35. Sainsbury, H. S. K.: Congenital funnel chest, Lancet 2:615, 1947.
36. Sauerbruch, E. F.: Die Chirurgie der Brustorgane (3d ed.; Berlin: Springer-Verlag, 1928), p. 735.
37. Sauerbruch, E. F.: Operative Beseitigung der angeborenen Trichterbrust, Dtsch. Z. Chir. 234:760, 1931.
38. Schoberth, H.: Die Trichterbrust, Ergeb. Chir. 43:122, 1961.
39. Vega Diaz, F., Pelous, A. N., Gonzales-Valdez, F., Grande, F. G. G., and Granados, A.: Pectus excavatum, Am. J. Cardiol. 10:272, 1962.
40. Wachtel, F. W., Ravitch, M. M., and Grishman, A.: The relation of pectus excavatum to heart disease, Am. Heart J. 52:121, 1956.
41. Wahren, H.: The use of a tibial graft as a retrosternal support in funnel chest surgery, Acta Chir. Scand. 99:568, 1950.
42. Weg, J. G., Krumholz, R. A., and Harkleroad, L. E.: Pulmonary dysfunction in pectus excavatum, Am. Rev. Respir. Dis. 96:936, 1967.
43. Williams, C. T.: Congenital malformations of the thorax; great depression of the sternum, Philos. Trans. R. Soc. Lond. 24:50, 1872.
44. Woods, R. M., Overholt, R. H., and Bolton, H. E.: Pectus excavatum, Dis. Chest 22:274, 1952.

Protrusion Deformities

Protrusion deformities of the sternum (pigeon breast, chicken breast, pectus carinatum) are substantially less common than the forms of pectus excavatum—the depression deformities of the sternum. The ratio of pectus carinatum to pectus excavatum in most series is 1 to 6 to 1 to 10.[1, 5, 15] During the time in which we have operated on some 400 patients with pectus excavatum, we have operated on some 31 patients with pectus carinatum.

Clinical Forms

Protrusion deformities are of two principal types, which differ in their appearance. The first, producing a *pouter pigeon breast*, is marked by prominent forward tilting of the manubrium, with what amounts to a manubriogladiolar

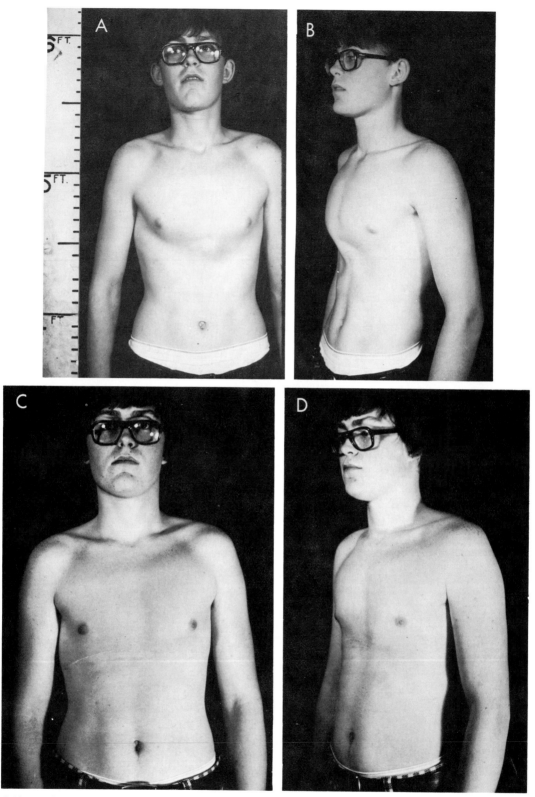

Fig. 41–11.—A 16-year-old boy with pectus carinatum. **A** and **B**, the abnormal prominence of the sternum is only partly apparent and is relative to the deep depression of the costal cartilages and ribs well lateral to the sternum. **C** and **D**, at 2 years after operation, the scar is inconspicuous. The excision of the incurved chondrocostal elements and the reefing sutures in the perichondrium (the resection having gone out into the bony rib in the four lower elements) have obliterated the depression. As occasionally is the case, the distal end of the sternum angled downward, and this was corrected by transverse anterior cuneiform sternotomy, allowing the distal end to be elevated and maintained in the corrected position by suture. Nothing else was done to the sternum itself. The combination of the elimination of the comparison between the sternum and the depressed costal cartilages, the traction on the sternum exerted by the tautened perichondrium and possibly the disappearance of the need for compensatory expansion of the chest in the midline has resulted in the restoration of a normal thoracic configuration.

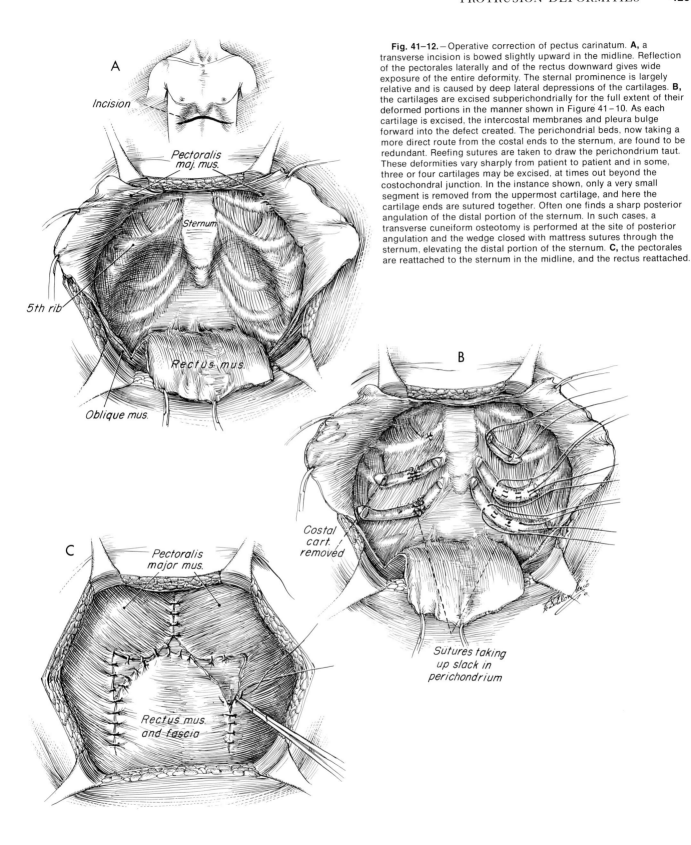

Fig. 41–12.—Operative correction of pectus carinatum. **A,** a transverse incision is bowed slightly upward in the midline. Reflection of the pectorales laterally and of the rectus downward gives wide exposure of the entire deformity. The sternal prominence is largely relative and is caused by deep lateral depressions of the cartilages. **B,** the cartilages are excised subperichondrially for the full extent of their deformed portions in the manner shown in Figure 41–10. As each cartilage is excised, the intercostal membranes and pleura bulge forward into the defect created. The perichondrial beds, now taking a more direct route from the costal ends to the sternum, are found to be redundant. Reefing sutures are taken to draw the perichondrium taut. These deformities vary sharply from patient to patient and in some, three or four cartilages may be excised, at times out beyond the costochondral junction. In the instance shown, only a very small segment is removed from the uppermost cartilage, and here the cartilage ends are sutured together. Often one finds a sharp posterior angulation of the distal portion of the sternum. In such cases, a transverse cuneiform osteotomy is performed at the site of posterior angulation and the wedge closed with mattress sutures through the sternum, elevating the distal portion of the sternum. **C,** the pectorales are reattached to the sternum in the midline, and the rectus reattached.

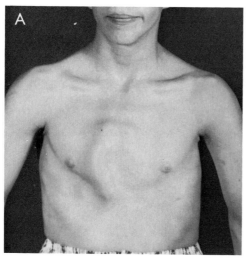
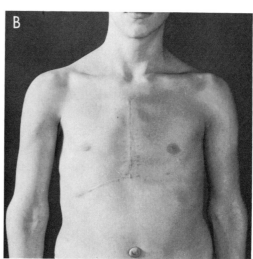

Fig. 41–13.—Atypical chest deformity, carinatum type. **A,** a boy of 15 with grotesque and socially disabling deformity of the chest wall consisting of bilateral costal cartilage and rib concavities; tilting, depression and rotation of the sternum, and extraordinary chondrosternal prominence on the right. **B,** after the first stage. The depressed costal cartilages on the right were excised subperichondrially and the redundant perichondrium reefed and some of the chondrosternal prominence excised. At the second operation, the sternum was rotated and its position corrected; and at the third stage, the left chondral depression was corrected.

prominence. Distal to this, the gladiolus inclines posteriorly and actually forms a type of pectus excavatum deformity, such that, in sagittal section, the sternum would show a Z-shaped configuration. This deformity usually is marked by abnormal fusion of all the sternal segments.[1, 5, 6] The sternum in these patients usually is broader than usual and the xiphoid occasionally bifid.

The deformity, more commonly thought of as pectus carinatum (Fig. 41–11) or pigeon breast, presents an obvious prominence of the sternum, largely of the corpus sterni, the manubrium being tilted little, if at all. A lateral depression of the ribs and costal cartilages to either side of the sternum accentuates the sternal prominence. In pectus carinatum, asymmetries and atypical deformities are common and may be bizarre.

These lateral depressions, or runnels, are deep enough to compress the heart and to reduce the thoracic volume substantially. The prominence of the sternum is largely relative, being accentuated by the lateral chondrocostal depressions and in part is compensatory to make up for the loss of intrathoracic space caused by the lateral depressions.[13]

The term pyramidal chest[10, 14] is used when the sternum angles steadily forward in a straight line from the manubrium to the xiphoid.

As with pectus excavatum, males are affected more frequently. Whereas pectus excavatum is seen commonly at birth, the various protrusion deformities usually are not recognized before the age of 3 or 4, and often escape attention until the early teens. The occurrence of pectus excavatum and pectus carinatum in the same family, its occasional occurrence, like pectus excavatum, in Marfan's syndrome and in patients with congenital heart disease and its occurrence[4] associated with congenital absence of the hand all suggest a congenital origin.[13]

Etiology

Although Brodkin[3] and Chin[5] have impugned failure of development of muscle in portions of the diaphragm, resulting in unequal pull, the evidence for this is unconvincing. We agree with Humbert,[8] who suggested that if there is excessively rapid growth of the ribs, it is a matter of chance whether they buckle so as to produce pectus excavatum or pectus carinatum.

Operative Correction

The pouter pigeon deformity is satisfactorily corrected by subperichondrial excision of the deformed cartilages and anterior cuneiform sternal osteotomies at the apices of the two angulations, with suture fixation.[11]

A number of operative procedures have been aimed at the correction of protrusion deformities. Lester[9] excised small portions of the involved cartilages subperiosteally, allowing redevelopment of the sternum in a depressed position. Chin[5] disengaged the xiphoid and reinserted it into a slot made for it in the sternum, at the level of the fourth costal cartilage, a procedure that, in small children, is said to pull the sternum back into proper position. Howard[7] has added Chin's procedure to that which we perform.

Our procedure for operative correction of the more common pigeon breast (Fig. 41–12) involves a subperichondrial resection of the deformed cartilages on both sides, with reefing sutures taking up the slack in the perichondrium, obliterating the lateral depressions. Ordinarily, nothing need be done to the sternum. In the occasional instance in which the distal sternum bends sharply backward, an anterior sternal osteotomy will allow this to be corrected. Large sternal bosses or a greatly thickened anterior cortex can be cut away with an osteotome. The results are uniformly satisfactory.

The variety of protrusion deformities probably is such that, even more than in depression deformities, a certain amount of ingenuity and individuality of approach in operative therapy is required (Fig. 41–13).

REFERENCES

1. Asp, K., and Sulamaa, M.: On rare congenital deformities of the thoracic wall, Acta Chir. Scand. 118:392, 1959/60.
2. Bianchi, C., Pizzoli, A., and Campacci, R.: Resultati a distanza. Su 20 casi di "Cifosi Sternale" trattati incruentemente, Fracastoro 61:779, 1968.
3. Brodkin, H. A.: Congenital chondrosternal prominence (pigeon breast). A new interpretation, Pediatrics 3:286, 1949.

4. Brodkin, H. A.: Pigeon breast—congenital chondrosternal prominence: Etiology and surgical treatment by xiphosternopexy, Arch. Surg. 77:261, 1958.
5. Chin, E. F.: Surgery of funnel chest and congenital sternal prominence, Br. J. Surg. 44:360, 1957.
6. Currarino, G., and Silverman, F. N.: Premature obliteration of the sternal sutures and pigeon-breast deformities, Radiology 70:532, 1958.
7. Howard, R.: Pigeon breast (protrusion deformity of the sternum), Med. J. Aust. 2:664, 1958.
8. Humberd, C. D.: Giantism of the infantilism type and its disclosure of the pathogenesis of pigeon breast and funnel chest, Med. Rec. 147:444, 1938.
9. Lester, C. W.: Pigeon breast (pectus carinatum) and other protrusion deformities of developmental origin, Ann. Surg. 137:482, 1953.
10. Peters, J. T.: Erklärung für das Zustandekommen des Pyramid-enförmigen Thorax, Klin. Wochenschr, 3:1535, 1924.
11. Ravitch, M. M.: Unusual sternal deformity with cardiac symptoms: Operative correction, J. Thorac. Surg. 23:138, 1952.
12. Ravitch, M. M.: The operative correction of pectus carinatum (pigeon breast), Ann. Surg. 151:705, 1960.
13. Ravitch, M. M.: *Congenital Deformities of the Chest Wall and Their Operative Correction* (Philadelphia: W. B. Saunders Company, 1977).
14. Szenes, T.: Thorax pyramidalis, Fortschr. Roentgenstr. 65:89, 1942.
15. Welch, K., and Vos, A.: Surgical correction of pectus carinatum (pigeon breast), J. Pediatr. Surg. 8:659, 1973.

Poland's Syndrome

HISTORY.—The name of Alfred Poland, who, as a medical student, reported a cadaver dissection of an incomplete form of this anomaly,[8] was given a hundred years later by Clarkson[2] to an anomaly that had, in fact, been described prior to Poland's report.[5, 7]

Poland described absence of the sternal and costal portions of the pectoralis major, absence of the pectoralis minor and absence of portions of the serratus magnus and external oblique, and a hand on which the middle phalanges were absent, and all the fingers except the middle finger showed webbing between the proximal phalanges. Duhamel[4] has termed this hand deformity brachysyndactyly. An extensive literature documents the range of abnormalities in this condition.[10] Absence or hypoplasia of the nipple and breast, hypoplasia of the subcutaneous fat, absence of the pectoralis minor, absence of varying lengths of cartilages or ribs II, III and IV or III, IV and V and hairlessness of the skin and axilla are classic. Hand deformity may be absent, less severe than that described or there may be an ectromelia. In addition, there may be vertebral deformities, or Sprengel's deformity. The etiology is not known, although, as I have pointed out,[10] a number of deformities have been reported resulting from pregnancies in which abortifacients had been used unsuccessfully. Alarming also, and possibly significant from the standpoint of etiology, is the fact that 3 children with this uncommon malformation have been reported to develop leukemia.[1, 6, 12]

In this section we are principally concerned with the chest wall aspects of Poland's syndrome. The deformity is made conspicuous by the combination of soft tissue and osteocartilaginous defects. If it is large, paradoxic respiration is prominent and occasionally has been the cause of symptoms, to the point of being described in some patients as a lung hernia.[11]

We have seen 28 patients with what we have recognized as variants of Poland's syndrome (Fig. 41–14), sent to us because of our interest in deformities of the chest wall. Fourteen had defects of ribs or cartilages or both and 8 patients were operated on. Results in 6 have been excellent and good or fair in the other 2.

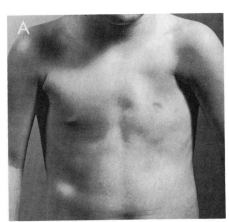

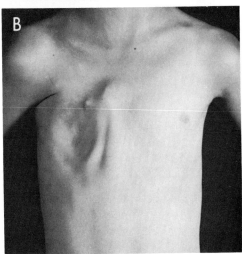

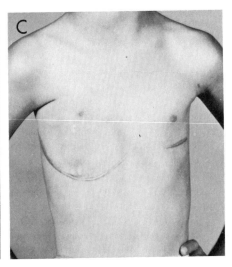

Fig. 41–14.—Syndrome of deficiency of 2d to 4th costal cartilages, absence of pectoralis minor and costal portion of pectoralis major, upward displacement of hypoplastic nipple and breast, hypoplasia of subcutaneous tissue—Poland's syndrome. This girl did not have any hand deformity. Most of our patients have been females. **A,** A.C., 2 years old. Satisfactory correction was achieved with rib grafts from the same side and a sheet of Teflon felt overlying the defect. **B** and **C,** P.J., 7 years old, with unsightly defect and conspicuous deformity. Paradoxic respiration was obvious, but there were no symptoms. The individual cartilaginous defects were bridged with bone grafts from a rib of the opposite side and the reconstruction reinforced with a sheet of Teflon felt. Absence of the costal portion of the pectoralis major still is obvious, but the chest has normal contour, the chest wall is solid and there is no paradoxic motion on respiration. The breast probably will develop but will be a fraction of the size of the opposite one. Cosmetic augmentation of the breast by prosthetic implant will be postponed until maturity.

In the first of our patients, an infant seen many years ago, we delayed operation, not being quite certain of the indications or of the corrective procedure to be used. The result was a progressively increasing deformity of the chest wall, so that we regretted the failure to perform a corrective operation. Since then, we have preferred to operate on these children at whatever age they were seen, whenever there was a substantial chondrocostal defect, both to relieve any paradox that might exist and to protect the intrathoracic viscera.

Operative Technique

In the operation for these deformities it is important to place the incision beyond the area of the defect (Fig. 41–15). The subcutaneous tissues are found thinned and the pectoral muscle replaced by a flimsy sheet of connective tissue. The operation to which we have come involves the use of rib grafts from the contralateral side. Splitting the rib with an oscillating saw permits the rib of even a small child to serve for two grafts. The pointed end of the rib placed across the defect is pressed medially into the edge of the sternum in a cavity made with a hemostat. Laterally, the graft overrides one of the denuded rib ends, to which it is fixed by through-and-through or circumferential sutures. We usually use two ribs, providing at least three grafts. To maintain the ribs in position, convex surface out, and to provide a normal contour, by making up for the absence of soft tissue, we place a sheet of Teflon felt over the defect. It is tautly sutured to the chest wall on all sides and sutured to the under-lying rib grafts.[9] In females, a mammary implant usually will be required after puberty to compensate for the substantial asymmetry of the two breasts or the absence of a breast on the affected side, and the chest wall reconstruction provides a firm base for the prosthesis.

REFERENCES

1. Boaz, D., Mace, J. W., and Gotlin, R. W.: Poland's syndrome and leukemia, Lancet 1:349, 1971.
2. Clarkson, P.: Poland's syndactyly, Guy's Hosp. Rep. 3:335, 1962.
3. Currarino, G., and Silverman, F.: Premature obliteration of the sternal sutures and pigeon-breast deformities, Radiology 70:532, 1958.
4. Duhamel, B., and Glicenstein, J.: Agénésis du grand pectoral et brachysyndactylie (syndrome de Poland), Chirurgie 101:233, 1975.
5. Froriep, R.: Beobachtung einese Falles von Mangel der Brust-drüse. Notizen aus dem Gebiete der Natur- und Heilkunde 23:254, 1839.
6. Hoefnagel, D., Rozycki, A., Wurster-Hill, D., Stern, P., and Gregory, D.: Leukaemia and Poland's syndrome, Lancet 2:1038, 1972.
7. Lallemand, L. M.: Éphémérides Medicales de Montpellier 1:144, 1826.
8. Poland, A.: Deficiency of the pectoral muscles, Guy's Hosp. Rep. 6:191, 1841.
9. Ravitch, M. M.: Atypical deformities of the chest wall—absence and deformities of the ribs and costal cartilages, Surgery 59:438, 1966.
10. Ravitch, M. M.: *Congenital Deformities of the Chest Wall and Their Operative Correction* (Philadelphia: W. B. Saunders Company, 1977).

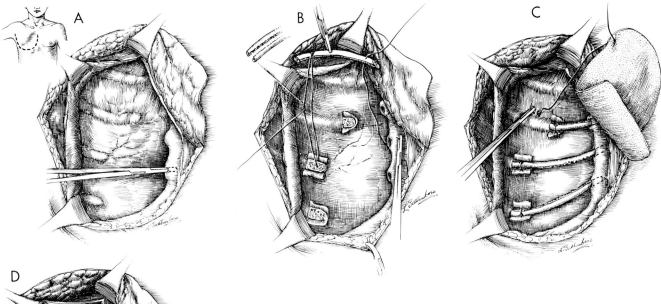

Fig. 41–15.—Poland's syndrome—operative technique. **A,** the curved incision is so placed that the entire line is well beyond the defect. Beneath the scanty subcutaneous fat there is a thin fascial layer, which is all that remains of the pectoralis major muscle. With this incised, one sees the gaps in the affected cartilages, or cartilages and ribs, and associated intercostal muscles. The fascial layer is easily separable from the pleura, which need not be entered. A hemostat is shown being bored into the edge of the sternum to create a pocket for the pointed end of a rib graft. **B,** one or two ribs are removed subperiosteally from the opposite side, through either the same incision or a separate one, and one or both are split with an oscillating saw. The ends of the defective cartilages or ribs are uncovered and freshened and the rib grafts sutured into place. The pointed medial end is pressed into the sternum and the lateral end sutured to the rib stumps. **C,** the grafts have been placed with their convexity forward. A sheet of prosthetic material is sutured so as to overlap the deformity on all sides. Marlex is satisfactory, but the thickness of Teflon is an advantage in these patients. **D,** the prosthesis is sutured beyond the margin of the defect under modest tension, and each rib is secured to the felt.

11. Rickham, P. P.: Lung hernia secondary to congenital absence of ribs, Arch. Dis. Child. 34:14, 1959.
12. Walters, T. R., Reddy, B. N., Bailon, A., and Vitale, L. F.: Poland's syndrome associated with leukemia, J. Pediatr. 82:889, 1973.

Rib Deformities in Diffuse Skeletal Disorders

In the past decade there have been separated out a number of disorders of the skeleton common to which is an inadequately formed thoracic cage, often to the point of incompatibility with life. The dramatic designation of thanatophoric (death-bearing) dwarfism first used by Maroteaux, Lamy and Robert[4] now has given way to the eponym Jeune's disease.[2, 3] In severe forms, the shortened horizontal ribs and narrow rigid thorax lead to death from respiratory insufficiency. The immobile narrow, cylindrical or even bell-shaped chest is pathognomonic. I have elsewhere[5] described the record of corrective operative attempts. Thus far, Waterston's patient[1] appears to be the only one to have survived operation in early infancy. We have operated on older children (2 years of age and 11 years of age) with deformities of this type in which there are very deep depressions, out almost to the axillary line. The 2-year-old child appeared to have a mild form of Jeune's disease; the older child had a similar deformity, but the underlying condition was a diffuse metaphyseal dysostosis.[5]

The single successful operation in early infancy was achieved by splitting the sternum and separating the two halves with bone grafts. Our own operations, done in older children, were directed to correcting the deep lateral costochondral depressions and eliminating and improving the respiratory mechanics.

REFERENCES

1. Barnes, N. D., Hull, D., Milner, A. D., and Waterston, D. J.: Chest reconstruction in thoracic dystrophy, Arch. Dis. Child. 46: 833, 1971.
2. Jeune, M., Beraud, C., and Carron, R.: Dystrophie thoracique asphyxiante de caractere familial, Arch. Fr. Pediatr. 12:886, 1955.
3. Jeune, M., Carron, R., Beraud, C., and Loaec, Y.: Polychondro-dystrophie avec blocage thoracique d'evolution fatale, Pediatrie 9:390, 1954.

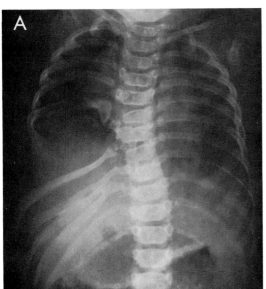

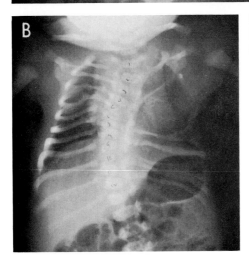

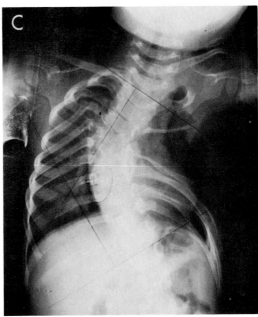

Fig. 41–16.—Absence of ribs. Numerous varieties of real or apparent absence of rib occur, with or without a chest wall bulge that can be interpreted as a lung hernia. **A,** an infant with a wide gap between ribs and a great soft tissue bulge. Actually there are 12 ribs, but some are deformed. These are associated with vertebral deformities. Osteotomies and approximation of the 6th and 7th ribs corrected the herniation and also the scoliosis. **B** and **C,** an infant with multiple absence of bony ribs on the left and abnormalities of bony ribs on the right. There was a large area of symptomatic, paradoxic respiration in the uncovered area. However, the most serious problem was vertebral. Note the large mass of fused bone on the right parallel to the vertebral column and striking progression of scoliosis in 16 months **(C).** Operation was advised, but declined.

4. Maroteaux, P., Lamy, M., and Robert, J-M.: La nanisme thanotophore, Presse Med. 75:2519, 1967.
5. Ravitch, M. M.: *Congenital Deformities of the Chest Wall and Their Operative Correction* (Philadelphia: W. B. Saunders Company, 1977).

Bizarre Rib Deformities

These vary from an abnormal prominence of a single costal cartilage, which is of cosmetic importance only, usually at the costal margin and which may be corrected by subperichondrial excision if the appearance is truly disturbing, to multiple anomalies of ribs and spine, both of which are serious (Fig. 41–16).

Patients with asymmetric deformities of the chest, in which all of the ribs on one side are sunken with some rotation of the sternum, seem to have a true unilateral costal deformity and not a variant of pectus excavatum. Because so many ribs are involved and the sternum may be rotated, a very extensive operation is required, and one technically difficult from the standpoint of maintaining fixation. We have had 3 such patients, 2 with excellent results and a third with a very rapid recurrence.[1]

REFERENCE

1. Ravitch, M. M.: *Congenital Deformities of the Chest Wall and Their Operative Correction* (Philadelphia: W. B. Saunders Company, 1977).

Tumors of the Chest Wall

Tumors of the chest wall proper are moderately uncommon in adults and distinctly more uncommon in children. The paramount observation is this: that malignant chest wall tumors are more common in children than benign chest wall tumors, and that a tumor in the chest wall of a child is more likely to be malignant than a tumor in the chest wall of an adult. Little appears to have been written dealing specifically with chest wall tumors in children. Gleanings from the collected reports of chest wall tumors in patients of all ages indicate that, of the benign tumors, chondromas of the ribs occasionally have been found in children (1 child of 11 years, of 31 collected by Harper[9]). Fonkalsrud[12] resected large osteochondromas from the rib of a 5½-year-old boy with "multiple exostoses in the long bones of the upper and lower extremities." In a 5-month-old boy they excised a large calcified aneurysmal bone cyst of the right rib posteriorly that had been growing rapidly from birth to the time of operation. Pathologic diagnosis was "embryonal aneurysmal bone cyst." Gaillard, Martinel, Berthoumieu and Eschapasse[6] reported a 9-year-old boy with a radiographically discovered calcified tumor at the anterior end of the fourth rib, which turned out to be an osteochondroma on the deep surface of the rib. We have had a similar case (Fig. 41–17). At least one osteoid osteoma has been reported. In 3 children, ribs have been found to be the seat of lesions of the lipoid histiocytoses. Of 10 giant cell tumors of the ribs reported by Buckles and Lawless,[3] 3 occurred in children 9, 11 and 14 years of age. Although only 1 of the 10 tumors was frankly malignant, 4 had invaded the soft tissues locally. The numbers in the various series are so small that no suggestion of the frequency of the various malignant chest tumors in children can be given.

Ewing's tumor of bone is, in general, a tumor of younger patients, and although the rib is one of its less common sites, the proportion of children with Ewing's tumor primary in the ribs appears to be somewhat higher than with this tumor in other bones. Here, as in other bones, the rapidly growing Ewing's tumor produces pain, fever, local heat and erythema, so that the lesion may be mistaken for an inflammatory process. The clinical outlook is bleak. Fonkalsrud's[12] 4-year-old girl with a painful mass in the left eighth rib, without other radiologic disease, had a biopsy-proved Ewing's sarcoma resected with the ribs above and below, as well as the pleura. She developed an abdominal mass 3 months later and, despite chemotherapy and radiotherapy, died 2 years after the original operation. In one series of 8 patients aged 6–59 with Ewing's tumor of the ribs, 4 were less than 30 years of age, 7 were dead and 1 still living with tumor.[18] On the other hand, in a 10-year-old girl with Ewing's tumor, Kinsella *et al.*[14] resected full thickness of the chest wall, including three ribs and portions of the lung. The patient was alive and free from obvious tumor 18 months later.

Sarcomas of various kinds comprise the principal group of malignant tumors of the chest wall in infancy and childhood. Most of them probably are chondrosarcomas,[17, 19, 21] although

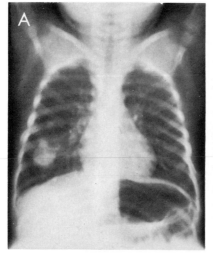
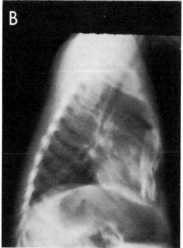

Fig. 41–17.—Osteochondroma of rib in a 3-year-old child with osteochondromata of ribs (note rib VII, left), scapula and long bones. The size the mass on the right already had reached, on the inner aspect of the rib where it could not be watched without repeated x-rays, led us to resect the tumor and involved costal element.

some of them have been diagnosed as osteogenic sarcomas and others are undifferentiated anaplastic sarcomas (Fig. 41–18).

It is important to remember about the chondrosarcomas that they appear deceptively benign histologically, even when they metastasize, and that any cartilaginous tumor of the flat bones of the chest wall, except an obvious osteochondroma, should be considered to be malignant.

From the M. D. Anderson Hospital[7] comes the report of an 8½-year-old boy with an unclassified sarcoma 4 cm in diameter, involving the seventh rib, for which 11 cm of ribs V, VI and VII were resected and the chest wall repaired with a Marlex prosthesis. He recovered easily from the operation but was dead of metastatic disease within 6 months.

Hopkins and Freitas[11] described what they considered to be two huge osteochondromas, one on either side, projecting into the thorax of a 3-month-old child, occupying 40% of the hemithorax on the left (8 cm diameter) and 50% on the right and causing dyspnea and cyanosis. The masses were removed in separate operations, taking one rib on the left and three on the right. There was no recurrence after 4 years. Nevertheless, the tumor probably was a chondrosarcoma. In another 3-month-old child, Hall and Ellison[8] resected an 8×10×15 cm mass reported to have been growing since birth. The child was well 6 years later. Polk *et al.*[19] reported a boy of 5 with a tumor involving one rib, previously abandoned as hopeless because of a massive pleural effusion. He was well 15 years after resection of the chest wall and irradiation for the chondrosarcoma. Winter and Tongen[22] reported a boy who, at age 3½, for an undifferen-

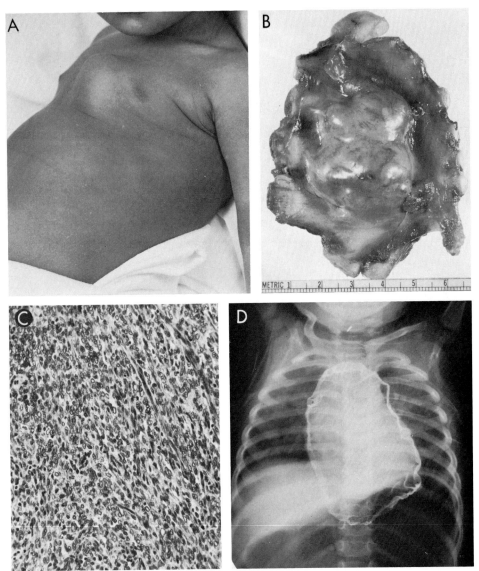

Fig. 41–18.—Undifferentiated sarcoma of ribs or sternum. A pea-sized lump was noted on the chest wall at age 2 or 3 months; at 13 months it was said to be "about as large as 3 almonds, over the ribs, just to the left of the lower end of the sternum." Growth since had been rapid. **A,** at 17 months, the mass, covering the lower chest anteriorly and most of the sternum, was 5.5 cm in diameter, projected outward some 3 cm, was rubbery, firm, fixed to the chest wall, not attached to the skin. Diagnosis was malignancy, probably chondrosarcoma. **B,** the resected specimen. Six cartilages were removed on either side, and bony rib included in two of those on the left. The entire gladiolus occupies the center. Note the internal mass, equal to the external mass, and covered by pleura. **C,** photomicrograph, showing highly cellular undifferentiated sarcoma, perhaps of periosteal origin. **D,** postoperative film, showing large tantalum sheet sutured in place. The child had little paradox and was thought to be doing well when she died abruptly 18 hours after operation. This was in 1951. Today we would use a firmer prosthesis, probably perform a tracheostomy and use mechanically assisted respirations for several days until confident the child could aerate effectively, although this baby showed no embarrassment.

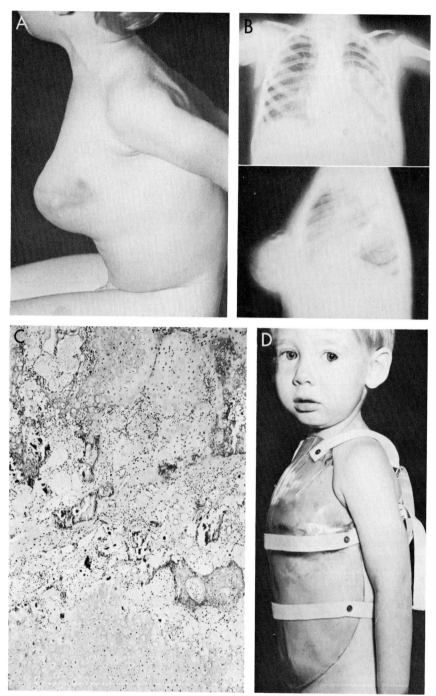

Fig. 41–19.—Chondrosarcoma of ribs and sternum. This boy was born with a cherry-sized mass just left of the sternum. The tumor grew steadily and was removed at age 9 months. Recurrence was obvious in 3 months, and tumor growth continued until hospitalization at age 2 years, when it was 10 × 10 cm and covered most of the anterior chest. **A,** the large tumor and scar of the first operation. The tumor was hard, fixed to chest wall and skin, extended from the 3d interspace to the costal margin and from the right side of the sternum to the left anterior axillary line. **B,** films showing the huge extent of the tumor and calcification within it. **C,** photomicrograph, showing chondrosarcoma. The entire mass was removed with overlying skin and underlying pleura, five ribs, distal portion of the sternum and a segment of the opposite costal margin. The free edge of the diaphragm was brought up to the ribs at the upper border of the defect and sutured there, turning the thoracic defect into an abdominal one. The specimen was 11 × 7 × 7 cm. The tumor had destroyed the ribs and cartilage in the area of the mass but still was covered by pleura on the undersurface. **D,** convalescence from this extensive procedure was uneventful. The heart was covered only by skin and fat, and a Plexiglas cuirasse was worn for protection. Two years later, during subcutaneous insertion of rib grafts across the defect, he suffered anoxic cardiac arrest. During only temporarily effective resuscitation by cardiac massage, the left chest was found to be free from tumor.

tiated sarcoma of the chest wall, had a wide chest wall resection, including two ribs. He survived an even larger resection for a local recurrence, a right lower lobectomy and a left lower lobe wedge resection for pulmonary metastases, then a third operation on the chest wall and spine for local recurrence. All operations were done in an 11-month period; and, on two occasions in this time, radon seeds were implanted in the chest wall. He was well 15 years later and had had a spinal fusion and Harrington rod correction of the severe scoliosis that had developed. The evidence is good that a number of these tumors were present at birth, that there is an occasional period of delay before rapid growth is manifest and that a number of patients who died might have been salvaged by an initially decisive and definitive operation instead of a period of observation or a temporizing limited procedure.

Desmoid tumors are rare in children and rarer still in extra-abdominal locations. Keeley *et al.*[13] operated successfully on a 5-year-old girl with large separate desmoids of the abdominal wall and chest wall. Bolanowski and Groff[2] reported a 10-year-old boy with a 3-month history of cough, weight loss and dyspnea, deviation of the trachea to the left and dullness and opacity over the entire area to the right chest. In the first operation, a huge extrapleural desmoid was peeled away from the anterosuperior chest wall. At a second operation, ribs II, III, IV and V anteriorly were resected and the defect covered with the normal muscle. The child was reported well 8 months later. Radically wide excisions appear to have been curative.

Treatment

A chest wall tumor in a child should be assumed to be malignant and should be treated initially by an en bloc full-thickness resection of the chest wall. Because of the risk of seeding with the tumor and because frozen section diagnosis of bone tumors is notoriously undependable, biopsy should not be performed and one should proceed with a radical resection. The skin incision should, if possible, be raised as a flap so that after the chest wall has been resected, the suture line will fall well beyond the defect, lest any failure of the suture line result in an empyema. If the tumor underlies the muscle belly of the latissimus or the pectoralis, the muscle, if not involved, may be retracted and spared. In the area of muscle attachments of the pectoralis or the serratus, the muscle must be removed with the tumor. An intercostal incision, at least one interspace above or below the first apparently normal rib beyond the tumor, will allow introduction of the finger to probe the pleural cavity to determine by palpation the apparent extent of the tumor. A block of chest wall then is removed, including muscle, bone or cartilage and pleura. If the tumor is close to or obviously involves the sternum, a wide resection of the sternum should be performed. The best hope for cure in most of these tumors lies in obtaining an adequate margin at the first operation; if there is any doubt, one should go an interspace higher or lower or carry the resection farther anteriorly or posteriorly. There is no room for compromise, even if both pleural cavities must be widely unroofed.[21]

With limited resections of the chest wall, particularly if heavy muscles have been preserved, no reconstruction is necessary. If a large segment of chest wall is resected, it is best to repair the defect in part with split-rib grafts from the contralateral side with or without an additional fascia lata or prosthetic repair. The prosthetic material with which we have the most experience for this purpose is Teflon felt, although we have also used Marlex with satisfaction. There is growing interest, in adults at least, in the replacement of the chest wall, after very large sternal resections, with acrylic prostheses, made and molded at the time, as neurosurgeons do for cranioplasty. Some surgeons have incorporated sheets of Marlex or metal mesh in these for easier suture to the surrounding tissues; others perforate the acrylic to allow tissue to grow into it.[5, 15] Stainless steel strips, in association with a prosthetic sheet, may be used to restore chest wall stability.[16] If the rib resection is such as to include the costal margin, we have, on a number of occasions, found it useful to shift the diaphragm to the upper margin of the defect, so that the large defect now becomes abdominal rather than thoracic (Fig. 41 – 19). This necessarily decreases the volume of the thorax but simplifies the reconstruction and eliminates the likelihood of any significant paradoxic respiration. Figures 41 – 18 and 41 – 19 illustrate tumors with which we have had experience, and in Chapter 44 is found an illustration (Fig. 44 – 14) of a neuroblastoma penetrating the chest wall and presenting as a chest wall tumor.

REFERENCES

1. Bergstrand, H.: Four cases of Ewing sarcoma in ribs, Am. J. Cancer 27:26, 1936.
2. Bolanowski, P. J. P., and Groff, D. B.: Thoracic wall desmoid tumor in a child, Ann. Thorac. Surg. 15:6, 1973.
3. Buckles, M. G., and Lawless, E. C.: Giant cell tumor of ribs, J. Thorac. Surg. 19:438, 1950.
4. Dorner, R. A., and Marcy, D. S.: Primary rib tumors, J. Thorac. Surg. 17:690, 1948.
5. Eschapasse, H., Gaillard, J., Costagliola, M., Martinel, C., Henry, E., and Berthoumieu, F.: Reparation de la paroi thoracique apres resection pour tumeur etendue, Ann. Chir. Thorac. Cardiovasc. 11:445–454, 1972.
6. Gaillard, J., Martinel, Ch., Berthoumieu, F., and Eschapasse, H.: Vraies et fausses tumeurs primitives de la paroi thoracique (a propos de 24 observations), Poumon Coeur 28:9, 1972.
7. Graham, J., Usher, F. C., Perry, J. L., and Barkley, H. T.: Marlex mesh as a prosthesis in the repair of thoracic wall defects, Ann. Surg. 151:4, 1960.
8. Hall, D. P., and Ellison, R. G.: Osteochondrosarcoma of the chest wall in a newborn infant, Am. Surg. 30:745, 1964.
9. Harper, F. R.: Benign chondromas of the ribs, J. Thorac. Surg. 9: 132, 1939.
10. Herbert, W. P.: Ewing's tumor of the rib: Report of two cases, J. Thorac. Surg. 5:189, 1935.
11. Hopkins, S. M., and Freitas, E. I.: Bilateral osteochondroma of the ribs in an infant: An unusual cause of cyanosis, J. Thorac. Cardiovasc. Surg. 49:247, 1965.
12. Joseph, W. L., and Fonkalsrud, E. W.: Primary rib tumors in children, Am. Surg. 38:338, 1972.
13. Keeley, J. L., De Rosario, J. L., and Schairer, A. E.: Desmoid tumors of the abdominal and thoracic walls in a child, Arch. Surg. 80:144, 1960.
14. Kinsella, F. J., White, S. M., and Koucky, R. W.: Two unusual tumors of the sternum, J. Thorac. Surg. 16:640, 1947.
15. Le Roux, B. T.: Maintenance of chest wall stability, Thorax 19: 397, 1964.
16. Le Roux, B. T., and Stemmler, P.: Maintenance of chest wall stability: A further report, Thorax 26:424, 1971.
17. O'Neill, L. W., and Ackermann, L. V.: Cartilaginous tumors of ribs and sternum, J. Thorac. Surg. 21:71, 1951.
18. Pascuzzi, C. A., Dahlin, D. C., and Clagett, O. T.: Primary tumors of the ribs and sternum, Surg. Gynecol. Obstet. 104:390, 1957.
19. Polk, J. W., *et al.*: Malignant lesions of the chest wall, Mo. Med. 58:217, 1961.
20. Ravitch, M. M.: , in Sabiston, D. C., and Spencer, F. C. (eds.), Gibbon's *Surgery of the Chest* (3d ed.; Philadelphia: W. B. Saunders Company, 1976).
21. Watkins, E., Jr., and Gerard, F. P.: Malignant tumors involving the chest wall, J. Thorac. Cardiovasc. Surg. 39:117, 1960.
22. Winter, R. B., and Tongen, L. A.: A malignant chest wall sarcoma with bilateral pulmonary metastases: A fifteen-year survival after multiple radical local excision and resection of bilateral pulmonary metastases and a successful treatment of scoliosis secondary to tumor surgery, Surgery 62:374, 1967.

42 Thomas M. Holder / Keith W. Ashcraft
Congenital Diaphragmatic Hernia

THIS CHAPTER covers most of the types of diaphragmatic defects of infants and children except for hiatal hernia (see Chap. 43).

HISTORY.—Ambroise Paré reported the first diaphragmatic hernia in 1597. It was of traumatic origin.[3] The first hernia of congenital origin was described by Riverius and is included in Bonetus's Sepulchretum of 1679. In 1761, Morgagni reviewed diaphragmatic hernia to that date, credited Stehelinus with noting the small lung in a fetus with diaphragmatic hernia and described a patient with the retrosternal hernia that now bears his name.[23] In 1848, Vincent Alexander Bochdalek described a congenital hernia through the posterior lateral part of the diaphragm, which he postulated resulted from an in utero rupture of a previously intact membrane in the lumbocostal triangle. Although this mechanism is not currently accepted, Bochdalek's name has for so long been associated with congenital posterolateral diaphragmatic hernia that the eponym Bochdalek hernia is accepted by general usage.[7, 49]

Aue performed a successful repair of congenital diaphragmatic hernia in 1902.[23] In 1925, Hedblom reviewed 378 cases of diaphragmatic hernia. He classified 44 hernias as "congenital." Twenty-two patients were children. Seventy-five percent of the untreated children failed to live beyond the first month of life.[27] He advocated early operation but his advice was generally unheeded.

Greenwald and Steiner[24] reviewed 82 children with diaphragmatic hernia reported between 1912 and 1929. Six of 11 patients operated on recovered. Forty-six were diagnosed at autopsy and most of the others died without operation. In 1941, Ladd and Gross[35] reported 12 survivors of 19 patients undergoing operation. In 1946, Gross[26] reported the first successful repair of a neonate less than 24 hours of age. By 1953, he reported 72 patients operated on for diaphragmatic hernia with only 8 deaths, of which 3 were due to associated anomalies.[25] Because of earlier current recognition and diagnosis of the condition and attempted operation in desperately ill neonates, that success rate has not been maintained.

Embryology

The diaphragm is complex in its embryogenesis. Coincident with its formation, the lung is rapidly developing and the gut returning to the abdominal cavity. The temporal relation of these events is important to the type and severity of anomaly produced.

The first component of the diaphragm to appear is the septum transversum, which forms from mesenchyme between the pericardium cranially and the coelom caudally. Dorsally, it joins the mediastinum containing foregut. Laterally, the pleural cavities connect with the pericardium and the peritoneal cavities. The caudal portion of the pleural membrane will separate the pericardium from the pleura. The pleuroperitoneal canal is narrowed by progressive lateral ingrowth of the more caudal pleuroperitoneal membrane. The posterolateral aspect of the diaphragm is the last to close—the site of the Bochdalek hernia. The left side usually closes later than the right. By 8–9 weeks of fetal life, the pleural and abdominal cavities are separated by the pleural and peritoneal membranes. An ingrowth of mesenchyme between the membranes provides the lateral musculature and the central tendinous portion of the diaphragm.

During the time the diaphragm is forming, the midgut is undergoing rapid elongation. Utilizing all available space, it herniates into the base of the umbilical cord. At about the 9th week, the gut returns to the abdominal cavity and rotates in a counterclockwise direction. This process usually is completed by the 10th week.

If the gut returns to the abdomen early or the closure of the pleuroperitoneal membrane is late or incomplete, the gut may herniate through the diaphragmatic defect. The normal rotation and fixation of the gut will not occur. No sac will separate abdominal viscera from thoracic viscera. If the pleuroperitoneal membrane has closed but the supportive structures of the diaphragm have not developed, a hernia sac will be present. With growth of the gut and other abdominal viscera that may have herniated into the chest, the developing lung is compressed. The abdomen loses much of its stimulus to enlarge.

The lung buds develop within the mediastinum at about the 4th week and begin to bulge into the future pleural cavity. The lungs do not fill the pleural cavity during the time the definitive bronchial tree is forming. All major bronchial buds are present before closure of the pleuroperitoneal canal, but segmental bronchi have not fully developed until about the 16th week. The "alveolar growth" period of the lung development is from 24 weeks to birth.[3, 23]

Morgagni retrosternal defects occur at the junction of the septum transversum, anterior chest wall and the lateral component of the diaphragm. The area is weak and defects result from retardation of fusion of the lower ribs and xiphisternum with the septum transversum at about the 7th week.[23]

Congenital *eventration* of the diaphragm is a result of a failure of development of muscle and not of lack of fusion of diaphragmatic components. It probably is related to the failure of migration of myoblasts along the phrenic nerves.

Posterolateral Congenital Diaphragmatic Hernia of Bochdalek

The posterolateral congenital diaphragmatic hernia of Bochdalek is by far the most serious of the diaphragmatic hernias. On occasion, it is the most urgent of all neonatal surgical emergencies, causing rapidly progressive and fatal respiratory distress. On other occasions, the lung is not markedly compromised, symptoms are minimal and occur later in childhood.

ANATOMY OF THE DIAPHRAGMATIC DEFECT.—There is a defect in the posterolateral aspect of the diaphragm, most often on the left side (Fig. 42–1) (83–94%),[13, 42] perhaps a result of later closure of the left pleuroperitoneal canal. Bilateral hernias are rare.[36]

A hernia sac may or may not be present. If present, it is very thin and usually consists of stretched pleura and peritoneum. The presence of a sac does not limit the amount of abdominal viscera that herniates into the chest. Nor does the presence of a sac favorably affect the outcome of patients operated on for this hernia. A sac was present in 62% of pa-

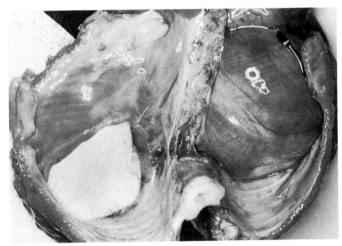

Fig. 42–1.—Bochdalek hernia, left, marked by gauze pack and viewed from above in postmortem photograph. There is no sac. A defect of this size can be closed directly without the need for prosthetic materials. Even posterolaterally, where the gauze and the defect seem to touch directly against the ribs, there usually will be found a rolled-up rim of diaphragmatic muscle.

tients reported by Johnson, Deaner and Koop,[30] whose preference for the thoracic approach may have accounted for an incidence higher than that reported by surgeons using the abdominal approach.

The diaphragmatic defect may be very small or quite large, involving most of the hemidiaphragm. Although a rim of muscle usually is present around the entire defect, sometimes there is no muscle laterally, adjacent to the chest wall. The posterior diaphragmatic musculature frequently is contracted beneath the pleura and peritoneum along the lower chest wall.

IN UTERO PATHOLOGIC ANATOMY.—A left hernia allows displacement into the chest of some or all of the following viscera: stomach, small bowel, ascending, transverse and descending colon, spleen, left lobe of the liver, pancreas, left kidney and adrenal (Fig. 42–2). The right-sided hernia usually contains liver and only a portion of the small and/or large intestine. The liver may have grown considerably after herniation and a deep indentation develops where the edges of the diaphragmatic defect have compressed it. This rim of diaphragm apparently does not interfere with the viability of the intrathoracic portion of the liver.

Incomplete rotation and fixation of the intestine occurs when the colon has herniated into the chest. Ladd's bands are infrequently seen in this condition. The abdominal cavity is small, since the abdominal viscera have taken up residence in the chest. This factor complicates surgical closure and will be discussed in detail under operative treatment.

The abdominal viscera in the chest cause a severe compression of the ipsilateral lung, a shift of the mediastinum and often marked reduction of the volume of the contralateral lung. The degree of compression of the lung affects pulmonary development. Hypoplasia of the lungs is a major factor affecting survival in neonates who are acutely symptomatic. Butler and Claireaux,[13] reporting the experience of the British Perinatal Mortality Survey, found that 13 babies dying of diaphragmatic hernia (without major associated anomalies) within 24 hours of birth had an average ipsilateral lung weight of 3.7 gm and a contralateral lung weight of 13.3 gm. The normal right lung weight for comparable size infants is 35 gm.

Histologically, the same authors found that the bronchi were distorted and showed side-to-side compression. There was a relative decrease in distal parenchyma. Alveoli and alveolar ducts were lined with cuboidal epithelium not normally present after the 13th week of gestation. Areechon and Reid[2] studied the histology of the lungs of 2 infants who died within 4 hours of birth of diaphragmatic hernia. They noted a relatively greater reduction in bronchioli than in bronchi, which had half the normal number of branchings. The arrest in development was irregular in distribution but the ipsilateral lung, particularly its lower lobe, was the most severely affected. The numbers of alveoli were not diminished but the size of each alveolus was reduced. The number of alveolar walls between the terminal bronchus and the pleura were normal. The ipsilateral lung of the most severely affected fetus did show reduction in both number and size of alveoli. "On the side of the hernia the stage of bronchial arrest corresponded to an intrauterine development of 10 to 12 weeks, on the contralateral to the development of 12 to 14 weeks."[2] DeLorimier et al.,[19] in lungs of lambs in which a diaphragmatic defect was produced in utero at 126 days of gestation, showed the alveoli and alveolar ducts to be small and lined with low cuboidal epithelium.

POSTNATAL PATHOPHYSIOLOGY.—Prior to birth, the lungs play no part in oxygenation of the fetus and the amount of pulmonary blood flow is of no major consequence. At parturition, the amount of functioning lung parenchyma,

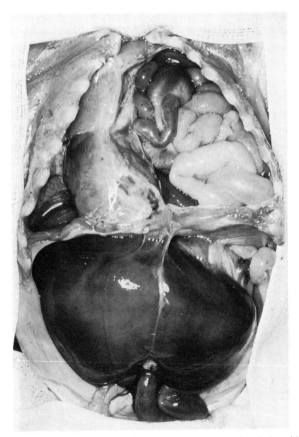

Fig. 42–2.—Bochdalek hernia. Postmortem appearance in a 1-day-old infant who had had increasing respiratory distress from birth and was dead on arrival. Almost the entire gastrointestinal tract and the spleen are in the left chest and the gut already is distended. The heart and mediastinum are displaced far to the right, where only a bit of the right lower lung is seen. The contracted nubbin of left lung is not visible.

the ability to ventilate the lung and the dynamics of pulmonary blood flow are fundamental to survival.

The neonate begins to swallow air with his first breath. As the herniated gut fills with swallowed air, it expands in the chest at the expense of the most compressible of the intrathoracic contents—the lungs. Pulmonary compression leads to decreased Pa_{O_2}, an increased Pa_{CO_2} and acidemia. These factors further increase pulmonary vascular resistance, increasing the right-to-left shunt through the ductus and/or patent foramen ovale. If the hernia is reduced and the lung expands, the process is reversed.

For the infant with hypoplastic lungs, the same neonatal hemodynamic and ventilatory disturbance occurs. Unfortunately, in such an infant, repair of the hernia will not allow survival if there is not sufficient pulmonary parenchyma to provide adequate oxygenation. It is not always possible to know preoperatively whether the physiologic alterations are due primarily to pulmonary compression or to compression plus hypoplasia.

Studies in newborn lambs in which a diaphragmatic hernia was created in utero show an elevated pulmonary artery pressure, increased ventricular end-diastolic pressure, increased atrial pressure and decreased left atrial oxygen saturation compared to controls. Cardiac output did not differ from controls but there was greater right-to-left shunting through the patent ductus arteriosus than with controls. There was a decrease in ipsilateral pulmonary blood flow and compliance was markedly reduced.[33] Hypoxia, hypercarbia and acidosis cause pulmonary vasoconstriction in the neonate and retard closure of the patent ductus arteriosus. Systemic hypoxia and acidemia complete a vicious circle, ultimately resulting in myocardial hypoxia and death. The same observations have been made in patients.[21]

The postnatal right-to-left shunt through the patent ductus results in a lower Pa_{O_2} in the descending aorta, compared to the proximal aorta. Right-to-left ductal shunting in "normal" neonates may be as high as 20%. The ductus arteriosus serves as a "vent" for the pulmonary circulation, and its closure leads to an increase in pulmonary artery and right heart pressure. If the ductus remains widely patent, it can reduce pulmonary blood flow and shunt so much desaturated blood into the systemic circulation as to produce severe tissue hypoxia and acidosis.[20]

The alveolar-arterial oxygen gradient is the result of shunting through the patent foramen ovale, the patent ductus arteriosus and within the lung by perfusion of underventilated parenchyma. There is not a direct correlation between the decreased Pa_{O_2}, increased Pa_{CO_2}, and acidemia and the degree of right-to-left shunting as measured by radial-descending aorta O_2 differences.[39]

CLINICAL PICTURE.—The incidence of posterolateral diaphragmatic hernia is reported as 1 in 12,500 live births[8] or 1 in 2200 total births (including stillbirths).[13] The sex incidence is reported as 1:1 by some and 2:1 (male:female) by others.[30, 38]

Polyhydramnios occurred in half of the stillborns and one-fifth of the live births reported by Butler and Claireaux.[13] All their stillborn babies and one-fourth of the live-born infants also had major associated anomalies, usually involving the central nervous system.

The onset of symptoms is related to the severity of the disease. The most severely affected babies are in respiratory distress at birth. Others, within minutes to hours after birth, develop increasing respiratory difficulty, with cyanosis, tachypnea and retractions. The abdomen in these infants usually is scaphoid as opposed to the customary rounded abdomen of the neonate (Fig. 42–3). The chest may be somewhat increased in anteroposterior diameter. Cyanosis, tachypnea, retractions, lethargy and even coma may be present. There are decreased to absent breath sounds on the involved (usually left) side of the chest with a shift of the heart sounds to the other chest. Rarely, bowel sounds are heard in the chest.

Those patients who have a later onset of symptoms usually have milder symptoms. Indeed, some patients have no symptoms in the neonatal period and may present much later with gastrointestinal rather than respiratory symptoms. Symptoms then tend to be dysphagia, vomiting, melena, cough, chest pain and recurrent respiratory infections.[34] Physical findings in this group of patients may be minimal, although some have decreased breath sounds on the involved side with shift of the heart to the opposite chest. Bowel sounds actually are heard in the chest in some of these patients, to the delight of those interested in unusual physical findings.

Many patients fall between these two extremes, although the majority present with respiratory symptoms in the first few days of life.

DIAGNOSIS.—Diagnosis usually is made by chest roentgenogram, which should also include the abdomen. Loops of gut in the chest establish the diagnosis. In the neonate, the heart most often is pushed well into the right chest and often only a small triangle of radiolucent lung is visible in

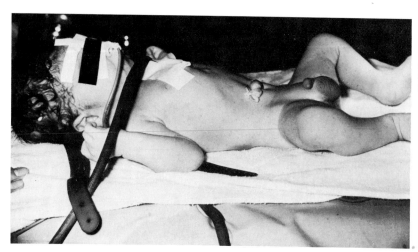

Fig. 42–3.—Bochdalek hernia in a neonate, showing the scaphoid appearance of the abdomen as a result of the herniation of a major part of the abdominal contents into the chest.

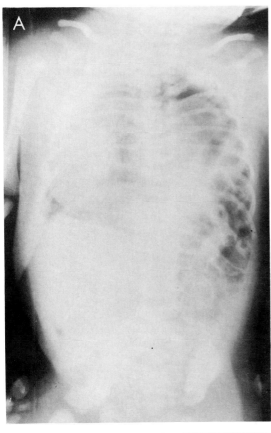

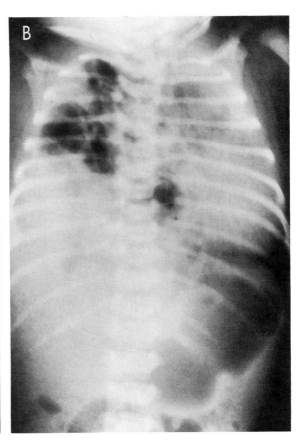

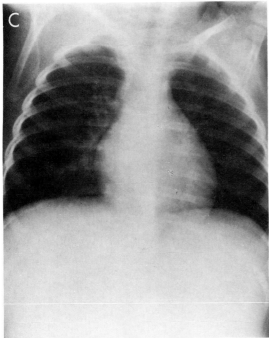

Fig. 42–4.—Bochdalek hernias, radiographic appearance. **A,** left-sided, characteristic appearance of a gas-filled left chest, and decreased amount of abdominal gas. The heart is shifted far to the right, and only a small triangle of lung at the right costophrenic angle represents aerated lung. (Compare with Fig. 42–2.) **B,** right-sided Bochdalek hernia (much less common than the left). Numerous loops of bowel in the chest displace the heart and the trachea far to the left. The air-filled viscus in the left abdomen is stomach. **C,** postoperative film of child in **B** shows essentially normal chest, although the right diaphragm has been slightly flattened by the repair.

the right costophrenic angle. The abdomen contains a paucity of bowel gas (Fig. 42–4).

The x-ray, if taken shortly after birth, before the gut contains much air, may be confusing. In this circumstance, the lungs often are poorly aerated. A repeat roentgenogram an hour later or after air is injected into the stomach often will clearly delineate gut in the chest (Fig. 42–5). If there still is a question of diaphragmatic hernia, a barium enema usually will show a portion of the colon through the posterolateral diaphragmatic defect into the chest. A significant finding in all films will be a decreased amount of abdominal gas. Radiopaque fluid injected into the peritoneal cavity has been

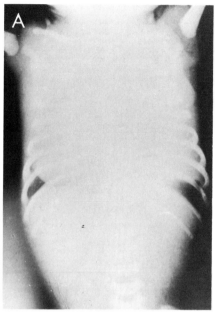 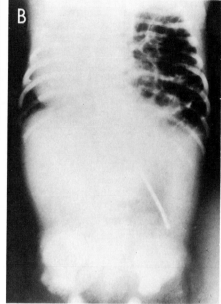

Fig. 42–5.—Bochdalek hernia in a newborn with serious respiratory distress. **A,** immediately after birth, one can distinguish only some air-filled lung in the right costophrenic sulcus. The air seen on the left, an interspace lower, probably already is in bowel. The heart, mediastinum and pleural contents are obscured. **B,** some minutes later, the x-ray is diagnostic. The small triangle of air seen at the left costophrenic angle is indeed initial swallowed air in the gut, and distended, air-filled gut fills the left hemithorax, pushing the mediastinal structures to the right lateral chest wall. The only aerated lung is seen in the right costophrenic angle. The nasogastric tube, placed as an immediate resuscitative measure to decompress the gastrointestinal tract and prevent the further aspiration of air, shows the esophagus well to the right of the midline, and the stomach still within the abdomen. The identical lung shadows on the right in the two films suggest that the mediastinal displacement is the result of pressure by the gut in intrauterine life, and at this point not yet materially affected by the presence of some air in the bowel. This child was operated on 5 hours after birth but did not survive.

helpful in the evaluation of a right-sided defect on occasion[51] but has no place in the diagnosis of the acutely symptomatic neonate.

DIFFERENTIAL CONSIDERATIONS.—Congenital cystic disease of the lung and staphylococcal pneumonia with pneumatoceles can both cause respiratory distress early in life and present an x-ray picture suggestive of diaphragmatic hernia (Fig. 42–6). The two former conditions have the usual amount of intestinal gas in the abdomen and there is no continuity of abdominal bowel gas with that in the chest. Barium studies of the intestinal tract are diagnostic.[14]

In the older patient, infant or child, whose symptoms are primarily gastrointestinal, an upper gastrointestinal series will show stomach and intestine, or both, above the diaphragm and delineate the portion of the diaphragm through which it passes into the chest.

ASSOCIATED ANOMALIES.—Hypoplastic lungs, malrotation of the intestine and patent ductus arteriosus frequently are associated with Bochdalek hernia. In Butler and Claireaux's survey[13] of perinatal deaths, 95% of stillborns and 21% of live-born children with Bochdalek hernia had major associated anomalies. The most frequent were central nervous system anomalies. In order of decreasing frequency, they were: anencephaly, Arnold-Chiari malformation, hydrocephalus and anencephaly. Congenital heart disease, genitourinary anomalies, esophageal atresia, omphalocele, hydronephrosis, cystic kidney and cleft palate also occurred in their patients.

Of the 76 patients who lived long enough to reach the Children's Hospital of Michigan, 13 had major associated anomalies and only 3 of these lived. Anomalies included congenital heart disease, esophageal atresia and duodenal obstruction. A number of other defects have been infrequently associated with diaphragmatic hernia. Major associated anomalies adversely affected the prognosis.[1]

PREOPERATIVE TREATMENT.—Therapy for the infant or child with Bochdalek diaphragmatic hernia who has no respiratory distress or symptoms is rather straightforward—reduction and repair of the hernia. However, the care of the majority of patients who do have respiratory distress is most challenging.

When the diagnosis of Bochdalek hernia is made in an infant with respiratory distress, the most important thing *not* to do is assist ventilation with a face mask. Such ventilation will force air into the stomach and intestine, increasing their volume in the chest at the expense of the already compromised lungs. A nasogastric tube should be introduced promptly to evacuate air from the stomach and prevent further air from accumulating. A sump tube works best. If preanesthetic ventilatory assistance is required, it *must* be given by endotracheal tube.

An umbilical artery catheter should be placed for pre- and postoperative monitoring of blood gases and pH. The initial determinations are helpful in preoperative management as well as prognosis. Boix-Ochoa[9] understandably found a grave outlook for his patients with initial Pa_{CO_2} over 100 mm Hg and a pH below 7. In Dibbins and Wiener's series, 11 of the 12 patients who died had an initial Pa_{CO_2} greater than 60 mm Hg.[21]

Determination of the right radial or temporal arterial blood gases obtained simultaneously with descending aorta values allows calculation of the degree of right-to-left shunting.[39, 41] The usual site of arterial blood sampling is the descending aorta distal to the ductus, via the umbilical artery catheter. Values obtained in this location will not necessarily represent the condition of the blood perfusing the

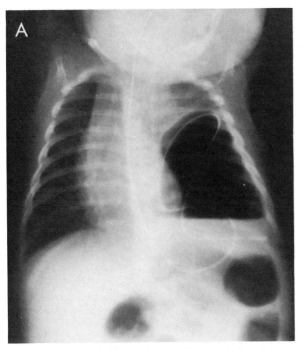

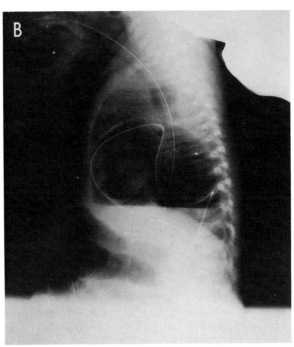

Fig. 42–6.—Bochdalek hernia. X-rays of a neonate in respiratory distress whose plain films originally suggested the diagnosis of congenital lung cyst. The PA **(A)** and lateral **(B)** views after a tube has been passed down through the esophagus show that the tube passes into the chest and into the area of radiolucency, proving that a diaphragmatic hernia is present and that the stomach is in the chest. The fact that the tube enters the chest two-thirds of the way to the lateral chest wall in the PA film and far posteriorly in the lateral film is conclusive evidence that the stomach has entered the chest through the classically located Bochdalek hernia.

brain, heart and eyes. In the presence of a right-to-left shunt through the ductus, the Pa_{O_2} gradient between ascending and abdominal aorta may be as high as 300 mm Hg.[39] This differential must be borne in mind when administering oxygen, particularly to the premature, who is more susceptible to retrolental fibroplasia.[41]

Assisted ventilation with 100% oxygen sometimes is necessary to support the baby's life. Response to this therapy has prognostic significance. If there is no improvement in Pa_{O_2}, the patient probably has hypoplastic lungs and little chance of survival.[9]

Careful attention to the neonate's body temperature is important because hypothermia increases oxygen consumption and contributes to acidosis. A thermo-neutral state decreases oxygen requirements in these infants, who are unable to meet even their minimal oxygen demand.

A sudden worsening of the patient's respiratory symptoms suggests a tension pneumothorax on the contralateral side, especially if the patient's ventilation is being assisted. This may require the prompt insertion of a chest tube without waiting for radiographic confirmation of pneumothorax.

Transportation of these desperately ill infants is a major problem. Unquestionably the infant's chance of survival, if the neonate has a viable pulmonary system, depends on the quality of the operation and of the intraoperative and postoperative management. Skillful care by the attending pediatrician during transportation may be the first step in ensuring survival. The baby should be kept warm, given oxygen and have the GI tract decompressed by sump suction. Those transporting the infant should have the ability and equipment to insert an endotracheal tube and ventilate the patient if the need arises. It may be necessary to diagnose and treat tension pneumothorax en route. The care during transportation of such an ill and extremely labile infant is a factor no less important in survival than a skillful anesthetic or operation.

Increasing the FI_{O_2} may correct hypoxia, and assisted ventilation reduce hypercarbia, if the lungs are not severely hypoplastic. Thus, both respiratory and metabolic acidosis will improve. Improvement of these will reduce the pulmonary vasoconstriction and reduce right-to-left shunting through the ductus. The use of intravenous sodium bicarbonate is of little value in respiratory acidosis, particularly if the Pa_{CO_2} is over 50 mm Hg, since the patient cannot then blow off the CO_2. THAM may be used in acidotic patients with Pa_{CO_2} greater than 50 mm Hg, since such patients are likely to be receiving ventilatory support. This obviates the most common complication of THAM—respiratory arrest.

Regardless of the degree of improvement with a period of intense preoperative care (which need not be long), operative correction should be undertaken promptly.

OPERATIVE TREATMENT.—Whether the procedure is emergency for respiratory distress or elective, endotracheal anesthesia is essential, since the pleural cavity will be entered. The umbilical artery catheter can be used for administration of fluids and drugs in the neonate, although intravenous administration is preferred. Blood transfusion rarely is needed. Operation should not be delayed for crossmatching.

Although abdominal, thoracic and thoracoabdominal incisions have all been advocated, we have a strong personal preference for the abdominal approach in the neonate, based on experience with all three incisions. The abdominal approach has the advantages of (1) easy reduction of the abdominal viscera, (2) good exposure for repair of the diaphragmatic defect without any pressure from the intestine, (3) easy exploration of abdominal viscera and treatment of associated anomalies, (4) gastrostomy can be readily accomplished and (5) the abdominal cavity may be enlarged, if necessary, by insertion of a prosthetic gusset in the wound. The advantages of the thoracic approach are: (1) good exposure of the diaphragm and (2) easy recognition and excision of a hernia sac. In the older child with primarily respiratory symptoms and the possibility of pulmonary-intestinal adhesions, the thoracic approach is better. For repair of a recurrent hernia (the abdomen now of adequate size), the thoracic approach is also best. For the neonate, however, thoracotomy has two overwhelming disadvantages. First, the reduction of the abdominal viscera back into the small abdominal cavity may be exceedingly difficult and result in undue trauma to them. Second, the diaphragmatic repair is done under considerable tension from the pressure of the reduced abdominal viscera—certainly not an optimal condition for a hernia repair of any kind.

An upper abdominal transverse or subcostal incision on the involved side provides the best exposure of the posterolateral diaphragmatic defect (Fig. 42–7). On opening the abdomen, the abdominal viscera that remain below the diaphragm are seen. The others reside in the chest. Reduction of these viscera is readily accomplished by gentle traction on the gut. A small retractor on the anterior lip of the defect is helpful in allowing air into the chest to break the negative pressure effect. The reduced viscera are placed on the abdominal wall for the moment.

Next, a careful search should be made for a sac. The sac may consist of only a layer of pleura or peritoneum and can be easily overlooked. The sac must be excised. A retained sac can collect fluid and form a cyst.[32] The ipsilateral lung is inspected and a chest tube is inserted through a chest wall stab wound prior to closure of the diaphragm. The advantages of postoperative chest tube drainage have been conclusively demonstrated by McNamara *et al.*[38]

The posterior rim of diaphragmatic muscle is covered by pleuroperitoneum and frequently not readily apparent. An incision laterally from the posterior medial diaphragmatic segment will uncover the muscle for repair. It usually is possible to approximate directly the anterior and posterior portion of the defect. A layer of horizontal mattress sutures of 2–0 silk imbricating one edge of the defect over the other is followed by a layer of interrupted simple sutures of the same material. This closure was advocated by Gross[25] and is our preference for the repair. Laterally there may be no muscle rim to the defect and the anterior musculature must be sutured directly to the chest wall. In this case, the chest wall sutures should go around the rib to provide a sound closure.

Rarely, the diaphragmatic defect is so large that there is insufficient musculature to bridge the defect for a primary closure. Simpson and Gossage[44] have used a muscle flap of anterior abdominal wall to fill this defect. The transverse and internal oblique muscles are separated from the external

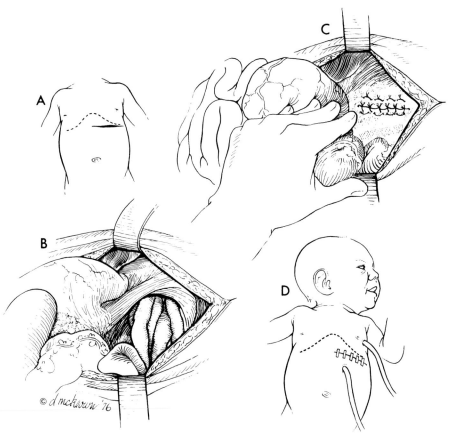

Fig. 42–7.—Bochdalek hernia, left—operative repair. **A,** transverse upper abdominal incision. **B,** the bowel is reduced by gentle traction on the gut. It may be necessary to slip a retractor under the edge of the diaphragmatic hernial ring to allow air to enter the chest and permit the bowel to be drawn down more easily. **C,** repair of the defect by imbricating one edge over the other with a series of horizontal mattress sutures of nonabsorbable material. The overlapping edge is tacked down with a second series of simple sutures.

It may be necessary to suture the diaphragm directly to the ribs by sutures passed around the appropriate ribs, but usually diaphragmatic muscle can be rolled from the most lateral portion of the defect, where, at first, it seems totally wanting. **D,** an intercostal tube is connected to 10 cm of water negative pressure. No attempt is made to inflate the lung. The gastrostomy tube initially serves to keep the intestinal tract deflated and later may be useful in feeding.

oblique and swung up as a pedicle to the existing diaphragmatic musculature. Their patient did well. We have preferred the use of a plastic prosthesis such as Marlex to fill the defect. As the patient grows, the prosthesis obviously does not. The result is a larger and larger portion of hemidiaphragm composed of functioning muscle pulled in from the sides.

The adrenal can easily be injured. In 15 of 17 deaths reported by Cook and Beckwith,[18] autopsy showed evidence of significant adrenal trauma. In some, the injury was deemed sufficient to render the gland nonfunctional in the postoperative period. They suggest that a relative adrenal insufficiency may play a part in some of the postoperative difficulties in these patients.

No effort is made to expand the ipsilateral lung to fill the pleural space. Ventilatory support is directed at simply providing adequate ventilation. Forceful ventilation usually will not expand the ipsilateral lung and may produce a contralateral tension pneumothorax. Indeed, because of the hypoplasia, the lung may be incapable of expansion.

Following the diaphragmatic repair, the duodenum is inspected. If there are constricting bands associated with malrotation, they are divided. Bill recommends that this be done in all patients as well as fixation of the cecum in the left abdomen. Other urgent visceral defects are sought and corrected.[12] A Stamm gastrostomy should be placed for postoperative gastrointestinal decompression.[28] The abdominal wall then is forcefully stretched in an effort to increase the size of the abdominal cavity and the abdomen is closed. If the intra-abdominal tension is excessive, a prosthetic gusset will enlarge the abdominal cavity for closure.[37, 43] Undue intra-abdominal tension interferes markedly with diaphragmatic excursions and reduces venous return. The repaired hemidiaphragm usually is flat due to the tension caused by repair of the defect. If the normal diaphragm is also elevated, due to increased abdominal pressure, and cannot descend with contractions, ventilation is severely limited. The abdominal cavity increases rapidly in size and the prosthesis usually can be removed and the abdomen closed in a week to 10 days.

POSTOPERATIVE CARE. — Postoperatively, the patients are kept warm in a high oxygen environment and given appropriate intravenous fluids. The gastrostomy tube is opened to dependent drainage and the chest tube connected to 10 cm of water negative pressure. The blood gases and pH are closely monitored. If the respiratory status is stable and satisfactory, no ventilatory assistance is needed. This would imply that any preoperative distress was the result of pulmonary compression.

If the patient has decreased Pa_{O_2}, increased Pa_{CO_2} and acidosis, respirator assistance through an endotracheal tube is necessary. In some patients, assistance is required for only a few hours and in others for several days. If there is a sudden worsening of the patient's condition, a contralateral pneumothorax should be suspected and treated by intercostal catheter. The ipsilateral lung expands to fill the thorax in a few hours in some patients and this usually suggests a good prognosis. In others, it may take a few days to 2 weeks for the lungs to expand to fill the chest cavity completely.

A repeated clinical observation, difficult to explain, is that a number of infants tolerate the operative procedure reasonably well and maintain a stable postoperative condition for a few hours. They then begin to have increasing hypoxia, hypercarbia and acidosis, with an increase in right-to-left shunting. Despite all therapeutic measures, they run a progressively downhill course and die. The explanation for this pattern is not clear. Presumably, patients with hypoplastic lungs should not do well early. Some investigators believe that the deterioration is due to increased pulmonary vasoconstriction, which leads to pulmonary hypertension, right-to-left shunting and increased hypoxia. These changes have been documented by cardiac catheterization.[17, 21] A number of pulmonary vasodilators have been used in an effort to decrease pulmonary artery pressure due to vasoconstriction. Drugs used include: priscoline, chlorpromazine, acetylcholine, morphine and corticosteroids. In some there has been a fall of pulmonary artery pressure, often accompanied by a fall in systemic pressure sufficient that right-to-left shunting actually was increased.[17, 21] Ligation of the ductus has not been successful in at least 1 patient.[17] Further investigation in this area is needed.

Berdon, Baker and Amoury[6] in 1968 concluded that the degree of hypoplasia of the lung varies considerably through a spectrum of minimal to very severe. With minimal hypoplasia, the patients do well, with severe hypoplasia there is not sufficient lung to sustain life. Between these extremes lie those with compromised pulmonary function whose survival depends on skillful respiratory support.

In the older infant and child, stretching the abdomen, gastrostomy and postoperative respiratory support are not often necessary. The postoperative care of these patients is similar to that after any other major operation.

RESULTS OF TREATMENT. — Results of treatment depend on the age and presenting symptoms. If the patients are those with gastrointestinal symptoms or those over several days of age, the outlook for survival, alleviation of symptoms and long-term results is excellent. For those neonates with a Bochdalek hernia in severe respiratory distress noted in the delivery room or in the first few hours of life, the outlook is grave. The over-all survival rate in any series, therefore, is dependent on the proportion of patients with severe respiratory distress early in life. Many series from children's hospitals do not include some of the patients with the most severe disease, since they do not live long enough to be transported to the pediatric surgical center. With a general acceptance of a more aggressive approach of recognition and therapy of neonates with respiratory distress and with better transport facilities, a larger proportion of the sicker infants is reaching these centers. Although the over-all survival no doubt has improved during the past 25 years, the percentage of survivors of recent series is not equal to the 87% survival reported by Gross[25] in 1953.

Combining (as best we can) the results of seven representative series[1, 9-11, 15, 30, 38] with a total of 410 patients with posterolateral diaphragmatic hernias, the following observations can be made. About half of the patients presented with severe respiratory distress in the immediate neonatal period (reported as first 24 or first 72 hours) and half of these died, 103 of 213. Selected recent portions of reported series totaling 64 patients with neonatal respiratory distress from diaphragmatic hernia indicate that with aggressive therapy, mortality fell to 31% (20 deaths).[9, 10, 38] Thus, modern concepts of treatment appear to have been of some value in increasing the survival rate of these very ill infants.

In the 197 patients in whom operation was not forced by respiratory symptoms in the first 72 hours, the survival rate was 93%. The outlook was best for those patients over 1 month of age.

The major cause of death is respiratory insufficiency, usually associated with hypoplastic lungs. Associated anomalies are also a frequent cause or contributing factor to mortality. Congenital heart disease is the most frequent. Contralateral pneumothorax, postoperative intestinal obstruction, sepsis and hemorrhage are also responsible for deaths.

Recurrence of the hernia is not common but can occur early in the postoperative period or within a few months.[10, 30] Recurrences should be repaired promptly.

Patients who survive do well clinically. The fate of the lung following repair is of interest but there are few long-term follow-up studies. The normal infant lung has the ability to grow after birth. Dunnill[22] has shown that there is a 10-fold increase in the number of alveoli from birth to adulthood, most of this taking place before 8 years of age. After 8 years, increase in lung volume is due to increase in size of alveoli.

Berdon, Baker and Amoury[6] could find no long-term radiologic abnormalities in patients who had insignificant pulmonary hypoplasia, i.e., that group who were not particularly ill in the neonatal period. Some of their patients with ipsilateral hypoplasia who survived developed emphysema of the involved lower lobe, as predicted by Areechon and Reid.[2] This was shown by late follow-up x-ray, and these emphysematous areas showed little blood flow as measured by lung scan. In some patients, however, the follow-up chest x-ray is normal (Fig. 42–8).

Wohl *et al.*[50] studied 17 patients, ages 6–19 years, who had been operated on during the first year of life for diaphragmatic hernia. Total lung capacity, vital capacity, forced expiratory volume and maximal expiratory flow volumes did not deviate from those of normal children. In 7 patients, radiospirometry revealed decreased perfusion of the ipsilateral lung. Lung volumes were normal, giving a decreased perfusion/volume ratio.

Chatrath *et al.*[16] studied 14 patients, ages 6 through 12 years, who had a Bochdalek hernia repaired in infancy. They found the lung volume components (functional residual capacity, residual volume and total lung capacity) to be normal. Indices of ventilatory function, forced expiratory volume and forced vital capacity, however, were decreased. This indicates emphysematous change.

Reid and Hutcherson[40] followed 30 patients with diaphragmatic hernia, 21 of whom were operated on in the neonatal period. Pulmonary function studies up to 21 years postoperatively showed a trend toward emphysema, with a high residual volume/total lung capacity ratio. Lung scans showed decreased perfusion to the ipsilateral lower lung. A disappointing observation was that 3 of their patients operated on as newborns were mentally retarded, presumably due to the initial hypoxia. None of their patients had increased respiratory infection or decreased exercise tolerance.

In summary, Bochdalek hernia may result in severe respiratory distress in the newborn. The degree of lung hypoplasia greatly affects the outcome of treatment. Vigorous pre- and postoperative respiratory support is a critical component of therapy. If the patient survives the postoperative period, the long-term outlook is excellent, although the hypoplastic lung may not reach normal function.

Retrosternal Hernias (Foramen of Morgagni)

Hernias through the retrosternal space of Morgagni constitute 2–4% of the larger series of diaphragmatic hernias reported.[3, 5, 11] These congenital hernias usually present much later and less dramatically than the Bochdalek hernias. The defect in the diaphragm often is small, allowing a smaller bulk of abdominal viscera to herniate into the chest. A sac almost always is present, which may limit the extent of herniation into the mediastinum or the chest. Symptoms produced by a small hernia into the mediastinum often are mild and do not come to medical attention. Morgagni hernias often are asymptomatic and discovered when an air-fluid level is noted in the lower mediastinum on routine chest x-ray. These hernias may be confused with eventration. On occasion, a Morgagni hernia is an incidental finding at laparotomy.

Some Morgagni hernias occur into the pericardium. The mass of gut herniated into the pericardium may produce serious or fatal compromise of cardiac output.

DIAGNOSIS.—The diagnosis of a Morgagni hernia may be established with a plain radiograph if a mass is seen extending into the anterior mediastinum from the abdomen (Fig. 42–8). Eighty percent of Morgagni hernias reported were found after the neonatal period.[4] The diagnosis may be definitely established by contrast gastrointestinal studies or by inverted contrast peritoneography.[48]

SURGICAL TREATMENT.—Surgical repair is indicated on diagnosis because of the risk of incarceration. The repair of

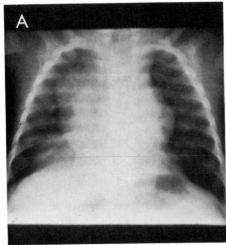
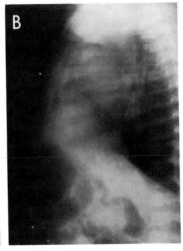

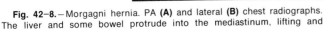

Fig. 42–8.—Morgagni hernia. PA **(A)** and lateral **(B)** chest radiographs. The liver and some bowel protrude into the mediastinum, lifting and distorting the cardiac silhouette. It usually is colon that enters the Morgagni hernial sac.

the Morgagni hernia probably is best accomplished by an upper abdominal incision. The viscera are easily reduced from this approach, the sac removed and the defect closed with interrupted sutures. Rarely are prosthetic materials necessary. The procedure carries only the basic mortality of laparotomy and general anesthesia.

Eventration

Diaphragmatic eventration is a congenital lesion characterized by incomplete development of the diaphragm. The pleura and the peritoneal layers are present but the muscular or fibrous diaphragm between them fails to develop properly, allowing for upward displacement of the attenuated diaphragm. Although some classifications include eventrations as congenital or acquired, it seems more logical to discuss eventrations as being congenital and to discuss under a separate section acquired malfunction of the diaphragm.

Diaphragmatic eventration may involve either the right or the left diaphragm or both. Partial defects in the diaphragm allowing for minor displacement of abdominal viscera into the thorax most often are located on the right whereas complete eventration usually is located on the left. Many children with complete eventration have other congenital abnormalities as well. If the eventration is large, interference with lung development may be nearly as striking as with a Bochdalek hernia. In these unusual instances, the child will present clinically much as if he had a Bochdalek hernia.

CLINICAL PICTURE. — Although about half of partial eventrations are asymptomatic, the other patients will manifest respiratory symptoms.[47] Recurrent infections, occasional wheezing, easy fatigability and dyspnea on exertion reflect poor ventilation. The degree of respiratory impairment depends on the extent of the eventration. The symptoms may be minimal to nearly disabling. Such symptoms may develop early in life or may follow the increase in intra-abdominal pressure associated with obesity.

Gastrointestinal symptoms may result from eventration of the diaphragm, particularly with complete eventration of the left hemidiaphragm. Gastric volvulus due to abnormalities in fixation have resulted in necrosis of the stomach.[31] More often, only postprandial pain and bloating are noted.

DIAGNOSIS. — Physical examination will reveal abnormalities in only a small number of patients with eventration because of the relatively mild disturbance in visceral location. With larger eventrations, dullness to percussion, interference with breath sounds, mediastinal shift and a scaphoid abdomen may be noted. Marked flaring of the lower costal margin during inspiration often is believed to be pathognomonic.[46] The inward pull of the diaphragm on the lower rib cage is not present to inhibit the spread of the ribs.

Chest roentgenograms usually show a smooth elevation of the hemidiaphragm, although at times there may be a localized elevation (Figs. 42–9 and 42–10). The differentiation of congenital eventration from acquired malfunction of the diaphragm is possible by fluoroscopy in many instances if the history is not of help. With eventration there will be either no movement or very slight downward movement of the diaphragm with inspiration. Both diaphragms must be observed simultaneously to determine whether they move synchronously or paradoxically.

Pneumoperitoneography using carbon dioxide or contrast peritoneography may be helpful in differentiating an eventration from a diaphragmatic hernia or a supradiaphragmatic mass lesion. The contrast study will define the position and integrity of the diaphragm.

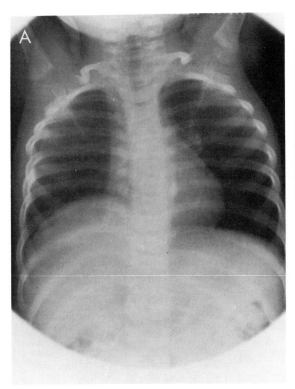 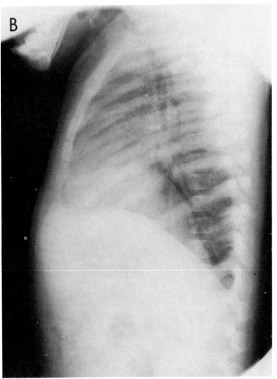

Fig. 42–9. — Eventration of the right diaphragm. PA **(A)** and lateral **(B)** radiographs. The right dome of the liver is elevated. This child was not operated on.

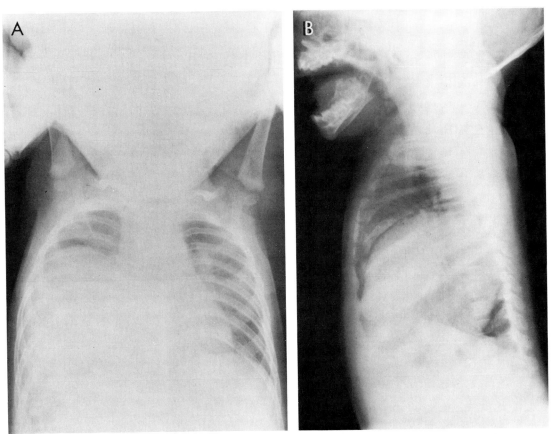

Fig. 42–10.—Complete eventration of a right diaphragm in a newborn, PA **(A)** and lateral **(B)** radiographs. The child was operated on, with resolution of his respiratory distress.

TREATMENT.—Operation is not necessary for asymptomatic eventrations, which are small and discovered later in life. Large eventrations should be plicated whether or not they are symptomatic. In general, patients with respiratory symptoms referable to the eventration should have the eventration plicated regardless of its size.

Clearing of the immediate pulmonary pathology should precede an operative attack on the eventration.

In those patients in whom the eventration has produced pulmonary symptoms, a thoracic approach provides the best exposure to avoid phrenic nerve injury during repair of the diaphragm. In those patients who have gastrointestinal symptoms or suspected gastric volvulus, an upper abdominal approach is suggested. Injury to branches of the phrenic nerve is more likely from this approach but evaluation of the stomach and intestine is necessary. In instances of bilateral anterior eventration, an upper abdominal approach is recommended because both diaphragms can be plicated at one operation. Posterior or bilateral large eventrations require individual thoracotomies, which may be done some days or weeks apart.

The operative treatment of eventration carries no mortal risk other than that of general anesthesia and laparotomy or thoracotomy.

Acquired Diaphragmatic Malfunction

Injuries to the phrenic nerve that result in malfunction of the diaphragm may occur as a result of birth trauma[45] or may follow cervical or thoracic operations. These are not congenital lesions, although they may occur at the time of birth.

Whether or not the paralyzed diaphragm interferes sufficiently with respiratory activity to produce symptoms really depends on the completeness of the phrenic palsy and the age of the patient. The newborn is a diaphragmatic breather. Diaphragmatic paralysis in the newborn often will be poorly tolerated because the mediastinum is very flexible. As the normal innervated hemidiaphragm contracts and lowers with inspiration, the paralyzed hemidiaphragm is drawn upward by negative intrathoracic inspiratory pressure and pushed up by positive intra-abdominal pressure. The mediastinal shift may be so great that it results in little air moving in and out of the trachea. Most of the air flow is back and forth from one lung to the other. The observation of this phenomenon on fluoroscopy is most impressive. In the older child, the mediastinum is rigid enough so that although the paradoxic motion of the hemidiaphragm is present there is little mediastinal shift. There may even be a net inspiratory effort on the paralyzed side if the accessory muscles of respiration are well enough developed to expand the rib cage and overcome the upward displacement of the diaphragm.

DIAGNOSIS.—Any neonate with respiratory distress deserves a chest x-ray. Significant disparity in level of one hemidiaphragm to the other should be suspect. Differential diagnostic consideration is between paralysis and eventration. As both hemidiaphragms and the mediastinum are observed at fluoroscopy, the paradoxic elevation of the paralyzed hemidiaphragm may be appreciated.

TREATMENT.—The treatment depends on the severity of the symptoms. Minimal or lessening respiratory distress

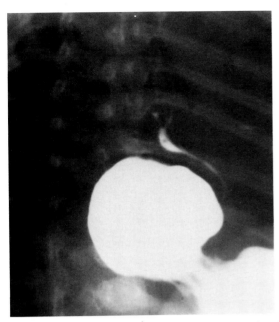

Fig. 42–11.—Paraesophageal hiatal hernia. Infant of 8 months with recurrent respiratory infection due to gastroesophageal reflux. The barium contrast studies confirm the distortion of the esophagus and the herniated portion of the stomach. Repair of the hernia and fundoplication prevented further aspiration pneumonitis.

does not warrant surgical treatment. In the infant whose symptoms are not severe, positioning in an infant seat at 60–75° will reduce pressure on the paralyzed diaphragm and improve ventilation. If intubation or ventilatory support is required or a borderline cardiorespiratory status is noted with little improvement over a brief period of observation in the hospital, plication of the diaphragm is indicated to lower and tighten the diaphragm, increasing space for the lung and decreasing paradox. This lesion should be approached transthoracically, since the branches of the phrenic nerve can be visualized and protected during the plication of nonabsorbable sutures radiating out from the hilum of the diaphragm, avoiding injury to the phrenic nerve branches as much as possible. Thus, should any diaphragmatic function return then, at least the paralyzed diaphragm will not interfere with respiration. In our experience, patients under the age of 8 months often require plication whereas after the age of 2 years it rarely is necessary.

RESULTS OF TREATMENT.—Marked improvement in ventilation should be expected. In our experience, the only child who did not respond well to plication of the diaphragm was a child of several months who had an undiagnosed neuromuscular disorder. In this patient, the diaphragmatic palsy was bilateral and appeared to be the earliest manifestation of his neuromuscular disease.

Paraesophageal Hiatal Hernia

The paraesophageal hiatal hernia only occasionally is associated with gastroesophageal reflux. Of major concern is the potential for incarceration or strangulation of the stom-

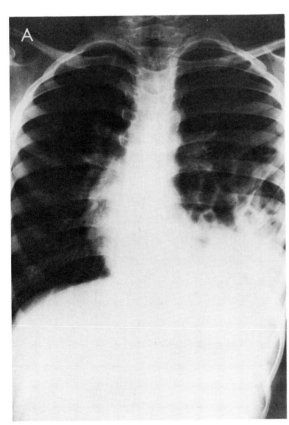

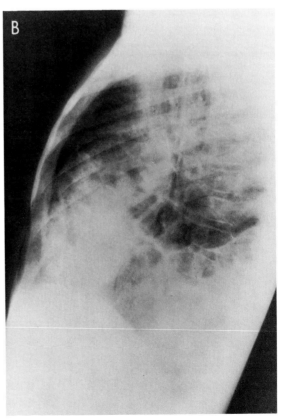

Fig. 42–12.—Traumatic diaphragmatic hernia in a child of 8 years, injured in an automobile accident. Fracture of the femur, lung contusion and a minor closed head injury were the initial problems. The patient was seen 7 months following this injury with respiratory infection and left chest pain. Chest x-ray revealed the above findings. At operation, the adhesions between lung and small intestine were divided and the 5-cm diaphragmatic defect was closed by direct suture.

ach or intestine. Regurgitation often is the presenting symptom, based on obstruction of the distal esophagus by the herniated stomach. If vomiting is not the presenting symptom, the diagnosis may be delayed until incarceration becomes manifest. On diagnosis, these hernias should be surgically repaired.

DIAGNOSIS. — The diagnosis of paraesophageal hiatal hernia may be suspected by plain x-ray showing a mediastinal air-fluid level, but contrast studies of the gastrointestinal tract usually are necessary for confirmation (Fig. 42–11).

SURGICAL TREATMENT. — Through an abdominal approach, the treatment consists of reduction of the hernia, closure of the defect, which usually will require closure of the hiatus as well, and fundoplication, more to prevent recurrence than as an antireflux procedure.

PROGNOSIS. — Both the hernia repair and the operative procedure to prevent gastroesophageal reflux should be nearly 100% successful in children. There will be the occasional patient who has suffered a catastrophic incarceration with strangulation and gangrene of the stomach, who may succumb. This, fortunately, is extremely rare in children.

Traumatic Hernia of the Diaphragm

As a result of one of the many forms of blunt trauma to the abdomen, an extremely high temporary pressure may be generated — enough to rupture the diaphragm. This occurs most commonly in automobile injuries, either where the child is a passenger or is a pedestrian.

Attention to other more pressing problems (head injury, pneumothorax and fractures) may allow the diaphragmatic rupture to be missed.[29] Its specific diagnosis may be obscured by the presence of other shadows in the hemithorax such as might be found with hemothorax or hemopneumothorax (Fig. 42–12). Once the patient's condition is stabilized, investigation to exclude the possibility of diaphragmatic rupture should be carried out. This may include gastrointestinal contrast studies and radioactive isotope scans of the liver and lungs. The left hemidiaphragm is ruptured more often than the right. These hernias should not be ignored, and regardless of whether symptoms are present following recovery from the acute injury, the hernia should be surgically approached and repaired. If there are no other serious injuries, or if there is respiratory distress or intestinal obstruction, the diaphragm is to be repaired immediately. It is wise to position the patient and plan the approach so that separate abdominal and thoracic incisions can be made or a combined incision made to repair such a hernia. Extensive adhesions between lung and intestine may have developed as a result of bleeding. Fatal incarceration, strangulation and necrosis may occur following traumatic diaphragmatic hernia if the lesion is not diagnosed and properly treated.

REFERENCES

1. Adelman, S., and Benson, C. D.: Bochdalek hernias in infants: Factors determining mortality, J. Pediatr. Surg. 11:569, 1976.
2. Areechon, W., and Reid, L.: Hypoplasia of lung with congenital diaphragmatic hernia, Br. Med. J. 1:230, 1963.
3. Baffes, T. G.: Diaphragmatic Hernia, in Benson, C. D., *et al.* (eds.), *Pediatric Surgery* (Chicago: Year Book Medical Publishers, Inc., 1962), Vol. 1.
4. Baran, E. M., Houston, H. E., Lynn, H. B., and O'Connell, E. J.: Foramen of Morgagni hernias in children, Surgery 62:1076, 1967.
5. Bentley, G., and Lister, J.: Retrosternal hernia, Surgery 57:567, 1965.
6. Berdon, W. E., Baker, D. H., and Amoury, R. A.: The role of pulmonary hypoplasia in the prognosis of newborn infants with diaphragmatic hernia and eventration, Am. J. Roentgenol. 103: 413, 1968.
7. Bochdalek, V. A.: Einige Betrachtungen über die Entstehung des angeborenen Zwerchfellbruches. Als Beitrag zur pathologischen Anatomie der hernien, Vjsche. prakt. Heilk. 19:89, 1848.
8. Bock, H. B., and Zimmerman, J. H.: Study of selected congenital anomalies in Pennsylvania, Public Health Rep. 82:446, 1967.
9. Boix-Ochoa, J., Peguero, G., Seijo, G., Natal A., and Canals, J.: Acid-base balance and blood gases in prognosis and therapy of congenital diaphragmatic hernia, J. Pediatr. Surg. 9:49, 1974.
10. Boles, E. T., Schiller, M., and Weinberger, M.: Improved management of neonates with congenital diaphragmatic hernias, Arch. Surg. 103:344, 1971.
11. Bonham-Carter, R. E., Waterston, D. J., and Aberdeen, E.: Hernia and eventration of the diaphragm in childhood, Lancet 1: 656, 1962.
12. Brennom, W. S., and Bill, A. H.: Prophylactic fixation of the intestine for midgut nonrotation, Surg. Gynecol. Obstet. 138:181, 1974.
13. Butler, N., and Claireaux, A. R.: Congenital diaphragmatic hernia as a cause of perinatal mortality, Lancet 1:659, 1962.
14. Campbell, D. P., and Raffensperger, J. G.: Congenital cystic disease of the lung masquerading as diaphragmatic hernia, J. Thorac. Cardiovasc. Surg. 64:592, 1972.
15. Cerilli, G. J.: Foramen of Bochdalek hernia: A review of the experience at Children's Hospital of Denver, Colorado, Ann. Surg. 159:385, 1964.
16. Chatrath, R. R., El Shafie, M., and Jones, R. S.: Fate of hypoplastic lungs after repair of congenital diaphragmatic hernia, Arch. Dis. Child. 46:633, 1971.
17. Collins, D. L., Travis, K. W., Turner, S. W., Pomerance, J. J., and Pappelbaum, S. J.: The significance of the pulmonary circulation in diaphragmatic hernia. Presented at the American Pediatric Surgical Association meeting, April, 1974.
18. Cook, R. C. M., and Beckwith, J. B.: Adrenal injury during repair of diaphragmatic hernia in infants, Surgery 69:251, 1971.
19. DeLorimier, A. A., Tierney, D. F., and Parker, H. R.: Hypoplastic lungs in fetal lambs with surgically produced congenital diaphragmatic hernia, Surgery 62:12, 1967.
20. Dibbins, A. W.: Neonatal diaphragmatic hernia: A physiologic challenge, Am. J. Surg. 131:408, 1976.
21. Dibbins, A. W., and Wiener, E. S.: Mortality from neonatal diaphragmatic hernia, J. Pediatr. Surg. 9:653, 1974.
22. Dunnill, M. S.: Postnatal growth of the lung, Thorax 17:329, 1962.
23. Gray, S. W., and Skandalakis, J. E.: *Embryology for Surgeons* (Philadelphia: W. B. Saunders Company, 1972).
24. Greenwald, G. M., and Steiner, M.: Diaphragmatic hernia in infancy and childhood, Am. J. Dis. Child. 38:361, 1929.
25. Gross, R. E.: *The Surgery of Infancy and Childhood* (Philadelphia: W. B. Saunders Company, 1953).
26. Gross, R. E.: Congenital hernia of the diaphragm, Am. J. Dis. Child. 71:579, 1946.
27. Hedblom, C. A.: Diaphragmatic hernia, JAMA 85:947, 1925.
28. Holder, T. M., Leape, L. L., and Ashcraft, K. W.: Gastrostomy: Its use and dangers in pediatric patients, N. Engl. J. Med. 286: 1345, 1972.
29. Holgersen, L. O., and Schnaufer, L.: Hernia and eventration of the diaphragm secondary to blunt trauma, J. Pediatr. Surg. 8: 433, 1973.
30. Johnson, D. G., Deaner, R. M., and Koop, C. E.: Diaphragmatic hernia in infancy: Factors affecting the mortality rate, Surgery 62:1082, 1967.
31. Katz, S. M., Holgersen, L. O., and Bishop, H. C.: Eventration of the diaphragm with gastric perforation, J. Pediatr. Surg. 9:411, 1974.
32. Kenigsberg, K., and Gwinn, J. L.: The retained sac in repair of posterolateral diaphragmatic hernia in the newborn, Surgery 57: 894, 1965.
33. Kent, G. M., Olley, P. M., Creighton, R. E., Dobbinson, T., Bryan, M. H., Symchych, P., Zingg, W., and Cummings, J. N.: Hemodynamic and pulmonary changes following diaphragmatic hernia in fetal lambs, Surgery 72:427, 1972.
34. Kirkland, J. A.: Congenital posterolateral diaphragmatic hernia in the adult, Br. J. Surg. 47:16, 1959.
35. Ladd, W. E., and Gross, R. E.: *Abdominal Surgery of Infancy and Childhood* (Philadelphia: W. B. Saunders Company, 1941).

36. Levy, J. L., Gunes, W. A., Louis, J. E., and Linder, L. H.: Bilateral congenital diaphragmatic hernias through the foramina of Bochdalek, J. Pediatr. Surg. 4:557, 1969.

37. Mahour, G. H., and Hays, D. M.: Ventral hernia coverage with silon after correction of congenital diaphragmatic hernia, J. Pediatr. Surg. 6:75, 1971.

38. McNamara, J. J., Eraklis, A. J., and Gross, R. E.: Congenital posterolateral diaphragmatic hernia in the newborn, J. Thorac. Cardiovasc. Surg. 55:55, 1968.

39. Murdock, A. I., Burrington, J. B., and Swyer, P. R.: Alveolar to arterial oxygen tension difference and venous admixture in newly born infants with congenital diaphragmatic herniation through the foramen of Bochdalek, Biol. Neonate 17:161, 1971.

40. Reid, I. S., and Hutcherson, R. J.: Long-term follow-up of patients with congenital diaphragmatic hernia, J. Pediatr. Surg. 11:939, 1976.

41. Rowe, M. I., and Uribe, F. L.: Diaphragmatic hernia in the newborn infant: Blood gas and pH considerations, Surgery 70:758, 1971.

42. Scheer, C. W., and Linville, J. L.: Congenital diaphragmatic hernia through foramen of Bochdalek, Arch. Surg. 91:823, 1965.

43. Simpson, J. S.: Ventral silon pouch: Method of repairing, Surgery 66:798, 1969.

44. Simpson, J. S., and Gossage, J. D.: Use of abdominal wall muscle flap in repair of large congenital diaphragmatic hernia, J. Pediatr. Surg. 6:42, 1971.

45. Stauffer, U. G., and Rickham, P. P.: Acquired eventration of the diaphragm in the newborn, J. Pediatr. Surg. 7:635, 1972.

46. Thomas, T. V.: Congenital eventration of the diaphragm, Ann. Thorac. Surg. 10:180, 1970.

47. Wayne, E. R., Campbell, J. B., Burrington, J. D., and Davis, W. S.: Eventration of the diaphragm, J. Pediatr. Surg. 9:643, 1974.

48. White, J. J., Oh, K. S., and Haller, J. A.: Positive-contrast peritoneography for accurate delineation of diaphragmatic abnormalities, Surgery 76:398, 1974.

49. White, J. J., and Suzuki, H.: Hernia through the foramen of Bochdalek: A misnomer, J. Pediatr. Surg. 7:60, 1972.

50. Wohl, M. E. B., Griscom, N. T., Schuster, S. R., Zwerdling, R. G., and Strieder, D.: Lung growth and function following repair of congenital diaphragmatic hernia, Pediatr. Res. 7:424, 1973.

51. Yeung, W. C., Haines, J. E., and Larson, S. M.: Diagnosis of posterolateral congenital diaphragmatic (Bochdalek) hernia by liver scintigram: Case report, J. Nucl. Med. 17:110, 1976.

43

The Esophagus

Congenital Esophageal Atresia and Tracheoesophageal Fistula

N. A. Myers / Eoin Aberdeen

"In recent years there has been no more dramatic advance in surgery than that which has taken place in the treatment of congenital atresia of the esophagus. In spite of innumerable attempts by many surgeons to correct this malformation by operative means, the abnormality was uniformly fatal throughout the world prior to 1939. In the decade following this, improvements in the surgical handling of babies with this anomaly have been so remarkable that in many centers a high proportion of these children now can be saved and can be provided with a satisfactory pathway for the transport of food to the stomach."—R. E. Gross[53]

History.—Congenital atresia of the esophagus without tracheoesophageal fistula was first described in 1670 by William Durston,[33] who observed the anomaly in one member of conjoined twins. The usual type of esophageal atresia accompanied by distal tracheoesophageal fistula was clearly portrayed in Thomas Gibson's[50] classic description (1697). The variations encountered in anomalies of the esophagus, usually accompanied by tracheoesophageal fistula, have been classified by many authors since the 1920s; perhaps the most used classification was presented in 1929 by Vogt.[142] The first operative attempt to correct the anomaly was made in 1888 by Steele[131] on a baby who obviously had atresia without an accompanying tracheoesophageal fistula. Ligation of the tracheoesophageal fistula as a step toward eventual correction of the anomaly was first used by Richter[119] in 1913. Although Keith[80] and Richter[119] envisaged the possibility of correction of the anomaly by an anastomosis of the two portions of the esophagus, a definitive operation of this type was not attempted until the late 1930s, when it was used independently by Lanman[93] and Shaw.[124] Late in the decade 1930–1940, a multiple-stage plan consisting of division or ligation of the tracheoesophageal fistula, gastrostomy and cervical esophagostomy usually was utilized. The first 2 patients to recover were operated on on successive days by Leven[94] and Ladd[89] in 1939 by this multiple-stage procedure. Each later had an esophagoplasty. However, the first baby to survive was born in 1935—a baby with esophageal atresia without an accompanying fistula. This patient had a gastrostomy performed but did not come to definitive esophageal replacement until 1949.[4] The first patient to survive a direct approach to the anomaly by division and closure of the tracheoesophageal fistula and simultaneous primary anastomosis of the two segments of the esophagus was operated on by Haight in 1941, and reported in 1943 by Haight and Towsley.[59] The first case of tracheoesophageal fistula unaccompanied by esophageal atresia was described by Lamb[90] in 1873 and the first survival was reported by Imperatori[78] in 1939.

Two particularly significant contributions to the literature in the 1960s were made by Ashcraft and Holder[4] relating "the story of esophageal atresia and tracheoesophageal fistula" and by Holder et al.[71] surveying the then current status of repair and results of treatment.

Whereas the early reports in the literature were essentially anecdotal,[5, 14, 41, 48, 67, 73, 77, 102, 104, 118, 129, 141, 146] recent articles have stressed the occasional occurrence of unusual types of anomaly,[7, 29, 126, 133] have included detailed reports and reviews[25, 86, 107, 136] and have been concerned with quality of survival and psychologic consequences in the family as a whole.[88]

The operative techniques that have been reported are summarized diagrammatically in Figure 43–1.

Incidence

Although the incidence of congenital atresia of the esophagus in reported series varies, Haight[56] pointed out that among infants born of residents of Washtenaw County, Michigan, the anomaly was recognized in 21 during a period of 30 years, which represented an incidence of 1 in 4425 live births. In 1974, Myers[108] reported an incidence of 1 in 4500 live births from a population of 3,500,000 in Australia, the data including information from a detailed perinatal survey.

The precise significance of genetic factors remains uncertain; however, sibling involvement has been described.[12, 61, 128] Two instances in siblings occurred during a 28-year period in a series of 104 patients admitted to the Royal Children's Hospital, Melbourne. The anomaly is also seen occasionally in one of twins; Haight[56] reported 11 such instances among the 288 infants in his series. Woolley et al.[147] reported the anomaly in both members of a pair of twins who appeared to be genetically identical.

Recently there have been reports[61] in two generations. Although such reports may be more frequent in the future, it would appear that this will be unlikely because the first survivor was born 38 years ago and the paucity of reports argues, thus far, against a heavy genetic influence.

Embryology

The embryology of congenital atresia of the esophagus with or without tracheoesophageal fistula is not clearly understood. The anomaly is known to originate in the interval between the end of the third week and the sixth week of fetal life.[130]

The cause of the anomaly must be multifactorial. When esophageal atresia and/or tracheoesophageal fistula occurs as an isolated anomaly, it is possible that mechanical factors may be responsible for the abnormal embryogenesis. The presence of vascular anomalies at the level of the atresia has been described by several authors who believe that the localized pressure thereby exerted on the developing esophagus is responsible for the loss of continuity. The tracheoesophageal fistula below the level of the obstruction is attributed to failure of complete closure of the laryngotracheal groove during this stage of development. Langman[91, 92] described several cases in which a fibrous cord, believed to be the remnant of an anomalous right subclavian artery, traversed the gap between the two segments of the esophagus. He believed also that an abnormally lengthy persistence of the primitive right-descending aorta may be a cause of esophageal atresia. In 5.1% of the cases seen by Haight,[56] an anomalous vessel, usually an anomalous right subclavian artery, was encountered at the level of atresia. Haight also

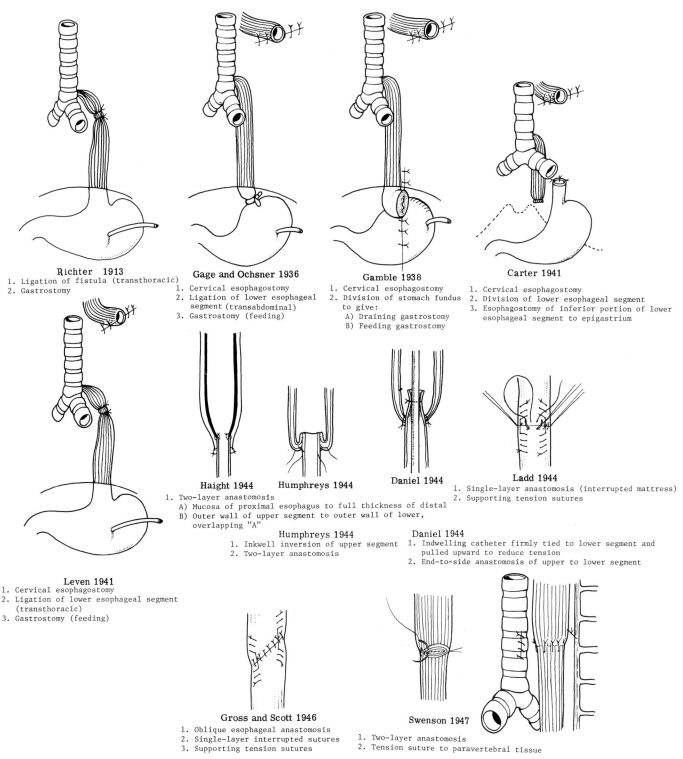

Richter   1913
1. Ligation of fistula (transthoracic)
2. Gastrostomy

Gage and Ochsner 1936
1. Cervical esophagostomy
2. Ligation of lower esophageal segment (transabdominal)
3. Gastrostomy (feeding)

Gamble 1938
1. Cervical esophagostomy
2. Division of stomach fundus to give:
   A) Draining gastrostomy
   B) Feeding gastrostomy

Carter 1941
1. Cervical esophagostomy
2. Division of lower esophageal segment
3. Esophagostomy of inferior portion of lower esophageal segment to epigastrium

Leven 1941
1. Cervical esophagostomy
2. Ligation of lower esophageal segment (transthoracic)
3. Gastrostomy (feeding)

Haight 1944   Humphreys 1944
1. Two-layer anastomosis
   A) Mucosa of proximal esophagus to full thickness of distal
   B) Outer wall of upper segment to outer wall of lower, overlapping "A"

Humphreys 1944
1. Inkwell inversion of upper segment
2. Two-layer anastomosis

Daniel 1944

Ladd 1944
1. Single-layer anastomosis (interrupted mattress)
2. Supporting tension sutures

Daniel 1944
1. Indwelling catheter firmly tied to lower segment and pulled upward to reduce tension
2. End-to-side anastomosis of upper to lower segment

Gross and Scott 1946
1. Oblique esophageal anastomosis
2. Single-layer interrupted sutures
3. Supporting tension sutures

Swenson 1947
1. Two-layer anastomosis
2. Tension suture to paravertebral tissue

Fig. 43–1.—Esophageal atresia. Techniques of repair, presented in historical progression. (*Continued.*)

commented that "A persisting fibrous cord like that described by Langman has been seen only rarely, and in such instances its size has been so small as to make it difficult to identify with certainty."

The association of esophageal atresia with other anomalies is well recognized. At times, the anomalies are multiple and in a few instances chomosomal aberrations can be rec-

ognized. It is not yet clear whether a common teratogen is responsible for the occurrence of multiple associated anomalies. A particularly interesting idea is the so-called VATER association,[9, 114] in which *V*ertebral anomalies,[13, 134] *A*nal anomalies, *T*racheo-*E*sophageal fistula with esophageal atresia, *R*enal anomalies[6] and *R*adial limb dysplasia are combined.

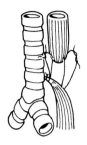
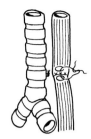
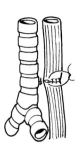
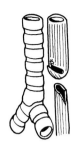
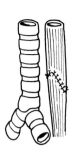

Sulamaa, Gripenberg and Ahvenainen 1951

SULAMAA, GRIPENBERG AND AHVENAINEN 1951-A

1. End of upper segment to side of lower segment anastomosis
2. Division of fistula after partial completion of anastomosis

Sulamaa, Gripenberg and Ahvenainen 1951

SULAMAA, GRIPENBERG AND AHVENAINEN, 1951-B

1. Tongue-like flap fashioned from upper segment (base is distal)
2. Lower segment enlarged by cutback
3. Single-layer interrupted suture anastomosis

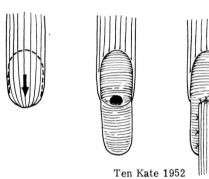
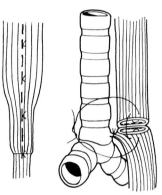
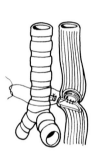
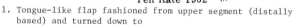

Ten Kate 1952

1. Tongue-like flap fashioned from upper segment (distally based) and turned down to
2. Envelop the lower segment in a two-layer overlapping anastomosis

Berman and Berman 1953

1. Fistula ligated in continuity
2. End of upper segment to side of lower segment anastomosis

Sanderud 1960

1. Division of fistula
2. End of upper segment to side of lower segment anastomosis

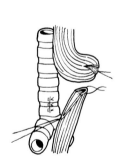
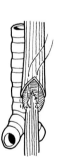
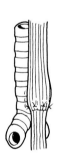
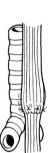
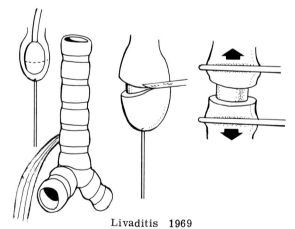

Humphreys and Ferrer 1964

1. Two-layer overlapping anastomosis (Haight-type)
2. Lower segment enlarged by cutback

Livaditis 1969

1. Pouch distended with balloon catheter
2. Circular incision of muscle layer only, 2 cm above end
3. Gentle traction with atraumatic clamps
(After Eraklis et al. 38a)

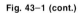

Fig. 43–1 (cont.)

Classification and Types of Anomaly

Many classifications have been suggested in the past and nearly all have involved the use of letters (Fritz,[42] Stephens, Mustard and Simpson[132]) or numbers (Ladd,[89] Gross[53]) or both (Vogt[142]). To avoid confusion, we prefer to adopt a descriptive classification. The important anomalies to be recognized are:

1. *Esophageal atresia with distal tracheoesophageal fistula (the common type)* (Fig. 43–2, A).

2. *Esophageal atresia with proximal tracheoesophageal fistula* (Fig. 43–2, B).

3. *Esophageal atresia with proximal and distal tracheoesophageal fistulas* (Fig. 43–2, C).

4. *Esophageal atresia (pure atresia)* (Fig. 43–2, D).

5. *Tracheoesophageal fistula (H-fistula)* (Fig. 43–2, E).

Unusual variations, of which the surgeon should be aware, have been described by:

Haight[56]—complete atresia of the esophagus at the junction of the middle and lower thirds.

Waterston *et al.*[143]—esophageal atresia with fistula as in the common type, but with atresia of the tracheoesophageal "fistula," close to its tracheal attachment.

Babbitt[8]—double fistula without atresia.

Knox[84]—tracheoesophageal fistula and esophageal diverticulum without accompanying atresia.

Humphreys *et al.*[76]—esophageal atresia with tracheoesophageal fistula, with multiple atresias of the lower esophageal segment.

Tuqan[139]—the common type with a fistula to the distal esophageal segment, but this distal segment itself being affected by stenosis.

Kluth[83] has assembled a detailed atlas of esophageal atresia and tracheoesophageal fistula in which the extensive bibliography is reproduced in diagrammatic form.

There is a remarkable similarity of the incidence of the various types of anomaly in the various reported series. Esophageal atresia with a tracheoesophageal fistula to the lower esophageal segment is the predominant anomaly in all. Thus, Haight[56] reported an 88.2% incidence of this anomaly. In 404 patients seen at the Royal Children's Hospital, Melbourne, during the period 1948–1977, the incidence was 86% (Fig. 43–3). Although in this series all these babies had air in the stomach on plain x-rays, absence of air does not exclude the possibility of a tracheoesophageal "fistula" between the trachea and lower esophagus.[23, 72, 143]

Associated Anomalies

Additional congenital anomalies frequently are present.[26, 49] The anomaly may be obvious or hidden; it may be simple or complicated; and it may or may not be life-threatening. For many babies with esophageal atresia, the associated anomaly greatly affects treatment and survival, especially so with cardiac anomalies, anorectal anomalies or other gut obstructions.

Inspection of the infant will disclose such anomalies as accessory auricles, cleft palate and imperforate anus. X-ray examination will indicate vertebral and rib anomalies and, in view of the relatively high incidence of urinary tract involvement, some authorities routinely advocate an excretory pyelogram. Should a cardiac anomaly be suggested, early consultation with a pediatric cardiologist is essential, and, in some, early cardiac investigation is obligatory. In babies with an anorectal anomaly it is essential to pass a tube into the stomach to exclude esophageal atresia. Our experience has paralleled that of Haight,[56] Waterston *et al.*[143] and others, indicating that between 30% and 40% of babies with esophageal atresia have significant other anomalies, and in a high proportion these are cardiovascular.[52] Piekarski and Stephens[112] reviewed the association and embryogenesis of tracheoesophageal and anorectal anomalies in 31 patients. Twenty-three had at least one other associated anomaly and in 23 of their series at least three of the VATER defects were found. They suggested that the high incidence of additional lesions is a reflection of generalized early damage to the mesenchymal tissue in the fourth week of gestation. They also suggested that similar embryologic mechanisms may occur and be affected similarly in both systems.

Symptomatology of Esophageal Atresia with or without Tracheoesophageal Fistula

The symptoms and signs of esophageal atresia, whether or not there is an accompanying tracheoesophageal fistula, depend primarily on esophageal obstruction and secondarily on respiratory tract complications. Lung malfunction may

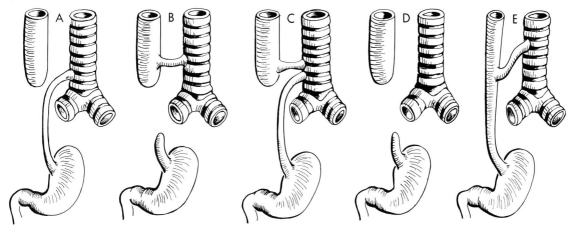

Fig. 43–2.—Anatomic patterns of esophageal atresia. **A,** with distal tracheoesophageal fistula. The most frequently encountered anomaly in all series. **B,** with proximal tracheoesophageal fistula. An uncommon anomaly; the abdomen is airless and the diagnosis may be "missed" unless contrast studies are used. **C,** with proximal and distal fistulas. A very uncommon anomaly. **D,** esophageal atresia without tracheoesophageal fistula. This anomaly almost invariably is associated with a "long gap" and esophageal replacement may be required. However, end-to-end esophageal anastomosis can be achieved in a proportion of patients. **E,** tracheoesophageal fistula without atresia. May present late. Associated with recurrent cough, pneumonia, etc. Surgical approach usually can be cervical.

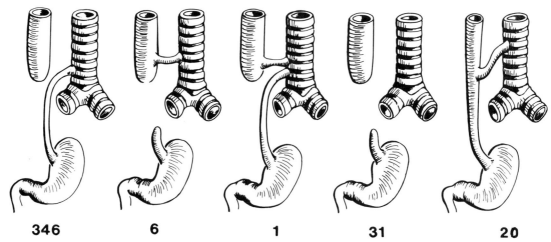

346   **6**   **1**   **31**   **20**

Fig. 43–3.—Congenital esophageal atresia. Distribution of 404 cases at Royal Children's Hospital, Melbourne, 1948–1977.

result from overflow of saliva from the blind esophageal segment, and aspiration, but when a fistula connects stomach to trachea, it is the regurgitation of gastric contents into the trachea that causes the most severe lung damage.[144]

In addition, many of the babies are premature and therefore likely to have idiopathic respiratory distress syndrome, which may complicate the clinical picture.

In the common type of the anomaly (with atresia and tracheoesophageal fistula to the distal esophageal segment), the clinical picture usually is classic. A history of polyhydramnios is frequent, and in one series was observed in about one-third of mothers bearing infants with the common type of the anomaly and in almost all mothers bearing infants with atresia without fistula.[144]

After birth, the baby remains "mucusy," may drool frothy mucus from the mouth and may have intermittent attacks of cyanosis. The abdomen usually is distended. Any feeding is immediately regurgitated, frequently in an explosive fashion, and this often is associated with a cyanotic episode. If diagnosis is delayed, increasing respiratory distress will develop as pneumonia becomes established and abdominal distention increases. Bile-stained aspirate from the pharynx or bile-stained "vomiting" may be observed. Ideally, the diagnosis is made at an early stage, either during the course of neonatal resuscitation or, more specifically, when a definite attempt is made to diagnose or exclude the presence of esophageal atresia in a baby born after a pregnancy complicated by polyhydramnios, since almost one-tenth of such

TABLE 43–1.—Method of Presentation of 288 Babies with Esophageal Atresia and Distal Tracheoesophageal Fistula (Including 1 Baby with an Associated Proximal Fistula)

"Mucusy"	163
"Vomiting" and/or "regurgitation"	25
"Unable to swallow"	3
Inability to pass a tube	21
Respiratory distress	18
Cyanotic attacks without feeding	15
Cyanotic attacks with feeding	16
Cyanosis with gavage feeding	2
Other anomalies (including multiple anomalies)	19
Failure of attempted gavage in a premature infant	3
Not clearly stated	3

pregnancies may involve infants with esophageal atresia.[121] The presence of other anomalies, particularly anorectal malformations, should alert the pediatrician or pediatric surgeon to the possibility of esophageal atresia.

When esophageal atresia occurs without a fistula, the clinical picture is similar, but respiratory features may be delayed, lung complications are much less frequent[144] and the abdomen tends to be scaphoid rather than distended.

Delay in diagnosis may postpone recognition of esophageal atresia until the second, third or even the fourth day of life. A continuing program of education of obstetricians, pediatricians, general practitioners, midwives, medical students and trainee nurses is essential in order to ensure early diagnosis. A baby has a better chance of survival when the diagnosis is made as soon as possible after birth.

Among nearly 300 babies with esophageal atresia and tracheoesophageal fistula of the common type, in 50% the presenting symptom was related to profuse oral and pharyngeal secretions requiring repeated aspiration. Thus, the "mucusy" baby is the most frequent alerting phenomenon; others are listed in Table 43–1.

Diagnosis

Esophageal atresia, with or without tracheoesophageal fistula, may be suspected cinically, but special investigation is required in order to prove the diagnosis. A firm catheter meets obstruction 10 cm from the gum margin; a plain x-ray frequently will demonstrate the air-filled upper esophageal pouch and x-ray of the abdomen will prove or disprove the presence of a tracheoesophageal fistula (Fig. 43–4). Final proof of the diagnosis of esophageal atresia can be obtained by the instillation of radiopaque material into the upper esophageal segment; this investigation is not obligatory and, in fact, some observers state categorically that it is contraindicated because it increases the morbidity and the risk of aspiration pneumonia.[86] The advantages of contrast studies of the upper pouch are threefold—the diagnosis of esophageal atresia is proved beyond doubt; differentiation from severe esophageal stenosis or traumatic submucosal perforation is possible; and an upper-pouch fistula can be detected.[30] However, the passage of a radiopaque catheter is sufficient in our view, unless clinical or x-ray evidence is equivocal. The surgeon should be present at the time of x-ray

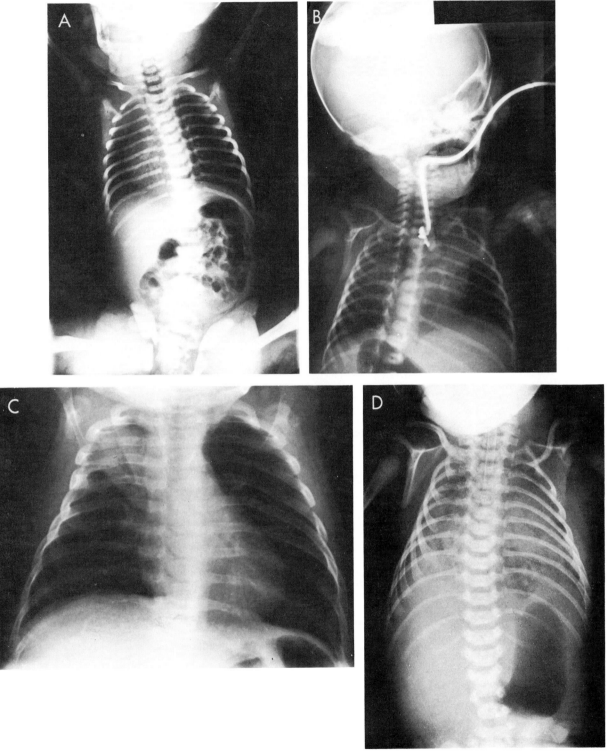

Fig. 43–4. — Esophageal atresia. Radiographic diagnosis of the most common (distal fistula) variety. **A,** plainly seen are the distended, gas-filled esophageal pouch ending at the level of T1, the absence of spinal anomalies, the overdistended left lung and abundant gas in the intestinal tract. With a large fistula, the stomach may be so hugely distended as to produce respiratory distress. **B,** x-ray shows that a *stiff* rubber catheter does not pass. If one wishes to insert radio contrast material, a few drops suffice and the material then is withdrawn by suction lest overflow into the lungs both cause pulmonary embarrassment and confuse the radiologic evaluation of the lungs after operation. **C,** aspiration pneumonia or atelectasis, particularly of the right upper lobe, as in this neonate, is common. Tracheal suction, gentle percussion and continuous pharyngeal suction usually lead to rapid clearance and prevent recurrence. **D,** the catheter passed from above stops at T3. There is diffuse pulmonary infiltration. There is no air beyond the stomach, alerting one to the presence of what is statistically the most common cause for this — duodenal atresia.

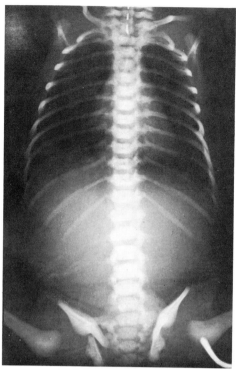

Fig. 43–5.—Esophageal atresia without fistula. The upper esophagus contains air; the abdomen is airless. The film always should be a "baby-gram" to show neck, chest, abdomen and pelvis.

screening, because investigation performed in his absence may have to be repeated.

Diagnostic study must include evaluation of all systems, with particular reference to the presence of pneumonia, the presence or absence of other congenital abnormalities and identification of chromosomal abnormalities. Clinical examination must take particular note of the perineum, the limbs and the facies. Modern cytologic techniques will enable early and accurate diagnosis of chromosomal anomalies if the clinical picture is not 100% diagnostic.

The x-ray examination of chest and abdomen, apart from indicating the presence, size and site of the air-filled upper pouch, permits evaluation of:

1. The skeletal elements—particularly the presence or absence of vertebral or rib anomalies.

2. The lung fields—with specific reference to areas of consolidation, atelectasis or emphysema.

3. The gastric and intestinal gas pattern—associated duodenal obstruction can be suspected or diagnosed. In the absence of a distal fistula, the abdomen is airless (Fig. 43–5) and therefore at this stage it is impossible to draw any conclusions regarding the intestinal tract. The stomach almost certainly will be small in the absence of a distal fistula and the surgeon should be aware of this when undertaking gastrostomy.

Differential Diagnosis

The classic clinical picture and radiologic findings usually permit an unequivocal diagnosis to be made.

Conditions that specifically enter into the differential diagnosis are:

1. All neonatal conditions producing respiratory distress.
2. Prematurity.

3. Congenital cardiac malformations.
4. Laryngoesophageal cleft.

Attention should also be paid to the newborn baby who "vomits," because not infrequently regurgitation of feeding is misinterpreted as true vomiting. For this reason, babies with esophageal atresia may, at times, be thought to have a simple feeding problem, gastroesophageal reflux or even intestinal obstruction. The aspiration from the pharynx or upper esophagus of fluid with an acid reaction does not preclude the diagnosis of esophageal atresia, and diagnostic delay has occurred when this finding has been misinterpreted, particularly when a long length of a soft catheter has been "passed" but actually has doubled up in the upper esophageal pouch or pharynx.

Management

The treatment of the baby with esophageal atresia requires great judgment as well as surgical skill. The management requires close cooperation among surgeon, neonatologist, intensive care therapist, anesthesiologist, radiologist, laboratory staff and nursing staff. The management must be concerned with the family as a whole, and especially the mother who still may be in an obstetric hospital, anxiously awaiting news and greatly needing emotional support. Any newborn emergency is a crisis for the family, and the manner in which the medical advisers meet this crisis may determine the ultimate emotional outcome and the human quality of the "surgical triumph."

In the baby with esophageal atresia, with or without a tracheoesophageal fistula, the three most important priorities in order are:

1. To save life.
2. To achieve alimentary continuity.
3. To preserve the esophagus.

Alimentary continuity can be achieved in a variety of ways, ideally by anastomosing the two esophageal segments and in an increasing proportion of patients this has proved to be possible. Nevertheless, some form of esophageal replacement will be required in some patients, and the surgeon responsible for the care of the baby with esophageal atresia must be familiar with the wide variety of techniques reported and must be prepared to vary the therapeutic program according to the specific problems and needs in the individual baby.

In general terms there are three basic ways in which the problem can be handled:

1. Primary anastomosis.
2. Delayed anastomosis.
3. Staged management.

PRIMARY ANASTOMOSIS.—This remains the aim of treatment of the fit baby with esophageal atresia and distal fistula, and with modern methods of preventing and treating respiratory failure it has become possible in an increasing number of patients. Primary anastomosis may be performed by the extrapleural or transpleural route, by end-to-end or end-to-side anastomosis and may or may not be combined with gastrostomy.

DELAYED ANASTOMOSIS.—The treatment of esophageal atresia is delayed when nonoperative or other operative measures are first used to improve the baby's condition. This program, which may include a gastrostomy for gastric drainage without commencement of feeding, is followed by early thoracotomy and correction of the anomaly. This approach is specifically designed for the baby presenting "late" with established pneumonia and also for the baby with coexisting

TABLE 43-2.—CORRELATION BETWEEN THERAPEUTIC GROUP AND PHASE OF TREATMENT
(NUMBERS OF PATIENTS)°

THERAPEUTIC GROUP	PHASE 1 1948-52	PHASE 2 1953-57	PHASE 3 1958-62	PHASE 4 1963-67	PHASE 5 1968-72	TOTAL
1. Primary anastomosis and immediate gastrostomy	—	—	3	2	3	8
2. Primary anastomosis; gastrostomy next day	4	—	—	—	—	4
3. Primary anastomosis	6	44	39	31	12	132
4. Primary anatomosis; gastrostomy for complications	3	2	13	9	6	33
5. Delay; gastrostomy followed by primary anastomosis	2	2	3	4	3	14
6. Primary anastomosis plus jejunal feeding tube	—	—	—	—	32	32
7. Primary anastomosis end-to-side	—	—	—	—	11	11
8. Staged management	1	1	8	19	5	34
TOTAL	16	49	66	65	72	268†

°From Myers.[108]
†One patient excluded because thoracotomy was not performed.

problems, such as hyperbilirubinemia, sepsis, metabolic disturbances, etc.

STAGED MANAGEMENT.—Here, the primary operation (gastrostomy and fistula division) permits feeding on the one hand and prevents aspiration on the other. In a few patients we have added cervical esophagostomy to keep the upper pouch empty. Staged management became increasingly popular when a critical evaluation of the factors affecting survival was made, particularly by Holder et al.,[71] by Koop and Hamilton[85] and by Waterston et al.[143] In the early years, staged management almost invariably involved cervical esophagostomy and gastrostomy, combined with division of the tracheoesophageal fistula. Subsequently, the method of staging by fistula division and gastrostomy, without cervical esophagostomy, was introduced, which has the advantage of preserving the esophagus and enabling alimentary continuity to be achieved later by esophageal anastomosis.

The infants who are most appropriately managed by staged procedures are those with one or more of the following factors:[2]

1. Prematurity.
2. Established pneumonia.
3. An associated life-threatening congenital anomaly.
4. A "long gap" between the two esophageal segments precluding primary anastomosis.
5. Deterioration during operation.

Although staged management still is required for some babies, its lessening place was emphasized by Myers[108] in 1974, from the experience at the Royal Children's Hospital, Melbourne.

That review enabled the following three conclusions to be reached:

1. Fistula division and gastrostomy had been lifesaving but had not been problem-free.
2. Modern techniques for the management of respiratory failure had so improved respiratory function that diminished lung function no longer was a necessary restraint on corrective operations.

3. Thoracotomy was well tolerated by very small babies.

This led to the decision to manage most babies, previously considered for staging, by primary esophageal anastomosis, with division of the fistula.

Staging remains an integral part of the treatment of nearly all babies who initially present with an airless abdomen—regardless of the presence or absence of an upper-pouch fistula.

A review of the experience at the Royal Children's Hospital, Melbourne, during a 25-year period from 1948 through 1972 enabled eight operative programs[108] to be recognized (Table 43-2). Obviously, as newer methods were introduced, the type of therapeutic program correlates with the period in which it was carried out.

Consideration always must be given to withholding surgical treatment under special circumstances; the usual indication will be the presence of multiple anomalies incompatible with normal life, but occasionally there will be clinical manifestations of a frank chromosomal abnormality, particularly trisomy E (see Tables 43-3 and 43-4).

The many factors that affect survival include transport, preoperative treatment and evaluation, choice of operation, postoperative treatment, recognition and management of complications and the nature of the individual anomaly.

TABLE 43-3.—ESOPHAGEAL ATRESIA WITH DISTAL TRACHEO-ESOPHAGEAL FISTULA (NUMBERS OF PATIENTS AND TREATMENT)

PHASE	TOTAL	OPERATED ON	NOT OPERATED ON
1. 1948-52	17	16	1
2. 1953-57	53	49	4
3. 1958-62	68	66	2
4. 1963-67	68	65	3
5. 1968-72	82	73	9
TOTAL	288	269	19

TABLE 43–4.—INDICATIONS FOR
WITHHOLDING OPERATION

INDICATION	NO. OF PATIENTS
Multiple anomalies	10
Trisomy E	4
Moribund	2
Down's syndrome	1
Gross hydrocephalus	1
Postmortem diagnosis	1
TOTAL	19

1. Transport

The baby with esophageal atresia frequently will need to be transported from the place of birth to a center with special facilities that will enable appropriate surgical treatment in the newborn period. Transport should be as expeditious as possible, and special care should be taken to ensure:

a) Adequate suction of the upper pouch to avoid aspiration into the respiratory tract, which may worsen an already dangerous situation. The patient should be inclined head up to discourage regurgitation (see later).

b) That the baby remains thermostable during the transport phase.

c) That oxygen is available.

2. Preoperative Treatment and Evaluation

Ideally, the baby is admitted, without delay, to an Intensive Care Unit, where a short period of observation should precede further interference, unless there is need for upper pouch suction or respiratory failure is evident or imminent, in which event immediate tracheal intubation will be required.

The immediate therapeutic measures are those applicable to all newborns (warmth, vitamin K, oxygen, etc.). There have been various opinions expressed regarding the most appropriate posture. To begin with, the baby should either lie flat or with the head end elevated. This is especially important when the abdomen is grossly distended or when other evidence indicates a large fistula. Later, it may be advisable to place the baby in the prone position, and at times the head-down position is indicated if upper pouch secretions are voluminous, and if the upper pouch is to remain undisturbed for any length of time.[20]

The principles of preoperative management are:

a) Specific care of the newborn with reference to maintenance of temperature, control of hypoprothrombinemia, restoration of homeostasis, recognition and management of physiologic disturbances, such as hypovolemia, hypoglycemia and hypocalcemia.

Dehydration is unlikely to be a problem and therefore intravenous fluids can be restricted to maintenance requirements. The ideal solution is 10% dextrose in 0.11% saline with added sodium bicarbonate if indicated.

b) Removal of upper pouch secretions. Two options are available: either intermittent aspiration of the upper pouch or continuous aspiration using a sump catheter (Replogle[117]). Both techniques have proved to be effective and the choice can be dictated by the experience of the medical and nursing staff.

c) Prevention and treatment of pulmonary disease. Stridor may indicate a significant degree of tracheomalacia and should alert the clinician to the possibility of dangerous

postoperative respiratory problems. The respiratory rate and the effort, degree of cyanosis, the nature and distribution of rales, abdominal distention and radiologic changes must all be evaluated. When, as frequently occurs, there is discrepancy between the clinical evaluation of "pneumonia" and the radiologic findings, more weight should be attached to the clinical evaluation.

If respiratory distress is severe, tracheal intubation may be necessary and, rarely, assisted ventilation may be required. These measures are used more often after operation.

Nursing the baby in a fully humidified atmosphere of up to 50% oxygen and attending to posture can combat the progressive deterioration in respiratory function that may result from a large distal fistula.

Special measures include the use of antibiotics and skilled physiotherapy.

d) Investigation. Investigation confirms the diagnosis, establishes the nature of the anomaly and determines treatment. Important investigations are: (1) Bacteriologic—cultures should be taken from the nose, pharynx, umbilicus and rectum, and from the blood, if indicated. (2) Biochemical—arterial blood samples are required to measure blood gases, and should be done in any infant whose respiratory function may be compromised. Venous blood is adequate for assessment of electrolyte balance (which is unlikely to be abnormal) and for assessment of the serum bilirubin level if the infant is jaundiced. (3) Hematologic—the blood type and Rh factor must be established and compatible blood cross-matched. The hemoglobin, the leukocyte count and the platelet count should be measured—the latter, in part, to establish a baseline. Thrombocytopenia suggests sepsis.

e) Decision regarding the timing of operation. It is impossible to be dogmatic regarding the timing of operation and each baby must be assessed individually. Correction of esophageal atresia and tracheoesophageal fistula is an elective emergency and in most instances will be performed within 12–18 hours of admission; the decision requires considerable judgment. A good general principle is to operate as soon as practicable if the presence of a large fistula is suspected, not to delay operation unduly in the baby in good condition, but to allow a short period for observation and evaluation in the "average" case.

3. Esophageal Atresia with Tracheoesophageal Fistula—Choice of Operation

Regardless of the exact program to be followed, certain general principles are essential if morbidity is to be lessened and mortality is to be avoided. These principles are:

a) Skilled anesthetic help.

b) Cooperation between surgeon and anesthesiologist, who should discuss the plan of management before and during operation.

c) Special measures to avoid heat loss and to monitor the baby's temperature during operation.

d) The need to individualize the operation according to the general status of the baby, the operative findings and the condition during operation.

There is a place for primary anastomosis without gastrostomy, in the opinion of many surgeons who reserve gastrostomy for later complications, such as anastomotic leak, severe stenosis or a recurrent tracheoesophageal fistula. However, it is the senior author's view that gastrostomy should be used universally—either as the first operative step (in some of those babies managed by a delayed approach) or at the time the anomaly is repaired. It is immaterial to this approach whether the anastomosis is end-to-end or end-to-side. Although staged management now is used less frequently in most centers, there always will be a need to stage the program in some babies. Furthermore, although cervical esophagostomy may be required occasionally and although there may be a place for gastric division as described by Gamble[45] in the 1930s and more recently by Meeker[106] and Randolph et al.,[115] it is generally agreed that staging is best performed by thoracotomy, division of the tracheoesophageal fistula, closure of the lower esophageal segment and gastrostomy. It is necessary to divide the fistula; ligation alone is likely to lead to disastrous recanalization of the fistula.

Gastrostomy has two objectives, particularly in the baby with esophageal atresia: to decompress the stomach and to permit feeding while the esophagus is healing, or before esophageal continuity has been achieved.[81] It is not possible for a gastrostomy to function in both of these ways at the same time unless special measures are adopted, and therefore it is therapeutically valuable to combine gastrostomy with the introduction of a transpyloric jejunal feeding tube, which permits both functions to be achieved. This can be referred to as a "double gastrostomy" (Fig. 43–6).

It is suggested that at present the following therapeutic programs are applicable in esophageal atresia with a distal tracheoesophageal fistula:

a) Thoracotomy, division of the tracheoesophageal fistula, axial esophageal anastomosis and a "double gastrostomy."

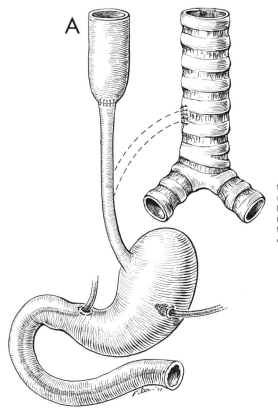
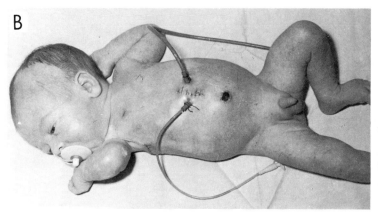
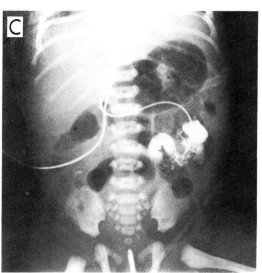

Fig. 43–6.—The "double gastrostomy," which permits aspiration of the stomach through one tube and jejunal feeding with the other. **A,** diagram of the situation after repair of esophageal atresia with distal tracheoesophageal fistula. **B,** the tube on the baby's right passes through the antrum into the jejunum. The tube on the baby's left is the conventional gastrostomy tube. **C,** injection of contrast material into the jejunal tube to confirm its location before feeding is begun. The "mushroom" of the radiolucent gastric catheter is barely visible.

b) Thoracotomy, division of the fistula, closure of the upper end of the lower esophageal segment and gastrostomy plus the introduction of a transpyloric jejunal feeding tube ("double gastrostomy"), i.e., staged management. The two main indications are a long gap between the two esophageal segments and deterioration during operation. The other indications no longer are so relevant.

c) Gastrostomy at the time of admission—followed by a thoracotomy in 24–28 hours or perhaps after a longer period. At thoracotomy, fistula division is performed and this may or may not be combined with axial anastomosis. Alternatively, the technique may take the form of fistula ligation with end-to-side anastomosis.

THORACOTOMY.—With the baby lying on the left side, the approach is either by rib resection—usually the fourth rib—or intercostal. Personal choice will indicate whether the approach is extrapleural or transpleural, as both routes have their advocates.[71] Accumulated evidence has shown that the margin of safety is greater with the extrapleural route, and this is the approach of choice. Should a pleural disruption occur during the course of dissection, it is best to alter the plan and approach the esophagus transpleurally. At times, under these circumstances, partial excision of the parietal pleura may prevent problems arising in the postoperative period from pleural "flap." The extrapleural approach will be especially valuable should the anastomosis leak and infection follow. This is much more likely to occur in the high-risk or low birth weight infant.

The incision, which begins at the level of the fifth rib posteriorly, is essentially horizontal, extending immediately below the angle of the scapula to the posterior axillary line. The extracostal muscles are incised and the scapula retracted upward. This allows the first rib to be palpated and the fourth rib to be identified by counting downward. The greater part of the fourth rib is resected and an extrapleural approach to the mediastinum follows. Dissection must be gentle and is facilitated by commencing posteriorly and bluntly dissecting with gauze swabs. As the pleura is freed, a small self-retaining retractor is introduced and pleural mobilization posteriorly continues until the azygos vein can be doubly ligated and divided. The endothoracic fascia then is gently separated, the lung, covered by the intact parietal pleura, is retracted forward and the following structures are identified—the trachea with the vagus nerve on its surface and the two esophageal segments. Not infrequently, both esophageal segments can be recognized rapidly, but on other occasions neither is visible. Under these circumstances, the upper segment can be identified if the anesthesiologist passes a catheter through the pharynx from above, pushing the upper esophageal pouch down until it comes into view. If any difficulty is experienced in identifying the lower esophageal segment, tracing the vagus nerve distally will help. The aorta may or may not be obvious. Sometimes a right aortic arch is present, or an anomalous right subclavian artery. One or the other may traverse the gap between the esophageal segments.

At this stage, the relative ease or difficulty or absolute infeasibility of primary anastomosis should be obvious. The lower esophageal segment is gently freed from its mediastinal bed and a sling placed around it. The junction between esophagus and trachea is identified and the tracheoesophageal fistula divided. The tracheal end of the fistula is oversewn with 5-0 atraumatic silk. To facilitate closure, initially a suture is introduced at either end of the fistula and one suture is continued to the other. A second "running"

suture then can be introduced deep to the first continuous suture to stabilize fistula closure.

The upper segment is mobilized by blunt dissection, reinforced by sharp dissection in the plane between the esophagus posteriorly and the trachea anteriorly.

All children who have been studied after surviving repair of esophageal atresia have shown at least an area of atonic esophagus in the region of anastomosis. Presumably this area of incoordinate esophagus may be the result of the denervation resulting from esophageal dissection. The implication is that dissection of both esophageal segments should be limited, but as a practical measure it is essential to mobilize the segments adequately if anastomosis is to be performed safely. As repeatedly stressed by Cameron Haight, because of the good vascularity and greater thickness of the wall of the upper esophagus, as compared with the lower, any gap between the two portions of the esophagus is overcome more by mobilization of the upper than of the lower esophagus.

Haight's[56] lucid description of the operative steps immediately prior to anastomosis cannot be bettered: "With traction on the two portions of the esophagus, an estimation is made of the ease or difficulty with which they can be approximated. If they come together readily, no further freeing of the lower esophagus is required. If it is apparent, however, that tension will be present in the anastomosis, the lower esophagus is then mobilized distally for a distance that is estimated to be sufficient to allow the two portions of the esophagus to be approximated subsequently without tension. The length over which the esophagus is freed at this stage of the operation depends on the previously measured distance between the two portions of the esophagus. If the distance is short or nil, the lower esophagus is isolated for only 2 or 3 cm. If the distance between the two portions of the esophagus is relatively great, i.e., 1.5–2.5 cm, the lower esophagus may need to be freed for at least 5 or 6 cm. One avoids freeing the lower esophagus completely over the portion of its circumference which faces the aorta, so that the arterial supply from the aorta is not interrupted. Also it is endeavored not to free the esophagus completely to the level of the diaphragm because of the possibility of producing an iatrogenic hiatal hernia."

End-to-end anastomosis of the two esophageal segments then is performed; various techniques have been described and Haight[56] himself continued to favor the telescopic type of anastomosis. However, there has been accumulating evidence suggesting that this type of anastomosis is more likely to be associated with a postoperative stricture, and evidence indicates that a well-performed one-layer anastomosis is quite safe.[71]

Because of the discrepancy in the size of the lumen of the two esophageal segments, and possibly some obvious ischemic changes at the upper end of the lower esophageal segment, it is wise to excise a few millimeters of the upper end of the lower esophageal segment. If this excision is made obliquely, it will also partially compensate for the discrepancy in caliber between the two segments.

The upper esophageal segment is distended by the pressure of a catheter passed from above and opened at its fundus. The contents are cultured. We utilize a one-layer anastomosis using 5-0 atraumatic silk sutures. The posterior layer of sutures is introduced first; a plastic catheter then is passed from above by the anesthetist and the anastomosis is completed over this catheter. The catheter is removed at the conclusion of the operation. The catheter keeps the lumen of the lower esophagus from collapsing during the anastomosis, it prevents the sutures from penetrating the opposite side of the anastomosis and it allows the sutures to be passed more certainly through the full thickness of the wall of the lower esophagus.

The anesthetist now gently reinflates the lungs. If reinflation is not gentle, pleural disruption can occur at this stage, or a pneumothorax may result from peripheral lung rupture following the period during which the lung has been collapsed.

A plastic catheter is introduced through a stab incision into the posterior mediastinum as a drain tube, connected to an underwater seal and the wound closed. If gastrostomy has not been performed previously, it is performed now.

If, despite extensive mobilization, the ends of the esophagus are too far apart to permit an anastomosis to be accomplished safely, the attempt at anastomosis must be abandoned. If life-threatening hypoxia and bradycardia develop during thoracotomy, the operation may have to be abandoned even earlier. Consideration may be given to cervical end-esophagostomy and later esophageal replacement, but at the time of the original operation we prefer to limit the procedure to division of the tracheoesophageal fistula and closure of the upper end of the lower esophageal segment. This then should be attached to the prevertebral fascia to prevent its retraction, and the site of attachment should be marked by the application of a silver clip. This will enable later radiologic evaluation of the gap between the two esophageal segments. A drain tube is introduced and the thoracotomy incision is closed. Gastrostomy, if not performed previously, is performed at this stage. A successful deferred anastomosis may well be possible at a later stage.

End-to-side anastomosis. Of the various types of anastomosis available there has in recent years been considerable interest in the end-to-side anastomosis, originally advocated by Sulamaa et al.[135] (who divided the fistula) and by Berman and Berman[11] (who left the fistula ligated but in continuity), and more recently popularized by Duhamel,[32] Ty, Brunet and Beardmore[140] and others. The technique involves ligation of the tracheoesophageal fistula, mobilization of the upper esophageal segment and a one-layer anastomosis between the opened distal end of the upper esophagus and the side of the lower esophagus below the site of ligation. Advantages claimed for this method are:

1. Stability of the anastomosis.
2. Increased size of anastomosis.
3. Preservation of blood supply to the lower esophageal segment.
4. Diminished disturbance of motility postoperatively.

This technique is not applicable in all cases, and the literature has many references to postoperative problems, particularly recurrent tracheoesophageal fistula. The technique may be made safe and satisfactory, as a review of a series of patients operated on by Kent[82] using this technique at the Royal Children's Hospital, Melbourne, has suggested, although Ein and Theman[36] reported 19 cases with 7 recurrent fistulas and additional leaks and strictures.

GASTROSTOMY.—In most instances, thoracotomy will be performed first. Then the baby will be gently moved from the lateral decubitus position to the supine position. A midline epigastric incision is made, the stomach delivered and circumferential silk sutures introduced well to the left so that the gastrostomy tube will lie below the liver edge and at an appropriate distance from the greater curvature. A short incision is made in the stomach within the circumferential

sutures. A self-retaining catheter of the Malecot type is introduced into the stomach and the sutures firmly drawn together and tied. A second set of circumferential sutures is placed a very short distance proximal to the pylorus. The stomach is incised at this point and a fine plastic catheter is threaded distally and its tip allowed to lie in the proximal jejunum some short distance from the duodeno-jejunal flexure (Fig. 43–6). The site of the tip of the catheter can be established by palpation, the right index finger being introduced into the abdomen below the transverse colon, or the proximal jejunum is delivered and the position of the catheter tip definitively established to be sure that it is not curled up. The principle of "double gastrostomy" that has been described must not be confused with gastric division, which has little or no place in the management of esophageal atresia.

The gastrostomy tube is brought out through a stab incision to the left of the midline and the transpyloric tube through a second stab incision to the right of the midline. Accurate fixation is essential. The abdominal incision is closed in layers. One now can decompress the stomach via the gastrostomy tube and feed the baby via the transpyloric tube.

4. Postoperative Management

The postoperative management must also include close observation to permit early recognition, and therefore early treatment, of complications.

CONTINUING CARE.—Those measures, commenced preoperatively and continued throughout operation, remain of vital importance in the postoperative period. Specifically, the baby must be kept warm, handled gently and maintained in a state of homeostasis.

It is important to monitor the vital signs during the first few days. Of particular importance are x-ray of chest, blood examination (hemoglobin level, leukocyte count and platelet count), evaluation of serum electrolytes and acid base balance, bacteriologic cultures of secretions or drainage.

Regardless of the operation performed, the baby may be embarrassed by pharyngeal secretions during the first few days, and continuing aspiration of the pharynx is necessary. If there has been an esophageal anastomosis, the suction tube must only be passed to a safe distance—say 8 cm—so that it will not reach, and possibly rupture, the anastomosis. To this end, an appropriate marker is placed on the side of the Isolette to warn the nursing attendants and guard against disaster.

Frequent discussion with the parents continues to be of great importance and every effort must be made to enable the mother to visit and hold her baby at the earliest opportunity.

RESPIRATORY CARE.—The baby with esophageal atresia and tracheoesophageal fistula may have severe respiratory tract disease preoperatively; postoperative respiratory failure is the most frequently encountered life-threatening problem and is due to the continuing pathologic processes present preoperatively—pneumonia, atelectasis—added to by the effects of pulmonary collapse during operation, the effects of the thoracotomy itself and a possible increase in airway secretions, with sepsis also possibly playing its part.

The respiratory problems, although multifactorial in origin, lead to the single common denominator of respiratory failure. Clinical evaluation must be reinforced by x-ray studies and blood gas estimations. The management of respiratory failure in infancy has altered considerably over recent years, due to both an increasing understanding of the underlying pathophysiologic mechanisms and the development of new techniques of treatment.

The value of nasotracheal intubation cannot be overestimated. Its lifesaving role has been quite obvious at the Royal Children's Hospital, Melbourne, and if an artificial airway is required it usually should be supplemented by constant positive airway pressure (CPAP) or intermittent positive pressure respiration (IPPR).

At this early stage it may not be clear whether airway obstruction is due to an intrinsic weakness in the tracheal wall—tracheomalacia. This may become clear only if the baby is in immediate distress after extubation.

Ordinarily, extubation is possible early. Following extubation, retention of secretions in the respiratory tract may require tracheal suction or reintubation.

FEEDING PROGRAMS.—When the technique has included gastrostomy and the introduction of a transpyloric tube, both tubes are initially allowed to drain freely for approximately 24 hours. Subsequently, the gastrostomy tube remains on free drainage, and, 36 hours later, hourly feedings through the transpyloric tube are commenced, with clear fluids initially, changing through half-strength expressed breast milk (EBM) to full-strength EBM.

On the fifth postoperative day, if a contrast study of the esophagus shows no fistula and no severe stenosis, the baby is weaned from the transpyloric tube feedings to gastrostomy feedings (Fig. 43–7). The transpyloric tube is removed on the eighth postoperative day, and any leak from the stomach is rare. Vomiting is not an infrequent problem—partly because the stomach has been kept empty during the postoperative period and partly because gastroesophageal reflux

is frequent. There may be some pylorospasm, and benefit can result from antispasmodic drugs; at times, pyloric stenosis may complicate the clinical picture and because of the difficulty of diagnosis there may be a delay in recognizing its presence.

In the robust baby, oral feedings usually are established rapidly and, ideally, breast feeding can also be established. If all is well, the gastrostomy tube is removed at the end of the third week.

If there is any suggestion of a leak at the anastomosis, the transpyloric tube should be left in situ until all is well; if the baby is small, if the anastomosis is narrow or is likely to stricture because it has leaked, if the baby has an associated cardiac anomaly or if the weight gain is poor, the gastrostomy tube should not be removed too early. If necessary, the baby can be sent home with a gastrostomy.

FURTHER OPERATIVE MEASURES IN STAGED MANAGEMENT.—Aspiration pneumonia must be prevented while the atresia remains and the upper pouch is intact. Since there now is no concern about a tracheoesophageal fistula pouring gastric juice into the trachea, the baby is nursed in the prone position with the head low[20] and the pharynx is aspirated intermittently or continuously, or by a combination of techniques. A Replogle[117] tube is used during the night during the first 2 weeks and during the day the upper pouch is aspirated regularly by intermittent suction. If all is well, the Replogle tube can be removed altogether and some babies will, in fact, learn to cough up their saliva with remarkable efficiency.

A second thoracotomy will be performed, in most instances when the baby weighs 2.5–2.7 kg. This almost inevitably will be a transpleural approach and although difficulties are to be expected, in almost all babies who have been

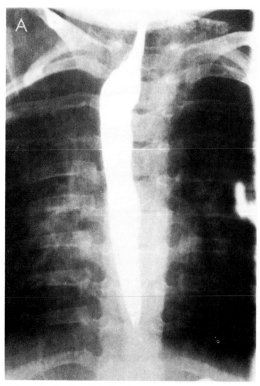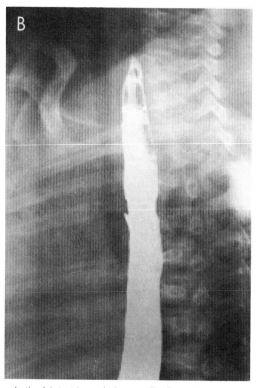

Fig. 43–7.—Esophageal atresia with distal tracheoesophageal fistula, postoperative barium swallow. **A,** same baby as in Figure 43–4, **A.** Barium swallow 1 month after operation. There is no narrowing, no obstruction and only the faintest irregularity over T3. **B,** early esophagogram in another infant in whom a near-perfect result still permits one to see the level of anastomosis at T2.

staged, end-to-end esophageal anastomosis can be achieved. To protect the anastomosis during the postoperative period, the transpyloric tube should be replaced. This usually can be achieved by passing a plastic tube through the gastrostomy stoma and manipulating it through the pylorus with the aid of x-ray image intensification. Technical problems during the second thoracotomy may include bleeding, adhesions and air leak from adherent lung. Patient and careful dissection will make these operative problems less likely.

In the unlikely event that end-to-end anastomosis proves impossible, the surgeon has two choices—to leave both esophageal segments in situ and consider a third thoracotomy later, or to proceed then and there to cervical esophagostomy and ultimate esophageal reconstruction.

5. Recognition and Management of Complications

i) Nonspecific complications—which may occur following any operation in the newborn period.

ii) Complications of an associated anomaly, particularly a cardiac lesion.

iii) Complications specific to esophageal atresia, which are:

a) Disruption of the anastomosis. This may range from insignificant to life-threatening. A small pseudodiverticulum from a contained leak and discovered incidentally on x-ray examination will regress spontaneously. Sometimes the resultant cavity is large and the x-ray alarming; nevertheless, progress usually results in disappearance of the cavity when the esophagus has healed (Fig. 43–8). Classically, with some disruption of the anastomosis, an esophagocutaneous fistula develops, not infrequently as early as the second postoperative day, but possibly not until the fourth or fifth postoperative day. Occasionally, the fistula may be as late as the tenth postoperative day. Saliva appears via the thoracotomy drain tube or, when the fistula develops late, will appear at the drain tube site or through the wound. If the lung remains fully inflated, the management is expectant, and the esophagocutaneous fistula will close spontaneously. When disruption is associated with frank sepsis, mediastinitis, empyema thoracis or both may develop.

If a sudden deterioration occurs in the condition of the baby, x-ray may show a pneumothorax, possibly under tension. This implies disruption of the esophageal anastomosis and may require immediate tube thoracostomy and improved mediastinal drainage, or even open thoracotomy to control the infection and the life-threatening mechanical interference with ventilation.

The diagnosis of anastomotic disruption and the precise cause are determined by clinical assessment, supplemented by x-ray examination and, if necessary, esophagogram.

b) Esophageal stricture. Some narrowing of the anastomotic site is almost inevitable; the degree of stenosis may vary from a minor constriction, which is merely a radiologic finding, through one producing dysphagia to complete occlusion at the anastomotic site. Stricture is more likely to develop when the anastomosis is made under tension, when sepsis complicates the postoperative picture or when in staged management the anastomotic region has been dissected twice. Ischemia of the esophageal segments or prematurity are possible contributory factors.[93]

Stricture is to be suspected if increasing difficulty in feeding develops, particularly from the third week onward. If a significant stricture is present radiologically, it should be dilated under direct vision. If antegrade dilatation is not effective, we use retrograde dilatation following the passage of a string. Resection and reanastomosis may salvage a baby with an intractable stricture. In a consecutive series at the Royal Children's Hospital, Melbourne, of 189 babies with esophageal atresia and distal tracheoesophageal fistula, 22 underwent successful resection for anastomotic stricture. Three of these patients also had a recurrent tracheoesophageal fistula.

Daily, home, parental antegrade dilatation of the esophagus with mercury-filled bougies has been utilized successfully in some babies, thus avoiding prolonged hospitalization.

c) Recurrent tracheoesophageal fistula. Haight[56] has pointed out that "the symptoms of a recurrent tracheoesophageal fistula are in some respect similar to those resulting from a tight stricture, in that the infant will choke and cough on swallowing, and pneumonitis will develop as a result of aspiration of the feedings." It is important, therefore, to exclude the presence of a stricture by appropriate examinations and to dilate a stricture if present.

The symptoms of a recurrent fistula may vary considerably according to the size of the fistula. With a fistula of very small diameter, coughing may occur only if the feeding is thin or very fluid.

Haight also pointed out that "diagnosis of a recurrent fistula is often difficult, and it may not be established with certainty even when the possibility is suspected."

The most reliable method of diagnosing a recurrent tracheoesophageal fistula is radiologic. Cineradiography, using a thin aqueous opaque medium, with the infant lying in the prone position has proved to be reliable in practice.[21] The vastly improved optical system of the Storz esophagoscope has made endoscopic evaluation much more reliable. In the past, introduction of methylene blue via an endotracheal tube while observing the esophagus via an esophagoscope enabled the diagnosis to be established. Passage of a ureteric catheter via a bronchoscope in the trachea has also confirmed the diagnosis, but the only method that can reliably exclude the diagnosis is the cineradiographic technique. The treatment is operative. In addition to dividing the recurrent tracheoesophageal fistula, it may be necessary to resect the adjacent area of the esophagus and perform a new anastomosis.

A recurrent tracheoesophageal fistula may not become manifest for several years following repair of esophageal atresia, and 2 patients in the Melbourne series were aged 10 years and 15 years when the diagnosis of a recurrent tracheoesophageal fistula finally was established.

Apart from the 3 patients operated on for stricture, who also had a recurrent tracheoesophageal stricture, in 5 others, reoperation was successfully performed for a recurrent tracheoesophageal fistula unassociated with a significant anastomotic stricture.

d) Recurrent and life-threatening respiratory obstruction. Babies with esophageal atresia and tracheoesophageal fistula may present with a wide variation in the degree of respiratory obstruction and may:

i) Develop stridor preoperatively.

ii) Have some stridor postoperatively.

iii) Usually have a typical brassy cough (referred to in the British parlance as the "TOF cough").

iv) Have episodic life-threatening respiratory obstruction, with episodes of apnea and cyanosis that appear some months after the repair operation.

The first indication that respiratory obstruction may be a problem after operation occurs when the early removal of the endotracheal tube is rapidly followed by dyspnea, cya-

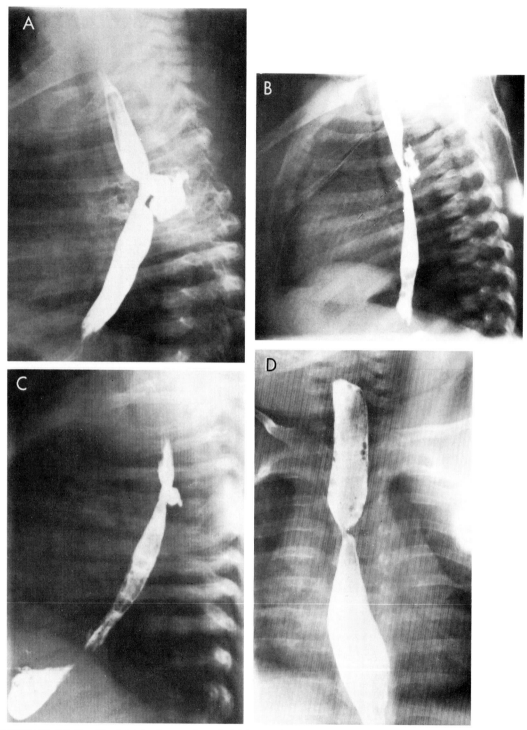

Fig. 43–8.—Esophageal atresia with distal tracheoesophageal fistula and leak. **A,** the esophagogram shows a "contained leak," a large pseudo-diverticulum, but no external fistula. **B** and **C** show progressive decrease in size of the extraluminal cavity. The child was well maintained by his jejunostomy feedings. **D,** the esophagus healed completely with an impressive stricture, successfully relieved by dilatation. Vigilance is required, since complete obliteration of such a dehisced anastomosis can occur quite rapidly. Dilatation cannot safely be performed while there remains a mediastinal cavity, but a swallowed string, recovered through the gastrostomy, will almost guarantee an ultimately successful dilatation.

nosis and bradycardia. It is not immediately possible to predict the natural history. If respiratory obstruction is mild, stridor is the only manifestation and needs no special treatment. If more severe, prolonged nasotracheal intubation may be required. If it is particularly severe, the baby's life may be in jeopardy immediately following extubation.

Despite many observations and reports, the precise cause of the respiratory obstruction is not always clear. We have found that gastroesophageal reflux is of some importance in some instances and when free reflux has been demonstrated, simple antireflux operation may suffice to prevent recurrence of the severe episodes of respiratory tract obstruction.

Similarly, such episodes may be associated with a stricture, and attention previously has been drawn to the possibility of a recurrent tracheoesophageal fistula. The disturbed motility that always is found in the midportion of the esophagus following repair must also be significant.

Recently, recognition of a problem first defined almost 30 years ago by Robert Gross has been re-emphasized. In 1963, Fearon and Shortreed[39] described a series of 69 patients with tracheal compression from an innominate artery, 9 of these patients having had previous repair of esophageal atresia. In 1966, Maurseth[105] reported a single case with the combined lesions. Filler et al.[40] and Benjamin et al.[10] have reported patients who developed severe respiratory obstruction with hypoxic attacks between birth and 7 months of age. Lateral x-ray of the chest showed that the air-filled trachea was compressed anteriorly at the level of the aortic arch. Tracheoscopy confirmed the slit-like compression of the midtrachea. Anterior fixation of the aortic arch relieved the tracheal obstruction, and convincing evidence of this is shown by Filler et al. with photographs taken through the bronchoscope before and after anterior suspension of the aortic arch.

Gross and Neuhauser[54] attributed this to an anomalously placed innominate artery. Mustard et al.[107a] reviewing an experience of 285 patients with innominate artery compression of the trachea, of whom 39 were treated by operation, demonstrated that the normally arising innominate artery can compress the trachea.

Presumably, this compression of the trachea is made more likely if the trachea is compressed posteriorly by a distended atonic esophagus.

The operative correction that Benjamin et al.[10] and Filler et al.[40] have found effective is essentially that described by Gross and Neuhauser[54] and by Mustard et al.[107a] The anterior mediastinum is approached laterally through the second right or left interspace. The thymus is dissected and the region of the innominate origin from the aortic arch is pulled forward by nonabsorbable mattress sutures in the adventitia of the aorta and innominate artery, or the sutures may be placed through the superior reflection of the pericardium. These sutures are attached to the anterior chest wall and firmly tied, thereby displacing the artery anteriorly and enlarging the tracheal lumen. The enlargement is confirmed at a later stage by tracheoscopy and the behavior of the patient postoperatively.

With a significant respiratory obstruction, the baby must be kept in the hospital, however long, until the problem has been solved. Prolonged nasotracheal intubation may be required; evaluation of the esophagus and the gastroesophageal junction is essential and abnormalities should be treated.

e) Other complications. Gastroesophageal reflux already has been mentioned and, at times, peptic esophagitis occurs, and may be a significant factor in anastomotic stricture.[113]

Episodes of foreign body impaction are not uncommon, at times related to stricture, but, more often than not, the result of a motility disorder in the midportion of the esophagus around the site of the anastomosis, which is not strictured. Animal studies on the effect of esophageal dissection on later esophageal motility are conflicting because of differences between animal species,[16, 60] but this constant finding in humans suggests that esophageal dissection should be no more than is necessary for anastomosis. Recurrent bronchitis as a consequence of overspill from the esophagus may also be a significant problem requiring appropriate treatment directed to the individual attack and to lessening the frequency of the attacks.

6. Treatment of the Long Gap

Although a "long gap" between the two esophageal segments is more likely to occur in esophageal atresia without tracheoesophageal fistula or in esophageal atresia with a proximal fistula, a significant "long gap" does occur in a small proportion of patients with a proximal atresia and a distal fistula—i.e., the common type.

The presence of a "long gap" may be suspected:

i) *Before birth*—if polyhydramnios is present. Although polyhydramnios may complicate all types of esophageal atresia, it is particularly common in atresia without fistula.[144] Prematurity is also a feature of this type of anomaly.

ii) *Clinically*—the scaphoid abdomen suggests atresia without fistula; the baby often is small for gestational age (SGA).

iii) *Radiologically*—the airless abdomen requires studies of the upper pouch. In the Melbourne series of 404 patients, the abdomen was "airless" on x-ray examination in 37, and in 6 of these (16%), an upper-pouch fistula was present. Without dye studies, the presence of such a fistula may not be diagnosed, and, in fact, in 2 of the 6 babies, the original diagnosis was atresia without fistula and there was considerable and dangerous delay in diagnosing the presence of the upper-pouch fistula. In the presence of a distal fistula, a high upper pouch demonstrated radiologically will alert the surgeon to the probability of encountering a "long gap."

A wide variety of techniques may be necessary in order to overcome a "long gap," and many of these techniques were reviewed at the International Symposium of Esophageal Atresia held in Bremen in 1974. The various techniques are applicable to all types of anomaly where a "long gap" is present. They are more likely to be required when the anomaly is of the less frequently encountered types—atresia without fistula or atresia with a proximal fistula.

Esophageal Atresia with Distal Tracheoesophageal Fistula

Even if a "long gap" is suspected on radiologic grounds, all such patients should have a thoracotomy performed. If anastomosis proves to be impossible, the fistula is divided and the upper pouch preserved, and gastrostomy performed (Fig. 43–9). At a later thoracotomy, end-to-end esophageal anastomosis usually is possible, and cervical end-esophagostomy should be necessary in only a few patients. Every effort should be made at the first operation to assess the situation before extensive mobilization of the upper pouch is carried out, to minimize scarring, which will complicate the second operation.

Esophageal Atresia without Fistula

In all reported series, "pure" esophageal atresia is a relatively uncommon anomaly. In the Melbourne experience, it represented approximately 7.5% of all types encountered.

If contrast studies exclude an upper-pouch fistula, gastrostomy alone then is performed. In order to assess the size of the stomach, to obtain information regarding the distal esophageal segment and to exclude distal obstruction, radiologic contrast studies of the stomach are carried out before the baby is fed. When the baby reaches the age of 1 month, both esophageal segments are evaluated with Bakes dilators or urethral sounds (Fig. 43–10). We have found primary anastomosis possible in a number of babies with isolated esophageal atresia. A retrospective study indicates that success is directly proportional to the original length of the upper

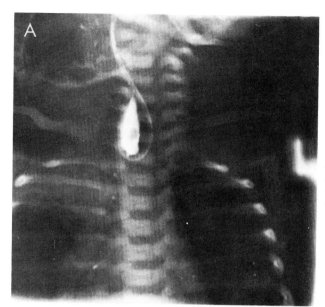

Fig. 43–9.—Esophageal atresia with distal fistula, demonstrated at operation to have a long gap and therefore staged by division of the fistula and gastrostomy. **A,** the initial diagnostic study. Catheter coiled in the esophageal pouch and a small volume of injected contrast material show the upper segment at T1. **B,** the clip marks the upper end of the distal segment after the fistula has been divided. Bougie was introduced as diagnostic study, indicating anastomosis was feasible. **C,** a satisfactory anastomosis was performed.

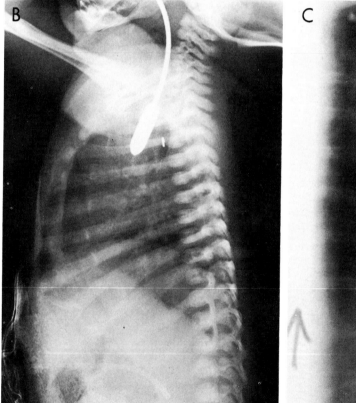

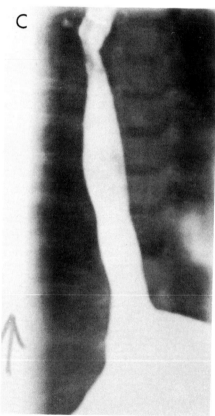

pouch. The most appropriate time for operation would appear to be when the baby is about 8 weeks of age. During this 8-week period, it is essential to protect the baby against aspiration pneumonia and the secretions must be aspirated from the upper pouch in the same way as in the baby with esophageal atresia and a distal fistula when the management is staged.

Gastrostomy is technically difficult in these babies because of the small size of the stomach; there is some advan-

tage in performing gastrostomy through a transverse rather than through a vertical abdominal incision, and following gastrostomy, when feeding is commenced, volumes initially should be small and increased gradually.

Many methods have been suggested to overcome the problem of the "long gap" between the two esophageal segments. These methods include:

i) Elongation of the upper pouch by means of bougienage[74] or a mercury-filled bag.[138]

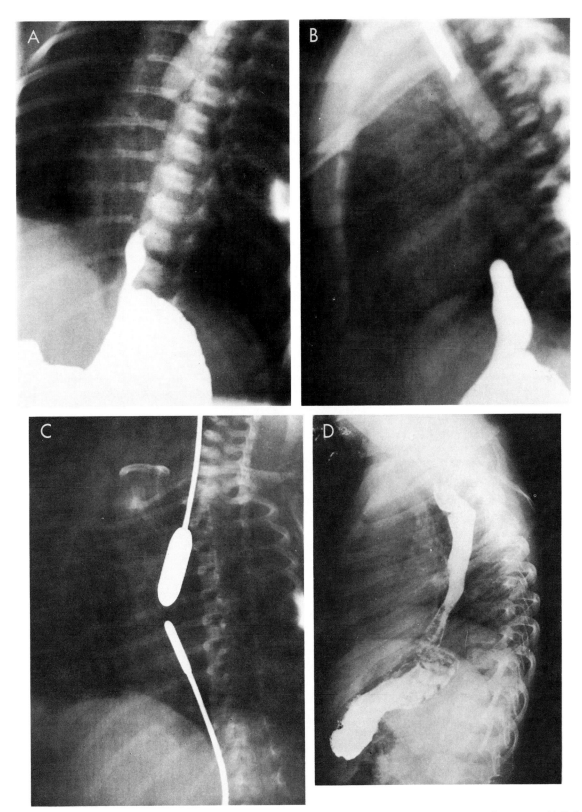

Fig. 43–10.—Esophageal atresia without fistula and with a "long gap." **A,** the baby has had a gastrostomy; reflux of barium shows the short distal esophagus. The solid rubber tip of a mercury-filled bougie pressing into the upper esophageal pouch shows the length of the gap (4½ vertebrae). **B** and **C,** with growth over several weeks, the gap has narrowed initially to 3 vertebrae and ultimately to minimal proportions, as shown following introduction of Bakes dilators to the point at which **(D)** anastomosis could be performed without undue difficulty.

ii) The Rehbein "olive and thread" technique.[116]

iii) Circular myotomy as described by Livaditis[96-101] and Eraklis *et al.*[38a]

iv) Azygoplasty.[43]

v) Self-fistulization.[122]

vi) Electromagnetic bougienage.[64, 65]

Many of these methods are potentially effective but, in many instances, natural growth will permit the "long gap" to be overcome and some evidence indicates that the esophageal segments grow at a faster rate than the thorax. Growth of the segments may be favorably influenced by the presence of some saliva in the upper pouch and by the pressure of free gastroesophageal reflux into the lower pouch.

Upper-pouch bougienage has its protagonists and antagonists. Introduction of this technique alerted pediatric surgeons to the possibility of avoiding cervical esophagostomy and subsequent esophageal replacement. "The best esophagus is the patient's own esophagus."

The circular myotomy technique of Livaditis[96, 101] (and as modified by Eraklis *et al.*[38]) has been used to lengthen the upper pouch with good results in the short term, but later esophageal function could be a problem, as found by Slim.[127] However, in some patients with esophageal atresia, replacement will be necessary and, in our experience, a gastric tube of the Gavriliu-Heimlich type from the greater curvature of the stomach gives satisfactory results.[3, 17, 23, 35, 46, 62]

Esophageal Atresia with Proximal Tracheoesophageal Fistula and Distal Atresia

Haight's[56] series did not include any such infants. Six cases occurred in the Melbourne series. Following early radiologic evaluation, the proximal tracheoesophageal fistula is divided and gastrostomy performed. If primary anastomosis has not been achieved, an attempt is made to perform end-to-end esophageal anastomosis, usually at about the age of 8 weeks. If it is not possible to achieve an esophageal anastomosis, cervical esophagostomy is performed with a view to esophageal replacement at a later stage, as for esophageal atresia without fistula.

Tracheoesophageal Fistula without Esophageal Atresia

The various reported series and cases show that most *tracheo*esophageal fistulas present in early infancy, a few in childhood and almost none in adult life whereas *broncho*esophageal fistulas rarely present in childhood, but nearly all present during the adult years. In the Royal Children's Hospital, Melbourne series of 29 patients with tracheoesophageal fistula and no atresia, 1 presented as late as the age of 3½ years.

The anatomic problem in isolated tracheoesophageal fistula is an "H" (or "Y") shaped communication between the esophagus and trachea—usually in the cervical region, but at times in the thorax.

The symptoms are coughing on feeding, spluttering with feedings, attacks of cyanosis and recurrent episodes of pulmonary collapse and pneumonia. A very significant physical sign is abdominal distention due to the presence of a large volume of gas in the stomach and bowel. X-ray may show an esophagus distended with air, an appearance not normally found.[137] The differential diagnosis includes all other causes of aspiration into the respiratory tract—particularly aspiration associated with gastroesophageal reflux or pharyngeal incoordination.

Having suspected the diagnosis, it is essential to withhold feedings; at times there is diagnostic confusion because oral feedings are replaced by gavage feedings and under these circumstances the symptoms may disappear. When the diagnosis has been suspected, the baby must be regarded as having a tracheoesophageal fistula until proved otherwise. Every effort must be made to establish the diagnosis as soon as possible. Radiologic examination—possibly needing to be repeated—is the most reliable method of demonstrating the presence of a fistulous communication between the esophagus and the trachea. Endoscopic examination, particularly using the newer forms of endoscopic equipment, will supplement the radiologic diagnosis. We have found that at times the use of a thick radiopaque substance—usually a barium compound—may demonstrate the fistula better than a thin medium.[66]

A simple clinical test that may alert the clinician to the diagnosis is to pass a catheter into the esophagus, holding the other end of the catheter under water; if a fistula is present, bubbles may escape with each respiratory excursion as the catheter tip passes the end of the fistula.

Treatment

Treatment of isolated tracheoesophageal fistula is operative closure of the fistula. Operation is again elective-emergency.

In most instances, the approach is cervical and preference is given to a right-sided cervical approach to avoid the thoracic duct.[1] The baby is positioned with the head and neck extended and the head turned well toward the left side. Through a transverse incision a short distance above the clavicle, the sternomastoid muscle is divided and dissection carried between the carotid sheath laterally and the esophagus and trachea medially. The recurrent laryngeal nerve is recognized and the fistula identified and surrounded by a sling. It then is divided, each end oversewn and closed with a nonabsorbable suture. Interposition of a small flap of fascia or muscle will lessen the risk of recurrence.

Is gastrostomy necessary? Opinions vary. In the Melbourne series of 20 patients, 2 have died—1 early in the series and another who developed a recurrent tracheoesophageal fistula and who did not have a gastrostomy. It was believed that a gastrostomy might have prevented this complication; therefore, gastrostomy now is performed routinely for this condition at the Royal Children's Hospital, Melbourne.

Eckstein *et al.*,[34] reporting 23 cases, found that when the diagnosis had been clearly made, simple division of the fistula without gastrostomy proved to be adequate, with all such patients surviving and giving good long-term results, even though abnormal esophageal motility was a frequent radiologic finding.[137]

Results of Treatment

Before 1940 there were but 3 survivals in babies born with esophageal atresia with or without tracheoesophageal fistula; from then on, an increasing number of survivals has been reported from an increasing number of centers, so that by the mid-1970s a very high percentage of babies is surviving. The mortality rate in "good-risk" babies now approximates zero; however, there still is a significant mortality in the "poor-risk" patient. Waterston *et al.*[143] made a major contribution when they pointed out that it is possible to divide the patients into three groups, according to risk factors:

GROUP A—birth weight over 2.5 kg and well.

GROUP B—i) birth weight 1.8–2.5 kg and well. ii) higher

TABLE 43–5.—CLASSIFICATION IN
RELATION TO SURVIVAL

CLINICAL GROUP	NO. TREATED	NO. SURVIVORS
A	102	94 (92%)
B	96	68 (71%)
C	71	27 (38%)
TOTAL	269	189 (70%)

birth weight, moderate pneumonia and/or an additional moderate congenital anomaly.

GROUP C – i) birth weight under 1.8 kg. ii) higher birth weight and severe pneumonia and/or an additional severe congenital anomaly.

Although it sometimes is difficult to distinguish marginal cases, this classification has the merits of clarity and simplicity. Two hundred sixty-nine babies with proximal atresia and distal fistula were classified into three groups following this grouping. These data are given in Table 43–5.

Other authors[51, 144] who have used this or a similar classification have shown similar proportions and results.

The survival figures at the Royal Children's Hospital, Melbourne, during the 25-year period reviewed (from 1948 to 1972) are indicated in Table 43–6. These figures indicate that, for all practical purposes, survival now is 100% in those patients classified as Group A or B. There still is a substantial mortality in Group C, but in a consecutive series of 57 unselected patients (1969–1973) there were 54 survivals—an unselected survival rate of 94%. Particular factors responsible for increased survival other than increasing surgical experience include over-all improved care of the newborn, modern methods of management of respiratory failure and, we believe, the technique of always performing gastrostomy and combining this with a transpyloric jejunal intubation.

Follow-up

In a long-term follow-up,[109] it is evident that there were problems and, inevitably, there always will be some problems. Attention was directed to the group of 72 patients who survived operation during the period 1948–1962, and it was possible to obtain a complete follow-up on 58 of these patients—more than 20 years in 15 patients, for 15–20 years in 28 patients and between 13 and 15 years in 15 patients. No patients in this group were managed by the currently used program, namely primary anastomosis combined with gastrostomy plus the introduction of a transpyloric jejunal feeding tube, and therefore a later review almost certainly will prove to be of great interest in comparing results following different surgical techniques.

TABLE 43–6.—SURVIVAL IN RELATION TO
PHASE OF TREATMENT AND CLINICAL GROUP

PHASE	GROUP A SURVIVAL	GROUP B SURVIVAL	GROUP C SURVIVAL
1. 1948–1952	33% (1)	50% (3)	14% (1)
2. 1953–1957	100% (7)	64% (18)	29% (4)
3. 1958–1962	76% (16)	59% (16)	28% (5)
4. 1963–1967	97% (29)	78% (14)	59% (10)
5. 1968–1972	100% (41)	100% (17)	47% (7)
6. 1973–1977	100% (17)	84% (16)	75% (12)
TOTAL: 73% (234)	93% (111)	73% (84)	45% (39)

Parentheses indicate number of survivals.

To measure the results of treatment is difficult. Inevitably there will be some difference in the frequency of review and in the interpretation placed on the x-ray findings by different radiologists. Nevertheless, it is possible to evaluate the long-term follow-up and the results of treatment using the following factors:

   i) The esophagus itself.
      a) Subjective function.
      b) Further treatment required.
      c) Radiologic assessment.
      d) Manometric studies.
   ii) The gastroesophageal junction. Was reflux or a hiatal hernia demonstrated?
   iii) The respiratory tract. How frequent were episodes of bronchitis and what was the change with the passing years?
   iv) Other anomalies that may or may not require treatment.
   v) The important areas of psychologic development, educational progress and the total emotional impact on the child and family, including siblings as well as parents.

Respiratory tract complications were studied by Dudley and Phelan[31] in long-term survivals of esophageal atresia at the Royal Children's Hospital, Melbourne, including patients presenting before and after 1963. One hundred of the 192 survivors of repaired esophageal atresia, aged 1 year and over on November 1, 1973, were reviewed to determine the frequency of respiratory complications. Seventy-eight children suffered from more than three attacks of bronchitis per year during the first 3 years of life and 48% of children more than 8 years of age were having three attacks per year. Episodes of cough persisting longer than 2 weeks were also common. These figures can be compared with the incidence for normal children in a city in northern England among whom less than 5% had more than three attacks of bronchitis each year at the age of 3 years and at 8 years of age less than 1% had three attacks of bronchitis per year.[107]

Dudley and Phelan suggested that recurrent aspiration of milk and food consequent on disordered esophageal motility was the major factor causing these respiratory complications. Recurrent respiratory tract complications, therefore, are important, but they are more prevalent in the first 8 years of life, with a peak incidence for multiple episodes of bronchitis occurring before the age of 3 years. The long-term follow-up study indicated that recurrent respiratory tract infections cease to be a problem in adolescence.

Dudley and Phelan[31] conclude by stating that if inhalation is the main cause of these respiratory problems, prevention may be possible if vagal branches of the esophagus can be preserved at the time of repair. Aspiration can be minimized by giving infants thickened feedings, keeping them in a semiupright position for 1 or 2 hours after feedings and by giving them a small drink of water after feedings. Children should also be encouraged to have a drink of water after meals and should not go to bed within 1–2 hours of eating or drinking.

The long-term follow-up indicated that dysphagia is a problem during the early years of life, but gradually this lessens. Nevertheless, it is apparent that many patients need to be careful when they eat and this care should continue throughout life. In a proportion of patients, further active treatment may be required—either dilatation or resection of a stricture. Occasional late deaths occur and these are particularly likely to be in connection with associated cardiac anomalies or chromosomal aberrations. In addition, in the Melbourne experience, there were two cot deaths and other series have reported similar deaths.

Burgess *et al.*[15] studied 9 patients aged 14–19 years, and although 8 of the 9 had arrived at a state of good swallowing and an absence of lung problems, 7 needed dilatation at some time in earlier years. All had normal pressure studies and all had functioning sphincters at the upper and lower ends of the esophagus, but all had an amotile area in the central esophagus.

Chrispin *et al.*[21] reported aspiration pneumonia and dysphagia in 14 patients up to 10 years after repair, none of whom had recurrent fistula or persistent stricture but all of whom had an absence of normal esophageal stripping waves as observed by fluoroscopy.

Shepard *et al.*[125] studied 20 children 1–11 years after repair and used cineradiography, manometry and endoscopy to correlate function with symptoms. All children had effective sphincteric action at each end of the esophagus, but all had an area of the esophagus without motor activity in the region of the anastomosis, and this immobile area was from 10% to 60% of the length of the esophagus. Ten were classified as having excellent functional results, 4 were good and 6 were fair, and improvement was observed with age.

Pieretti *et al.*[113] reviewed 217 survivors operated on in Toronto between 1958 and 1973. Stenosis of varying degrees was noted in 77 (35%). Of these, 15 had stenoses that were not improved by repeated dilatation, and all showed evidence of gastroesophageal reflux, accompanied by a demonstrable hiatal hernia in 9. An antireflux operation proved successful in all, and the stricture did not recur in any. Studies on the Toronto series had been among the first to show that a deficient swallowing ability of the esophagus was more often the cause of postoperative dysphagia and respiratory infection than was esophageal stricture.[28]

To summarize the follow-up of patients with repaired esophageal atresia, it is evident that although esophageal function is not normal, although dysphagia is an early problem, although the children are subject to recurrent respiratory infections in the early years of life, although there are demonstrable radiologic changes and although there are manometric abnormalities, the end result of treatment is by and large very satisfactory.

Summary

The management of the baby with esophageal atresia and tracheoesophageal fistula can be a most satisfying experience for the infant, his family and the pediatric surgeon. Equally, problems and frustrations beset the surgeon, the baby and the baby's family.

Among the problems requiring further investigation are:

i) The need to identify the cause of the faulty embryogenesis and the genetic implications for these families.

ii) Problems associated with the "long gap" and efforts to avoid esophageal replacement.

iii) Problems associated with life-threatening respiratory tract obstruction from tracheal compression.

iv) Should all patients have a gastrostomy?

v) Are the advantages claimed for gastrostomy combined with a transpyloric jejunostomy tube valid? If so, should this be performed routinely in all babies?

vi) What are the long-term results of end-to-side anastomosis, particularly in relation to esophageal motility and the frequency of respiratory tract infection?

Laryngotracheoesophageal Cleft

A persisting cleft between the upper ends of the respiratory tract and esophagus allows easy communication between the two structures. The cleft may vary in length from being, at the shortest, less than the length of the arytenoid cartilages, between which the cleft lies, or may extend, at the longest, the entire length of the trachea. Descriptive titles have varied from cleft larynx to laryngotracheoesophageal cleft or persistent esophagotrachea. Fewer than 40 cases have been described, and successfully treated cases may not exceed 10 in number since the first report of success by Pettersson[111] in 1955. A detailed review of the literature was published in 1974 by Burroughs and Leape.[18] Seven cases have been described with an associated esophageal atresia and tracheoesophageal fistula. Diagnosis may be difficult, and even experienced bronchoscopists have missed the diagnosis, because the cleft may not be identified readily, although the newer bronchoscopes probably will improve diagnosis. Fourteen cases have been identified at autopsy, mostly in the earlier years of pediatric surgery. The clinical presentation may be identical with that of esophageal atresia and tracheoesophageal fistula, which may be an additional lesion in about one-fifth of cases. Mahour *et al.*[103] reported such a combination, but with two proximal and one distal tracheoesophageal fistulas successfully corrected. Diagnosis should be made by cineradiography with the technique described for tracheoesophageal fistula or by direct inspection by laryngoscopy or bronchoscopy. The possibility of this diagnosis should be considered in every newborn who develops respiratory distress on feeding. The operative repair of the cleft has proved to be difficult, most requiring long periods in the hospital, and all successful cases have had tracheostomy performed and used for several years in most cases. Multiple operations often have been necessary.[47, 63] (See also Chap. 29.)

REFERENCES

1. Aberdeen, E.: Congenital Tracheo-oesophageal Fistula without Oesophageal Atresia, in Rob, C., and Smith, R. (eds.), *Operative Surgery* (2d ed.; London: Butterworths, 1968), Vol. 2, p. 363.
2. Abrahamson, J., and Shandling, B.: Esophageal atresia in the underweight baby: A challenge, J. Pediatr. Surg. 7:608, 1972.
3. Anderson, K. D., and Randolph, J. G.: The gastric tube for esophageal replacement in children, J. Thorac. Cardiovasc. Surg. 66:333, 1973.
4. Ashcraft, K. W., and Holder, T. M.: The story of esophageal atresia and tracheoesophageal fistula, Surgery 65:332, 1969.
5. Ashley, J. D., Jr.: Congenital atresia of the esophagus with tracheo-esophageal fistula, Radiology 36:621, 1941.
6. Atwell, J. D., and Beard, R. C.: Congenital anomalies of the upper urinary tract associated with esophageal atresia and tracheoesophageal fistula, J. Pediatr. Surg. 9:825, 1974.
7. Azimi, F., and O'Hara, A. E.: Congenital intraluminal mucosal web of the esophagus with tracheo-esophageal fistula, Am. J. Dis. Child. 125:92, 1973.
8. Babbitt, D. P.: Double tracheoesophageal fistula without atresia. Report of a case, N. Engl. J. Med. 257:713, 1957.
9. Barry, J. E., and Auldist, A. W.: The VATER association: One end of a spectrum of anomalies, Am. J. Dis. Child. 128:769, 1974.
10. Benjamin, B., Cohen, D., and Glasson, M.: Tracheomalacia in association with congenital tracheoesophageal fistula, Surgery 79:504, 1976.
11. Berman, J. K., and Berman, E. J.: Congenital atresia of the esophagus with tracheo-esophageal fistula. A simplified method of restoring continuity of the esophagus, Am. J. Surg. 86:436, 1953.
12. Blank, R. H., Prillaman, P. E., Jr., and Minor, G. R.: Congenital esophageal atresia with tracheoesophageal fistula occurring in identical twins, J. Thorac. Cardiovasc. Surg. 53:192, 1967.
13. Bond-Taylor, W., Starer, F., and Atwell, J. D.: Vertebral anomalies associated with esophageal atresia and tracheoesophageal fistula with reference to the initial operative mortality, J. Pediatr. Surg. 8:9, 1973.

14. Brennemann, J.: Congenital atresia of the esophagus, with report of three cases, Am. J. Dis. Child. 5:143, 1913.

15. Burgess, J. N., Carlson, H. C., and Ellis, F. H., Jr.: Esophageal function after successful repair of esophageal atresia and tracheoesophageal fistula. A manometric and cinefluorographic study, J. Thorac. Cardiovasc. Surg. 56:667, 1968.

16. Burgess, J. N., Schlegel, J. F., and Ellis, F. H., Jr.: The effect of denervation on feline esophageal function and morphology, J. Surg. Res. 12:24, 1972.

17. Burrington, J. D., and Stephens, C. A.: Esophageal replacement with a gastric tube in infants and children, J. Pediatr. Surg. 3:246, 1968.

18. Burroughs, N., and Leape, L. L.: Laryngotracheoesophageal cleft: Report of a case successfully treated and review of the literature, Pediatrics 53:516, 1974.

19. Carter, B. N.: An operation for the cure of congenital atresia of the esophagus, Surg. Gynecol. Obstet. 73:485, 1941.

20. Castilla, P., Irving, I. M., Rees, G. J., and Rickham, P. P.: Posture in the management of esophageal atresia: Variations on a theme by Dr. E. B. D. Neuhauser, J. Pediatr. Surg. 6:709, 1971.

21. Chrispin, A. R., Friedland, G. W., and Waterston, D. J.: Aspiration pneumonia and dysphagia after technically successful repair of oesophageal atresia, Thorax 21:104, 1966.

22. Cohen, D. H.: Personal communication.

23. Cohen, D. H., Middleton, A. W., and Fletcher, J.: Gastric tube esophagoplasty, J. Pediatr. Surg. 9:451, 1974.

24. Daniel, R. A., Jr.: Congenital atresia of the esophagus: With tracheo-esophageal fistula, Ann. Surg. 120:764, 1944.

25. David, T. J., and O'Callaghan, S. E.: Oesophageal atresia in the south west of England, J. Med. Genet. 12:1, 1975.

26. David, T. J., and O'Callaghan, S. E.: Cardiovascular malformations and oesophageal atresia, Br. Heart J. 36:559, 1974.

27. Dennis, N. R., Nicholas, J. L., and Kouar, I.: Esophageal atresia: Three cases in two generations, Arch. Dis. Child. 48:980, 1973.

28. Desjardins, J. G., Stephens, C. A., and Moes, C. A. F.: Results of surgical treatment of congenital tracheo-esophageal fistula, with a note on cinefluorographic findings, Ann. Surg. 160:141, 1964.

29. Donahoe, M. D., and Hendren, W. H.: The surgical management of laryngotracheoesophageal cleft with tracheo-esophageal fistula and esophageal atresia, Surgery 71:363, 1972.

30. Dudgeon, D. L., Morrison, C. W., and Woolley, M. M.: Congenital proximal tracheoesophageal fistula, J. Pediatr. Surg. 7:614, 1972.

31. Dudley, N. E., and Phelan, P. D.: Respiratory complications in long-term survival of esophageal atresia, Arch. Dis. Child. 51:279, 1976.

32. Duhamel, B.: *Technique Chirurgicale Infantile* (Paris: Masson et Cie, 1957).

33. Durston, W.: A narrative of monstrous birth in Plymouth October 22, 1670; together with the anatomical observations taken thereupon by William Durston, Doctor in Physick, and communication to Dr. Tim Clerk, Philos. Trans. R. Soc. V: 2096, 1670.

34. Eckstein, H. B., Aberdeen, E., Chrispin, A., Nixon, H. H., Waterston, D. J., and Wilkinson, A.: Tracheo-oesophageal fistula without oesophageal atresia, Z. Kinderchir. 9:43, 1970.

35. Ein, S. H., Shandling, B., Simpson, J. S., and Stephens, C. A.: A further look at the gastric tube as an esophageal replacement in infants and children, J. Pediatr. Surg. 8:859, 1973.

36. Ein, S. H., and Theman, T. E.: A comparison of the results of primary repair of esophageal atresia with tracheoesophageal fistulas using end-to-side and end-to-end anastomoses, J. Pediatr. Surg. 8:641, 1973.

37. Engel, M. A., Vos, L. J. M., De Vries, J. A., and Kuijjer, P. J.: Esophageal atresia with tracheo-esophageal fistula in mother and child, J. Pediatr. Surg. 5:564, 1970.

38. Eraklis, A. J., and Gross, R. E.: Esophageal atresia: Management following an anastomotic leak, Surgery 60:919, 1966.

38a. Eraklis, A. J., Rossello, P. J., and Ballantine, T. V. N.: Circular esophagomyotomy of upper pouch in primary repair of long-segment esophageal atresia, J. Pediatr. Surg. 11:709, 1976.

39. Fearon, B., and Shortreed, R.: Tracheobronchial compression by congenital cardiovascular anomalies in children. Syndrome of apnea, Ann. Otol. 72:949, 1963.

40. Filler, R. M., Rossello, P. J., and Lebowitz, R. L.: Life-threatening anoxic spells caused by tracheal compression after repair of esophageal atresia: Correction by surgery, J. Pediatr. Surg. 11:739, 1976.

41. Flood, H. C.: Congenital obstruction of the esophagus, Atlant. Med. J. 30:537, 1926.

42. Fritz, E.: Eine seltene Misbildung der oberen Luftwege (Teilweiser Mangel der Luftröhre, Verschlus des Kehlkopfes und Ösophagotrachealfistel), Virchows Arch. (Pathol. Anat.) 289:264, 1933.

43. Fufezan, V., Veleanu, C., Duica, C., Habenicht, E., and Socolius, M.: The use of azygo-oesophagoplasty in the treatment of oesophageal atresia, Kind. Chir. (supp.) 134, 1975.

44. Gage, M., and Ochsner, A.: The surgical treatment of congenital tracheo-esophageal fistula in the new-born, Ann. Surg. 103:725, 1936.

45. Gamble, H. A.: Tracheo-esophageal fistula. Description of a new operative procedure and case report, Ann. Surg. 107:701, 1938.

46. Gavriliu, D.: Aspects of Esophageal Surgery, in *Current Problems in Surgery* (Chicago: Year Book Medical Publishers, Inc., October, 1975).

47. Geiger, J. P., O'Connell, T. J., Jr., Carter, S. C., Gomez, A. C., and Aronstam, E. M.: Laryngotracheal-esophageal cleft, J. Thorac. Cardiovasc. Surg. 59:330, 1970.

48. Gengenbach, F. P., and Dobos, E. I.: Congenital tracheo-oesophageal fistula, J. Pediatr. 19:644, 1941.

49. German, J. C., Mahour, G. H., and Woolley, M. M.: Esophageal atresia and associated anomalies, J. Pediatr. Surg. 11: 299, 1976.

50. Gibson, T.: *The Anatomy of Humane Bodies Epitomized* (6th ed.; London: Awnsham and Churchill, 1703).

51. Glasson, M. J., Dey, D. L., and Cohen, D. H.: Oesophageal atresia: Results of treatment, Med. J. Aust. 1:69, 1971.

52. Greenwood, R. D., and Rosenthal, A.: Cardiovascular malformations associated with tracheoesophageal fistula and esophageal atresia, Pediatrics 57:87, 1976.

53. Gross, R. E.: *Surgery of Infancy and Childhood* (Philadelphia: W. B. Saunders Company, 1953).

54. Gross, R. E., and Neuhauser, E. B. D.: Compression of the trachea by an anomalous innominate artery. An operation for its relief, Am. J. Dis. Child. 75:570, 1948.

55. Haight, C.: Congenital atresia of the esophagus with tracheoesophageal fistula. Reconstruction of esophageal continuity by primary anastomosis, Ann. Surg. 120:623, 1944.

56. Haight, C.: The Esophagus, in Mustard, W. T., *et al.* (eds.), *Pediatric Surgery* (2d ed.; Chicago: Year Book Medical Publishers, Inc., 1969), Vol. 1, p. 357.

57. Haight, C.: Some observations on esophageal atresia and tracheoesophageal fistulas of congenital origin, J. Thorac. Surg. 34:141, 1957.

58. Haight, C.: The management of congenital esophageal atresia and tracheoesophageal fistula, Surg. Clin. North Am. 41:1281, 1961.

59. Haight, C., and Towsley, H. A.: Congenital atresia of the esophagus with tracheoesophageal fistula. Extrapleural ligation of fistula and end-to-end anastomosis of esophageal segments, Surg. Gynecol. Obstet. 76:672, 1943.

60. Haller, J. A., Jr., Brooker, A. F., Talbert, J. L., Baghdassarian, O., and Vanhoutte, J.: Esophageal function following resection. Studies in newborn puppies, Ann. Thorac. Surg. 2:180, 1966.

61. Hausmann, P. F., Close, A. S., and Williams, L. P.: Occurrence of tracheoesophageal fistula in three consecutive siblings, Surgery 41:542, 1957.

62. Heimlich, H. J.: Reversed gastric tube (RGT) esophagoplasty for failure of colon, jejunum and prosthetic interpositions, Ann. Surg. 182:154, 1975.

63. Hendren, W. H.: Repair of laryngotracheoesophageal cleft using interposition of a strap muscle, J. Pediatr. Surg. 11:425, 1976.

64. Hendren, W. H., and Hale, J. R.: Electromagnetic bougienage to lengthen esophageal segments in congenital esophageal atresia, N. Engl. J. Med. 293:428, 1975.

65. Hendren, W. H., and Hale, J. R.: Esophageal atresia treated by electromagnetic bougienage and subsequent repair, J. Pediatr. Surg. 11:713, 1976.

66. Hiller, H.: Personal communication.

67. Hirsch, I. S.: Congenital atresia of the esophagus, report of two cases, JAMA 76:1491, 1921.

68. Holder, T. M.: Transpleural versus retropleural approach for repair of tracheoesophageal fistula, Surg. Clin. North Am. 44: 1433, 1964.

69. Holder, T. M., and Ashcraft, K. W.: Esophageal Atresia and Tracheo-Esophageal Fistula, in *Current Problems in Surgery* (Chicago: Year Book Medical Publishers, Inc., August, 1966).

70. Holder, T. M., and Ashcraft, K. W.: Esophageal atresia and tracheoesophageal fistula, Ann. Thorac. Surg. 9:445, 1970.

71. Holder, T. M., Cloud, D. T., Lewis, J. E., Jr., and Pilling, G. P.:

Esophageal atresia and tracheoesophageal fistula. A survey of its members by the surgical section of the American Academy of Pediatrics, Pediatrics 34:542, 1964.

72. Holt, J. F., Haight, C., and Hodges, F. J.: Congenital atresia of the esophagus and tracheo-esophageal fistula, Radiology 47:457, 1946.

73. Howard, R.: Oesophageal atresia with tracheo-oesophageal fistula: Report of six cases with two successful oesophageal anastomoses, Med. J. Aust. 1:401, 1950.

74. Howard, R., and Myers, N. A.: Esophageal atresia: A technique for elongating the upper pouch, Surgery 58:725, 1965.

75. Humphreys, G. H., and Ferrer, J. M., Jr.: Management of esophageal atresia, Am. J. Surg. 107:406, 1964.

76. Humphreys, G. H., Hogg, B. M., and Ferrer, J.: Congenital atresia of esophagus, J. Thorac. Surg. 32:332, 1956.

77. Huntington, J. L., Young, J. H., and Foot, N. C.: Report of a case of congenital atresia of the oesophagus, Boston Med. Surg. J. 180:354, 1919.

78. Imperatori, C. J.: Congenital tracheoesophageal fistula without atresia of the esophagus. Report of a case with plastic closure and cure, Arch. Otolaryngol. 30:352, 1939.

79. Ten Kate, J.: A method of suturing in operations for congenital oesophageal atresia, Arch. Chir. Neerl. 4:43, 1952.

80. Keith, A.: A demonstration on constriction and occlusions of the alimentary tract of congenital or obscure origin, Br. Med. J. 1:301, 1910.

81. Kent, M.: Transpyloric Jejunal Feeding Tubes in Neonatal Surgery, in Proceedings of the Paediatric Surgical Congress, Melbourne, Vol. 2, p. 394, 1970.

82. Kent, M.: Personal communication.

83. Kluth, D.: Atlas of esophageal atresia, J. Pediatr. Surg. 11:901, 1976.

84. Knox, G.: Congenital tracheoesophageal fistula without esophageal atresia, Surgery 30:1016, 1951.

85. Koop, C. E., and Hamilton, J. P.: Atresia of the esophagus: Increased survival with staged procedures in the poor-risk infant, Ann. Surg. 162:389, 1965.

86. Koop, C. E., and Hamilton, J. P.: Atresia of the esophagus: Factors affecting survival in 249 cases, Z. Kinderchir. 5:319, 1968.

87. Koop, C. E., Schnaufer, L., and Broennle, A. M.: Esophageal atresia and tracheoesophageal fistula: Supportive measures that affect survival, Pediatrics 54:558, 1974.

88. Koop, C. E., Schnaufer, L., Thompson, G., Haecker, T., and Dalrymply, D.: The social, psychological and economic problems of the patient's family after successful repair of oesophageal atresia, Z. Kinderchir. 17:125, 1975.

89. Ladd, W. E.: The surgical treatment of esophageal atresia and tracheoesophageal fistulas, N. Engl. J. Med. 230:625, 1944.

90. Lamb, D. S.: A fatal case of congenital tracheo-esophageal fistula, Phila. Med. Times 3:705, 1873.

91. Langman, J.: Esophageal atresia accompanied by a remarkable vessel anomaly, Arch. Chir. Neerl. 4:39, 1952.

92. Langman, J.: Esophageal atresia and esophago-tracheal fistula, Acta Neerl. Morphol. 6:308, 1949.

93. Lanman, T. H.: Congenital atresia of the esophagus. A study of thirty-two cases, Arch. Surg. 41:1060, 1940.

94. Leven, N. L.: Congenital atresia of the esophagus with tracheoesophageal fistula. Report of successful extrapleural ligation of fistulous communication and cervical esophagostomy, J. Thorac. Surg. 10:648, 1941.

95. Lister, J.: The blood supply of the oesophagus in relation to oesophageal atresia, Arch. Dis. Child. 39:131, 1964.

96. Livaditis, A., et al.: Esophageal end-to-end anastomosis, Scand. J. Thorac. Cardiovasc. Surg. 6:206, 1972.

97. Livaditis, A.: End-to-end anastomosis in esophageal atresia. A clinical and experimental study, Scand. J. Thorac. Cardiovasc. Surg. (Supp. 2), 1969.

98. Livaditis, A.: Esophageal atresia; a method of overbridging large segmental gaps, Z. Kinderchir. 13:298, 1973.

99. Livaditis, A., Bjorck, G., and Kangstrom, L. E.: Esophageal myectomy. An experimental study in piglets, Scand. J. Thorac. Cardiovasc. Surg. 3:181, 1969.

100. Livaditis, A., and Ivemark, B.: Esophageal anastomosis in piglets. Histologic and microangiographic aspects of the early phases of healing, Scand. J. Thorac. Cardiovasc. Surg. 3:174, 1969.

101. Livaditis, A., Okmian, L., Bjorck, G., and Ivemark, B.: Esophageal suture anastomosis. An experimental study in piglets, Scand. J. Thorac. Cardiovasc. Surg. 3:163, 1969.

102. McClellan, R. H., and Elterich, T. J.: Atresia of esophagus with tracheo-esophageal fistula, Am. J. Dis. Child. 26:373, 1923.

103. Mahour, G. H., Cohen, S. R., and Woolley, M. M.: Laryngotracheoesophageal cleft associated with esophageal atresia and multiple tracheoesophageal fistulas in a twin, J. Thorac. Cardiovasc. Surg. 65:223, 1973.

104. Mathieu, A., and Goldsmith, H. E.: Congenital atresia of the esophagus with tracheo-oesophageal fistula, Am. J. Surg. 22:233, 1933.

105. Maurseth, K.: Tracheal stenosis caused by compression from the innominate artery, Ann. Radiol. (Paris) 9:287, 1966.

106. Meeker, I. A.: In Hays, D. M., Woolley, M. M., and Snyder, W. H.: Changing techniques in the management of esophageal atresia, Arch. Surg. 92:611, 1966.

107. Miller, F. J. W., Court, S. D. M., Walton, W. J., and Knox, E. G.: *Growing Up in Newcastle upon Tyne* (London: Oxford University Press, 1960).

107a. Mustard, W. T., Bayliss, C. E., Fearon, B., Pelton, D., and Trusler, G. A.: Tracheal compression by the innominate artery in children, Ann. Thorac. Surg. 8:312, 1969.

108. Myers, N. A.: Oesophageal atresia: The epitome of modern surgery, Ann. R. Coll. Surg. Engl. 54:277, 1974.

109. Myers, N. A.: Large gap between the segments, Kind. Chir. (supp. 65), 1975.

110. Myers, N. A.: Oesophageal atresia with distal tracheo-oesophageal fistula—a long-term follow-up, Prog. Pediatr. Surg. 10:15, 1977.

111. Pettersson, G.: Inhibited separation of larynx and the upper part of trachea from oesophagus in a newborn, Acta Chir. Scand. 110:250, 1955.

112. Piekarski, D. H., and Stephens, F. D.: The association and embryogenesis of tracheo-oesophageal and anorectal anomalies, Prog. Pediatr. Surg. 9:63, 1976.

113. Pieretti, R., Shandling, B., and Stephens, C. A.: Resistant esophageal stenosis associated with reflux after repair of esophageal atresia: A therapeutic approach, J. Pediatr. Surg. 9:355, 1974.

114. Quan, L., and Smith, D. W.: The VATER association. Vertebral defects, Anal atresia, T-E fistula with esophageal atresia, Radial and Renal dysplasia: A spectrum of associated defects, J. Pediatr. 82:104, 1973.

115. Randolph, J. C., Tunell, W. P., Lilly, J. R., and Altman, R. P.: Gastric division: A surgical adjunct in selected problems with esophageal anomalies, J. Pediatr. Surg. 6:657, 1971.

116. Rehbein, F., and Schweder, N.: Reconstruction of the esophagus without colon transplantation in cases of atresia, J. Pediatr. Surg. 6:746, 1971.

117. Replogle, R. L.: Esophageal atresia: Plastic sump catheter for drainage of the proximal pouch, Surgery 54:296, 1963.

118. Reynolds, R. P., and Morrison, W. W.: Congenital malformations of the esophagus, Am. J. Dis. Child. 21:339, 1921.

119. Richter, H. M.: Congenital atresia of the oesophagus; an operation designed for its cure. With a report of two cases operated upon by the author, Surg. Gynecol. Obstet. 17:397, 1913.

120. Sanderud, A.: Treatment of oesophageal atresia: A modification in technique, Acta Chir. Scand. 119:339, 1960.

121. Scott, J. S., and Wilson, J. K.: Hydramnios as an early sign of oesophageal atresia, Lancet 2:569, 1957.

122. Shafer, A. D., and David, T. E.: Suture fistula as a means of connecting upper and lower segments in esophageal atresia, J. Pediatr. Surg. 9:669, 1974.

123. Shaw, H. L. K.: Congenital atresia of the esophagus, Am. J. Dis. Child. 20:507, 1920.

124. Shaw, R.: Surgical correction of congenital atresia of the esophagus with tracheo-esophageal fistula. Case report, J. Thorac. Surg. 9:213, 1939.

125. Shepard, R., Fenn, S., and Sieber, W. K.: Evaluation of esophageal function in postoperative esophageal atresia and tracheoesophageal fistula, Surgery 59:608, 1966.

126. Sheth, N. P.: Tracheo-oesophageal fistula with oesophageal atresia and oesophageal stenosis in the distal segment, Asian Assoc. Paed. Surgeons, Article 128, 1976.

127. Slim, M. S.: Circular myotomy of the esophagus: Clinical application in esophageal atresia, Ann. Thorac. Surg. 23:62, 1977.

128. Sloan, H., and Haight, C.: Congenital atresia of the esophagus in brothers, J. Thorac. Surg. 32:209, 1956.

129. Smith, E. D.: The treatment of congenital atresia of the esophagus, Am. J. Surg. 37:157, 1923.

130. Smith, E. I.: The early development of the trachea and esophagus in relation to atresia of the esophagus and tracheoesophageal fistula, Contrib. Embryol. Carnegie Inst. Wash. #245, 36:41, 1957.

131. Steele, C.: Case of deficient oesophagus, Lancet 2:764, 1888.

132. Stephens, C. A., Mustard, W. T., and Simpson, J. S., Jr.: Con-

genital atresia of the esophagus with tracheo-esophageal fistula, Surg. Clin. North Am. 36:1465, 1956.

133. Stephens, G., and Stephens, H. B.: H-type tracheo-oesophageal fistula complicated by oesophageal stenosis, J. Thorac. Cardiovasc. Surg. 59:325, 1970.

134. Stevenson, R. E.: Extra vertebrae associated with esophageal atresias and tracheoesophageal fistulas, J. Pediatr. 81:1123, 1972.

135. Sulamaa, M., Gripenberg, L., and Ahvenainen, E. K.: Prognosis and treatment of congenital atresia of the esophagus, Acta Chir. Scand. 102:141, 1951.

136. Swenson, O., et al.: Repair and complications of esophageal atresia and tracheo-esophageal fistula, N. Engl. J. Med. 267:960, 1962.

137. Thomas, P. S., and Chrispin, A. R.: Congenital tracheo-oesophageal fistula without oesophageal atresia, Clin. Radiol. 20:371, 1969.

138. Thomasson, B. H.: Congenital esophageal atresia: Mercury bag stretching of the upper pouch in a patient without tracheoesophageal fistula, Surgery 71:661, 1972.

139. Tuqan, N. A.: Annular stricture of the esophagus distal to congenital tracheoesophageal fistula, Surgery 52:394, 1962.

140. Ty, T. C., Brunet, C., and Beardmore, H. E.: A variation in the operative technic for the treatment of esophageal atresia with tracheo-esophageal fistula, J. Pediatr. Surg. 2:118, 1967.

141. Vinson, P. P.: Congenital strictures of the esophagus, JAMA 80:1754, 1923.

142. Vogt, E. C.: Congenital esophageal atresia, Am. J. Roentgenol. 22:463, 1929.

143. Waterston, D. J., Bonham-Carter, R. E., and Aberdeen, E.: Oesophageal atresia: Tracheo-oesophageal fistula. A study of survival in 218 infants, Lancet 1:819, 1962.

144. Waterston, D. J., Bonham-Carter, R. E., and Aberdeen, E.: Congenital tracheo-oesophageal fistula in association with oesophageal atresia, Lancet 2:55, 1963.

145. Weiss, E.: Congenital atresia of esophagus, with esophagotracheal fistula, JAMA 80:17, 1923.

146. Willard, H. G.: Congenital atresia of the esophagus, JAMA 78:649, 1922.

147. Woolley, M. M., Chinnock, R. F., Paul, R. H.: Premature twins with esophageal atresia and tracheo-esophageal fistula, Acta Paediatr. 50:423, 1961.

Congenital Esophageal Stenosis and Esophageal Diaphragm (Membrane or Web)

N. A. MYERS / EOIN ABERDEEN

SEVERE STENOSIS of the esophagus is even more a burden for a child and his family than it is for an adult. The child who cannot swallow normally has difficult social adjustments to make, and may avoid eating in front of any but his family and close friends. The child's mother also is stressed, at times to the limits of endurance, as she sees her specially prepared offerings regurgitated by the anguished child, and if the child is not growing well, the mother will be even more tormented by the feelings of guilt that so readily attack parents of children with severe congenital anomalies.

Until about 40 years ago it was assumed that esophageal obstructions occurring in the very young were all congenital. Diagnostic terms were used loosely, and one cannot make an index search of the literature for esophageal atresia much before 1913, because all cases were termed esophageal stenosis. Even such a great scholar and embryologist as Sir Arthur Keith,[11] writing in 1910, did not distinguish between "atresia" (without passage or perforation) and "stenosis" of the esophagus (although the word atresia had been precisely used in the mid-nineteenth century to describe congenital heart anomalies with complete obstruction).

The diagnostic problem with the esophagus is that reflux esophagitis can occur early and can cause an esophageal stricture, even within days of birth in rare instances.[23] Reflux esophagitis may be much more severe in infants and children than in adults, causing severe fibrosis and shortening of the esophagus as well as strictures, diaphragms and webs. Trauma to the esophagus by swallowed chemical or foreign body may also result in a stricture causing esophageal obstruction, and this is more likely to occur in mentally retarded children, especially ones living in an institution. On the other hand, a congenital stricture may be the site at which a swallowed foreign body or food may impact.

The recognition of the natural history of reflux esophagitis and the role of esophageal hiatal hernia was a major advance in surgery. Philip Allison, especially, was one who directed the attention to the anatomy of the hiatus and who emphasized that a short esophagus usually was an acquired condition and not, as many had presumed, a congenital one.[1] Methods of diagnosing hiatal hernia became much more precise, and it was appreciated that reflux esophagitis was not always associated with a hiatal hernia (although the gastroesophageal junction may be higher than normal) and that hiatal hernia can be present without significant reflux.

As the role of esophageal reflux became more widely appreciated, it was commonly proposed that almost all stenotic lesions of the esophagus were acquired and very few were congenital. The pendulum of popular surgical belief has swung back in the past few years from the extreme view that true congenital stenosis hardly ever occurred, but it is recognized that stenosis of the esophagus that is undeniably congenital is uncommon.

Two forms of esophageal stenosis about which there can be little dispute as to their congenital origin have been reported more recently. One is the stenosis associated with abnormal tissue rests in the esophageal wall containing respiratory tissue such as cartilage and ciliated epithelium.[17] Deiraniya,[2] when reporting two such cases in 1974, referred to 12 other cases from 9 reports in the German and English language literature. That this lesion probably is much underreported is suggested by the report by Ohkawa et al.,[16] who described 5 cases from their own experience. The barium swallow may show a gradual tapering of the esophagus or may show an abrupt narrowing. The lesion most often is at the distal end of the esophagus, but may appear anywhere in the lower third. Ishida et al.,[9] reporting 3 cases in 1969, observed that esophageal stenosis has been reported with tracheobronchial remnants other than cartilage in two reports, and these patients had been operated on in late middle age, in contrast to those who had cartilage included in the abnormal tissue rests, nearly all of whom were operated on in the first years of childhood. Most of these have had normal swallowing in the first months of life until solids were introduced into the diet during infancy, an observation also made by Gross.[4] Esophagoscopy may not reveal any abnormalities.[13]

Most of these patients presented with isolated lesions, but Deiraniya reported the first such in association with esophageal atresia and tracheoesophageal fistula.[20] His second patient also had a hiatal hernia associated with the embryologic abnormality, which is more likely to confuse than help the differential diagnosis in future cases.

The treatment, resection of the short affected segment and primary anastomosis, generally has been successful in the reported cases.

The second type of congenital stenosis of the esophagus depends, for the recognition of its congenital nature, on the similarity of the deformity to the more commonly occurring esophageal atresia of the newborn. Since the atresia must present within the first few days of life (and survival is possible only if effective treatment is available) there has been no reason to question the congenital origin of esophageal atresia. Even though patients with esophageal stenosis may first present during later infancy or the first years of childhood, if their deformity varies greatly from the normal anatomy and closely resembles the appearance of a common form of esophageal atresia, it is reasonable to presume that it is of congenital origin. Jewsbury[10] described a case with gross anatomy very similar to the common type of esophageal atresia plus tracheoesophageal fistula, except that the upper and lower esophageal segments were joined by a natural canal connecting the fistula to the upper pouch, which it joined at the side, asymmetrically, so this was an example of congenital stenosis with fistula. Patients have been described without fistula whose anomaly resembles an atypical esophageal atresia, in which the lower segment attaches as though the fistula were joined asymmetrically to the upper pouch of the esophagus rather than to the trachea. The result was a narrow canal of esophagus with a bulging area of esophagus just above, which could be labeled a diverticulum.[15, 19] Such examples of stenosis obviously would seem to be congenital, and another obvious congenital stenosis is that which occurs in the lower esophageal segment of a newborn with the common form of esophageal atresia and fistula.[20] Congenital esophageal stenosis may also occur with tracheoesophageal fistula without esophageal atresia.[14]

The spectrum of esophageal atresia varies from a true partial, or almost total, agenesis of the esophagus, with the esophageal segment separated by a distance varying from large to small, to forms in which the esophageal segments are juxtaposed, either directly end to end (in which case the esophagus may appear normal when inspected from the outside) or the segments are overlapping and meet side to side. The segments may be separated by the full thickness of the esophageal wall or only by a thin diaphragm of mucous membrane. (The range of variations is displayed diagrammatically in a masterly review of the literature by Kluth.[12]) If the diaphragm of mucous membrane is not complete, the lesion is one of congenital stenosis. To prove that a stenosis is congenital and not acquired may be difficult but is required for precise diagnosis and proper treatment. In general, the earlier in the child's life that the lesion presents and the higher its location in the esophagus the more likely is the lesion to be congenital in origin. The histology of the membrane and adjacent esophagus may not necessarily define the difference between a congenital and an acquired cause.

The long-term response to conservative management may be a final factor to consider in deciding whether the cause is congenital or acquired. If a single or a few dilatations of a diaphragm or web of mucous membrane in an infant are sufficient to permit normal swallowing for many years, the likelihood of the lesion being a congenital diaphragm membrane or web is much increased. The stricture associated with reflux esophagitis in children very rarely will be cured permanently by dilatation.

Diagnosis and Differential Diagnosis

Any child who presents with chronic dysphagia and/or frequent vomiting, especially after meals, should have a radiologic investigation. Swallowing of contrast medium should be studied using the image intensifier, fluoroscopy and cineradiography. A good radiologic study will also indicate if there is lack of coordination in the region of the pharynx causing repeated aspiration into the trachea and whether the esophagus has a normal stripping wave. It may show a

stenosed area or even a diaphragm, will show function of the gastroesophageal junction and identify gastroesophageal reflux. Reliable interpretation of these findings requires a special interest and experience in the child's esophagus.

Esophagoscopy is the other important diagnostic tool. The newer esophagoscopes with the Hopkins lens system permit a much better visualization of the esophagus than was possible with previous equipment and give better visualization than the flexible gastroscope. Lesser degrees of stenosis will be apparent only if a wide-bore esophagoscope is passed, so distending the esophagus above the stricture as to make the stricture more apparent. Radiologic study should precede esophagoscopy because a form of blind pouch may lie just below a stricture and, if not identified beforehand, may lead to esophageal perforation during the examination.

Treatment of Congenital Esophageal Stricture

Almost any child with dysphagia from a congenital stenosis requires surgical relief—either by dilatation or by operation. If reflux esophagitis is present and is the cause of the stenosis, this must be dealt with, and treatment is described in this chapter under Hiatal Hernia and Gastroesophageal Reflux. Occasionally, esophagitis may be associated with a truly congenital stricture.[2]

In general terms, excision is required if ectopic tissue rests in the esophagus are the cause of the stenosis or if the degree of deformity is severe.[20] The aim of excision is to create an esophagus with an even and adequate diameter through its length. If excision is not clearly indicated, the alternative is dilatation of the stricture. Repeated dilatations have been used for acquired stricture, both those following reflux esophagitis and those following esophageal anastomosis. Let it be recognized that ring strictures of the esophagus, almost as much as ring strictures of the urethra, have forced surgeons to recognize one of the uncomfortable principles of surgery—the natural history of maturing scar tissue; scar tissue contracts during the phase of maturation unless fixed in an isometric state, and, having matured, scar tissue no longer contracts. Mature scar tissue rings may be broken by acute dilatation, but, having been broken, the ends will again be joined by maturing scar tissue with its innate tendency to contract. Mature scar tissue can be acutely elongated or stretched only with great difficulty, but can be progressively stretched over a longer period. Maturation of scar tissue usually takes about 6–9 months.

Single membranes of an obstructing mucosal diaphragm have been effectively treated by a single or a few dilatations, because the surrounding esophageal wall is not scar tissue and has an adequate diameter.[3] More often, repeated dilatations are necessary.[22] The dilatation may be made through an esophagoscope (which involves a general anesthetic). The risks of esophageal perforation are small but significant, and even an experienced endoscopist may cause an occasional esophageal perforation. Retrograde dilatation has established a safer record in the management of the difficult stricture and we quote the excellent description of the management of the tight stricture by Ravitch in the Second Edition of this book.[18]

"TREATMENT.—Early experiences with the impossibility of finding the lumen in the area of the edematous obstruction, whether tubular or due to a diaphragm, and mishaps with esophageal perforation on attempted bougienage, led us to adopt a relatively simple and effective method of treating these patients.

"Once the diagnosis has been established by appropriate

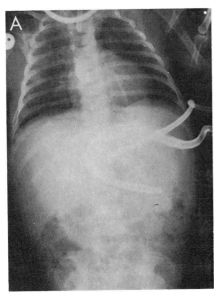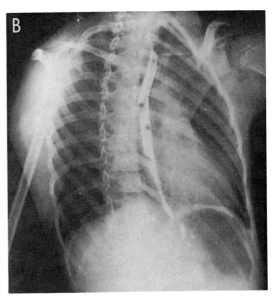

Fig. 43–11.—Congenital esophageal stenosis. A 3-week-old infant with 10-day history of increasing dysphagia culminating in apparent total occlusion. **A,** a catheter passed through the mouth met an obstruction in the midesophagus, and Lipiodol fills the proximal esophagus in a pouch ending at T1. Esophagoscopy showed what appeared to be a web type of obstruction with a tiny crescentic opening at one portion. Gastrostomy was done, and

after 10 days of constant esophageal catheter suction and no oral feedings, the child could swallow a string readily. The esophagus was dilated with graduated plastic beads pulled through on a string, replaced by a Salzer bougie as soon as it could be passed. There was no tendency to recurrence. **B,** barium swallow 3 years later shows no evidence of obstruction or of hiatal hernia. The child has been well.

barium swallows, if a bougie does not fall easily into the stomach, a gastrostomy is performed and nothing is given by mouth for a week or 10 days, while a catheter with constant suction keeps the esophagus empty. At the end of a week, a spool of fine silk thread is suspended above the baby's head and the end of the thread passed into the baby's mouth. As the baby chews and swallows, the thread finds its way through the stenosis and into the stomach, where it is readily fished out, either with a crochet needle or with a suction tip. A heavy silk thread now is drawn after the fine silk, through the mouth and out the gastrostomy, and tied into an endless loop. Into this loop are spliced sections of thread on which there have been formed olive-shaped beads of cellulose acetate, varying from barely perceptible thickenings of the thread to beads 6 or 8 mm in diameter or larger. These are pulled through the mouth, down the esophagus, through the stricture and out the gastrostomy, or back and forth, in progressively larger sizes. When, after several days, the largest bead passes without difficulty, the daily dilatations are replaced by dilatations every second and every third day, until it is proved that there is no tendency to restricture (Fig. 43–11). As soon as the esophagus will readily accept a Hurst (mercury-filled) or Salzer (shot-filled) bougie, the string is removed and the gastrostomy allowed to close. There has been little tendency to restricture; and after several months of precautionary weekly, followed by bimonthly, calibrations of the esophagus with bougies, treatment may be discontinued. Actually, once the larger sizes of the plastic beads have been pulled through the stricture, one may begin to use bougies, either the flexible woven, olive-tipped variety or the Salzer, Hurst, shot- or mercury-filled rubber catheters. In most patients with congenital stenosis, as opposed to patients with inflammatory stricture, particularly those that occur after anastomoses, a few dilatations are all that are needed, and there is little or no tendency to restricture. The Tucker soft rubber threaded dilators, essentially tapered tubes of solid rubber with threads incorporated in their cen-

ters, serve equally well for dilatation by this method. A thread is passed via the nose and pulled out from the gastrostomy. Holinger, one of the pioneers in this field, emphasized with his colleagues[8] the need to continue dilatation for 1 year in caustic strictures, and at times such a long program of treatment may be required for severe congenital stricture managed by intermittent dilatation."

Other methods of management include alteration of the scar tissue in escharotic strictures by drugs given systemically, but this work still is in the experimental stage. Local injection of steroids has been useful,[7] especially in infants with anastomotic strictures, and may help avoid the major operation of esophageal resection or replacement.

Intraesophageal stents have also been used experimentally and in patients with caustic strictures,[5] but stents should not be placed so that the gastroesophageal junction is made incompetent. We have had personal experience of very severe esophagitis appearing quite suddenly in the midesophagus 3 months after such placement of a stent, and similar experience has been reported by others.[6]

The long-term outlook seems to be good. Once a period of a year or more of normal swallowing has been achieved, recurrence of the stenosis is very unusual.

REFERENCES

1. Allison, P. R.: Peptic ulcer of the oesophagus, Thorax 3:20, 1948.
2. Deiraniya, A. K.: Congenital oesophageal stenosis due to tracheobronchial remnants, Thorax 29:720, 1974.
3. Gilat, T., and Rozen, P.: Fiberoptic endoscopic diagnosis and treatment of a congenital esophageal diaphragm, Am. J. Dig. Dis. 20:781, 1975.
4. Gross, R. E.: *The Surgery of Infancy and Childhood* (Philadelphia: W. B. Saunders Company, 1953), p. 103.
5. Hill, J. L., Norberg, H. P., Smith, M. D., Young, J. A., and Reyes, H. M.: Clinical technique and success of the esophageal stent to prevent corrosive strictures, J. Pediatr. Surg. 11:443, 1976.
6. Holden, M. P., and Wooler, G. H.: Mousseau-Barbin tubes for benign strictures of the oesophagus, Thorax 26:619, 1971.

7. Holder, T. M., Ashcraft, K. W., and Leape, L.: The treatment of patients with esophageal strictures by local steroid injections, J. Pediatr. Surg. 4:646, 1969.
8. Holinger, P. H., Johnston, K. C., Potts, W. J., and daCunha, F.: The conservative and surgical management of benign strictures of the esophagus, J. Thorac. Surg. 28:345, 1954.
9. Ishida, M., Tsuchida, Y., Saito, S., and Tsunoda, A.: Congenital esophageal stenosis due to tracheobronchial remnants, J. Pediatr. Surg. 4:339, 1969.
10. Jewsbury, P.: An unusual case of congenital oesophageal stricture, Br. J. Surg. 58:475, 1971.
11. Keith, A.: Constrictions and occlusions of the alimentary tract of congenital or obscure origin, Br. Med. J. 1:301, 1910.
12. Kluth, D.: Atlas of esophageal atresia, J. Pediatr. Surg. 11:901, 1976.
13. Kumar, R.: A case of congenital oesophageal stricture due to a cartilaginous ring, Br. J. Surg. 69:533, 1962.
14. Moysen, Fr.: Sténose oesophagienne congénitale et fistule trachéo-oesophagienne cervicale, Ann. Chir. Infant 11:179, 1970.
15. O'Bannon, R. P.: Congenital partial atresia of the esophagus associated with congenital diverticulum of the esophagus. Report of a case, Radiology 47:471, 1946.
16. Ohkawa, H., Takahashi, H., Hoshino, Y., and Sato, H.: Lower esophageal stenosis in association with tracheobronchial remnants, J. Pediatr. Surg. 10:453, 1975.
17. Paulino, F., Roselli, A., and Aprigliano, F.: Congenital esophageal stricture due to tracheobronchial remnants, Surgery 53:547, 1963.
18. Ravitch, M. M.: Esophageal Stenosis and Stricture, in Mustard, W. T., et al. (eds.), Pediatric Surgery (2d ed.; Chicago: Year Book Medical Publishers, Inc., 1969) Vol. 1, p. 382.
19. Sidaway, M. E.: Duplication of the oesophagus, Ann. Radiol. 7: 400, 1964.
20. Takayanagi, K., Komi, K., and Li, N.: Congenital esophageal stenosis with lack of the submucosa, J. Pediatr. Surg. 10:425, 1975.
21. Tuqan, N. A.: Annular stricture of the esophagus distal to congenital tracheoesophageal fistula, Surgery 52:394, 1962.
22. Valerio, D., Jones, P. F., and Stewart, A. M.: Congenital oesophageal stenosis, Arch. Dis. Child. 52:414, 1977.
23. Waterston, D. J.: Die Behandlung der Oesophagusstenose, Langenbecks Arch. Chir. 316:695, 1966.

Corrosive Strictures of the Esophagus

J. ALEX HALLER, JR.

INGESTION OF powerful corrosive agents usually is a suicide attempt in teen-agers and adults and an accident in younger children. Management of an acute burn is controversial and treatment of the resultant esophageal stricture is extremely difficult. The public health problem of poison ingestion continues despite eloquent pleas, beginning with Chevalier Jackson in 1902, for passage of legislation to hamper the access by children to dangerous materials. The Federal Caustic Act of 1927 required labels that warned of danger; but, as pointed out by Leape *et al.*,[2] altering packages to make them unattractive, with smaller volumes or with safety caps does not protect against accidental ingestion by those who cannot read.

Incidence

Counting all chemical ingestions that could be responsible for esophageal stricture, Leape *et al.*[2] estimate 5000 cases in children each year. Holinger's[1] series recorded 78% occurring in children ages 1–5 years, with a 2:1 predominance of males, which shifts to a female predominance with

suicidal attempts in teen-agers. Children constitute 80–85% of instances of corrosive chemical ingestion in most series.[3-5]

Etiology and Pathophysiology

Strong alkalis, primarily sodium hydroxide, are responsible for the greatest number of severe strictures,[3, 6] but many common agents, such as bleach,[7] nonphosphate detergents,[8] clinitest tablets,[9] sodium carbonate (washing soda)[4] and ammonia[1] may cause corrosive injury to the esophagus. Acid burns of the esophagus produce coagulation necrosis, which impedes deeper penetration into the esophageal wall, and are more likely to cause damage to the stomach or duodenum.[10] Of special interest to physicians caring for children are clinitest tablets, which are commonly accessible, attractive in appearance and come in easily opened screw top bottles. These tablets stick to the esophagus and produce strictures that are unusually difficult to dilate and usually require resection.[9]

The degree of burn from ingested corrosive agents depends on the duration of contact and the concentration of the caustic material.[11] The injury may be categorized by the depth of burn as superficial or deep. Superficial burns have erythema, edema, vesiculation or superficial ulceration.[1] Deep burns involve the entire esophageal wall and may extend into the adjacent mediastinum or into the pleural or peritoneal cavity.

Healing of the lesion may be divided into three phases:[12] (1) Acute necrosis with coagulation of intracellular protein: cell death invokes an intense inflammatory reaction. This is associated with vascular thrombosis and hemorrhage and lasts 1–4 days. (2) Ulceration-granulation phase. The eschar sloughs, exposing an ulcerative base. Inflammatory edema reaches its maximum; neovascularization and fibroblast proliferation begin and collagen deposition occurs during this phase (5th–14th day). The structural integrity of the esophagus is weakest during this period. (3) Cicatrization and stricture formation. The collagen begins to contract and adhesions form; there is replacement of muscle by dense scar. Re-epithelialization occurs over the 14–90-day period and maturation of the scar may continue for months.

Diagnosis

An irrefutable history of ingestion of a corrosive substance and evidence of burns on inspection of the lips, tongue, oropharynx, hands, face, neck and chest are essential. Substernal, back and abdominal pain may indicate perforation. Stridor, dyspnea and hoarseness are suggestive of concomitant aspiration. Dysphagia is frequent and may be due in part to spasm, but has a large component of inflammatory edema, which may lead to obstruction and secondary aspiration pneumonia.

Treatment

It is generally agreed that early esophagoscopy is essential for precise therapy.[9, 12-17] Esophagoscopy should be performed under general anesthesia by an experienced endoscopist. Patients with impending airway obstruction should not be endoscoped but should be started immediately on antibiotics and steroids. The potential of instrument perforation is obviated if endoscopy is discontinued as soon as any esophageal burn is seen, although some authors have reported a high percentage of complications.[3] As many as 71%[16] of patients suspected of ingesting corrosives and having oropharyngeal burns will not have esophageal injury and the incidence is variously reported as 50%,[12] 44%[15, 17] and 25%.[18] Ten percent to 15% of patients with esophageal burns have no oropharyngeal burns.[3, 13, 18, 19] Esophagoscopy provides some knowledge of the extent of the burn, but it is difficult to assess the depth of the burn. Full-thickness burns do not always lead to stricture,[20] and, although it has been stated that strictures may occur with intact esophageal musculature,[21] this rarely, if ever, occurs.[20] It is impossible to decide the extent of damage from esophagograms in the first 24 hours. Severe esophageal dysfunction may occur without morphologic stricture.[20] By the time significant changes have occurred in the esophagus, as demonstrated by x-ray, it is too late to institute preventive therapy.

Although some authors advocate the use of a neutralizing solution and gastric lavage,[13] children who accidentally ingest caustic solutions will immediately regurgitate and therefore are unlikely to have significant residual caustic in the stomach. Induced vomiting or lavage may compound the original injury.

The following protocol for the management of children with caustic ingestion has been used at Johns Hopkins Hospital since 1963.

For Acute Burns in Children (< 48 hours):
a) Detailed history; identify caustic agent.
b) Place patient on "nothing by mouth."
c) Start an intravenous line, type and crossmatch.
d) Notify ENT and pediatric surgery services.
e) Obtain signed operation permit for esophagoscopy.
f) Obtain hematocrit and urinalysis.
g) Check heart and lungs for general anesthesia.

Admit
a) Chest film on admission.
b) Esophagoscopy within 12 hours after admission.
c) Esophageal cinefluoroscopy within 24 hours, if possible.

If No Esophageal Burn:
a) Care for mouth burn.
b) Discharge.
c) Return to ENT clinic in 1 month.
   1. No esophageal symptoms: Return in 1 year.
   2. Suggestive esophageal symptoms: Cine-esophagography and dilatation, as indicated.

If Esophagus is Burned:
a) Immediate steroids (must be within 48 hours); dose—2 mg/kg/day of prednisone (or equivalent).
b) Antibiotics—ampicillin for 10 days.
c) IV fluids—until patient can swallow saliva (usually within 48 hours).
d) Clear liquids after c)—advance to soft diet, as tolerated.
e) Repeat cinefluoroscopy 3 weeks after burn.
   1. If significant stricture:
      aa) Stop steroids.
      bb) Begin dilatations.
   2. If no stricture:
      aa) Stop steroids.
      bb) Follow monthly in ENT clinic for 1 year.

The combined experience using this treatment protocol at Johns Hopkins Hospital and Jackson Memorial Hospital includes 235 children with ingestion, of whom 69 (29%) were proved to have esophageal burns. Eight (12%) of these children developed strictures, 5 of which required prolonged dilatations. The remainder of the entire group have normal

esophageal function and none has required esophageal replacement.

Routine early bougienage, originally advocated by Salzer[22] and advised by Gellis and Holt,[23] Marchand[24] and Moody and Garrett,[25] is not believed to be indicated by others whose experimental models demonstrate increased risk of perforation and no decrease in stricture formation. Additionally, young children may have psychologic trauma with repeated dilatations; this seems unacceptable if other effective modes of therapy can be used. The inflammatory response is decreased by the use of steroids, and subsequent fibroplasia may be inhibited if steroid therapy is initiated in the first 48 hours.[26] Experimental studies suggest a reduced incidence of postburn stricture with this regimen.[27] Similar effects were noted in the clinical trials of Borja et al.[3] (10–13%) and Cardona and Daly[14] (9%) in comparison to the data on bougienage by Desportes and Ray[28] (80%) and Alford and Harris[29] (50%). Signs of esophageal or gastric perforations contraindicate steroid therapy. Other authors have advocated the use of antibiotics[26, 27] to help prevent pulmonary and mediastinal infection during treatment. Gram-positive organisms are most often responsible for infection. Citron et al.[32] and Dafoe and Ross[12] have suggested the use of an oral solution combining steroids, anesthetic and antibiotics. We believe that children who are able to swallow without difficulty should be started on early oral feedings for the beneficial self-bougienage involved in swallowing food. Recent reports advocating the use of esophagus splints have been extremely interesting, and Reyes and Hill[34] have reported no strictures in experimental full-thickness esophageal burns with the use of an intraluminal stent in the esophagus for 3 weeks.

Madden et al.[35] described experimental use of beta aminoproprionitrile, a powerful lathyrogen, in combination with bougienage to correct established corrosive strictures, but no clinical evaluations have been reported.

Ritter et al.[36] and Gago et al.[37] have advised the use of emergency esophagogastric resection in treatment of liquid caustic ingestion. Their experience is limited to 7 patients. They advocate gastric lavage and if an alkaline aspirate persists, laparotomy is in order. If the stomach appears burned, an esophagogastrectomy should be performed. If the stomach does not appear burned, they advise esophagectomy. In response to those articles, Ashcraft[38] reported no esophagogastric perforations in 20 children with liquid caustic ingestion, suggesting that the ingested volume may be less in children, consequently causing less severe damage, but he agreed that gastrostomy might be indicated, since the incidence of stricture is so high.

Complications

Corrosive stricture is the most frequent complication of caustic burns of the esophagus and, despite current therapy, will occur in 10–20% of ingestions of caustic solutions. The percentage is much higher with liquid lye.[2] Webb et al.[31] state that strictures will occur in all third degree burns. Maintenance of function in a strictured esophagus is largely dependent on esophageal dilatation (Fig. 43–12). Periodic retrograde dilatation is the safest form of chronic stricture therapy. If a gastrostomy is performed for retrograde dilatation, it should be positioned low on the fundus and the tube brought out well below the costal margin. Morgan and Harkins[39] have used a silicone rubber string, which causes no alar erosion and facilitates passage of the bougies.

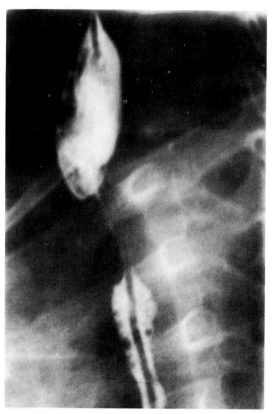

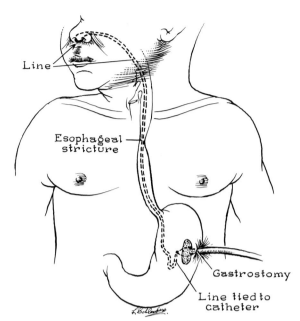

Fig. 43–13.—Internalized modification of esophageal retrieval line. After dilatation, the retrieval line is passed around the nasal septum and both ends are drawn into the stomach, where they are tied to the gastrostomy catheter. This results in an almost completely internalized line that is protected, well tolerated and easily retrieved for subsequent use with the dilatations.

Fig. 43–12.—A 5½-year-old child accidentally ingested oven cleaner and was observed at another hospital for 6 weeks, without specific treatment. Four months later, he was referred to Johns Hopkins Hospital for failure to thrive. His high thoracic esophageal stricture has responded to retrograde dilatation, with increasingly longer intervals between dilatations. It is not anticipated that reconstruction will be necessary.

We have used an internalized modification that obviates the erosion and prevents harassment by peers (Fig. 43–13). In our hands, Hurst or Maloney mercury-filled dilators are too flexible to dilate tight strictures by antegrade dilatation. String-guided Mixter bougies may involve considerable delay and discomfort in swallowing the string. Lilly and McCaffrey[41] have described a method using a fiberoptic esophagoscope to introduce a wire guide for Eder-Puestow stringless dilators and have been successful in 3 patients.

Holder *et al.*[42] and Mendelsohn and Maloney[43] have reported the successful use of triamcinolone intralesional injections for treatment of short strictures, thus allowing dilatation in a limited series of patients who had been refractory to bougienage.

If repeated dilatation is required, some form of esophageal bypass may become necessary. The psychologic and physical trauma associated with multiple dilatations may significantly affect a young patient's psychosocial development. The merits of jejunal, left or right colon or stomach as esophageal substitutes are discussed in this chapter under Esophageal Replacement, but we believe that colon is better in children than jejunum or stomach.

Fistulous communication between the esophagus and the tracheobronchial tree is a rare but devastating complication.[44] Twenty patients have been reported with peptic ulceration of the lower esophagus 20–50 years after a corrosive burn. These were believed to be secondary to shortening of the esophagus by scar contractions. Treatment may require

resection with interposition as the treatment of choice. The incidence of carcinoma of the esophagus arising from lye stricture is 1000 times that of the general population and therefore immediate endoscopic and radiologic evaluation should be done for inability to dilate a chronic stricture or progressive stenosis on esophagograms.[45] Malignant changes occur 15–40 years after the lye ingestion. Negative biopsies are inconclusive, since the stenosis limits access by esophagoscopy. A somewhat better prognosis with this scar carcinoma has been attributed to an anatomic barrier that may be imposed by the dense scar tissue.

REFERENCES

1. Holinger, P.: Management of esophageal lesions caused by chemical burns, Ann. Otol. Rhinol. Laryngol. 77:819, 1968.
2. Leape, L. L., Ashcraft, K. W., Scarpelli, D. G., and Holder, T. M.: Hazard to health—liquid lye, N. Engl. J. Med. 284:578, 1971.
3. Borja, A. R., Ramsdell, H. T., Thomas, T. V., and Johnson, W.: Lye injuries of the esophagus—analysis of ninety cases of lye ingestion, J. Thorac. Cardiovasc. Surg. 57:534, 1969.
4. Kernodle, G. W., Taylor, G., and Davison, W. C.: Lye poisoning in children, Am. J. Dis. Child. 73:935, 1948.
5. Hardin, J. C., Jr.: Caustic burns of the esophagus: A ten-year analysis, Am. J. Surg. 91:742, 1956.
6. Owens, H.: The importance of various chemicals as etiologic agents in stricture formation, Arch. Otolaryngol. 60:482, 1954.
7. Weeks, S. R., and Ravitch, M. M.: Esophageal injury by liquid chlorine bleach: Experimental study, Pediatrics 74:911, 1968.
8. Lee, J. F., Simonowitz, D., and Bloch, G. E.: Corrosive injury of the stomach and esophagus by nonphosphate detergents: An experimental study, Am. J. Surg. 123:652, 1972.
9. Burrington, J. D.: Clinitest burns of the esophagus, Ann. Thorac. Surg. 20:400, 1975.
10. Steigmann, F., and Dolehick, R. A.: Corrosive acid gastritis, N. Engl. J. Med. 254:981, 1956.
11. Kruz, H.: On the treatment of corrosive lesions in the oesophagus. An experimental study, Acta Otolaryngol. (supp.) (Stockh.) 102:1, 1952.
12. Dafoe, C. S., and Ross, C. A.: Acute corrosive oesophagitis, Thorax 24:291, 1969.

13. Kinnman, J. E. G., Lee, B. C., Lee, C. W., and Shin, H. I.: Management of severe lye corrosion of the oesophagus, J. Laryngol. Otol. 83:899, 1969.

14. Cardona, J. C., and Daly, J. F.: Current management of corrosive esophagitis, Ann. Otol. Rhinol. Laryngol. 80:521, 1971.

15. Bikhazi, H. B., Thompson, E. R., and Shumrich, D. A.: Caustic ingestion: Current status—a report of 105 cases, Arch. Otolaryngol. 89:112, 1969.

16. Haller, J. A., Jr., Andrews, H. G., White, J. J., Tamer, M. A., and Cleveland, W. A.: Pathophysiology and management of acute corrosive burns of the esophagus: Results of the treatment in 285 children, J. Pediatr. Surg. 6:578, 1971.

17. Jones, R. J., and Samson, P. C.: Esophageal injury, Ann. Thorac. Surg. 19:216, 1975.

18. Yarington, C. T., Bales, G. A., and Frazer, J. P.: A study of management of caustic and esophageal trauma, Ann. Otol. Rhinol. Laryngol. 73:1130, 1964.

19. Oppenheim, P., and Owen, F. B., Jr.: Early esophagoscopy in the treatment of corrosive esophagitis, GP 34:134, 1965.

20. Butler, C., Madden, J. W., Davis, W. M., and Peacock, E. E.: Morphologic aspects of experimental esophageal lye strictures. Pathogenesis and pathophysiologic correlations, J. Surg. Res. 17:232, 1974.

21. Burford, T. G., Webb, W. R., and Ackerman, L.: Caustic burns of the esophagus and their surgical management: A clinicoexperimental correlation, Ann. Surg. 138:453, 1953.

22. Salzer, H.: Early treatment of corrosive esophagitis, Klin. Wochenschr. Wien 33:307, 1920.

23. Gellis, S. S., and Holt, L. E.: The treatment of lye ingestion by the Salzer method, Ann. Otol. Rhinol. Laryngol. 51:1086, 1942.

24. Marchand, P.: Caustic strictures of the esophagus, Thorax 10:171, 1965.

25. Moody, F. G., and Garrett, J. M.: Esophageal achalasia following lye ingestion, Ann. Surg. 170:175, 1969.

26. Johnson, E. E.: A study of corrosive esophagitis, Laryngoscope 73:1651, 1963.

27. Haller, J. A., Jr., and Bachman, K.: The comparative effect of current therapy on experimental caustic burns of the esophagus, Pediatrics 34:236, 1964.

28. Desportes, W., and Ray, E. S.: Lye burns of the esophagus treated with steroid therapy: Rupture of the esophagus following bougienage, Arch. Otolaryngol 70:130, 1959.

29. Alford, B. R., and Harris, H. H.: Chemical burns of the mouth, pharynx and esophagus, Ann. Otol. Rhinol. Laryngol. 68:122, 1959.

30. Cleveland, W. W., Chandler, J. R., and Lawson, R. B.: Treatment of caustic burns of the esophagus, JAMA 186:262, 1963.

31. Webb, W. R., Koutras, P., Echer, R., et al.: An evaluation of steroids and antibiotics in caustic burns of the esophagus, Ann. Thorac. Surg. 9:95, 1970.

32. Citron, P. B., Pincus, I. J., Geohas, M. C., and Haverback, B. J.: Chemical trauma of the esophagus and stomach, Surg. Clin. North Am. 48:1303, 1968.

33. Balasegram, M.: Early management of corrosive burns of the esophagus, Br. J. Surg. 62:444, 1975.

34. Reyes, H. M., and Hill, J. L.: Modification of the experimental stent technique for esophageal burns, J. Surg. Res. 20:6570, 1976.

35. Madden, J. W., Davis, W. M., Butler, C. H., et al.: Experimental esophageal lye burns in correcting established strictures: Beta aminoproprionitrile and bougienage, Ann. Surg. 178:277, 1973.

36. Ritter, F. N., Gago, O., Kirsh, M., Kormon, R. M., and Orvald, T. O.: The rationale of emergency esophagogastrectomy in the treatment of liquid caustic burns of the esophagus and stomach, Arch. Otolaryngol. 80:513, 1971.

37. Gago, O., Ritter, F. N., Martel, W., Orvald, T. O., Delevan, J. W., Dieterle, R. V. A., Kirsch, M. M., Kahn, D. R., and Sloan, H.: Aggressive surgical treatment for caustic surgery of the esophagus and stomach, Ann. Thorac. Surg. 13:243, 1972.

38. Ashcraft, K.: Letter to the Editor, Ann. Thorac. Surg. 14:221, 1972.

39. Morgan, W. W., and Harkins, G. A.: Silicone rubber tubing as a guide in dilating chronic esophageal stricture in children, J. Pediatr. Surg. 7:412, 1972.

40. Golladay, E. S., and Tepas, J. J.: An improved method for retaining a nasogastric retrieval line for children undergoing chronic esophageal dilatation. (Submitted for publication.)

41. Lilly, J. O., and McCaffrey, J.: Esophageal stricture dilatation. A new method adapted to fiberoptic esophagoscope, Am. J. Dig. Dis. 16:1137, 1971.

42. Holder, T. M., Ashcraft, K. W., and Leape, L.: The treatment of patients with esophageal stricture by local steroid injection, J. Pediatr. Surg. 4:646, 1969.

43. Mendelsohn, H. J., and Maloney, W. H.: The treatment of benign strictures of the esophagus with cortisone injection, Ann. Otol. Rhinol. Laryngol. 79:900, 1971.

44. Amoury, R. A., Hrabovsky, J. C., Leonidas, J. N., and Holder, T. M.: Tracheoesophageal fistula after lye ingestion, J. Pediatr. Surg. 10:273, 1975.

45. Lansing, P. B., Ferrante, W. A., and Ochsner, J.: Carcinoma of the esophagus at the site of lye stricture, Am. J. Surg. 118:108, 1969.

Hiatal Hernia and Gastroesophageal Reflux

JUDSON G. RANDOLPH

SURGEONS AND PEDIATRICIANS have become increasingly aware of the clinical manifestations of gastroesophageal reflux in the young patient. There appear to be two distinct forms of this malady, with clinical manifestations differing markedly in the infant and the older child. In the early months of life, the vomiting associated with gastroesophageal reflux produces the nutritional consequences of delayed growth and development.[24, 25, 35, 42] Recurrent respiratory infections secondary to aspiration may be frequent and severe.[32, 33, 36, 38] In the majority of infants, these symptoms resolve spontaneously as valvular competence at the gastric cardia develops during the second year of life.[7, 18]

In 1947, Berenberg and Neuhauser focused attention on infants with gastroesophageal reflux without hiatal hernia, coining the well-known term "chalasia" (relaxation) for this condition.[7, 39] Following their observation that gastroesophageal reflux spontaneously disappears by 12–15 months of age, pediatricians everywhere have confirmed that propping babies in infant seats controls the reflux. Some infants diagnosed as having chalasia are patients with small hiatal hernias. Since the symptoms, effects and treatment are similar in the two conditions, anatomic distinctions between neuromuscular failure of the esophagocardiac valve mechanism (chalasia) and projection of gastric mucosal folds above the diaphragm (hiatal hernia) are not important. There are no reliable criteria for predicting those babies who will spontaneously develop valvular function at the esophagogastric junction and those who will continue to be symptomatic. In older children, the symptoms of dysphagia, substernal burning and eructation are similar to complaints attributed to hiatal hernia in adults.

The treatment of gastroesophageal reflux emphasizes the differences between the two age groups of patients. Antacids are ineffective in the treatment of infants and preadolescent children with gastroesophageal reflux. The upright position is used as the treatment of both infants and older patients. In adults, the objective is symptomatic improvement whereas in infants postural therapy often will prevent vomiting until reflux disappears spontaneously. In adolescents and adults, such spontaneous resolution of symptoms does not occur. Whether those infants whose gastroesophageal reflux has improved spontaneously will be more susceptible to the development of hiatal hernia in adult life has not been established. It is important, however, to identify that group of infants who suffer from pernicious gastroesophageal reflux whose vomiting is not controlled by postural therapy.

Etiology

The etiology of hiatal hernia and gastroesophageal reflux in infancy and childhood is not well understood. Some authors believe that congenital shortening of the esophagus produces a hernia.[53] At operation, however, the fact that the herniated gastric cardia can be brought easily below the diaphragm in most instances argues against this concept.[5] Roviralta[46] has coined the term "phrenico-pyloric syndrome," postulating functional pyloric obstruction as the basis for gastroesophageal reflux. A poorly developed right diaphragmatic crus,[11] an inadequate tethering effect of the left gastric artery[12] and lax phrenico-esophageal ligaments[5] have also been suggested as causative factors in the congenital form of hiatal hernia. At present, however, a single explanation for incompetence of the gastroesophageal junction in infants and children remains unproved.

Esophageal Manometry Studies

In 1956, using manometric methods, Fyke, Code and Schlegel[29] demonstrated the presence of lower esophageal sphincter function under the control of the central nervous system. These investigators also demonstrated that the sphincter was important in preventing reflux from the stomach. The normal pressure of the lower esophageal sphincter ranges from 15 to 25 mm Hg above the resting intragastric pressure. Pressure in the lower esophagus equilibrates with that of the stomach when swallowing is initiated. It has been shown that the resting pressure of the lower esophageal sphincter in infants with chronic reflux is uniformly lower than that in control infants.

Since the original studies by Code and his co-workers,[29] the accuracy of esophageal manometry has been refined by DeMeester and Skinner[48] in the adult, by Benz *et al.*[6] in children and by Ament and Euler in infants.[24]

Using a perfusion technique especially adapted for infants, Ament studied 40 babies with chronic vomiting. In 7 patients who failed to respond to a controlled 6-week medical regimen, a mean pressure in the lower esophageal sphincter of 11.0 mm Hg was recorded. In 31 patients who did well on the same regimen, a significantly higher average pressure of 21.0 mm Hg was recorded.

Radiologic Considerations

An accurate esophagogram is essential in the diagnosis of gastroesophageal reflux.[18, 21, 24, 30] Considerable patience may be needed to demonstrate a small hiatal hernia or gastroesophageal reflux. If the first study is normal but clinical symptoms remain, a second examination is appropriate, particularly cineradiography. In an effort to explain the higher incidence of pathologic gastroesophageal reflux and hiatal hernia in England than that seen in the United States,[22, 28] Darling studied those radiologic maneuvers used at the Hospital for Sick Children in London.[21] He then adopted their techniques for study of his patients. Cineradiographs, special positioning, refeeding small amounts of contrast material after coating the esophagus with barium swallow and the use of the horizontal-supine position markedly increased the detection of abnormal reflux. Fisher has demonstrated the value of scintiscanning techniques to diagnose and quantify gastroesophageal reflux.[26]

Endoscopy

Esophagoscopy is not essential for all patients. In most clinical reports, about 60% of children have been esophago-scoped.[14, 32, 36] Diagnostic esophagoscopy is undertaken (1) when there is definite evidence of esophagitis by x-ray or by clinical observations (bleeding or pain), (2) in the face of a poor response to nonoperative therapy and (3) as a preliminary to operative correction of reflux.

Gastric Secretory Studies

Studies in infants have demonstrated profound effects on gastric secretion in various disease states. For example, babies with a major loss of intestine have highly significant elevations in gastric acid production. However, in 11 infants with gastroesophageal reflux ranging in age form 9 days to 10 weeks, values for gastric volume, pH, total acid and the rate of acid production were comparable to those of normal infants.[3] There is no evidence that hiatal hernia or gastroesophageal reflux in infants is associated with gastric hyperacidity.

Clinical Findings

Infants

The signs and ultimate morbidity of gastroesophageal reflux in infants are primarily related to insufficiency of nutritional intake as a result of repeated vomiting. A clinical picture evolves that merges with other ill-defined feeding problems of this age group. Aspiration and recurrent pneumonia occur in 15–30% of babies with gastroesophageal reflux. Esophagitis is rare. The diagnoses at the time of admission to the hospital of patients who subsequently are found to have gastroesophageal reflux vary widely (Table 43–7). The list emphasizes the spectrum of diagnostic entities that such patients may mimic; included are: pneumonia, asthma, vascular ring, H-type tracheoesophageal fistula, pyloric stenosis and congenital heart disease. Even more striking are patients seen after protracted gastroesophageal reflux. By presenting a picture of inanition and underdevelopment, these patients may mimic sepsis, hypothyroidism, lead intoxication or chronic brain syndrome. Some babies may present with anemia associated with chronic blood loss from esophagitis, but episodes of major upper gastrointestinal hemorrhage are rare. The diagnosis of pathologic gastrointestinal reflux should be considered in all infants with (1) unexplained persistent vomiting, (2) failure of anticipated growth and weight gain, (3) repeated respiratory infections, (4) apneic spells and (5) anemia.[25, 36, 38, 43]

Vomiting.—Vomiting is the major consequence of gastroesophageal reflux, and well over 90% of infants present with this symptom. In 60% of the cases, regurgitation of feedings begins in the first week of life. The vomiting has been characterized as an effortless regurgitation of undigest-

TABLE 43–7.—ADMITTING DIAGNOSES IN
HOSPITALIZED CHILDREN° SUBSEQUENTLY
SHOWN TO HAVE GASTROESOPHAGEAL REFLUX

Feeding problem	13
Pneumonia	7
Pyloric stenosis	7
Anemia	6
Peptic ulcer	6
Milk allergy	4
GE reflux/hiatal hernia	3
Other	6
TOTAL	52

°Children's Hospital, Washington, D. C.

ed food occurring when the infant is recumbent. However, of the infants studied in our own institution, only a few showed this distinctive pattern. Fifty percent of our patients vomited projectilely and raised the question of hypertrophic pyloric stenosis. Hematemesis is rare, but coffee-ground vomitus was found in 6% of our patients.

FAILURE TO THRIVE.—The term "failure to thrive" has been applied rather generally in pediatric parlance to infants whose weight gain, growth and general development have been below the expected norm. In such patients, weight gain and over-all physical development may be subnormal for years. In a series of 20 infants discovered to have gastroesophageal reflux as the basis for their failure to thrive, all were below the tenth percentile in weight and growth.[35] Regurgitation of feedings was present in varying degrees in most of these patients. Included in this group were babies admitted with an erroneous presumptive diagnosis of hypothyroidism and lead intoxication, diagnoses suggested by the starving, listless appearance of these infants.

RECURRENT ASPIRATION AND PNEUMONITIS.—The respiratory complications of gastroesophageal reflux occur in approximately 20% of patients. Seven of 52 infants treated in our hospital for gastroesophageal reflux had pneumonia and in 4 patients there had been repeated hospitalizations for pneumonia. Tentative diagnoses of congenital heart disease, asthma, vascular ring and H-type tracheoesophageal fistula were entertained before the true cause was established.

BLEEDING.—Anemia associated with hiatal hernia results from chronic blood loss secondary to peptic esophagitis. Frank hematemesis occurred in only 2 of the 52 patients from our institution, but 11 children had occult blood in the vomitus or the stool. Six of these patients were sufficiently anemic to require blood transfusions. In this group, the complications of pernicious reflux tended to obscure the underlying disease. Only after radiographic demonstration of the gastroesophageal reflux was the etiology of the anemia unmasked and subsequently cured by appropriate therapy.

Children

In children 2 years of age and older, the symptoms and consequences of gastroesophageal reflux are similar to those seen in adult patients.[12-15, 27] The interesting exception is Sandifer's syndrome, wherein children angulate and twist the neck, so closing the esophagus and preventing vomiting.[50] Children and adolescents with gastroesophageal reflux are more likely to show radiologic and endoscopic evidence of gastric herniation at the hiatus. They complain of substernal burning, eructation and upper abdominal discomfort. Children suffering from gastroesophageal reflux with or without hiatal hernia seem to develop strictures more frequently than do adults.[10, 14, 41] It is uncommon that a child or adolescent will suffer from recurrent pulmonary problems secondary to aspiration. However, gastroesophageal reflux and aspiration may be related to asthma or the development of chronic bronchiectasis in childhood, and these potential relationships have been overlooked in some patients.[23] Major hemorrhage from esophagitis is rare in children and adolescents, but occult bleeding may be persistent and debilitating.[36] Gastroesophageal reflux should be considered in the differential diagnosis of children with chronic iron-deficiency anemia. Older children now can be studied with pH and pressure studies in evaluating their need and suitability for operation.

Nonoperative Treatment

A regimen of frequent feeding and the maintenance of an upright posture greater than 60 degrees has controlled the symptoms of more than 80% of infants who suffer with gastroesophageal reflux.[2, 7, 12, 44] Depending on the severity of symptoms, the upright position can be varied from 1 hour after every feeding to 24 hours a day. In the malnourished, weak, underweight baby with reflux, a carefully executed and monitored program of intensive medical management should be carried out in the hospital for 3 weeks. If this controlled regimen reverses the infant's inanition, the regimen can be continued safely in the home environment. On the other hand, if 3 weeks of carefully conducted hospital therapy cannot control vomiting and produce definite weight gain, operative correction should be undertaken. In the less severely afflicted infant, a period of 3 months of home care can be used to determine the efficiency of nonoperative therapy. Dietary control has little to offer children, but restriction of feeding after 6 P.M. to aid in gastric emptying before sleeping appears useful.[24] Elevation of the head of the bed using 8-inch blocks is helpful in controlling reflux at night. The use of anticholinergic drugs in an effort to decrease gastric secretion has been advocated by some. These compounds, however, have also been shown to reduce the pressure in the lower esophagus and to diminish gastric motility.[48] Since such effects actually may increase reflux, we have never used them in the management of our patients.

Indications for Operation

The indications for surgical correction of gastroesophageal reflux in infants are based primarily on failure of the medical regimen. The exception is found in those patients who exhibit a major dislocation of the stomach into the chest. With such anatomic derangement, the inevitable consequences are predictable and include dysphagia, malnutrition, stricture and pressure of the herniated stomach on intrathoracic structures. Operation always is recommended for this group.

The criteria used for the selection of infants for operation have been defined[43] as: (1) persistent vomiting after a sustained rigorous medical regimen, plus one of the following; (2) absent or poor weight gain over an extended period of observation; (3) severe nutritional depletion requiring hospitalization, with no response to 3 weeks of intense medical treatment; (4) recurrent pneumonia; (5) gastrointestinal bleeding from esophagitis; (6) major displacement of the stomach into the chest (Fig. 43–14 and 43–15); (7) stricture (Fig. 43–16); (8) serious family disruption by the incessant vomiting. This last item is necessarily the most controversial and hinges on assessment by the physician caring for the patient and the patient's family; as such, it is a rare indication for operation.

For most older children, at least 6 months of continuous, carefully supervised conservative treatment should be undertaken before a decision for operation is reached. As in adult patients, there are specific exceptions to this period of therapy, which include: (1) symptomatic esophagitis uncontrolled by the medical regimen; (2) esophageal stricture; (3) translocation of a major portion of the stomach into the chest; and (4) pulmonary problems resulting from aspiration. The need for operation varies from 15% to 30% of those pediatric patients identified as having pathologic gastroesophageal reflux. Carcassonne of Marseilles[15] operated on 46 infants and children in a series of 154 patients seen with symptomatic reflux. Cahill, Aberdeen and Waterston[14] reported

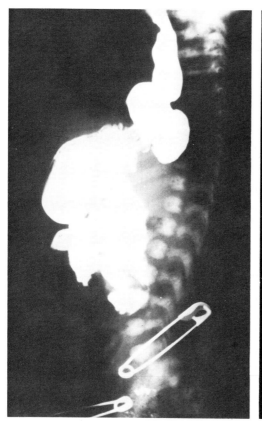

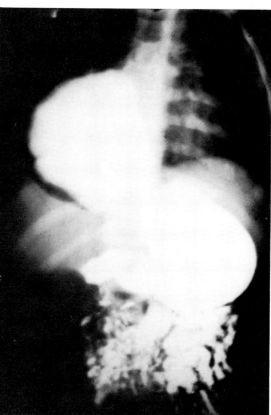

Fig. 43–14 (*left*).—Sliding hiatal hernia. Esophagogram in a 3-day-old infant. This infant was admitted for massive vomiting. Major displacement of the stomach into the chest is an indication for prompt operation.

Fig. 43–15 (*right*).—Paraesophageal hernia. Contrast x-ray study in a 9-

month-old infant. The cardia is below the diaphragm but most of the body of the stomach lies in a paraesophageal hernia sac adjacent to the pericardium. Operation should be advised for such patients. Obstruction, bleeding or strangulation can all occur.

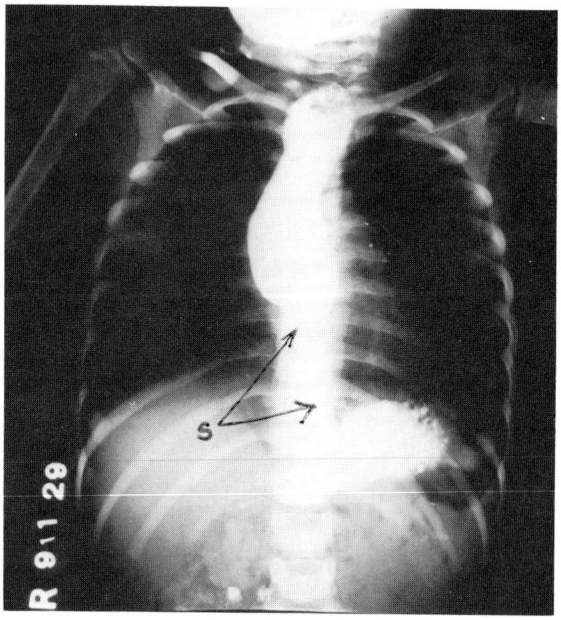

that 102 children were selected for operation from 755 from London and its environs who were diagnosed with hiatal hernia and reflux.

Surgical Treatment

Although there is no argument as to the objective of the operation, namely elimination of reflux, there is considerable controversy as to the best procedure to accomplish this goal. Skinner and Belsey[47] have listed the four functions of the normal cardia, believing that all of these should be preserved or enhanced by surgical repair: (1) to permit the unimpeded passage of food; (2) to prevent the reflux of acid, peptic or pancreatico-biliary secretions into the esophagus; (3) to permit the voluntary eructation of air trapped in the stomach; (4) to permit gastric evacuation by vomiting when necessary. Until recent years, most children with hiatal hernia and/or gastroesophageal reflux were treated with the basic Allison[1] repair. Recurrences after this procedure have led to other approaches. The three operations used in children are, in order of frequency: (1) Nissen fundoplication,[40] (2) Boerema gastropexy[9] and (3) Belsey Mark IV repair.[5] As yet, the Hill[31] repair has not been used extensively in children. The aim of all procedures is the creation of an intra-abdominal segment of esophagus and the fixation of the stomach in its normal position beneath the diaphragm.

Thoracic vs Abdominal Approach

In infants and children, successful repair of an uncomplicated hiatal hernia can be accomplished with equal ease

Fig. 43–16.—Reflux esophagitis and stricture. A 4-month-old baby who now shows relatively little herniation. The esophagus is strictured below and dilated above.

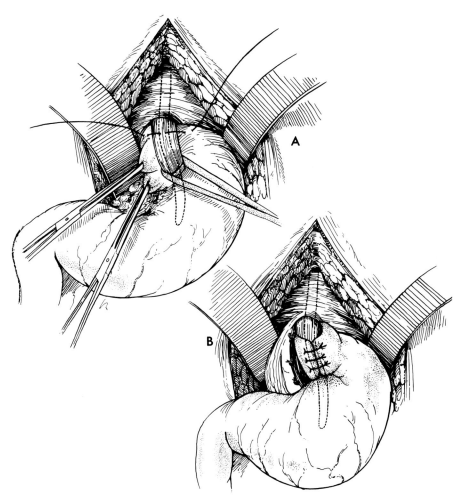

Fig. 43–17.—Nissen fundoplication. **A,** the first suture has been placed to draw the fundus around the gastroesophageal junction. Note that the suture passes through esophageal muscle. **B,** completed fundoplication.

through the chest or through the abdomen. Proponents of the thoracic route maintain that this approach permits assessment of the distal esophagus for external evidence of disease. The chest affords a more direct approach in patients with stricture, who may require revision or resection of the diseased esophagus. The advocates of an abdominal approach point out that infants and young children tolerate the abdominal approach well, the exposure is excellent and allows accurate evaluation of the esophagogastric junction and anatomic relationships around the hiatus. The left lobe of the liver is easily reflected. The abdominal approach also affords ready access for pyloroplasty in those children who also have outlet obstruction. Additionally, a gastrostomy, sometimes needed for uninterrupted alimentation of the depleted infant, is readily performed through the abdomen.

The Nissen Fundoplication (Figs. 43–17 and 43–18)

The Nissen operation is conceptually sound, technically simple to perform and mechanically effective. Through an upper abdominal incision, 2 or 3 cm of esophagus are dissected free and drawn into the abdomen. One or two sutures are placed posteriorly in the crura to narrow the aperture. A catheter of appropriate size (#20 for infants, #24 for children) is passed into the stomach from above and the repair then is carried out around the esophagus with the tube in place. With a tape around the cardia to provide traction, the fundus is passed behind the esophagus and brought around it as a collar. The anterior and posterior portions of this collar

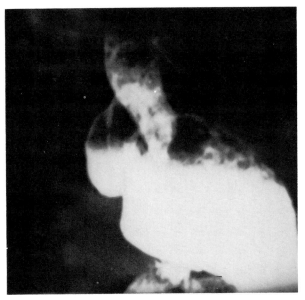

Fig. 43–18.—Nissen fundoplication—barium study. Note valve effect of the fundus around the cardia.

are sutured to the esophagus and to each other using three or four nonabsorbable sutures. The esophageal bite is important to prevent the newly constructed gastric valve from sliding up and down. An additional suture uniting the esophagus, fundus and diaphragm is useful for anchoring the valve below the diaphragm.

The Boerema Gastropexy

The important features of the Boerema operation are: (1) mobilization of the left liver lobe to obtain adequate exposure of the esophageal hiatus; (2) reduction of the hernia into the abdomen; and (3) approximation of the fibers of the lesser curvature of the stomach against the right anterior abdominal wall. To accomplish this, a row of five or six nonabsorbable seromuscular sutures are placed just anterior to the lesser curvature. The stomach is retracted caudally and the sutures are carried to the right side of the linea alba and tied with the knots on the anterior surface of the aponeurosis. It is essential that the lesser curvature be fixed to the abdominal wall under considerable tension.

The Belsey Mark IV Operation (Fig. 43–19)

Through a thoracic incision, the distal esophagus and proximal stomach are carefully dissected free. Two or three sutures are placed in the crura to be tied after the remainder of the repair has been completed. Two rows of vertical mattress sutures are used to invert the esophagus downward into the stomach. The proximal stomach thus is pulled upward, creating a valvular mechanism around the distal

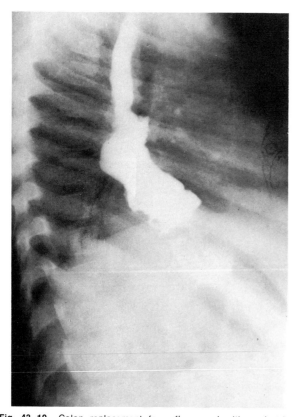

Fig. 43–19.—Colon replacement for reflux esophagitis and stricture. This child had a severe stricture treated by hernia repair and repeated esophageal dilatations. Progression of the stricture ultimately required resection and replacement. An effective antireflux operation usually will make such replacement unnecessary.

esophagus. The sutures pass through the diaphragm, the fundus and then the esophagus. A spoon retractor is used to allow proper placement of key sutures and to reposition the valve beneath the diaphragm as the sutures are tied down. The crural sutures then are tied, creating a posterior buttress against which the abdominal segment of the esophagus can be compressed.

Pyloroplasty

Patients with partial gastric outlet obstruction and delayed emptying of the stomach may benefit from concomitant pyloroplasty. Authors have varied in their opinion as to the necessity for this measure. Ament has had no patient in whom pyloroplasty was recommended at the time of hiatal hernia repair.[24] Delayed gastric emptying, albeit a somewhat subjective impression of the radiologist, has been identified in 25% of our patients of all ages. In these children, a concomitant pyloroplasty has been performed.[42, 43] Johnson has not found this in his patients.[33] A few children with this finding on postoperative gastrointestinal x-ray study have required pyloroplasty as a secondary procedure several weeks to a month later.

Results of Repair

The incidence of recurrence seems to be higher in children than in adults. Skinner and Belsey of Bristol report a recurrence rate of 58% in 19 children operated on under 2 years of age.[47] In the series of infants under a year of age from Washington Children's Hospital there were 4 recurrences in 31 patients (13%).[43] Carcassonne *et al.* of Marseilles reported 3 deaths and 4 strictures that required a second operation in 46 patients.[15] However, this group reported no recurrences when the Nissen procedure was combined with the Boerema gastropexy. Vos and Boerema of the Netherlands report 25 of 27 children with a normal x-ray after gastropexy.[51] Two had minimal reflux and 1 patient developed an esophageal stenosis that led to his death. Johnson *et al.*, of Salt Lake City reporting 55 children of all ages, achieved good results in 51 using the Boerema gastropexy.[33]

In infants, burping may be difficult after a successful repair. The "gas bloat" syndrome follows the Nissen repair in occasional patients; this unpleasant consequence of successful valve construction is marked by abdominal distention and an inability to vomit. Patients may require gastric aspiration for relief; these occurrences usually cease 2 or 3 months after operation. Operation for gastroesophageal reflux is successful in infants and children. Symptoms are controlled and normal growth is achieved. The operative procedures described above all seem to be equally effective in the hands of surgeons experienced in their use.

Treatment of Esophageal Stricture

The incidence of esophageal stricture varies widely in reported series. There is an unexplained prevalence of strictures in the patient material reported in Europe not seen in the United States.[14] Most strictures will respond to repeated esophageal dilatation if the gastroesophageal reflux is surgically eliminated. If the stricture is unyielding, either resection or a plastic procedure on the esophagus is recommended. The Thal seromuscular patch operation is well suited to children.[50a] For this operation, the esophagus and upper stomach are mobilized as in the Belsey procedure. An incision is made into the lumen of the esophagus beginning above the stricture and carried downward onto the fundus of the stomach. A portion of the fundus is folded over the defect and sutured so that the serosa of the stomach presents on the inner surface of the esophagus. There is a significant incidence of recurrent stricture following Thal's original operation, unless full fundoplication to eliminate reflux is carried out simultaneously, as advocated by Woodward.[52]

Some strictures are so extensive or accompanied by such inflammation that resection of the distal esophagus is necessary. In these patients, re-establishment of the continuity is best accomplished by utilizing a short segment of colon (see Fig. 43–19). This approach offers the best protection against recurrent reflux and esophagitis. After resection of the involved portion of the esophagus, a segment of colon is transposed on its vascular pedicle, through the hiatus. An anastomosis is created between the colon and the middle portion of the esophagus below the aortic arch; the distal colon segment is joined to the upper stomach. Following this type of reconstruction, reflux is minimal. The colon clears mucous secretions quite well and the complication rate is low. Direct anastomosis of the stomach to the midesophagus re-creates the reflux problem, invites esophagitis, causes some degree of pulmonary compression and is not to be performed.

In summary, gastroesophageal reflux is a common finding in infants. In the early months of life, reflux can be controlled by postural therapy; thereafter, the reflux disappears. In some babies, conservative therapy is ineffective and malnutrition and respiratory problems supervene. For such patients, operation is advised. In older children, complaints, pathology and surgical decisions are similar to those found in adult patients.

REFERENCES

1. Allison, P. R.: Reflux esophagitis, sliding hiatal hernia, and the anatomy of repair, Surg. Gynecol. Obstet. 92:419, 1951.
2. Astley, R., and Carre, I. J.: Gastroesophageal incompetence in children with special reference to minor degrees of partial thoracic stomach, Radiology 62:351, 1954.
3. Avery, G. B., Randolph. J. G., and Weaver, T. H.: Gastric response to specific disease in infants, Pediatrics 38:874, 1966.
4. Baue, A. E., and Belsey, R. H.: The treatment of sliding hiatal hernia and reflux esophagitis by the Mark IV technique, Surgery 62:396, 1967.
5. Belsey, R.: Surgery of the Diaphragm, in Brown, J. M. (ed.), *Surgery of Children* (Baltimore: The Williams & Wilkins Company, 1963), p. 762.
6. Benz, L. J., *et al.*: A comparison of clinical measurements of gastroesophageal reflux, Gastroenterology 62:1, 1972.
7. Berenberg, W., and Neuhauser, E. B. D.: Cardio-esophageal relaxation (chalasia) as a cause of vomiting in infants, Pediatrics 5:414, 1950.
8. Bettex, M., and Kuffer, F.: Long-term results of fundoplication in hiatus hernia and cardio-esophageal chalasia in infants and children: Report of 112 consecutive cases, J. Pediatr. Surg. 4:526, 1969.
9. Boerema, I., and Germs, R.: Fixation of the lesser curvature of the stomach to the anterior abdominal wall after repositioning of the hernia through the esophageal hiatus, Arch. Chir. Neerl. 7:351, 1955.
10. Boix, O. J., and Rehbein, F.: Esophageal stenosis due to reflux oesophagitis, Arch. Dis. Child. 40:197, 1965.
11. Botha, G. S. M.: Gastroesophageal region in infants. Observations on anatomy, with special reference to closing mechanism and partial thoracic stomach, Arch. Dis. Child. 33:78, 1958.
12. Brown, F. V., *et al.*: Medical and surgical management of esophageal hiatus hernia in children, Bol. Med. Hosp. Infant. Mex. 41:17, 1963.
13. Burke, J. B.: Partial thoracic stomach in childhood, Br. Med. J. 2:787, 1959.
14. Cahill, J. L., Aberdeen, E., and Waterston, D. J.: Results of surgical treatment of esophageal hiatus hernia in infancy and childhood, Surgery 66:597, 1969.
15. Carcassonne, J., Bensoussan, A., and Aubert, J.: The management of gastroesophageal reflux in infants, J. Pediatr. Surg. 8:574, 1973.
16. Carré, I. J.: Natural history of partial thoracic stomach ("hiatus hernia") in children, Arch. Dis. Child. 34:344, 1959.
17. Carré, I. J.: Postural treatment of children with partial thoracic stomach ("hiatus hernia"), Arch. Dis. Child. 35:569, 1960.
18. Carré, I. J., and Astley, R.: Gastroesophageal junction in infancy: Combined cineradiographic and manometric study, Thorax 13:159, 1958.
19. Chrispin, A. R., and Friedland, G. W.: Functional disturbance in hiatal hernia in infants and children, Thorax 22:422, 1967.
20. Cravioto, J., Delicardie, E. R., and Birch, H. G.: Nutrition, growth, and neuro-integrative development: An experimental and ecologic study, Pediatrics 38:319, 1966.
21. Darling, D. B.: Hiatal hernia and gastroesophageal reflux in infancy and childhood: Analysis of the radiologic findings, Am. J. Roentgenol. 123:724, 1975.
22. Darling, D. B., Fisher, J. H., and Gellis, S.: Hiatal hernia and gastroesophageal reflux in infants and children: Analysis of incidence in North American children, Pediatrics 54:450, 1974.
23. Dees, S. C.: The role of gastroesophageal reflux in nocturnal asthma in children, N. C. Med. J. 35:230, 1974.
24. Euler, A. R., and Ament, M. E.: Gastroesophageal reflux in children: Clinical manifestations, diagnosis, pathophysiology, and therapy, Pediatr. Ann. 5:678, 1976.
25. Filler, R. M., Randolph, J. G., and Gross, R. E.: Esophageal hiatus hernia in infants and children, J. Thorac. Cardiovasc. Surg. 47:551, 1964.
26. Fisher, H. S., *et al.*: Gastroesophageal (GE) scintiscanning to detect and quantitate GE reflux, Gastroenterology 70:301, 1976.
27. Forshall, I.: Cardio-esophageal syndrome in childhood, Arch. Dis. Child. 30:46, 1955.
28. Friedland, G. W., Dodds, W. J., Sunshine, P., and Zboralske, F. F.: Apparent disparity in incidence of hiatal hernia in infants and children in Britain and United States, Am. J. Roentgenol. 120:305, 1974.
29. Fyke, F. E., Code, C. F., and Schlegel, J. F.: The gastroesophageal sphincter in healthy human beings, Gastroenterologia 86:135, 1956.
30. Hiebert, C. A., and Belsey, R.: Incompetency of the gastric cardia without radiological evidence of hiatus hernia, J. Thorac. Cardiovasc. Surg. 42:352, 1961.
31. Hill, L. D.: An effective operation for hiatal hernia, Ann. Surg. 166:681, 1967.
32. Jewett, T. C., and Waterston, D. J.: Surgical management of hiatal hernia in children, J. Pediatr. Surg. 10:757, 1975.
33. Johnson, D. G., Herbst, J. R., Oliveros, M. A., and Stewart, D. R.: Evaluation of gastroesophageal reflux surgery in children, Pediatrics 59:62, 1977.
34. Kamal, I., and Guiney, E. J.: The treatment of hiatus hernia in children by anterior gastropexy, J. Pediatr. Surg. 7:641, 1972.
35. Lilly, J. R., LoPresti, J., and Randolph, J. G.: Hiatal hernia in infants, South. Med. J. 60:545, 1967.
36. Lilly, J. R., and Randolph, J. G.: Hiatal hernia and gastroesophageal reflux in infants and children, J. Thorac. Cardiovasc. Surg. 55:42, 1968.
37. Listerud, M. D.: Details of interest and controversy in the anatomy of the esophageal hiatus and hiatal hernia, Surg. Clin. North Am. 44:1211, 1964.
38. McNamara, J. J., Paulson, D. L., and Urschel, H. C.: Hiatus hernia and gastroesophageal reflux in children, Pediatrics 43:527, 1969.
39. Neuhauser, E. B. D., and Berenberg, W.: Cardio-esophageal relaxation as cause of vomiting in infants, Radiology 48:480, 1947.
40. Nissen, R., and Rossetti, M.: *Die Behandlung von Hiatushernien und Reflux-Oesophagitis mit Gastropexie und Fundoplication* (Stuttgart: Georg Thieme Verlag, 1959).
41. Pieretti, R., Shandling, B., and Stephens, C. A.: Resistant esophageal stenosis associated with reflux after repair of esophageal atresia: A therapeutic approach, J. Pediatr. Surg. 9:355, 1974.
42. Randolph, J. G.: Pedicle pyloroplasty, J. Pediatr. Surg. 6:388, 1971.
43. Randolph, J. G., Lilly, J. R., and Anderson, K. D.: Surgical treatment of gastroesophageal reflux in infants, Ann. Surg. 180:479, 1974.
44. Ravitch, M. M.: Chalasia and Achalasia of the Esophagus, in Benson, C. D., *et al.* (eds.), *Pediatric Surgery* (Chicago: Year Book Medical Publishers, Inc., 1962), p. 299.

44a. Ravitch, M. M.: Personal communication.

45. Rohatgi, M., Shandling, B., and Stephens, C. A.: Hiatus hernia in infants and children: Results of surgical treatment, Surgery 69:456, 1971.

46. Roviralta, E.: *Les Vomissements du Nourrison* (Paris: Flammarion, 1952).

47. Skinner, D. B., and Belsey, H. R.: Surgical management of esophageal reflux and hiatus hernia: Long-term results with 1030 patients, J. Thorac. Cardiovasc. Surg. 53:33, 1967.

48. Skinner, D. B., and DeMeester, T. R.: Gastroesophageal Reflux, in *Current Problems in Surgery* (Chicago: Year Book Medical Publishers, Inc., January, 1976).

49. Strawczynski, H., Beck, I. T., McKenna, R. D., and Nickerson, G. H.: Behavior of lower esophageal sphincter in infants and its relationship to gastroesophageal regurgitation, Pediatrics 64:17, 1964.

50. Sutcliffe, J.: Torsion spasms and abnormal postures in children with hiatal hernia (Sandifer's syndrome), Prog. Pediatr. Radiol. 2:190, 1969.

50a. Thal, A.: A unified approach to surgical problems of the esophagogastric junction, Ann. Surg. 168:542, 1968.

51. Vos, A., and Boerema, I.: Surgical treatment of gastroesophageal reflux in infants and children: Long-term results in 28 cases, J. Pediatr. Surg. 6:101, 1971.

52. Woodward, E. R., and Hollenbeck, J. I.: The treatment of peptic-esophageal stricture with combined fundic patch-fundoplication, Ann. Surg. 182:472, 1975.

53. Wylie, W. G., and Field, E. C.: The etiology of intermittent oesophageal regurgitation and haematemesis in infants, Arch. Dis. Child. 21:218, 1946.

Replacement of the Esophagus

JUDSON G. RANDOLPH / KATHRYN D. ANDERSON

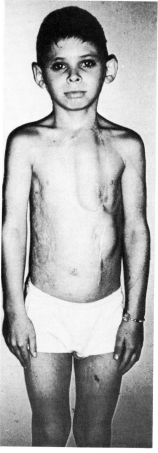

Fig. 43–20.—An early survivor born with esophageal atresia, reconstructed by antethoracic skin tube, linked with free skin graft, bridging the gap between upper esophagus and stomach. (From Gross, R. E.[20])

HISTORY.—The challenge of esophageal replacement has occupied surgeons since 1877, when Czerny[12] described cervical esophagectomy with reconstruction. Historically, skin tubes,[7, 20] various intestinal conduits[41, 51] and transposition of the stomach into the thorax[49] have been used for esophageal replacement. The first attempt at replacement of the esophagus by an antethoracic skin tube was by Bircher in 1894.[7] Following his attempts there were a number of reports in the Russian and German literature using this technique and modifications. In 1934, Ochsner and Owens[39] found 32 cases in which skin was used to reconstruct the esophagus, but few of these patients were children. Among the earliest children to receive antethoracic skin tubes were the rare survivors of esophageal atresia and tracheoesophageal fistula reported by Ladd, Lanman and Gross.[20] The skin conduits were used to bridge the gaps between the exteriorized esophageal pouch and the stomach (Fig. 43-20) and were performed in many stages. A useful surgical procedure at that time, the development of safe intrathoracic techniques ultimately made the antethoracic skin tube obsolete. Another approach was to advance the stomach into the thorax or even to the neck for anastomosis to the esophagus. This procedure has found frequent use in adult patients as a method of reconstruction after esophageal resection for malignancy. In the child, the volume occupied by the displaced stomach significantly restricts ventilation, and gastric distention can be disastrous. Furthermore, the inevitable gastroesophageal reflux in this location has led to peptic esophagitis, stricture and overflow of gastric acid into the tracheobronchial tree in children in whom this method of esophageal substitution has, therefore, been abandoned. A variety of synthetic tubular prostheses[6, 30, 42] have been used as esophageal substitutes in experimental models without significant success.

Segments of jejunum have been advocated for esophageal replacement, beginning with Roux[41] in 1907 and continued by Yudin[51] and by Merendino.[36] The principal disadvantages of this technique are related to the serpentine looping of excess jejunum brought up to the neck to allow the mesenteric vessels to be free from tension. Peptic ulceration of jejunal loops has occurred near the anastomosis with the stomach. Although some surgeons continue to use small bowel interposition successfully in children, this method has not achieved wide usage.[14]

Colon interposition originally was used for esophageal substitu-

tion in adult patients after resection for cancer.[29, 34] In 1955, Dale and Sherman[13] demonstrated the effectiveness of the colon for esophageal reconstruction in children. The colon continues to be the most widely used method of esophageal replacement in children.[21, 27, 31, 37, 50] However, in specific clinical circumstances, the colon may be unsuitable. In these instances, the reversed gastric tube, suggested by Jianu,[28] developed by Gavriliu[18] and popularized in the United States by Heimlich,[23, 24] has proved to be a satisfactory alternative for esophageal reconstruction in adults and in children.[2, 9, 43]

Indications

In children, the two most common indications for esophageal substitution are congenital esophageal atresia and caustic esophageal stricture. In most babies with isolated esophageal atresia, the distal segment of the esophagus is virtually absent. An increasing number of patients have been reported in whom successful primary esophageal anastomosis has been achieved after the upper and lower pouches have been dilated or stretched[22] (see Congenital Esophageal Atresia and Tracheoesophageal Fistula earlier in this chapter). Nevertheless, in many infants born with isolated esophageal atresia and in occasional infants with atresia and tracheoesophageal fistula, the distance between the upper and lower pouches precludes primary anastomosis. For such patients, an esophageal substitution procedure is required.

Esophageal stricture secondary to the ingestion of corro-

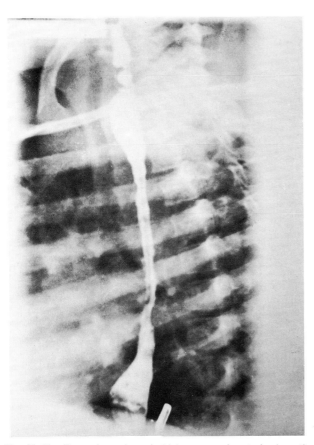

Fig. 43-21.—X-ray of esophageal stricture secondary to lye ingestion; esophageal replacement required.

sive materials is the second major indication for esophageal replacement (Fig. 43-21). Although most caustic esophageal strictures can be managed by repeated esophageal dilatations, there are many children in whom dilatation fails to produce an adequately functioning esophagus. Rarely, reflux esophagitis will produce such severe strictures that replacement of a portion of the esophagus is required.[5, 47] Recent advances in the technique of portosystemic shunts[1, 10] in small children have all but eliminated the necessity for esophageal replacement for hemorrhage from esophageal varices.

Aims in Selection of an Esophageal Substitute

In esophageal replacement, the following criteria are paramount: (1) the substitute esophagus must function as an efficient conduit from mouth to stomach to satisfy the nutritional needs of the child; (2) reflux of gastric acid into the conduit must be minimized or, if reflux occurs, the substitute esophagus itself must be resistant to gastric acid; (3) ventilatory mechanics must not be impaired by the bypass; (4) the operative procedure must be technically adaptable to small children; (5) placement of the conduit must be such that the child has little or no external deformity.

Timing of Operation

Although major surgical procedures can be carried out safely in the newborn period, there seems little merit in performing an esophageal replacement at this time. There is a severe potential disadvantage to having an infant swallow into an immobile conduit before he is able to sit unsupported. Because the aperistaltic bypass empties only by gravity, the recumbent infant is at risk from aspiration. Since an infant's nutritional requirements can be temporarily met by gastrostomy feedings, the recommended time for esophageal substitution is at 8-12 months or when the infant's weight is close to 20 pounds. By this time, an infant usually can sit alone and the risk of aspiration is diminished.

The Colon

The colon functions as a satisfactory conduit for passage of food and is considered by many surgeons to be the organ of choice for esophageal substitution. Overflow from the colon segment into the trachea is unusual and can largely be avoided by training the children to eat slowly in the upright position. The colon is readily accommodated in the chest. Although gastric reflux with ulceration of the unprotected mucosa and stricture formation are complications that have been noted in children,[26] these are not common sequelae. The right or left colon can be used with equal success; antiperistaltic and isoperistaltic arrangements seem to function equally well. Long-term follow-up studies have confirmed the ability of a properly constructed colon interposition to support nutrition in a growing child.

In planning for coloesophagoplasty, a barium enema is obtained to observe the rotation of the colon, its anatomic configuration and the presence of any anomalies or occult disease. A clear liquid or an elemental diet is given for 48 hours prior to operation, and a standard mechanical preparation of the bowel is carried out immediately prior to operation. Parenteral antibiotics are begun 24 hours before the procedure.

Operative Technique for Colon Interposition

A transverse incision, dividing both rectus muscles above the umbilicus, provides excellent exposure of the entire colon. Sufficient mobilization of both right and left colon is carried out to allow detailed assessment of the entire blood supply. Vascular clamps are placed on the right colic and ileocolic vessels to isolate the middle colic artery, and the right colon is carefully observed for signs of ischemia before these vessels are divided and the terminal ileum transected. The transverse colon is again transected the required measured distance distal to the middle colic artery. Ileocolic anastomosis and appendectomy are performed. An opening is made in the hepatogastric ligament so that the right colon with its vascular pedicle can be passed behind the stomach without kinking the middle colic artery (Fig. 43-22). After making an incision in the left side of the neck above the jugular notch, a retrosternal tunnel is created by blunt dissection. The tunnel must be adequate to admit the colon segment and its vascular pedicle without compromise. The colon segment then is drawn carefully through the tunnel and brought out the cervical incision (see Fig. 43-22). When using the right colon, it is easiest to orient it in an isoperistaltic manner with the most proximal colon in the neck. The lower end of the colon is anastomosed to the proximal stomach,[5, 13] eliminating redundancy in the colon insofar as possible. The cecum or terminal ileum is anastomosed to the mobilized upper esophagus using a single layer of interrupted nonabsorbable sutures. If there is any question regarding the adequacy of blood supply, the upper colonic segment is exteriorized in the neck and anastomosis deferred for 7-10 days. Pyloroplasty often is performed in conjunction with coloesophagoplasty.[21, 32]

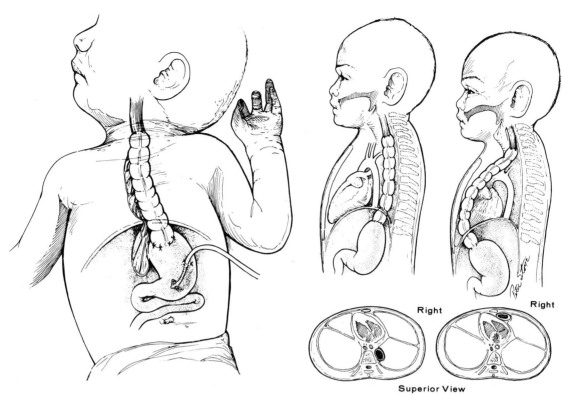

Fig. 43–22.—Colon esophagoplasty; the colon may be placed in a retrosternal or retrohilar position with equal success. (From Randolph, J. G.: Surgical Problems of the Esophagus, in Sabiston, D., and Spencer, F. (eds.): *Gibbon's Surgery of the Chest* [3d ed.; Philadelphia: W. B. Saunders Co., 1976.])

Retrohilar transposition of the transverse and left colon on a pedicle of left colic artery was first described by Waterston.[50] In his original description, the entire procedure was performed through a thoracic approach, the diaphragm being incised peripherally to expose the abdominal contents. Separate abdominal and thoracic incisions may be used, however. After mobilization and division of the middle colic artery, the left colon is transposed isoperistaltically on the vascular pedicle of the left colic artery. The colon is drawn posterior to the stomach and pancreas and through an incision in the diaphragm, posterolateral to the esophageal hiatus. The colon segment is placed behind the hilum of the left lung, and the upper end is brought into the neck by tunneling through Sibson's fascia posterior to the subclavian vessels and lateral to the carotid sheath. If the colon interposition is being performed for esophageal atresia, the distal colonic anastomosis may be made to the short lower esophageal remnant. A gastrostomy always is performed.

After coloesophagoplasty, the patient should be kept in a semiupright position. Appropriate antibiotics are administered systemically for 10 days. Gastrostomy feedings usually are begun on the fifth day. A barium swallow should be obtained at 10 to 12 days to confirm the integrity of the anastomosis before oral feedings are begun.

Results

Since the first reports of colon transposition in children there has been a steady improvement in the morbidity and mortality. In a report by Gross and Firestone[21] there was only 1 death in 47 patients. Other authors have reported similar low mortality rates.[4, 26, 46, 48, 50] The incidence of immediate and long-term complications, however, remains signif-

icant in all hands. Fortunately, most of these can be treated satisfactorily or are self-limiting. Salivary fistula from the upper anastomosis is the most common postoperative complication.[4, 8, 32, 38, 44, 46] Such fistulas usually close spontaneously and only rarely require formal operative repair.[4, 46] Anastomotic stricture is not uncommon, particularly if a salivary leak has occurred.[4, 15, 44] The occasional stricture at the distal anastomosis is particularly troublesome because dilatation at this level is mechanically difficult and operative revision often is necessary.[4, 8, 21, 44] The most serious complication of colon bypass is compromise of the vascular supply to the colon, with consequent ischemia and necrosis. This error may result from misjudgment of the adequacy of the vascular arcade of the transposed colon, from inadvertent interruption of anomalous venous supply, from compression of the segment in the various apertures in its new course or from excessive tension. Major ischemia or infarction requires immediate removal of the conduit. Minor degrees of ischemia, even though insufficient to produce frank necrosis of the colon segment, can result in fibrosis and shortening.[33] Additional conduit length in such cases may be obtained by multiple linear, transverse incisions in the seromuscular coat along the teniae.[33] This maneuver permits elongation of the colon and may salvage a foreshortened colon.

Aspiration of material from the colon into the trachea, as a consequence of delayed colonic emptying,[44] is aggravated by the recumbent position. Propping up the child and elevation of the head at night may be necessary for many months postoperatively.[4] Lesser degrees of gastroesophageal reflux into the colon conduit can occur because of absence of a sphincter mechanism at the gastrocolonic junction. Persistent gastric reflux into the colon conduit

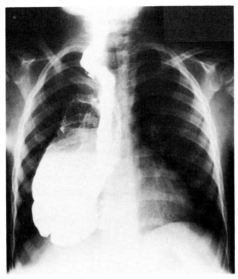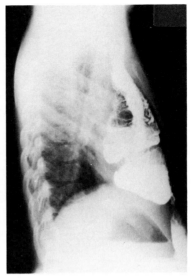

Fig. 43–23.—Transposed colon with marked redundancy and characteristic cascading of barium through the conduit. Nutrition and swallowing normal.

suggests the need for pyloroplasty if delayed emptying is demonstrated.[21, 32]

Peristalsis in the colonic segment is largely ineffective and food is conducted into the stomach by gravity.[8, 40, 44] Sieber and Sieber[45] studied transposed colon segments manometrically and concluded that the colon is without active peristaltic waves. Distally, no pressure barrier was identified to prevent gastrocolic reflux. The intrathoracic colon may assume a markedly redundant configuration postoperatively (Fig. 43–23), which may contribute to delayed emptying of the conduit, thereby increasing the risk of regurgitation and aspiration. This redundancy may be observed incidentally in the absence of symptoms.[29, 44, 48]

Colon interposition has proved to be an effective method of substituting for a diseased or absent esophagus.[4, 21, 26, 44] Several major centers have reported their long-term follow-up of children who have had colon interposition, and these results represent an accumulation of some 190 children with follow-up ranging from 1 year to as long as 16 years[4, 15, 21, 32, 44, 46, 48] (Table 43–8). Waterston followed 53 patients for up to 16 years[4]; of these, 44 patients were classified as having a good or excellent result. These children were all eating normal diets and their weight curves were normal. Schiller et al.[44] reported an 11-year follow-up on 24 patients. Nineteen of these children had good to excellent results; all patients were able to eat a regular diet, although none ate rapidly and regurgitation was demonstrated with swallowing in the recumbent position. In an earlier report from the same institution, Othersen and Clatworthy[40] reported that the children were in the lower percentile of their growth curves; but, in the later report, growth was reported as normal. Thus, although patients may be in the lower percentiles of growth, catch-up growth later restores them to normal weights. This catch-up growth is demonstrated even in the few patients who have had prolonged problems with diarrhea or malabsorption.[32] Redundancy of the transposed colon is not uncommon but does not seem to be associated with delayed growth.

TABLE 43–8.—LONG-TERM FOLLOW-UP OF PATIENTS WITH COLON INTERPOSITION

AUTHOR	NUMBER OF PATIENTS	LENGTH OF FOLLOW-UP (YEARS)	RESULTS AND COMMENTS
Gross and Firestone[21] (Boston)	47	1–12	"Normal" weight gain. Only 1 patient considered underweight. All patients ate slowly but swallowed well
Louhimo et al.[32] (Finland)	7	1–5	5/7 early growth failure. All had malabsorption; exhibited "catch-up growth" after 3 or 4 years
Singh and Rickham[46] (Liverpool)	12	1–7	Normal weight curves
Schiller et al.[44] (Columbus)	24	Up to 11	Lower percentiles of weight, but normal growth curves. Three patients with persistent diarrhea but normal growth. 19/24 excellent or good; 5/24 fair or poor
Waterston[50] (London) 1955–1971	53	1–16	Weight curves normal. 44/53 excellent or good
German and Waterston[19] (London) 1970–1976	21	Up to 6	14/21 weight curves normal (in 3d–25th percentiles). 14/21 excellent or good; 2/21 fair; 2/21 poor

Strictures of the cervical anastomosis often resolve with time, and dilatation rarely is necessary on a long-term basis. Gastrocolonic reflux remains a hazard, and ulceration of the conduit as a result of reflux must be regarded as a lifelong potential problem.[26, 35] In addition, malignancy of the transposed colon segment may occur, although if a major cause of colonic cancer is absorption of carcinogens during the slow passage through the colon at the end of this digestive process, the intrathoracic colon might be expected to be spared.

The Gastric Tube

Certain clinical situations exist in which the colon is not suitable for an esophageal substitute. These are: (1) an associated high imperforate anus, (2) a poorly developed marginal artery or other abnormality of the vascular arcade, (3) anomalies of the colon itself. To address the shortcomings of the colon in certain clinical circumstances, gastric tube bypass has been applied in children as well as in adults.[2, 9, 11] For the past several years, we have used the gastric tube as the primary substitute for the esophagus. The indications in 15 children are listed in Table 43–9. The gastric tube serves as an eminently satisfactory conduit for food. Reflux of gastric contents into the tube is not of great concern, since the tube is gastric. The ease of constructing the conduit and the reliable vascular supply add to the attraction of this method of substitution. Satisfactory maintenance of nutrition has been confirmed in follow-up evaluation.[2, 11, 17]

Operative Technique

To construct a tube from the greater gastric curvature, it is essential that the entire length of the left gastroepiploic artery, its junction with the right gastroepiploic artery and the right gastroepiploic artery, to the pylorus, be identified and preserved. The right gastroepiploic artery is divided approximately 2 cm proximal to the pylorus. The gastric tube is begun at the point of arterial division by incising the stomach on its greater curvature. The anterior and posterior walls of the stomach then are cut parallel to the greater curvature (Fig. 43–24, A). The flap so created is fashioned into a tube and sutured around a catheter of appropriate size (18 to 24 French) (Fig. 43–24, B). The tube is constructed with an inner mucosal layer of 3-0 absorbable sutures and an outer serosal layer of interrupted 3-0 nonabsorbable sutures. The suture line is interrupted for the initial several centimeters

at its distal (cervical) end so that trimming the tube after construction will not disrupt a continuous suture line. The tube is cut from the stomach and sutured in stages to minimize blood loss; the greater curvature of the stomach is also closed in stages as the tube construction progresses. It is necessary to remove the spleen. The tube readily reaches the neck (Fig. 43–24, C). Like the colon, the gastric tube may be placed substernally or brought through the chest behind the root of the left lung. Creation of a substernal tunnel is accomplished exactly as described above under colon bypass. If the retrohilar position is selected, a left thoracotomy is necessary. A 2-cm incision is made in the diaphragm posterolateral to the esophageal hiatus and the gastric tube drawn through. The vascular pedicle should be protected from kinking and twisting as the tube is passed from the abdomen into the chest and placed behind the lung. Two or three seromuscular sutures anchor the gastric tube to the diaphragm on its thoracic surface. Working through a cervical incision, Sibson's fascia is exposed, a tunnel created in the thoracic inlet posterior to the subclavian vessels and the gastric tube delivered into the neck without torsion. Anastomosis between the gastric tube and the esophagus may be carried out primarily or may be delayed. It is preferable to do the entire procedure in a single stage, since gastric contents refluxing onto the neck can cause both maceration and inflammation of the skin, making subsequent dissection difficult. However, if there is any question about the integrity of the blood supply to the upper end of the tube or if the tube is very edematous after the long procedure,[16] the operation should be staged. The cervical anastomosis between the esophagus and the gastric tube is performed in two layers. The neck incision is drained. The gastrostomy should be re-established.

In the event that the left gastroepiploic artery is not suitable for vascular supply of the tube, this vessel can be divided high on the greater curvature and the tube constructed in the reverse direction on a vascular pedicle originating with the right gastroepiploic artery.[11, 17] In this instance, after creation of the gastric tube, the stomach is rotated posteriorly so that the tube can be delivered into the neck.

Postoperative Management

Gastrostomy feedings are begun after 5 days. Oral feedings can be given on the tenth day if a barium swallow demonstrates integrity of the tube. If the cervical anastomosis has been delayed, the gastric tube can be appraised by inserting a catheter into the stoma and instilling barium into the tube; the cervical anastomosis then is performed 10–14 days after the major procedure, and oral liquids can be started 5 days later.

Results

Contrast studies confirm that the gastric tube serves as an efficient and rapid conduit from mouth to stomach. Furthermore, it retains its tubular shape without development of the redundancy and dilatation often seen in colon segments (Fig. 43–24, D). After 1–3 months, the stomach regains adequate volume to allow a return to regular feeding. Although almost universally present, reflux is not a major problem. It has been shown that reflux can be prevented entirely if a 6-cm segment of the gastric tube remains in the abdomen.[25] This may be difficult to achieve when the entire esophagus is replaced. Like the colon, the gastric tube is aperistaltic and children do not empty the gastric tube well in a recumbent position. Nonetheless, nutritional require-

TABLE 43–9.—GASTRIC TUBE FOR ESOPHAGEAL REPLACEMENT

PATIENT	DIAGNOSIS	AGE	COMMENT
1	Lye stricture	4 years	"Failed" colon
2	Lye stricture	5 years	
3	Lye stricture	3 years	
4	Lye stricture	3 years	Lost to follow-up
5	Esophageal atresia	8 months	
6	Esophageal atresia	8 months	
7	Esophageal atresia	8 months	
8	Esophageal atresia	1 year	Death*
9	Esophageal atresia	1 year	
10	Esophageal atresia	18 months	
11	Esophageal atresia	4 years	"Failed" colon
12	Esophageal atresia	1 year	
13	Lye stricture	3 years	
14	Lye stricture	2 years	
15	Esophageal atresia	1 year	

*Death at 18 months from unrecognized perforation of tube by bougie.

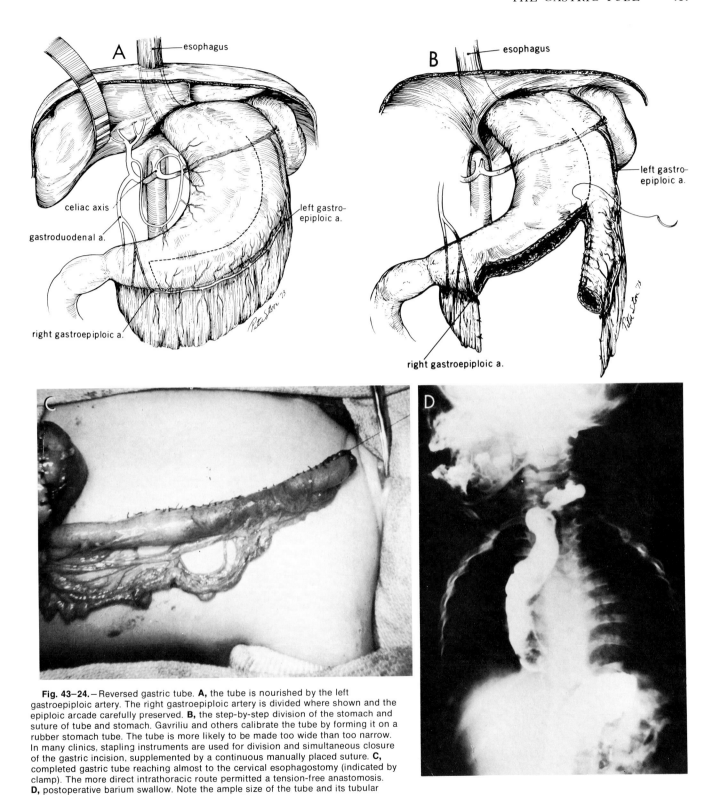

Fig. 43–24.—Reversed gastric tube. **A,** the tube is nourished by the left gastroepiploic artery. The right gastroepiploic artery is divided where shown and the epiploic arcade carefully preserved. **B,** the step-by-step division of the stomach and suture of tube and stomach. Gavriliu and others calibrate the tube by forming it on a rubber stomach tube. The tube is more likely to be made too wide than too narrow. In many clinics, stapling instruments are used for division and simultaneous closure of the gastric incision, supplemented by a continuous manually placed suture. **C,** completed gastric tube reaching almost to the cervical esophagostomy (indicated by clamp). The more direct intrathoracic route permitted a tension-free anastomosis. **D,** postoperative barium swallow. Note the ample size of the tube and its tubular shape. (From Anderson, K. D., and Randolph, J. G.[3])

ments are satisfied in most patients. Although most of our patients are in the lower percentiles for growth, each child's weight curve is satisfactory and developmental landmarks have been normally achieved.

Deaths from this procedure are unusual.[2, 11, 17] In the Children's Hospital National Medical Center series of 15 pa-

tients, 1 patient died 10 months postoperatively when dilatation of a cervical anastomotic stricture resulted in an unrecognized perforation. Salivary fistulas resulting from minor leaks at the cervical anastomosis are not uncommon; but, in our series, all but one closed spontaneously. One gastric tube leaked into the chest, and this was managed satisfacto-

TABLE 43–10.—GASTRIC TUBE FOR
ESOPHAGEAL REPLACEMENT—COMPLICATIONS

	TYPE	TREATMENT
Major	Gastric outlet obstruction	Pyloroplasty
	Stricture	
	(a) Cervical anastomosis	Revision of anastomosis
	(b) Diaphragmatic hiatus	Death from unrecognized perforation during dilatation
	Leak of gastric tube in chest	Spontaneous closure without stricture
	Perforation of gastric tube in chest during dilatation	Thoracotomy and closure of perforation
Minor	Leak—cervical anastomosis	
	(a) Temporary (4)	Healed spontaneously
	(b) Persistent (1)	Operative closure
	Ulcer in tube	Healed spontaneously

rily by chest tube drainage; the fistula closed spontaneously. Stricture of the cervical anastomosis is infrequent and will respond, in most instances, to several dilatations.[2, 11, 17] Peptic ulcer development within the gastric tube has been observed.[3] In these cases, redundancy or narrowing of the tube caused stasis, leading to prolonged contact of the mucosa with gastric acid (Table 43–10).

Summary

Both the colon and gastric tubes are established for esophageal substitution in children. The colon has enjoyed the greatest popularity and its value has been well established by long-term follow-up. The gastric tube is equally satisfactory from a functional point of view and short-term complications are perhaps less prominent than in the colon. Longer follow-up, so far, has fulfilled the early promise; and, in some major institutions, the gastric tube now is the first procedure for esophageal substitution.

REFERENCES

1. Altman, R. P.: Portal decompression by interposition mesocaval shunt in patients with biliary atresia, J. Pediatr. Surg. 11:809, 1976.
2. Anderson, K. D., and Randolph, J. G.: The gastric tube for esophageal replacement in children, J. Thorac. Cardiovasc. Surg. 66:333, 1973.
3. Anderson, K. D., Randolph, J. G., and Lilly, J. R.: Peptic ulcer in children with gastric tube interposition, J. Pediatr. Surg. 10:701, 1975.
4. Azar, H., Crispin, A. R., and Waterston, D. J.: Esophageal replacement with transverse colon in infants and children, J. Pediatr. Surg. 6:3, 1971.
5. Belsey, R.: Reconstruction of the esophagus with left colon, J. Thorac. Cardiovasc. Surg. 49:33, 1965.
6. Berman, E. F.: Plastic esophagus, Sinai Hosp. J. Balt. 1:40, 1952.
7. Bircher, E.: Ein beitrag zur plastichen bildung eines neuen oesophagus, Zentralbl. Chir., Dec. 21, 1907.
8. Blanchard, H., Roy, C. C., Perreault, G., *et al.*: Retrosternal esophageal replacement in 18 children, Can. J. Surg. 15:137, 1972.
9. Burrington, J. D., and Stephens, C. A.: Esophageal replacement with a gastric tube in infants and children, J. Pediatr. Surg. 3:246, 1968.
10. Clatworthy, H. W., Jr., and Boles, E. T., Jr.: Extrahepatic portal bed block in children. Pathogenesis and treatment, Ann. Surg. 150:371, 1959.
11. Cohen, D. H., Middleton, A. W., and Fletcher, J.: Gastric tube esophagoplasty, J. Pediatr. Surg. 9:451, 1974.
12. Czerny, V.: Neue Operationen, Zentralbl. Chir. 4:443, 1877.
13. Dale, W. A., and Sherman, C. D.: Late reconstruction of congenital esophageal atresia by intrathoracic colon transplantation, J. Thorac. Surg. 29:344, 1955.
14. Dave, K. S., Holden, G. H., Holden, M. P., Bekassy, S. M., and Ionescu, M. I.: Esophageal replacement with jejunum for nonmalignant lesions, Surgery 72:466, 1972.
15. De Boer, A.: The retrosternal colonic esophageal substitute in children, Surg. Clin. North Am. 44:1449, 1964.
16. Ein, S. H.: Personal communication.
17. Ein, S. H., Shandling, B., Simpson, J. S., and Stephens, C. A.: A further look at the gastric tube as an esophageal replacement in infants and children, J. Pediatr. Surg. 8:859, 1973.
18. Gavriliu, D., and Georgescue, L.: Esophagoplastic direction a material gastric, Rev. Stiintelor Med. (Bucharest) 3:33, 1955.
19. German, J. C., and Waterston, D. J.: Colon interposition for the replacement of the esophagus in children, J. Pediatr. Surg. 11:227, 1976.
20. Gross, R. E.: *The Surgery of Infancy and Childhood* (Philadelphia: W. B. Saunders Company, 1955).
21. Gross, R. E., and Firestone, F. N.: Colonic reconstruction of the esophagus in infants and children, Surgery 61:955, 1967.
22. Hays, D. M., Woolley, M. M., and Snyder, W. H.: Changing techniques in the management of esophageal atresia, Arch. Surg. 92:611, 1966.
23. Heimlich, H. J.: Elective replacement of the oesophagus, Br. J. Surg. 53:913, 1966.
24. Heimlich, H. J., and Winfield, J. M.: The use of a gastric tube to replace or bypass the esophagus, Surgery 37:549, 1955.
25. Henderson, R. (in discussion), Anderson, K. D., and Randolph, J. G.: Gastric tube for esophageal replacement in children, J. Thorac. Surg. 66:333, 1973.
26. Holder, T. H.: Personal communication.
27. Holder, T. H.: Transpleural versus retropleural approach for repair of tracheoesophageal fistula, Surg. Clin. North Am. 144:1443, 1964.
28. Jianu, A.: Gastrostomie u. oesophagoplastik, Dtsch. Z. Chir. 118:383, 1912.
29. Kelling, G.: Oesophagoplastik mit hilfe des querkolon, Zentralbl. Chir. 33:34, 1911.
30. Lister, J., Altman, R. P., and Allison, W. A.: Prosthetic substitution of thoracic esophagus in puppies, Ann. Surg. 162:812, 1965.
31. Longino, L. A., Woolley, M. M., and Gross, R. E.: Esophageal replacement in infants and children with use of a segment of colon, JAMA 171:1187, 1959.
32. Louhimo, I., Pasila, M., and Visakorpi, J. K.: Later gastrointestinal complications in patients with colonic replacement of the esophagus, J. Pediatr. Surg. 4:663, 1969.
33. Lynn, H. B.: Simple method of elongating a colonic segment for esophageal replacement, J. Pediatr. Surg. 8:391, 1973.
34. Mahoney, E. B., and Sherman, C. D.: Total esophagoplasty using intrathoracic right colon, Surgery 35:936, 1954.
35. Malcolm, J. A.: Occurrence of peptic ulcer in colon used for esophageal replacement, J. Thorac. Cardiovasc. Surg. 55:763, 1968.
36. Merendino, K. A., and Dillard, D. H.: The concept of sphincter substitution by an interposed jejunal segment for anatomic and physiological abnormalities at the esophagogastric junction; with special reference to reflux esophagitis, cardiospasm and esophageal varices, Ann. Surg. 142:486, 1955.
37. Neville, W. E., and Clowes, G. H. A., Jr.: Colon replacement of the esophagus in children for congenital and acquired disease, J. Thorac. Cardiovasc. Surg. 40:507, 1960.
38. Nicks, R.: Colonic replacement of the esophagus, Br. J. Surg. 54:124, 1967.
39. Ochsner, A., and Owens, N.: Antethoracic esophagoplasty for impermeable stricture of the esophagus, Ann. Surg. 100:1055, 1934.
40. Othersen, H. B., and Clatworthy, H. W.: Functional evaluation of esophageal replacement in children, J. Thorac. Cardiovasc. Surg. 53:55, 1967.
41. Roux, C.: L'oesophago-jejuno-gastrostomie. Nouvelle operation par retrecissement infranchissable de l'oesophage, Sem. Med. 27:37, 1907.
42. Salama, F. D.: Prosthetic replacement of the esophagus, J. Thorac. Cardiovasc. Surg. 70:739, 1975.
43. Sanders, G. B.: Esophageal replacement with reversed gastric tube, JAMA 181:944, 1962.
44. Schiller, M., Frye, T. R., and Boles, E. T.: Evaluation of colonic replacement of the esophagus in children, J. Pediatr. Surg. 6:753, 1971.
45. Sieber, A. M., and Sieber, W. K.: Colonic transplants as esophageal replacement. Cineradiographic and manometric evaluation in children, Ann. Surg. 168:116, 1968.

ACHALASIA OF THE ESOPHAGUS **489**

ACHALASIA OF THE ESOPHAGUS 489

46. Singh, A., and Rickham, P. P.: Subtotal colonic replacement of the oesophagus in infancy, Br. J. Surg. 58:377, 1977.
47. Skinner, D. B., and DeMeester, T. R.: Gastroesophageal Reflux, in *Current Problems in Surgery* (Chicago: Year Book Medical Publishers, Inc., January, 1976).
48. Soave, F.: Intrathoracic transposition of the transverse colon in complicated oesophageal atresia, Prog. Pediatr. Surg. 4:91, 1972.
49. Sweet, R. H.: Transthoracic resection of the esophagus and stomach for carcinoma, Ann. Surg. 121:272, 1945.
50. Waterston, D.: Colonic replacement of esophagus (intrathoracic), Surg. Clin. North Am. 44:1441, 1964.
51. Yudin, S. S.: The surgical construction of 80 cases of artificial esophagus, Surg. Gynecol. Obstet. 78:561, 1944.

Achalasia of the Esophagus

JUDSON G. RANDOLPH

ACHALASIA is a motor disturbance of uncertain etiology characterized by failure of the cardia to relax during swallowing. Although relatively rare in either adult or child, large series of patients have been reported that include as many as 5% of cases in children.[10-12, 18] Infants as young as 2 weeks have been diagnosed with this disorder. Three reports[2, 14, 20] of 2 or more affected siblings in one family have also been reported. Achalasia should be included in the differential diagnosis of infants and children whose complaints center around regurgitation, rumination, failure to thrive and recurrent upper respiratory infections.[15, 16]

In 1888, Einhorn[3] first described a muscular obstruction at the esophagogastric junction. In 1904, von Mikulicz[21] suggested spasm of the cardia as the cause of the obstruction and first introduced the term cardiospasm.

The term achalasia (*a* — without + *chalasia* — relaxation) means failure of relaxation and was first used by Hurst and Rake[8] in 1930. The symptoms, physiologic changes and radiologic findings all are directly dependent on failure of the distal esophagus to relax. This, in turn, impedes the passage of solids and eventually liquids. After a period of time, proximal dilatation of the esophagus occurs.

The etiology of achalasia is not known. In 1927, Rake reported a decrease in the number of ganglion cells, which other workers have since confirmed,[4, 17] but the observation is not universally made. The appearance of achalasia in Chagas' disease, in which trypanosomes destroy ganglion cells in many locations of the body, lends support to the theory of ganglion cell dysfunction.[9] However, biopsies in other well-documented cases of achalasia have shown normal ganglion cells. Alvarez[1] has compared achalasia to Hirschsprung's disease, and Higgs and Ellis[7] have suggested that the primary lesion may occur in the nuclei of the vagal nerves supplying the esophageal wall. This theory is supported by the fact that response in the vagal postsynaptic cholinergic fibers is preserved even in advanced cases of achalasia.

The diagnosis of achalasia rests on a barium swallow, which demonstrates the dilated proximal esophagus tapering smoothly into a "parrot's beak" ending in an apparently tight esophagogastric stricture (Fig. 43–25). Lack of peristalsis in the esophagus and failure of the lower sphincter to relax after deglutition are identifiable by fluoroscopy[22] and by

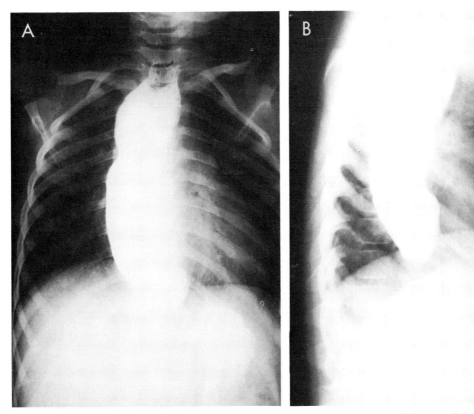

Fig. 43–25.—Achalasia. **A,** AP view of esophageal swallow in a 9-year-old child with longstanding symptoms of dysphagia and recurrent aspiration pneumonia. **B,** lateral view of same patient.

esophageal motility studies. Manometry has assumed importance in diagnosing those early cases in which the esophagus has not yet become dilated. There is no actual mechanical obstruction or stricture in patients with achalasia; the area of radiologic narrowing always is found to be soft and pliable and will readily accept a large bougie. Esophagoscopy usually is unnecessary in adults and has not proved to be useful for diagnosis in children. If, however, there is any question of associated esophagitis, this must be confirmed at esophagoscopy before treatment is undertaken.

Like its etiology, the treatment of achalasia is controversial. Although dilatation has been practiced since Thomas Willis first described achalasia in 1674, ordinary bougienage produces only transient and temporary relief. Mechanical dilators are available, but these devices are dangerous and their use is beset with complications.[13] Permanent relief requires forceful disruption of the lower esophageal muscle with mechanical, pneumatic or hydrostatic pressure. The most common method of achieving this involves the placement of a rubber balloon across the gastroesophageal junction, under fluoroscopic control, and inflating it under measured pressure with water or air.

The rate of improvement after dilatation is surprisingly consistent for most large series, ranging from 60% to 70%. However, in a series of 15 children with achalasia reported by Tachovsky, Lynn and Ellis,[18] 8 of the 15 were treated with dilatation an average of 8 times each with no permanent relief. The longest period of symptomatic relief was just under 3 years, and all the patients ultimately required operation. For any infant with achalasia, forceful dilatation would be difficult to regulate. Thus, operation is the only treatment that can be recommended in these small subjects.

Successful operative therapy for achalasia was introduced in 1913 by Heller,[6] who described a transthoracic anterior and posterior esophagomyotomy. In 1923, Zaaijer[23] showed that an anterior myotomy alone was all that was required to relieve the obstruction. Although it was originally reserved for dilatation failures, most surgeons now recommend this operation as the definitive treatment for patients with achalasia.[4, 16a, 18] Gastroesophageal reflux and esophagitis may follow the Heller procedure because of the obligatory dissection of the esophageal hiatus. There now is unanimity of opinion among surgeons that the extramucosal muscle-splitting procedure should be coupled with a reconstruction of the hiatus or a formal antireflux operation.

In an extensive experience with both modes of therapy, Ellis and Olsen[4] found a 94% initial success rate with the modified Heller procedure compared to a 65% success rate with hydrostatic dilatation. All children ultimately were treated operatively. With a mean follow-up of 7 years, 12 children were classified as showing excellent results, 1 was judged good, 1 fair and 1 lost to follow-up. The 2 patients classified less than excellent were followed far into adulthood and operated on 10 and 40 years after the onset of symptoms.

In summary, achalasia is a rare condition in infants and uncommon in children. It must be differentiated from other esophageal problems such as gastroesophageal reflux, centrally caused motility disturbances, duplications and congenital stenosis. In all infants and young children, surgical correction is the treatment of choice.

REFERENCES

1. Alvarez, W.: A simple explanation for cardiospasm and Hirschsprung's disease, Gastroenterology 13:422, 1949.
2. Dayalan, N., Chettur, L., and Ramakrishnan, M.: Achalasia of the cardia in siblings, Arch. Dis. Child. 47:115, 1972.
3. Einhorn, M.: A case of dysphagia with dilatation of the esophagus, Med. Rec. Ann. 34:751, 1888.
4. Ellis, F. H., Jr., and Olsen, A. M.: *Achalasia of the Esophagus.* Major Problems in Clinical Surgery series. (Philadelphia: W. B. Saunders Company, 1969), Vol. IX.
5. Heitmann, P., and Wienbeck, M.: The immediate effect of successful pneumatic dilatation on esophageal function in achalasia, Scand. J. Gastroenterol. 7:197, 1972.
6. Heller, E.: Extramukose Cardioplastik beim chronischen Cardiospasmus mit Dilatations des Oesophagus, Mitt. Grenzgeb. Med. Chir. 27:141, 1913.
7. Higgs, B., and Ellis, F.: The effect of bilateral supradorsal vagotomy on canine esophageal function, Surgery 58:828, 1965.
8. Hurst, A., and Rake, G.: Achalasia of the cardia: So-called cardiospasm, Q. J. Med. 23:491, 1930.
9. Koberle, F.: Enteromegaly and cardiomegaly in Chagas disease, Gut 4:399, 1963.
10. Moersch, H.: Cardiospasm in infancy and in childhood, Am. J. Dis. Child. 38:294, 1929.
11. Olsen, A., Holman, C., and Andersen, H.: Diagnosis of cardiospasm, Dis. Chest 23:477, 1953.
12. Payne, W., Ellis, F., and Olsen, A.: Treatment of cardiospasm (achalasia of the esophagus) in children, Surgery 50:731, 1961.
13. Payne, W. S., and Olsen, A. M.: Motor Disturbances of Deglutition, in *The Esophagus* (Philadelphia: Lea & Febiger, 1974).
14. Polonsky, L., and Guth, P.: Familial achalasia, Digest. Dis. 15:291, 1970.
15. Redo, S., and Bauer, C.: Management of achalasia in infancy and childhood, Surgery 53:263, 1963.
16. Schultz, E.: Achalasia in children as a cause of recurrent pulmonary disease, J. Pediatr. 59:522, 1961.
16a. Steichen, F., Heller, E., and Ravitch, M.: Achalasia of the esophagus, Surgery 47:846, 1960.
17. Swenson, O., and Economopoulos, C.: Achalasia of the esophagus in children, J. Thorac. Cardiovasc. Surg. 41:49, 1961.
18. Tachovsky, T., Lynn, H., and Ellis, H.: The surgical approach to esophageal achalasia in children, J. Pediatr. Surg. 3:226, 1968.
19. Vantrappen, G., Hellemans, J., Deloof, W., Valembois, P., and Vanderbroucke, J.: Treatment of achalasia with pneumatic dilatations, Gut 12:268, 1971.
20. Vaughan, W., and Williams, J.: Familial achalasia with pulmonary complications in children, Radiology 107:407, 1973.
21. von Mickulicz, J.: Zur Pathologie und Therapie des Cardiospasms, Dtsch. Med. Wochenschr. 30:17, 1904.
22. Willich, E.: Achalasia of the cardia in children, Pediatr. Radiol. 1:229, 1973.
23. Zaaijer, J.: Cardiospasm in the aged, Ann. Surg. 77:615, 1923.

Diverticulum of the Esophagus

MARK M. RAVITCH

Pharyngoesophageal Diverticulum

IN ADULTS, the common posterior midline pharyngeal diverticulum, presenting essentially as a mucosa-submucosa-covered hernia in the diamond-shaped area of muscular weakness above the cricopharyngeus fibers, obviously is an acquired lesion. Lahey and Warren[9] carefully described the pathogenesis and development of such pharyngeal diverticula.

In rare instances, congenital diverticula at this level have been reported in children. They are true diverticula with complete muscular walls. The reported instances have manifested themselves in newborn infants by a clinical picture simulating that of atresia of the esophagus. The infants regurgitate mucus and formula, and cough with feedings, but usually without cyanosis. Contrast material fills a pouch high in the thorax and overflows into the trachea, none entering the stomach. There is gas in the stomach. A catheter passed from above enters the diverticulum rather than the esophagus. The 2 patients of Brintnall and Kridelbaugh[1] were operated on for presumed esophageal atresia, the diverticulum then being discovered and treated definitively. The first died of mediastinitis after excision of the diverticulum; the second died during exploration, with established pneumonia of both lungs. In both instances, the lesion was a true diverticulum, composed of the full thickness of pharyngeal wall, including muscle. Duhamel's[2] first patient was a 3-day-old infant with salivation, strangulation and cyanosis. On endoscopy, an opening was seen behind and to the left of the pharyngoesophageal junction. Lipiodol swallow demonstrated a long sac behind the esophagus, descending in the posterior mediastinum to the third dorsal vertebra. The infant died soon after. Autopsy disclosed a diverticulum opening out of the hypopharynx. A second child had an almost identical lesion, discovered only on endoscopy. The diverticular pouch was longer and narrower, and after endoscopy symptoms disappeared. His third patient had a diverticulum arising from the upper portion of the piriform sinus and passing anteriorly. This child died of asphyxia after a successful operation for atresia of the right colon. The patient of Rouchy, Crézé and Courtillé[17] was a 24-hour-old full-term infant, presenting with difficulty in respiration and salivating abundantly. The diagnosis of esophageal atresia seemingly was confirmed by high obstruction to passage of a catheter and radiologic evidence of a blind esophageal sac. The infant died 24 hours after gastrostomy and proved to have a diverticulum of the hypopharynx behind the esophagus. Review of the films showed a thin stream of contrast material in the esophagus proper.

Rush and Stingily[18] reported on a baby who lived for 20 days with severe respiratory distress. When he cried, a small, soft, fluctuant swelling appeared above the clavicle. This increased day by day until at the time of death it was 7 × 5 cm. Aspirated through the neck, it yielded air and pus. At autopsy, a large sac was found that led by a narrow isthmus to the esophagus through an opening in the posterolateral portion at the level of the cricoid. The narrow sac filled with air, became infected and the combination caused obstruction and regurgitation, which led to pneumonia and death.

Laurent et al.[10] treated a neonate with dysphagia and respiratory distress. A large diverticulum, in the usual relationships of a Zenker diverticulum, displaced the esophagus and trachea. The diverticulum had a muscular wall. As it was resected there came into view an esophagotracheal fistula. The infant died.

Traumatic Pseudodiverticulum of the Pharynx in the Newborn

After the presentation of three cases by Ekloff[4] in 1968 before the European Society of Radiology, Girdany, Sieber and Osman[5] reported two more cases of traumatic perforation of the posterior pharyngeal wall in neonates, with the subsequent creation of a pseudodiverticulum, causing an obstruction mistaken for esophageal atresia, and a serious mediastinitis. A catheter may pass preferentially through the perforation for a short distance. Barium outlines the pouch. The two 1973 cases of Edison and Holinger[3] in the newborn and the two later cases of Osman and Girdany[15] in older infants suggest that maintenance of a nasogastric tube and treatment with antibiotics may be all that is required. Sieber successfully closed the pharyngeal perforation in one of his patients, although, in any case, a prolonged period of dysphagia appears likely.

The cause of the injury has been passage of a suction catheter in most cases, an obstetrician's finger in one, a father's finger in another. Messer et al.,[12] reporting from Strasbourg in 1973, found five other reported cases and reported what they thought to be a congenital diverticulum, since the child was born at home, unattended, but the "diverticulum" was in a mass of mediastinal inflammatory tissue and there was no epithelium in the resected specimen.

Diverticulum of the Esophagus Associated with Stenosis

It seems likely that congenital diverticulum of the thoracic esophagus at or above the level of the carina is another variation of those tracheoesophageal anomalies, the most common of which is classic esophageal atresia with tracheoesophageal fistula.

Robb[16] successfully excised a thoracic esophageal diverticulum in a boy of 11. It was associated with what appeared to be a congenital tracheoesophageal fistula. O'Bannon[14] found at autopsy in a newborn a diverticular pouch at the level of the third thoracic vertebra just proximal to a narrow congenital esophageal stenosis. Knox[8] reported an esophageal diverticulum with a tracheoesophageal fistula and without esophageal stenosis in a case somewhat similar to Robb's, and TenKate[19] reported a case similar to O'Bannon's. Grant and Arneil's[6] second case was similar to these — in a newborn presenting as an instance of tracheoesophageal fistula with esophageal atresia. The diverticulum at the level of the carina filled with Lipiodol that did not pass into the esophagus. A catheter could be passed into the

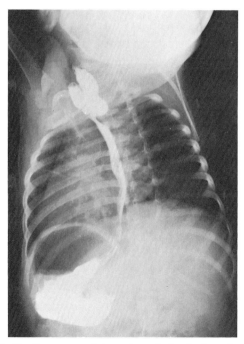

Fig. 43–26.—True congenital esophageal diverticulum. A 2-year-old girl was subject to respiratory infections from birth, with recurrent febrile episodes, cough and expectoration. Progressive dysphagia appeared at 15 months. The oblique roentgenogram shows the large diverticular sac arising low in the cervical esophagus. At operation, the sac was found to arise posteriorly and extend behind the esophagus to a level below the clavicle. The communication with the esophagus was about 2.5 cm in diameter. The excised sac consisted of a full thickness of esophageal wall, thus representing a true diverticulum. True congenital diverticula of the esophagus, of which this was the single example at the Johns Hopkins Hospital, are rare. (Courtesy of Dr. A. R. Nelson.[13])

esophagus to the diverticulum but no farther. A transthoracic resection of the diverticulum, on the day of birth, met with immediate success, and the child was discharged home swallowing well on the 15th day. He died elsewhere at the age of 9 weeks with multiple lung abscesses.

Meadows[11] described communicating esophageal duplication in 2 patients, one looking much like an ordinary epiphrenic diverticulum but containing duodenal and pancreatic tissue, the other one tubular and communicating at its lower end. Two other children (2 months and 10 years of age) had symptomatic epiphrenic diverticula.

True Congenital Diverticulum of the Esophagus

True diverticula of the esophagus proper, unassociated with any suggestion of tracheoesophageal anomaly, probably are the rarest of all esophageal anomalies. There are several reports of children with signs of recurrent respiratory infection and progressive dysphagia.[6, 7, 13] Nelson's[13] patient was successfully operated on at the age of 2 by Blalock through a cervical incision, although the diverticulum could not be totally excised through this approach (Fig. 43–26). The 8-year-old patient of Jackson and Shallow[7] died of empyema. Grant and Arneil[6] operated on their patient at age 5. He had had stridor since birth and some dysphagia from the time he began to take solid food. Radiologic studies at age 10 months had shown a large diverticulum rising high in the cervical esophagus. The operation was performed through a left supraclavicular incision, and the large sac was found to communicate widely with the esophagus on its posterior aspect 2 cm below the pharyngoesophageal junction. A one-stage resection was completed successfully.

REFERENCES

1. Brintnall, E. S., and Kridelbaugh, W. W.: Congenital diverticulum of the posterior hypopharynx simulating atresia of the esophagus, Ann. Surg. 131:564, 1950.
2. Duhamel, B.: Deux cas de diverticules congenitaux de l'oesophage cervical: Considérations sur le diagnostic des malformations congenitales de l'oesophage, Arch. Fr. Pediatr. 6:499, 1949.
3. Edison, B., and Holinger, P. H.: Traumatic pharyngeal pseudo-diverticulum in the newborn infant, J. Pediatr. 82:3, 1973.
4. Ekloff, O., Lohn, G., and Okmean, L.: Submucosal perforation of the esophagus in the neonate, Acta Radiol. 8:187, 1969.
5. Girdany, B. R., Sieber, W. K., and Osman, M. Z.: Traumatic pseudodiverticulums of the pharynx in newborn infants, N. Engl. J. Med. 280:237, 1969.
6. Grant, J. C., and Arneil, G. C.: Congenital diverticulum of the esophagus, Surgery 46:966, 1959.
7. Jackson, C., and Shallow, T. A.: Diverticula of the esophagus: Pulsion, traction, malignant, and congenital, Ann. Surg. 83:1, 1926.
8. Knox, G.: Congenital tracheoesophageal fistula without esophageal atresia, Surgery 30:1016, 1951.
9. Lahey, F. H., and Warren, K. W.: Esophageal diverticula, Surg. Gynecol. Obstet. 98:1, 1954.
10. Laurent, Y., Schuermans, J., and Brombart, M.: Poche pharyngoesophagienne postérieure et fistule oesotracheal chez un nouveau-né, Acta Gastroenterol. Belg. 24:618, 1961.
11. Meadows, J. A., Jr.: Esophageal diverticula in infants and children, South. Med. J. 63:6, 1970.
12. Messer, J., Krivosic, R., Krug, J. P., Berger, J., Willard, D., and Buck, P.: Diverticules et pseudo-diverticules du pharynx simulant chez le nouveau-né une atrésie de l'oesophage, Pediatrie T. 28:1, 1973.
13. Nelson, A. R.: Congenital true esophageal diverticulum: Report of a case unassociated with other esophagotracheal abnormality, Ann. Surg. 145:258, 1957.
14. O'Bannon, R. P.: Congenital partial atresia of esophagus associated with congenital diverticulum of the esophagus: Report of a case, Radiology 47:471, 1946.
15. Osman, M. Z., and Girdany, B. R.: Traumatic pseudodiverticulums of the pharynx in infants and children, Ann. Radiol. 16:3, 1973.
16. Robb, D.: Congenital tracheoesophageal fistula without atresia but with esophageal diverticulum, Aust. N. Z. J. Surg. 22:120, 1952.
17. Rouchy, R., Crézé, J., and Courtillé, P.: Diverticule congenital de l'oesophage chez un nouveau-né, Bull. Fed. Soc. Gynecol. Obstet. 6:105, 1954.
18. Rush, L. V., and Stingily, C. R.: Congenital diverticulum of the esophagus: Case report, South. Med. J. 22:546, 1929.
19. TenKate, J.: Congenital diverticulum of oesophagus, Arch. Chir. Neerl. 4:277, 1952.

44   Mark M. Ravitch / David C. Sabiston

Mediastinal Infections, Cysts and Tumors

Anatomy

The mediastinum is the portion of the thoracic cavity bounded anteriorly by the sternum, posteriorly by the vertebral column and on either side by the medial surfaces of the right and left pleurae. The thymus, heart, pericardium and the great vessels, trachea, right and left main bronchi, esophagus, vagus nerve, phrenic nerve, sympathetic nerve trunks and the thoracic duct are all in the mediastinum. For anatomic descriptive purposes, the mediastinum has been divided more or less arbitrarily into four subdivisions (Fig. 44–1). This is of some clinical significance in view of the observation that the various inflammatory and neoplastic processes have their genesis in specific anatomic divisions and on this account cause differing symptoms.

The *superior mediastinum* is located above the plane connecting the fourth thoracic vertebra with the sternomanubrial junction. Normally, it contains the arch of the aorta, the innominate, carotid and subclavian arteries, the pulmonary arteries and veins, superior vena cava, innominate and subclavian veins, most of the thymus gland, the phrenic nerves and an extensive plexus of lymph nodes and communicating lymphatic vessels.

The *anterior mediastinum* is bounded in front by the ster-

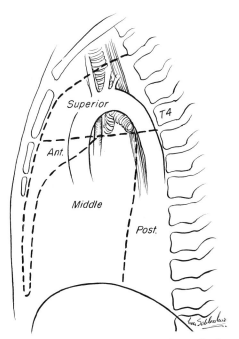

Fig. 44–1.—Diagram of the divisions of the mediastinum.

num and behind by the pericardium. It extends above to the margin of the superior mediastinum and below to the diaphragm. It contains the remainder of the thymus, numerous lymph nodes and some fatty tissue. The anterior portion of the diaphragm, adjacent to this space, occasionally is the site of a congenital defect (foramen of Morgagni) through which abdominal viscera may herniate.

The *middle mediastinum* is occupied by the heart and pericardium, lymph nodes and lymphatic vessels.

The *posterior mediastinum* is bounded behind by the vertebral column, in front by the posterior aspect of the pericardium, above by the superior mediastinum, with which it is continuous, and below by the diaphragm. Within it are found the trachea, esophagus, thoracic duct, descending aorta, vagus and phrenic nerves, the sympathetic nerve trunks and numerous lymph nodes with their associated lymphatic channels.

Infections of the Mediastinum

ACUTE MEDIASTINITIS.—The mediastinum offers no anatomic barriers to the spread of infection within it, and any kind of suppurative mediastinitis is a grave condition. Bacterial invasion of the mediastinum may follow (1) perforation of the pharynx, esophagus or trachea by disease, ingested foreign bodies, endoscopic injury, penetrating wounds or blunt force in compression injuries of the chest; (2) thoracic and cervical operations complicated by wound infection or suture-line leaks; (3) retropharyngeal or cervical infections breaking through the containing cervical fascia and extending downward, and (4) rupture of suppurative mediastinal lymph nodes.

Mediastinal infection generally evokes a severe systemic response manifested by pain, dyspnea, high fever and striking tachycardia. Infections involving the superior mediastinum, with accompanying edematous compression of the great veins, may result in duskiness and edema of the head

and neck. Infections of the posterior mediastinum do not usually cause localizing signs, unless escape of air from esophagus or trachea produces mediastinal emphysema, which appears on the roentgenogram, or dissects upward into the neck, producing crepitation in the supraclavicular fossa. The roentgenogram in acute mediastinitis demonstrates a widened mediastinum and sometimes a pleural thickening or a pleural effusion, which may be a sterile, sympathetic or irritative effusion or may represent actual empyema from direct extension of the suppurative process.

Although the use of antibiotics has sharply decreased the incidence and mortality from mediastinitis, antibiotic therapy alone is not to be relied on except in the less severe infections and those in which treatment has been instituted very early. Incision and drainage is the safest treatment for most suppurative processes, and those in the mediastinum constitute not an exception but an outstanding indication. An esophageal perforation, for instance, is hazardous chiefly if continued leakage occurs into the undrained mediastinum.

Infection of the anterior mediastinum resulting from an accidental wound, rupture of the lymph nodes or complication of intrasternal therapy or biopsy can be adequately drained through the space left by excision of the third or fourth left costal cartilage.

A supraclavicular incision provides access to the superior mediastinum, the approach being between the esophagus and trachea medially and the carotid sheath laterally. Occasionally, posterior mediastinal infections may be drained adequately by this route, but for more dependent drainage, the extrapleural and paravertebral resection of an appropriate rib provides direct access to the area of origin of the infection for those cases not best approached transpleurally.

TUBERCULOSIS.—Mediastinal tuberculosis is one of the more common causes of significant hilar lymphadenopathy in childhood. The mediastinal disease represents the result of lymphatic drainage from primary lesions in the pulmonary parenchyma, extending to the nodes along the trachea and bronchi. Although the nonspecific systemic effects of tuberculosis may be present, more often than not symptoms may be few or absent despite striking radiologic changes. A positive tuberculin skin reaction and evidence of a primary pulmonary lesion in the roentgenogram suggest the tuberculous origin of the mediastinal node enlargement. Not rarely, the parenchymal lesion is inconspicuous or not demonstrable radiographically. Calcification in the parenchymal lesion or the nodes is pathognomonic. The involved nodes usually are in the middle and posterior mediastinum surrounding the main bronchi and trachea and, although usually predominantly on the side of the pulmonary disease, frequently are bilateral.

At times, the mediastinal nodes enlarge so greatly as to compress or erode into the bronchus and produce atelectasis (Fig. 44–2, *A* and *C*). More commonly, the slow scarring of nodes as the process heals leads to a gradual and late bronchial obstruction from the cicatricial process, producing atelectasis and repeated episodes of infection at a time when the tuberculous process is itself inactive.[2] This is the common cause of the middle lobe syndrome, usually seen in middle or late adult years, but occasionally in childhood (Fig. 44–2, *C*). Unrelieved atelectasis from this cause, complicated by repeated infections behind the obstruction, with or without the additional radiologic demonstration of bronchiectasis,[6] requires lobectomy. Figure 44–3 illustrates a rare instance of acute, life-threatening compression of the

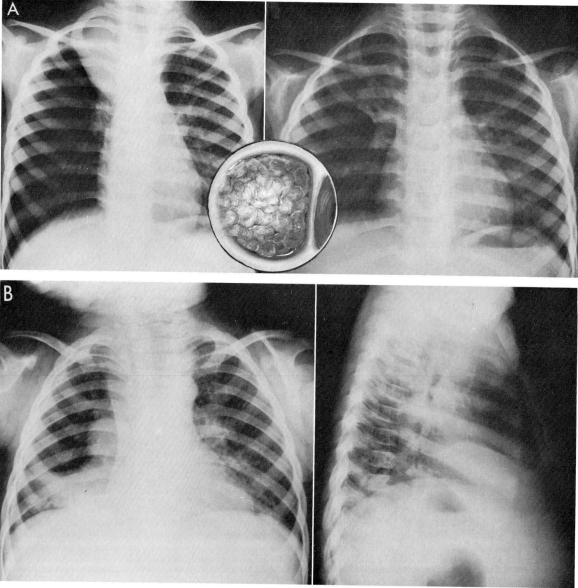

Fig. 44–2.—Mediastinal tuberculosis. **A,** atelectasis of right upper lobe in a 2½-year-old boy. *Left,* the dense shadow looks remarkably like a tumor, particularly since shift of the trachea is prevented by the enlarged paratracheal nodes. *Inset* shows the right main bronchus occluded by granulation tissue, which was removed through the bronchoscope. *Right,* 9 days later, the companion film shows the degree of re-expansion. He made good recovery. Atelectasis in tuberculosis often results from a combination of extrabronchial compression and erosion, with endotracheal obstruction. **B,** rupture into pleural cavity in a 1-year-old boy. Anteroposterior *(left)* and lateral roentgenograms show enlarged mediastinal nodes, generally broadened mediastinal shadow, thickened pleura *(left)* and encapsulated interlobar fluid *(right).* He was not apparently ill. Tuberculin reaction was positive, and a guinea pig inoculated with pleural aspirate died of tuberculosis. The boy recovered and 7 years later had only a healed and calcified primary focus on the right. *(Continued.)*

trachea by a tuberculous abscess of the mediastinum. Emergency decompression was successful. Except for such rare instances, the treatment of tuberculous mediastinal disease usually is nonoperative, although nontuberculous obstructive sequelae require operation more often than is generally supposed. Joly *et al.*[3] did, however, report on 8 children with large mediastinal tuberculous masses who did not respond to a year's therapy. Thoracotomy, evacuation and resection of the masses were undertaken in the absence of tracheal compression. All of the children did well.

Mediastinal granuloma due to histoplasmosis may simulate mediastinal tuberculosis.[1, 7] Woods[8] reports a 4-year-old

child with tracheal obstruction by a mediastinal granuloma due to *Histoplasma capsulatum,* a noncalcified mass in the right superior mediastinum, which displaced and compressed the trachea. Evacuation and partial resection of the granulomatous mass relieved the obstruction, and the child did well. Pate and Hammon[4] reported 4 children with mediastinal fibrosis producing the superior vena cava syndrome and evidence that this was on the basis of histoplasmosis. All 4 were operated on successfully. Of the 93 primary mediastinal masses seen at the Children's Hospital of Pittsburgh from 1956 to 1975, 1 was due to histoplasmosis. This was a 6 × 4 cm anterior mediastinal mass in an asymp-

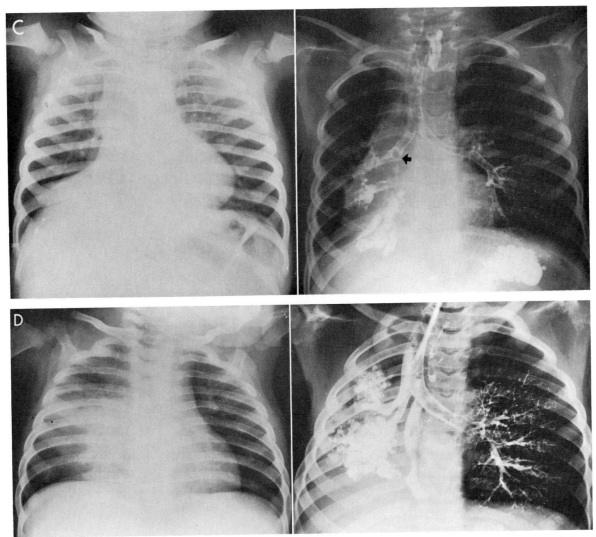

Fig. 44–2 (cont.).—C, bronchial obstruction and atelectasis (RLL, RML). *Left,* at age 21 months, this child had a positive reaction to 0.01 mg OT and tubercle bacilli on gastric lavage. The dense triangular shadow at the right base is due to occlusion of the intermediate bronchus by nodes outside it and possibly to bronchial erosion with concomitant endobronchial disease. *Right,* 4 years later. Bronchogram shows narrowing (*arrow*) of intermediate bronchus, atelectasis and bronchiectasis of lower and middle lobes and calcified nodes in right paratracheal region. He did well after right middle and lower lobectomy and a year later was successfully treated for tuberculous meningitis. **D,** bronchial obstruction and atelectasis (RUL, RML, RLL).

The child was exposed from birth to a tuberculous mother. *Left,* at 17 months she was tuberculin-positive and had marked enlargement of bronchial lymph nodes on the right and extensive parenchymal shadow. *Right,* 5 years later. This degree of mediastinal shift with entire trachea, esophagus and heart in right hemithorax had been present since age 3. There is severe saccular bronchiectasis throughout the right lung. Most of the bronchial obstruction had long since disappeared, and when the lung was removed to control the secondary infection, no residual tuberculous activity was found. The child did well. (Courtesy of Dr. J. B. Hardy.)

tomatic 6-year-old boy whose histoplasma skin tests and serum titers were positive. The mass was resected, followed by a 2-week course of amphotericin B. He did well.

SARCOID.—Sarcoidosis is observed occasionally in children.[5] The scarcity of reports makes it difficult to state the relative frequency of the clinical manifestations in children, but both pulmonary and mediastinal lesions appear to be prominent in childhood disease. As in adults, the uveal tract, skin, bones and viscera have been involved. Uveitis, cervical node enlargement or cutaneous nodules on the face of a child with mediastinal lymph nodes suggest the possibility of sarcoid, although the same association of lesions is seen in tuberculosis. The tuberculin and Nickerson-Kveim tests may differentiate the two diseases. In a boy of 15 with a history of fatigability and blurring of vision, the specific diagnosis was made by biopsy of a cervical lymph node (Fig. 44–4), although no cervical nodes were abnormally palpable.

REFERENCES

1. Gayboski, W. A., *et al.:* Surgical aspects of histoplasmosis, Arch. Surg. 87:590, 1963.
2. Hardy, J. B., and Brailey, M.: *Tuberculosis in White and Negro Children* (Cambridge, Mass.: Harvard University Press, 1958), Vol. 1.
3. Joly, H., *et al.:* Traitement chirurgical de certaines adenopathies mediastinales tuberculeuses, Presse Med. 71:2731, 1963.
4. Pate, J. W., and Hammon, J.: Superior vena cava syndrome due to histoplasmosis in children, Ann. Surg. 161:778, 1965.
5. Reeves, R. J., Baylin, G. J., and Jones, P. A.: Boeck's sarcoid in children, South. Med. J. 41:295, 1948.
6. Thomas, D. E., and Winn, D.: Middle lobectomy for tuberculosis in childhood, J. Thorac. Cardiovasc. Surg. 39:175, 1960.

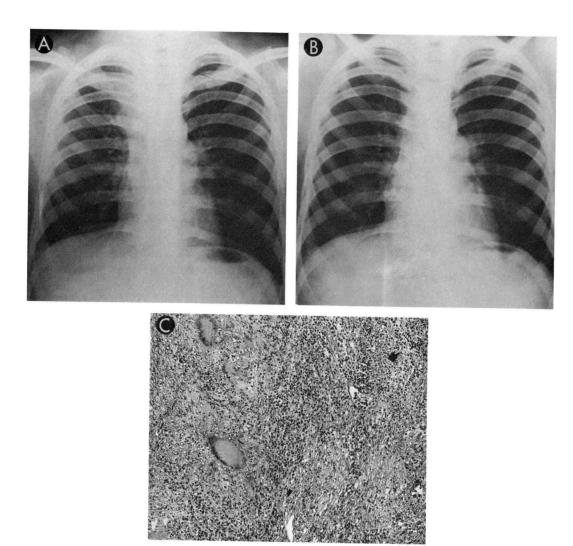

Fig. 44–3.—Mediastinal tuberculosis; tracheal compression. **A,** chest film of 8-year-old boy shows a lesion in right upper mediastinum. He had been well until 6 days previously, when he had dyspnea, which progressed. Severe tracheal obstruction was obvious. Emergency thoracotomy was required for excision and evacuation of a mass of necrotic nodes and tuberculous pus. Such a lesion is very unusual. **B,** chest film after 1 year of streptomycin therapy shows clearing of the lesion. **C,** photomicrograph of the mediastinal abscess shows typical appearance of tuberculosis with giant cells, epithelioid reaction and caseation. Acid-fast organisms were demonstrated in the sections.

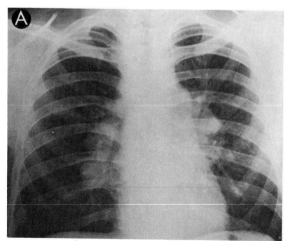

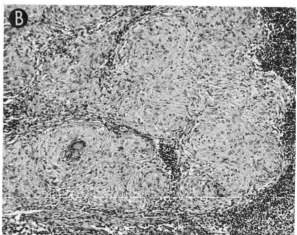

Fig. 44–4.—Sarcoid of mediastinal nodes. Boy of 15 with history of fatigability and blurring of vision. Diagnosis was made by the finding of specific lesions in a small cervical node removed by biopsy, although no cervical nodes were abnormally palpable. **A,** there are bilateral hilar masses. Similar nodes higher in the mediastinum would have been more characteristic of sarcoid. This appearance cannot be distinguished from tuberculosis. **B,** photomicrograph shows hard tubercles and giant cells typical of sarcoid. No Schaumann refractile bodies are seen. Six years later the mediastinal nodes had disappeared and he seemed well.

7. Williams, K. R., and Burford, T. H.: Surgical treatment of granulomatous paratracheal lymphadenopathy, J. Thorac. Cardiovasc. Surg. 48:13, 1964.
8. Woods, L. P.: Mediastinal histoplasma granuloma causing tracheal compression in a 4-year-old child, Surgery 58:448, 1965.

Thymus

The thymus normally occupies the anterior and superior mediastinum. It is composed chiefly of lymphatic tissue, with the characteristic Hassall's corpuscles of apparent epithelial origin. A good deal has been learned about the nature of the cells of the thymus and particularly of the part that thymocytes play in the immune defenses. For a time there was some interest in thymectomy in association with renal transplantation, but that practice has now largely been abandoned. The association of thymectomy with myasthenia gravis dates back to Blalock's 1939 paper,[5] reporting the removal of the thymus for a thymoma in a patient with myasthenia gravis, whose myasthenia was thereby relieved. The first deliberate thymectomies for myasthenia gravis were reported 2 years later.[4] A quarter century since, enthusiasm for thymectomy has waxed and waned, the results have not

been predictable and its proper place in the treatment of myasthenia gravis still has not been established. Inasmuch as on the order of 25% of patients are relieved from symptoms and dependence on cholinesterase inhibitors by thymectomy, and in another 50% symptoms are well controlled under medication, the operation would appear still to have a place. Myasthenia does present in early childhood. The youngest patient on whom we have operated—without striking benefit—was 4 years of age. Sutin[15] has performed thymectomy for myasthenia in an infant of 2 years. The removal of the thymus can be accomplished either through a median sternotomy or through a cervical incision, first proposed at the turn of the century[16] and only recently revived in the United States.

Aberrant positioning of the thymus, with or without cyst formation, may attract attention. In some instances, the thymus has been sufficiently enlarged to present as a cervical tumor.[1, 2, 14] In most such cases, one sees and feels a soft, bulging mass in the suprasternal fossa, made prominent when the child cries. The mass may be found at operation to extend into the superior mediastinum or may be entirely cervical. In fact, the normal thymus frequently extends up

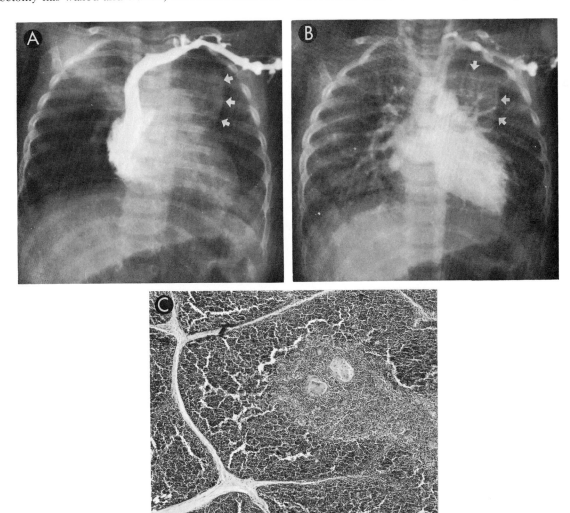

Fig. 44–5.—Enlarged thymus. Thymic enlargement ordinarily is asymptomatic, but the radiologic picture may suggest mediastinal tumor, and operation may be required in doubtful instances. This patient, 6 months old, was being studied because of a cardiac murmur. The plain film showed a large, smoothly rounded mediastinal shadow on the left. **A** and **B,** early and later views in the angiocardiographic series. *Arrows* indicate the mediastinal mass. Angiocardiographic demonstration of both right and left sides of the heart without abnormality clearly indicates that the mass is of nonvascular origin. **C,** the excised mass proved to be an enlarged thymus. The photomicrograph shows normal thymic tissue with characteristic Hassall's corpuscles.

into the neck on either side—perhaps 80% of the time.[10] Obviously, a considerably enlarged thymus extending from the mediastinum up into the neck would be in a strategic position to obstruct the trachea. This was, of course, the common basis for the irradiation of the "enlarged thymus" in infancy, which, disastrously, much later yielded a crop of patients with papillary carcinoma of the thyroid gland. However, from time to time, children appear of whom it can at least be said that they had enlarged thymuses and upper respiratory difficulty that disappeared concomitantly with the thymectomy.[13] At times, a large anterior mediastinal mass that cannot surely be called thymus presents a problem. Corticosteroids—in infants—may shrink the gland.

Injection of gas into the mediastinum has been used by some. In the end, some of these children will be operated on (Fig. 44–5).

A number of children have been reported with thymic cysts. Cervical thymic cysts usually present as masses in the anterior cervical triangle, but of the four cervical and two anterior mediastinal thymic cysts that Beiger and McAdams[3] reported from the Cincinnati Children's Hospital, one of the cervical cysts presented as an enlarging posterior pharyngeal mass. Lamesch[8] of Luxembourg, reporting an 11-year-old boy with a fluctuant mass "the size of a grapefruit" lying under the anterior border of the left sternocleidomastoid muscle that proved to be a thymic cyst, collected 24 addi-

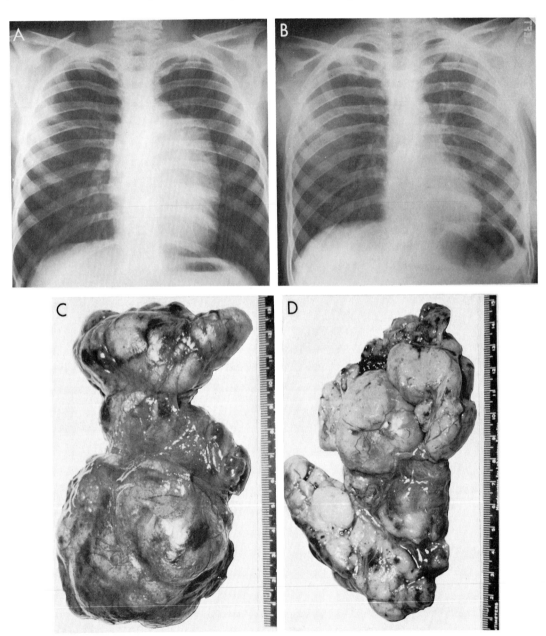

Fig. 44–6.—Benign thymoma. A boy of 11 had x-ray study because of mild cough. **A,** preoperative posteroanterior roentgenogram shows the left border of the heart superiorly to be continuous with a dense mass, thought on fluoroscopy to be anterior to and separable from the heart, so that angiocardiography was not required. **B,** postoperative posteroanterior roentgenogram shows the cardiac silhouette returned to normal. He was well 3 years later. **C** and **D,** operative specimen. The large, firm, lobulated, anterior mediastinal mass was readily dissected through a left anterior thoracotomy. (Median sternotomy is equally satisfactory for resection of thymic tumors and may be required for thymomas with a large cervical component.) Sections showed characteristic features of benign thymoma. (Courtesy of Dr. J. E. Lewis, Jr.)

tional cases in children from 3½ months of age. The cysts are lined by epithelium, often ciliated, there are lymphocytes in the lining, and, in the wall, cholesterol crystals and granulomas are common, and thymic tissue always is present—relatively normal in appearance—containing Hassall's corpuscles, etc. Ectopic thymic tissue has presented as a radiographic mass in the posterior mediastinum in a 9-week-old infant.[12] Thymomas occur in childhood, both benign and malignant[11] (Fig. 44–6).

Whether in the chest[17] or in the neck, the thymic cysts, otherwise asymptomatic, may undergo rapid expansion, either from hemorrhage into them or in association with respiratory infections, and then may produce symptoms.

Thymo-lipoma is a rare benign tumor composed of fat and thymic tissue intermixed. Moigneteau and colleagues,[9] of Nantes, found a total of 48 reported cases. Their own patient was a 9-year-old boy who had vague symptoms and a large mediastinal shadow that continued to grow slowly under observation. He finally was operated on successfully after 10 full years of observation. The tumors are large, lobulated, delicately encapsulated, almost entirely composed of fat, with here and there recognizable thymic tissue elements.

Perhaps the most confusing lesion of the thymus is that called granulomatous thymoma, of which we have had 1 at the Children's Hospital of Pittsburgh. The term originally was applied to lesions of the thymus, which had the appearance of the nodular sclerosing form of Hodgkin's disease, even though the Reed-Sternberg cells often were atypical and exceedingly difficult to find. These patients characteristically presented without mediastinal or peripheral lymph nodes or lesions to suggest Hodgkin's disease. The results in patients who have had "granulomatous thymomas" simply resected even when, apparently, a complete extirpation could be performed, and who have not had radiotherapy, have been disastrous. It has become progressively more clear, in fact, that this is another manifestation of Hodgkin's disease, whether it actually begins in the thymus or not, or whether the thymic cells actually participate in some way in the disease or not.[6, 7]

REFERENCES

1. Arnheim, E. E., and Gemson, B. L.: Persistent cervical thymus gland: Thymectomy, Surgery 27:603, 1950.
2. Behring, C. H., and Bergman, F.: Thymic cyst of the neck, Acta Pathol. Microbiol. Scand. 59:45, 1963.
3. Beiger, R. C., and McAdams, A. J.: Thymic cysts, Arch. Pathol. 82:535, 1966.
4. Blalock, A., Harvey, A. M., Ford, F. R., and Lillienthal, J. L., Jr.: Treatment of myasthenia gravis by removal of thymus gland; preliminary report, JAMA 117:1529, 1941.
5. Blalock, A., Mason, M. F., Morgan, H. J., and Riven, S. S.: Myasthenia gravis and tumors of the thymic region, Ann. Surg. 110:544, 1939.
6. Fechner, R. E.: Hodgkin's disease of the thymus, Cancer 23:16, 1969.
7. Katz, A., and Lattes, R.: Granulomatous thymoma, or Hodgkin's disease of the thymus? A clinical and histologic study and a re-evaluation, Cancer 23:1, 1969.
8. Lamesch, A., Capesius, C., and Theisen-Aspesberro, M. C.: Cervical thymic cysts in infants and children, Z. Kinderchir. Grenzgeb. 14:2, 1974.
9. Moigneteau, C., Cornet, E., Mmes. Gordeef, A., Dubigeon, P., Delajarte, A., and Guillement, J. M.: Le thymo-lipome, J. Chir. (Paris) 1:94, 1967.
10. Noback, G. J.: Contribution to topographic anatomy of thymus gland: With particular references to its changes at birth and in period of newborn, Am. J. Dis. Child. 76:102, 1948.
11. Oelsnitz, G. von der: Thymustumoren im Kindesalter, Langenbeck's Arch. Klin. Chir. 322:1247, 1968.
12. Saade, M., Whitten, D. M., Necheles, T. F., Leape, L., and Darling, D.: Posterior mediastinal accessory thymus, J. Pediatr. 1:71, 1976.
13. Sealy, W. C., Weaver, W. L., and Young, W. G., Jr.: Severe airway obstruction in infancy due to thymus gland, Ann. Thorac. Surg. 1:4, 1965.
14. Simons, J., Robinson, D. W., and Masters, F.: Cervical thymic cyst, Am. J. Surg. 108:578, 1964.
15. Sutin, G. J., Hewitson, R. P.: Myasthenia gravis in a 2-year-old treated by thymectomy, S. Afr. Med. J. 40:1002, 1966.
16. Veau, V., and Olivier, E.: Aberration du thymus: Technique—resultats, Presse Med. 18:257, 1910.
17. Zanca, P., Chuang, T. H., DeAvila, R., and Galindo, D. L.: True congenital mediastinal thymic cyst, Pediatrics 36:615, 1965.

Tumors in Mediastinal Lymph Nodes

LYMPHOSARCOMA. — In the majority of instances, this lesion of the lymph nodes in the anterior mediastinum is a *secondary* one in children whose primary lesion is cervical, but primary mediastinal lesions occur. Characteristically, the anterior mediastinum is involved. The chest film of an 11-year-old boy with rather sudden onset of superior vena caval obstruction is shown in Figure 44–7. The ultimate prognosis in these children is bleak, although considerable symptomatic relief often can be achieved and an occasional cure may follow a combination of operative therapy, irradiation and chemotherapy.

HODGKIN'S DISEASE. — Primary involvement of the mediastinum in Hodgkin's disease is rare in childhood. The lesions in such instances are localized primarily in the anterior mediastinum. The therapy and prognosis of Hodgkin's disease are undergoing hopeful changes with the appreciation of the classification of the forms of Hodgkin's disease, the staging by biopsy, lymphangiography and splenectomy, following the lead of Kaplan and others.

LEUKEMIA. — Occasionally this may involve the mediastinum primarily, and lymphadenopathy in this location may appear before characteristic changes in the peripheral blood. Irradiation and systemic administration of antimetabolites may produce remarkable temporary regressions.

Mediastinal Cysts and Tumors

Cysts and tumors of the mediastinum are not rare in infancy and childhood, and extraordinarily large tumors have been removed successfully. The clinical manifestations of these masses are essentially those of expanding, space-occupying lesions and reflect their location. The symptoms most frequently encountered are chest pain, cough, respiratory distress, hemoptysis, dysphagia and weight loss. Bronchial or tracheal compression may result in desperate dyspnea requiring urgent thoracotomy.[1, 16, 21, 33, 42] Remarkably enough, a number of these cysts and tumors, even when large, are asymptomatic and show only incidentally on chest roentgenograms. Table 44–1 shows the various types in 320 mediastinal cysts and neoplasms seen at the Mayo Clinic,[8, 43] the Johns Hopkins Hospital,[15, 35] the Children's Hospital of Pittsburgh[2] and Indiana University.[20] The usual sites of the more common lesions are diagrammed in Figure 44–8.

Diagnostic studies, important in the preoperative evaluation of these patients, include, in addition to posteroanterior, lateral and oblique roentgenograms, a barium swallow and infrequently bronchography. In children with mediastinal lesions, it is not often that esophagoscopy or bronchoscopy will be required. Occasionally, angiocardiography is useful when the question arises as to origin of a mass from the heart or great vessels. Sonography can differentiate between solid and cystic tumors, and the current competition between sonography and computer-assisted tomography has not yet resolved the appropriate place of each, although either may be spectacularly revealing in a given instance. Precise diag-

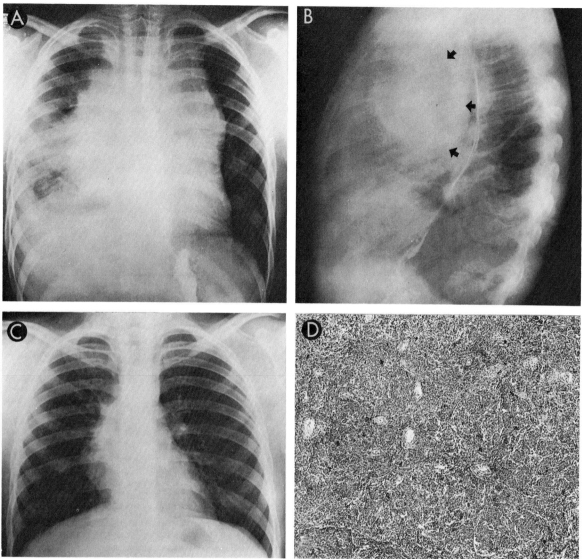

Fig. 44–7.—Lymphosarcoma. Occasionally, lymphosarcoma begins primarily in the anterior mediastinum and may conceivably justify attempts at operative removal before irradiation and chemotherapy. More often, mediastinal lymphosarcoma is only an episode in a diffuse disease. This boy of 11 developed signs of superior vena cava obstruction. **A,** plain film shows bilateral mediastinal and some pulmonary opacification. **B,** lateral roentgen-ogram shows the bulk of the lesion in the anterior mediastinum. The massive and infiltrating neoplasm could not be extirpated. **C,** irradiation caused marked clinical improvement and obvious clearing of mediastinal enlargement, but the child ultimately died. **D,** photomicrograph of the mediastinal lesion shows closely packed small cells and absence of any germinal centers.

nosis before operation may not be possible. The presence of gastric mucosa in enteric cysts has led to their successful diagnosis by technetium pertechnetate scanning.[12, 26] Since some mediastinal tumors have malignant potentialities and most others sooner or later will cause symptoms by virtue of their location, it is our position that all mediastinal tumors and cysts should be removed whenever they are discovered, even though there are no symptoms.

Cysts of Foregut Origin

A variety of epithelium-lined cysts occur in the mediastinum.

ENTERIC CYSTS.—Called also enterogenous cysts, gastrogenous cysts and esophageal duplications (see also Chap. 87), these cysts are found in the posterior mediastinum.

They are muscle-walled, spherical or tubular, have the external appearance of bowel and may be lined by any type of alimentary tract epithelium, or even by ciliated epithelium, since portions of the embryonal foregut are lined by ciliated epithelium. The muscle is arranged in layers, complete with myenteric plexuses (Fig. 44–9). Very commonly, cervical or upper thoracic vertebral anomalies, particularly hemivertebrae, are associated (Figs. 44–10 and 44–11),[9, 11, 44] and not rarely the same patients have intra-abdominal enterogenous cysts.[3, 32, 41] In rare instances, the cyst may be attached to or communicate with the spinal canal.[4] Neurologic symptoms due to spinal cord compression have been relieved by transthoracic excision of intrathoracic and intraspinal components[31] or by separate laminectomy and thoracotomy.[40] Among the most fascinating aspects of the posterior mediastinal enteric cysts is their occasional connection with

TABLE 44–1.—Incidence of Cysts and Primary Neoplasms of the Mediastinum in Infancy and Childhood°

		INDIANA	JOHNS HOPKINS	MAYO	PITTS-BURGH	TOTAL	%
Neurogenic tumors	Ganglioneuroma	2	6	16	11	105	33.0
	Ganglioneuroblastoma	1	–	2	6		
	Neuroblastoma	4	8	11	23		
	Neurofibroma	2	3	7	–		
	Neurofibrosarcoma	–	–	1	1		
	Ganglioneurosarcoma	–	1	–	–		
Teratoid cysts and tumors	Teratoma—incl. "dermoid" cysts	3	8	21	4	37	11.57
	Teratocarcinoma	1	–	–	–		
Thymic lesions	Normal thymus	–	–	–	1	25	8.0
	Thymic hyperplasia	6	8	2	1		
	Thymic cysts	–	–	2	4		
	Thymic tumors	–	–	–	1		
Thyroid	Thyroid	–	–	1	–	1	
Cysts of fore-gut origin	Enteric cysts (esoph. dupl.)	3	6	7	11	48	15.0
	Bronchogenic cysts	8	2	5	6		
Sequestered lung	Sequestered lung	–	1	–	1	2	
Pericardial cysts	Pericardial cysts	–	1	–	1	2	
Vascular malformations and tumors	Hemangioma	1	4	3	5	22	7.0
	Lymphangioma (incl. hygroma)	3	–	6	–		
	Hemangiopericytoma	–	–	1	–	4	
	Hemangioendothelioma	1	–	–	–		
	Angiosarcoma	–	–	2	–		
Lymphomas	Lymphosarcoma	1	4	9	8	31	10.0
	Hodgkin's disease	2	4	–	3		
Lipoidoses	Letterer Siewe's disease	–	2	–	–	2	
Miscellaneous	Miscellaneous malignancies	1	10	1	2	14	4.0
Benign connective tissue tumors	Lipoma	–	1	–	1	5	
	Fibroma	–	2	–	1		
Granulomas	Tbc.	–	5	–	–	16	5.0
	Sarcoid	3	3	3	–		
	Histoplasmosis	–	–	–	1		
	Histiocytosis X	–	–	–	1		
	Miscellaneous	–	–	5	–	5	
	TOTAL	42	79	105	93	320	

°One hundred five cases from the Mayo Clinic,[8, 43] 42 cases from Indiana University;[20] 80 cases from Johns Hopkins Hospital;[15, 35] 93 cases from the Children's Hospital of Pittsburgh.[2] Heidelberg series[19] of 59 cases shows similar proportions in the major groups: 14 neurogenic tumors, 18 teratoid tumors, 9 cysts, 6 tumors of vascular origin, but 15 assorted carcinomas and sarcomas represent an unusually high proportion, if these were all primary and unclassifiable tumors.

the alimentary canal.[25] Such apparently purely mediastinal cysts may penetrate through the diaphragm to end blindly in the abdomen[37] or may connect with the jejunum (see Fig. 44–10) or duodenum, so that barium and air may enter the long mediastinal diverticulum (see Fig. 44–11). As a rule, enteric cysts are closely associated with the esophagus but may be readily dissected away except in rare cases, unlike similar cysts associated with the bowel. Ordinarily, they have no communication with the lumen of the esophagus and, therefore, being lined with secretory epithelium, fill with fluid, attain a large size and cause symptoms in infancy or early childhood. They are more than twice as common on the right as on the left side and, if long enough, show a recognizable constriction due to compression by the azygos vein (see Fig. 44–10). Because they frequently are lined by gastric mucosa, which secretes an extremely acid solution, peptic ulceration of these cysts occurs, with resultant substernal pain, erosion into lung, bronchus or esophagus, and hemorrhage.[32] Fatal hemorrhage into the bronchial tree has been recorded[26] and partial pulmonary resection[26] or pneumonectomy[30] has been lifesaving in some cases.

Mediastinal cysts of foregut origin of the other two types discussed below are less likely to fill with secretions and expand and cause symptoms from compression or erosion, so that they are not so often discovered in early years.[18, 25, 27, 29]

BRONCHOGENIC CYSTS.—The second type and perhaps the most common, taking all ages, usually is lined by respiratory epithelium, occasionally with cartilage and a little smooth muscle in its wall, and never with a well-formed muscular wall and myenteric plexus, as seen in the first type.[18, 28] Bronchogenic cysts may be located within the lung or, more commonly, along or fused with the main bronchi and only occasionally communicate with the bronchial lumen; if they do, the radiographic appearance suggests a pulmonary cyst. They have been reported within the pericardial sac and to have caused death from pressure.[6] Bronchogenic cysts often are not demonstrable radiologically except for compression of the trachea or bronchus. In a collective review of 31 cases in infants and children, Opsahl and Berman[29] found that 25 patients had symptoms. In 14, the lesion was seen on x-ray films and operation undertaken—successfully in 12. The 11 symptomatic children who were not operated on died. Of 10 infants with bronchogenic cysts reported from the Children's Hospital of Boston,[10] 7 were in severe or moderate respiratory distress. In

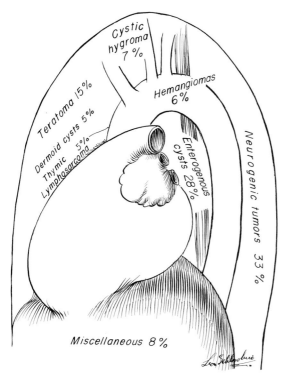

Fig. 44–8.—Mediastinal cysts and tumors. Sites of distribution of lesions in children, 320 cases from Johns Hopkins,[15, 35] Mayo Clinic,[8, 43] Indiana University[20] and Children's Hospital of Pittsburgh[2] series. Neurogenic tumors, occurring entirely in the posterior mediastinum, form the largest group. Teratomas and dermoids in the anterior mediastinum and the posterior mediastinal cysts of foregut origin (duplications of the esophagus and bronchogenic cysts) are the other two most common groups of lesions. The lymphomas are all in the anterior mediastinum.

form (including the 3 fatal cases), the presence of a mediastinal mass was not recognized, and 2 died without operation, the cyst being found only at autopsy. Like others, Eraklis and colleagues[10] comment on the occasional difficulty, at operation, of finding the cyst hidden in the structure-filled mediastinum.

ESOPHAGEAL TYPE.—The third type of mediastinal cyst of foregut origin is extremely closely associated with the esophagus, and frequently actually is intramural, but contains a ciliated epithelial lining, cartilage in the wall, no intestinal mucosa, no significant amount of muscle in the wall and has no associated vertebral abnormality.

Maier[27] divided the bronchogenic cysts into five groups—paratracheal, carinal, hilar, paraesophageal and miscellaneous. Although the theory of abnormal budding from the respiratory tract readily seems to explain the first groups, it is not as ready an answer to the formation of those cysts that are associated with the esophagus or occur behind it and are attached to the vertebrae. These, like the enterogenous cysts, obviously derive from the primitive foregut, but the precise mode of origin is a subject for speculation.

Treatment.—The cysts of these three groups cause symptoms by virtue of their size and location and, in the case of the enteric cysts, because of peptic ulceration. Resection is required for all of them, and total extirpation usually is possible. One should be aware of the possibility of transdiaphragmatic extension of the enteric cysts, and of abnormally coursing pulmonary or other vessels, particularly with bronchogenic cysts. Occasionally, dense adherence to esophagus

or bronchus or trachea may make total removal of a cyst difficult or impossible. One then may choose to peel the mucosa of the cyst away from the attached structure, leaving the nonepithelial portions of the wall. Chemical cauterization has been utilized but is hazardous and uncertainly effective. In an earlier day, Ladd advised marsupialization—establishment of an external fistulous tract. This would not be acceptable today. Internal drainage of an enteric cyst into the esophagus has been used, but in a cyst with gastric mucosal lining would lead to peptic ulceration and the inevitable sequel of hemorrhage or stricture.

Cystic Hygroma (Lymphogenous Cyst)

These multilocular, thin-walled cysts containing lymphatic fluid and dilated lymphatic channels are congenital and characteristically appear in the posterior triangle of the neck (see Chap. 36). Extension of a portion of the process into the mediastinum is not uncommon. Rarely, the lesion arises primarily in the mediastinum; Gross and Hurwitt[14] found 3 instances of this type in 112 patients with cystic hygroma. Total extirpation of the mediastinal portion of a cervical hygroma or of one primarily arising in the mediastinum may not always be possible, but removal of all the grossly recognizable tissue will relieve the symptoms of pressure and prevent the occurrence of infection in the cyst in association with respiratory infections. It would seem that if all of the cyst is removed and no gross tumor is left behind, the remnants may be permanently encased in scar tissue and cause no further symptoms. The results of operation are excellent, and the risks are nonspecific.

Pericardial Cysts (Coelomic Cysts)

In the roentgenogram, these cysts usually appear in the cardiophrenic angle as delicate spherical shadows attached to the pericardium. They are thin walled, lined by flattened mesothelium, contain clear fluid and may be effortlessly removed. The cysts are asymptomatic and are removed principally to establish their innocent nature. Their occurrence in a child is rare. Such a lesion in a 6-year-old child represents the only childhood example of this type in the records of the Armed Forces Institute of Pathology. We note 2 in our collected series.

A variety of miscellaneous mediastinal cysts occur. Shidler and Holman[38] described a 4-month-old infant with respiratory distress since birth who had a mesothelium-lined cyst containing clear fluid located between the aorta and vena cava. An unusual transpericardial approach proved to be successful.

Tumors of Neurogenic Origin

The tumors of neurogenic origin that occur in infancy and childhood are of three principal histologic and clinical types. All arise in the posterior mediastinum, usually in the more cephalad portion, and present a characteristically dense, sharply circumscribed radiologic appearance.[2] The benign tumors—ganglioneuroma and neurofibroma—may grow to very large size without producing symptoms until Horner's syndrome or marked displacement of the trachea attracts attention. The neuroblastoma, the only malignant tumor of the three, may cause pain from involvement of nerve trunks or may cause symptoms from distant metastases, and occasionally may erode through the chest wall, producing a visible mass (see Fig. 44–14).

Neurinomas, which are not rare in older patients and may

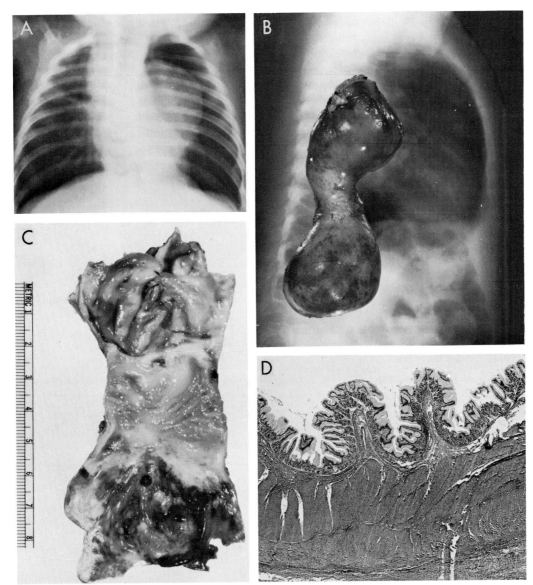

Fig. 44–9.—Mediastinal cyst of foregut origin (enteric cyst). A boy of 4 months had a 3-week history of severe respiratory distress. **A,** the plain film shows a moderately dense, sharply rounded and discrete mass projecting into the left hemithorax. **B,** in the lateral film the mass was seen to be entirely in the posterior mediastinum. The specimen, here superimposed on the roentgen picture, was readily excised. The bulbous caudal portion extended below the diaphragm, which constricted the midportion of the tubular thick-walled structure, whose external appearance was that of bowel. There was no communication with the gastrointestinal tract. **C,** the interior of the cyst had thick, velvety mucosa with recognizable gastric rugae. The cyst was filled with turbid yellow fluid. **D,** photomicrograph of the lining shows characteristic gastric rugae.

occur along the intercostal nerves, even anteriorly, do not seem to develop in children.

There may be clinical and radiologic clues to the nature of these tumors, as indicated below, but in the absence of one or another of these indicative differences it is not possible to make a specific differential diagnosis without operation.[27]

GANGLIONEUROMA.—This is the most common neurogenic mediastinal tumor of childhood, and most ganglioneuromas reported have occurred in infants or children. It is discovered in infants more commonly than is the neurofibroma. The tumors tend to reach very large size, are discrete, well encapsulated and offer no difficulty in removal, unless they have reached so great a size that this in itself consitutes a problem.[17] The characteristic histologic feature (Fig. 44–12)

is the typical ganglion cell, indicative of the origin of these tumors from the ganglions of the sympathetic chain. At least one ganglioneuroma, with an intraspinal extension (dumbbell or hourglass tumor), has been reported. Varying amounts of fibrous tissue are seen within the tumor, and sometimes younger forms of sympathetic cells, so that at times a ganglioneuroma may not be a tumor of a pure cell type, and some of these tumors have malignant potentials, based on a greater admixture of younger sympathetic cells. Such ganglioneuroblastomas should be treated by irradiation following operative removal. In a 5-year-old girl[39] presenting with an almost 3-year history of watery diarrhea, a large mediastinal tumor seen on x-ray and proved to be a pure ganglioneuroma, with no neuroblastomatous elements, both the tumor and the serum showed high levels of vasoac-

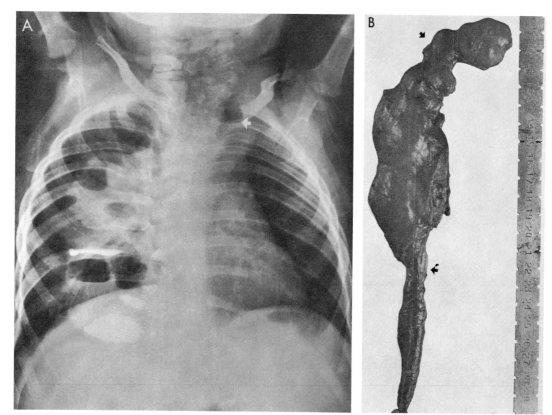

Fig. 44–10.—Mediastinal foregut cyst communicating with small intestine. A 1-year-old boy with a 1-week history of high fever and frequent vomiting, dyspnea, cyanosis and evidence of pulmonary infection. He had had other such bouts previously. **A,** film taken during a barium meal shows multiple cervical and upper thoracic vertebral anomalies, multiple gas-filled shadows in the right hemithorax, some in the apex of the left chest *(arrow)* and several deposits of barium above the diaphragm. At other stages in the barium study, almost the entire area of opacity and gas in the right chest was filled with barium. **B,** operative specimen. The mass was entirely posterior mediastinal. *Upper arrow* shows the site of constriction by the azygos vein; *lower arrow,* the point where the cystic structure passed through the dia-phragm. The caudal end communicated with the lumen of the jejunum in its first loop at the mesenteric border, passing between leaves of the mesentery. The sac contained fluid with an acid reaction. Microscopic sections showed gastric mucosa predominating in the upper half of the specimen and small intestinal mucosa predominating in the lower half, although there were areas of both in each portion. It is well to be aware of such transdiaphragmatic communications. Preoperative confusion with diaphragmatic hernia is obviously possible; approaches to the two lesions are somewhat different, particularly for surgeons who prefer the abdominal approach for hernia. (Courtesy of Dr. J. Snodgrass.)

tive intestinal peptide (VIP), and diarrhea was relieved despite incomplete removal of the tumor.

NEUROFIBROMA.—The neurofibromas that arise from nerves in the posterior mediastinum—intercostal, phrenic, vagus or sympathetic—may occur as isolated tumors or as part of the neurofibromatosis of Recklinghausen's disease. In the latter instances, the family history, the presence of the pigmented cutaneous stigmata and the usual multiplicity of lesions all point to this diagnosis (Fig. 44–13) (see Chap. 135). Dumbbell tumors or associated scoliosis are pathognomonic suggestions of the nature of a given tumor in the posterior mediastinum. In such instances, the intervertebral foramina are enlarged and the costovertebral articulations may be displaced. At operation, the tumors usually are sufficiently large, in the area in which intercostal nerves and sympathetic trunks are both located, that frequently it is not possible to be certain of the precise origin of the tumor. Furthermore, in neurofibromatosis, plexiform neurofibromas (rankenneurom) are common, with apparent extensions of the tumor along the sheaths of numerous small nerves, so that total extirpation is impossible. In such cases, one must be content with resection of the principal mass. Although malignant degeneration of neurofibromas is common and to be feared, it takes place mainly or entirely in tumors of large size.

NEUROBLASTOMA.—The neuroblastoma is a malignant tumor of sympathetic origin arising from what is conceived to be an immature precursor of the ganglion cell (Fig. 44–14). The majority of neuroblastomas in infancy are found in association with the adrenal gland. When large, such tumors not infrequently extend through or behind the diaphragm into the thorax. Neuroblastomas occurring primarily within the mediastinum and not associated with abdominal tumors are not excessively rare. The presence in the urine of elevated levels of the catecholamines is diagnostic. Although the radiologic appearance frequently suggests a sharply circumscribed lesion, operation usually discloses fairly diffuse infiltration into the soft tissues and involvement of the adjacent ribs and vertebral bodies without evidence of encapsulation. Despite this, vigorous attempts at operative eradication, with removal of the involved portions of the thoracic wall and electrocauterization of the tumor bed, followed by postoperative irradiation, have resulted in a significant number of apparently indefinite survivals. At the Columbus, Ohio, Children's Hospital,[23] 19 of 134 patients with neuroblastoma or ganglioneuroblastoma had dumbbell

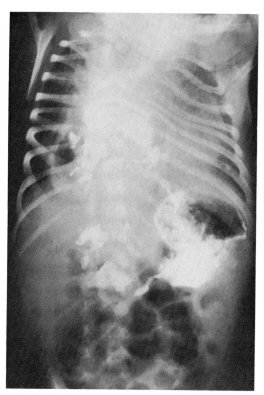

Fig. 44–11.—Mediastinal foregut cyst; neonatal distress, spinal communication. An infant of 1 month had been cyanotic and dyspneic since birth. Roentgen studies showed rachischisis of lower cervical and upper thoracic segments, with marked widening of interpeduncular spacing and abnormal segmentation. The esophagus was displaced anteriorly. In the GI series, the gas- and fluid-filled cystic shadows posterior to the heart are seen to connect with the intestine. At operation, several dilated loops of a bowel-like structure lay in the posterior mediastinum. The caudal end arose from the jejunum, with which it communicated. The mediastinal structure was excised and its infradiaphragmatic attachment to the bowel divided. After 4 uneventful days the baby became acutely ill and *Escherichia coli* was cultured from blood and cerebrospinal fluid. At autopsy, the cephalic end of the cyst was found to communicate with the spinal canal through a bony defect in the T1 vertebra. The remaining portion of the cyst formed an abscess sac communicating with the spinal canal. There was severe meningitis. This is a clear example of persistence of all the elements of the neuro-enteric-canal-residua malformation. (Courtesy of Children's Hospital of Detroit.)

tumors; 9 were abdominal tumors, 9 were thoracic and 1 was cervical, and almost all had neurologic deficits. After two-stage operation and postoperative irradiation, 11 of 17 followed more than 2 years were well. In the series from the Children's Hospital of Boston there were 27 children with mediastinal neurofibroma seen over 22 years; 2 children presented with paraplegia. The planned treatment was resection (thought complete in only 8 cases), irradiation and chemotherapy (nitrogen mustard). Twenty-three of the 27 children are alive, without evidence of tumor, 2–10 years after operation; the 2 paraplegic children have had almost complete return of function. All 19 infants and 50% of the older children were survivors.[13] As with the abdominal neuroblastomas, the period of risk formula seems to hold. The best results are in the youngest infants, and the probability of cure is soonest established in them. The postoperative irradiation inevitably injures several vertebrae sufficiently and shortens the length of the trunk, and, together with resection of posterior rib segments—necessary in some chil-

dren—may lead to scoliosis, so that the children must be followed with this in mind.

Treatment.—It is estimated that some 20% of neurogenic tumors of the mediastinum are malignant. The neuroblastomas are malignant from the start, and the neurofibromas have a potentiality for malignant degeneration that has been claimed to be as high as 40%.[22] All of these tumors can grow to enormous size, in mass alone constituting a threat to life, and at this point create technical difficulties for the surgeon. The tumors should be removed when first recognized. A formal posterolateral thoracotomy affords the best exposure, although occasionally with small tumors, a rib resection over the tumor provides direct and satisfactory access. The neurofibromas and ganglioneuromas, which usually are sharply encapsulated, may be removed without much difficulty unless great size has led to extensive vascular connections. If dumbbell intraspinal extensions are recognized before operation, laminectomy for removal of the intraspinal portion usually is performed first. The neuroblastomas require en bloc chest wall resection and a vigorous effort at removal or destruction of the tumor, followed by irradiation and chemotherapy (see Fig. 44–14).

Teratomas and Dermoid Cysts

Second in frequency only to the mediastinal tumors of neurogenic origin, these embryologic malformations contribute some of the largest and most unusual mediastinal tumors. The term dermoid cyst usually is applied to tumors composed entirely of ectodermal derivatives. The typical dermoid is a thick-walled fibrous sac lined by squamous epithelium in which are seen the various skin appendages, the sac being filled with hair and occasionally teeth and the typical caseous detritus.

Teratomas, which may be solid or cystic, contain derivatives of all three embryonic germ layers. In addition to cartilage and bone, glial tissue is a characteristic component, together with all manner of epithelial structures and many bizarre types of glandular tissue. In fact, it has become apparent that if careful search is made in the wall of most dermoid tumors, whether of the mediastinum or of the ovary, at least a small portion of the wall may be found to contain a solid tumor in which there are derivatives of the other two germ layers. The tumors almost invariably are found in the anterior mediastinum (Figs. 44–15 and 44–16), occasionally within the pericardium. They may reach enormous size, bulging out into one hemithorax or the other, and when the great size and long duration of the tumor have caused a bulging of one side of the chest wall, the clinical diagnosis of teratoma or dermoid may be made with some assurance on inspection of the patient. Only an occasional tumor is recognized to be malignant at birth, but perhaps 20–25% of the solid teratomas have been called malignant. The criteria of malignancy, based in a few cases solely on histologic evidence within the primary tumor, are somewhat uncertain in view of the bizarre admixture of various elements, so that the actual incidence of malignancy proved by the ultimate clinical behavior of the tumors is a little lower than the figures given. When malignancy occurs, almost invariably it is in the form of carcinoma rather than sarcoma, and usually of an adeno- or papillary type of carcinoma. Death comes from direct extension and pulmonary and other metastases. Symptoms of the benign tumors are caused by displacement of the trachea, esophagus or heart and great vessels or by infection within the cyst and erosion into the pleural cavity

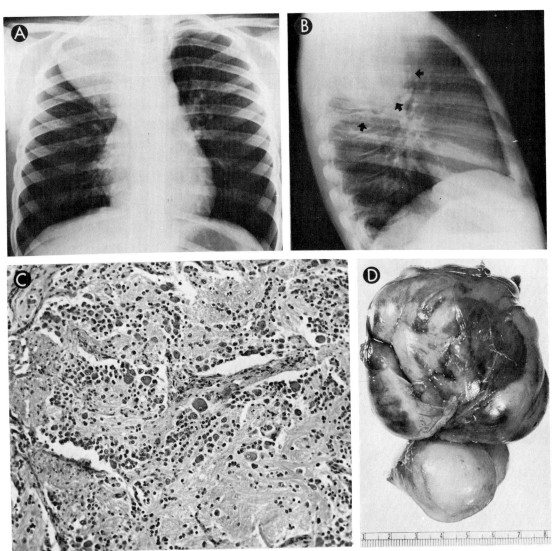

Fig. 44–12.—Ganglioneuroma of mediastinum. A boy of 6 had severe chronic cough. **A** and **B,** roentgenograms show a discrete, dense, rounded tumor filling the posterior mediastinum. Tumors of neurogenic origin invariably are in the posterior mediastinum, usually in the cephalad portion. **C,** photomicrograph shows characteristic ganglion cells, almost in pure culture, although the few small, round, hyperchromatic cells may represent younger forms in the sympathetic series. A varying amount of neurofibrillary structure is found in these tumors. **D,** operative specimen. The lobulated tumor was readily removed. The attachments were few, loose and not vascular.

or trachea. The coughing up of hair in such instances is a pathognomonic sign. Until either infection or malignant degeneration has occurred, the tumors are quite readily removable.[22, 28, 34] As in other mediastinal tumors, their discovery is the indication for their removal because malignancy may be present or may develop and because continued growth of the tumor leads to serious symptoms from pressure and displacement of mediastinal structures. In addition, infection of these tumors or erosion into other structures may produce dangerous consequences and greatly complicate the problem of operative removal.

Miscellaneous Neoplasms

A wide variety of additional neoplasms and cysts of all kinds have been described in the mediastinum, usually in isolated case reports.[36, 45] These include hemangiomas, lipomas,[24] embryonal rhabdomyosarcomas (Fig. 44–17), osteochondromas, pheochromocytomas[7] and a group of anaplastic carcinomas and sarcomas.

In addition to the lesions discussed in this chapter, it must be remembered that a number of other conditions that occur in the mediastinum require consideration in the differential diagnosis. These include intrathoracic goiter, aneurysms of the pulmonary artery and other congenital anomalies of the great vessels and diaphragmatic hernia of any of the several types. Although differentiation often may be made on clinical and roentgenologic grounds, frequently only operation discloses the final diagnosis.

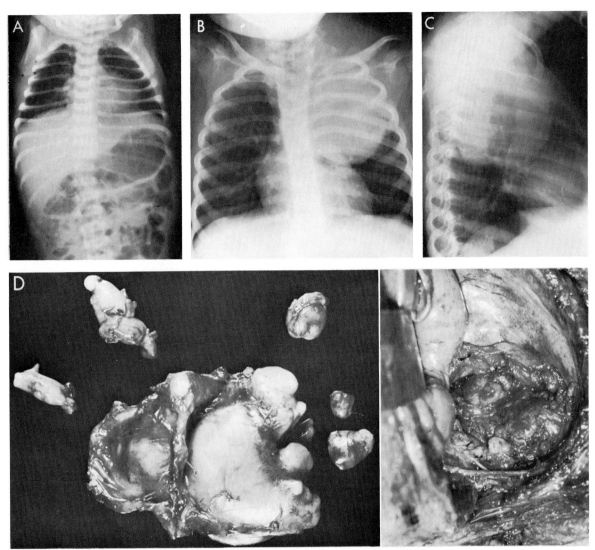

Fig. 44–13.—Mediastinal neurofibroma; von Recklinghausen's disease. This 2½-year-old child was one of 8 siblings. The father and one of his brothers have frank von Recklinghausen's disease. The mother has no stigmata. Seven of the 8 children have obvious neurofibromatosis. All have multiple areas of cutaneous pigmentation and at least subcutaneous nodules. Four have had large tumors operated on. **A,** roentgenogram in neonatal period shows no obvious tumor. **B,** at age 2½, during routine study of all the siblings, the chest film shows an enormous asymptomatic left supraclavicular tumor, uniformly dense and sharply circumscribed. **C,** the intrathoracic tumor is so large that it would be difficult to say that it arose in the posterior mediastinum, although obviously it is closely applied to the paravertebral gutter. This growth in the short life of the child is remarkably rapid and cause for concern. At operation, the firm spherical mass was found to have numerous pseudopod-like projections posteromedially and posterosuperiorly, extending into the mediastinum and neck. There was no hourglass spinal tumor and no direct invasion by the mass, extension being by innumerable nerve-like connections from 1 to 15 mm in diameter ramifying in all directions. These were amputated as far from the tumor as possible. Postoperatively, the child had Horner's syndrome. Microscopic sections showed plexiform neurofibroma. **D:** *left,* gross specimen, view of the flattened posterior aspect with its pleural covering peeled back, showing a number of the processes, which extended into the neck and mediastinum. These were amputated close to the tumor; then additional portions were removed from the tumor bed after delivery of the tumor. *Right,* the tumor bed, showing the upper half of the thorax now empty and the stubs of tumor processes extending into the neck and mediastinum before they were excised.

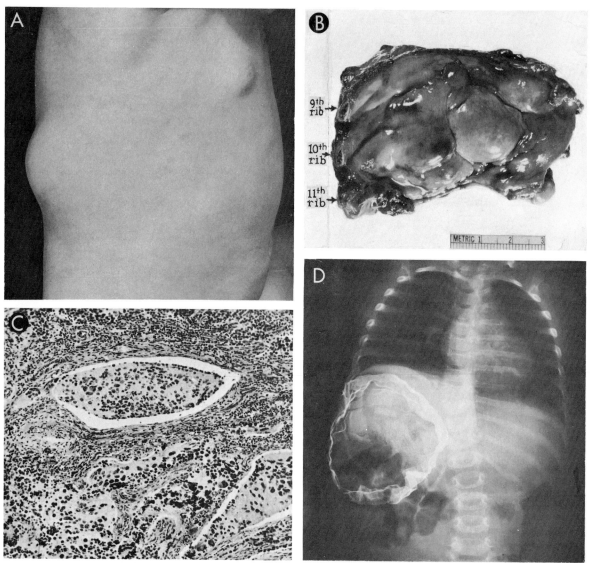

Fig. 44–14.—Neuroblastoma of mediastinum, presenting as a chest wall tumor in a baby of 8 months. **A,** the tumor caused a visible bulge in the posterior axillary line. It was fixed to the deep tissues. **B,** operative specimen, pleural aspect. The diffusely spreading, not localized character of the tumor is obvious. A full-thickness block of all tissues of the chest wall, except skin and fat, was removed. Almost certainly, the tumor infiltrated between the vertebrae. The tumor bed was coagulated with electrocautery. **C,** the tumor is composed largely of very young cells of the sympathetic series and therefore qualifies as a sympathicoblastoma, but here and there occasional ganglion cells were found. Official diagnosis was ganglioneuroblastoma.

Presence of a solid plug of tumor in a vein, plainly visible here, led to an incorrectly gloomy prognosis. **D,** the diaphragm was moved to the 8th rib, the upper border of the operative defect, and the resultant large ventral hernia repaired with tantalum mesh. This film, made some months later, shows the tantalum to be largely fragmented. The patient presented a large hernia. We no longer use metallic mesh, preferring Teflon felt. The child was free from tumor 10 years later, but resection and heavy irradiation resulted in severe scoliosis. Thoracic neuroblastoma tends to have a good prognosis.[13]

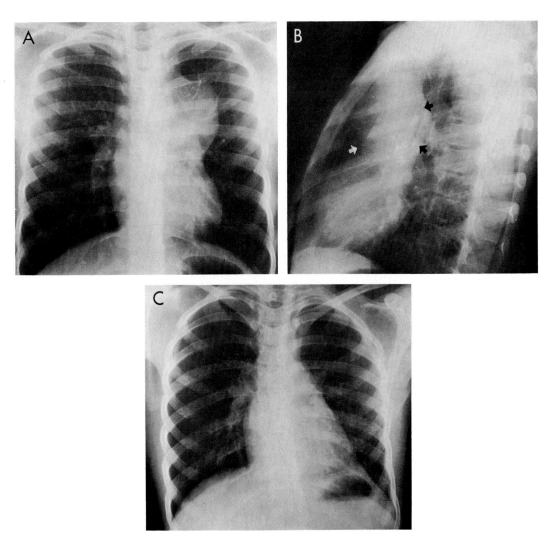

Fig. 44–15.—Teratoma of mediastinum. An 11-year-old girl had no symptoms but repeated episodes of dizziness, possibly attributable to superior vena cava obstruction, although she had no symptoms of the superior vena cava syndrome. In general, this syndrome appears only with malignant tumors and occasional chronic sclerosing mediastinal infections. **A** and **B,** preoperative roentgenograms show the fairly dense, somewhat irregularly nodular mass in the anterior mediastinum projecting into the left hemithorax. **C,** posteroperative film, after uneventful removal of the benign cyst, shows an essentially normal chest.

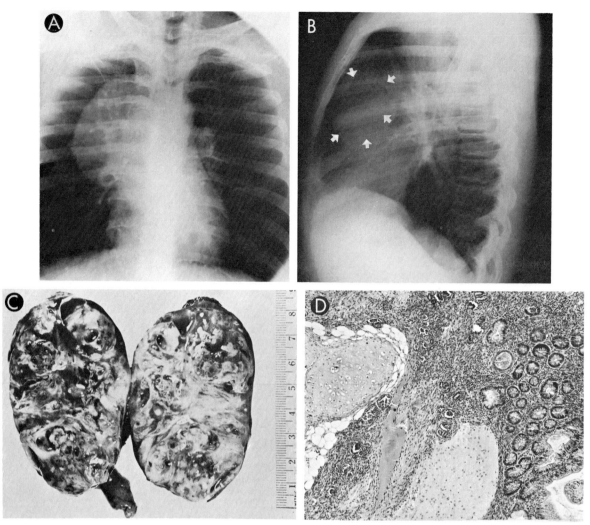

Fig. 44–16.—Mediastinal teratoma. A boy of 12 had a 6-month history of occasional pains in the right chest. Teratomas may reach great size without causing symptoms except those due to displacement or compression of mediastinal structures, and occasionally are so large and have been present for so long in the growing chest wall that the chest bulges asymmetrically on the side of the tumor. **A** and **B,** plain films show the large mass of somewhat varying density in the anterior mediastinum extending into the right hemithorax. **C,** gross specimen shows areas of varied consistency, but aside from a few frank cysts, this is a solid tumor. **D,** photomicrograph shows the melange of histologic structures characteristic of teratomas—cartilage on the left, glial tissue bottom center, various types of fibrous tissue, glandular structures and fat. But when malignancy occurs (20–25%) it is almost invariably epithelial and usually adenocarcinoma.

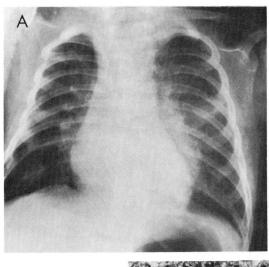 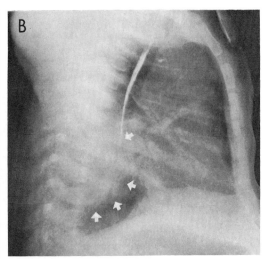

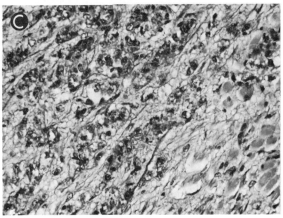

Fig. 44–17. — Embryonal rhabdomyosarcoma. A 2-month-old boy had intermittent fever and rapidly progressive paralysis of the lower extremities. **A,** plain film shows the shadow of a mediastinal mass on the left. **B,** lateral film shows the lesion to be located posteriorly. **C,** photomicrograph of specimen removed at operation for biopsy study only. A few muscle fibers are identifiable in the lower right corner. The extremely anaplastic and embryonal tumor was thought to be probably rhabdomyosarcoma. (Courtesy of Dr. J. E. Lewis, Jr.)

REFERENCES

1. Alshabkhoun, S., Starkey, G. W. B., and Asnes, R. A.: Bronchogenic cysts of the mediastinum in infancy, Ann. Thorac. Surg. 4:532, 1967.
2. Bar-Ziv, J., and Nogrady, M. B.: Mediastinal neuroblastoma and ganglioneuroma: The differentiation between primary and secondary involvement on the chest roentgenogram, Am. J. Roentgenol. 125:2, 1974.
3. Beardmore, H. E., and Wigglesworth, F. W.: Vertebral anomalies and alimentary duplication, Pediatr. Clin. North Am. p. 457, May, 1958.
4. Bentley, J. F. R., and Smith, J. R.: Developmental posterior enteric remnants and spinal malformations: The split notochord syndrome, Arch. Dis. Child. 35:76, 1960.
5. Bower, R.: Personal communication, 1977.
6. Dabbs, C. H., Berg, R., and Peirce, E. C., II: Intrapericardial bronchogenic cysts, J. Thorac. Surg. 34:718, 1957.
7. Edmunds, L. H., Jr.: Mediastinal pheochromocytoma, Ann. Thorac. Surg. 2:745, 1966.
8. Ellis, F. H., Jr., and DuShane, J. W.: Primary mediastinal cysts and neoplasms in infants and children, Am. Rev. Tuberc. 74: 940, 1956.
9. Elwood, J. S.: Mediastinal duplication of the gut, Arch. Dis. Child. 34:474, 1959.
10. Eraklis, A. J., Griscom, N. T., and McGovern, J. G.: Bronchogenic cysts of the mediastinum in infancy, N. Engl. J. Med. 281:1150, 1969.
11. Fallon, M., Gordon, A. R. G., and Lendrum, A. C.: Mediastinal cysts of foregut origin associated with vertebral abnormalities, Br. J. Surg. 41:520, 1954.

12. Ferguson, C. C., Young, L. N., Sutherland, J. B., and Macpherson, R. I.: Intrathoracic gastrogenic cyst—preoperative diagnosis by technetium pertechnetate scan, J. Pediatr. Surg. 8:827, 1973.
13. Filler, R. M., Traggis, D. G., Jaffe, N., and Vawler, G. F.: Favorable outlook for children with mediastinal neuroblastoma, J. Pediatr. Surg. 7:136, 1972.
14. Gross, R. E., and Hurwitt, E. S.: Cervicomediastinal and mediastinal cystic hygromas, Surg. Gynecol. Obstet. 87:599, 1948.
15. Haller, J. A., Mazur, D. O., and Morgan, W. W., Jr.: Diagnosis and management of mediastinal masses in children, J. Thorac. Cardiovasc. Surg. 68:385, 1969.
16. Haller, J. A., Shermeta, D. W., Donahoo, J. S., and White, J. J.: Life-threatening respiratory distress from mediastinal masses in infants, Ann. Thorac. Surg. 19:364, 1975.
17. Hamilton, J. P., and Koop, C. E.: Ganglioneuromas in children, Surg. Gynecol. Obstet. 121:803, 1965.
18. Hardy, L. M.: Bronchogenic cysts of the mediastinum, Pediatrics 4:108, 1949.
19. Hecker, W. Ch., Rüter, E., and Vogt-Moykopf, I.: Beitrag zur Klinik kindlicher Mediastinaltumoren: Analyse von 59 Fällen, Thoraxchirurgie 15:392, 1967.
20. Heimburger, I. L., and Battersby, J. S.: Primary mediastinal tumors of childhood, J. Thorac. Cardiovasc. Surg. 50:92, 1965.
21. Hurwitz, A., Conrad, R., Selvage, I. L., Jr., and Orbeton, E. A.: Hypertrophic lobar emphysema secondary to a paratracheal cyst in an infant, J. Thorac. Cardiovasc. Surg. 51:412, 1966.
22. Kent, E. M., et al.: Intrathoracic neurogenic tumors, J. Thorac. Surg. 13:116, 1944.
23. King, D., Goodman, J., Hawk, T., Boles, E. T., and Sayers, M. P.: Dumbbell neuroblastomas in children, Arch. Surg. 110:888, 1975.

24. Kleinhaus, S., and Ducharme, J. C.: Mediastinal lipoma in children, Surgery 66:790, 1969.
25. Leider, H. J., Snodgrass, J. J., and Mishrick, A. S.: Intrathoracic alimentary duplications communicating with small intestine, Arch. Surg. 71:203, 1955.
26. Macpherson, R. I., Reed, M. H., and Ferguson, C. C.: Intrathoracic gastrogenic cysts: A cause of lethal pulmonary hemorrhage in infants, J. Can. Assoc. Radiol. 24:362, 1973.
27. Maier, H. C.: Bronchogenic cyst of the mediastinum, Ann. Surg. 127:476, 1948.
28. Morrison, I. M.: Tumors and cysts of the mediastinum, Thorax 13:294, 1958.
29. Opsahl, T., and Berman, E. J.: Bronchogenic mediastinal cysts in infants, Pediatrics 30:376, 1962.
30. Page, U. S., and Bigelow, J. C.: A mediastinal gastric duplication leading to pneumonectomy: A case report, J. Thorac. Cardiovasc. Surg. 54:291, 1967.
31. Piramoon, A. M., and Abbassioun, K.: Mediastinal enterogenic cyst with spinal cord compression, J. Pediatr. Surg. 9:543, 1974.
32. Rhaney, K., and Barclay, G. P. T.: Enterogenous cysts and congenital diverticula of the alimentary canal with abnormalities of the vertebral column and spinal cord, J. Pathol. Bacteriol. 77:457, 1959.
33. Ribet, M., Callafe, R., Prost, M., and Lequien, P.: Emphyseme obstructif par kyste bronchogenique comprimant la bronche chez l'enfant, Ann. Chir. Thorac. Cardiovasc. 13:124, 1974.
34. Rusby, N. L.: Dermoid cysts and teratomata of the mediastinum, J. Thorac. Surg. 13:169, 1944.
35. Sabiston, D. C., Jr., and Scott, H. W., Jr.: Primary neoplasms and cysts of the mediastinum, Ann. Surg. 130:777, 1952.
36. Saini, V. K., and Wahi, P. L.: Hourglass transmural type of intrathoracic lipoma, J. Thorac. Cardiovasc. Surg. 47:600, 1964.
37. Shepherd, M. P.: Thoracic, thoraco-abdominal and abdominal duplication, Thorax 20:82, 1965.
38. Shidler, F. P., and Holman, E. F.: Mediastinal tumors, Stanford Med. Bull. 10:217, 1952.
39. Swift, P. G. F., Bloom, S. R., and Harris, F.: Watery diarrhea and ganglioneuroma with secretion of vasoactive intestinal peptide, Arch. Dis. Child. 50:896, 1975.
40. Tarnay, T. J., Wittig, H. J., Lucas, R. V., Jr., and Warden, H. E.: Chronic and recurrent atelectasis in children, Surgery 62:520, 1967.
41. Veeneklaas, G. M. H.: Pathogenesis of intrathoracic gastrogenic cysts, Am. J. Dis. Child. 83:500, 1952.
42. Weichert, R. F., III, Lindsey, E. S., Pearce, C. W., and Waring, W. W.: Bronchogenic cyst with unilateral obstructive emphysema, J. Thorac. Cardiovasc. Surg. 59:287, 1970.
43. Whittaker, L. D., and Lynn, H. B.: Mediastinal tumors and cysts in the pediatric patient, Surg. Clin. North Am. 53:893, 1973.
44. Willich, E.: Thorako-abdominale magenduplikatur, Kinderchirurgie 5:115, 1967.
45. Wilson, J. R., and Bartley, T. D.: Liposarcoma of the mediastinum, J. Thorac. Cardiovasc. Surg. 48:486, 1967.

45   DALE G. JOHNSON

Endoscopy

THE FIELD OF ENDOSCOPY—direct inspection and manipulation inside hollow organs or body cavities—has evolved from the shaped tin tube with a wax candle light, used by Bozzini in 1806, to our modern instrumentation involving a variety of miniaturized telescopes and sophisticated flexible fiberoptic devices.

Bronchoscopy

Killian's work in 1898, using cocaine anesthesia, hollow metal tubes and the reflected light of an electric globe, established him as the father of bronchoscopy. A few years later, Jackson established the first school for bronchoesophagology in the United States.[1]

Instrumentation

Rigid, hollow tubes of variable design and diameter have been the standard equipment of the bronchoscopist for many years. Supplemental optical telescopes have also been utilized for some time, but the more recent development of the Hopkins rod-lens system (Fig. 45–1),[2] with miniaturization of the telescope diameter, high resolution, magnification and wide-angle view, has greatly expanded the application of endoscopy in pediatric surgery.

At present, the Storz* line of pediatric bronchoscopes offers the widest range of capability in infants and children. Bronchoscope sheaths of appropriate length and diameter are available for the smallest premature infant to the adult. Miniaturized biopsy forceps or grasping tools can be manipulated through an instrument channel while ventilation is maintained through a closed circuit and the viewing telescope is in place. Selective suctioning can also be accomplished with sharp and magnified visual control. For problems requiring a larger foreign body forceps, the telescope can be removed for work without optical magnification through the main channel.

The Storz infant urethral resectoscope has also proved to be very useful for endoscopic resection of granuloma and some types of stenosis in the upper airway of infants.[5]

Flexible fiberoptic bronchoscopes at present have little or no application in small infants. The diameter of even the smallest of these instruments (4 mm) approaches the infant's total airway diameter, and the fiberscopes have no channel for ventilation. In larger children and adolescents it is possible to pass the smaller size flexible bronchoscopes through an endotracheal tube, with airway control through a side arm adapter. Even so, the small (or absent) instrument channel limits the amount of manipulation or suctioning that can be performed. The flexible bronchoscope does offer the advantage of easy direction into the upper lobes or the segmental bronchi, but, in children, the flexible instrument seldom can be directed into an orifice inaccessible to the rigid bronchoscope simply because the outer diameter remains too large. Limited foreign body manipulation with flexible grasping instruments can be achieved through the flexible endoscope, but airway foreign bodies rarely are a problem in older children, in whom the flexible bronchoscope can be introduced.

Technique

Bronchoscopy in infants and children is most effectively and safely performed in the operating room under general anesthesia. The airway should be controlled with a semiclosed system, and continuous cardiac monitoring is essential. Rapid and repeated blood gas monitoring is also useful during difficult manipulations or for complicated endoscopic resections. The examination of the airway should be a sterile procedure, particularly in small infants.

The "sniffing" position provides proper positioning for bronchoscopy. This is obtained by flexion of the head and neck on the anterior chest, with subsequent moderate hyperextension of the head on the forward-flexed neck. Introduction of the bronchoscope is facilitated by initial exposure of the vocal cords. As the tongue and epiglottis are lifted forward, the blade of the laryngoscope should be advanced slightly into the vallecula to open and elevate the epiglottis farther. A common error in infants involves too deep insertion, because the larynx is situated at a higher level than in the adult.

The point of smallest diameter in the infant trachea is at the cricoid level just below the cords. If the bronchoscope does not pass easily at this point, the sheath should be replaced for one of smaller diameter. Once the bronchoscope is in the upper trachea, a flexible side arm can be attached to the anesthesia machine for semiclosed system ventilation. Fogging of the telescope can be avoided by prewarming of the instrument in warm water and by placing a thin layer of antifoam on the tip of the lens before insertion. An alternative system involves the use of an antifog sheath that passes a small stream of air under positive pressure around the telescope to prevent fogging and fouling with secretions.

SPECIAL TECHNIQUES.—The sharp and magnified view provided by the rod-lens telescope adds greatly to the precision and ease of foreign body manipulation in the airway. Once the foreign object has been grasped, it is necessary to withdraw the entire bronchoscope to effect removal. Some foreign bodies are more easily grasped by a device with spring hooks in a flexible sheath. This can be passed through the instrument channel while the telescope is in place. Other foreign bodies are too friable for retrieval by the hooks or an alligator jaw and must be handled with larger forceps

*K. Storz Endoscopy Co., Tuttlingen, West Germany. Distributor: K. Storz Endoscopy America, Inc., 658 S. San Vicente Blvd., Los Angeles, California 90048.

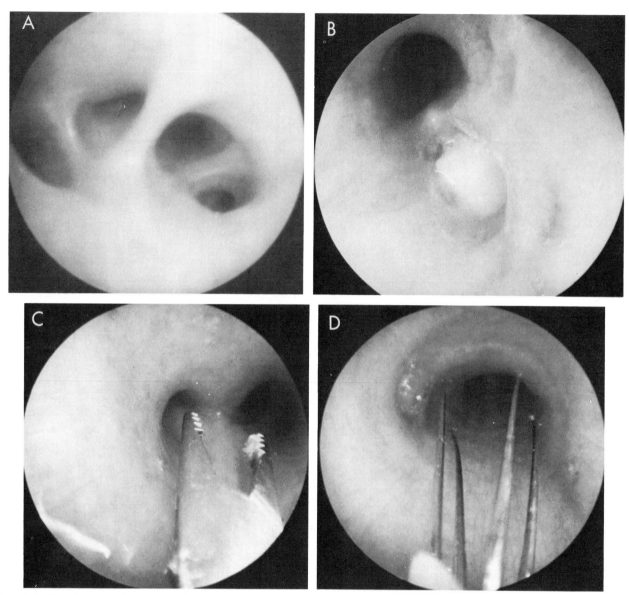

Fig. 45–1.—Bronchoscopic views. **A,** middle lobe and basal segmental bronchial orifices in a 2-week-old infant, as seen with the Hopkins rod-lens telescope. **B,** peanut fragment in right main bronchus. **C,** the flexible alligator forceps appears larger than the bronchus because it is closer to the viewing telescope. Actually, this instrument can be used to retrieve foreign bodies lodged below the origin of the upper lobe on either side. **D,** a flexible multi-pronged grasping tool has been passed down the instrument channel of the child-size bronchoscope. Manipulation of a foreign body within the bronchus is facilitated by the magnified view through the rod-lens telescope.

passed through the main channel after the telescope has been removed. When foreign bodies are lodged at the bronchus intermedius on the right or at the junction of the lower and upper lobe bronchi on the left, a Fogarty no. 3 embolectomy balloon catheter can be very useful. The balloon is passed beyond the foreign body under direct vision, inflated and then withdrawn to displace the object upward into the main bronchus or trachea or even into the bronchoscope. If the foreign body has been displaced into the more proximal airway, it then can be removed with one of the grasping instruments.

Occasionally an infant with a foreign body will have an airway too small for passage of the 3.5–30-cm sheath beyond the carina. For detailed visualization deeper within the airway it then is useful to use a shorter 3.5–20-cm sheath in combination with the 30-cm telescope and a rubber adapter at the proximal end. The telescope can be extended beyond the sheath, following suctioning of the deeper airway through the open channel, for visualization into the segmental bronchi. Deep extractions can again be performed with the Fogarty balloon catheter.

Indications

Acute inflammatory disease of the upper airway seldom requires endoscopic investigation. A clinical history of acute onset of stridor leaves a differential diagnosis of infection or foreign body. Acute infectious croup may be mimicked by foreign body in the hypopharynx, producing irritation and secondary edema of the larynx, but foreign body problems usually are associated with more acute onset plus a history of ingesting or aspirating some object. X-rays may show the

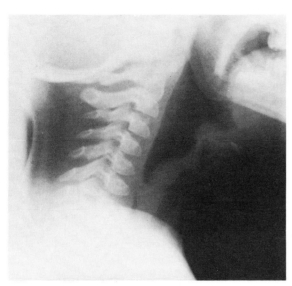

Fig. 45–2.–Epiglottitis. The swollen epiglottis and edematous aryepiglottic folds can be seen on a lateral neck view with soft tissue technique. Endoscopic manipulation usually is to be avoided in the presence of acute inflammation such as this.

acute subglottic edema associated with infectious croup, an enlarged epiglottis with epiglottitis (Fig. 45–2) or direct evidence of a foreign object. Endoscopic manipulation usually is contraindicated in the early stages of infectious croup or epiglottitis.

A problem seen with increasing frequency, however, is the apparent infectious croup in a small infant with a history of previous airway intubation or manipulation for respiratory support in the newborn period. Such infants may have delayed onset of postintubation subglottic stenosis, which becomes manifest as an apparent infectious croup months after discharge from an intensive care unit. The stridor does not disappear in such infants with usual therapy or after the usual time interval, and identification of the underlying subglottic stenosis can be achieved only by endoscopic visualization.

Laryngomalacia is one of the more common congenital obstructive lesions of the upper airway and is characterized by an inspiratory stridor or croaking, often increasing during the first 6–12 months of life. Onset of symptoms may occur during the first week of life, however. Progression in the degree of obstruction, secondary to instability and inspiratory prolapse of the supraglottic structures into the airway, may require tracheostomy, but this is not commonly the case. Growth of the larynx subsequently brings stability to the arytenoids and false cords, with a spontaneous decrease and disappearance of symptoms. Diagnosis can be made with a laryngoscope, but endoscopic evaluation of the larynx and trachea should be performed to rule out any lower lesions that might also present with the common symptom of stridor. The epiglottis in a child with laryngomalacia has a characteristic folded "omega" shape, and the prolapse of the supraglottic structures can easily be seen on inspiration.

Vocal cord paralysis is an important cause of stridor in infants, and may follow birth trauma or operative manipulation in the chest or neck. Unilateral vocal cord palsy following a transcervical division of a tracheoesophageal fistula or construction of a cervical esophagostomy for esophageal atresia has occurred. Proper diagnosis of airway obstruction secondary to cord palsy depends on laryngoscopic evaluation of

cord movement before the infant is deeply anesthetized. Bronchoscopy then is performed to be certain that the respiratory distress is not from some more distal obstruction in the respiratory tract. As the bronchoscope passes through the larynx, the airway obstruction is relieved, confirming that the obstruction is at the level of the larynx.

Foreign bodies in the upper airway usually are manifested by sudden choking, dyspnea, voice change and occasionally death from asphyxia. Partial airway obstruction may also result from a large foreign body lodged in the upper esophagus, causing posterior compression of the trachea. Foreign bodies occasionally become lodged above the cricoid and beneath the cords because of the narrower cricoid diameter. Removal is extremely urgent and difficult in this situation. Some foreign bodies in the trachea are more safely pushed down into the right main bronchus to allow recovery of gas exchange before the extraction is attempted.

Laryngeal trauma may cause obstruction from edema and hematoma or from actual cartilaginous fracture or disruption. Temporary tracheostomy nearly always is required for treatment, but careful endoscopic evaluation is important for assessing the damage and planning subsequent management.

Post-tracheostomy obstructions in infants are common and almost always mechanical in nature. Careful endoscopic evaluation of the airway will reveal most decannulation problems to be associated with granuloma or cartilaginous deformity. The granulomas can be managed fairly easily by endoscopic resection, and the cartilaginous deformities usually can be handled by direct tracheal reconstruction (Fig. 45–3).[4]

Postintubation subglottic stenosis is being seen with increasing frequency as smaller and sicker infants are salvaged through the aid of mechanical ventilation in newborn intensive care units. The stenosis nearly always occurs at the subglottic cricoid level and usually is manifested by the baby's inability to tolerate removal of the endotracheal tube. In such cases, tracheostomy is necessary, reserving for later the attack on the subglottic stenosis. A number of infants who have been decannulated successfully develop stridor and significant upper airway obstructions several months

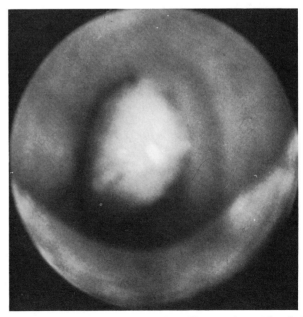

Fig. 45–3.–Post-tracheostomy granuloma. The granuloma at the site has partially occluded the tracheal lumen.

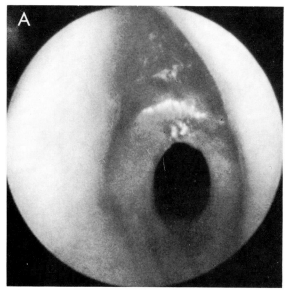

Fig. 45–4.—Subglottic stenoses following intubation. **A,** diaphragm-like subglottic stenosis below vocal cords in an infant of 9 months. She had endotracheal intubation for 3 days as a newborn for correction of esophageal atresia. Symptoms of progressive inspiratory stridor prompted endoscopic evaluation 9 months after she had been successfully decannulated. Three tracheal dilatations at 14-day intervals produced little improvement. Endoscopic resection of the web without a distal tracheostomy was easily accomplished. Subsequent tracheoscopy revealed a normal lumen, and the patient has remained without symptoms. **B,** severe postintubation subglottic stenosis in an infant who was asymptomatic for 8 months after successful endotracheal decannulation. She was re-evaluated because of apparent intractable croup. Temporary tracheostomy was required because the subglottic lumen was less than 2.0 mm. The transverse bar was removed by endoscopic resection. Two subsequent staged quadrant resections were performed endoscopically at the cricoid level. Triamcinolone injection and two dilatations were followed by successful tracheal decannulation. A minor recurrence of stridor 6 months later was again treated by a single resection with injection and dilatation. Repeat tracheostomy was not required and the patient remains asymptomatic 2 years later.

later (Fig. 45–4). Endoscopic evaluation may reveal a tracheal lumen at the cricoid level less than 2 mm in diameter. Management of this problem is complicated, but the recently described endoscopic resection of the stenosis in small infants[5] has facilitated early decannulation and eliminated many of the problems with long-term tracheostomy care or with the more complicated reconstructive attempts using intraluminal stents. Our own experience involves 20 such cases wherein properly timed and staged endoscopic resections of subglottic scar either greatly shortened the duration of maintenance of the tracheostomy or eliminated the need for tracheostomy altogether. Technical aspects of the resection must be followed precisely to avoid electrothermal injury and further scarring of the tracheal lumen.

Isolated "N" type tracheoesophageal fistula presents with recurrent coughing and aspiration associated with feedings. Diagnosis often can be made by barium esophagogram, but frequently the fistula does not fill and the diagnosis remains in question. Tracheoscopy with a 30-degree telescope to examine the posterior tracheal wall is definitive for ruling in or out the presence of a tracheoesophageal fistula (Fig. 45–5). If the fistula is identified in the usual location a few centimeters above the carina, it is useful to pass a small catheter through the fistula by way of the instrument channel in the scope. This aids subsequent identification of the fistula at dissection through a cervical or thoracic exposure.

Laryngotracheoesophageal cleft is a complex malformation involving a failure of partitioning between the upper airway and the esophagus. The cleft may be short, involving only the larynx, or it may extend all the way down to the thoracic inlet. The literature is replete with examples of missed diagnosis because of inadequate endoscopic evaluation. One report records 9 previous bronchoscopies before the correct diagnosis was identified.[3] Diagnosis with modern instrumentation is straightforward and precise (see Chap. 29).

Selective suctioning of bronchial segments in children with *cystic fibrosis* or in certain situations following major surgical procedures can be done with precision using the infant bronchoscopes and optical telescopes. In larger children with chronic pulmonary infection or cystic fibrosis,

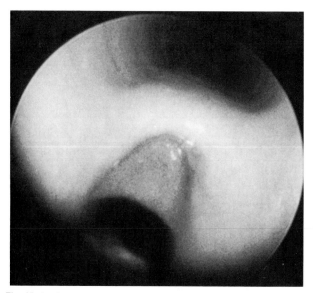

Fig. 45–5.—Tracheoesophageal fistula. A #5 ureteral catheter can be seen in a tracheoesophageal fistula located just below the thoracic inlet and 2–3 cm above the carina. The catheter was left in the fistula to facilitate exposure and division of the tracheoesophageal communication through a low, transverse incision in the right side of the neck.

the flexible fiberoptic scope occasionally is more versatile for this purpose.

Complications

Modern endoscopic equipment has reduced the incidence of complications associated with bronchoscopy, largely because the surgeon can see and manipulate within the airway with a high degree of precision. The forceful passage of a scope too large for the infant's airway may lead to subglottic edema and significant airway obstruction following the endoscopic procedure. Perforation of the trachea or bronchus is possible with an endoscope, and the resulting pneumothorax or pneumomediastinum, if undiscovered, can be fatal. The introduction of infection through poor technique and contaminated instruments can also have serious consequences. Finally, inadequate control of ventilation or partial mechanical obstruction of the airway during instrumentation can result in cerebral hypoxia and cardiac arrest. Successful management involves skill, the right instrumentation, caution, physiologic monitoring and the close cooperation of a pediatric anesthesiologist.

Endoscopy of the Upper GI Tract

A volunteer professional sword swallower provided Kussmaul in 1870 with the opportunity to describe the first esophagoscopy. Using the reflected light of a lamp for illumination, Kussmaul passed a hollow rigid tube through the mouth, pharynx and esophagus into the stomach of his cooperative subject. Thus began the practice of hollow tube esophagoscopy, which, with modification in lighting systems, remains a valuable part of endoscopic management today.

Mikulicz in 1881 introduced the gastroscope, consisting of a number of small optical units coupled together with articulated joints. In 1897, Kelling invented a flexible metal esophagoscope. The year following, in 1898, he invented a gastroscope, the lower third of which could be flexed to 45 degrees and with an objective window that could be rotated a full 360 degrees. He utilized a miniature electric globe that was built together with a prism. In 1936, Schindler worked with Wolf, an optical physicist and manufacturer, to design a semiflexible gastroscope incorporating a rubber finger at the working end. The system contained more than 48 lenses and used an electric globe for illumination. The present generation of endoscopes for the upper GI tract was initiated by Hirschowitz *et al.* in 1958 with the introduction of flexible fiberglass gastroscopes.[1]

Esophagoscopy

The development of the flexible fiberoptic gastroscope has in no way eliminated the usefulness, and for some conditions the superiority, of the rigid esophagoscope. This is particularly true in pediatric patients, and the pediatric endoscopist should have available a variety of instruments to use as indicated in specific situations. The flexible scopes are essential for visualization of the stomach and the duodenum, and for some diagnostic problems in the esophagus they are also superior. The flexible scopes are equipped with convenient suction, insufflation and irrigating mechanisms that can be operated during continuous viewing, and this is a great advantage. However, the flexible scopes are clearly inferior for foreign body extraction and for management of strictures. The biopsy channel is so small that the biopsies usually contain only fragments of mucosa and are difficult to interpret. In addition, the color transmission of the fiber bundle tends to attenuate the natural bluish hue of prominent varices, producing an orange-red coloration resembling that of normal mucosal folds. Finally, the flexible scopes are difficult to sterilize. Concern remains about the possibility of transmitting hepatitis, and, for the present, flexible fiberoptic esophagoscopy is considered contraindicated in patients who are HAA-positive.

TECHNIQUE.—Although sedation with topical anesthesia nearly always is preferable for upper GI endoscopy in adults, general anesthesia is preferable for children. The patient's cooperation is required for endoscopy under local anesthesia and frequently this is not possible to obtain in a frightened child. General anesthesia minimizes psychic trauma, increases the safety of the manipulation and makes endoscopy much easier for the surgeon.

The supine position with the neck forward and the head extended on the neck is satisfactory for most esophagoscopy in children. When using a rigid scope, it is useful to have an assistant straighten out the dorsal curve by placing both hands beneath the patient's lower dorsal spine during manipulation of the lower third of the esophagus. The lateral position with the left side up is also satisfactory, and particularly so if flexible endoscopy is being performed with a need to examine the duodenum.

The open rigid esophagoscope is introduced under direct vision into the back of the pharynx with the lip of the beveled portion anterior. The lip of the scope then is used to elevate gently the larynx and to open the cricopharyngeus. The patient's mandible and maxilla are supported with the left hand, using the thumb and index finger around the esophagoscope as with a pool cue. The right hand is used to manipulate the scope like a pencil. The scope should not be advanced unless the lumen of the pharynx or esophagus is clearly visualized straight ahead. If the cricopharyngeus does not open up with elevation by the lip of the scope against the posterior portion of the larynx, the esophageal lumen should be identified by passage of a soft rubber catheter as a lumen finder. The scope then is passed over this catheter into the upper esophagus under direct vision. A view of the esophageal lumen should be maintained as the scope is advanced through the gastroesophageal junction into the stomach. More detailed inspection then can be obtained as the scope is withdrawn.

The Storz rigid esophagoscope with the viewing telescope is even simpler to pass. The suction catheter can be used as a lumen finder, and a detailed view of the esophageal wall can be obtained during both the advance and withdrawal of the esophagoscope by positioning the flexible suction catheter just ahead of the viewing telescope. A disadvantage of this scope is its smaller diameter. Air insufflation to eliminate mucosal folds will compensate for this, but the procedure involves rather cumbersome manipulation. For infants and children, the 4-mm, 30-cm scope is the most convenient. The infant 20-cm scopes are really too short for satisfactory examination of the gastroesophageal junction.

Initial passage of the flexible esophagogastroscope commonly is done blindly in the sedated adult patient who can cooperate by swallowing. In an anesthetized child it may be simpler to pass through the cricopharyngeus under direct vision. Occasionally this presents difficulty, but ordinarily the cricopharyngeal lumen can be identified by insufflation through the air channel of the scope. Extreme hyperextension of the head may make the passage through the pharynx difficult, and a more natural and relaxed position is preferable. A bite protector for the fiberscope should be used in case the patient becomes light and tightens the mandible. We have used the Olympus GIF-P, which has an outside diameter of 7.2 mm at the tip, and a forward-viewing 65-degree lens. This scope has only two-way control of the tip through a 150-degree arc each way, but it can be used in infants a few weeks of age. Manipulation is somewhat more difficult than with the larger adult scopes having four-way control. For newborns and prematures, the smaller Olympus flexible fiberoptic bronchoscope (BF-B2) with two-way control can also be used. This endoscope has a channel adaptable for either suction or insufflation but not both simultaneously—a disadvantage. The Olympus Company recently has marketed a pediatric instrument with four-way control and improved optical resolution (GIF-P2). The forward-viewing angle is 85 degrees with an outer diameter at the tip of 9.0 mm. This is the preferable instrument for flexible fiberoptic endoscopy beyond the newborn period.

Following esophagoscopy, patients usually are restricted to clear liquids and observed for signs of possible perforation. If the procedure has been performed carefully under direct vision all the way, the likelihood of perforation is almost nil. The more common sites of perforation, usually with rigid scopes, are in the posterior pharynx, the lower third of the esophagus or the stomach. Perforations also occur during dilatation of strictures, and the area of a dilated stricture should be examined carefully with the optical telescope or the flexible fiberscope before the procedure is terminated. Occult perforation usually is associated with pain, rapid onset of fever and sometimes prostration. Chest x-ray usually shows mediastinal widening or air, if the perforation is intrathoracic (Fig. 45–6).

A recent survey has revealed a perforation rate of 0.03% in 221,410 cases of an upper GI endoscopy.[8] An earlier report recorded a rate of 0.1% for rigid esophagoscopes and 0.093% with flexible instruments.[6] These percentages involve adult patients. My personal experience in infants involves one

perforation following dilatation of an anastomotic stricture. A linear split through the scar was identified immediately with the flexible scope, and the problem was managed successfully by simple extrapleural drainage. An additional 172 infants and children have received upper GI endoscopy in the past 5 years without complication (Fig. 45–7).

INDICATIONS.—The management of *esophageal stricture,* acquired or congenital, represents one of the major indications for esophagoscopy in the childhood age group. Stricture of varying degree is a relatively frequent occurrence following anastomosis of the esophagus for esophageal atresia. Esophagoscopy is useful to visualize the anastomosis or to perform direct-vision antegrade esophageal dilatation. Esophagoscopy is also useful to position a catheter or string through a stricture and into the stomach. Subsequently this can be attached to Tucker dilators for retrograde dilatation. The Storz esophagoscopes with the viewing telescope are most useful for dealing with upper esophageal anastomotic problems in small infants. Once the anatomy is carefully inspected, the telescope can be removed and dilatations or other manipulations can be performed through the open lumen of the scope. The flexible scope is cumbersome for this application because it has no open channel through which instrumentation can be performed.

Anastomotic problems following colon interposition for esophageal atresia, on the other hand, are more safely and easily evaluated with the flexible fiberscope. This is because the interposed colon segment often is tortuous, and it is difficult or dangerous to pass a rigid scope in this situation.

Caustic burns of the esophagus may require a variety of instruments for evaluation. In the acute burn stage, the cricopharyngeus and upper esophagus can be seen in more detail and with more safety using the Storz rigid scope and the viewing telescope. Evaluation of the lower esophagus with this instrument is not quite so satisfactory, however, because of the tortuosity of the lumen of the esophagus and

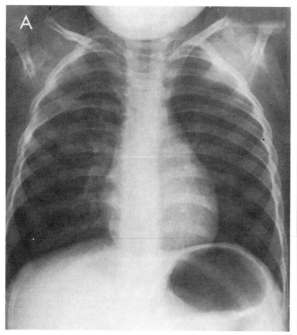 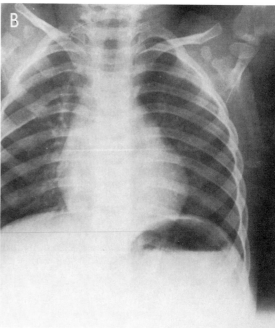

Fig. 45–6.—Esophageal perforation. Chest films before **(A)** and 4 hours after **(B)** esophagoscopy with dilatation of a stricture. Mediastinal widening with air collection in the upper mediastinum can be seen on the right. This signifies esophageal perforation. The child was successfully treated by prompt extrapleural drainage.

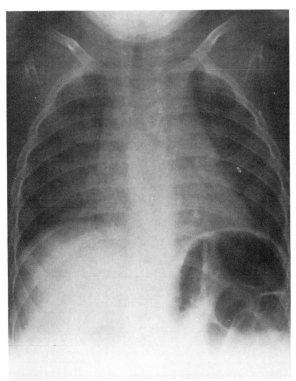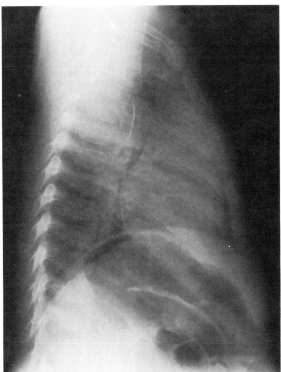

Fig. 45–7.—Invisible metallic foreign body in esophagus. The aluminum soda pop can top, which has perforated the esophagus and lodged against the aorta, can be seen on edge in the lateral view. It is not visible on the PA film. It was successfully removed by extrapleural thoracotomy.

because it is more difficult to inflate the esophagus with this rigid instrument. The flexible scope is very satisfactory in such patients. The flexible scope is also very satisfactory in the upper esophagus if it is passed under direct vision through the cricopharyngeus rather than blindly. If the esophagus is overinflated with the flexible scope, the mucosa becomes flattened out and it may be more difficult to detect mucosal injury. In addition, the slight color distortions through the fiberoptic bundle add to the problem in discriminating superficial burns of the esophageal mucosa. Once the stricture has become chronic, the flexible scope is very good for evaluation, but the rigid scope is more useful for antegrade dilatations. For difficult problems where dilatation must be performed under direct vision, the larger-lumen modified Jezberg or Negus esophagoscope is necessary to allow passage of dilators through the main channel of the scope.

Foreign bodies in the esophagus also require a variety of instruments. The simple vegetable matter foreign body above a chronic stricture is most easily extracted through a large-lumen rigid scope such as the modified Jezberg scope. Objects of metal or plastic may be less readily identified and should first be localized with the flexible scope or with a rigid scope and telescope. It is worth noting that the aluminum zip top on a soda pop can, exclusive of the ring, is not radiopaque in the esophagus except when viewed on edge. Even then, it appears as only a very faint crescent-shaped line. We have recovered one such object from the esophagus, using the Storz system with telescope, when the object had been missed on two previous rigid esophagoscopies. A second patient was referred to us following negative rigid esophagoscopy, cervical esophagotomy and thoracic esophagotomy. A red-colored plastic guitar pick then was recovered endoscopically from a flap in the esophageal mucosa. The superb view provided by the rod-lens telescope made this possible. Manipulation of instruments for grasping a foreign body usually is simpler through a rigid scope, but newer grasping instruments have been devised so that objects such as pins and embedded coins can be removed successfully with the flexible instrument. Open safety pins in the esophagus can be grasped by the spring, passed into the stomach, turned around and removed with ease. Most coins in the esophagus, however, do not require endoscopy at all. They can be removed very simply under fluoroscopy with the use of a balloon catheter passed beyond the coin, inflated and then withdrawn with the coin ahead of the balloon (Fig. 45–8).

Evaluation of *disordered function* of the lower gastroesophageal sphincter or for the presence of reflux is best performed with the flexible scope. Inflation of the esophagus with air allows one to see the lower gastroesophageal sphincter open and close. In the case of achalasia, the sphincter fails to open. One gets a much better idea of the resistance of this sphincter and of the dilated esophagus above by using the flexible scope. Gastroesophageal reflux can be evaluated in a limited way with this technique, but esophagoscopy in the anesthetized child does not provide a good representation of the sphincter function under normal conditions. Further evaluation of gastroesophageal reflux is aided by passage of the flexible scope into the stomach for retrograde viewing of the gastroesophageal sphincter function from below.

Identification of *reflux esophagitis* when the esophagitis is early is difficult by esophagoscopy. Advanced esophagitis or stricture is easily identified with the flexible scope or with the optical telescope and the rigid instrument. Where no ulcers are present, however, evaluation of esophagitis is not accurate in the early stages. A color change from the pink-

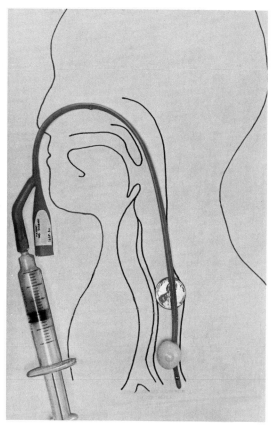

Fig. 45–8.—Coins in the esophagus usually can be removed in the x-ray department using a balloon catheter and fluoroscopic control of the manipulation.

yellow of the normal esophagus to a deeper red occurs with superficial esophagitis, but this often is difficult to appreciate with the intense light from the fiber source. Color distortion through the fiberoptic bundles also makes this more difficult. A cobblestone appearance of the mucosa with patchy erythema, easy friability and bleeding on contact may be associated with early erosive esophagitis, but precision of diagnosis depends for the most part on mucosal biopsy. Multiple mucosal biopsies can be obtained through the flexible scope, but the specimens obtained with the tiny forceps are very superficial and the evidence still may be inconclusive. When necessary, deeper specimens should be obtained using a larger forceps through an open rigid instrument or with a blind biopsy capsule manipulated through the open instrument or under fluoroscopic control.

The identification of *esophageal varices* is said to be roughly 85% accurate with the flexible fiberscope.[7] The nearly constant insufflation of air distends the esophagus and compresses the mucosa. This tends to obscure smaller varices, which may be identified more frequently with open tube esophagoscopy. Also, the color transmission of the fiber bundle tends to diminish the natural bluish hue of prominent varices. Magnification may account for further error because the magnified image produced by the fiberoptic endoscope is not uniform and depends in large measure on the distance of the image from the instrument. Normal mucosal folds lying close to the instrument may have the appearance of varices. Nevertheless, the ease and safety of examination using the flexible scope makes this instrument very useful in experienced hands. Varices sometimes have a

grayish white color and can be identified if the examination is careful and unhurried. An additional advantage of the flexible scope relates to the capability of passing it through the cardia into the fundus of the stomach. A retrograde view of cardioesophageal varices then can be obtained. It is usual to lavage the stomach with iced saline prior to endoscopy for bleeding because a large amount of clot in the stomach will prevent intragastric manipulation and observation. Esophageal varices can also be identified using the rigid scope with the optical telescope, but this system eliminates the useful intragastric observation.

Gastroduodenoscopy

Gastroduodenoscopy is possible in infants and children only with the newer flexible fiberscopes. The technique of insertion is the same as that for flexible esophagoscopy. Once the fiberscope has been passed into the stomach, it should be manipulated in a systematic fashion to examine the entire surface of the stomach mucosa. This involves a retrograde view of the gastroesophageal junction and fundus as well as a careful view of the pylorus and antrum. The flexible scopes in the smaller pediatric sizes are the forward-viewing upper GI panendoscopes. In larger children, it is possible to pass the adult side-viewing gastroscope, but satisfactory examination can be obtained with the forward-viewing scopes, the newest of which (Olympus GIF-P2) provides an 85-degree-angle view. Cannulation of the papilla of Vater is possible only with a side-viewing duodenoscope, and the smallest child in our experience on whom pancreatic duct cannulation has been performed successfully was a 40-pound 5-year-old.

INDICATIONS.—The applications of gastroscopy in infants and children are infrequent, but endoscopic evaluation has been useful in a few specific circumstances. The diagnosis of antral or prepyloric web sometimes is difficult to make radiographically. Gastroscopy has been useful in our experience both to confirm and exclude this diagnosis. Gastroscopy has proved to be useful to evaluate the presence or absence of peptic ulceration of the stomach or duodenum, bleeding from gastritis and bleeding from gastric varices. Evaluation of the stomach sometimes is part of the esophageal evaluation in cases of caustic ingestion. If no burns are seen in the esophagus, the stomach is also examined. Furthermore, gastroscopy has proved to be valuable in a rare child with stomal problems associated with previous operation for peptic ulcer. Gastric tumors, duplications or hemangiomas might serve as additional rare indications for gastroscopy. We have diagnosed one child with a communicating gastric duplication that was embedded in the head of the pancreas. This lesion caused pain on gastric filling and was not demonstrated clearly by previous upper GI series, but was seen endoscopically.

Laparoscopy

Laparoscopy is a well-established technique for evaluation of abdominal and pelvic conditions in adults. It has been used infrequently in infants and children, but the recent development of the Hopkins rod-lens optical system has made this a practical procedure for a few specific conditions.

Laparoscopy involves the endoscopic visualization of the contents of the peritoneal cavity. This is accomplished by introduction of a small telescope through the anterior abdominal wall after the prior establishment of a pneumoperitoneum. Although possible to perform under local anesthesia in adults, the procedure is much more satisfactory with general anesthesia in infants and children.

TECHNIQUE.—A special pneumoperitoneum needle (Veress[9]) is introduced just lateral to the midline above or below the umbilicus, after first palpating to make certain that the bladder is not distended and so will not be punctured. The Veress needle contains a spring-loaded cannula, which protrudes beyond the beveled needle tip as soon as the peritoneum is punctured. This prevents perforation of underlying viscera. CO_2 or N_2O is introduced through the cannula to produce pneumoperitoneum and provide a space for introduction of the laparoscopy cannula and telescope. The gas is most safely introduced by means of an insufflating device that has a reducing valve, a flowmeter and a continuous-pressure meter. Intra-abdominal pressures in an infant should not exceed 15–20 mm Hg, and even these pressures must be reduced if there is any interference with respiration.

Once an adequate pneumoperitoneum has been established, the needle is removed. A tiny skin incision of 4–5 mm then is made for insertion of the laparoscopy cannula. The cannula trocar is withdrawn and replaced with the viewing telescope. The pneumoperitoneum does not escape because of a valve system in the cannula. If instrumentation or biopsy of pelvic or abdominal organs is to be performed under direct vision, it may be necessary to insert a second cannula for the biopsy instrument.

INDICATIONS.—Visualization of internal genitalia for diagnosis of intersex problems is very satisfactory with laparoscopy and may save the child an exploratory operation.

Examination of the liver is also satisfactory with laparoscopy, and in some cases the visualization of the dome of the liver is superior to that obtained by open laparotomy. Endoscopic visualization of the liver is useful for a selective liver biopsy in case of tumor nodules, for second-look operations in case of liver malignancy and occasionally for evaluation of cysts or tumors of the liver.

Laparoscopy has limited use in evaluation of the small bowel, mesentery or retroperitoneum. The bowel can be seen from the surface, but only a fragmentary and incomplete view of the intestine can be obtained. Often the appendix can be visualized, and this may be useful in some chronic pain syndromes where one wishes to avoid an exploratory laparotomy.

In the past 5 years, we have performed laparoscopy three times for evaluation of intersex problems, twice for chronic pain syndromes in preadolescents and three times for selective biopsy or evaluation of liver nodules. In each case, the information obtained was useful in management. Three additional infants with obstructive jaundice were laparoscoped early in our experience. The information obtained did not obviate a subsequent laparotomy, and we no longer consider laparoscopy for evaluation of this problem.

REFERENCES

1. Berci, G.: History of Endoscopy, in Berci, G. (ed.), *Endoscopy* (New York: Appleton-Century-Crofts, 1976).
2. Berci, G., and Kont, L. A.: A new optical system in endoscopy with special reference to cystoscopy, Br. J. Urol. 41:564, 1969.
3. Jahrsdoerfer, R. A., Kirchner, J. A., and Thaler, S. U.: Cleft larynx, Arch. Otolaryngol. 86:108, 1967.
4. Johnson, D. G., and Jones, R.: Surgical aspects of airway management in infants and children, Surg. Clin. North Am. 56:263, 1976.
5. Johnson, D. G., and Stewart, D. R.: Management of acquired tracheal obstructions in infancy, J. Pediatr. Surg. 10:709, 1975.
6. Katz, D.: Morbidity and mortality in standard and flexible gastrointestinal endoscopy, Gastrointest. Endosc. 15:134, 1969.
7. Schapiro, M.: Flexible Fiberoptic Esophagoscopy, in Berci, G. (ed.), *Endoscopy* (New York: Appleton-Century-Crofts, 1976).
8. Silvis, S., *et al.*: Endoscopic complications, JAMA 235:928, 1976.
9. Veress, J.: Neues Instrument zur Ausführung von Brust-oder Bauchhöhlenpunktionen, Dtsch. Med. Wochenschr. 41:1480, 1938.

46 MARK M. RAVITCH

Congenital Malformations and Neonatal Problems of the Respiratory Tract

Neonatal Respiratory Distress

CYANOSIS OR DYSPNEA in the newborn signals the need for precise and expeditious investigation and treatment. Apart from congenital heart disease there is a wide variety of conditions causing respiratory distress in the newborn on a mechanical basis, which, by definition, makes such emergencies problems for surgical relief. The surgical aspects of dyspnea are emphasized in this section. The underlying conditions accounting for noncardiac dyspnea are discussed in greater detail in the sections on diaphragmatic hernia, esophageal atresia and tracheoesophageal fistula, mediastinal tumors, endoscopy, chylothorax, pulmonary agenesis, abnormal tracheobronchial communications, anomalies of pulmonary vessels, congenital cystic disease of the lung, pneumonia and empyema.

In general, the causes of respiratory distress that concern the surgeon are those due to obstruction of the airway, those due to pulmonary collapse or displacement and those due to parenchymal disease or insufficiency. Frequently, two, or even three, of these mechanisms occur simultaneously, as in diaphragmatic hernia through Bochdalek's foramen, in which the ipsilateral lung may be grossly hypoplastic, the

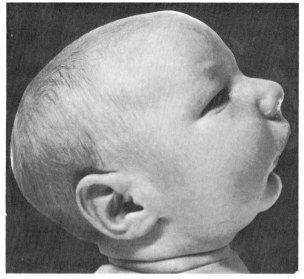 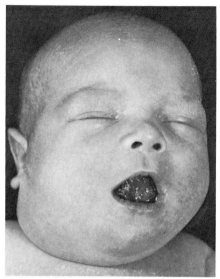

Fig. 46–1 (left).—Pierre Robin syndrome. This newborn had respiratory difficulty, especially during feedings. Gavage through a small plastic feeding tube and positioning to extend the neck with the child in lateral position tided the patient over for several weeks until the condition was better tolerated. At times, it is necessary to advance the tongue, preferably by a plastic procedure on the mucous membrane.

Fig. 46–2 (right).—Lymphangioma infiltrating the neck, floor of the mouth

and tongue, causing respiratory obstruction (preoperative view). Removal was undertaken at age 1 week. Widespread extension into trachea, larynx, esophagus, floor of the mouth and mediastinum made complete removal impossible. Tracheostomy was necessary postoperatively, and radiotherapy was given. Three years later, most of the neck deformity was gone, but the tongue was still enlarged and covered by cysts.

contralateral lung undeveloped and both compressed by the distended herniated intrathoracic intestine.

The infant with an obstructed upper airway (Figs. 46–1 and 46–2) will show cyanosis and rapid labored respirations, stridor and marked suprasternal and intercostal inspiratory retractions. Examination of the neck, nose, mouth and throat, or laryngoscopy, may disclose the obstructing lesion. PA and lateral films of both the chest and the head and neck are essential. If the evidence for principal airway obstruction is good and no obstructing lesion has been found in the upper airway, bronchoscopy may well be required.

Stridor or severe inspiratory retractions do not accompany the dyspnea due to pulmonary displacement or parenchymal inadequacy. Respirations are rapid and labored, the degree of cyanosis depending on the amount of compromised pulmonary tissue. Physical examination and chest radiographs ordinarily will indicate the nature of the underlying problem. Obstruction to a main bronchus or lobar bronchus may produce either distention or collapse of the lung or lobe and the breathing is more like that of pulmonary insufficiency than of obstruction. With partial bronchial obstruction there may be wheezing.

DIAGNOSIS.—The physical examination, including laryngoscopy and bronchoscopy as indicated, and PA and lateral films of the chest and of the head and neck usually will establish the likely diagnosis and indicate the appropriate therapy. In the presence of obstructive breathing, the neck is rapidly examined, a finger passed into the mouth and the baby tested to see whether relief from the dyspnea may be obtained by hyperextension of the neck. If the obstruction is oropharyngeal and respiratory distress is severe, a pharyngeal airway or endotracheal tube may be the first step in treatment. The x-rays are viewed for shadows bulging into the pharynx, for forward, lateral or posterior displacement of the trachea, air in the soft tissues, mediastinum or pleural cavity, displacement of the heart and mediastinum, degree

of aeration of both lungs, position of the diaphragms (Figs. 46–3 and 46–4), malformations of the bony framework of the chest wall, areas of opacification or radiolucency in the pulmonary parenchyma. Not infrequently, an area of radiolucency may present a diagnostic problem in differentiating

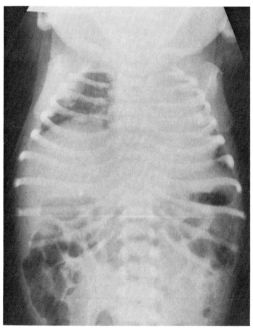

Fig. 46–3.—Right diaphragmatic paralysis due to phrenic nerve injury during a difficult delivery. Dyspnea and cyanosis were present from birth. Elevation of the diaphragm with mediastinal shift and cardiac displacement leaves little aerated lung. Oxygen therapy and semiupright positioning relieved symptoms, and in several weeks the child could leave the hospital. Ultimate outlook should be good, although regeneration of the nerve is unlikely.

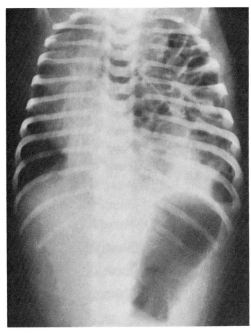

Fig. 46–4.—Diaphragmatic hernia on the left, causing progressively severe cyanosis and dyspnea in this 2-day-old child. Loops of bowel collapsed the left lung, herniating across the mediastinum to the opposite side. Only the gas-filled stomach remains in the small abdominal cavity. Immediate laparotomy with reduction of bowel and repair of the defect in the foramen of Bochdalek was done. Recovery was uneventful.

between a congenital lung cyst, lobar emphysema, pneumatocele and tension pneumothorax or diaphragmatic hernia. Classically, a tension pneumothorax (Fig. 46–5) will show the compressed lung at the hilum, a depressed diaphragm and a sharp costophrenic sulcus and no lung markings in the clear hemithorax. In lobar emphysema (see Fig. 46–6),

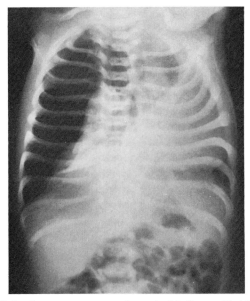

Fig. 46–5.—Spontaneous pneumothorax in this 3-year-old child caused sudden, very severe respiratory distress. The collapsed lung is seen at the right hilus. The tension pneumothorax has herniated the anterior mediastinum, compressing the opposite lung. Immediate insertion of an intercostal catheter through a trocar, with closed drainage, relieved symptoms, and sealing of the leak with re-expansion of the lung was complete in 24 hours.

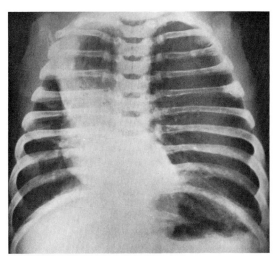

Fig. 46–6.—Lobar emphysema involving left upper lobe, causing increasing dyspnea and cyanosis at age 14 days. Diminished breath sounds were noted over the left chest, with mediastinal shift to the right. This film shows herniation of the mobile anterior mediastinum. A filmy web of lung markings in the radiolucent area suggests emphysema rather than lung cyst. Immediate lobectomy led to uneventful recovery. No specific cause of obstruction was found in the resected specimen.

the distended lobe, almost invariably upper, may fill the entire chest, but one usually will see a rounded lower border of the radiolucent shadow, some lung markings in the area of radiolucency and frequently the shadow of the compressed lower lobe. A congenital lung cyst with a ball valve mechanism presenting as a tension cyst occurs almost exclusively in the lower lobes. Like a lobar emphysema, it should show a rounded lower and lateral border, may show the compressed and collapsed upper lobe and should show no lung markings in the area of radiolucency (Fig 46–7). A postpneumonic pneumatocele distended by the same mechanism may be radiologically indistinguishable from a lung cyst, although it may occur in any lobe and may, like the lung cyst, be multiple. Bilateral disease almost categorically excludes the possibility of congenital lung cyst.

OBSTRUCTION OF THE AIRWAY.—The airway may be obstructed anywhere along the respiratory system from the nasal choanae to the smaller bronchi. The obstruction may be complete or partial, intrinsic or extrinsic. Congenital tracheomalacia, in which collapse of the airway causes an extremely troublesome problem, occasionally requires very long-term intubation or tracheostomy. A number of operative procedures have been suggested to stiffen the trachea.

CHOANAL ATRESIA.—The newborn infant is a nose breather and bilateral choanal atresia may produce alarming respiratory difficulty. Cyanosis at rest, inability to feed because of cyanosis and respiratory difficulty, and relief by crying, suggest the diagnosis. Symptoms are relieved by insertion of a nasopharyngeal airway tube. The operative treatment of choanal atresia is described in Chapter 29.

PIERRE ROBIN SYNDROME.—Mandibular hypoplasia and relative or actual macroglossia and posterior displacement of the tongue, frequently with cleft palate, lead to obstruction of the upper airway by the tongue (see Fig. 46–1). Maintaining the child in the face-down position relieves dyspnea and may be the sole treatment required, or traction on the tongue or operative advancement may be used.

Tumors of the neck and floor of the mouth commonly ob-

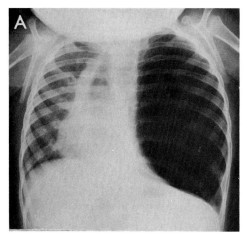 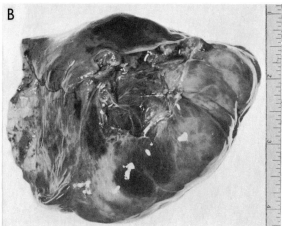

Fig. 46–7.—Congenital cystic disease of the lung—tension cyst in a year-old infant who had repeated attacks of respiratory infection and dyspnea from age 5 months, and 2½ months of continuous hospitalization. **A,** roentgenogram shows marked displacement of heart and mediastinum to the right by the air-filled cyst. The cyst edge can be seen in the costophrenic sulcus and medially in the cardiophrenic angle on the left. **B,** operative specimen. The left hemithorax was filled by a large, round, smooth, bluish thick-walled air-containing cyst. Pleural surfaces were smooth and shiny. The cyst was evacuated but refilled rapidly with air, necessitating its deflation during operation by needle and demonstrating a flap-valve mechanism. The cyst occupies the entire lower lobe except for a small fringe of diaphragmatic portion anteriorly. The upper lobe, a tiny compressed nubbin displaced into the mediastinum, expanded nicely and filled the hemithorax. The cyst wall was lined by low cuboidal epithelium. The child had no further difficulty.

struct by displacement of the tongue, by bulging into the pharyngeal airway, by compression or displacement of the trachea or by actual invasion of the epiglottis, larynx or trachea, as is particularly seen in hemangiomas or lymphangiomas (see Fig. 46–2). (See also Figs. 34–1 and 36–7.) We have seen desperate neonatal obstruction from a congenital goiter, from hemangioma of the thyroid and from lateral cervical teratomas. Infants may seem to tolerate a considerable degree of dyspnea relatively well but are prone to collapse suddenly from the fatigue of the exertion or from a sudden increase in the obstruction caused by manipulation and examination. Any degree of dyspnea in an infant should be viewed with concern, analyzed as rapidly and precisely as possible and the appropriate decision made for endoscopic intubation, tracheostomy or operative relief.

INTRATHORACIC TRACHEAL OBSTRUCTION.—Mediastinal lesions of all kinds may produce critical tracheal or bronchial compression, with or without displacement. Haller,[13] in a period of 3 years, treated 5 infants, 4 of them newborns, for life-threatening respiratory distress from mediastinal masses. There were two bronchogenic cysts, one teratoma, one enteric cyst and one far-advanced neuroblastoma. Mediastinal cysts of foregut origin, causing respiratory obstruction, are principally bronchogenic cysts, which tend to lie close to the trachea or major bronchus, but occasionally the much larger enteric duplications may cause tracheal or bronchial compression. The bronchogenic cysts are particularly treacherous because, often being small and buried in the mediastinum, they may not show discrete shadows on the x-ray and may, in fact, be difficult to find in the mediastinum at operation. It is not always clear from the chest films and from examination whether, in the presence of an overdistended lung on one side and an opacified lung on the other, we are dealing with primary overdistention of one lung and compression and collapse of the other or primary collapse of one lung and compensatory overdistention of the other. We have known a bronchogenic cyst to compress the right main bronchus with collapse and compensatory overdistention of the left lung, the upper lobe of which was mistakenly removed for what was thought to be lobar emphysema.

Congenital vascular rings may obstruct the trachea, and the diagnosis may be suggested in an infant whose stridor and obvious tracheal obstruction are significantly relieved when the head is held hyperextended (see Chap. 57).

Other vascular malformations or anomalies may compress the trachea or the bronchus. A large patent ductus arteriosus may compress the left main bronchus[18, 29] and can even produce lobar emphysema relieved by division of the ductus.[29] An anomalous or enlarged pulmonary artery may cause tracheobronchial obstruction.[4] The section on anomalies of the pulmonary vessels deals with the problem of the aberrant left pulmonary artery with a circumtracheal course.

Congenital lobar emphysema is the result of obstruction to a lobar bronchus, almost invariably an upper lobar bronchus. Lobar emphysema may cause desperate respiratory distress early in the neonatal period. The lesion generally is confined to a single lobe, usually upper (see Fig 46–6). The most common mechanical factor seems to be bronchial collapse due to abnormalities or absence of the cartilage, as in 22 of 28 of the cases from Great Ormond Street.[21] It is generally recognized that the mortality of the condition is 50% if untreated and that death may occur fairly rapidly, although, in some children, dyspnea does not begin for weeks or months after birth and the condition then may be tolerated for some time. Except in those instances in which there is an obvious external compressing lesion, the treatment has been removal of the distended lobe. The failure to find an intrinsic bronchial lesion in all cases may be due to inadequate pathologic search or to the unavoidable fact that the intrinsic cartilaginous lesion of bronchus may have been destroyed by clamping, transection and suture, so that no lesion is left for the pathologist to find.[27] The patient reported by Murray, Talbert and Haller,[28] who was cured by bronchotomy and removal of a mucus plug, is almost unique. Murray's review of 166 patients showed an operative mortality of 7% – 12 patients, of whom 3 had congenital heart disease, 1 had postoperative pneumothorax, 1 had aspiration of mucus, 1 had severe infection and 4 had brain damage from preoperative hypoxia. Three of the deaths were due to diffuse emphysema following operation. Lobectomy in the infant is technically extraordinarily simple and well tolerated. There is some uncertainty about the ultimate pulmonary function of patients who have had an upper lobectomy for lobar emphysema in infancy. Sloan's studies in 6 children suggest that they may not have altogether normal function.[6] However, given the high mortality of nonoperative treatment, there would appear to be little choice. The few patients recovering without operation tend to have persistent emphysema.[27] Fischer, Potts and Holinger[8] reported from as far back as 1952 from the Children's Memorial Hospital in Chicago 11 resections with no death and a single death in 33 reported resections. This is more likely representative of the actual risk. Needle aspiration of the emphysematous lobe has been suggested as definitive treatment, but pneumothorax is a hazard[16] and the ultimate outlook is uncertain. Murray's review cites 4 instances of fatal consequences of attempted aspiration of the emphysematous lobes and many nonfatal mishaps. Roghair[33] reported 2 children with modest dyspnea from what appears clearly to have been lobar emphysema, who received no treatment, were followed into adult life and then were found to have perfectly normal x-rays and to be asymptomatic.

The occasional patient with symptoms persisting after lobectomy may have similar areas of cartilage deficiency in other bronchi.

Dyspnea, diminished excursion of the affected side with decreased breath sounds and hyperresonance in a child who is increasingly cyanotic demand prompt immediate roentgen study of the chest. A radiolucency in the lung fields, usually either upper or apparently involving an entire hemithorax, with a shift of the mediastinum, suggests lobar emphysema or congenital lung cyst. The appearance of scattered lung markings in the area of radiolucency and the recognition that the collapsed lobe is lower rather than upper differentiate emphysema from lung cyst.

Hislop and Reid[14] from the Brompton in London, the latter already having played such an important role in demonstration of the underdevelopment of the pulmonary parenchyma in diaphragmatic hernia, in 1970 demonstrated in 3 children who had what appeared to be straightforward lobar emphysema a new condition that they called polyalveolar lobe with emphysema. Painstaking step sections of the lung and quantitative examination of the pulmonary structures demonstrated that although the lungs had, in fact, trapped air, the histologic criteria of emphysema were wanting, the alveoli were not hyperinflated and that, in fact, what one had was a large increase in the number of alveoli without any increase in the number of bronchioles or of pulmonary arteries.[9] Part of the hyperlucency seen in the radiographs they attributed to the decreased vascularity resulting from a relative paucity of arteries. There was some abnormality in the bronchial cartilages, and they pointed out that in these patients (as one occasionally sees clinically) a segment of the lobe might escape the changes. In the United States, in 1973, Munnell, Lambird and Austin[26] in Oklahoma reported another case of polyalveolar lobe also demonstrated by quantitative microscopic studies of the lung section.

The emphysema due to foreign bodies, or inflammatory swelling of the bronchial lining, usually is less severe and more often occurs in the older infant and child. Bronchoscopy, not indicated for suspected neonatal lobar emphysema, and likely to be as hazardous as valuable in the newborn, obviously is required when an aspirated foreign body is suspected.

Many very young infants with rapidly ballooning lobar emphysema present such emergencies that delay of operation is dangerous and unjustified, and there are numerous reports of successful lobectomy in the first 24 hours of life. Lobectomy is the treatment of choice, and since the upper lobe almost always is the lobe involved, an anterolateral thoracotomy in the third or fourth interspace suffices. During induction of anesthesia, positive pressure may further overinflate the lobe and reduce respiratory exchange to such a degree that rapid thoracotomy and delivery of the overdistended lobe are required to relieve the intrathoracic compression and save the infant. The patient of Gross and Lewis[11] probably was the first operated on. Occasionally the condition is bilateral, and on several occasions a second lobe has had to be removed.[19]

Sloan's[6] long-term follow-up and physiologic evaluation of 6 patients perhaps is the only one of its kind. The children had all grown and developed normally and were leading active lives, some of them competing in sports. However, pulmonary function tests demonstrated decreased vital capacity, thought to be proportional to the amount of lung removed, with a normal or slightly increased total lung volume, suggesting a compensatory response accomplished by overdistention of the remaining lung.

As might be expected, 9 of the 28 patients with lobar emphysema from the Hospital for Sick Children, Great Ormond Street, with its huge load of patients with congenital heart disease, had major congenital cardiac defects, and 3 of them died of congenital heart disease. All 9 had the emphysematous portion of the lung resected—in 2, the ductus was divided concomitantly and in 1, the ductus was ligated, the emphysematous lobe was not resected but required to be rapidly resected early in the postoperative period. In 2 children with severe congenital cardiac lesions, 1 with tetralogy of Fallot, the other with coarctation, the pre-existing lobar emphysema left undisturbed at the cardiac operation, lobectomy was required within 24 hours of the cardiac operation. Congenital lung cyst can produce a tension cyst from a flap valve mechanism (see Fig. 46–7) but usually without the severity seen in lobar emphysema. Cystic adenomatoid hyperplasia may result in severe respiratory embarrassment from the size of the mass of abnormal tissue,[2, 38] and respiratory distress has been reported as well with extralobar sequestrations.[34] Congenital pulmonary cystic lymphangiectasis may so distort and compress the lung as to be incompatible with survival.[17]

Pulmonary Displacement

Compression and mediastinal shift with accompanying respiratory distress may result from abnormal elevation of the diaphragm or the presence in the thoracic cavity of air, fluid or mass.

Paralysis of the diaphragm, usually due to birth injury, results in a striking and uniform elevation of the hemidiaphragm, compression of the ipsilateral lung and mediastinal shift (see Fig. 46–3). Infrequently, the respiratory distress may be so great that it may be necessary to imbricate the diaphragm, taking out the slack and thus flattening it and restoring room for pulmonary expansion.[32] Phrenic nerve injury may occur as the only birth injury or may be associated with other evidences of traumatic delivery. The diagnosis is suspected by physical examination of the dyspneic child and the x-ray is pathognomonic. Eventration of the diaphragm, if an extensive enough area of diaphragm replaced by a thinned-out membrane balloons into the thorax, may produce pulmonary compression in the same way. Diaphragmatic hernia through Bochdalek's foramen produces some of the more serious respiratory difficulties seen in the neonate, and on two bases, of which the least important, particularly in infants dyspneic at birth, is the interference with respiration caused by the mass of abdominal contents herniated into the chest. The most important cause of respiratory distress in babies with diaphragmatic hernia is the hypoplasia of both lungs. In the immediate postnatal period, the rapidity and severity of the respiratory distress suggest the diagnosis and a scaphoid abdomen and a dull percussion note of the chest and mediastinal displacement may make the diagnosis even before radiographic examination. Immediate gastric intubation and constant suction are required to remove whatever fluid may be present in the stomach and to prevent the further passage of air into the herniated intestinal tract. The magnitude of the dyspnea is such that these children frequently require tracheal intubation and artificial respiration almost from birth (see Fig. 46–4).

Fluid effusions occur in the neonate for a variety of reasons, and, if they are large enough, may be cause for dyspnea. Chylothorax usually requires a few days or weeks to become manifest, almost invariably is unilateral and the dyspnea is slowly progressive. Catheter drainage usually is curative (see the next section).

A handful of infants have been described, desperately dyspneic or apneic at delivery and requiring intubation and artificial respiration, who proved to have bilateral pleural effusions. The treatment is bilateral tube thoracostomy. In the 1961 case of Stephan and Otto,[36] a single bilateral thoracentesis, yielding a total of 75 ml of clear fluid, sufficed for relief. In this case, the fluid was thought not to be chyle and its source was undetermined. In the 1973 report by Doolittle, Ohmark and Egan,[7] bilateral catheter drainage had to be resorted to and, in all, a total of 1000 ml of fluid was drained from the pleural cavities over the first 23 days of life. Although gross fat could not be seen in the fluid after feedings, the chemical analysis of fluid and the large numbers of lymphocytes in it suggested that it was, in fact, chyle.

Pneumothorax, pneumomediastinum and pneumopericardium of the newborn frequently are associated with neonatal respiratory distress and constitute a fascinating problem both in their treatment and in the analysis of their pathogenesis. The evidence suggests that careful routine radiographic examination would disclose on the order of 0.5% of newborn infants to have air in the pleural cavity.[5] Air in the anterior mediastinum alone may be seen even more frequently. Macklin's 1939 suggestion[23] and a subsequent analysis of the problem have provided the generally accepted explanation. The first breaths of a newborn briefly create an enormous pressure difference between the atmospheric pressure inside the aerated alveolus and the pressure in the surrounding lung. If initial expansion of the lung is rapid and smooth, the period of these extreme pressure differences is so small that rupture of the alveolus does not occur. In the patient with aspiration of meconium, amniotic fluid or blood, atelectasis of portions of the lung leads to prolongation of the high pressures across aerated alveoli and leads to their rupture.[5] The rupture of the alveolus is within the pulmonary

Fig. 46–8.—Neonatal pneumopericardium. A 1900-gm infant transferred to Cook County Hospital, Chicago, at 2 hours of age for respiratory distress, hyaline membrane disease. At 22 hours of age, he required intubation and constant positive airway pressure. At 40 hours of age, he suddenly became cyanotic and apneic and was revived by aspiration of the left pneumothorax. Twenty hours later, while on respirator, he developed bradycardia and cyanosis; the heart sounds were muffled and subsequently inaudible. Cardiac tamponade was suspected and diagnosed by the films shown in **A** and **B.** Subxiphoid aspiration of 15 cc of air relieved the symptoms. He was weaned from the respirator on the 6th day and discharged from the hospital well at 42 days. (Courtesy of T. F. Yeh.)

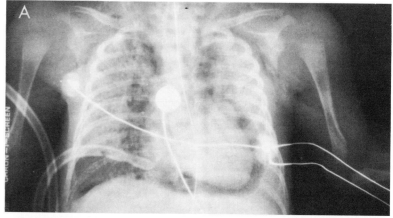

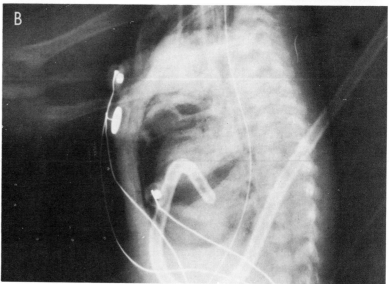

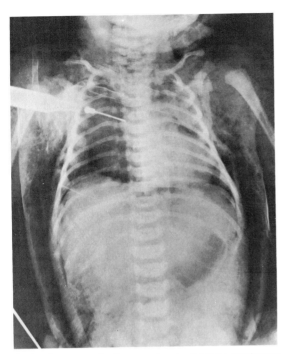

Fig. 46–9.—Pneumomediastinum and subcutaneous emphysema in a newborn who required resuscitation, which was given by mouth-to-mouth insufflation. It was noted that "each time the doctor blew into the child's mouth, the child got bigger." Tubes were put into the anterior mediastinum and both pleural cavities. The air absorbed, and the child left the hospital well.

parenchyma and usually not on the pleural surface. Air dissects along the cardiovascular sheaths to the lung root into the mediastinum, the pleural space[23] and even into the pericardium[39] and the soft tissues of the neck[39] (Fig 46–8). Pneumothorax and pneumomediastinum are particularly common in prematures with respiratory distress syndrome, in children with respiratory distress of any sort, even postmature babies, and, as might be expected, in children receiving artificial respiration[3, 24, 30, 35] (Fig. 46–9). A specific association with severe renal malformations, particularly renal agenesis, was suggested by Stern *et al.*[37] but dismissed in a careful study by Lucaya, Gil and Moreiras,[22] who suggested that it was due entirely to the frequency of assisted respirations in the delivery room.

If the film of a child with respiratory distress shows pneumothorax, the safest plan is to insert a small plastic catheter leading to underwater drainage. Air in the mediastinum, anterior to the heart, seen in lateral films in asymptomatic children may be much more common than is appreciated. So long as the child is, in fact, asymptomatic, the air need not be aspirated and small pneumothoraces in children who are not in distress may be taken as an indication for careful observation of the child without immediate catheter drainage. Obviously, tension pneumothorax or pericardial tamponade allows no temporizing, requires catheter drainage of the pleural cavity and at least aspiration of the pericardium. Bilateral pneumothorax occurs occasionally and obviously increases the hazard.

Pulmonary Deficiency

The function of the lungs themselves may be at fault. Failure of the lungs to expand appropriately or neonatal respiratory difficulty from neonatal aspiration may require tracheal section or bronchoscopic aspiration.

The Jeune syndrome, with its small, bell-shaped thorax and its short horizontal ribs, may cause fatal respiratory inadequacy (see p. 427).

The respiratory distress syndrome in the neonate (hyaline membrane distress), most common in distressed prematures and children born of cesarean section, is manifested by progressive tachypnea and dyspnea, often beginning within an hour or two of birth. The introduction of positive airway pressure-assisted respirations through an intratracheal tube has made an enormous difference in the previously high mortality of these children.

In the respiratory distress syndrome, a number of observations[12, 15, 25] have demonstrated that in the presence of low arterial tension, the ductus may fail to close and that its persistent patency may be associated with heart failure, gravely aggravating the respiratory distress. Operative interruption of the ductus has resulted in relief from the cardiac failure and increased cure rate of the respiratory distress syndrome. Obviously, these terribly ill infants would represent very specific indications for pharmacologic closure of the ductus once the utility and safety have been confirmed (see p. 630). The respirator management of babies with RDS may cause pulmonary interstitial emphysema,[20] the air from ruptured alveoli following the vascular sheaths and producing a recognizable pattern of multiple sharply defined lucencies radiating from the pulmonary hila. The resulting overdistention of the lung further complicates the baby's respiratory difficulty. At times, the accumulation of air is unilobar and resulting in the hugely overdistended lobe, resection of which has been lifesaving.[9, 10]

Clearly, any condition that leads to neonatal aspiration will result in dyspnea, and among these are esophageal atresia, which may also produce dyspnea if a large tracheoesophageal fistula results in massive abdominal distention.

Spontaneous rupture of the esophagus has, in each of the 13 cases analyzed in the paper by Aaronson, Cywes and Louw,[1] been manifested by intense dyspnea with a tension pneumothorax, hydrothorax or hydropneumothorax. The onset of symptoms was within a few minutes of birth to 48 hours; the children were for the most part otherwise normal and had had uneventful births. Catheter drainage alone has been uniformly fatal, and repair, from either the abdominal or the transpleural approach has been successful in 7 of the 8 infants in whom it was undertaken.

REFERENCES

1. Aaronson, I. A., Cywes, S., and Louw, J. H.: Spontaneous esophageal rupture in the newborn, J. Pediatr. Surg. 10:459, 1975.
2. Benatre, A., Laugier, J., Rolland, J. C., Delvert, B., Vandooren, M., and Desbuquois, G.: Malformation pulmonaire kystique asphyxiante du nouveau-né, Arch. Fr. Pediatr. 27:821, 1970.
3. Bomsel, F., and Larroche, J. Cl.: L'emphysème interstitiel pulmonaire du nouveau-né, J. Radiol. Electrol. 53:505, 1972.
4. Borg, S. A., Young, L. W., and Roghair, G. D.: Congenital avalvular pulmonary artery and infantile lobar emphysema. A diagnostic correlation, Am. J. Roentgenol. 125:412, 1975.
5. Chernick, V., and Avery, M. E.: Spontaneous alveolar rupture at birth, Pediatrics 32:5, 1963.
6. DeMuth, G. I., and Sloan, H.: Congenital lobar emphysema: Long term effects and sequelae in treated cases, Surgery 59:601, 1966.
7. Doolittle, W. M., Ohmark, D., and Egan, E. A.: Congenital bilateral pleural effusions: A cause for respiratory failure in the newborn, Am. J. Dis. Child. 125:435, 1973.
8. Fischer, W., Potts, W. J., and Holinger, P. H.: Lobar emphysema in infants and children, J. Pediatr. 41:4, 1952.
9. Fletcher, B. D., Outerbridge, E. W., and Dunbar, J. S.: Pulmonary interstitial emphysema in the newborn, J. Can. Assoc. Radiol. 21:273, 1970.
10. Fletcher, B. D., Outerbridge, E. W., Youssef, S., and Bolande, R. P.: Pulmonary interstitial emphysema in a newborn infant treated by lobectomy, Pediatrics 54:808, 1974.

11. Gross, R. E., and Lewis, J. E.: Defect in the anterior mediastinum, Surg. Gynecol. Obstet. 80:549, 1945.

12. Gupta, J. M., van Vliet, P. K. J., Fisk, G. C., and Wright, J. S.: Ductus ligation in respiratory distress syndrome, J. Thorac. Cardiovasc. Surg. 63:642, 1972.

13. Haller, J. A., Shermeta, D. W., Donahoo, J. S., and White, J. J.: Life-threatening respiratory distress from mediastinal masses in infants, Ann. Thorac. Surg. 19:364, 1975.

14. Hislop, A., and Reid, L.: New pathological findings in emphysema in childhood. 1. Polyalveolar lobe with emphysema, Thorax 25:682, 1970.

15. Horsley, B., Lerberg, D. B., Allen, A. C., Zuberbuhler, J. K., and Bahnson, H. T.: Respiratory distress from patent ductus arteriosus in the premature newborn, Ann. Surg. 177:806, 1973.

16. Korngold, H. W., and Baker, J. M.: Nonsurgical treatment of unilobar obstructive emphysema of the newborn, Pediatrics 14:206, 1954.

17. Laurence, K. M.: Congenital pulmonary cystic lymphangiectasis, J. Pathol. Bacteriol. 70:325, 1955.

18. Leape, L. L., Ching, N., and Holder, T. M.: Lobar emphysema and patent ductus arteriosus. Development of emphysema while under observation, Pediatrics 46:97, 1970.

19. Leape, L. L., and Longino, L. A.: Infarcted lobar emphysema, Pediatrics 34:246, 1964.

20. Leonidas, J. C., Hall, R. T., and Rhodes, P. G.: Conservative management of unilateral pulmonary interstitial emphysema under tension, J. Pediatr. 87:776, 1975.

21. Lincoln, J. C. R., Stark, J., Subramanian, S., Aberdeen, E., Bonham-Carter, R. E., Berry, C. L., Path, M. C., and Waterston, D. J.: Congenital lobar emphysema, Ann. Surg. 1:55, 1971.

22. Lucaya, J., Gil, M. D., and Moreiras, M.: Pneumothorax and/or pneumomediastinum in newborn infants with renal malformations, Ann. Radiol. 19:103, 1976.

23. Macklin, C. C.: Transport of air along sheaths of pulmonic blood vessels from alveoli to mediastinum, Arch. Intern. Med. 64:913, 1939.

24. Mansfield, R. B., Graham, C. B., Beckwith, J. B., Hall, D. G., and Sauvage, L. R.: Pneumopericardium and pneumomediastinum in infants and children, J. Pediatr. Surg. 8:601, 1973.

25. May, R. L., Meese, E. H., and Timmes, J. J.: Congenital lobar emphysema: Case report of bilateral involvement, J. Thorac. Cardiovasc. Surg. 48:850, 1964.

26. Munnell, E. R., Lambird, P. A., and Austin, R. L.: Polyalveolar lobe causing lobar emphysema in infancy, Ann. Thorac. Surg. 16:624, 1973.

27. Murray, G. F.: Collective review. Congenital lobar emphysema, Surg. Gynecol. Obstet. 124:611, 1967.

28. Murray, G. F., Talbert, J. L., and Haller, J. A.: Obstructive lobar emphysema of the newborn infant, J. Thorac. Cardiovasc. Surg. 53:886, 1967.

29. Pierce, W. S., deParedes, G. C., Friedman, S., and Waldhausen, J. A.: Concomitant congenital heart disease and lobar emphysema in infants, Ann. Surg. 172:951, 1970.

30. Ponte, C., Remy, J., Bonte, C., Lequien, P., and Lacombe, A.: Pneumothorax et pneumomediastins chez le nouveau-né, Arch. Fr. Pediatr. 28:817, 1971.

31. Potts, W. J., Holinger, P. H., and Rosenblum, A. H.: Anomalous left pulmonary artery causing obstruction to right main bronchus, JAMA 155:1409, 1954.

32. Riker, W. L.: Neonatal Respiratory Distress, in Mustard, W. T., et al. (eds.), *Pediatric Surgery* (2d ed.; Chicago: Year Book Medical Publishers, Inc., 1969), Vol. 1, p. 439.

33. Roghair, G. D.: Nonoperative management of lobar emphysema, Radiology 102:125, 1972.

34. See, G., Dayras, J. Cl., and Echle, L.: Gêne respiratoire du nouveau-né provoquée par une séquestration pulmonaire extralobaire, Ann. Pediatr. 21:211, 1974.

35. Shawker, T. H., Dennis, J. M., and Gareis, J. W.: Pneumopericardium in the newborn, Am. J. Roentgenol. 116:3, 1972.

36. Stephan, W. K., and Otto, M. L.: Report of a previously unrecognized cause of neonatal asphyxia, JAMA 176:133, 1961.

37. Stern, L., Fletcher, B. D., Dunbar, J. S., Levant, M. N., and Fawcett, J. S.: Pneumothorax and pneumomediastinum associated with renal malformations in newborn infants, Am. J. Roentgenol. 116:785:1972.

38. Wille, L., and Wurster, K.: Congenital cystic adenomatoid pulmonary hamartoma in a newborn infant, Z. Kinderheilk. 11:1, 1974.

39. Yeh, T. F., Vidyasagar, D., and Pildes, R. S.: Neonatal pneumopericardium, Pediatrics 54:4, 1974.

Chylothorax

SUDDEN ACCUMULATION of chyle in the thorax or abdomen occurs at three periods of life: (1) in the neonatal period, (2) in later childhood, when it usually is due to trauma, either accidental as in compression injuries to the chest or by direct operative injury to the thoracic duct, and (3) later in life, when, in addition to trauma, neoplastic and inflammatory obstructions of the thoracic duct lead to extravasation.

SPONTANEOUS CHYLOTHORAX.—A newborn infant or one in the first month of life presenting with dyspnea, mediastinal displacement and a collection of fluid filling one hemithorax, usually the right, may, in the absence of any evidence of infection, be assumed to have a chylothorax. It has been shown[2] that ligation of the superior vena cava in dogs and cats will cause a chylous pleural effusion in 50% of the animals, and it seems reasonable to suppose that abrupt rises of venous pressure in the course of delivery or during resuscitative attempts immediately after delivery should result in thoracic duct rupture. The extravasated chyle presently ruptures from the mediastinum into the pleural cavity. In a number of instances, operation has disclosed one or several fistulas between the thoracic duct and the pleural cavity. It is probable that some such openings represent congenital fistulas. At birth, the fluid is clear, serous and turns milky only after feedings are begun. Diagnosis is made on the finding of a sterile fluid, white cells in which are predominantly lymphocytes and whose fat content is higher than that of plasma, protein content half that of plasma and electrolyte content the same as that of plasma. Globules of fat may be seen microscopically and stained.[8]

The very small number of reported cases—5 from the Mayo Clinic,[11] 16 in Boles and Izant's[3] review and 38 in Tischer's[13] review (which failed to find the 2 cases reported here in the first edition)—merely indicates that most clinics see few such cases, and that most of the individual instances are not reported. Eleven of the 16 patients reviewed by Boles and Izant had effusion and respiratory distress within the first 5 days of life, and 5 of the 11 were in respiratory distress within hours of birth. Given the observed rate of reaccumulation of chyle, this suggests that in some of these infants the chyle might have been present in the pleural cavity before birth, having leaked through such a fistulous orifice as has been described. We have seen a child with a chylous effusion in the peritoneal cavity—chylous ascites—that caused troublesome distention and respiratory distress from the elevated diaphragm immediately after delivery—obviously an antenatal ascites. It is of more than passing interest that the effusion occurred on the right side of 11 of Boles' 16 patients and was bilateral in 1.

In the chylothorax of the neonatal period, aspiration seems to be all the treatment required (Fig. 46–10). Some patients respond to two or three thoracenteses yielding a total of only several ounces of fluid. The greatest total amount of fluid aspirated from a child who recovered was the 1955 ml aspirated in 27 thoracenteses over 30 days by Boles and Izant.[3] Both patients of Randolph and Gross[10] were operated on successfully, but in only 1 was it thought that the chylous leaks were closed and the proximal thoracic duct ligated successfully. The 2 patients we saw at the Harriet Lane Home, both with right-sided effusions, responded

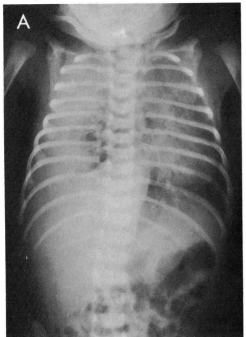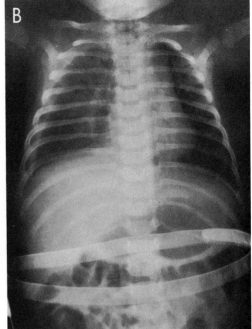

Fig. 46–10.—Spontaneous chylothorax in the neonate. This 22-day-old baby had had respiratory distress for 10 days. Three aspirations on successive days totaling 61 ml of characteristic creamy white chyle relieved her symptoms and there was no reaccumulation. She remained well. **A,** initial film before aspiration. The entire right hemithorax is filled with opaque fluid. The heart is displaced against the left chest wall; the right lung is the small nubbin compressed against the mediastinum. **B,** after aspiration, the lung is almost fully expanded but for a little evidence of fluid or thickened pleura at the periphery.

in a few days to aspiration and presented no therapeutic problem. Among Tischer's[13] 38 collected cases in the first 3 months of life there were 6 deaths in the 10 cases seen in 1944 or earlier, none of them in patients treated operatively. In the 28 subsequent cases there were 2 deaths, both in infants with bilateral effusions in the immediate postnatal period, 1 treated with bilateral tube drainage, 1 not treated. Of the 26 survivors seen since 1944, only 4 were operated on. Nutrition may become a serious problem in children requiring repeated thoracentesis, because of the loss of both protein and fat.[4] The successful management of chylous ascites by feeding a diet of medium chain triglycerides, which pass from the intestine directly into the portal circulation, now has been reported in infants with iatrogenic chylothorax.[6, 8] Reinfusion of the aspirated chyle is feasible and has been done, but at times with catastrophic reactions.

TRAUMATIC CHYLOTHORAX.—The principal experience with traumatic chylothorax has been afforded after thoracic operations and, in particular, the Blalock operation for tetralogy of Fallot performed on the left side. Although Shumacker and Moore[12] assumed an aggressive attitude toward these lesions and operated promptly to ligate the thoracic duct proximal to the fistula, Maloney and Spencer,[9] with an experience of 13 cases of traumatic chylothorax seen on the cardiac surgery service of Johns Hopkins Hospital, found that 11 of the 13 patients responded readily to repeated aspiration. Only 2 required operative ligation of the duct, both of whom survived.

There is general agreement now that underwater seal catheter drainage to keep the lung expanded and promote its adherence to the chest wall is the soundest therapy. If drainage persists in quantities beyond the tolerance of the child and shows no sign of diminishing, or is persisting after 2 or 3 weeks, one is justified, whether for neonatal or iatrogenic chylothorax, in ligating the thoracic duct just above the diaphragm through a right thoracotomy. This, however, rarely is necessary. Intravenous alimentation obviously will have a place in the treatment of these children.

Chylothorax may also be associated with diffuse lymphangiomatosis or lymphangiectasis with a variety of presentations. Congenital lymphangiomatosis of bone, fortunately rare, has been uniformly fatal. Although the tissues are widely involved, the diffuse bone lesions, demonstrable radiologically, are a prominent feature. Involvement of the lungs leads to chylothorax, frequently bilateral. Death usually is due to infection.[5, 6] Berberich et al.[1] of Seattle report a 3½-year-old child with lymphangiomatosis and chylothorax and massive drainage of chyle after thoracostomy. Lymphangiogram demonstrated two thoracic ducts and pooling of contrast material at the level of T10. Medium chain triglycerides diet was ineffective. At right thoracotomy, cystic lymph-filled lesions were found over the mediastinal pleura and "a spongy malformation 7 cm in length at the level of the aortic hiatus." The parietal pleura was stripped, the right thoracic duct was ligated, the mediastinal lymphatic malformation excised and sutures placed to occlude the left duct. Chylous drainage erased. Subsequently, this patient had a pathologic fracture and a bout of staphylococcal pneumonia. The observation was made that during the prolonged initial period of tube drainage, humoral and cell mediastinal immunity were seriously lowered and returned to normal after operation.

REFERENCES

1. Berberich, F. R., Bernstein, I. D., Ochs, H. D., and Schaller, R. T.: Lymphangiomatosis with chylothorax, J. Pediatr. 87:941, 1975.
2. Blalock, A., Cunningham, R. S., and Robinson, C. S.: Experi-

mental production of chylothorax by occlusion of superior vena cava, Ann. Surg. 104:359, 1936.

3. Boles, E. T., and Izant, R. J., Jr.: Spontaneous chylothorax in the neonatal period, Am. J. Surg. 99:870, 1960.
4. Burdette, W. J.: Management of chylous extravasation, Arch. Surg. 78:815, 1959.
5. Fessard, Cl., Boulesteix, C., Roudil, Ch., Grynblat, N., Fondimare, A., Dumas, R., Jean, R., and Dailly, R.: Ascite chyleuse, chylothorax et ectasies capillaires intra-osseuses, Arch. Fr. Pediatr. 31:489, 1974.
6. Gershanick, J. J., Jonsson, H. T., Jr., Riopel, D. A., and Packer, R. M.: Dietary management of neonatal chylothorax, Pediatrics 53:400, 1974.
7. Gutierrez, R. M., and Spjut, H. J.: Skeletal angiomatosis: Report of three cases and review of the literature, Clin. Orthop. 85:82, 1972.
8. Kosloske, A. M., Martin, L. W., and Schubert, W. K.: Management of chylothorax in children by thoracentesis and medium-chain triglyceride feedings, J. Pediatr. Surg. 9:365, 1974.
9. Maloney, J. V., Jr., and Spencer, F. C.: The nonoperative treatment of traumatic chylothorax, Surgery 40:121, 1956.
10. Randolph, J. G., and Gross, R. E.: Congenital chylothorax, Arch. Surg. 74:405, 1957.
11. Roy, P. H., Carr, D. J., and Payne, W. S.: The problem of chylothorax, Mayo Clin. Proc. 42:457, 1967.
12. Shumacker, H. B., Jr., and Moore, T. C.: Surgical management of traumatic chylothorax, Surg. Gynecol. Obstet. 93:46, 1951.
13. Tischer, W.: Der Chylothorax im ersten Trimenon, Z. Kinderchir. 5:43, 1967.

Pulmonary Agenesis

THERE MAY BE complete agenesis of both lungs, one lung, a lobe or lobes. Minetto *et al.,*[3] in their exhaustive review of the subject, divided the lesions into bilateral pulmonary agenesis, unilateral pulmonary agenesis, pulmonary aplasia, pulmonary hypoplasia and lobar aplasia. Agenesis has been known to exist for several hundred years; Morgagni described it in 1762. In 1907, Von Eiken first made the clinical diagnosis correctly. In 1928, Boenninger first made the diagnosis on the basis of bronchography, and in 1940 Stokes and Brown first confirmed the diagnosis bronchoscopically.

Bilateral pulmonary agenesis is the rarest malformation, of which some half dozen cases have been reported. The children are not necessarily stillborn and may make respiratory efforts. The trachea may be entirely wanting, or a portion of it may be preserved with or without an associated esophageal anomaly. Cardiac anomalies usually are associated.

Thirty instances of *unilateral pulmonary agenesis,* 17 on the left and 13 on the right, were collected by Minetto and his colleagues. Although about half the infants with pulmonary agenesis as their principal lesion die in infancy or early childhood, the reported cases have included patients aged 60–70 dying of other causes. Skeletal, cardiac and other visceral anomalies commonly are associated. Respiratory symptoms—dyspnea, cyanosis, harsh breathing—are common, and even the children who survive frequently show retarded development. Although in some instances the chest on the affected side may be less well developed, it is striking that more often the outward appearance of the thorax does not suggest absence of a lung. The flattening of the chest and narrowing of the interspaces that occur after pneumonectomy are not usually found in pulmonary agenesis. Presumably this is due to the fact that from early intrauterine life, the heart has been completely displaced into the hemithorax left empty by pulmonary agenesis, and the thorax is,

in a sense, filled. The mediastinum is markedly shifted and the percussion note over the affected side is flat. Roentgenograms show a dense homogeneous shadow on the affected side, with the heart entirely in that hemithorax. The clinical story of respiratory difficulty, with the roentgenogram showing a massive mediastinal shift, often is interpreted as massive atelectasis. Bronchoscopy shows absence of one major bronchus, and bronchography confirms this observation (Fig. 46–11). Collected series suggest a predilection for the left side and for males. As might be expected, absence of the right lung is associated with more symptoms and a shorter life expectancy than absence of the left lung.

The cause of death has been a source of considerable discussion, particularly when other significant anomalies are not found and in view of the fact that in perhaps half the reported cases, pulmonary agenesis has been compatible with normal life. The patients who died usually had a history of severe dyspnea, frequently with wheezing and cough. A few had obvious pulmonary infection in the sole lung. Maier and Gould[2] operated on a 10-week-old infant who had been born prematurely and had been subject to frequent and severe bouts of respiratory distress, thought to be due to pressure on the trachea. The child often had held her head in an extended position and tended to tire while feeding. At operation, the trachea was found compressed and deviated by an abnormally coursing aorta lying unusually far toward the right. It was not possible to relieve the compression and displacement, and the infant died. Maier suggested that such kinking of trachea or bronchus, plain at the operating table, obscure at autopsy, might account for some deaths. Hendren,[1] in a very similar case, when fixation of the aorta to the sternum failed to give relief, reoperated and resected the portion of left main bronchus made malacic by aortic compression and then, in a third operation, divided the aortic arch and inserted a Dacron graft, allowing the aortic arch to widen, thus for the first time successfully relieving the tracheal compression. The child died of sepsis. Anomalies of lobation and of the bronchovascular patterns of the remaining lung have been reported[4] but the remaining lung is not decreased in size and should be adequate to sustain life. Reid,[5] in a characteristically painstaking morphologic study of the left lung in a child with agenesis of the right lung, who had died at 3 months of repeated attacks of pneumonia, made no mention of the relation of pulmonary artery and bronchus but found a reduction of bronchial branches in the left lung and an even less developed pulmonary artery, while the alveoli were so increased in number, although small in size, as to represent an alveolar population appropriate for two normal lungs at 3 months.

Minetto counted 93 reports of patients with *pulmonary aplasia,* a condition in which, once more, the lung is absent but there is a rudimentary bronchial stump. The carina is normal, seen bronchoscopically. The main bronchus on the affected side may end blindly or may show a tentative division into several branch bronchi. The symptoms, prognosis and state of the contralateral lung are essentially the same as in total agenesis.

Pulmonary hypoplasia, as analyzed by Minetto, composes a heterogeneous group of conditions, including an underdeveloped lung in association with a diaphragmatic hernia, hypoplastic lung with absence of a pulmonary artery and a globular malformation in which a mass of poorly differentiated pulmonary tissue is attached to a malformed and underdeveloped bronchus.

Lobar aplasia has been reported some 30-odd times. It may be unilobar or bilobar. A combination of absence of the

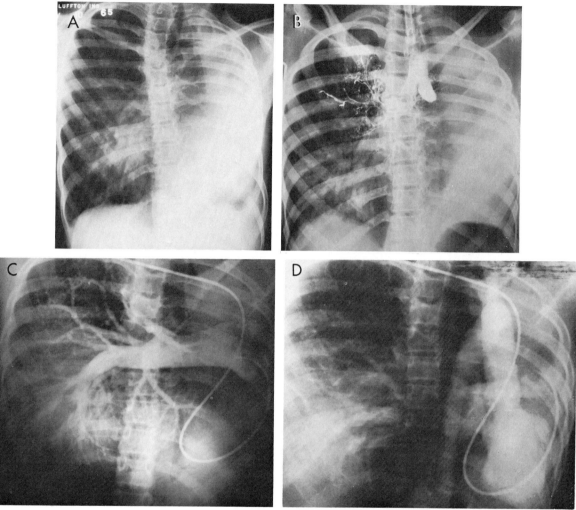

Fig. 46–11.—Agenesis of the left lung. A 12-year-old girl had profound pectus excavatum (see Fig. 41–5), ectromelia of the hand and disabling dyspnea rapidly progressive for the past 2 years. **A,** posteroanterior film, showing the heart in the left chest, mediastinal hernia into the left chest and opacity of unknown nature in the left upper chest. **B,** bronchogram, showing only a stump of the left main bronchus. This was also observed broncho-scopically, when the right main bronchus showed a yielding external compression, as if by a vessel. **C,** angiocardiogram; catheter in right pulmonary artery. There is no evidence of a left pulmonary artery. **D,** angiocardiogram; left heart phase. The left ventricle and ascending and descending aorta are clearly visible. Some of the opacity remains unaccounted for—possibly thymus. (From Ravitch and Matzen.[4])

right upper lobe and right middle lobe is the most common single type. The heart is markedly displaced to the side of the agenesis, and repeated pulmonary infections seem to be common in patients in this group. If the bronchial connections to the remaining lobe, or lobes, on the affected side are adequate and if angiocardiography shows normal pulmonary vasculature there is no treatment to be offered. If the bronchi are inadequate, or if no pulmonary artery or an extremely small one is found to the remaining lobe, a resection may relieve the symptoms.

REFERENCES

1. Harrison, M. R., and Hendren, W. H.: Agenesis of the lung complicated by vascular compression and bronchomalacia, J. Pediatr. Surg. 10:813, 1975.
2. Maier, H. C., and Gould, W. J.: Agenesis of the lung with vascular compression of the tracheobronchial tree, J. Pediatr. 143:38, 1953.
3. Minetto, E., Galli, E., and Boglione, G.: Agenesia, aplasia, ipoplasia polmonare, Minerva Med. 49:4635, 1958.
4. Ravitch, M. M., and Matzen, R. N.: Pulmonary insufficiency in pectus excavatum associated with left pulmonary agenesis, congenital clubbed feet and ectromelia: Improvement following operation, Dis. Chest 54:58, 1968.
5. Ryland, D., and Reid, L.: Pulmonary aplasia—a quantitative analysis of the development of the single lung, Thorax 26:602, 1971.

Abnormal Tracheobronchial Communications and Variations in Lobation

ABNORMAL TRACHEAL COMMUNICATION.—The most common abnormality of this type is certainly that associated with esophageal atresia (see Chap. 43).

The single most common anomalous bronchial origin associated with symptoms is so-called ectopic tracheal bronchus (trifurcation of the trachea), which usually arises on the right side. It is thought sometimes to represent an apical segmental bronchus arising separately proximal to the carina and at other times to be truly supernumerary. The eparterial

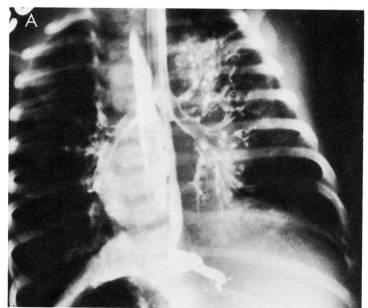
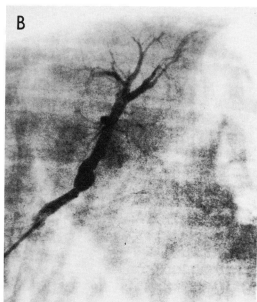

Fig. 46–12.—Congenital bronchobiliary fistula. **A,** roentgenogram of the chest following endoscopic catheterization and injection of contrast material into a congenital bronchobiliary fistula arising from the right main-stem bronchus in a 3-week-old girl. **B,** communication with the biliary tree demonstrated in a Polaroid x-ray film made at operation after injection into the distal end of the tract. This infant had bilious vomiting initiated by coughing and associated with pneumonia and right middle lobe atelectasis. The diagnosis had been established by aspiration of bile from the anomalous orifice in the right main-stem bronchus. The patient is well 7 years following division and ligation of the fistula. (Courtesy of William K. Sieber.)

bronchus of a number of animal species arises from the trachea separately, and the situation then appears to be not unlike that seen in these patients. The abnormally arising pulmonary segments frequently are the site of repeated pulmonary infection, which requires resection for relief.[3] Roshe[4] described an unusual variant in which there were one tracheal bronchus and two additional separate bronchi of the upper lobe, one arising essentially from the trachea at the origin of the right main bronchus and the other just below it. Each of the three segments had an anomalous pulmonary vein draining into the superior vena cava. Resection of the three segments cured the repeated attacks of pulmonary infection. The abnormal pulmonary venous drainage had not been anticipated.

BRONCHOBILIARY FISTULA.—A fascinating anomaly of tracheobronchial communication is that in which there is a congenital bronchobiliary fistula. Sieber,[5] of the Children's Hospital of Pittsburgh, reported a 3-week-old baby with a cough productive of green sputum from birth. The suspected bronchobiliary fistula was demonstrated at bronchoscopy when a catheter was passed into an anomalous orifice just to the right of the carina, injected Dionosil outlining a tract (Fig. 46–12, *A*) passing down through the diaphragm into the liver. At operation, the 5-mm inside diameter fistula was seen to originate just to the right of the carina, and perforated the diaphragm just to the right of the esophageal hiatus. A 2-cm section of the tract was excised and the child did well. Intraoperative injection through the lower end of the fistula outlined the intrahepatic biliary tree (Fig. 46–12, *B*). In the almost identical lesion in the 14-month-old child of Stigol *et al.,*[6] the tract was histologically like bronchus proximally and "like esophagus" distally. The tract in Weitzman's[7] child was similar distally. Sieber and his colleagues analyzed the 5 previous cases. All coughed yellow or green sputum from birth and had repeated pulmonary problems.

BRONCHOPULMONARY FOREGUT MALFORMATIONS.—In this category I have chosen to include only those anomalies in which an essentially normal lung is connected by its bronchus to the esophagus or stomach (Fig. 46–13). Extralobar sequestration (q.v.), on the left, may have such an esophagogastric origin of the bronchus, but, for the present at least, we are inclined to believe that to be a rather different lesion, with a different embryopathic basis, although some disagree.[1, 2] Heithoff and colleagues,[2] reporting 2 cases of bronchopulmonary foregut malformation of their own, 24 reported cases and 3 additional ones from the Children's Hospital of Pittsburgh, for a total of 29, have presented the most useful analysis of the problem. The right main bronchus arose from the esophagus in 10, the left lower lobe bronchus in 11 and other lobar bronchi in the remainder. The gastrointestinal communication was with the lower esophagus or cardioesophageal junction in 24, the gastric fundus in 3 and the mid or upper esophagus in 2. The diagnosis often was made only after months or years (up to 18) of pulmonary symptoms. Females were affected twice as often as males. Systemic arteries supplied the affected lobe or lung in 17; 1 had both a systemic and a pulmonary artery. The most useful diagnostic measure was the esophagogram. Associated anomalies were common—diaphragmatic hernia, vertebral, gastrointestinal and cardiac. The 5 deaths in the 23 patients operated on were ascribed to the associated malformations. The treatment was resection of the involved lobe or lung in all cases. It is not beyond the bounds of possibility that if the anomaly is recognized in the first day or two of life, before the inevitable infection results, at least in a case in which the main bronchus arises from the esophagus, the bronchus might be sutured to the trachea and the lung preserved.

VARIATIONS IN LOBATION.—The lingular segment of the left upper lobe occasionally is entirely separated, as if it were a left middle lobe, and other segments may be so de-

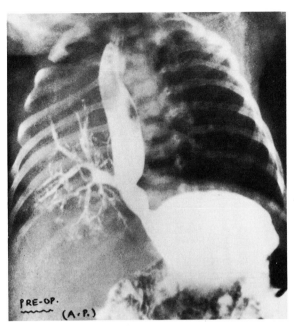

Fig. 46–13.—Anomalous origin of the right main bronchus from the esophagus; esophagogram in a 3-week-old infant with persistent cough and pneumonia involving the entire right lung. This infant died of progressive respiratory insufficiency at 1 year of age. (Courtesy of William K. Sieber.)

marcated. The azygos lobe on the right side is not an abnormality of lobation but a radiographic phenomenon created by the passage of the azygos vein in a sulcus in the posterior aspect of the left upper lobe and can be diagnosed from the characteristic, almost vertical shadow of the vein in the plain x-ray film. The condition causes no symptoms and requires no treatment.

REFERENCES

1. Gerle, R. D., Jaretzki, A., III, Ashley, C. A., and Berne, A. S.: Congenital bronchopulmonary foregut malformation, N. Engl. J. Med. 278:1414, 1968.
2. Heithoff, K. B., Sane, S. M., Williams, H. J., Jarvis, C. J., Carter, J., Kane, P., and Brennom, W.: Bronchopulmonary foregut malformations. A unifying etiological concept, Am. J. Roentgenol. 126: 46, 1976.
3. Marks, C.: The ectopic tracheal bronchus: Management of a child by excision and segmental pulmonary resection, Dis. Chest 50: 652, 1966.
4. Roshe, J.: Bronchovascular anomalies of the right upper lobe, J. Thorac. Cardiovasc. Surg. 50:86, 1965.
5. Sane, S. M., Sieber, W. K., and Girdany, B. R.: Congenital bronchobiliary fistula, Surgery 69:599, 1971.
6. Stigol, L. C., Traversaro, J., and Trigo, E. R.: Carinal trifurcation with congenital tracheobiliary fistula, Pediatrics 37:89, 1966.
7. Weitzman, J. J., Cohen, S. E., Woods, L. O., Jr., and Chadwick, D. L.: Congenital bronchobiliary fistula, J. Pediatr. 73:329, 1968.

Anomalies of the Pulmonary Vessels

A VARIETY OF ANOMALIES of the pulmonary vasculature are of significance, particularly in respect to their relation to the lungs and quite apart from those considerations related to cardiovascular surgery.[3]

Anomalous Systemic Arteries Supplying the Lung

In the discussion of congenital cystic disease of the lung, of lower accessory lung and of bronchopulmonary foregut malformations, instances are mentioned in which these conditions are associated with one or several large arteries from the descending thoracic aorta, or the abdominal aorta, entering the periphery of the lung. In some of these cases there is no pulmonary artery; in others, both types of arterial circulation exist.

Hypoplastic Lung with Anomalous Systemic Arteries

Maier[10] reported a 12-year-old girl with moderate dyspnea and diminished volume of the right lung. Angiocardiography showed a small right pulmonary artery. At operation, two large systemic arteries were found perforating the diaphragm and supplying the right lung. The vessels were divided and the patient was relieved from symptoms. A 14-year-old boy with frequent respiratory infections, cough, sputum and dyspnea had an anomalous bronchial architecture.[10] At operation, no pulmonary arteries or veins supplying the right lung were found. A number of arteries entered the lung from the diaphragm, and venous drainage was into the superior vena cava. The lung was removed, with relief from symptoms.

Absence of the Pulmonary Artery to One Lung

Patients with this anomaly show some reduction in the volume of the abnormal lung and absence of the normal hilar vascular shadows. The mediastinum is displaced toward the anomalous lung and the contralateral lung is overdistended and emphysematous. Maier reported such an instance in a boy of 9 with recurrent pulmonary infection. There was no pulmonary artery. The pulmonary veins were normal. The arterial supply was from a systemic vessel descending along the trachea and entering the right upper lobe. Absence of the pulmonary artery is more common on the right than on the left. A number of such patients have been seen, some with symptoms of pulmonary infection sufficient to warrant resection. Ferencz,[2] in her excellent review, reported 25 collected cases of absence of one pulmonary artery in patients with otherwise normal hearts. At least 4 had definite abnormalities of the bronchopulmonary pattern, and only 1 was known to have anomalous pulmonary venous return. Hemoptysis was the most serious symptom and at times was severe, presumably caused by excessive inflow of blood into the lung from systemic channels. Three of the 25 had bronchiectasis; none had lung cysts or sequestrations.

Aberrant Left Pulmonary Artery

Respiratory obstruction from compression of the trachea by a vascular ring due to a double aortic arch or other anomaly of the great vessels is well known (see Chap. 57). Less well known is compression of the trachea by an aberrant left pulmonary artery looping around the trachea from the right side. Among the 15 cases reviewed by Jacobson *et al.*[6] there were only 3 survivals, 2 after division, relocation and resuture of the vessel and 1 without operation. Potts *et al.*[12] have beautifully illustrated the operation in their report of the first successful operative relief (Fig. 46–14). By the time of N. K. Yong's report of 2 cases,[15] the literature contained reports of 35, including one[9] corrected by division, translocation and resuture of the right main bronchus. From Chil-

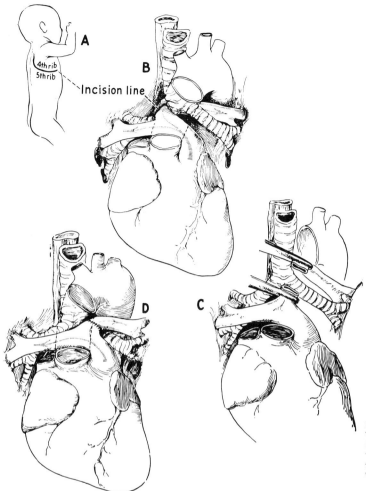

Fig. 46–14.—Tracheobronchial obstruction by aberrant left pulmonary artery. **B,** the pulmonary artery passes to the right of the trachea, compressing the right main bronchus, trachea, or both, on its course around and behind the trachea to the left. **C,** transection and rerouting of the left pulmonary artery anterior to the left main bronchus. **D,** the completed reconstruction. (From W. J. Potts *et al.*[12])

dren's Memorial Hospital in Chicago, Koopot *et al.*[8] reported 5 cases of anomalous left pulmonary artery encircling the trachea and right main bronchus, passing then behind the trachea to the left lung. All 3 treated by division of the pulmonary artery and resuture anterior to the trachea survived. They found 64 reported cases of the anomaly, 24 surviving. Phelan and Venables'[18] 4 unoperated patients ultimately recovered.

Congenital Pulmonary Arteriovenous Fistula

This condition is uncommon but, because of its clinical interest, a substantial number of instances have been reported.[13, 17] It consists of a direct communication within the lung between a pulmonary artery and vein. Occasionally the feeding artery is systemic.[1, 7] The connection usually is in the form of an aneurysmal sac, sometimes quite small but at other times several centimeters in diameter. Of great importance is the fact that the lesions may be multiple and may occur in more than one lobe and in both lungs. They may be associated with obvious telangiectases of the lung (Fig. 46–15). The cases occur sporadically, but Glenn *et al.*[4] reported instances in siblings, and the father of our patient, reported by Sloan and Cooley,[14] had an almost identical lesion. Pulmonary arteriovenous fistulas occur with particular frequency in patients with hereditary hemorrhagic telangiectasia (Rendu-Osler-Weber disease), and perhaps a sixth

of the reported cases of pulmonary arteriovenous aneurysms have been associated with this syndrome. Somewhat less than a quarter of the cases have been discovered in childhood; almost all of the others have been diagnosed early in adult life, the symptoms in most cases going back to childhood. Some of the arteriovenous aneurysms suggest cavernous hemangiomas, but others are relatively simple sacs with direct and obvious arterial and venous connections. The walls are extremely thin. The arterial and venous branches supplying and draining the aneurysm may be quite large and conspicuous enough to show on a plain roentgenogram. In some instances, the arterial supply has been from an aberrant systemic artery.[16] In 1974, from the Mayo Clinic, Dines and colleagues[1] surveyed 63 cases seen over 20 years. In only 3 was a systemic blood supply responsible. Hereditary telangiectasia affected 48 of the 63 patients. Of the 63, 36 were operated on. The prognosis was bad in the cases of Rendu-Osler-Weber's hereditary telangiectasia because of the increased incidence of multiple fistulas, both in the lung and elsewhere, and increased rate of fistula growth and increased frequency of complications from the fistulas.

SYMPTOMS.—The physiologic disturbances produced by pulmonary arteriovenous fistulas depend on the shunt of unoxygenated blood into the peripheral circulation. The shunts may be of very great volume and commonly are suffi-

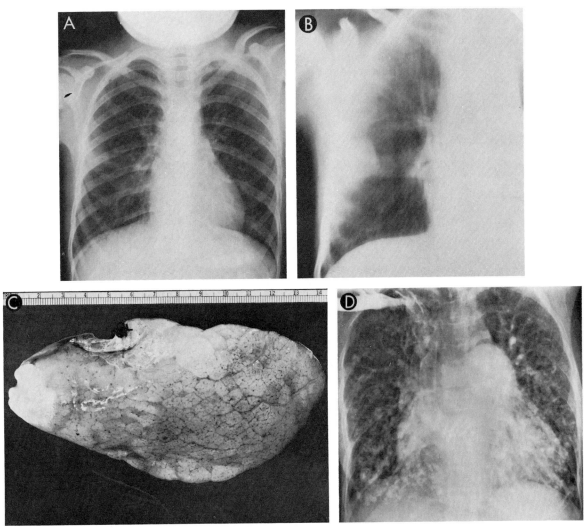

Fig. 46–15.—Pulmonary arteriovenous fistulae. Child seen at 8 years with polycythemia, cyanosis and dyspnea, temporarily relieved by right middle lobectomy but ultimately developing high-output cardiac failure. **A,** plain film shows a peripheral opacity on the right at the level of the third anterior interspace. **B,** laminagram shows clearly the spherical body of the arteriovenous sac and distinctly outlines the feeding and draining pulmonary vessels. **C,** operative specimen, right middle lobe. At operation, the entire right lung was found to be dotted with numerous telangiectatic and heman-gioma-like lesions from 2–3 mm to 1–1.5 cm in size. Some of the larger ones were slightly raised and palpable. The large aneurysmal arteriovenous communication was in the right middle lobe. The specimen was photographed after injection of radiopaque material into the pulmonary artery. The lobulated white area at the posterior tip of the middle lobe is the aneurysmal sac. A pneumonectomy was not performed because of the possibility that similar lesions existed on the other side. **D,** angiocardiogram 8 years after middle lobe resection. (See text.)

ciently large to cause clinical cyanosis and to result in unsaturation and anoxemia of a degree to stimulate the bone marrow to produce striking polycythemia. The child illustrated in Figure 46–15 was first correctly diagnosed by a hematologist to whom the patient had been sent with a diagnosis of polycythemia vera. Cardiac enlargement occurs in some patients but as a rule is not severe. However, Hall and his colleagues[5] successfully resected the left lower lobe in a 6-day-old infant with cardiomegaly, tachycardia, tachypnea and intense cyanosis. The lobe was found to be replaced by a huge arteriovenous malformation. Dyspnea is the most common symptom. Epistaxis probably reflects the presence of similar telangiectases in the nasal mucosa. Cerebral symptoms are common, presumably due to anoxemia or to thrombosis in association with the polycythemia. Brain abscesses occur as in other lesions with right-to-left vascular shunting. Hemoptyses are frequent and severe and occasionally exsanguinating. Fatal hemorrhage has occurred from rupture of an aneurysm into the pleural cavity, the aneurysms almost always being at the surface of the lung.

PHYSICAL EXAMINATION.—Abnormal murmurs commonly are heard over the site of the aneurysms, and occasionally a thrill has been palpated. Cyanosis and clubbing are almost invariable, and associated telangiectases or hemangiomas of the skin and mucous membranes have been seen in almost half the patients.

RADIOLOGIC FINDINGS.—The aneurysms themselves usually are visible on the plain film as rounded or lobulated discrete densities connected to the hilus by the cord-like vessels (see Fig. 46–15, A). Pulsation of the mass frequently can be noted under the fluoroscope. Laminography sharply outlines the sac and its vessels (see Fig. 46–15, B). Angiocardiography is the most definitive roentgenologic procedure and almost invariably shows the arterial and venous supply and the aneurysmal sac.

TREATMENT.—The lesions are sufficiently dangerous in themselves to warrant operation on diagnosis. The symptomatic patients, those with severe polycythemia, with cyanosis and dyspnea or history of hemoptyses, obviously require operation. The operation is simple enough and sufficiently free from specific hazard to be equally advisable on a prophylactic basis for patients with diagnosed arteriovenous fistula who have few or no symptoms.

Because of the frequent multiplicity of the lesions, the propensity of previously insignificant lesions to increase in size with the passage of time and the possibility that small lesions, radiologically invisible, exist in the other lung, as little pulmonary tissue as possible should be removed. At times, it is feasible to excise the aneurysmal sac and its vessels without excising any lung tissue at all,[11] and in other instances it may be possible to perform wedge or segmental resections. When telangiectases are found, the probability that they exist in the contralateral lung is sufficiently good so that these should be ignored and only the principal aneurysm excised. The immediate result of excision is excellent in terms of mortality, relief from symptoms and physiologic restoration to a normal condition. The resection involves no specific hazard. The ultimate prognosis depends on the existence or development of other systemic shunts in the lung or of other manifestations of hereditary telangiectasia. In this respect, the case shown in Figure 46–15 is of interest.

The child underwent middle lobe resection for an AV fistula at age 8, when she presented with a 16-month history of fatigability, progressive cyanosis and dyspnea and development of clubbing of the fingers. The hemoglobin was 17.5 gm, red blood cells 6.1 million and hematocrit 53.2. Eight years after middle lobe resection, she seemed essentially well except for cyanosis on exertion beginning 4 years following operation. Dyspnea on exertion then began to return and increased progressively, with cyanosis and fatigability. In 1955, she was hospitalized with headache and stiff neck. Two brain abscesses were drained, one right frontal, one right parietal. She returned in 1957 because of attacks of paroxysmal nocturnal dyspnea and severe cyanosis. She now had pulsating vascular swellings over the right external malleolus and the mandible. Because of occasional hematemesis, a barium study was undertaken, which showed a gastric ulcer.

The progressive high-output failure made it imperative to learn whether her pulmonary arteriovenous fistulas were limited to the right lung, in which case a completion of the pneumonectomy might be considered, or whether they involved the left lung as well, in which case she would be beyond operative assistance.

The angiogram (Fig. 46–15, D) shows numerous arteriovenous fistulas in both lungs. Those in the right lung are somewhat larger and more impressive than those on the left, but the involvement on the left side is sufficiently great to make completion of the right pneumonectomy useless. Note the great enlargement of the right side of the heart and the huge pulmonary arteries. The left side of the heart is large also.

The diffuseness of this lesion puts the patient beyond the hope of rescue by operative intervention, and she is doomed to die of cardiac failure if one of the other hazards of her condition does not prove fatal before that occurs.

REFERENCES

1. Dines, D. E., Arms, R. A., Bernatz, P. E., and Gomes, M. R.: Pulmonary arteriovenous fistulas, Mayo Clin. Proc. 49:461, 1974.
2. Ferencz, C.: Congenital abnormalities of pulmonary vessels and their relation to malformation of the lung, Pediatrics 28:993, 1961.
3. Findlay, C. W., Jr., and Maier, H. C.: Anomalies of the pulmonary vessels and their surgical significance, Surgery 29:604, 1951.
4. Glenn, F., Harrison, C. S., and Steinberg, I.: Pulmonary arteriovenous fistula occurring in siblings: Report of two cases, Ann. Surg. 138:886, 1953.
5. Hall, R. J., Nelson, W. P., Blake, H. A., and Geiger, J. P.: Massive pulmonary arteriovenous fistula in the newborn, Circulation 31:762, 1965.
6. Jacobson, H. J., II, Morgan, B. C., and Humphreys, G. H., II:
7. Keszler, P., and Kollar, L.: Anéurisme intralobaire d'une artère d'origine aortique à destination pulmonaire traitée par lobectomie, Ann. Chir. Thorac. Cardiovasc. 9:529, 1970.
8. Koopot, R., Nikaidoh, H., and Idriss, F. S.: Surgical management of anomalous left pulmonary artery causing tracheobronchial obstruction, J. Thorac. Cardiovasc. Surg. 69:239, 1975.
9. Lochard, J., Vert, P., and Chalnot, P.: Trajet aberrant de l'artère pulmonaire gauche comprimant l'origine de la bronche souche droite, Ann. Chir. Thorac. Cardiovasc. 2:458, 1963.
10. Maier, H. C.: Absence or hypoplasia of a pulmonary artery with anomalous systemic arteries to the lung, J. Thorac. Surg. 28:145, 1954.
11. Parker, E. F., and Stallworth, J. M.: Arteriovenous fistula of the lung treated by dissection and excision without pulmonary excision, Surgery 32:31, 1952.
12. Potts, W. J., Holinger, P. H., and Rosenblum, A. H.: Anomalous left pulmonary artery causing obstruction to right main bronchus, JAMA 155:1409, 1954.
13. Schumacker, H. B., Jr., and Waldhausen, J. A.: Pulmonary arteriovenous fistulas in children, Ann. Surg. 158:713, 1963.
14. Sloan, R. D., and Cooley, R. N.: Congenital pulmonary arteriovenous aneurysm, Am. J. Roentgenol. 70:183, 1953.
15. Tan, P. M., Loh, T. F., Yong, N. K., and Sugai, K.: Aberrant left pulmonary artery, Br. Heart J. 30:110, 1968.
16. Watson, W. L.: Pulmonary arteriovenous aneurysm, Surgery 22:919, 1947.
17. Yater, W. M., Finnegan, J., and Giffin, H. M.: Pulmonary arteriovenous fistula (varix): Review of the literature and report of two cases, JAMA 141:581, 1949.
18. Phelan, P. D., and Venables, A. W.: Management of pulmonary artery sling: A conservative approach, Thorax 33:67, 1978.

Aberrant left pulmonary artery, J. Thorac. Cardiovasc. Surg. 39:602, 1960.

Congenital Cystic Disease of the Lung

DISCUSSIONS OF CYSTIC DISEASE of the lung are handicapped by a number of factors. The older authors, particularly, often confused undoubtedly acquired cystic formations, such as bronchiectasis and the pneumotocele of staphylococcal pneumonia, with congenital conditions. Among the undoubted congenital cystic conditions of the lung there are a number of varieties, and simultaneous discussion of these without clear differentiation of the types, particularly in any consideration of embryologic mechanisms, still further confuses the issue.

We will consider bronchogenic cysts, "true" congenital lung cysts, congenital cystic adenomatoid malformation of the lung, miscellaneous congenital cystic malformations and lower accessory lobe.

Bronchogenic Cysts

These are unilocular, round, thick-walled cysts lined by ciliated respiratory epithelium, located in the mediastinum or close to the major bronchi but not communicating with them. They probably represent early malformations dating to the time of closure of the primitive foregut, and are dealt with in Chapter 44, in the discussion of mediastinal cysts and tumors. Biancalana[4] has described an intrapulmonary unilocular cyst, without a bronchial communication, which he considers to be an intrapulmonary bronchogenic cyst (see Chap. 44).

True Congenital Lung Cysts

ETIOLOGY.—The congenital nature of lung cysts is evident from the fact that they have been seen in infants only a few hours old, that cysts in babies only a few hours or weeks old have been found to be lined by tall ciliated columnar epithelium (Fig. 46–16, B), that they are associated with

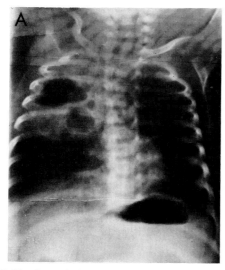
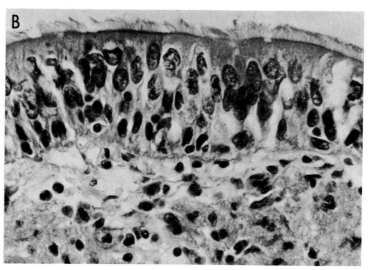

Fig. 46–16. – Congenital cystic disease of the lung. Infection in a 13-week-old infant with 3-week history of cough. At operation, cysts were found to involve the upper lobe, to which the middle lobe was fused; both were removed. The upper lobe was occupied by a pus-filled multilocular cyst 5.5 cm in greatest diameter. **A,** preoperative roentgenogram, showing a number of separate air sacs in the opacified right upper lobe. **B,** photomicrograph of the cyst lining, consisting of tall columnar ciliated bronchial epithelium. There were a few mucous glands in the cyst wall and a thin layer of smooth muscle between the basement membrane and fibrous wall of the cyst. In some areas there was acute inflammation. The child was well and grew normally after operation. It is inconceivable that ciliated epithelium of this kind could have come to line an acquired lesion in this infant's short preoperative life.

other abnormalities such as trilobed left lungs and aberrant systemic arteries arising from the aorta and inserting into the periphery of the involved lobe (Plate II, *A*, p. 1467 and Fig. 46–17, *B*) and that, in some of them, abnormal epithelial formations have been found, suggesting hamartomatous structures (see Fig. 46–19). At this point in the experience with lung cysts in children there no longer is discussion as to whether they are congenital or acquired, and debate instead centers on the embryogeny of these malformations. Nevertheless, it is important to note that most students agree that very few significant lung cysts are found in autopsies on stillborn babies. This probably can be explained by the assumption that the epithelial clefts that exist are neither large nor conspicuous until dilated in vivo by air or by accumulations of the mucus they secrete. The cysts of which we speak invariably communicate with the bronchus, as demonstrated by air in their cavities, anthracotic pigment in their walls or the admission of contrast medium during bronchographic study. From the standpoint of the thoracic surgeon interested in pediatric problems, the condition is not rare, and our own experience exceeds 20 cases.

CLINICAL PICTURE. – Because the cysts communicate with the bronchial air passages, they almost inevitably become infected. Infection may occur within the first weeks of life (see Fig. 46–16) and may be severe, or it may develop quite suddenly years later. A number of our patients with multilocular cysts were treated for years for bronchiectasis (see Fig 46–17). It is not at all uncommon for a large unilocular cyst to become infected and to be diagnosed as a lung abscess or empyema. Three of our patients were sent to us when their "empyema" cavities failed to collapse under long-continued intercostal tube drainage (Fig. 46–18), and we operated on 1 of our own patients with the thought that he had a lung abscess. In him, the presence of a systemic artery from the aorta to the left lower lobe and the well-preserved respiratory epithelium lining the cavity made the diagnosis. The failure of a lung cyst to collapse under tube drainage is characteristic. Not rarely, large thin-walled cysts

distend with air that is trapped by a flap valve mechanism, so that tension cysts develop and necessitate attention because of the resultant respiratory embarrassment. Cysts of the kind under discussion may be unilobar or multilobar and occur somewhat more often in the lower lobes than in the upper lobes and as frequently on one side as on the other. An entire lung may be occupied by cysts. We have not had a patient with proved bilateral congenital cystic disease, and, faced with a picture suggesting bilateral cystic disease, we would be inclined to search carefully for evidence of cystic fibrosis of the pancreas with resultant bronchiectasis.

Clubbing of the fingers rarely if ever is associated with congenital lung cysts. Metastatic infections apparently have not been described. Rupture of the cyst into the pleural cavity with empyema, or tension pneumothorax, also seems not to occur, except as the result of diagnostic aspiration. Hemoptysis is seen, but infrequently. Womack and Graham[43] in 1942 suggested the possibility of carcinoma arising in such a cyst. Bauer[2] reported an unequivocal instance, and several others are on record. Cysts in every way resembling those under discussion have at times become symptomatic only in adult life or have been incidental findings at autopsy in patients who had been entirely asymptomatic. Nevertheless, the rule is for the cysts to cause symptoms early in life, either from distention and pulmonary insufficiency or from infection and resultant cough, sputum production, fever and malnutrition. In general, congenital lung cysts are not associated with anomalies elsewhere in the body, cystic or otherwise.

DIFFERENTIAL DIAGNOSIS. – Congenital diaphragmatic hernia, also seen chiefly on the left side, may suggest congenital cystic disease of the lung with multiple fluid levels and areas of opacity. Displacement of the mediastinum, intestinal obstruction and severe dyspnea are not usual with cystic disease. Postpneumonic pneumatoceles, after staphylococcal or other pneumonia, may be indistinguishable from the cavities of lung cysts, particularly if the history is undependable and a series of films is not available. If a pneumato-

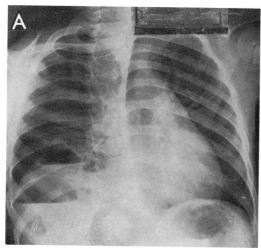

Fig. 46–17.—Congenital cystic disease of the lung simulating bronchiectasis. A 6½-year-old boy with repeated attacks of pulmonary infection variously diagnosed as pneumonia and bronchitis since age 9 months. Nocturnal cough and morning sputum had been constant. He had intermittent bouts of dyspnea and noisy respirations. Bronchiectasis had been diagnosed. Repeated bronchoscopic aspirations gave no relief and he was referred for consideration of operation. **A,** roentgenogram showing several large fluid levels at the right base. **B,** at operation, the right lower lobe was found to be firm and covered by old inflammatory tissue. A large systemic vessel, apparently arising from the distal aorta and about the size of a lead pencil, entered the convexity of the posterolateral surface of the lower lobe. In normal position was the usual pulmonary arterial branch to the lower lobe. The lobe is almost entirely replaced by numerous large cysts, many intercommunicating and all filled with glairy mucopus. In addition to the large cysts seen on the roentgenograms, there are numerous smaller ones.

cele is suspected, one should delay operation for several weeks, looking for gradual disappearance of the lesion. A cyst under tension may be indistinguishable from lobar emphysema, but in either case treatment is urgent and surgical. On the right side, a mediastinal foregut remnant (esophageal duplication) communicating through the diaphragm to the bowel, hence containing air, may be confusing, although its shadow should be separable from that of the lung.

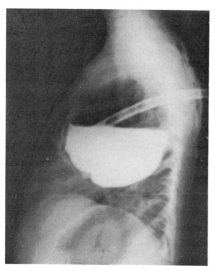

Fig. 46–18.—Congenital cystic disease of the lung misdiagnosed as empyema. A 3-year-old boy with history of severe respiratory infection at age 14 months and repeated subsequent infections, always in the right lung. At age 2, rib resection and drainage were performed for suspected empyema after pus was aspirated from the cavity. There had never been any sputum. The wound had drained constantly since. A second rib resection and catheter drainage had failed to affect the size of the cavity. At operation, a smooth-walled cyst was found in the right lung, which was dissected from the remainder of the upper lobe and removed. Despite the 11 months of drainage, the cyst was lined by well-preserved epithelium varying from tall ciliated, evenly columnar cells to pseudostratified columnar epithelium.

PATHOLOGY AND EMBRYOGENESIS.—The cysts usually are lined by respiratory epithelium whose tall columnar character and delicate cilia may be well preserved, even after repeated infection and drainage. On the other hand, some cysts, even in small infants, show signs of erosion and granulation tissue as the result of infection, and these cysts may be lined by pseudostratified squamous epithelium. It is uncommon for lung abscesses to become lined by ciliated epithelium, the epithelium lining an old abscess usually being squamous. It has been reported, however, that such cavities can be lined by ciliated epithelium, and this has been alleged to be the source of the epithelium in cysts called congenital. Since this is a process that requires many months for development, it cannot be regarded as the mechanism of the appearance of ciliated epithelium in the cysts of children days or weeks old.

The cyst walls may contain odd bits of bronchial cartilage and smooth muscle but rarely mimic bronchial architecture in any systematic way. Abnormal proliferations of mucus-secreting glands or of respiratory epithelium may suggest adenomas or hamartomas (Fig. 46–19). In our report[36] of such an instance in 1949, we suggested that this was merely a variation of the pathologic picture and further evidence that congenital cystic disease of the lung is indeed congenital. The condition has since been christened *congenital cystic adenomatoid malformation* of the lung.[3, 7, 21, 22] The reviews by Holder and Christy[21] and Belanger *et al.*,[3] both appearing in 1964, listed 32 and 34 published reports. Craig, Kirkpatrick and Neuhauser[8] thought, as do we, that there is a spectrum of congenital cystic disease varying from cysts with no adenomatosis through cysts with incidental adenomatosis to adenomatosis with incidental cysts. The excised left lower lobe of Holder's successfully operated on 7-day-old infant with adenomatosis contained no cysts. The case of Ch'in and Tang,[7] relieved by lobectomy, had been associated with generalized anasarca, which has been seen in other cases. Aslam,[1] in a 9-day-old baby with tachypnea from birth and developing anasarca, removed "a massive tumorlike lower lobe of the left lung, which occupied the whole of

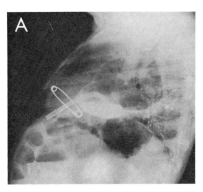

Fig. 46–19.—Cystic adenomatoid malformation of the lung. An 11-year-old boy, known to have had a cystic area in the lung since he was a year old. A tube thoracotomy was performed at age 5, during an attack of "pneumonia" and high fever. The tube had been worn continuously for 6 years, with constant discharge of glairy fluid and an obvious bronchial fistula. **A,** roentgenogram after Lipiodol was injected into the cyst through the catheter shows free communication with the bronchial tree. When the cyst was dissected away from the chest wall and the external opening clamped off, a flap-valve mechanism was demonstrated. The entire left lower lobe was removed and found to be occupied by a large unilocular, fibrous-walled cyst with smooth lining. **B,** the cyst is lined by bronchial epithelium with tall ciliated columnar cells and mucous glands beneath the lining. Masses of malformed cells and frond-like processes of mucous glands project into the lumen. **C,** hamartomatous malformation of mucous glands in the lung are seen at a distance from the cyst wall. (From Ravitch and Hardy.[36])

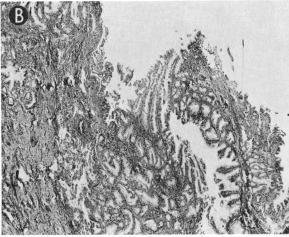

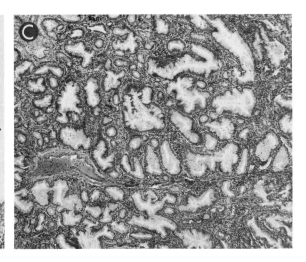

the left hemithorax and part of the right . . ." and was supplied by a systemic artery and vein, as well as a pulmonary artery and vein. The lesion was a cystic adenomatoid malformation in which systemic arteries to the lung are not usually found. The anasarca cleared. Thus, the histologic picture, the frequent location in upper lobes and the absence in these cases of anomalous systemic arteries supplying the affected lobe all argue for the establishment of congenital cystic adenomatoid malformation of the lungs as at least a special subgroup of cases within the category of congenital cystic disease.

Most interesting, and important from the standpoint of the surgeon, in the usual congenital cystic disease of the lung are the anomalous systemic vessels arising from the descending aorta or the abdominal aorta and entering the lung away from the hilus[15, 34, 37] (Fig. 46–20). These served

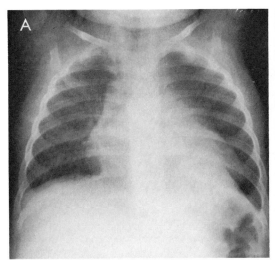

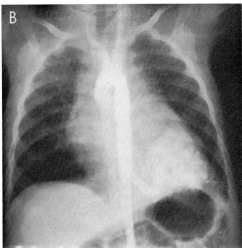

Fig. 46–20.—Congenital cystic disease of the lung. A child of 6 months with repeated history of pulmonary infection. **A,** roentgenogram shows a peculiar triangular opacity in the left lung in the supradiaphragmatic area behind the heart. It was suggested that this might be a "sequestered" lobe. **B,** a catheter aortogram demonstrates a very large branch of the lower thoracic aorta, not much smaller than the aorta itself, feeding directly into the lung. At operation, several systemic arteries were found going into the lower lobe, which was carneous and contracted, with normal-appearing bronchus, pulmonary artery and vein. Resection was followed by uneventful recovery.

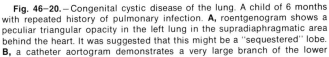

Pryce[34, 35] as the basis for his theory of *pulmonary sequestration*, the assumption being that these abnormal arteries have exerted traction on a portion of the lower lobe, divorcing it in varying degrees from its anatomic association with the remainder of the lower lobe. The theory fails to explain the development of the forms of cystic disease that occur without any vascular abnormality. Instances are on record of fatal hemorrhage resulting from avulsion of one of these abnormal aortic branches in the course of delivery of a cystic lobe by an unsuspecting operator. The arteries may be single or multiple and in our experience have been up to 6–8 mm in diameter (see Plate II, *A*). The systemic arteries usually are associated with diminution or abnormality of pulmonary arterial supply to the affected lobe, and there may be a systemic venous outflow (through the azygos system) as well as pulmonary venous outflow. Boyden[5] thinks that the arterial anomaly is essentially a coincidence, and others[13] fail to be attracted to Pryce's theory of primacy of the arterial malformation. Nevertheless, the term sequestration is firmly fixed, and congenital cystic disease of the lungs is equated by most with intralobar sequestration (for extralobar sequestration, see later).

Abbey Smith's[42] logical analysis suggests that, in the fetus, the development of cystic disease, particularly in the posterior section of the basal segment of the left lower lobe, is associated with insufficient or inadequate pulmonary arterial inflow. In these circumstances, he has proposed that there persist and enlarge vessels from the aorta, still present at this early embryonic stage. He has pointed out that such an aberrant systemic artery rarely if ever is seen in the absence of the pulmonary changes of sequestration. In another of the careful morphologic studies from the Brompton of lung anomalies, Hislop, Sanderson and Reid[20] further analyzed the effect of vascular anomalies on lung structure.

TREATMENT.—The treatment of congenital lung cysts is removal of the cyst or the involved segment, lobe or lobes. The large unilocular cysts that distend with air may, in some instances, be peeled away from the lobes in which they arise without sacrifice of any significant amount of pulmonary tissue. Lobes that are the seat of multilocular communicating cysts of varying sizes that contain much mucus as well as air usually require lobectomy. Operation is specifically advised, even in the absence of symptoms, in the knowledge that symptoms almost invariably will develop, and that operation on a healthy child with an uninfected cyst or system of cysts is safer than operation on a child who is chronically ill and has a grossly infected lung. The only death in a child with cystic disease in the Johns Hopkins series was in 1939, when a child of 8 months was sent home to be "built up" and to return in 2 years but died of "pneumonia" a month after discharge. There are numerous reports of lobectomies in the first weeks of life, and Minnis[28] successfully removed a lower lobe of an infant on the first day of life for cystic disease of the left lower lobe. Preoperative sputum cultures will help to guide antibiotic therapy. The aortogram, demonstrating anomalous systemic arterial supply to the involved lobe, both confirms the diagnosis and forewarns the surgeon (see Fig. 46–20), but need not be a required part of a preoperative study.

We do not think that there is any place for preliminary drainage of infected cysts. In the presence of a dangerously overexpanded cyst, venting it with a needle may be necessary while preparations for operation are being made. Ordinarily, the accumulation of air within a congenital cyst is gradual, and the respiratory embarrassment does not suddenly become extreme except in the presence of superimposed contralateral pulmonary infection. Localized congenital emphysema in the newborn, on the other hand, may lead to rapid development of respiratory distress. Pneumatoceles after staphylococcal pneumonia may, at times, distend with great rapidity to produce alarming symptoms. The treatment of lobar emphysema is lobectomy and of tension pneumatoceles, catheter drainage.

PROGNOSIS AFTER PULMONARY RESECTION IN CHILDHOOD.—It is a truism of thoracic surgery that, technically, pulmonary resection in infants is infinitely easier than pulmonary resection in adults because of the elasticity of the hilar structures and the absence of scar and matted lymph nodes.[6, 9, 28] It has been thought that the infant can respond to pulmonary resection with an actual increase in the number of his respiratory units and so perhaps suffer less in terms of loss of functioning respiratory tissue than the older child or adult. Engle[12] suggested that in children under the age of 5, new acini and alveoli are formed after pulmonary resection, but that beyond that age, lung growth is achieved principally by enlargement of existing alveoli. Reid,[38] our most knowledgeable student of the subject, states, in essence, that the issue still is unresolved, that airway multiplication normally occurs only before birth and that "alveolar multiplication beyond the normal does not occur after birth." There now is ample experience with lobectomy and pneumonectomy in infants and children who have gone on to an asymptomatic early adult life.

The function of the residual lung after pulmonary resection early in life has been investigated.[26] In puppies, it has been shown that functional pulmonary diffusing surface is restored from 9 to 12 months after pulmonary resection. This is thought to be both by hyperplasia and by "regeneration" of alveoli in the growing animal. Pneumonectomy in the adult animal leads to an increase of the air space without a corresponding increase of the functional alveolar capillary diffusing surface. Some evidence of emphysema in pneumonectomized puppies developed after a number of years.[14] The early studies by Lester, Cournand and Riley[25] and by Peters *et al.*[32] of children who had had pneumonectomies and a healthy remaining lung showed that residual air was increased in some, ventilatory capacity was adequate for extreme physical demands and that maximal breathing capacities were at least as great as the expected normal for one lung. More recent studies by Filler[14] and Giammona *et al.*[17] support the earlier observations. Filler studied 15 adolescents who had had bisegmentectomy, lobectomy or bilobectomy for post-tuberculous bronchiectasis. Subjects with bisegmentectomy showed no impairment of pulmonary function, even when measured by bronchospirometry; the remaining patients had slight decreases of lung volume and physiologic evidence of hyperdistention of the remaining lung parenchyma without evidence of bronchial obstruction and without effect on maximal breathing capacity. The respiratory function of the lung was unimpaired. Bronchospirometry showed decrease of lung volume and pulmonary perfusion on the side operated on quantitatively proportional to the extent of resection. Distention of the remaining lobe or lobes was proportionately greater in the upper than in the lower lobectomies. Peters and his colleagues compared their studies of 11 patients under 16 at the time of pulmonary resection with those of patients operated on between the ages of 16 and 21. The results in the younger group were excellent, except for 4 with residual disease. These 4 were rated as having good results, with slight exertional dyspnea.

Of the 12 older patients, 6 had excellent results, 5 good and 1 fair. And, of these, 3 had persistent bronchiectasis. The children operated on at a younger age had lower residual volume-lung capacity ratios and higher maximal breathing capacities, suggesting to Peters that hyperplasia rather than overdistention occurred in the remaining lung of the younger group. Most of the resections were done for bronchiectasis, only two for lung cysts in the young group and one in the older group, so the possibility of disease in the remaining lung affects these studies. In children with certainly normal residual lung, even slighter defects might be found. Giammona *et al.* studied 8 children who had had pneumonectomy at age 1–15 years and at intervals of 2–15 years after operation. Most of the patients had been operated on for bronchiectasis, only 2 for lung cyst. Their observations demonstrated moderate overinflation of the lung with minimal restriction of respiratory function. The carbon monoxide diffusion capacity was affected. The ratio of pulmonary capillary blood volume to pulmonary arterial blood volume was increased, suggesting overdistention of the pulmonary capillary bed after pneumonectomy. Pulmonary arterial pressure was high normal at rest and elevated with exercise. Pulmonary arterial resistance was normal at rest and with exercise. In sum, pulmonary resection is well tolerated by children, and, in the absence of disease in the remaining pulmonary parenchyma, is associated with minimal physiologic and clinical changes, at least into early adult life.

Pulmonary Lymphangiectasis

Other and rare types of cystic formations are the inconsequential pleural, thin-walled cysts that communicate with lymphatic vessels and are thought to be congenital cystic dilatations of the pulmonary lymphatics.[29] Occasionally, small cysts of the pleural mesothelium occur. However, congenital lymphangiectasis is a serious disease, half of the time associated with cardiac malformations,[16, 31] especially anomalous venous return.[16, 39] Although Virchow presented the first description of a case, only recently has the condition been reported with any frequency, most publications dating from Laurence's[23] report of 10 cases. Respiratory distress and cyanosis appear soon after birth; the condition affects both lungs and ordinarily is fatal in the neonatal period.[18, 23] The roentgenogram may show a ground glass or reticular opacity, but at its most striking suggests a chest full of soap bubbles. The condition is bilateral, thus not amenable to operative relief by resection. Since the large cardiac surgical experience with anomalous venous return far exceeds the number of cases of pulmonary lymphangiectasis, it is not likely that venous obstruction plays an etiologic role, although Rywlin and Fojaca[39] report an infant dying 1 hour and 40 minutes after birth, in whom pulmonary lymphangiectasis was associated with a blind common pulmonary vein. Laurence[23] and Giedion, Muller and Molz[18] reported identical cases of infants who died after a few hours of desperate respiratory distress. The roentgenogram in Giedion's case showed a striking appearance, as of a chest full of soap bubbles. In both infants there was diffuse pulmonary lymphangiectasis.

A variety of pathologic processes occasionally cause cystic degeneration of the lung. Lung abscess and bronchiectasis have been mentioned. Cysts have been reported also in several of the lipoid histiocytoses.[29] We have seen a child with papillomatosis of the larynx and trachea in whom the papillomatosis extended down into her smaller bronchi, with resultant destruction of the lungs by the formation of cysts lined with these papillomas.[30, 41]

Lower Accessory Lobe (Extralobar Pulmonary Sequestration)

The lower accessory lobe is a rare and characteristic anomaly, probably embryologically significant in connection with the possible development of the forms of lung cysts. Characteristically, the accessory lobe is a rounded, smooth, soft mass lying between the dome of the diaphragm and the inferior surface of the lung, almost always on the left. It is covered by what appears to be smooth, glistening visceral pleura. The accessory lobe is not attached to the lung, is not air-containing and is nourished by an artery directly from the aorta. Histologically, the accessory lobe displays a variety of epithelial structures suggesting alveoli and bronchi with occasional areas of cartilage. The lung itself usually is normal in its anatomic conformation and division into lobes.

These anomalies usually are noted as asymptomatic radiographic shadows or may cause symptoms by compression of the lower lobe. Occasionally, such a sequestered accessory lobe has been found within the pericardium[10] or beneath the diaphragm. They have been removed as mediastinal tumors of unknown nature. Operation presents no technical problems.[11, 24] In most instances, the pedicle of such a lobe reaches into the mediastinum in close relation to the esophagus. In the cases of Louw and Cywes[27] and of Rubin *et al.*[37] there was an epithelium-lined communication between the esophagus and the sequestered lobe. Boyden[5] had previously suggested, on the basis of a patient operated on by Bill in whom a similar but solid pedicle was found, that extralobar pulmonary sequestrations probably are the result of an abnormal embryonic diverticular outpouching of the esophagus. Louw and others have pointed out the frequent association of diaphragmatic hernia with this lesion. The lung whose sole bronchus arises from the esophagus,[19] occasionally reported as a sequestration, is discussed under abnormal tracheobronchial connections (p. 531). This malformation more probably is related to the mechanisms producing esophageal atresia and tracheoesophageal fistula than to those producing sequestration of the lung.

REFERENCES

1. Aslam, P. A., Korones, S. B., Richardson, R. L., and Pate, J. W.: Congenital cystic adenomatoid malformation with anasarca, JAMA 212:622, 1970.
2. Bauer, S.: Carcinoma arising in a congenital lung cyst, Dis. Chest 40:552, 1961.
3. Belanger, R., LaFleche, L. R., and Picard, J. L.: Congenital cystic adenomatoid malformation of the lung, Thorax 19:1, 1964.
4. Biancalana, L.: Die lungenzysten, Thoraxchirurgie 11:511, 1964.
5. Boyden, E. A., Bill, H. A., and Creighton, S. A.: Presumptive origin of a left lower accessory lung from an esophageal diverticulum, Surgery 52:323, 1962.
6. Burnett, W. E., and Caswell, H. D.: Lobectomy for pulmonary cysts in a 15-day-old infant, with recovery, Surgery 23:84, 1948.
7. Ch'in, K. Y., and Tang, M. Y.: Congenital adenomatoid malformation of one lobe of a lung with general anasarca, Arch. Pathol. 48:221, 1949.
8. Craig, J. M., Kirkpatrick, J., and Neuhauser, E. B.: Congenital cystic adenomatoid malformation of the lung in infants, Am. J. Roentgenol. 76:516, 1956.
9. Crossett, E. S., and Shaw, R. R.: Pulmonary resection in the first year of life, Surg. Gynecol. Obstet. 97:417, 1953.
10. d'Abreu, A. L.: *A Practice of Thoracic Surgery* (London: Edward Arnold, Ltd., 1958).
11. DeBakey, M., Arey, J. B., and Brunazzi, R.: Successful removal of lower accessory lung, J. Thorac. Surg. 19:304, 1950.
12. Engle, S.: *Lung Structure* (Springfield, Ill.: Charles C Thomas, Publisher, 1962).

13. Ferencz, C.: Congenital abnormalities of pulmonary vessels and their relation to malformation of the lung, Pediatrics 28:993, 1961.
14. Filler, J.: Effects on pulmonary function of lobectomy performed during childhood, Am. Rev. Respir. Dis. 80:801, 1964.
15. Findlay, C. W., Jr., and Maier, H. C.: Anomalies of the pulmonary vessels and their surgical significance, Surgery 29:604, 1951.
16. France, N. E., and Brown, R. J. K.: Congenital pulmonary lymphangiectasis. Report of 11 examples with special reference to cardiovascular findings, Arch. Dis. Child. 46:528, 1971.
17. Giammona, S. T., et al.: The later cardiopulmonary effects of childhood pneumonectomy, Pediatrics 37:79, 1966.
18. Giedion, A., Muller, W. A., and Molz, G.: Angeborene Lymphangiectase der Lungen, Helv. Paediatr. Acta 22:170, 1967.
19. Hanna, E. F.: Bronchoesophageal fistula with total sequestration of the right lung, Ann. Surg. 159:599, 1964.
20. Hislop, A., Sanderson, M., and Reid, L.: Unilateral congenital dysplasia of lung associated with vascular anomalies, Thorax 28: 435, 1973.
21. Holder, T. M., and Christy, M. G.: Cystic adenomatoid malformations of the lung, J. Thorac. Cardiovasc. Surg. 47:590, 1964.
22. Kwittken, J., and Reiner, L.: Congenital cystic adenomatoid malformation of the lung, Pediatrics 30:759, 1962.
23. Laurence, K. M.: Congenital pulmonary cystic lymphangiectasis, J. Pathol. Bacteriol. 70:325, 1955.
24. Leahy, L. J., and MacCallum, J. D.: Cystic accessory lobe, J. Thorac. Surg. 20:72, 1950.
25. Lester, C. W., Cournand, A., and Riley, R. L.: Pulmonary function after pneumonectomy in children, J. Thorac. Surg. 11:529, 1942.
26. Longacre, J. J., Carter, B. N., and Quill, L. M.: An experimental study of some of the physiological changes following total pneumonectomy, J. Thorac. Surg. 6:237, 1937.
27. Louw, J. H., and Cywes, S.: Extralobar pulmonary sequestration communicating with the esophagus and associated with a strangulated congenital diaphragmatic hernia, Br. J. Surg. 50:102, 1962.
28. Minnis, J. F., Jr.: Congenital cystic disease of the lung in infancy, J. Thorac. Cardiovasc. Surg. 43:262, 1962.
29. Moffat, A. D.: Congenital cystic disease of the lungs and its classification, J. Pathol. Bacteriol. 79:361, 1960.
30. Moore, R. L., and Lattes, R.: Papillomatosis of the larynx and bronchi, Cancer 12:117, 1959.
31. Noonan, J. A., Walters, L. R., and Reeves, J. T.: Congenital pulmonary lymphangiectasis, Am. J. Dis. Child. 120:314, 1970.
32. Peters, R. M., et al.: Respiratory and circulatory studies after pneumonectomy in childhood, J. Thorac. Surg. 20:484, 1950.
33. Peters, R. M., Wilcox, B. R., and Schultz, E. H., Jr.: Pulmonary resection in children: Long-term effect on the function and lung growth, Ann. Surg. 154:652, 1964.
34. Pryce, D. M.: Lower accessory pulmonary artery with intralobar sequestration of lung: A report of seven cases, J. Pathol. Bacteriol. 58:457, 1946.
35. Pryce, D. M., Sellors, T. H., and Blair, L. G.: Intralobar sequestration of lung associated with an abnormal pulmonary artery, Br. J. Surg. 35:18, 1947.
36. Ravitch, M. M., and Hardy, J. B.: Congenital cystic disease of the lung in infants and children, Arch. Surg. 59:1, 1949.
37. Rubin, E. H., et al.: Intralobar pulmonary sequestration—aortographic demonstration, Dis. Chest 50:561, 1966.
38. Ryland, D., and Reid, L.: Pulmonary aplasia—a quantitative analysis of the development of the single lung, Thorax 26:602, 1971.
39. Rywlin, A. M., and Fojaca, R. M.: Congenital pulmonary lymphangiectasis associated with a blind common pulmonary vein, Pediatrics 41:931, 1968.
40. Shannon, M. P., Grantmyre, E. B., Reid, W. D., and Wotherspoon, A. S.: Congenital pulmonary lymphangiectasis, Pediatr. Radiol. 2:235, 1974.
41. Singer, D. B., Greensburg, S. D., and Harrison, G. M., Papillomatosis of the lung, Am. Rev. Respir. Dis. 94:777, 1966.
42. Smith, R. A.: Some controversial aspects of the intralobar sequestration of the lung, Surg. Gynecol. Obstet. 114:57, 1962.
43. Womack, N. A., and Graham, E. A.: Developmental abnormalities of the lung and bronchogenic carcinoma, Arch. Pathol. 39: 301, 1946.

47
Infectious Diseases of the Lungs and Pleura

Pneumonia and Empyema

MARK M. RAVITCH

HISTORY.—The fact that pulmonary infections were followed by empyema and that this required external drainage for cure was known to the ancients. Hippocrates, Paul of Aegina, Fabricius and other ancient authorities were concerned with the optimal time and manner of drainage of the empyema. Laufranc used the cautery to perforate the chest and to drain the empyema. One of Vesalius' celebrated cases was a cure of empyema. The first formal thoracotomy for empyema in modern times is ascribed to Kuster, in 1889. Graham conclusively demonstrated the dangers of early open thoracotomy for empyema in the resultant pneumothorax and collapse; and thereafter, until the antibiotic era, discussion as to therapy largely centered on the relative advantages of open drainage and the various types of closed drainage, and the optimal time for utilization of these measures.

Pathogenesis

Empyema thoracis, or accumulation of pus within the pleural cavity, occurs from (1) hematogenous spread in children with septicemia, (2) direct or lymphatic extension from inflammatory or suppurative processes within the lung or (3) contamination of the pleural cavity by external trauma, operation or operative sequelae. In addition to the systemic signs of infection, the children show varying degrees of tachypnea and cyanosis. If the collection of fluid is large, the intercostal spaces may bulge and there may be a striking mediastinal shift. Neglected empyemas may rupture outward through the chest wall (empyema necessitatus), through the lung and the bronchial tree or through the diaphragm. In ancient times, external drainage of empyema was recognized as no more than an anticipation of this process.

Incidence and Mortality

Twenty years ago, it appeared that postpneumonic empyema in infants and children was a vanishing disease of historical interest only. Writing in 1961 for the first edition, we stated: ". . . if it were not for the children with staphylo-

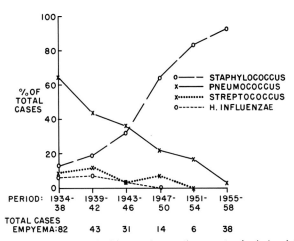

Fig. 47–1.—Empyema: incidence of causative agents. Analysis of 214 cases of empyema among 10,632 diagnosed cases of pneumonia at the Harriet Lane Home of the Johns Hopkins Hospital, Jan. 1, 1934, to Dec. 31, 1958 (see Table 47–1 for time periods according to drug therapy). Empyema had almost disappeared in the 4-year period 1951–54, when 6 cases were seen, 5 staphylococcal, 1 pneumococcal. In the final period there are almost as many cases as in the initial period, 1939–42, but due entirely to an upsurge in occurrence of staphylococcal pneumonia and empyema among infants. Empyema from streptococcus and *H. influenzae* is no longer seen.

coccal empyema, medical students and interns might rarely see a case of empyema, except perhaps on a traumatic or a postoperative basis." We did not realize it then, but the story told by Figure 47–1, reproduced from the first edition, represented the end of a trend and not the beneficent effects of antibacterial chemotherapy and antibiotic therapy. That the use of these agents did, in fact, affect the clinical picture, occurrence and relative incidence of the forms of bacterial pneumonia is clear enough from Figure 47–1 and Table 47–1. The effect of the various antibacterial agents over the period of the study can be summarized somewhat as follows. With the advent of sulfonamides, the need for hospitalization was not affected but the total mortality from both pneumonia and empyema dropped somewhat. The introduction of penicillin sharply decreased the need for hospitalization of children with pneumonia but the mortality from empyema and pneumonia among those who were admitted to the hospital did not change, and essentially the only change in mortality occurred during period V, when there were no deaths from empyema although the mortality rate for pneumonia still was 13% (see Table 47–1). The percentage of the empyema patients under 2 years of age underwent a steady increase from the beginning of the study, when the figure was 55%, through the final period, when 89% of the chil-

dren were 2 years of age. This reflects the predominant affinity of staphylococcal pneumonia and empyema for infants. In period V, during which chlortetracycline was introduced, there were only 6 cases of empyema, 1 due to pneumococcus and 5 to staphylococcus. In the final period, 1955 through 1958, despite no change in the total number of pneumonia patients seen or hospitalized or in the incidence of pneumonia in children under 2, there were 38 cases of empyema, an increase of incidence to 14% of the hospitalized cases. Thirty-five cases were due to staphylococcus, and of the 38 cases, 34 (89%) occurred in patients under age 2. There were no deaths due to pneumococcus after 1947, no deaths due to streptococcus after 1939 and no case of streptococcal empyema after 1948. Infection due to *Hemophilus influenzae* was not seen after 1944.

In the 1934–38 period, the death rate from staphylococcal empyema was 55%. It must be admitted that here, as in other cases of empyema of various kinds, multiple manifestations of the infectious process were seen often and contributed to the deaths that occurred. The death rates from staphylococcal empyema in the successive periods of study were 25%, 0%, 11%, 0% and, in period VI (1955–58), with a sudden upsurge of staphylococcal empyemas, 15%.

The effect of widespread antibacterial therapy appears to have been to decrease the need for hospitalization of children with pneumonia and to eliminate almost entirely the incidence of empyema due to pneumococcus, streptococcus and *H. influenzae*. This was accompanied by a sharp increase of empyemas due to the staphylococcus, almost all in infants (Table 47–2). Although the increase of staphylococcal pneumonia and empyema may have been the inevitable effect of the proper widespread therapeutic use of antibacterial agents, a general feeling prevailed that indiscriminate use of antibiotics far beyond the specific indication for serious infections may have aggravated the preferential overgrowth of staphylococcus in a large section of the population, thereby accounting for the changes in incidence noted. This rather pat explanation was rudely upset when, almost as soon as it was written, the incidence of staphylococcal pneumonia very sharply decreased. This has been a worldwide phenomenon, and once more the total number of postpneumonia empyemas seen in our hospitals is very small.

We continue to see occasional cases of staphylococcal pneumonia and empyema, but what amounted to the worldwide pandemic of staphylococcal pneumonia in infants in the middle 1950s has not recurred thus far, although the staphylococcus remains the most common cause of postpneumonic empyema in childhood.[4]

A report from the Columbus (Ohio) Children's Hospital[2] of their experience in the decade 1960–1970 covered 69

TABLE 47–1.—Mortality among Hospitalized Patients with Pneumonia and Empyema

PERIOD	CASES HOSPITALIZED	NO. OF CASES	DEATHS	MORTALITY, %
I: 1934–38 (presulfonamide)	Pneumonia	864	77	9
	Empyema	82	24	29
II: 1939–42 (sulfonamides)	Pneumonia	958	58	6
	Empyema	43	5	12
III: 1943–46 (penicillin)	Pneumonia	506	54	10
	Empyema	31	5	16
IV: 1947–50 (penicillin and streptomycin)	Pneumonia	205	26	13
	Empyema	14	2	14
V: 1951–54 (penicillin, streptomycin, and chlortetracycline)	Pneumonia	276	36	13
	Empyema	6	0	0
VI: 1955–58 (polyantibiotic)	Pneumonia	266	41	15
	Empyema	38	4	11

TABLE 47–2.—PRIMARY STAPHYLOCOCCAL
PNEUMONIA AT HARRIET LANE HOME OF
THE JOHNS HOPKINS HOSPITAL, 1955–58:
MORTALITY BY AGE GROUPS

AGE RANGE	CASES	MORTALITY, %
0–3 months	25	17
4–12 months	21	5
1–6 years	14	0
Over 6 years	0	0
TOTALS	60	8

cases of empyema in children—only 10 per year. Cultures were positive in 75%, and, of these, 80% were due to staphylococcus (28 cases), 3 to pneumococcus, 3 to beta-hemolytic streptococcus and 1 to pseudomonas. Sixty per cent of the cases were in infants. The over-all mortality was 7%; the mortality after the introduction of methicillin in 1963 was 3.2%.

Treatment of Empyema

The acceptance of Graham's work after World War I on the respiratory dynamics involved in open drainage of empyema in the presence of an unfixed mediastinum, and the general understanding, after World War II, of the importance of full pulmonary expansion in the treatment of suppurative collections in the chest rendered obsolete the old polemics. In their place has come a rational understanding of the relative indications for tube thoracostomy and open thoracotomy.

It always has been possible to treat an occasional patient with empyema successfully by means of repeated aspiration, with or without instillation of antibiotics. This method is substantially less certain to cure than drainage, likely to require considerably more time and probably causes more discomfort to the patient. In any case, a substantial number of patients so treated ultimately will require a drainage procedure, and there is the risk that in the meantime the pleural exudate will have thickened sufficiently so that it may not be possible to expand the lung. The degree of success in the treatment of empyema should be gauged by the rapidity with which the patient is cured of his suppurative disease and the rapidity with which the hemithorax begins to function normally. Treatment, therefore, combines appropriate systemic antibiotics and effective drainage.

In the face of a frank empyema or a large and probably infected effusion in association with pneumonia, it is our practice at once to institute intercostal tube drainage running to an underwater seal, usually with additional negative pressure. This may be done as soon as the collection of fluid is found. Since open pneumothorax is not produced, no risk is involved. The largest catheter that the intercostal space can accommodate should be used. If too large a catheter is used, the pressure of the ribs will occlude it. In older children, the familiar trocar thoracotomy set is used. Since we customarily utilize negative pressure drainage, we are not as concerned as formerly about techniques to avoid admission of air. In infants, after a skin incision has been made, the catheter, grasped in a hemostat, may be pressed through the chest wall into the pleura. In patients of all ages, trocar thoracotomy (and rib resection and open drainage) are performed under infiltration anesthesia. The catheter is inserted posterolaterally in the lowest interspace through which pus has been aspirated, preferably not so far posteriorly as to cause discomfort in the supine position. Formation of empyema in unusual locations requires insertion of the catheter accord-

ingly. From this point on, so long as the patient continues to improve, as measured by subsidence of fever, tachycardia and dyspnea and decrease in the size of the cavity on repeated measurement and roentgen study, no more need be done. The tube is removed when the cavity is reduced to a sheath around the tube. If at any time the patient's condition reaches a plateau short of disappearance of the empyema cavity and complete restoration of the clinical condition to normal, a rib resection and open drainage should be performed at once.

Chronic empyema, in which the lung cannot be made to expand, occasionally may require decortication—the removal of the fibrinous rind over the parietal and visceral pleura. The deforming collapse procedures of the Schede and other types should never be required in children.

Staphylococcal Pneumonia and Empyema

The special nature of staphylococcal pneumonia and its complications and the likelihood that with another cyclic swing it will become common again justify specific consideration of its clinical course and management. Staphylococcal pneumonia primarily attacks infants; approximately one-fourth of the cases are seen in the first year of life, and there is a direct relationship between age and mortality (see Table 47–2). The history usually is of sudden onset of a respiratory infection with extremely rapid progression. At times, within a few hours of onset, the child may manifest tachypnea, fever, dyspnea, cough and cyanosis. The violent respiratory efforts may lead to abdominal distention, elevating the diaphragm and increasing dyspnea. The physical signs are those associated with any pneumonic infection. Usually, staphylococcus can be obtained from cultures of material from the nasopharynx or of pleural fluid obtained by thoracentesis before antibiotic therapy is begun, even when only a little thin fluid is present, and obviously will be cultured in the presence of a frank empyema.

RADIOGRAPHIC CHARACTERISTICS.—A pulmonary infiltrate is present in all these patients, and in our experience is bilateral in approximately 10%. In 67 patients with staphylococcal pneumonia observed at the Harriet Lane Home of the Johns Hopkins Hospital,[5] pleural effusion or empyema occurred in 72%. Radiographic visualization of air within the lung parenchyma as excavations or pneumatoceles or within the pleural cavity as pneumothorax (Figs. 47–2 and 47–3) and evidence of a bronchial fistula in the latter are said to be pathognomonic of staphylococcal pneumonia. Frequently it is assumed that this is a new phenomenon and peculiar to staphylococcal pneumonia and staphylococcal empyema. Actually, in our experience, there have been observed various radiolucent shadows presumed to be parenchymal in occasional pneumococcal and other empyemas. Pyopneumothorax was seen in the Harriet Lane Home in the study period 1934–1958 in at least 23 instances of pneumonia and empyema due to organisms other than staphylococcus, principally pneumococcus.[4] In the same period there were 24 instances of pyopneumothorax with staphylococcal empyema. The presence, therefore, of a pneumatocele and particularly of pyopneumothorax, although suggestive of a staphylococcal infection, should not be taken as conclusive evidence. The origin of these pneumatoceles probably is explained by abscess formation in the bronchial wall and erosion through the bronchus with direct leakage of air into the parenchyma through a flap-valve defect rather than as the result of a parenchymal abscess with tissue destruction. The delicate bronchial tissues of infants are fairly readily de-

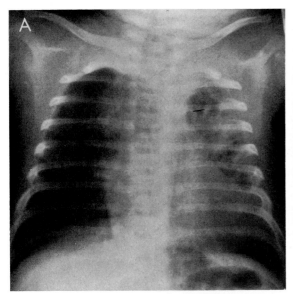
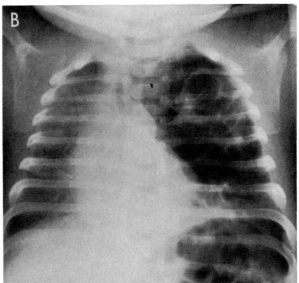
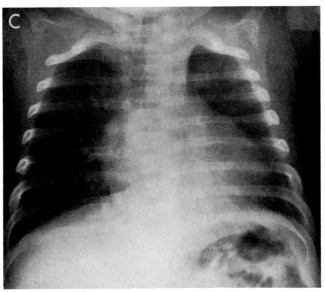

Fig. 47–2.—Staphylococcal pneumonia and tension pneumothorax. **A,** in a profoundly ill infant, the left lung is mottled and numerous small areas of radiolucency can be seen. There is some pulmonary infiltration in both upper lobes. **B,** without having reached very large size, one of the pneumatoceles ruptured into the left pleural cavity. There are tension pneumothorax and displacement of the mediastinum to the right. Although most of the left lung is collapsed and there is a herniation of air across the mediastinum, several of the pneumatoceles remain distended and visible. **C,** tube thoracotomy and negative pressure drainage have expanded the lung and relieved the respiratory embarrassment. The pulmonary infiltration has almost completely disappeared.

stroyed, even by the less vigorously histolytic enzymes of organisms other than the staphylococcus.

TREATMENT.—Massive doses of antibiotics rank first in the treatment of staphylococcal pneumonia. The pattern of resistance of the organisms and the effectiveness of antibiotics changes constantly. Currently we use methicillin as the first-line drug.

Three principal indications for surgical intervention may be mentioned: (1) *Massive effusion* with respiratory distress, which may occur with astonishing rapidity and require catheter drainage under negative pressure. (2) *Tension pneumothorax,* which is treated in the same way. The tension pneumothorax may develop as a more or less anticipated complication of a pre-existing pneumatocele or may result from rupture of a subcortical abscess and a bronchial leak without an obvious pneumatocele. (3) *Rapid expansion of a pneumatocele,* treated by insertion of an intercostal catheter into the pneumatocele, and suction drainage. In occasional sick infants, pneumatoceles form and expand with great suddenness. There is hardly any condition in which hour-to-hour observation and a sense of urgency for immediate treatment is as strongly required as in staphylococcal pneumonia. Pneumatoceles on one side or the other, or both, may increase in size with great rapidity, causing dyspnea with or without rupture into the pleural cavity and pneumothorax. We have performed as many as five tube thoracotomies in one infant before finally bringing the condition under control. The mere existence of a pneumatocele is not an indication for insertion of a catheter. We reserve this for the very

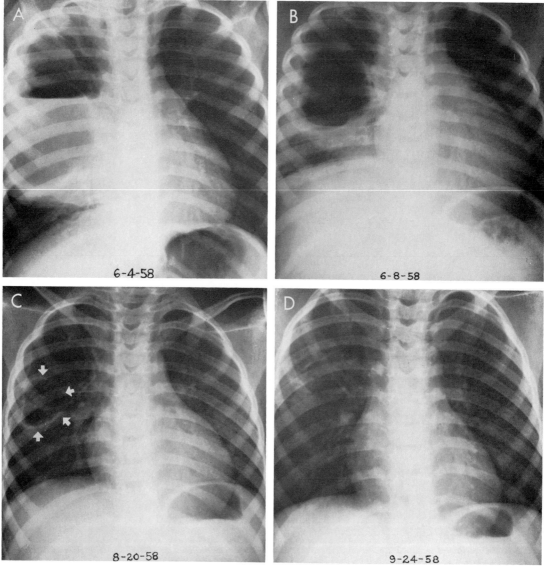

Fig. 47–3.—Staphylococcal pneumonia and pneumatoceles. This infant was admitted with staphylococcal pneumonia. Rapid increase of dyspnea was accompanied by expansion of a previously small pneumatocele, which partially filled with fluid. Catheter drainage brought immediate relief and ultimate cure. **A,** the huge pneumatocele occupies most of the right chest; there is a fluid level across its midportion. One might be pardoned for uncertainty as to whether this represented a pneumatocele with fluid level or a pyopneumothorax. The sharp curved outline of the lower portion of the opacity and absence of fluid in the costophrenic sulcus suggest that the air and fluid are in a pneumatocele within the pulmonary parenchyma. **B,** an intercostal catheter has evacuated the fluid. The pneumatocele is decreasing in size and the lower lobe has begun to expand. **C,** the catheter has been removed and the pneumatocele allowed to disappear slowly. **D,** 15 weeks after onset of the pneumonia, the pneumatocele has finally disappeared. It is probable that, had the catheter been left in the pneumatocele and negative pressure applied for a longer time, the pneumatocele would have collapsed more rapidly.

large or rapidly expanding pneumatoceles. Even when the infection itself has been brought under control and when the child is afebrile, comfortable, no longer dyspneic and eating well, the pneumatocele may expand and cause mechanical distress. It is not at all rare for an infant to leave the hospital with a small persistent pneumatocele that requires weeks for complete disappearance. At times, such a cyst will begin to expand and require readmission of the child for catheter decompression. Occasionally, an infant is seen in whom the original pneumonia was unremarked at home and whose pneumatocele now must be distinguished from the sac of a congenital lung cyst.[3] If there is any clinical likelihood that the parenchymal air collection represents a pneumatocele,

thoracotomy should be postponed for a period of observation to allow the suspected pneumatocele to recede.

RESULTS OF TREATMENT.—In the 67 cases mentioned previously, intercostal drainage was used in 28 (41.8%). In 15 patients, the intercostal catheter was inserted to release a tension pneumothorax following rupture of a pneumatocele. With the early use of drainage by an intercostal catheter, rib resection rarely is necessary for open drainage. Such a procedure was used only once in this series.

Staphylococcal pneumonia may be superimposed on a severe underlying disease such as cystic fibrosis of the pancreas, congenital biliary atresia or agammaglobulinemia, gravely altering the prognosis of the disease. The 7 patients with such complicating disease died. The over-all mortality in the 60 patients with primary staphylococcal pneumonia was 8%, but in the 25 patients in the first 3 months of life there was a 17% mortality. None of the 14 children over 1 year of age died.

A remarkable series of 6 consecutive cases of staphylococcal pneumonia complicated by staphylococcal pericarditis in children 7 months to 6 years of age is reported from Beirut by Slim et al.[6] The 3 originating in their own hospital represented 10% of their 30 cases of staphylococcal pneumonia; 5 of the 6 required open pericardial drainage. All survived.

Asp, Pasila and Sulamaa[1] of Helsinki, where staphylococcal pneumonia still was common in 1964, presented a startlingly different therapeutic approach. In 20 very sick children, 3 weeks to 5 years of age with staphylococcal pneumonia and pyopneumothorax, usually under tension, with accompanying mediastinal shift, they performed an immediate open thoracotomy. Pus and fibrin were evacuated, the lung decorticated and bronchial fistulas sutured. All 20 children recovered, although 3 required a second operation. Hospital stay was 1–3 months. This approach is radically contrary to our belief that in staphylococcal empyema catheter drainage with negative pressure is all that is required and that open thoracotomy should be reserved for the rare failure with catheter drainage.

REFERENCES

1. Asp, K., Pasila, M., and Sulamaa, M.: Treatment of pyopneumothorax in infants and children, Acta Chir. Scand. 128:715, 1964.
2. Cattaneo, S. M., and Kilman, J. W.: Surgical therapy of empyema in children, Arch. Surg. 106:564, 1973.
3. Potts, W. J., and Riker, W. L.: Differentiation of congenital cysts of the lung and those following staphylococcic pneumonia, Arch. Surg. 61:684, 1950.
4. Ravitch, M. M., and Fein, R.: The changing picture of pneumonia and empyema in infants and children: A review of the experience at the Harriet Lane Home from 1934 through 1958, JAMA 175: 1039, 1961.
5. Sabiston, D. C., Jr., et al.: The surgical management of complications of staphylococcal pneumonia in infancy and childhood, J. Thorac. Cardiovasc. Surg. 38:421, 1959.
6. Slim, M. S., Rizk, G., and Uwaydah, M.: Mediastinal complications of staphylococcal infection in childhood: Experience with six consecutive cases, Surgery 69:755, 1971.

Bronchiectasis

KENNETH J. WELCH

HISTORY.—Bronchiectasis was well described by Laennec in 1810, a time when this disease was uniformly fatal. In 1905, Jackson first demonstrated abnormalities of bronchial architecture with nebulized bismuth powder. In 1922, Sicard and Forestier introduced iodized oil (Lipiodol).[1]

Early pulmonary resections were carried out with use of mass ligatures. The mortality rate was in the range of 25% due to hemorrhage from erosion of vessels at the hilus and development of bronchopleural fistula.

Churchill and Belsey,[11] in work later amplified by Blades and Kent,[6] recommended individual ligation and division of the structures at the pulmonary hilus. Jackson and Huber[31] introduced the concept of segmental anatomy, outlined the bronchovascular segments and devised the system of classification that is in current use (Fig. 47–4). Overholt and Langer[38] developed the technique for resection of individual pulmonary segments, limiting resection to the area of disease and sparing adjacent parenchyma. Bloomer et al.[7] prepared injection specimens demonstrating the various types of bronchopulmonary disease.

Refinements of x-ray technique and anatomic resection have extended the scope and accuracy of surgical intervention. Mortality in partial resection of the lung in children is less than 1% in capable hands.

Etiology

The most common cause of bronchiectasis in childhood is pulmonary infection, in the past particularly when complicating pertussis and measles. It occurs in tuberculosis as a result of bronchial obstruction or parenchymal damage. Bronchiectasis secondary to hereditary or congenital disorders and to aspiration or inhalation of foreign bodies accounts for most other cases. Children with cystic fibrosis now commonly survive into the second decade of life through prolonged prophylactic broad-spectrum antibiotic therapy. An increasing number require pulmonary resection for bronchiectasis or uncontrolled bleeding.

The etiology of bronchiectasis in 308 children seen at Children's Hospital Medical Center, Boston, from 1940 to 1976 is shown in Table 47–3 and from the literature in Table 47–4. The etiology of bronchiectasis in patients operated on from 1940 to 1965 arranged in 5-year periods is shown in Figure 47–5. From 1940 to 1945, the leading cause of bronchiectasis was pneumonia, followed by assorted infections, pertussis and the usual causes of bronchiectasis seen today. A similar pattern was seen from 1945 to 1950, when even more children were encountered with advanced disease. From 1950 to 1955 there was a reduction of the number of cases over-all and the virtual disappearance of the postpneumonic form of bronchiectasis and of bronchiectasis following pertussis. The period 1955–1960 witnessed the further reduction of postpneumonic bronchiectasis of any bacterial variety and the emergence of patients with cystic fibrosis. Since then, cystic fibrosis has led the list, and there has been an increased number of cases due to foreign body, congenital anomalies and hereditary or poorly understood autoimmune disorders. Various conditions deserve special mention.

PNEUMONIA.—It is probable that most patients acquire bronchiectasis in the first year of life (80 of 209 in one series, with 75% of patients under age 5). With early antibiotic therapy, the postpneumonic group is rapidly shrinking. Among 1894 pertussis patients, 87 developed pneumonia with at least transient cylindrical dilatation of the secondary bronchi.[18] These changes appear to be reversible. Blades and Dugan[5] called this pseudobronchiectasis.

ALLERGY.—About 20% of patients with bronchiectasis have associated sinusitis or other evidence of allergy. The bronchiectatic focus may trigger recurring attacks of asthma. Following removal of the destroyed pulmonary segment (4 patients), the asthmatic attacks were ameliorated. Recent attention has been focused on extrinsic allergic alveolitis associated with bronchopulmonary aspergillosis.[45] Clinical presentation is severe asthma with infiltrates and local destruction.

The condition was first reported by Hinson et al.[28] They recognized a form of proximal bronchiectasis with normal caliber distally. Tissue damage is thought to be due to precipitation mediated by Arthus III reaction. The causal agent usually is A. fumigatus. Aspergilloma has been reported.[42]

Aspergillus colonization of the lung may occur on a variety of backgrounds, including tuberculosis, sarcoidosis, bronchiectasis, lung abscess and pulmonary infarction.

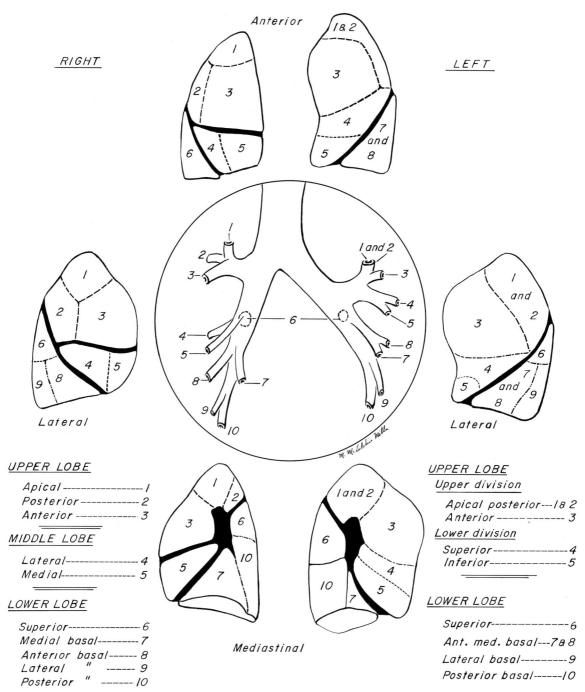

Fig. 47–4.—Pulmonary segmental anatomy. (After Jackson and Huber.[31])

IMMUNE DEFICIENCY.—We have seen agammaglobulinemia in 5 boys with the congenital form and in 1 girl with an acquired deficiency evident at age 8.[47] All had recurring pneumonia, bronchiectasis, chronic sinusitis and otitis. Two patients underwent pulmonary resection, with a total of five lobes removed; both children are alive at age 17 and 19. The others died. Congenital or surgical absence of the thymic gland, inadequacy of lymphatic tissue throughout the body, congenital neutropenia and immunosuppression are also associated with bronchiectases. We have had 5 such patients.

FOREIGN BODIES.—Opaque foreign bodies are readily recognized, and usually are recovered endoscopically before irreversible lung changes occur. Vegetable foreign bodies are difficult to diagnose. Grasses travel in ratchet fashion to the periphery of the lung. Weeks or months may pass before segmental or lobar suppuration leads to the diagnosis. Bronchial secretions aspirated during diagnostic studies always should be stained and examined for vegetable fibers.

Eight of 32 patients with bronchiectasis due to a foreign body had inhaled timothy grass (*Phleum pratense*); 7 re-

TABLE 47–3.—ETIOLOGY OF BRONCHIECTASIS IN CHILDHOOD: CHILDREN'S HOSPITAL MEDICAL CENTER, BOSTON, 1940–1976

CATEGORY	CASES	%
1. Bronchiectasis secondary to infection	145	47
a) Following pneumonia	71	
b) Associated with nonspecific infection	28	
c) Following pertussis	22	
d) Associated with asthma	16	
e) Complicating tuberculosis	4	
f) Following measles	3	
g) Following scarlet fever	1	
2. Bronchiectasis secondary to cystic fibrosis	85	17
3. Bronchiectasis secondary to hereditary or congenital disorders	42	13
a) Anatomic pulmonary anomalies	15	
b) Kartagener's triad	9	
c) Agammaglobulinemia (congenital)	5	
d) Immune deficiency	5	
e) Cardiovascular anomalies	4	
f) "Congenital" bronchiectasis	3	
g) Pulmonary vascular anomaly	1	
4. Bronchiectasis secondary to aspiration	36	12
a) Foreign body	23	
b) Blood	8	
c) Liquid feeding	5	
TOTAL	308	

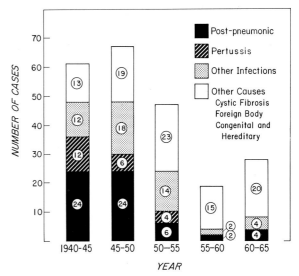

Fig. 47–5.—Changing etiology of bronchiectasis encountered in 224 pulmonary resections at Children's Hospital, Boston, from 1940 to 1965.

quired lobectomy (Fig. 47–6). We have discussed the peculiarities in terms of localization in the right lower lobe and the intensity of the granuloma reaction. Jackson[30] encountered 35 such patients. Since our original report in 1948,[48] 3 of 5 additional patients have required lobectomy. Wooley[52] added 3 cases. Seventeen cases of "empyema necessitatis" have been reported, with extrusion of the foreign body.[30]

KARTAGENER'S SYNDROME.—We have encountered 10 children with Kartagener's triad of situs inversus, sinusitis and bronchiectasis[34] (Fig. 47–7). Five have undergone lobectomy. Holmes *et al.*[29] reported 13 patients, of whom 7 required lobectomy. In 1962, Kartagener and Straki[34] collected 334 cases; they observed that 20% of patients with situs inversus have bronchiectasis Nickamin[37] reported the condition in the newborn. Afzelius and associates[1, 2, 10] and Pedersen[39] have found a genetic axonemal defect involving production, assembly or attachment of the dynein arms to cilia as well as to sperm tails in patients with Kartagener's syndrome. Dynein arms are responsible for the bending movements of cilia and sperm tails. The disorder produces slow to

TABLE 47–4.—ETIOLOGY OF BRONCHIECTASIS IN CHILDHOOD[°]

CAUSE	CASES
Postpneumonic	127
Mucoviscidosis	70
Pulmonary tuberculosis	53
Foreign body aspiration	31
Congenital bronchovascular defect	26
Allergy (sinusitis-asthma)	18
Exanthems	13
Miscellaneous causes (Kartagener's syndrome; agammaglobulinemia)	13
Undetermined	6
TOTAL	357

[°]From the literature.

absent mucociliary transport as measured by tracheobronchial clearance and immotile spermatozoa. Males with the disorder are sterile, females are not; 2 women with the disorder have borne apparently healthy children. Both the bronchiectasis and sinusitis in this syndrome are due to a lack of ciliary movements of the respiratory epithelium. These findings have been confirmed in our institution by Gerald[24] in 6 patients to date; both sexes are affected equally. Brush biopsy of the posterior nasopharynx provides material for electron microscopy. Two patients with situs inversus totalis had normal cilia.

About 12% of children with dextrocardia though not Kartagener's syndrome develop bronchiectasis, but 25% of the siblings of individuals with dextrocardia develop bronchiectasis with the heart in the normal position.[17]

Fonkalsrud *et al.*[21] reviewed the manifestations of situs inversus in 37 children. Half the patients had major cardiac lesions, tetralogy of Fallot being the most common. One patient had Kartagener's triad and required pulmonary resection. Thirteen patients had atelectasis and recurring bronchopneumonia.

WILLIAMS-CAMPBELL SYNDROME.—Bronchiectasis in this condition seems to be due to a genetic defect with cartilage rings of little stability. Williams and Campbell[50] reported universal bronchiectasis associated with cartilage deficiency in 5 children, with 15 additional cases to 1972.[36]

MIDDLE LOBE SYNDROME.—In the middle lobe syndrome,[15, 27] pneumonitis, bronchial obstruction and atelectasis most frequently are due to extrinsic compression from mediastinal nodes (Fig. 47–8). Wilkinson encountered this in primary tuberculosis. In 5 of 20 patients resected, the right middle lobe was involved. The right middle lobe was removed in 5 of 30 recent resections for bronchiectasis. Persistent or recurrent middle lobe collapse requires lobectomy. The right middle lobe syndrome also occurred in 4 children with pectus excavatum (Fig. 47–9).

CYSTIC FIBROSIS.—Cystic fibrosis now is the leading cause of bronchiectasis in children requiring pulmonary resection; 54 resections have been performed to date at our institution, 35 since 1965 (see Surgical Management of the

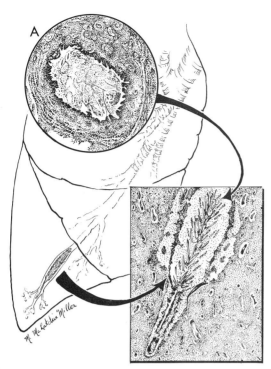
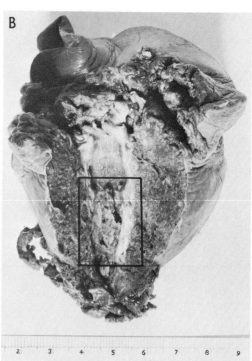

Fig. 47–6.—Bronchiectasis: foreign body (timothy grass head) aspiration. **A,** by ratchet progression, the timothy head advances into the periphery of the right lower lobe. Inset drawings were made from thin section photomicrographs. The grass fibers may at times be seen in stains of material aspirated during bronchoscopy. **B,** resected right lower lobe showing extensive destruction and bronchiectasis. The timothy head is readily seen in the outlined area.

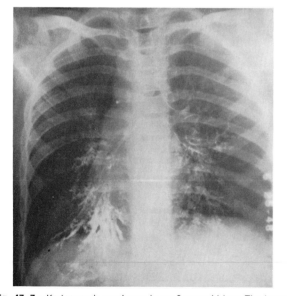

Fig. 47–7.—Kartagener's syndrome in an 8-year-old boy. The bronchogram shows complete situs inversus. The left lung is in the right hemithorax, and the lingular branch of the upper lobe, particularly the lower division, is involved in the bronchiectatic process. The left lower lobe in the right hemithorax shows bronchiectasis in all divisions. Sinus films showed pansinusitis. At operation, the basal portion of the lower lobe in the right chest was firm, purple, mottled, and the lingular segment of the upper lobe atelectatic. Lower lobe and lingula were removed. (Courtesy of Dr. M. M. Ravitch.)

Pulmonary Complications of Cystic Fibrosis later in this chapter).

TUMORS.—In children, endobronchial tumors as a rule are benign adenomas, carcinoids or cylindromas, which ultimately obstruct a major bronchus and destroy the lung distally (see Chap. 48). Wellons *et al.*[49] recently reported 2 cases and found an additional 54 in the literature (Fig. 47–10) (see Chap. 48). As with other cases, diagnosis was delayed due to erroneous interpretation of the secondary manifestations, pneumonitis, fever or wheezing.

DEFORMITIES.—On occasion, extreme forms of scoliosis, pectus excavatum (see Fig. 47–9), pectus carinatum, mixed anterior thoracic deformities and those produced by somite disturbance in the dorsal region are associated with bronchiectasis. This results from displacement of mediastinal structures, compression of main-stem bronchi, an inefficient thoracic cage and inadequate drainage of the lower lobes following infection. Nine such patients in our series have required lobectomy.

Symptoms

The most common complaint in symptomatic bronchiectasis is cough. In "dry" bronchiectasis, paroxysms of coughing occur from irritation of the bronchial passages by temperature change or miscellaneous irritants. In the "wet" variety, cough is associated with production of sputum. Patients with bronchiectasis characteristically have recurring prolonged respiratory infections. Generally, the sputum is thick and tenacious, yellow-green and often copious. Coughing often is induced by changes of position, interrupts children at play and while they sleep. Hemoptysis, usually encountered at some stage of the disease, can vary from streak-

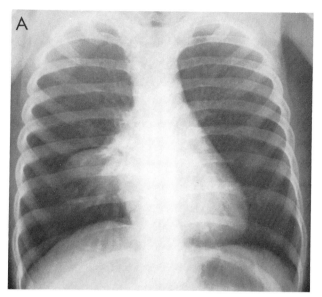

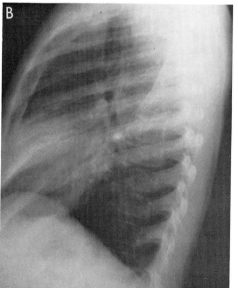

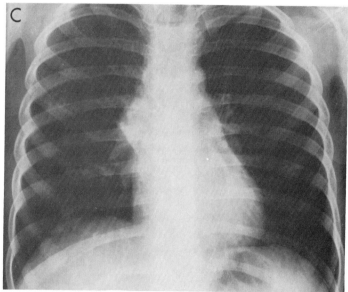

Fig. 47–8.—Right middle lobe syndrome (nontuberculous, postpneumonic). A 6-year-old girl with history of recurring localized pulmonary infection from her first year. **A,** anterior projection, showing typical distribution of the area of absorption atelectasis in middle lobe segments 4 and 5. **B,** lateral view, identifying area of atelectasis. The fissures are now concave, indicating a burned-out process with functional destruction of this lobe. At operation, the middle lobe was shrunken, fibrotic and airless. **C,** roentgenogram 1 month after right middle lobectomy showing residual evidence of hilar dissection. The patient was asthmatic and was substantially improved.

ing of the sputum to exsanguinating or suffocating hemorrhage. Paroxysms of coughing eventually lead to vomiting in younger children. Sometimes out of proportion to the degree of involvement, many patients have dyspnea due to bronchospasm and shunting. We no longer see metastatic brain abscess and amyloidosis. The incidence of pulmonary osteoarthropathy varies. Strang[46] reported 51% in 209 children.

Diagnosis

The diagnosis of bronchiectasis is suggested by a history of pneumonia in early life or by any historical fact or clinical finding pointing to the various causes discussed above.

X-RAY EXAMINATIONS.—As a rule, plain anteroposterior and lateral films of the chest are not diagnostic of bronchiec-

tasis. In most cases, an increase of bronchovascular markings is evident at the hilus. A downward and outward streaking or, at times, frank segmental or lobar atelectasis may be observed. Any x-ray change in the lower lung fields is suggestive. In all suspected cases, early diagnostic bronchoscopy and bronchography are indicated.

BRONCHOSCOPY AND BRONCHOGRAPHY.—In children, general anesthesia is required. Secretions should be aspirated into a standard Lukens collector. A full range of grasping forceps and maneuverable catheters should be available.

All segments of the bronchial tree should be mapped. Direct aspiration of bronchiectatic cavities provides better filling and avoids harmful spill into contralateral bronchi. The ideal bronchogram should resemble a leafless tree. A good deal of distribution is accomplished by the patient's

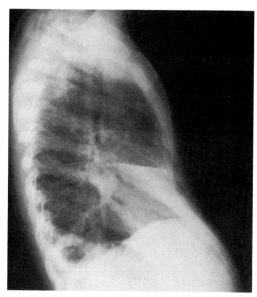

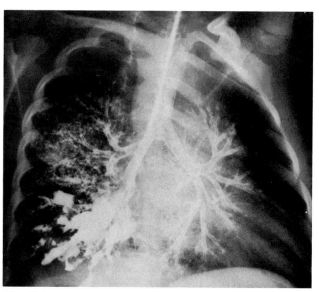

Fig. 47–9.—Right middle lobe syndrome with recurring pneumonia and atelectasis in a 4-year-old boy with pectus excavatum. He had a total of 6 pneumonic episodes always involving the right lung and on 3 occasions with atelectasis of the right middle lobe. The condition is thought to be due to compression of the right middle lobe bronchus by the retrodisplaced sternum and right costal cartilages. There has been no recurrence since operative correction of the pectus excavatum.

Fig. 47–11.—Bronchiectasis. Bronchogram showing saccular and cylindrical bronchiectasis of the right lower lobe due to recurring pneumonia.

own ventilation. The bronchi should not be overfilled to the extent of "putting leaves on the tree." Overfilling of the bronchi, particularly in tiny babies, may lead to anoxia as well as obscure radiographic features. A minimal amount (5–15 ml) of Dionosil is instilled. Spot films capture the bronchographic picture when it is clearest. It usually is possible to obtain satisfactory bronchial details of all five lobes (Fig. 47–11). No operation should be performed prior to complete mapping of all lobes and segments, and probably not for 7–10 days after the study.

PULMONARY FUNCTION STUDIES.—In the case of extensive bilateral disease, when a total of as much as one lung in various segmental combinations must be removed, pulmonary function studies are mandatory. Xenon scans for ventilation and perfusion and pulmonary artery flow patterns and rates using technetium sulfur now permit highly accurate determinations of total and differential pulmonary function in children of any age by noninvasive techniques. Children under age 5 are unable to cooperate to any degree in conventional pulmonary function studies. Older children should be studied by conventional pulmonary function techniques, including the determination of workload with upright exercise.

Bacteriology

The flora in bronchiectasis is diverse and constantly changing. Careful culture technique is important at the time of bronchoscopy in order to gain the most information in this regard. In the gram-positive series, pneumococci, hemolytic streptococci and *Staphylococcus aureus* are found in that order. Fortunately, most respond to presently available antibiotics. In patients who have had prolonged and complex antibiotic therapy, gram-negative organisms appear, including *Escherichia coli, Aerobacter aerogenes, Hemophilus influenzae,* pseudomonas, *Proteus vulgaris* and, on occasion, *Klebsiella.* If the process has reached the putrid stage, fusospirochetal organisms are added. If broad-spectrum antibiotics have been used over a long period, as in patients with cystic fibrosis, there is overgrowth of *Candida albicans* and *Aspergillus.*

Treatment

MEDICAL MANAGEMENT.—Nonoperative management has greatly altered the prognosis in patients with extensive bilateral disease,[19, 20] but its long-term value is limited by the development of antibiotic allergy in a certain percentage of patients and by the eventual emergence of resistant organisms. In patients with established bronchiectasis of known anatomic distribution, it can at best be considered a palliative form of therapy. The young patient with gross anatomic disease, adequate pulmonary reserve and without major associated disease should have the advantage of a definitive

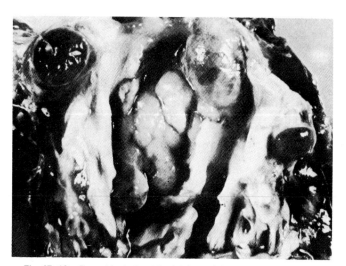

Fig. 47–10.—Bronchiectasis of the left lower lobe produced by endobronchial obstruction, in this instance by a bronchial adenoma. Such lesions are often located in the lower reaches of main-stem bronchi. Because of the rarity of primary pulmonary neoplasms in children, they are seldom identified until the lobe has been totally destroyed.

resection. The choice of antibiotics in preoperative preparation is based on culture and sensitivities. Long-term treatment usually produces resistant strains and more dangerous organisms.

Ampicillin 50 mg/kg/24 hr may be given preoperatively and throughout the postoperative course. If gram-negative organisms are present, amoxicillin 25 mg/kg/24 hr should be substituted. For *Klebsiella*, cefazolin (Amcef-Kefzol) 50 mg/kg/24 hr IV is used. Tetracycline is of particular value in cystic fibrosis and may be given in amounts up to 50 mg/kg/24 hr for long periods.

SURGICAL TREATMENT. — In addition to general supportive care aimed at putting the patient in the best possible condition prior to resection, certain specific steps should be undertaken. All patients will benefit to some degree from postural drainage for 15 minutes 3 times daily before each meal.

Additional aids in preoperative preparation include the use of Mucomist (acetylcysteine, 1–4 ml of a 10% solution q.i.d. as aerosol). For an expectorant, we prefer glyceryl-guaiacolate. Preoperative instruction in breathing exercises using all of the muscles of respiration is of great value in children old enough to understand and cooperate.

INDICATIONS FOR RESECTION. — Indications for resection include harassing cough, productive sputum, hemoptysis, toxicity, fever, weight loss and bronchographic evidence of localized irreversible lung destruction. These children usually are presented for resection between ages 5 and 15.

AREAS FOR RESECTION. — There obviously is a limit to the amount of pulmonary tissue that can safely be resected. Of considerable importance is the work of Bremer,[9] subsequently supported by Reed,[41] which showed that young children are capable of pulmonary new growth. This coincides with the universal experience that infants and children can stand extensive pulmonary resection, including pneumonectomy, exceptionally well[40] (see p. 540).

Pulmonary resection in infants and young children is compensated for by multiplying and remodeling to fill the space available as a result of the resection. Clinically, this is apparent to age 4. There is relative increase in the size of the primary and secondary bronchi. Following resection there is an increase in the number of alveoli in remaining ipsilateral units to age 8. Animal studies following segmental and lobar excisions of the lung fail to demonstrate increase of lung volume by the manufacture of complete new units.[41] Bilateral procedures for bronchiectasis were done infrequently at Boston Children's Hospital and the Mayo Clin-

ic.[13, 26] In our recent experience, only 1 of 37 patients required bilateral resection (Table 47–5). Reports from Europe still indicate greater vulnerability to chronic respiratory infection, and bilateral procedures are performed 14 times more often than in the United States.[19, 22] Strang[46] found bilateral disease in 28% of 290 patients.

The basal segments of the lower lobes are involved most frequently; the superior segments of the lower lobes usually are free from disease except with cystic fibrosis and tuberculosis. With disease of the left basal segments, the lingula is involved in 80% of cases. With diseased basal segments on the right, the right middle lobe is involved in 60%.

The right middle lobe has been called the homologue of the lingular division of the left upper lobe and often is involved and resected with the right lower lobe. An example of postpneumonic bronchiectasis involving the left lower lobe and lingula is shown in Figure 47–12.

The anatomic distribution of lung segments resected for bronchiectasis in children is shown in Table 47–6.[4, 16, 22, 26, 51]

Decision as to the extent of resection generally is made before operation and should be based on bronchographic evidence. Frankly consolidated carneous-appearing pulmonary tissue can be recognized and obviously must be resected, but segments that show gross saccular bronchiectasis radiographically may appear surprisingly normal on inspection and palpation at the time of operation.

Technique of Pulmonary Resection

LEFT LOWER LOBECTOMY AND LINGULECTOMY. — With the patient in the lateral position, an incision is made the entire length of the seventh interspace (Fig. 47–13, A). The schematic drawing (B) indicates the segmental distribution of the diseased area as seen in the lateral projection. C shows the arrangement, at each pulmonary hilus, of branches of the pulmonary artery, pulmonary vein and segmental bronchi, which customarily are divided in that order. The line of demarcation between the overinflated dorsal segments of the left upper lobe and the collapsed fibrotic lingula are illustrated in D. It usually is more convenient to remove the left lower lobe before lingulectomy (E). The lower lobe is freed by division of the pulmonary ligament and is drawn superiorly and medially to permit isolation and division of its bronchovascular supply. F, following removal of the left lower lobe, segmental resection of upper lobe segments 4 and 5 is completed, with preservation of the interlobar vein. This serves as an anatomic guide to complete removal of the lingula. G, the bronchial stumps are closed with simple end-on 4-0 Proline sutures for the lingula and end-on sutures backed up with several horizontal mattress sutures for the left lower lobe. These closures should be made flush with the walls of the parent bronchi. Anatomic variations in the removal of other lobes and segments is beyond the scope of this section.

Postoperative Management

Freedom from complications after pulmonary resection in children depends on careful attention to the maintenance of full expansion of the remaining lobe or segments. This is achieved by constant suction through intercostal catheters with 20–40 cm of water negative pressure and replacement of these catheters as indicated by accumulations of fluid and air in the postoperative roentgenograms. We maintain a moist atmosphere with a vaporizing device. Children must be strongly encouraged to cough. Intratracheal aspiration

TABLE 47–5. — LOBECTOMY AND/OR SEGMENTAL RESECTION FOR BRONCHIECTASIS, CHILDREN'S HOSPITAL MEDICAL CENTER, BOSTON, 1945–1977 (278 RESECTIONS, 226 PATIENTS)

Postpneumonic	96
Cystic fibrosis°	54
Foreign body	34
Mixed infections or mycotic	29
Pertussis	22
Hereditary-congenital	19
Thoracic deformity	9
Immune deficiency	7
Tumor	4
Allergy	4
TOTAL	278

°No deaths following partial pulmonary resection for bronchiectasis due to causes other than cystic fibrosis. Seven deaths in 54 resections for cystic fibrosis, none since 1970.

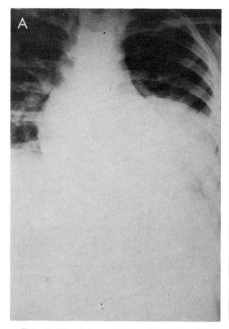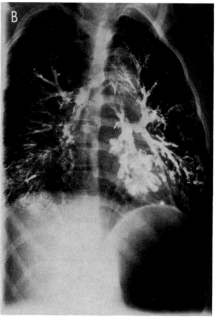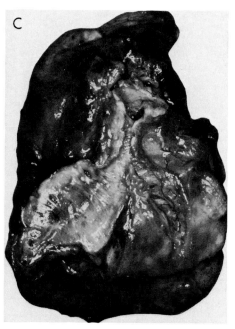

Fig. 47–12.—Advanced bronchiectasis—irreversible changes in the left lower lobe and lingular segment of the left upper lobe following bacterial infection. **A,** roentgenogram showing complete opacification of left lower lung field. **B,** bronchogram showing extensive saccular bronchiectasis of left lower lobe with involvement of lingular division of the left upper lobe. Postpneumonic bronchiectasis occurs most frequently in these areas. **C,** hemisected specimen of resected left lower lobe showing a huge bronchiectatic cavity and parenchymal destruction.

should be used as vigorously as in adults, using fresh sterile catheters for each aspiration. Breathing exercises are resumed as soon after operation as possible. Tracheostomy, rarely required except in cystic fibrosis patients, is in them performed electively 5 days before pulmonary resection. Antibiotics are given for 1 week following operation.

Results of Surgical Treatment

Cooley *et al.*[13] pointed out that pulmonary resection for bronchiectasis can be accomplished in children with 1% mortality but stated that long-term results were disappointing and the complication rate high. Such an adverse experience is not widely agreed on, and it is generally believed that operation should be done at any age when there is irreversible bronchial destruction and symptomatic difficulties are of sufficient degree.[19, 51] Lobectomy can be performed in patients under 1 year with a satisfactory low mortality.[14, 35]

Segmental resection has found its place in the operative treatment of young adults with bilateral disease and is used with increasing frequency in this age group because removal of pulmonary tissue can be compensated for only by overdistention. In the younger child, it has its most frequent application in lingulectomy. Overholt and Langer[38] reported

TABLE 47–6.—PULMONARY RESECTION FOR BRONCHIECTASIS, CHILDREN'S HOSPITAL MEDICAL CENTER, BOSTON, 1966–1977*

LLL	12	Cystic fibrosis	27
RLL	12	Immune deficiency	7
RUL	9	Foreign body	6
RML	7	Mixed infections	5
Lingula	5	Genetic (Kartagener)	2
Segmental	4	Bronchial anomaly	2
LUL	4		
TOTALS	53		49

*Bilateral resection 4 patients.

100 segmental resections for bronchiectasis. Among them were 85% with multiple segments, 60% had lingular involvement and 45% right middle lobe involvement.

Surgical treatment of bronchiectasis at Children's Hospital Medical Center, Boston, during the period 1945–1977 is summarized in Table 47–5 and from 1966 to 1977 in Table 47–6. Much earlier, extending back to 1934, pneumonectomy was performed in 10 children, with a mortality of 40%. This reflects the far-advanced bilateral disease encountered in that period. Surgical resection was an act of desperation. A pneumonectomy in a child with contralateral disease as well is not performed today. Three deaths followed lobectomy in children with cystic fibrosis and end-stage disease with pulmonary insufficiency.[43] We have had no deaths following partial resections for bronchiectasis due to causes other than cystic fibrosis from 1940 to 1978.

Jaubout *et al.*[32] reported 97 pulmonary resections in children for bronchiectasis, with no deaths. Foster *et al.*[23] reported pulmonary resection in 55 children, with 1 death. This group included 11 patients with tuberculosis, in contrast to the 4 in our series. Sealy *et al.*[44] reported 140 resections during the period 1954–1964, with 1 death. Seventy patients with localized disease were completely relieved from respiratory symptoms. An equal number of patients had multisegmental disease and 80% were greatly improved after resection. Bourie and Lichter,[8] in a 10-year survey of bronchiectasis in New Zealand (1952–1962), operated on 125 patients; 91 had unilateral and 68 had bilateral resections. There was 1 death following 165 resections. Complications occurred in 93 patients; 39 had collapse, 3 pneumothorax, 2 bronchopleural fistula, 6 empyema and 4 serous effusion. Satisfactory results were reported, with 55% classified as excellent and 42% as good. Clark[12] surveyed bronchiectasis in 116 Scottish children, with 2 deaths. No complications were encountered in 89 children. Pneumothorax occurred in 4, sterile effusion in 5, empyema in 1 and bronchopleural

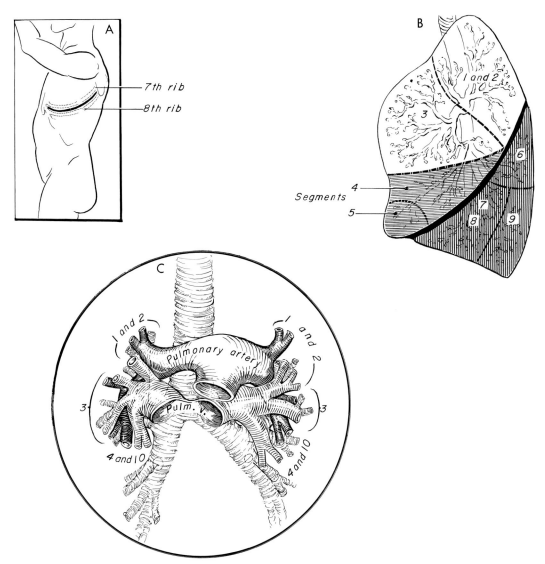

Fig. 47–13.—Technique of left lower lobectomy and lingulectomy, the most common resection for bronchiectasis (in 85% of cases of left lower lobe bronchiectasis, the lingula is involved). **A,** full posterolateral thoracotomy resection is rarely necessary in children. **B,** segments to be resected in children with unilateral disease. Segmental resection is infrequent, although the superior segment of the lower lobe (6) is often uninvolved. **C,** relation of hilar structures. The lingular bronchus arises as the lowest upper lobe bronchus or directly from the main bronchus opposite the bronchus of the superior segment of the lower lobe, as the lingular artery is opposite the artery of the superior segment. *(Continued.)*

fistula in 1. Repeated bronchograms were made to learn whether bronchiectasis is a progressive disease. In 46 children there was no change. In 27, the disease worsened in unresected areas. In 6 patients, new bronchiectatic areas developed. This study contradicts the statement of Churchill and Belsey[11] that the full extent of the disease is seen at the time of first bronchoscopy.

Conclusion

Adequate medical treatment of pneumonic infection prevents the development of bronchiectasis in most cases. The milder grades that do develop often are reversible. Although more severe cases can be kept under medical control for a number of years and may even improve at puberty, medical control thereafter is difficult to sustain as the patient is ravaged by recurring pulmonary infection, with gradual loss of pulmonary reserve and compliance. The full symptom complex often reappears in the second and third decades, with worsening bronchographic picture and chronic toxicity. While the decreasing incidence of bronchiectasis from most causes has made lung resection less common than formerly, the operative risk has been lowered significantly.

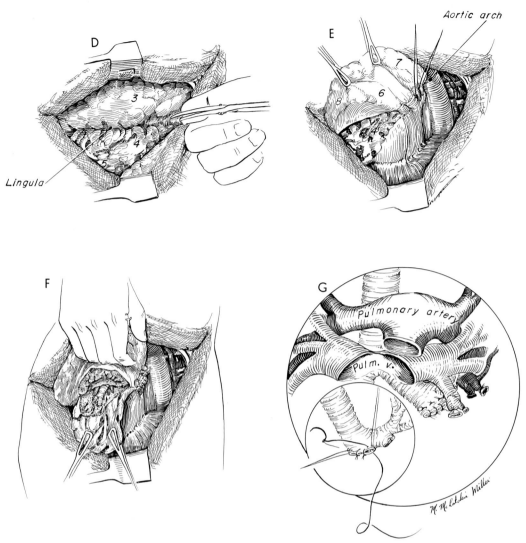

Fig. 47–13 *(cont.).* – **D,** the collapsed lingula *(4)* is readily distinguished from the anterior segment *(3).* **E, F** and **G,** the pulmonary ligament is divided, as succulent nodes are dissected away, the inferior pulmonary vein secured and the lower lobe bronchus divided serially as the periphery is clamped and the central cut end sutured as it is cut. Inflation of the upper lobe permits separation of the attachment to the lower lobe by sharp or blunt dissection.

The lingular artery is secured, the lingular bronchus occluded with a vascular clamp and the lung inflated to identify the bronchus beyond question. The bronchus is divided and the lingula stripped from the remainder of the upper lobe on the intersegmental plane, bleeders and air leaks being carefully sutured.

REFERENCES

1. Afzelius, B. A., *et al.:* Lack of dynein arms in immotile human spermatozoa, J. Cell Biol. 66:225, 1975.
2. Afzelius, B. A.: A human syndrome caused by immotile cilia, Science 193:317, 1976.
3. Anderson, H. A., and Moersch, H. J.: *Diseases of the Chest* (Springfield, Ill.: Charles C Thomas, Publisher, 1959).
4. Baffes, T. C., and Potts, W. J.: Pulmonary resection in infants and children, Pediatr. Clin. North Am. 1:709, 1954.
5. Blades, B., and Dugan, D. J.: Pseudo-bronchiectasis, J. Thorac. Surg. 13:40, 1944.
6. Blades, B., and Kent, E. M.: Individual isolation and ligation in pulmonary resection, J. Thorac. Surg. 10:84, 1940.
7. Bloomer, W. E., Liebow, A. A., and Hales, M. R.: *Surgical Anatomy of the Bronchovascular Segments* (Springfield, Ill.: Charles C Thomas, Publisher, 1960).
8. Bourie, J., and Lichter, I.: Surgical treatment of bronchiectasis: Ten-year survey, Brit. M. J. 2:908, 1965.
9. Bremer, J. L.: The fate of remaining lung tissue after pneumonectomy or lobectomy, J. Thorac. Surg. 6:336, 1937.
10. Camner, O., Mossberg, B., and Afzelius, B.: Evidence for congenitally nonfunctioning cilia in the tracheobronchial tract in two subjects, Am. Rev. Respir. Dis. 112:802, 1975.
11. Churchill, E. D., and Belsey, R.: Segmental pneumonectomy in bronchiectasis: The lingular segment of the left upper lobe, Ann. Surg. 109:481, 1939.
12. Clark, N. S.: Bronchiectasis in childhood, Br. Med. J. 1:80, 1963.
13. Cooley, J. C., *et al.:* Surgical treatment of bronchiectasis in children, JAMA 158:1007, 1955.
14. Crossett, E. S., and Shaw, R. R.: Pulmonary resection in the first year of life, Surg. Gynecol. Obstet. 97:417, 1953.
15. Dees, S. C., and Spock, A.: Right middle lobe syndrome in children, JAMA 197:8, 1966.
16. Diamond, S., and Van Loon, E. L.: Bronchiectasis in childhood, JAMA 118:771, 1942.
17. Dickey, L. B.: Kartagener's syndrome in children, Dis. Chest 23:657, 1953.
18. Fawcitt, J., and Parry, H. E.: Lung changes in pertussis and measles in childhood, Br. J. Radiol. 30:76, 1957.
19. Field, C. E.: Prognosis of bronchiectasis in childhood, Arch. Dis. Child. 36:587, 1961.
20. Field, C. E.: Bronchiectasis in childhood. Prophylaxis, treatment and progress, Pediatrics 4:239, 1949.

21. Fonkalsrud, E. W., Tompkin, R., and Clatworthy, H. W.: Manifestations of situs inversus in infants and children, Arch. Surg. 92:791, 1966.
22. Ford, F. J.: The course of bronchiectasis in childhood, Glasgow Med. J. 291:19, 1948.
23. Foster, J. H., Jacobs, J. K., and Daniel, R. A.: Pulmonary resection in infancy and childhood, Ann. Surg. 153:658, 1961.
24. Gerald, P.: Personal communication.
25. Glausser, E. M., Cook, C. D., and Harris, G. B. C.: Bronchiectasis: A review of 187 cases in children, with follow-up pulmonary function studies in 58, Acta Paediatr., Supp. 165, 1966.
26. Gross, R. E.: *The Surgery of Infancy and Childhood* (Philadelphia: W. B. Saunders Company, 1951), p. 785.
27. Hatch, H. B., and Buchell, B. C.: Middle lobe syndrome in children, Am. Rev. Tuberc. 76:291, 1957.
28. Hinson, K., Moon, A. J., and Plummer, N. S.: Bronchopulmonary aspergillosis. Review and report of 8 cases, Thorax 7:317, 1952.
29. Holmes, L. B., Blennerhassett, J. B., and Austen, K. F.: A reappraisal of Kartagener's syndrome, Am. J. Med. Sci. 255:13, 1968.
30. Jackson, C.: Grasses as foreign bodies in the bronchus, Laryngoscope 62:897, 1952.
31. Jackson, C. L., and Huber, J. F.: Correlated applied anatomy of the bronchial tree and lungs with a system of nomenclature, Dis. Chest 9:319, 1943.
32. Jaubout, M. deB., Mollard, P., and Garbit, J. L.: Traitement chirurgical des dilatations des bronches chez l'enfant, Ann. Pediatr. 41:758, 1965.
33. Kartagener, M.: Zur Pathogenese der Bronchiectasien: Bronchiectasen bei Situs viscerum inversus, Beitr. Klin. Tuberk. 83:489, 1933.
34. Kartagener, M., and Straki, P.: Bronchiectasis with situs inversus, Arch. Pediatr. 79:163, 1962.
35. Mendez, F. L., Jr., Leahy, L. C., and Butsch, W. L.: Some aspects of bronchiectasis in infants, J. Thorac. Surg. 24:50, 1952.
36. Mitchell, R. E.: Congenital bronchiectasis due to deficiency of bronchial cartilage (Williams-Campbell syndrome). A case report, J. Pediatr. 87:230, 1975.
37. Nickamin, S. J.: Kartagener's syndrome in the newborn, JAMA 161:966, 1956.
38. Overholt, R. H., and Langer, L.: A new technique for pulmonary segmental resection, Surg. Gynecol. Obstet. 84:257, 1947.
39. Pedersen, H.: Absence of Axonemal Arms of Immobile Human Spermatozoa, in Coutino, E. M., and Fuchs, F. (eds.), *The Physiology and Genetics of Reproduction* (New York: Plenum Publishing Corporation, 1974).
40. Pierce, W. S.: Pulmonary resection in infants younger than one year of age, J. Thorac. Cardiovasc. Surg. 61:875, 1971.
41. Reed, L.: Personal communication.
42. Safirstein, B. H.: Aspergilloma consequent to allergic bronchopulmonary aspergillosis, Am. Rev. Respir. Dis. 108:940, 1973.
43. Schuster, S. R., et al.: Pulmonary surgery for cystic fibrosis, J. Thorac. Cardiovasc. Surg. 48:765, 1964.
44. Sealy, W. C., et al.: The surgical treatment of multisegmental and localized bronchiectasis, Surg. Gynecol. Obstet. 123:80, 1966.
45. Slavin, R. G.: Immunologically mediated lung diseases—"extrinsic allergic alveolitis" and allergic bronchopulmonary aspergillosis, Postgrad. Med. 59:137, 1976.
46. Strang, C.: The fate of children with bronchiectasis, Ann. Intern. Med. 44:630, 1956.
47. Suhs, R., et al.: Hypogammaglobulinemia with chronic bronchitis or bronchiectasis: Treatment of 5 patients with long term antibiotics, Arch. Intern. Med. 116:29, 1965.
48. Welch, K. J., and Carter, M. D.: Bronchiectasis following aspiration of timothy grass: Report of 8 cases, N. Engl. J. Med. 238:832, 1948.
49. Wellons, H. A., et al.: Bronchial adenoma in childhood, Am. J. Dis. Child. 130:301, 1976.
50. Williams, H., and Campbell, P.: Generalized bronchiectasis associated with deficiency of cartilage in the bronchial wall, Arch. Dis. Child. 35:182, 1960.
51. Wissler, H., and Hatz, M. L.: Prognosis of bronchiectasis in childhood, Helv. Paediatr. Acta 12:475, 1958.
52. Wooley, P. V.: Grass "inflorescences" as foreign bodies in the respiratory tract, J. Pediatr. 46:704, 1955.

Lung Abscess

KENNETH J. WELCH

HISTORY.—During the period 1930–1945, 159 patients with lung abscess were seen at Children's Hospital Medical Center, Boston. At that time, the over-all mortality hovered around 40% with combined medical and surgical therapy, usually two-stage drainage. In 1939, Neuhoff and Touroff[21] reported favorable results of an aggressive one-stage surgical attack—rib resection, unroofing of the abscess cavity and packing. Monaldi established the value of intracavitary suction in selected cases. In 1948, Glover and Clagett[12] demonstrated the value of pulmonary resection, reporting a reduction of mortality to the range of 18%. They also pointed out the ravages and complications resulting from failure to intervene at the appropriate time, with loss of valuable adjacent lung parenchyma. In a significant number of patients, brain abscess developed.[33]

Lung abscess is a destructive, suppurative process in one or more lung segments caused by tissue invasion by pyogenic organisms. The infection usually is polymicrobic, frequently anaerobic and in part fusospirochetal.[6]

Much of the recent literature indicates that lung abscess now is a combined medical and surgical disease.[4, 13, 30, 32] Conflicts in estimates of mortality and morbidity are explained by the fact that lung abscess has a different outlook depending on etiology, ranging from excellent when primary and due to aspiration to poor when secondary and pyemic. Most adult surgical series are concerned with lung abscess deriving from aspiration and poor oral hygiene, bronchogenic carcinoma and tuberculosis. Most medical reports deal with acute nonspecific or aspiration lung abscess.[8] There is no recent survey of lung abscess in children. A review of our material reveals that 31 patients were operated on for lung abscess from 1960 to 1977; all survived.

The etiology of lung abscess in children is quite different from that encountered in adults (Table 47–7).

Diagnosis

A history suggesting any of the conditions listed in Table 47–7, followed by an acute illness with cough, production of sputum, chest pain, hemoptysis, fever, leukocytosis, anemia and weight loss suggests lung abscess. The frequency of

TABLE 47–7.—ETIOLOGY AND PATHOGENESIS OF LUNG ABSCESS IN CHILDREN

1. Aspiration abscess
    a) Acute nonspecific
    b) Foreign body
2. Specific pulmonary infections
    a) Staphylococcus
    b) *Klebsiella pneumoniae*
    c) *Mycobacterium tuberculosis*
    d) *Entamoeba histolytica*
    e) Salmonella
    f) Fungi (botryomycosis, aspergillosis, candidiasis, actinomycosis)
    g) Helminthes (echinococcus)
3. Secondary infection of congenital lung cyst or sequestrated lobe
4. Septic infarction
5. Diffuse parenchymatous disease of unknown etiology
    a) Cystic fibrosis
    b) Honeycomb variety of Hamman-Rich syndrome
6. Immune deficiency, congenital neutropenia and immunosuppression
7. Benign pulmonary neoplasm
8. Miscellaneous conditions (hydrocarbon ingestion, infected traumatic lung cysts)

TABLE 47–8.—SYMPTOMS IN 70 PATIENTS
WITH LUNG ABSCESS

SYMPTOMS	NO. OF PATIENTS	%
Cough	61	87
Productive sputum	52	74
Chest pain	36	51
Hemoptysis	36	51
Weight loss	25	36
Fever	25	36
Chills	16	23
Night sweats	11	16

specific complaints is listed in Table 47–8. In the early stage, the condition cannot be distinguished by x-ray from segmental or lobar consolidation from any cause and is essentially a pneumonic process. Ultimately, confluent lobular infarction results in breakdown of lung parenchyma, and at some point there is sudden communication with the parent bronchus, indicated by harassing cough and profuse expectoration. Children under age 5 who swallow the purulent material do not produce sputum. Hemoptysis appears, and coincident with the evacuation of septic material there are rapid defervescence and abatement of toxicity. X-ray study now reveals a thick-rimmed spherical cavity with a smooth outline and air-fluid level. Planigrams are helpful in estimating the location and thickness of the abscess wall and the maturity of the process. Serial x-rays reveal the effectiveness of medical therapy over a period of 6–8 weeks. Bronchoscopic aspiration and culture permits identification of the bacterial offender. Cultures should be planted under aerobic and anaerobic conditions as well as on Sabouraud's medium to identify fungi. The stained sediment may disclose vegetable fibers inhaled as a foreign body. Infection with acid-fast organisms must be excluded. Bronchoscopy is helpful, both for diagnosis and to clear away thick secretions from the parent bronchus.

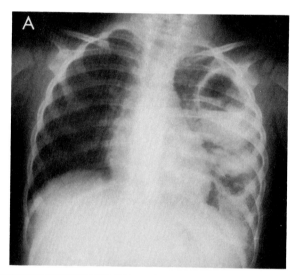

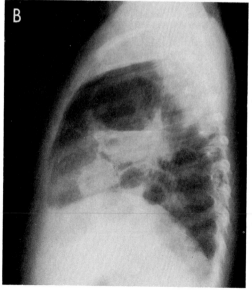

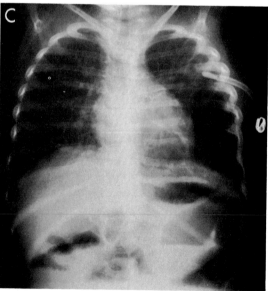

Fig. 47–14.—Lung abscess following staphylococcal pneumonia. **A,** roentgenogram of a 15-month-old girl with an expanding mature abscess of the left upper lobe that did not respond to antibiotic therapy. **B,** lateral view showing air-fluid level and location of the process in the second apical posterior and anterior segments of the upper lobe. The process was controlled by Monaldi intracavitary suction, obviating the need for pulmonary resection. **C,** roentgenogram 1 month later showing obliteration of abscess cavity and a few unresolved cysts in the lower lung field.

Varieties of Lung Abscess

ACUTE NONSPECIFIC ASPIRATION ABSCESS.—The development of aspiration abscess requires one of several conditions: (1) Suppression of the cough reflex that may occur with anesthesia or sedating or narcotizing drugs; a central nervous system lesion such as trauma, neoplasm or epilepsy; or the anoxia associated with semidrowning. (2) Inhalation of septic material, most commonly clotted blood and infected tissue associated with nasopharyngeal operations (tonsillectomy), vomitus, debris from carious teeth or purulent drainage- from chronic sinusitis. (3) Esophageal functional or obstructive disorders with overflow of saliva and ingested food and liquids into the airway.

The site of the aspiration abscess is determined by the position of the child at the moment of inhalation. In a supine patient, the right lung will be involved, the material becoming lodged in the apical segment of the right lower lobe. When the patient is on the right side, the posterior segment of the right upper lobe will be maximally involved. With the patient on the left side, the most commonly involved area is the posterior segment of the left upper lobe. If the child is face down at the time of inhaling the foreign material, as in resuscitation from drowning, the maximally involved areas will be the right middle lobe or the lingula of the left upper lobe—the most anterior. During the period of recovery from anesthesia, the child should be kept on the right side and face down. Heavy sedation is not ordered until the patient has responded sufficiently to understand the spoken voice, and the first word by the recovery room attendant should be "cough."

Organisms recovered from patients with aspiration abscess are nondescript and ordinary residents of the nasopharynx and upper intestinal tract. Most common are Vincent's organisms and spirochetes followed by Bacteroides, *E. coli* and anaerobic streptococcus. These in combination account for the odor and bad taste of sputum in putrid lung abscess.

LUNG ABSCESS DUE TO SPECIFIC PULMONARY INFECTIONS.—*Staphylococcus.*—Lung abscess due to staphylococcus was common in infancy (Fig. 47–14) but is seen today only in debilitated patients.[17]

Klebsiella pneumoniae.—Friedländer's pneumonia is a virulent, often fatal type of pulmonary infection. It usually is seen in the infant who has undergone major surgery and has been "covered" by antibiotics, usually gentamicin and clindamycin. An entire lobe usually is involved with massive slough. The usual end result is lobectomy.

Actinomycosis.—We have had 1 child with lung abscess due to *Actinomyces israelii.* This unusually destructive fungus disregards normal tissue barriers and extends uninterruptedly across lung, pleura and chest wall, forming intercommunicating abscesses and eventual skin sinuses. Pus contains sulfur granules.

Tuberculosis.—One child, age 9, had reinfection type tuberculosis with conversion of the right upper lobe to a honeycomb of abscesses of uniform size (Fig. 47–15).

Entamoeba histolytica.—The diagnosis of amebic abscess of the lung will not be made unless one suspects the true etiology and pursues the diagnosis with warm stage preparations and cultures of excretions from the gastrointestinal tract and secretions from the lung. The pleuropulmonary complications of amebiasis were presented in the classic paper by DeBakey and Ochsner.[10] The sputum characteristically resembles anchovy paste. The infection does not re-

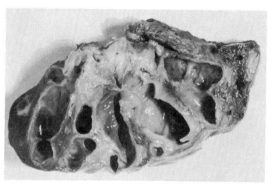

Fig. 47–15.—Lung abscess with reinfection or adult-type pulmonary tuberculosis. Surgical specimen of right upper lobe resected from a 9-year-old boy. Note multiple abscess cavities of uniform size, so-called honeycomb destruction, of the entire lobe.

spond to antimicrobial agents. When the etiology of lung abscess cannot be explained, the patient should be given a trial course of emetine or chloroquine. Two cases of pulmonary amebic abscess without hepatic involvement have been described.[24] Multiple cerebral abscesses complicating pulmonary amebiasis in children have been reported by Hughes[16] and Bachy.[2]

Salmonella.—Lung abscess may occur many weeks after clinical salmonellosis. The gastrointestinal symptoms usually are so violent as to require hospitalization because of acute dehydration, blood loss and toxicity. Following mucosal destruction, the organisms spread to the lungs and other organs in a septicemic phase. Similarly, lung abscess in children due to *Yersinia enterocolitica* has been described by Norris *et al.*[23] and Sebes.[26]

Echinococcus (hydatid cyst).—The disease seldom is seen in the United States, but now must be kept in mind in view of rapid shifts in world populations. It is endemic throughout much of South America. There are curved irregularities within the cavities that can be demonstrated by tomography, and a nearly certain diagnosis usually can be made from x-ray examination, the Casoni skin test and serum flocculation tests. Treatment consists of enucleation or appropriate pulmonary resection. Our 2 cases involved the left upper lobe in 1 and the left lower lobe in 1 (Fig. 47–16). Recent cases of pulmonary hydatid disease in children have been reported by Amir-Jahed.[1]

DIFFUSE PARENCHYMATOUS DISEASE OF UNKNOWN ETIOLOGY.—Cystic fibrosis affects primarily the parenchymatous organs, pancreas, spleen, salivary glands and lung. On occasion, because of impaired drainage and bronchial stenosis, confluent bronchopneumonia will convert to a lung abscess (Fig. 47–17). Two patients required resection for lung abscess. Botryomycosis occurred in each.[18]

A second widespread pulmonary disorder is the honeycomb variety of the Hamman-Rich syndrome. Lung abscess in many lobes results from diffuse interstitial fibrosis. The disease ordinarily is fatal in not more than 6 months. Recently, a group of patients has been encountered who are thought to represent a subtype of the Hamman-Rich syndrome. The disease has a more protracted course, with involvement of all lobes and segments. Resection is contraindicated; diagnosis can be made only by lung biopsy.

MISCELLANEOUS CAUSES.—Immune deficiency caused by thymic absence, agammaglobulinemia, congenital neutropenia or immunosuppression has created a new wave of

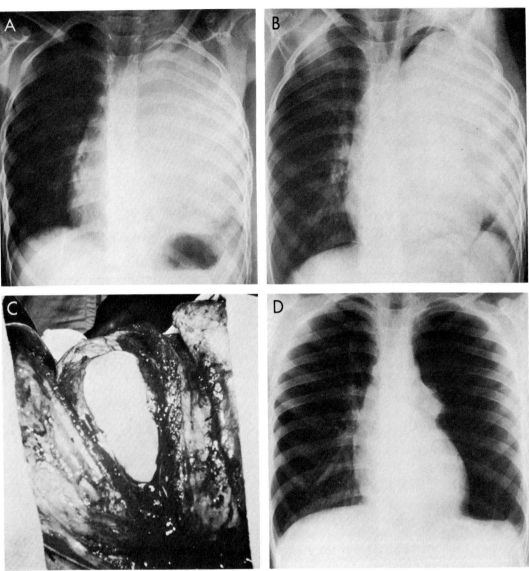

Fig. 47–16.—Hydatid cyst of the lung. Echinococcal disease of the left upper lobe in a 9-year-old Macedonian boy with cough, chest pain, moderate weight loss and low-grade fever. A pleural fluid culture showed no growth. Skin tests for tuberculosis, coccidioidomycosis and histoplasmosis were negative. The Casoni intradermal test was equivocal. Serum hemagglutination and flocculation tests for hydatid disease were negative. Liver scan was normal and scan of the left lung showed low perfusion. **A,** PA roentgenogram showing a white-out of the left hemithorax without displacement of mediasti-

nal structures. **B,** induced pneumothorax clearly defines the intrapulmonary lesion. **C,** the left thoracic cavity has been opened widely. The operative photograph shows the hydatid cyst as a football-sized unilocular process, marble white in color. Without further manipulation, the cyst was allowed to deliver itself by inflation of the left lung. There were no macroscopic daughter cysts. The specimen was found to contain a liter of clear fluid and sandy granules identified as scoleces. Left upper lobectomy was performed. **D,** roentgenogram obtained 6 months after operation.

interest in lung abscess. The usual rules of conservatism and prolonged medical therapy do not apply. Lung abscess in such patients is multifocal, often due to aspergillosis, and is enormously destructive.[11, 29] Our 5 most recent cases requiring surgical intervention fell in this category.

Medical Treatment

The mainstay of medical treatment is the intensive use of appropriate intravenous antibiotics over a period of several weeks. Penicillin has been effective in 95% of patients with acute nonspecific or primary lung abscess. Mitchell[20] recommends 6 million to 12 million units of penicillin G per day IV for 2–4 weeks, later reduced to 4 million units given by mouth for 4–6 weeks. Bartlett has recommended clindamy-

cin rather than penicillin G for aspiration or primary lung abscess; however, 15% of children develop pseudomembranous colitis.[3] For penicillin-sensitive individuals, cefazolin (Amcef-Kefzol) 50 mg/kg/24 hr IV is recommended, later shifting to erythromycin by mouth 30–50 mg/kg/24 hr. For cases due to pure staphylococcus, methicillin (Staphcillin) 100 mg/kg/24 hr is given IV for up to 6 weeks. For lung abscess due to Klebsiella, cefazolin (Amcef-Kefzol) 50 mg/kg/24 hr per day IV combined with kanamycin 15 mg/kg/24 hr is recommended. New strains encountered at our institution are resistant to clindamycin and gentamicin. Flippin cured 21 of 25 patients with primary lung abscess by administering penicillin G on an ambulatory basis 750 mg q.i.d. Most authorities agree that intravenous antibiotics for 2–4 weeks is the preferred method of treatment.[4, 13, 19] In

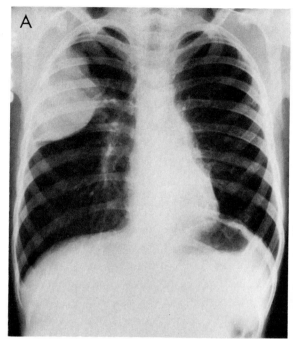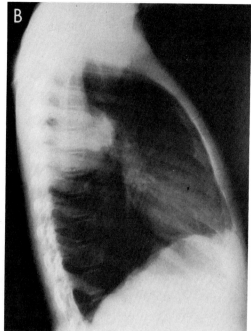

Fig. 47–17. — Lung abscess in a 10-year-old boy with cystic fibrosis. **A,** anteroposterior roentgenogram showing a large area of homogeneous density. The lesion involved the apical and posterior segments of the right upper lobe. There was no communication with the parent bronchi. **B,** lateral roentgenogram showing the further limits of the process. Pleural symphysis permitted external drainage in this child. With bronchoscopy and vigorous medical therapy, most lung abscesses in cystic fibrosis eventually will evacuate their contents into the tracheobronchial tree. Mycetoma involving the midlung can be managed conservatively unless progressive expansion results in atelectasis or air trapping in adjacent lobes or segments.

lung abscess, multiple antibiotics are undesirable because of the rapid emergence of resistant organisms. It has been recommended that once treatment has begun, sputum be discarded rather than change antibiotics based on culture and sensitivities in a polymicrobial situation. Antibiotic treatment should be continued for 1 week beyond x-ray disappearance of the lesion. Most recent reports suggest a diminishing role for surgery in the treatment of lung abscess. Weiss[31] reports 60 patients with 71 cavities. All were followed to disappearance. On medical treatment alone, 13% were healed in 2 weeks, 44% in 4 weeks and 70% at 3 months. Right upper lobe cavities were slower in closing than in other locations. Six of 71 cavities persisted, yet the patients remained asymptomatic, the cavities did not refill and operation was not required. Bartlett and Finegold[4] have stressed the importance of anaerobic pulmonary infections, reporting 70 cases of lung abscess, with a 14% mortality, and 358 additional cases from the literature. Organisms identified were: Bacteroides, Fusobacterium, spirochetes, anaerobic streptococcus, actinomyces and clostridia. Again, the mainstay of treatment was penicillin G in massive doses.

A valuable adjunct to antibiotic therapy is postural drainage to encourage coughing for three 15-minute periods daily. Positioning of the patient depends on the location of the cavity. The patient is taught to sleep in the appropriate position with the foot of the bed on blocks. The respiratory therapist encourages children to cough and applies cupped percussion over the involved lobe or segments several times a day. Bronchoscopy is of special value in children who remain toxic or are too young to understand the importance of and reason for coughing. Expectorants, vapor and mucolytic agents have established value.

Gradually, fever and toxicity diminish. The sputum measured daily becomes reduced in amount and improved in quality. Coincident with this, the size of the abscess cavity diminishes. A time limit must be placed on medical therapy, usually between 2 and 3 months. Later, the process converts to a chronic lung abscess. The cavity becomes larger and the walls remain separated and thickened. Ultimately there is squamous metaplasia with ingrowth of epithelium, making spontaneous closure impossible. Failure to intervene surgically at this point will result inevitably in the late complications of lung abscess (Table 47–9).

Surgical Treatment

There is no question that the vast majority of lung abscesses in otherwise intact children will be cured by intensive appropriate antibiotic therapy. Today there seldom is any indication for open thoracotomy for drainage. Resection is indicated for failure of complete resolution under antibiotic therapy, for unremitting hemoptysis,[27] bronchial stenosis, bronchiectasis distal to the abscess or in other lobes and segments and "recurrence" of the abscess in situ after apparent medical control. Earlier intervention will be required in

TABLE 47–9.—COMPLICATIONS OF CHRONIC
LUNG ABSCESS

GENERAL	PULMONARY
1. Bacterial resistance	1. Empyema
2. Resistant anemia	2. Pneumothorax
3. Septicemia	3. Bronchopleural fistula
4. Mediastinitis	4. Bronchiectasis
5. Brain abscess	5. Recurring in situ abscess
	6. Recurring pneumonia, ipsilateral or contralateral
	7. Pulmonary insufficiency

patients who are immunodefective or immunosuppressed or have important underlying medical conditions that cannot be improved or completely eliminated, such as transplant patients, patients with lymphoma, inflammatory bowel disease, adolescent diabetes, collagen disease and white cell deficiency. Mortality with lung abscess still is close to 20% in this group. When there is pyemic seeding, mortality is doubled. Bronchoscopy is therapeutic as well as diagnostic (Fig. 47–18). All patients with lung abscess should be bronchoscoped. Proximal bacteriology usually is inaccurate and a reliable culture must be obtained from within the abscess cavity or at the lobe orifice. With repeated suctioning, the success of medical therapy with antibiotics can be greatly enhanced and the time shortened. A further role of bronchoscopy has been stressed by Groff *et al.*[15] They reported 5 children with lung abscess treated by transbronchial drainage utilizing the Cordis venous catheter armed with a stylet. This catheter was introduced through the side arm of a Portex endotracheal tube. By changing the position of the patient, any of the lobe orifices can be entered. One patient had abscesses involving the left upper and left lower lobes. Another had a right lower lobe abscess. Both patients were treated satisfactorily with this technique. Three additional patients ultimately required resection for granulomatous

TABLE 47–10.—ETIOLOGY OF SURGICALLY TREATED LUNG ABSCESS, CHILDREN'S HOSPITAL MEDICAL CENTER, BOSTON, 1960–1977

Aspiration abscess		9
Specific infections		13
Fungi	6	
Staphylococcus	2	
Hydatid cyst	2	
E. coli	1	
Klebsiella	1	
Tuberculosis	1	
Immune deficiency		4
Infected lung cyst		2
Cystic fibrosis		2
Benign tumor		1
TOTAL		31

disease, Aspergillus mycetoma and progressive distal bronchiectasis. Tinel supports the transbronchial drainage concept of Groff, reporting 5 children with lung abscess. In his opinion, 3 were incorrectly resected. Two were drained using a flexible bronchoscope and a Selectocath.[28] Further experience has been reported by Connor[9] and in Scandina-

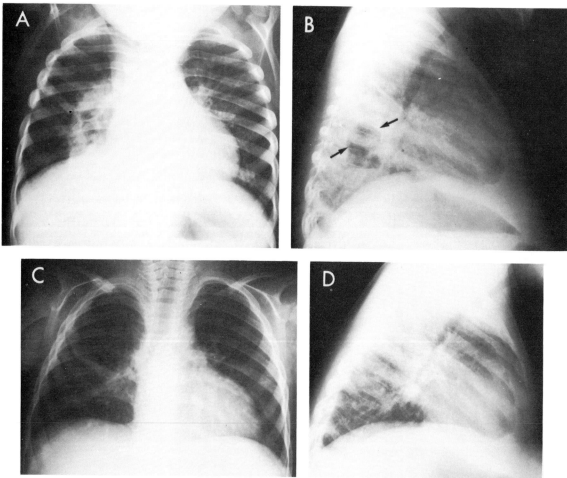

Fig. 47–18.—Lung abscess in a 4-year-old child with congenital neutropenia. **A,** PA roentgenogram showing an abscess involving the right upper lobe. After 2 weeks of antibiotic therapy there was little improvement. **B,** lateral projection showing the air-fluid level of the abscess cavity. The patient was successfully treated by transbronchial drainage, which also provided the specific bacterial diagnosis—*Klebsiella.* **C,** following drainage of the abscess and treatment with gentamicin there is complete disappearance of the abscess, with only mild reactive peribronchitis at the hilus. **D,** lateral projection shows complete clearing of the abscess. Transbronchial drainage is of particular value in children who have inherited immune deficiency or immune suppression.

TABLE 47–11.—SURGICAL TREATMENT OF
LUNG ABSCESS, CHILDREN'S HOSPITAL MEDICAL CENTER,
BOSTON, 1960–1977

Therapeutic bronchoscopy	27
Lobectomy	15
Transbronchial drainage	5
Segmental resection	4
Thoracotomy drainage	3
Monaldi drainage	2
TOTAL	56

via.[11] From this experience, it would seem reasonable to attempt internal drainage prior to resection. However, resection therapy for lung abscess should not be withheld in the patient who has an unresolved and unimproving process after more than 2 months of medical and other adjunctive therapy.

The etiology of the lung abscesses in our patients requiring surgical treatment is indicated in Table 47–10 and the surgical procedures performed are shown in Table 47–11. Our recent experience tends to confirm the observations of Groff that an intermediate role for the surgeon may be in guiding the radiologist in the transbronchial drainage of lung abscess. When medical treatment fails, conservative resection of the lobe or segments involved in the lung abscess must realistically follow. Complications were few and unimportant in our 31 children so treated in the modern era.

REFERENCES

1. Amir-Jahed, A. K.: Clinical echinococcosis, Ann. Surg. 182:541, 1975.
2. Bachy, A.: Lung and cerebral abscesses in amebiasis, J. Pediatr. 88:364, 1976.
3. Bartlett, J. G.: Treatment of aspiration pneumonia and primary lung abscess. Penicillin G. vs. clindamycin, JAMA 234, 935, 1975.
4. Bartlett, J. G., and Finegold, S. M.: Anaerobic pleuropulmonary infections, Medicine 51:413, 1972.
5. Bernhard, W. F., Malcolm, J. A., and Wylie, R. H.: Lung abscess: A study of 148 cases due to aspiration, Dis. Chest 43:620, 1963.
6. Brock, R. C.: *Lung Abscess* (Springfield, Ill.: Charles C Thomas, Publisher, 1952).
7. Bujak, J. S., *et al.:* Nocardiosis in a child with chronic granulomatous disease, J. Pediatr. 83:98, 1973.
8. Collins, H. A., Guest, J. L., and Daniel, R. A.: Primary lung abscess, J. Thorac. Cardiovasc. Surg. 47:383, 1964.
9. Connor, J. P.: Transbronchial catheterization of pulmonary abscesses, Ann. Thorac. Surg. 19:254, 1975.
10. DeBakey, M. E., and Ochsner, A.: Pleuropulmonary complications of amebiasis, J. Thorac. Surg. 5:225, 1936.
11. Editorial: Bilateral pulmonary aspergilloma—intracavitary instillation of antifungal agents, Scand. J. Respir. Dis. 57:163, 1976.
12. Glover, R. P., and Clagett, O. T.: Pulmonary resection for abscess of lung, Surg. Gynecol. Obstet. 86:385, 1948.
13. Gopalakrishna, K. V.: Primary lung abscess: Analysis of 66 cases, Clev. Clin. Q. 42:3, 1975.
14. Groff, D. B., and Marquis, J.: Treatment of lung abscess by transbronchial catheter drainage, Radiology 107:61, 1973.
15. Groff, D. B., *et al.:* Primary lung abscess in childhood, J. Med. Soc. N. J. 71:649, 1974.
16. Hughes, F. B.: Multiple cerebral abscesses complicating hepatopulmonary amebiasis, J. Pediatr. 86:95, 1975.
17. Ieviev, V. S.: Lobectomy in a male infant for staphylococcal destruction of the lung, Vestn. Khir. 115:90, 1975.
18. Katznelson, D., *et al.:* Botryomycosis, a complication of cystic fibrosis, Pediatrics 4:53, 1949.
19. Levine, M. M.: Anaerobic (putrid) lung abscess in adolescence, Am. J. Dis. Child. 130:77, 1976.
20. Mitchell, R. S.: Lung Abscess, in Baum, G. L. (ed.), *Textbook of Pulmonary Disease* (Boston: Little, Brown and Company, 1974).
21. Neuhoff, H., and Touroff, A. S. W.: Acute putrid abscess of the lung, J. Thorac. Surg. 9:439, 1939.
22. Nonoyama, A., *et al.:* Surgical treatment of empyema and pulmonary abscess in young children, J. Jpn. Assoc. Thorac. Surg. 22:954, 1974.
23. Norris, J. F., *et al.:* Enterococcal lung abscess. Medical and surgical treatment, Chest 65:688, 1974.
24. Nunnally, L. C., and Cole, F. H.: Left pulmonary amebic abscess: Two cases, Arch. Surg. 86:621, 1963.
25. Reed, W. P.: Indolent pulmonary abscess associated with Klebsiella and Enterobacter, Am. Rev. Respir. Dis. 107:1055, 1973.
26. Sebes, J. I.: Lung abscess due to *Yersinia enterocolitica*, Chest 69:546, 1976.
27. Thoms, N. W., *et al.:* Life-threatening hemoptysis in primary lung abscess, Ann. Thorac. Surg. 14:347, 1972.
28. Tinel, W. P.: In discussion of Groff, D. B., *et al.*[15]
29. Varkey, B., *et al.:* Pulmonary aspergilloma. A rational approach to treatment, Am. J. Med. 61:626, 1976.
30. Waterman, D. H., Domm, S. E., and Rudgers, W. K.: Lung abscess—a medicosurgical problem, Am. J. Surg. 89:995, 1965.
31. Weiss, W.: Cavity behavior in acute, primary, nonspecific lung abscess, Am. Rev. Respir. Dis. 108:1273, 1973.
32. Weiss, W., and Flippin, H. F.: Treatment of acute nonspecific lung abscess, Arch. Intern. Med. 120:8, 1967.
33. Wolcott, M. W., Coury, O. H., and Baum, G. L.: Changing concepts in the therapy of lung abscess: A twenty-year survey, Dis. Chest 10:1, 1961.

Pulmonary Tuberculosis

KENNETH J. WELCH

PULMONARY TUBERCULOSIS is caused by inhalation of *Mycobacterium tuberculosis*, var. hominis, described by Koch in 1882. The current system of classification includes: 1 Tb exposure tuberculin negative. II Tuberculosis infection, without disease, tuberculin positive. III Tuberculosis infection, with disease. IV Mycobacterial disease (other).[40, 57]

Despite a steady decrease in the total incidence of tuberculosis in the United States, the disease remains prevalent in the lower socioeconomic groups. Three hundred eighty-one cases of primary tuberculosis in children recently were registered in Massachusetts—about 5% of adult cases.[49] Among these, 90% were pulmonary and 10% were extrapulmonary. The percentage of positive tuberculin reactors of high-school age decreased from 90% in 1930 to approximately 20% in 1960 and is unchanged today.[56] At the same time, below the age of 15 years, a gradual reduction in death rate has taken place.[38] Deaths still occur in children under 5 and in adolescent girls when clinical diagnosis is delayed and appropriate antibacterial therapy is not undertaken. The most virulent and destructive form of the disease is seen in nonwhites.

Modern chemotherapy provides the tools to control, sterilize and cure most cases of pulmonary tuberculosis in children and to eliminate all extrapulmonary lesions. The disease remains common as the consequence of large shifts of rural populations into crowded urban areas. Case-finding must be pursued vigorously in all children's hospitals both for the active treatment of the child and for the protection of members of the hospital staff and the community.[51] Pulmonary tuberculosis still ranks high in the list of causes of disability and death in children, on a global basis.[26] An active tuberculosis registry combined with selective BCG immunization and prophylactic combined antituberculous therapy of certain high-risk individuals can break the epidemiologic chain and lead to an over-all decrease in the incidence of this disease. The American Thoracic Society has recommended that certain high-risk groups receive 1 year of isoniazid therapy.[10] These include household contacts of patients with active tuberculosis, skin test reactors with negative sputum and a chest x-ray consistent with tuberculosis who have not previously received adequate chemotherapy, persons whose skin tests have converted within 2 years, skin test reactors receiving prolonged adrenocorticoid or immunosuppressive therapy and those who have leukemia, Hodgkin's disease, diabetes mellitus or silicosis.

DIAGNOSIS.—Symptoms of pulmonary tuberculosis are unreliable. A routine tuberculin test must be performed on all children with a history of exposure and on those over 6 years of age. The intradermal Mantoux test is preferred, using a 5 TU dose of polysorbate 80 stabilized PPD (purified protein derivative). The test must be repeated annually thereafter. The multiprong Tine disk is popular and used for large-scale screening.[26] Tuberculin reactivity is impaired in conditions in which cellular immunity is impaired—lymphoproliferative disorders, sarcoidosis, steroid therapy, miliary tuberculosis, immunosuppression and concomitant measles. Numerous febrile illnesses are capable of diminishing tuberculin sensitivity. For a variety of reasons, approximately 20% of patients may give an inappropriate response to tuberculin testing.[2]

PREVENTION.—Newborn children of tuberculous mothers must be separated from the source of contact for 12 weeks. If the placenta is involved, these infants must have a tuberculin test and chest x-ray. If the reaction to the tuberculin test is positive, they must be given isoniazid (INH) for 1 year. Measles immunization is mandatory during antituberculous chemotherapy.[48] If the tuberculin reaction is negative, primary prophylaxis or secondary prophylaxis with BCG vaccination is advised.[19, 53] Vaccination is most commonly used in population groups with a high incidence of tuberculous infection. Rigid conditions are established for BCG vaccination. They include a negative Mantoux test and a negative chest film within the 2 weeks before vaccination, which is performed by the multiple puncture disk method of Rosenthal.[58] After 12 weeks, both the Mantoux test and the chest x-ray are repeated. The tuberculin reaction now should be positive; if not, the vaccination should be repeated. Major intrathoracic complications may follow revaccination of an infant or child with a positive tuberculin reaction. BCG creates an antigenic explosion in regional and mediastinal lymph nodes, which may perforate into a bronchus with fatal results. The major effort in the United States and Canada has been toward diagnosing, isolating and treating children at high risk, rather than vaccination.[10]

Primary Pulmonary Tuberculosis: Childhood Type

Two to 10 weeks after open tuberculosis contact, the previously tuberculin-negative child becomes tuberculin-positive. At the site of localization, usually in the central or peripheral areas of the lung, exudation occurs, shortly followed by enlargement of the regional bronchial, hilar and mediastinal lymph nodes. This pattern has been called the childhood or primary type of tuberculosis. Pulmonary tuberculosis occurring in older children usually represents reinfection from either endogenous or exogenous organisms and has been called the adult, or chronic, type. It is a different pathologic entity, involves the apical and posterior areas of the upper lobes and requires a different surgical approach.

In the childhood type, the spontaneous course of the disease usually is in the direction of healing of the parenchymal lesion and decrease of the mediastinal and hilar lymphadenopathy. Healing of the primary focus occurs with fibrosis and calcification, producing the x-ray stigma or Ghon complex. Hematogenous dissemination is rare today, occurring either as miliary spread or as meningitis. Dissemination under combined antibacterial therapy is less than 0.5%.

Although the tendency in the primary complex is toward healing, other patterns can develop. There may be progressive parenchymal disease with caseation pneumonia. Enlarged caseous bronchial nodes may produce segmental obstruction and on occasion may rupture into the bronchus, producing obturation obstruction or an endobronchial ulcerative process with mechanical sequelae. Massive perforation into the airway has caused asphyxiation.[17]

In a child below the age of 5, a positive Mantoux reaction indicates primary tuberculosis even in the absence of symptoms. Despite the relatively good prognosis, it is recommended that these children be treated for 1 year with isoniazid (INH). They are not considered infectious and are not restricted. A chest x-ray is obtained at 3 months and at the end of 1 year, with annual chest x-rays from then on. Any child whose tuberculin reaction converts from negative to positive within 1 year should be treated similarly; such conversion is the reason for annual tuberculin testing of all children. This group must be observed closely at puberty, especially girls. The child over 6 with a positive tuberculin reaction and no known contact can be observed without treatment.

PLEURISY WITH EFFUSION.—Lincoln et al.[32] reviewed 202 cases of pleurisy with effusion, all with a positive tuberculin reaction (Fig. 47–19). Pleurisy with effusion is not usually associated with a serious prognosis. Clinical manifestations may be a mild systemic reaction, dyspnea from large effusions or, rarely, high fever. Fibrothorax develops in 4% of untreated patients; 5% later have chronic pulmonary tuberculosis. Of Lincoln's 202 patients, before the availability or utilization of modern antimicrobial therapy, 26 had hematogenous spread.

Pleural effusion requires thoracentesis for diagnosis, and on rare occasions repeated taps may be necessary to relieve compression. The effusion usually is absorbed as progress is made in the control and healing of the underlying parenchymal lesion.

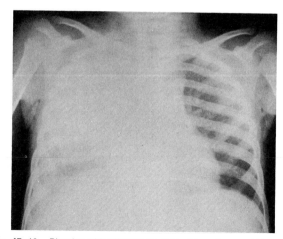

Fig. 47–19.—Pleurisy with effusion developed in a 5-year-old boy within 4 months of onset of primary tuberculosis. Diagnostic thoracentesis or aspiration of massive collections may be required, but less than 4% of such instances require decortication.

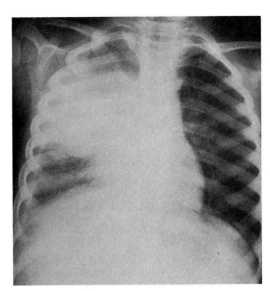

Fig. 47-20.—Mediastinal tuberculosis. Massive hilar and mediastinal lymph node reaction with obstruction of the right upper lobe bronchus. In the presence of stridor or evidence of impending perforation, operation should be considered. Steroids may speed up resolution of the process. In this case, under full chemotherapy these nodes completely disappeared in 4 months.

Tuberculous pleurisy with effusion is actively treated with isoniazid (INH) 15 mg/kg/24 hr and ethambutol 15 mg/kg/24 hr for 2 years. In addition, prednisone, 1 mg/kg/day in 4 doses, is given until the effusion clears.[10]

TUBERCULOUS HILAR LYMPHADENOPATHY.—The node reaction in primary tuberculosis may be massive (Fig. 47-20). The right middle lobe is earliest and most frequently compromised by nodal matting and constriction. The "middle lobe syndrome" was first described by Brock, as reported by Lindskog and Spear.[35] The early lesion is overinflation (obstructive emphysema) followed by resorption

atelectasis. If atelectasis persists for several months, the lobe fails to re-expand. In the same way, basal segments of the lower lobes may be involved. Many young adults with arrested tuberculosis have well-tolerated residual atelectasis at the lung base. Development of symptomatic bronchiectasis requires surgical intervention. Weber reports 25 cases of atelectasis in 235 children with primary tuberculosis. Bronchoscopy relieved the atelectasis in 20 patients; 5 developed bronchiectasis.[6]

Massive nodal enlargement occurs in 11% of children with the primary complex. Chesterman[9] estimated that less than 0.5% require operation. There is little unanimity about surgical intervention to relieve nodal enlargement.[1, 16, 18, 28] Attitudes vary from nonintervention to aggressive and frequent bronchoscopy and attempted evacuation of these nodes endoscopically or by open operation. Instances are recorded of asphyxial deaths associated with node perforation or tracheal compression. Massive collections of nodes high in the chest may cause stridor or superior caval obstruction. Considerable risk attends any extensive mediastinal procedure for the removal or evacuation of large nodal masses, and all that is required is a decompressing procedure.

Like the rapid clearing of effusion and the healing of endobronchial ulcerations, nodal enlargement will subside under treatment with isoniazid (INH) and ethambutol. The use of steroids has been recommended.[39, 47]

Although there are isolated examples in which nodal evacuation is indicated, healing and involution occur so consistently that thoracotomy rarely is required (see p. 493).

ULCERATIVE ENDOBRONCHITIS.—It is not our practice to bronchoscope children solely for a positive sputum culture. Bronchoscopy is indicated if signs of bronchial obstruction develop, when the lesion may be demonstrated directly or by bronchography. The therapy is prednisone 1 mg/kg/day for 6-12 weeks during full INH and ethambutol coverage. The condition is seen as a progression of primary tuberculosis and in the older child with the adult or chronic type of reinfection tuberculosis.

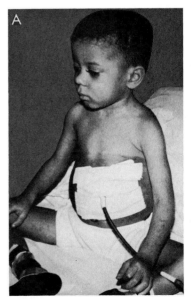
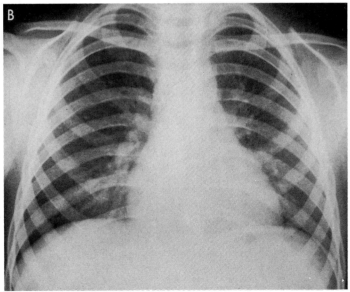

Fig. 47-21.—Mediastinal tuberculous bronchoesophageal fistula. In this 4-year-old child, the spontaneous fistula followed erosion of caseous mediastinal tuberculosis into the right main bronchus and esophagus. Swallowing resulted in flooding of the right lung. **A,** treatment consisted of gastrostomy and antibacterial therapy without thoracotomy. **B,** chest film after 3 months of antibacterial therapy showing the fistula closed and complete clearing of the right lung with disappearance of most of the enlarged nodes.

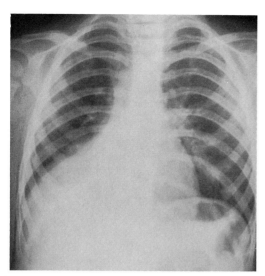

Fig. 47–22. – Mediastinal tuberculosis. Right lower lobe collapse persisting after adequate antibacterial therapy. After 21 months there are no clinical signs or symptoms of secondary bronchiectasis. Conservatism is recommended in treatment of this lesion.

Pulmonary resection should not be attempted in the presence of active ulcerative endobronchitis.[33] Twelve patients observed by Lincoln healed completely and none required resection. Five additional children with perforation into a bronchus healed without resection.[56] No local manipulation other than removal of obstructing granulation tissue appears to be of significant value.[44] Late operations may be required because of segmental complications produced by proximal bronchial strictures. Webb *et al.*[55] pointed out that after several months of therapy, none of 51 patients showed evidence of endobronchial disease.

BRONCHOESOPHAGEAL FISTULA. – The unusual occurrence of bronchoesophageal fistula was commented on by Danino *et al.*,[12] who referred to 670 cases collected by Monserrat, of which 41 were due to tuberculosis. They described a case in a boy of 7 who had a communication between the esophagus and the posterior basal segment of the right lower lobe. He was treated by right lower lobectomy and esophageal suture. We have encountered 3 similar cases, most recently in 1974. All healed with medical treatment without resort to pulmonary resection or closure of the fistula (Fig. 47–21).

ATELECTASIS. – Atelectasis of a lobe or segment can result from extrabronchial compression of large reactive hilar nodes (Fig. 47–22). An initial area of atelectasis can convert to obstructive emphysema. Occasionally, this proceeds to perforation of the caseous node into a bronchus. At this stage, therapeutic bronchoscopy has an important role in clearing away the debris and reopening the involved area.

Medical Treatment

Antibiotics and Chemotherapy

Specific antimicrobial chemotherapeutic agents and antibiotics have radically altered the treatment and prognosis of pulmonary tuberculosis. Irreversible parenchymal disease now can be eradicated surgically with the aid of these drugs. In a field changing rapidly as new drugs, new dosages, new schedules and new combinations are tried, several generalizations apply: (1) Combination drug therapy is preferable to single drug therapy. (2) Prolonged therapy is less likely to produce resistant organisms than is interrupted and resumed therapy. (3) In serious complications, a triple drug regimen is used from the outset. (4) All antituberculous drugs now available are potentially toxic.

ISONIAZID (INH). – Isoniazid is the mainstay of all treatment programs for primary prophylaxis and for patients with active parenchymal disease. It is used in all patients except those few who are hypersensitive to the drug, those whose organisms are resistant to INH and those who develop hepatotoxicity in the form of clinical hepatitis. INH usually is used alone in the treatment of uncomplicated primary tuberculosis. In progressive primary tuberculosis, INH is combined with ethambutol. It is combined with ethambutol and streptomycin as triple therapy in miliary tuberculosis and tuberculous meningitis.

Toxicity. – Isoniazid is neurotoxic in adults and adolescents but rarely so in young children. Adolescents are given pyridoxine one-tenth the amount of INH concurrently. INH is hepatotoxic in some individuals, usually in a subclinical form with elevated SGOT levels. INH is discontinued with levels above 250. It always is discontinued with clinical hepatitis.

Dosage. – Twenty mg/kg/day, maximum of 500 mg by mouth.

STREPTOMYCIN. – Used largely as one component of triple therapy. It must be given by intramuscular injection, usually in patients with poorly controlled disease requiring hospitalization.

Toxicity. – Streptomycin is neurotoxic to the eighth cranial nerve, producing vestibular disturbance or nerve deafness. Patients must be regularly tested for hearing acuity and coordination. Short-term use of the drug is recommended.

Dosage. – Twenty mg/kg/day, maximal dose 1 gm, and given twice a day IM for 1 month only.

ETHAMBUTOL. – This is being used more commonly in children, although it is not officially recommended for use under age 12. It is far better tolerated and is less toxic than PAS, which it has largely supplanted.

Toxicity. – Retrobulbar neuritis with loss of vision has been reported. All patients should have an ophthalmology consultation before starting ethambutol therapy. There should be periodic checks on visual acuity and green color perception.

Dosage. – Fifteen mg/kg/day by mouth.

RIFAMPIN. – Rifampin has been spectacularly successful in the rapid conversion of positive sputum and the rapid control of diffuse spreading parenchymal disease. It should not be used in any routine situation and must be reserved for patients who are not doing well with other combined therapy or for patients who have resistant mycobacteria. Overuse of rifampin undoubtedly will reduce its effectiveness.

Toxicity. – Rifampin is hepatotoxic, as is INH. It is also myelosuppressive, especially involving the white cell series.

Dosage. – Ten to twenty mg/kg/day. Single dose daily, maximum 600 mg by mouth.

PREDNISONE. – Usually given in combination with other drugs. Its greatest effectiveness lies in the rapid lysis of fever and toxicity and the rapid disappearance of pleural effusion, mediastinal node enlargement and ulcerative endobronchitis in primary tuberculosis. It is used for short periods only and usually not long enough to produce adrenal suppression.

Dosage.—One mg/kg/day by mouth for periods of up to 1 month with tapering.

MISCELLANEOUS DRUGS.—Ethionamide, pyrazinamide, viomycin, cycloserine and kanamycin. These constitute second-line drugs and are used for conventional intolerance or organism resistance.[10]

Surgical Treatment

HISTORY.—Doyen performed lobectomies in growing children with pulmonary tuberculosis in 1939. In 1951, Ross[43] reported 7 lobectomies and 6 pneumonectomies. In 1952, Rubin and Mishkin[45] reported 30 resections, with 2 deaths.

Boyd and Wilkinson[3] reported 250 pulmonary resections in children in 1954; 8% were for tuberculosis (20 cases).

Igini *et al.*[22] reported 25 resections for tuberculosis in children in 1960. Leading indications were bronchiectasis (11 patients) and cavitary disease (14 patients). There were 2 deaths.

In 1961, Webb *et al.*[55] performed 51 resections for tuberculosis. Ten were performed for primary tuberculosis and 40 for reactivation

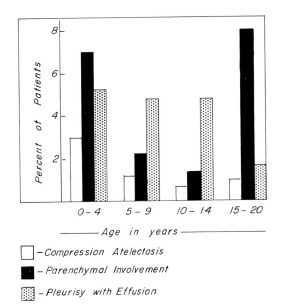

Fig. 47–24.—Pulmonary complications by age groups in 874 untreated patients with pulmonary tuberculosis. (From Lotte *et al.*[36])

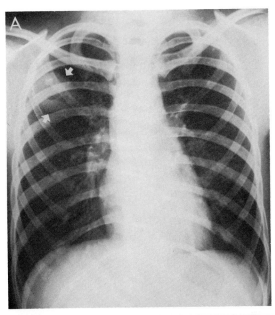

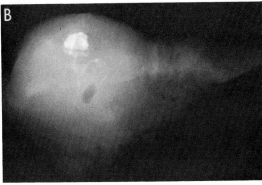

Fig. 47–23.—Tuberculoma of right upper lobe. **A,** a round, circumscribed area of opacity with a focus of calcification and immediately beneath it an irregular small cavity *(arrows).* The rest of the lung field is clear. Acid-fast bacilli were identified in gastric washings. The lesion did not respond to antibacterial therapy. (Courtesy of Dr. R. Overholt.) **B,** x-ray of the resected right upper lobe again shows the tuberculoma-like lesion. It correlates well with the preoperative film **(A).**

tuberculosis. Indications for operation were: in primary tuberculosis, large cavity, 2; persistent tuberculous pneumonia, 4; symptomatic bronchiectasis, 1; and persistent collapse, 3. In reactivation tuberculosis, 18 resections were performed for residual cavities, 11 for fibroid lung and 10 for bronchiectasis. In all, there were 7 pneumonectomies, 28 lobectomies and 16 segmental resections. There were no deaths.

A conservative approach was taken by Cameron *et al.*[8] in 409 patients with primary childhood tuberculosis encountered to 1957. Five ultimately were treated by lobectomy.

In most cases, primary tuberculosis is a self-limited disease. About 2 years must follow the initial primary infection before the adult type of disease can develop. During this period, most patients come under full control. There is no convincing evidence that collapse of basal segments without superimposed mixed-organism bronchiectasis requires resection (Fig. 47–22). Resection is indicated for secondary bronchiectasis, chronic fibrosed lung and tuberculoma illustrated by the following case.

H. C., an 8-year-old girl, was found to have a circular homogeneous density opposite the second rib on the right (Fig. 47–23, *A*). The lesion enlarged, with evidence of central cavitation. Acid-fast bacilli were identified on gastric aspiration studies. The tuberculin reaction was positive. There was no response to medical therapy. The lesion was interpreted as a moderately advanced process resembling a tuberculoma. Right upper lobectomy was performed (Fig. 47–23, *B*). There was moderately active tuberculous endobronchitis of the apical segmental bronchus. There were other caseous nodules in the lower lobe.

The complications of primary pulmonary tuberculosis in various age groups occurring within 2 years of onset in 895 untreated patients observed by Lotte *et al.*[36] are shown in Figure 47–24. Brailey[5] reported a similar experience in untreated patients. This is in sharp contrast to treated patients recently reported by Hsu,[20] who followed 712 children to inactive status. Seven patients required operation.

Reinfection Pulmonary Tuberculosis: Adult Type

From 2 to 20 years following the original infection, patients may develop the adult type of tuberculosis with involvement of the posterior and apical portions of the upper lobes. This occurred in 7% of 622 children with known primary tuberculosis. It differs from the childhood disease, in that there is fibrocaseous pneumonia with central cavitation, the formation of a fibrous shell and eventual healing. For demonstrated fibrocaseous foci, with or without cavitation, after an appropriate period of uninterrupted therapy, resection has much to offer. It has been estimated that 20% of adolescents with reinfection tuberculosis have upper lobe cavitation. Failure to resect the involved segments in apparently quiescent cases leaves viable organisms in caseous foci and makes these children vulnerable to reinfection throughout life.

Except for resection, operative procedures utilized in adults are not satisfactory when applied to young children, and other procedures today find infrequent application even in adults.

With evidence of unilateral residual cavitary disease after 18–24 months of chemotherapy and in the absence of endobronchial ulceration, resection is the procedure of choice, if possible under cover of a previously unused drug. Segmental resection, although theoretically desirable to preserve lung parenchyma, should not be performed in chil-

dren because it opens up planes of infection, inviting spread to remaining lung tissue, and is associated with a high complication rate, notably empyema and bronchopleural fistula.[7] For the same reason, there are few indications for wedge resection, although both now are made safer by the use of stapling procedures.

INDICATIONS FOR PULMONARY RESECTION.[46, 52]—These include: (1) An open cavity with or without positive sputum after 6 months of combined drug therapy. (2) Residual caseous nodules, fibrocaseous disease or caseous nodose disease. Tubercle bacilli must be considered to be resident in such lesions, and the child is exposed to a high risk of relapse. (3) Irreversible destructive lesions such as bronchiectasis and bronchostenosis with hemoptysis, a positive sputum and total disorganization of a lobe or segment demonstrated by bronchography. (4) Recurrent or persistent hemorrhage. (5) An unexpandable lobe with chronic encapsulated empyema. (6) Nodular disease with resistant organisms and intermittent positive sputum.

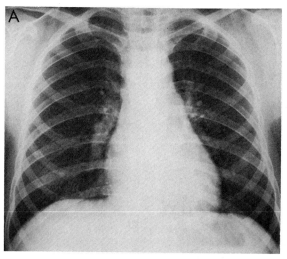

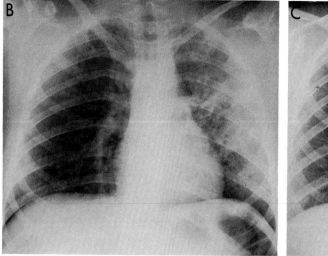

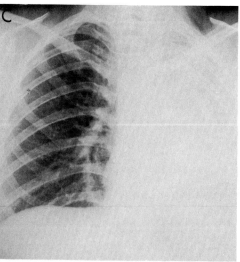

Fig. 47–25.—Tuberculosis of reinfection or adult type, with severe diabetes mellitus. **A,** a small focus of tuberculosis can be identified in the left lung. At this time, the patient was 13 years old and had had diabetes since age 10. **B,** 1 year later, the entire left lung is involved by caseous and nodular tuberculosis. There is no evidence of contralateral spread. **C,** left pneumonectomy was performed, after a short period of drug therapy, because of the poor outlook with medical therapy alone. The mediastinum is maintained in relatively good position by a left oleothorax. (Courtesy of Dr. R. Overholt.)

CONTRAINDICATIONS TO PULMONARY RESECTION.[46, 52] — There are four clear contraindications: (1) Inadequate pulmonary reserve. (2) Extensive bilateral disease. (3) Involvement of an entire lung where active areas will be opened up in a plane of optimal resection. (4) The presence of another fatal disease.

At times, the need for operative intervention may be influenced by the presence of other disease. The outlook is poor in diabetic children with the adult form of pulmonary tuberculosis (Fig. 47–25, A and B).

A distressing but rare complication following resection is reactivation and dissemination of disease, usually to the opposite side. The presence of bilateral disease ordinarily contraindicates pulmonary resection. In late adolescence, a limited tailored thoracoplasty may be necessary on one side with resection on the other. Rivarola *et al.*[42] reported that 10% of their patients required bilateral operation, with a mortality of 15%.

There has been a steady decrease in the number of resections for reinfection tuberculosis. Operative mortality has fallen to 2.1%.[29, 52] About 85% of patients followed for 2–5 years have had no reactivation.[38]

CONCLUSIONS. — Since the advent of modern antibacterial therapy, we have witnessed the disappearance of medical collapse therapy and the virtual disappearance of surgical collapse therapy.[23] Resection still is indicated for the occasional lesions that do not come under medical control. Provided that the surgical procedure is performed under full antibacterial control, with insistence on preoperative sputum conversion, pulmonary resection for tuberculosis can be performed with a mortality and complication rate only slightly in excess of that for other inflammatory lung conditions. It probably always will be required for cavernous, nodular, bronchiectatic and carnified residua. An increasing number of children will be encountered with granulomatous pulmonary lesions due to atypical mycobacteria, no longer considered tuberculosis, which now account for 9% of all admissions for acid-fast pulmonary infections.[11, 25]

REFERENCES

1. Adler, D., and Richards, W. F.: Consolidation in primary pulmonary tuberculosis, Thorax 8:223, 1953.
2. BCG vaccination in Massachusetts, N. Engl. J. Med. 288:521, 1973.
3. Boyd, E. L., and Wilkinson, F. R.: Pulmonary resection in childhood tuberculosis, Dis. Chest 26:442, 1954.
4. Brailey, M. E.: Epidemic Aspects of Harriet Lane Study, in Commonwealth Fund: *Tuberculosis in White and Negro Children* (Cambridge, Mass.: Harvard University Press, 1958), Vol. 2, p. 26.
5. Brailey, M. E.: Prognosis in white and colored tuberculous children, Am. J. Public Health 33:343, 1943.
6. Brashear, R. E.: Atypical mycobacteria: A factor to consider in lung disease, Postgrad. Med. 58:117, 1975.
7. Brewer, L. A.: Tuberculous Empyema and Bronchopleural Fistula in Clinical Tuberculosis, in Pleutae, K. H., and Radner, D. B. (eds.), *Clinical Tuberculosis* (Springfield, Ill.: Charles C Thomas, Publisher, 1966).
8. Cameron, J. K., Hay, J. D., and Temple, L. S.: A critical examination of the role of surgery in the treatment of primary pulmonary tuberculosis in children, Thorax 12:329, 1957.
9. Chesterman, J. T.: The surgery of primary pulmonary tuberculosis in children, Thorax 12:159, 1957.
10. Committee on Therapy, American Thoracic Society, National Tuberculosis and Respiratory Disease Association and Center for Disease Control: Joint Statement on the preventive treatment of tuberculosis, Am. Rev. Respir. Dis. 104:460, 1971.
11. Corpe, R. F., and Liang, J.: Surgical resection in pulmonary tuberculosis due to atypical *Mycobacterium tuberculosis*, J. Thorac. Cardiovasc. Surg. 40:93, 1960.
12. Danino, E. A., Evans, C. J., and Thomas, J. H.: Tuberculous bronchoesophageal fistula in a child, Thorax 10:351, 1955.
13. Delarre, N. C., and Gale, G. L.: Surgical salvage in pulmonary tuberculosis, Ann. Thorac. Surg. 18:38, 1974.
14. East African/British Medical Research Councils: Controlled clinical trial of four short course (6-month) regimens of chemotherapy for treatment of pulmonary tuberculosis. Second report, Lancet 1:1331, 1975.
15. Giraud, P., et al.: Indications and results of excisional surgery in primary tuberculosis in children, Rev. Tuberc. (Paris) 25:1261, 1961.
16. Giraud, P., et al.: Traitement chirurgical de complications graves de la primo-infection, Pediatrie 9:557, 1954.
17. Gorgenyi-Gottche, O. G., and Kassay, D.: Importance of bronchial rupture in tuberculosis of endothoracic lymph nodes, Am. J. Dis. Child. 74:166, 1947.
18. Hardy, J. B., Proctor, D. F., and Turner, J. A.: Bronchial obstruction and bronchiectasis complicating primary tuberculosis infection, J. Pediatr. 41:740, 1952.
19. Heimbeck, J.: Vaccination sous-cutanée et cutanée au BCG 1926–1948, Sem. Hop. Paris 25:771, 1949.
20. Hsu, K. H.: Isoniazid in the prevention and treatment of tuberculosis. A 20-year study of the effectiveness in children, JAMA 229:528, 1974.
21. Huish, D. W.: The surgical treatment of pulmonary tuberculosis in childhood and adolescence, Thorax 11:186, 1956.
22. Igini, J. P., Fox, R. T., and Less, W. M.: Resection for pulmonary tuberculosis in infants and children, Dis. Chest 37:176, 1960.
23. Johnston, R. F., and Wildrick, K. H.: "State of the Art" Review. The impact of chemotherapy on the care of patients with tuberculosis, Am. Rev. Respir. Dis. 109:636, 1974.
24. Jones, E. M., and Howard, W. L.: Treatment of tuberculosis in children, Pediatrics 17:146, 1955.
25. Jones, J. D.: Surgery of Pulmonary Tuberculosis Caused by Unclassified Acid-fast Mycobacteria, in Pleutae, K. H., and Radner, D. B. (eds.), *Clinical Tuberculosis* (Springfield, Ill.: Charles C Thomas, Publisher, 1966).
26. Kendig, E. L.: Tuberculosis, in Gellis, S. S., and Kagan, B. M. (eds.), *Current Pediatric Therapy* (Philadelphia: W. B. Saunders Company, 1974).
27. Kendig, E. L.: Tuberculosis, in Gellis, S. S., and Kagan, B. M. (eds.), *Current Pediatric Therapy* (Philadelphia: W. B. Saunders Company, 1968).
28. Laff, H. I., Hurst, A., and Robinson, A.: Importance of bronchial involvement in primary tuberculosis of childhood, JAMA 146:778, 1951.
29. Langston, H. T., Baker, W. L., and Pyle, M. M.: Surgery in pulmonary tuberculosis, Ann. Surg. 164:573, 1966.
30. Lefrak, S. S., et al.: Chemoprophylaxis of tuberculosis, Arch. Intern. Med. 135:606, 1975.
31. Levitan, M., and Zelman, M.: Excisional therapy of pulmonary tuberculosis in children, Am. J. Dis. Child. 79:30, 1950.
32. Lincoln, E. M., Davies, P. A., and Bovornkitti, S.: Tuberculous pleurisy with effusion in children, Am. Rev. Tuberc. 77:271, 1958.
33. Lincoln, E. M., et al.: Endobronchial tuberculosis in children, Am. Rev. Tuberc. 77:39, 1958.
34. Lincoln, E. M., and Sewall, E. M.: *Tuberculosis in Children* (2d ed.; New York: McGraw-Hill Book Company, Inc., 1963), p. 3.
35. Lindskog, G. E., and Spear, H. C.: Middle lobe syndrome, N. Engl. J. Med. 253:489, 1955.
36. Lotte, A., et al.: The treatment of primary tuberculosis in childhood, Pediatrics 26:641, 1960.
37. McConville, J. H., and Rapoport, M. I.: Tuberculosis management in the mid-1970s, JAMA 235:172, 1976.
38. Myers, J. A.: Prognosis in treatment of tuberculosis among children, Dis. Chest 44:27, 1963.
39. Nemir, R. L., et al.: Prednisone as an adjunct in the chemotherapy of lymph nodes in bronchial tuberculosis in childhood, Am. Rev. Respir. Dis. 95:402, 1967.
40. Oatway, W. H., et al.: Diagnostic Standards and Classification of Tuberculosis (New York: American Thoracic Society, 1975).
41. Rifampicin or ethambutol in the routine treatment of tuberculosis, Br. Med. J. 4:568, 1973.
42. Rivarola, C. H., Norton, L. W., and Levene, N.: Bilateral

resection for cavitary pulmonary tuberculosis, J. Thorac. Cardiovasc. Surg. 50:277, 1965.

43. Ross, C. A.: Pulmonary resection for tuberculosis in children, Thorax 6:375, 1951.
44. Rothman, P. E., Jones, J. C., and Peterson, H. G.: Endoscopic and surgical treatment of pulmonary tuberculosis in children, Am. J. Dis. Child. 99:315, 1960.
45. Rubin, M., and Mishkin, S.: Resection for pulmonary tuberculosis in children and adolescents, Surg. Gynecol. Obstet. 95:751, 1952.
46. Sloan, H., and Milnes, R.: Pulmonary Resection for Tuberculosis, in Steele, J. D. (ed.), *Surgical Management of Pulmonary Tuberculosis* (Springfield, Ill.: Charles C Thomas, Publisher, 1957).
47. Smith, M. H. D.: The role of adrenal steroids in the treatment of tuberculosis, Pediatrics 22:774, 1958.
48. Starr, S., and Berkovitch, S.: Effects of measles gamma globulin and vaccine measles on the tuberculin test, N. Engl. J. Med. 270:386, 1964.
49. Steiner, M., and Cosio, A.: Primary tuberculosis in children, N. Engl. J. Med. 274:755, 1966.
50. Steiner, R., *et al.*: "Primary drug resistance" in children, Am. Rev. Respir. Dis. 110:98, 1974.
51. Stewart, C. J.: Tuberculosis infection in a paediatric department, Br. Med. J. 1:30, 1976.
52. Strieder, J. W., Laforet, E. G., and Lynch, J. P.: Surgery of pulmonary tuberculosis, N. Engl. J. Med. 276:960, 1967.
53. Strom, L.: Vaccination against tuberculosis, Am. Rev. Tuberc. 74:28, 1956.
54. *Symposium on Childhood Tuberculosis*, Brit. J. Dis. Chest (London: Baillière, Tindall & Cox, 1960).
55. Webb, W. R., Wofford, J. L., and Strauss, H. K.: Resectional therapy for pulmonary tuberculosis in children, Surgery 51:270, 1962.
56. Weber, A. L., Bird, K. T., and Janower, M. L.: Primary tuberculosis in childhood, with particular emphasis on changes affecting the tracheobronchial tree, Am. J. Roentgenol. 103:123, 1968.
57. Weg, J. G.: Diagnostic standards of tuberculosis—revised, JAMA 235:1329, 1976.
58. Wilson, J. M., *et al.*: Tuberculosis in Eskimo children. A comparison of disease in children vaccinated with bacillus Calmette-Guérin and nonvaccinated children, Am. Rev. Respir. Dis. 108:559, 1973.

Surgical Management of the Pulmonary Complications of Cystic Fibrosis

SAMUEL R. SCHUSTER/MARSHALL Z. SCHWARTZ

Pulmonary Resection in Cystic Fibrosis

CYSTIC FIBROSIS is an autosomal recessive disease that affects the exocrine glands primarily, the pathologic changes in which result in the production of chemically abnormal secretions by the nonmucus-producing glands, while the mucus-secreting glands produce a highly viscid mucus.[1-4] The abnormally viscid secretions[7] of these glands act to obstruct pulmonary bronchi and bronchioles, producing the severe pulmonary structural changes so characteristic of this disease.[1] These present as areas of atelectasis, or of bronchiectasis with microabscesses, and result in cough, marked sputum production and febrile episodes.[5] In most patients, the pathologic processes described above are generalized and involve most areas of the lung. A few patients, however, present with a localized area of more severe pulmonary involvement. These isolated local areas of more severe disease are likely to result in an acute exacerbation of symptoms and to cause an accelerated progression of the deteriorative changes in the remainder of the lung.

On initial considerations, patients with a progressive pulmonary disease such as cystic fibrosis appear to be unlikely candidates for pulmonary resection. If, however, one accepts the principle of providing palliation and an improved quality of life, even in patients whose primary disease is incurable, there are a few carefully selected patients who can benefit from pulmonary resection.[6, 8, 9] The goal of these surgical efforts is to improve the patient's quality of life by resecting areas of severe localized disease.

Patient Selection

Only those patients should be considered as operative candidates who show roentgenographically a localized area of lung with disease advanced far beyond that in the rest of the lung. The advanced lesion may involve a segment, a lobe or an entire lung. In most instances, the areas in question are atelectatic and almost always bronchiectatic. Histologic examination frequently demonstrates multiple microabscesses.

Once such a patient is identified, studies should be done to make the following determinations:

1. Is the area of increased pathology affecting the patient's state of well-being? Is it likely to hasten the progression of pulmonary involvement through the entire lung?
2. Is this process reversible?
3. Can the patient withstand thoracotomy and pulmonary resection?

Our experience at Children's Hospital Medical Center, Boston, provides the basis for making the above determinations. A total of 51 patients have undergone one or more pulmonary resections for localized parenchymal disease. Two other patients had resections for uncontrollable hemorrhage. In addition, there were 3 patients who had pulmonary resections performed elsewhere but subsequently were followed at CHMC. The average age of the patients was 9.5 years and the interval from recognition of localized changes to resection was 2.5 years. Most patients had received good to excellent home care management and regular clinical and x-ray follow-up. Their home care management included broad-spectrum antibiotics, postural drainage, physiotherapy and expectorants. This group of patients had developed localized areas of severe pulmonary disease that often caused a significant increase in cough and sputum production and resulted in limitation of activity. The over-all effect was to retard growth and weight gain, and resulted in a deterioration in the quality of life. We have the very strong conviction, based on our experience,[6-8] that resection of these areas of severe localized disease has led to a slowing in the over-all progression of the pulmonary involvement.

Pulmonary function tests, including ventilation and perfusion xenon scans, should be done to help determine, by quantitative methods, whether or not these patients are capable of withstanding thoracotomy and resection. In our own series, the usual battery of pulmonary function studies has not, on the whole, been of critical value in providing this information. Since most of these studies require the cooperation of the patient, they cannot be used in the younger patients. Furthermore, one should anticipate considerable variability in the results of pulmonary function tests, depending on the effectiveness of the patient's tracheal toilet measures on any given day. The most helpful quantitative information is obtained from the xenon ventilation and perfusion scans. In virtually all instances, those areas of lung resected made no significant contribution to the patient's over-all ventila-

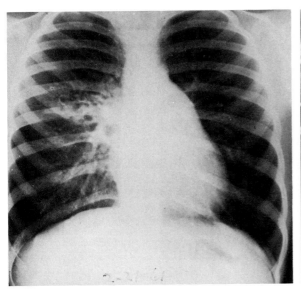

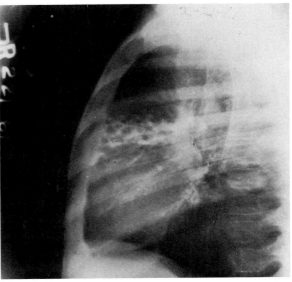

Fig. 47–26.—Cystic fibrosis—segmental disease. A patient with relatively good lung fields except for clearly evident bronchiectatic changes limited to the anterior segment of the right upper lobe. Coincident with the ap-

pearance of these changes, there was a striking increase in the severity of symptoms. This patient survived 13 years following resection of the anterior segment, carrying on with normal activities until shortly prior to death.

tory capacity. In the final analysis, the best criterion for determining the patient's capacity to withstand thoracotomy is a clinical evaluation of the level of activity maintained by the patient on a program of good medical therapy.

Bronchoscopy rarely is helpful preoperatively. Although we have used it in 64% of our patients for both diagnostic and therapeutic purposes, we rarely have been able to reexpand an area of atelectasis in patients with cystic fibrosis.

Bronchography as a preoperative study is also rarely indicated. On infrequent occasions, one may wish to evaluate the lung that is not going to be resected. Bronchography of the severely affected section of lung is unnecessary, since the disease is clearly evident on an ordinary chest roentgenogram. Since the information obtained is frequently of little value, the added morbidity associated with bronchography

in these patients makes the study undesirable as a routine procedure.

Sputum cultures should routinely be obtained preoperatively and commonly are positive for staphylococcus and/or pseudomonas.

Figure 47–26 shows a patient with limited segmental disease who responded well to pulmonary resection.

Figure 47–27 is typical of the majority of patients who have undergone resection. There was a single lobe involved in a severe process of atelectasis and bronchiectasis. The lobe contained multiple microabscesses.

Figure 47–28 shows total destruction of one lung whereas the sparing of the other lung is striking. Six patients with this degree of pulmonary involvement have had pneumonectomy. Such patients often show the most striking improvement following resection.

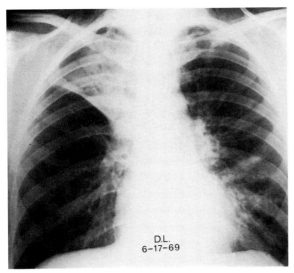

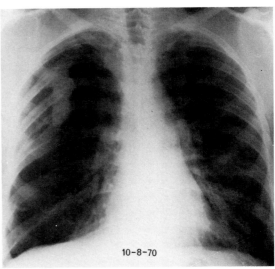

Fig. 47–27.—Cystic fibrosis—lobar disease. Patient typical of most patients in this series with chronic right upper lobe atelectasis and bronchiectasis. The second x-ray shows the relatively normal appearance 16

months following resection of the upper lobe. The patient was carrying on with normal activities.

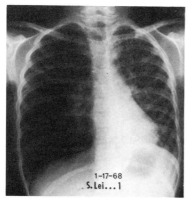 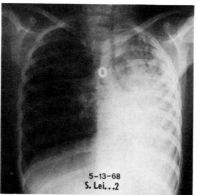 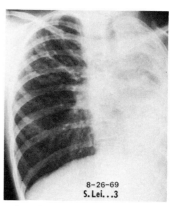

Fig. 47–28. — Cystic fibrosis — involvement of an entire lung. The first x-ray demonstrates beginning significant changes occurring in the left lung, with contraction of the left lung and shift of the mediastinum to the left. The same patient is seen in the second x-ray 4 months later with striking deterioration. There has been total destruction of the left lung. There was no ventilatory contribution by that lung. The third x-ray shows the same patient 1 year after left pneumonectomy. Here, severe chronic cough and production of mucopurulent sputum had been markedly alleviated.

Preoperative Preparation

All patients should be on a vigorous medical program prior to operation. Each patient is admitted 1–2 weeks earlier for a "cleanout." This includes the use of intravenous antibiotics, extensive physiotherapy and the establishment of a tracheostomy 5–7 days prior to thoracotomy. The routine use of this tracheostomy in all cystic fibrosis patients undergoing pulmonary resection has been instrumental in improving their management and decreasing their postoperative morbidity.

Preoperative tracheostomy is recommended for the following reasons:

1. The patient must be given time to adjust both physically and psychologically to the presence of the tracheostomy prior to thoracotomy.

2. These patients very frequently develop subcutaneous emphysema in association with the establishment of a tracheostomy. The interval between tracheostomy and thoracotomy allows time for the subcutaneous emphysema to subside.

3. The patient learns to manage the tracheostomy and to speak with this device in place.

4. The tracheostomy enhances the patient's preoperative preparation by providing ready access for pulmonary suction.

5. Most important, the tracheostomy provides access for postoperative tracheal toilet, which otherwise would be very difficult in the face of the pain associated with thoracotomy and in the presence of highly viscid mucopurulent secretions.

There have been no major untoward problems associated with the tracheostomy.

Operative Considerations

All thoracotomies in patients with cystic fibrosis are done with the patient prone. The chest is entered through a posterior periscapular incision as described by Overholt. This permits all bronchial secretions during operation to drain into the trachea, whence they can be readily suctioned by the anesthesiologist, and avoids spilling large volumes of mucopurulent secretions into the dependent lung during the course of resection.

These patients all have strikingly hyperplastic peribronchial lymph nodes with increased vascularity of all tissues secondary to the many bronchial artery-pulmonary artery anastomoses. There is a foreshortening of the hilar structures and numerous vascular adhesions between the parietal and visceral pleura.

Postoperative Care

Postoperatively, we stress intravenous antibiotics, vigorous pulmonary therapy, careful tracheal toilet via the tracheostomy and early ambulation. The routine use of postoperative intermittent positive-pressure breathing is to be avoided. Assisted respiration should be utilized only when necessary to maintain adequate ventilation and then only for as brief a time as possible. Early in our experience, the use of IPPB resulted in dissemination of pulmonary infiltrates in a patient who was an ideal candidate for operation and had been doing very well up to that point.

Table 47–12 shows the anatomic distribution of resections in our series. Lobectomy is the most common procedure, the right upper lobe being the one most frequently resected. Severe lower lobe involvement in this series

TABLE 47–12.—PULMONARY RESECTIONS

LEFT SIDE		RIGHT SIDE			
Pneumonectomy	3	Pneumonectomy	3	Middle lobe and anterior segment upper lobe	1
Upper lobe	3	Upper lobe	9		
Lower lobe	4	Middle lobe	8	Middle lobe and superior segment lower lobe	1
Lingula	1	Lower lobe	4	Superior segment lower lobe	1
Lower lobe and lingula	3	Upper and middle lobes	4	Anterior segment upper lobe	1
Lingula and superior segment lower lobe	1	Middle and lower lobes	3	Upper lobe and superior segment lower lobe	1
TOTALS	15				36

TABLE 47-13.—RESULTS OF PULMONARY RESECTION
IN CYSTIC FIBROSIS

EXCELLENT	GOOD	FAIR	UNSATISFACTORY	POOR
8 (16%)	23 (45%)	11 (21%)	4 (8%)	5 (10%)

Excellent: Symptom-free and full activity
Good: Definite decrease in symptoms, increased sense of well-being
Fair: Mild decrease in symptoms, increased sense of well-being
Unsatisfactory: Unchanged
Poor: Increase in symptoms or death as a result of operation

Seven deaths occurred within 90 days of pulmonary resection, all before 1970. There have been no deaths since. One death was after pneumonectomy, the others after resection of at least one lobe; none of the 7 patients had a preoperative tracheostomy. Two of these patients (not included in the table) were operated on for severe and unremittent hemoptysis before our program of bronchial artery embolism.

usually was limited to the superior segment of the lower lobe. That segment often has been resected along with the upper lobe. On the left side, involvement of the upper lobe alone is less characteristic. There were 6 pneumonectomies, equally divided between the right and left.

Results

Evaluation of the results of pulmonary resection has been based on the patient's ability to carry on with activity and the evidence of a state of well-being. The results have been categorized as excellent, good, fair, unsatisfactory and poor. An excellent result indicates a patient who is symptom free and can carry on with full activity. A good result indicates a definite decrease in symptoms with an increased sense of well-being. A fair result indicates a mild decrease in symptoms with an increased sense of well-being. Unsatisfactory indicates an unimproved patient. A poor result indicates an increase in symptoms or a patient who died as a result of the operative procedure.

Table 47-13 shows a distribution of results. There were 16% with an excellent result, 45% had a good result, 21% a fair result, 8% an unsatisfactory result and 10% had a poor result. In our judgment, those patients who fall in the excellent, good or fair category had benefited significantly from the operation—83% of the patients. The advantages of improved patient selection and management are far more evident when it is noted that there have been no poor or unsatisfactory results since 1968.

Based on the above findings, we believe that a carefully selected group of patients with cystic fibrosis will benefit from resection of localized areas of severe pulmonary disease if the principles described above are pursued.

REFERENCES

1. di Sant'Agnese, P. A.: Bronchial obstruction with lobar atelectasis and emphysema in cystic fibrosis of pancreas, Pediatrics 12:178, 1953.
2. di Sant'Agnese, P. A., Darling, R. C., Perera, G. A., et al.: Abnormal electrolyte composition of sweat in cystic fibrosis of the pancreas, Pediatrics 12:549, 1953.
3. di Sant'Agnese, P. A., and Talamo, R. C.: Pathogenesis and physiopathology of cystic fibrosis of the pancreas: Fibrocystic disease of the pancreas (mucoviscidosis), N. Engl. J. Med. 277:1287, 1344, 1399, 1967.
4. Hirschorn, K., Bowman, B. H., Nadler, H. L., et al.: Cystic Fibrosis, Genetic Factors, in Mangos, J. A., and Talamo, R. C. (eds.), *Cystic Fibrosis. Projections Into the Future* (New York: Stratton Intercontinental Book Corporation, 1976), pp. 275-310.
5. Holsclaw, D. S.: Common pulmonary complications of cystic fibrosis, Clin. Pediatr. 9:346, 1970.
6. Kulczycki, L. L., Craig, J. M., and Shwachman, H.: Resection of pulmonary lesions associated with cystic fibrosis of the pancreas, N. Engl. J. Med. 257:203, 1957.
7. Lorin, M. I., Denning, C. R., and Mandel, I. D.: Viscosity of exocrine secretions in cystic fibrosis: Sweat, duodenal fluid and submaxillary saliva, Biorheology 9:27, 1972.
8. Mearns, M. B., Hodson, C. J., Jackson, A. D. M., Haworth, E. M., Sellars, T. H., Sturridge, M., France, N. E., and Reid, L.: Pulmonary resection in cystic fibrosis. Results in 23 cases, 1957-1970, Arch. Dis. Child. 47:499, 1972.
9. Schuster, S. R., Shwachman, H., Harris, G. B. C., and Khaw, K-T.: Pulmonary surgery for cystic fibrosis, J. Thorac. Cardiovasc. Surg. 48:750, 1964.

Pneumothorax in Cystic Fibrosis

Pneumothorax is the most frequent complication secondary to the pathologic pulmonary changes in cystic fibrosis and occurs most frequently in the older patient.[1-4] A survey of the reports regarding pneumothorax in cystic fibrosis from four clinics (Table 47-14) illustrates the frequency of this problem.[6] The average age at appearance of this complication varies from 13¾ years to 22 years. Its incidence is relatively low, except for a single report that comes from an adult clinic. The majority of cases occur spontaneously, although in occasional instances there are specific events, such as trauma and the use of intermittent positive-pressure breathing, which may induce the problem. We see some 12 patients a year with cystic fibrosis and pneumothorax, a fourth of whom have had a previous pneumothorax.

Pneumothorax seems to occur with equal frequency in both lungs and is recurrent in many patients. The associated symptoms are sudden onset of chest pain and shortness of breath. There do occur a number of silent episodes in which the pneumothorax has been detected by routine chest x-ray, and only retrospectively has the patient recognized or admitted a progressive increase in shortness of breath.

The typical cystic fibrosis patient with pneumothorax is a teen-ager, moderately ill with far-advanced diffuse bilateral pulmonary disease. Many patients have had frequent episodes of pulmonary infiltrations prior to the pneumothorax and the recurrence rate after the first pneumothorax is almost 45%. In our own series of 45 cases reported in 1969, 15 patients died while hospitalized for this problem.

Treatment

Since the patients who develop pneumothoraces have far-advanced diffuse bilateral disease, they rarely are candidates for treatment by open thoracotomy and parietal pleurectomy. A variety of methods have been used in an attempt to obliterate the pleural space to avoid recurrent pneumothorax. Instillations of silver nitrate and atabrine solutions, and sterile talc have been used. These have not dependably obliterated the pleural space and have, on occasion, produced unacceptable pain and pleural effusion.

A significant percentage of the patients present with an unchanging pneumothorax and minimal symptoms. In these patients, we have advocated a period of watchful waiting for 48-72 hours. Partial collapse of the lung with the air leak seems to help in sealing that leak. Following this period of observation, the pneumothorax is aspirated by means of a small catheter. After evacuation of the pneumothorax, the patient is observed for several hours and x-rays repeated. In many instances there will have been no further air leak and therefore no further therapy is indicated. The patient who develops recurrent pneumothorax should have a chest tube inserted for water seal suction.

Those patients who have significant symptoms related to the pneumothorax should, of course, have immediate insertion of a chest tube, which then is placed to underwater seal

TABLE 47–14.—PNEUMOTHORAX IN CYSTIC FIBROSIS

CLINIC	YR. OF REPORT	YR. OF SURG.	NO. PTS.	AVERAGE AGE	NO. EPISODES	MALE	F.	RT.	L.	BILAT.	% OF CASES AT TIME OF REPORT	INCIDENCE
Boston	1969	1950–1969	46	14⁵/₁₂	88	34	12	38	42	8	14/46	2.5%
NIH	1969	1960–1969	15	15	32	8	7	16	15	1	5/15	3.8%
Minn. Babies' N. Y.	1968	1953–1967	20	13⁹/₁₂	36	9					5/20	2.8%
London	1970	1964–1969	7	22	8					3		14.0%

Since 1970, we continue to see about 12 children a year with pneumothorax complicating cystic fibrosis; of them, a quarter have had pneumothorax previously.

suction. Some patients with a very large air leak may require more than one chest tube connected to high negative pressure suction (30–40 cm).

Ultimately, virtually all pneumothoraces can be managed using a chest tube and it is a rare patient who will require more extensive therapy such as thoracotomy and pleurectomy.[5]

REFERENCES

1. Boat, T. F., di Sant'Agnese, P. A., Warwick, W. T., and Handwerger, S. A.: Pneumothorax in cystic fibrosis, JAMA 209:1498, 1969.
2. Fanconi, G., and Metaxas-Buhler, M.: Spontanpneumothorax bei pankreas-fibrose mit bronchiektasien, Helv. Paediatr. Acta 7:289, 1947.
3. Holsclaw, D. S.: Common pulmonary complications of cystic fibrosis, Clin. Pediatr. 9:346, 1970.
4. Lifschitz, M. I., Bowman, F. O., Denning, C. R., and Wylie, R. H.: Pneumothorax as a complication of cystic fibrosis, Am. J. Dis. Child. 116:633, 1968.
5. Mitchell-Heggs, P. F., and Batten, J. C.: Pleurectomy for spontaneous pneumothorax in cystic fibrosis, Thorax 25:165, 1970.
6. Shwachman, H.: Cystic fibrosis, Curr. Probl. Pediatr. 8:1, Aug. 1978.

Major Hemoptysis in Patients with Cystic Fibrosis

Major hemoptysis, a late complication of cystic fibrosis, is increasing in frequency because of the current greater longevity of patients with this disease.[4]

In 1975, Fellows *et al.*[3] reported on selective bronchial arteriography in 6 patients with cystic fibrosis and massive hemoptysis. They made the observation that arteriographic findings correlated with bronchoscopic observations. Since that time, selective bronchial arteriography has been performed in 18 patients with cystic fibrosis at Children's Hospital Medical Center, Boston. Initially, these studies were simply to verify the bleeding site. The 7 most recent patients have also had definitive treatment of hemoptysis by embolism of the bronchial arteries.[11]

Arteriography has been done under local anesthesia percutaneously from the femoral artery using preshaped polyethylene ultrathin-wall catheters.

Embolism was achieved by injection of small pieces of Gelfoam (1 × 1 × 2 mm) peripherally into the bronchial artery involved in the hemorrhage. The artery was filled from the periphery proximally until it had been completely occluded. The selective bronchial arteriograms were well tolerated, there was little or no pain and no complications occurred, although sometimes there was coughing. It is well to bear in mind the potential hazard of compromising an accessory spinal artery by direct injection or injection into an artery that communicates with the anterior spinal artery. Instances of transverse myelitis have been reported.

Pathogenesis

In patients with bronchiectasis, Liebow, Hales and Lindskog[5] demonstrated that there was great enlargement and tortuosity of the bronchial arteries and many anastomoses between these vessels and the pulmonary arteries. Macroscopic bronchopulmonary shunts were shown by Liebow *et al.*[5] and Marchand *et al.*[7] In the presence of emphysema, bronchiectasis, lung abscess, tuberculosis and neoplasms there have been demonstrated increased anastomoses between the bronchial and pulmonary arteries, with enlargement of these small vessels and a concomitant increase in bronchial artery flow. In 1938, Wood and Miller,[10] in subacute and chronic tuberculosis, showed that the bronchial arteries became dilated, tortuous and established new ramifications.

The inflammatory changes occurring in cystic fibrosis resemble those present in tuberculosis, with a concomitant increase in peribronchial granulation tissue, the site of many

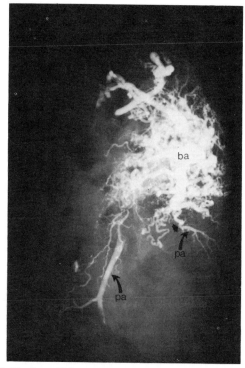

Fig. 47–29.—Bronchial arteriogram in cystic fibrosis. This arteriogram clearly demonstrates the greatly enhanced bronchial arterial supply to the region of the right upper lobe, with increased size of vessels, marked tortuosity and a number of direct shunts between the bronchial artery *(ba)* and the pulmonary arteries *(pa)*.

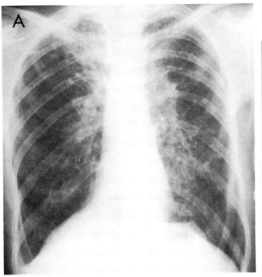
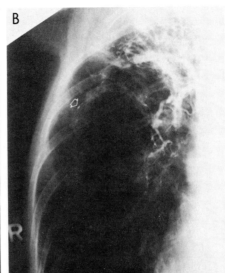

Fig. 47–30.—Enlargement and tortuosity of bronchial arteries in cystic fibrosis patient. **A,** parenchymal and vascular (bronchial) markings in cystic fibrosis. This x-ray is characteristic of the appearance found in many of the patients with far-advanced diffuse pulmonary involvement who develop major hemoptysis. Our bronchial arteriographic studies have convinced us that many of the shadows previously thought to represent intrinsic pulmonary parenchymal changes in fact represent a marked increase in size and number of bronchial vessels as seen in Figure 47–28. **B,** cystic fibrosis–bronchial arteriogram. This arteriogram demonstrates that many of the shadows seen in the plain chest roentgenogram, originally thought to represent parenchymal changes, actually are concentrations of hypertrophied and tortuous bronchial arteries and collaterals.

of the bronchopulmonary shunts.[8] These anastomoses become larger and more numerous with increasing severity of the disease and lead to dilatation and tortuosity of the bronchial arteries,[6] with rupture of these vessels into a bronchus. The classic arteriogram is demonstrated in Figure 47–29, which shows marked increase of the bronchial arterial supply to the region of the right upper lobe, with increased size of vessels, marked tortuosity and a number of bronchopulmonary shunts.

Hemoptysis

Hemorrhage occurs as a result of the erosion of the enlarged, thin-walled bronchial vessels, which appear during the course of the development of the bronchopulmonary anastomoses. Massive pulmonary hemorrhage appears most commonly in those patients with far-advanced, diffuse pulmonary involvement. The characteristic chest x-ray of a patient who is likely to develop hemoptysis as a result of diffuse bilateral severe disease is seen in Figure 47–30, *A*. As a result of our bronchial arteriographic studies, we now realize that many of the shadows previously thought to represent intrinsic pulmonary parenchymal changes in fact represent a marked increase in size and number of bronchial vessels, as demonstrated in the arteriogram of the same patient (Fig. 47–30, *B*).

Localization and Treatment

With rare exceptions, the plain chest roentgenogram is not very helpful. Since most of these patients have far-advanced bilateral pulmonary disease there rarely is a specific site of more severe involvement that can clearly be recognized on the chest x-ray as the source of hemorrhage.

Bronchoscopy remains the most reliable means of localizing the site of hemoptysis. This procedure should be avoided when the patient is bleeding massively. It almost always is possible to control the major hemoptysis for a period of time by sedation and bed rest. Bronchoscopy is best done

when the patient still is bringing up small amounts of blood-streaked sputum but not enough blood so that the entire bronchial tree will be flooded with it. Under these conditions, the orifice from which the blood is coming almost always can be identified. We have found it very helpful to cor-

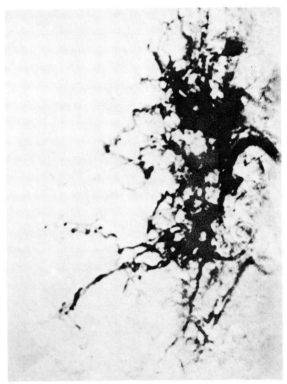

Fig. 47–31.—Cystic fibrosis–bronchial arteriogram–subtraction film. A striking demonstration of the large and tortuous bronchial vessels seen in a typical bronchial arteriogram of a patient with cystic fibrosis and major hemoptysis.

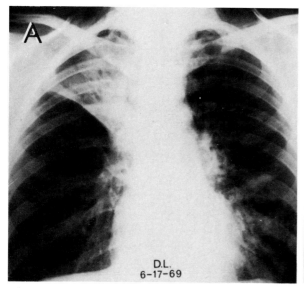
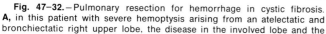
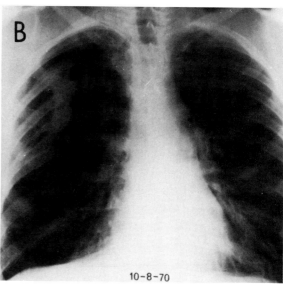

Fig. 47–32.—Pulmonary resection for hemorrhage in cystic fibrosis. **A,** in this patient with severe hemoptysis arising from an atelectatic and bronchiectatic right upper lobe, the disease in the involved lobe and the slight involvement of the remainder of the lung led to the resection of the right upper lobe. **B,** the child did well.

relate our bronchoscopic observations with selective bronchial arteriography. There has been a striking correlation between the site identified as the origin of the hemoptysis by bronchoscopy and the presence of the markedly dilated, tortuous and increased number of bronchial vessels and bronchopulmonary anastomoses. A striking demonstration of these large and tortuous bronchial vessels is seen in Figure 47–31, a subtraction study of a bronchial arteriogram.

There are three possible modes of intervention:

1. *Surgical resection* of the pulmonary segment or lobe from which the blood is coming rarely is a possibility, since most patients with this complication have diffuse, far-advanced pulmonary disease and are poor candidates for thoracotomy. Despite the fact that it is the rare patient in whom one would electively pursue this course there are occasional instances when hemorrhage is persistent and the surgeon is forced to proceed with resection to avoid having the patient drown in his own blood. It is for this reason that it is important to identify the area of lung that is bleeding in the event that resection becomes necessary as an emergency procedure. We have done resections for hemorrhage in 2 patients who clearly demonstrated local lesions as the source of hemorrhage with relatively little change in the remainder of the lung. The child whose x-rays are shown in Figure 47–32 had severe pulmonary hemorrhage and an atelectatic right upper lobe. Although the remainder of the lung showed some of the chronic changes associated with this disease, it was in relatively good condition. There was no further hemorrhage following resection of the right upper lobe.

2. *Angiographic embolization* of the artery that is bleeding. This almost always is a bronchial artery that has eroded into a bronchus. The bleeding is arterial and because of the dilated, thin-walled character of the bronchial arteries they

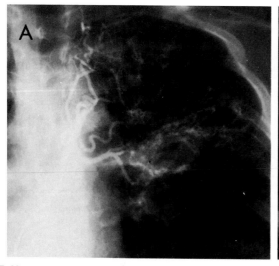
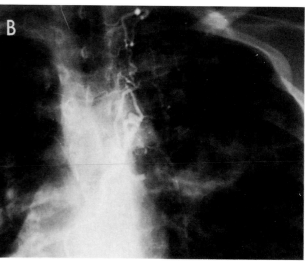

Fig. 47–33.—Bronchial arteriograms in a patient with bleeding from the left upper lobe. **A,** before gelfoam embolism. **B,** after embolism. The film clearly shows sharp occlusion of the previously patent bronchial artery to the left upper lobe bronchus.

TABLE 47–15.—HEMOPTYSIS IN CYSTIC FIBROSIS: RESULTS OF EMBOLISM

NO.	PT.	AGE	BRONCHOS-COPY	NO. OF EMBOLISMS	RESULT	FOLLOW-UP
1	LF	20	+	R (1)	Good	10 mo
2	PK	24	+	R & L (3)	Good	1 mo (died) resp. failure
3	RB	22	+	R (1)	Good	1 yr
4	AF	18	+	R (1)	Good	3 mo
5°	DL	23	+	L (2)	Good	3 wk left upper lobectomy
6	KO	18	+	R (1)	Good	3 wk (died) resp. failure
7	HZ	24	+	R (1)	Good	10 mo

°Situs inversus.

are the most likely vessels to bleed. Remy[9] has demonstrated in 104 patients that hemoptysis can be effectively treated by embolization of bronchial arteries. His series included only 1 patient with cystic fibrosis. Our own experience in 7 patients demonstrates that this is an effective method of managing massive hemoptysis in these debilitated patients. Figure 47–33 demonstrates pre- and postembolization bronchial arteriograms in a patient with left upper lobe hemorrhage. The postembolization view (Fig. 47–33, *B*) clearly shows the absence of filling of the peripheral portion of the two principal bronchial arteries that were supplying the dense area in the left upper lobe.

3. *Ligation and division of the bronchial arteries.* Our initial attempt at direct control of the hemorrhage in a patient with massive hemoptysis with cystic fibrosis was in a 22-year-old male who was having frequent repeated episodes of major pulmonary bleeding. Bronchoscopy revealed the bleeding to be coming from the right upper lobe, and angiography verified this by demonstrating the typical bronchial arterial findings in this area. The patient was noted to have two main bronchial arteries that took their origin from the usual site in the descending thoracic aorta. Each was larger than normal, the right bronchial artery significantly larger than the left. The two vessels were divided at their origin from the descending aorta through a left thoracotomy incision. This patient has had no further significant hemoptysis in the 22 months since that procedure. Despite this successful treatment, we have since elected to pursue a less invasive form of therapy—angiographic embolization of the bleeding bronchial arteries. This experience does demonstrate the efficacy of surgical division of the bronchial artery if angiographic embolization is not available or is not successful.

Table 47–15 shows a summary of our experience. Each patient had a preangiographic bronchoscopy, which demonstrated a positive correlation with the angiographic findings. Both the right and left main bronchial arteries were occluded by emboli during the initial procedure in 1 patient, the right main bronchial artery only in 3, the right upper bronchial artery in 1 and the left upper bronchial artery in 1. Bleeding stopped in all patients, although 2 of the 7 patients had recurrent massive hemoptysis within 7 and 10 days. Their hematocrit drops were 8.9% and 7.2%, respectively. Both patients required multiple embolism procedures before the massive hemoptysis ceased.

One patient died from respiratory failure 4 weeks after embolism. Another patient died as a result of hepatic failure 3 weeks after embolism. The remaining 5 patients had no recurrence in the 3-week to 12-month follow-up period. Despite cessation of hemorrhage following embolism in 1 of these patients, the decision was made to resect her left upper lobe because of severe bronchiectatic changes that resulted in large amounts of mucopurulent sputum. This patient also has situs inversus in addition to cystic fibrosis. Comparison of earlier pulmonary function tests and arterial blood gas studies with sequential studies postembolization in 6 patients did not show any unexpected changes. Three of these patients had xenon lung scan studies. There were no unexpected ventilation perfusion or equilibration changes.

There were no significant complications of the bronchial artery embolisms, although 3 patients developed a temperature elevation above 101° and chest pain within 3 days. The duration of these findings was less than 72 hours.

REFERENCES

1. Botenga, A. S. J.: The role of bronchopulmonary anastomosis in chronic inflammatory processes of the lung: Selective arteriographic investigation, Am. J. Roentgenol. 104:829, 1968.
2. Feigelson, H. H., and Ravin, H. A.: Transverse myelitis following selective bronchial arteriography, Radiology 85:663, 1965.
3. Fellows, K. E., Stigol, L., Schuster, S., Khaw, K. T., and Shwachman, H.: Selective bronchial arteriography in patients with cystic fibrosis and massive hemoptysis, Radiology 114:551, 1975.
4. Holsclaw, D. S., Grand, R. J., and Shwachman, H.: Massive hemoptysis in cystic fibrosis, J. Pediatr. 76:829, 1970.
5. Liebow, A. A., Hales, M. R., and Lindskog, G. E.: Enlargement of the bronchial arteries and their anastomoses with the pulmonary arteries in bronchiectasis, Am. J. Pathol. 25:211, 1949.
6. Mack, J. F., Moss, A. J., Harper, W. W., *et al.*: The bronchial arteries in cystic fibrosis, Br. J. Radiol. 38:422, 1965.
7. Marchand, P., Gilroy, J. C., and Wilson, V. H.: Anatomical study of bronchial vascular system and its variations in disease, Thorax 5:207, 1950.
8. Moss, A. J., Desilets, D. T., Higashino, S. M., *et al.*: Intrapulmonary shunts in cystic fibrosis, Pediatrics 41:438, 1968.
9. Remy, J., Armand, A., Fardon, H., Grand, R., and Viosin, C.: Treatment of hemoptysis by embolization of bronchial arteries, Radiology 122:33, 1977.
10. Wood, D. A., and Miller, M.: Role of dual pulmonary circulation in various pathologic conditions of lungs, J. Thorac. Surg. 7:649, 1938.
11. Schuster, S. R., and Fellows, K. E.: Management of major hemoptysis in patients with cystic fibrosis, J. Pediatr. Surg. 12:889, 1977.

Tumors of the Lung

A VARIETY OF NEOPLASMS affect the lungs in childhood. In the majority of cases, pulmonary involvement with tumor is the result of metastatic spread. However, in a small but significant group, the children present with primary lesions.

Primary Tumors

Bronchial Adenoma

Bronchial adenomas probably are the most common primary lung tumors in childhood. Wellons *et al.*[19] found 56 reports of bronchial adenoma in children aged 4–16 years and added 2 additional cases. We have treated 2 children with bronchial adenoma in the past 12 years. These tumors are recognized as low-grade adenocarcinomas that arise from different cell types within the bronchial mucosa.[6] They are classified histologically as carcinoids, cylindromas, mucoepidermoid tumors and bronchial mucous gland adenomas. The carcinoid tumor is the most common and accounts for 80–85% of all adenomas.

In most cases, the adenoma grows in a primary or secondary bronchus and classically produces recurrent cough, hemoptysis and pulmonary infection, symptoms similar to those of a retained foreign body. In most cases, symptoms have been present for 2–12 months before diagnosis.[18] However, in some children, diagnosis has been delayed for as long as 4 or 5 years, the wheezing from the bronchial obstruction having been considered to be due to bronchial asthma. Bronchiectasis may develop in the lung distal to the obstruction, especially in children with longstanding bronchial obstruction and severe pulmonary infections. Rarely, the adenoma is situated in the periphery of the lung and no specific symptoms are noted.

In the usual case, chest x-ray obtained at the time of initial symptoms shows a pulmonary infiltrate or atelectasis distal to the obstruction with no evidence of a mass (Fig. 48–1). Persistence of the radiographic abnormalities or recurrence of the findings at the same site should raise the possibility of an obstructing endobronchial lesion. Although pulmonary tomography can aid in demonstrating the presence of an intrabronchial lesion, bronchoscopy is necessary for diagnosis. Typically, the carcinoid adenoma appears pink and friable and bleeds profusely. As a result, biopsy must be performed with care and the surgeon must be prepared to take emergency measures to control hemorrhage. The mucoepidermoid and cylindromatous adenomas are less vascular and better circumscribed. Bronchography can be of value in estimating the degree of bronchiectasis distal to the obstruction, a factor that may be important in deciding whether or not diseased lung can be salvaged.

Although carcinoid tumors can produce serotonin, the carcinoid syndrome has not been documented in children with bronchial carcinoid. However, hyperserotonemia and elevated urinary 5HIAA without the carcinoid syndrome have been noted in some cases. A search for abnormal serotonin secretion should be made in each case, since serial measurements can be used to evaluate the adequacy of treatment.

Bronchoscopic removal of the adenoma is not recommended as definitive treatment for bronchial adenoma, since most of these tumors grow through the bronchial wall. In Verska and Connolly's review,[18] bronchial adenoma was removed at bronchoscopy in 4 children. Two had recurrence requiring further therapy, 1 developed a bronchial stricture that required pneumonectomy and the fourth was lost to follow-up. A review of 20 adults with bronchial adenoma treated by endoscopic resection showed 2 operative deaths due to hemorrhage and 2 late deaths due to recurrent pneumonia. Complete removal was achieved in only 4 patients and an average of 15 bronchoscopies per patient was required for control.[17] Another obvious disadvantage of bronchoscopic removal is that assessment of regional lymph node involvement is not possible.

Most adenomas require pulmonary resection for complete removal. Lobectomy is recommended for a lesion localized to a lobar bronchus or peripheral lung. More extensive resections ranging from bilobectomy to pneumonectomy are necessary when an adenoma in a main bronchus extends into a lobar bronchus or extraluminally to adjacent structures (see Fig. 48–1). Sleeve resection of the involved bronchus should be considered for the small adenoma confined to a central bronchial segment, provided that recurrent infection has not destroyed the distal lung. Verska and Connolly[18] successfully performed a sleeve resection of the bronchus in a 12-year-old and had a good result at 1 year. The findings of Boyd and his associates[2] indicate that sleeve resection for bronchial adenoma often is feasible for older patients.

About 5% of bronchial adenomas reported in childhood have shown evidence of malignancy: local invasion or metastases to regional lymph nodes.[19] Carcinoids and cylindromas appear to be more invasive than the mucoepidermoid tumors. In most series that contain patients of all ages, surgical treatment of bronchial adenoma has resulted in a 90% 10-year survival.[12] These tumors are also potentially lethal in childhood. At least 2 of the children described in the literature have died of metastatic disease.[19] One patient in our experience had recurrent adenoma that invaded the diaphragm, pericardium and lung 7 years following initial right middle lobectomy. Despite additional operation, he eventually died. Radiation therapy should be considered for trial in those children in whom complete removal of the tumor is impossible. Cylindromas occurring in other sites respond rapidly to irradiation in most instances, and carcinoid tumors have shown encouraging responses to irradiation.[8]

Bronchogenic Carcinoma

In contrast to its frequency in adults, carcinoma of the lung is very rare in children. In a recent review of the world

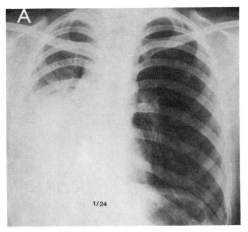

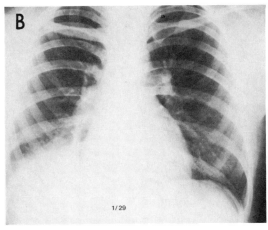

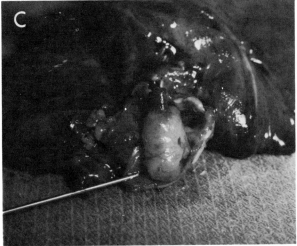

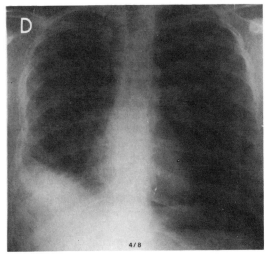

Fig. 48–1.—Bronchial adenoma in a 10-year-old girl who had several episodes of hemoptysis. **A,** chest x-ray on Jan. 24 showed collapse and in-flammation of the right middle and lower lobes, which improved **(B)** on anti-biotics by Jan. 29. Bronchoscopy, performed because of persistent symp-toms, demonstrated an endobronchial tumor in the intermediate bronchus. **C,** at operation, middle and lower lobectomy was necessary for complete removal. The well-circumscribed bronchial adenoma (mucoepidermoid type) can be seen in the resected specimen at the tip of the probe. **D,** a satisfactory chest x-ray 2 months after operation (April 8). The child remains well 8 years after operation.

literature, Niitu *et al.*[14] found 39 cases in children from 5 months to 16 years of age. The occurrence of a coexistent congenital malformation of the lung in 3 of 16 children suggests a possible causal relationship.[4] The histologic patterns are similar to those seen in adults, although incidence differs with each histologic type. Undifferentiated carcinoma and adenocarcinoma are the most frequent variants. Squamous cell carcinoma is present in only 15% of cases.[14]

Unfortunately, in most cases, findings that lead to a correct diagnosis do not occur until the disease is widespread. Cough and dyspnea from pleural effusion and extremity or back pain from bone metastases are the most common presenting symptoms. Resection of bronchogenic carcinoma for cure has not been possible for most children. However, if the tumor is discovered at an earlier stage, the outlook is not hopeless. Of 10 patients reported from Japan, 5 had complete removal of tumor by lobectomy or pneumonectomy. Three were free from tumor 3, 6 and 8 years later.[14]

Other Tumors

A variety of malignant neoplasms have been found to arise in the lung in isolated cases.[5] In the past 20 years, we have

seen individual cases of children with neurofibrosarcoma, embryoma, mesothelioma, fibrosarcoma, rhabdomyosarcoma and endothelial sarcoma originating in the lung. For localized lesions, lobectomy or pneumonectomy can be curative. More aggressive surgical therapy is warranted for lesions that extend from the lung to adjacent structures in the thorax. Chemotherapy and radiation should also be considered for the majority of these children, who will be found to have extensive local disease.

Cartilaginous tumors, usually classified as hamartoma or chondroma, probably are the most common benign pulmonary neoplasms. These tumors usually are found in the periphery of the lung and are composed of fibrous tissue, fat, bronchial epithelium and cartilage. They usually are detected incidentally on x-ray and rarely cause symptoms. Limited resections are sufficient for cure. Occasionally, these lesions arise in or near a major bronchus[16] and cause symptoms from bronchial obstruction. Postlethwait's report[15] of 13 cases suggests that, in such cases, bronchoscopic removal of these benign lesions is safe and practical when the distal lung is not irreparably damaged.

In a review of histiocytoma of the lung, a lesion that probably is a neoplasm, Dubilier *et al.*[7] reported 7 cases in children. Although histiocytoma appears to have malignant potential when growing in other locations, these authors conclude that in the lung it is a benign neoplasm and can be eradicated by wide local excision that includes a margin of uninvolved lung.

The pulmonary nodule accidentally discovered in an x-ray should be resected after infectious processes—tuberculosis, coccidioidomycosis, histoplasmosis—have been ruled out. It may be a malignant tumor and not a hamartoma.

Metastatic Tumors

Wilms' Tumor

Pulmonary metastases, present at initial diagnosis or developing later in the course of the illness, occur in about half of the children with Wilms' tumor.[3] In most cases, a standard treatment protocol is followed. Initial therapy includes radiation therapy (1500 rads to both lungs) and chemotherapy (actinomycin D and vincristine). Additional radiation is given to sites of persistent tumor. Resection is undertaken when radiography indicates tumor persistent or recurrent after treatment, provided that complete removal is technically possible. Occasionally, a metastatic nodule has been excised through a thoracoabdominal approach when encountered during the removal of a primary tumor. In the past 10 years, we have operated on 6 children with Wilms' tumor metastases, 5 of whom represented failures of radiation and chemotherapy. In these children, 1–5 separate metastatic nodules were removed either by wedge resection (single or multiple) or by lobectomy. Three are long-term survivors.[1] If an aggressive multidisciplinary attack is utilized, more than 50% of all children with pulmonary metastases from Wilms' tumor can be salvaged.[3]

Osteogenic Sarcoma

Pulmonary metastases from this tumor are very common and, until recently, approximately 80% of patients developed fatal pulmonary lesions within 2 years of diagnosis. However, since the introduction of adjuvant high-dose methotrexate chemotherapy, the incidence of pulmonary metastases following amputation or excision of the primary tumor has been reduced to about 30%. Even macroscopic pulmonary lesions have disappeared in some patients with high-dose methotrexate therapy.[9]

In the past, pulmonary resection for metastatic osteogenic

sarcoma was offered only to a very select group of patients. Although gross lesions could be removed, most patients still succumbed because microscopic tumor deposits at other sites in the lung eventually became evident. Operation was considered only when the patient had a long disease-free interval after amputation, and then only for a solitary metastasis or when, at most, 2 or 3 lesions were present in one lung. Now that a chemical agent is available that can eliminate microscopic subclinical disease, the role of surgery is being re-evaluated at our institution and others.[13] Presuming that gross tumor deposits in the lung can be eliminated by operation, and microscopic tumor deposits can be eliminated by chemotherapy, a new protocol is in progress in which pulmonary resection is undertaken for children with pulmonary nodules that do not disappear with high-dose methotrexate therapy and for those with metastases that appear during adjuvant chemotherapy. Even children with multiple lesions and those with bilateral disease are candidates for pulmonary resection.[10]

In the past 3 years, pulmonary metastases have been treated operatively in 15 children. Seven were our own patients who developed pulmonary lesions while on adjuvant high-dose methotrexate therapy and 8 were referred here when pulmonary metastases developed. Since most children had more than one metastatic nodule, and since we wished to preserve as much lung tissue as possible (especially in the event that further resection might become necessary), nodules were removed by wedge resection rather than by lobectomy or pneumonectomy. Twenty-seven thoracotomies were performed in the 15 children. Eight children presented with bilateral metastases and 2 separate operations were required initially. Additional resections were necessary in 4 children in whom a new lung metastasis became evident 3–9 months later. Most patients had 1–5 nodules per lung, but 1 child had 21 on the left and 15 on the right. Following operation in 10 children, irradiation was given to both lungs (1500 rads), with additional irradiation to localized areas of residual disease. Despite intensive radiation therapy and chemotherapy before and after operation, few surgical complications were noted. Evacuation of a hemothorax was necessary in 1 child and drainage of a localized empyema was required in another. Early results of this program are encouraging. To date, 2 of 15 patients show no evidence of disease 18 months and 2 years following resection of pulmonary metastases. Five others treated more recently have no evidence of disease, but still are receiving

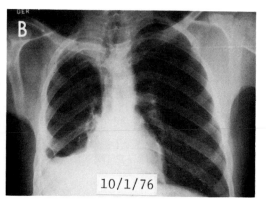

Fig. 48–2.—Metastatic osteogenic sarcoma in an 18-year-old boy who had a left above-knee amputation for osteogenic sarcoma in November of 1973. **A,** he was referred with pulmonary metastases on the right on 10/29/74. At thoracotomy, a large metastatic mass invading the middle and lower lobes, diaphragm and pericardium was found. After middle and lower lobectomy and partial resection of the diaphragm and pericardium, no gross tumor remained. Postoperative radiation therapy was given and courses of chemotherapy with high-dose methotrexate were continued for 18 months. **B,** 2 years after operation (10/1/76), he was alive and well without evidence of metastatic disease.

chemotherapy. Three patients have died of osteogenic sarcoma and 5 others are alive but with evidence of disease. Pulmonary metastases have not recurred in 2 of these children. It appears that wedge resection and chemotherapy can salvage at least some patients with metastatic pulmonary lesions that have been uniformly fatal in the past (Fig. 48–2).

Other Tumors

Resection plays an important role in the management of some children with isolated lung metastases from a variety of neoplasms.[1] In many instances, these lesions represent residual or resistant disease following chemotherapy and radiation therapy.

Operations to eradicate metastatic lung lesions have varied in extent from wedge resection to pneumonectomy. To control primary lung cancer, it is agreed that lobectomy or pneumonectomy is necessary because these tumors involve the major bronchi and pulmonary lymphatics. However, in metastatic cancer, tumor masses usually are located peripherally, and to minimize loss of lung tissue, most surgeons have chosen to excise these nodules by wedge resection when technically possible. We have reviewed our experience with wedge resection for pulmonary metastases and have found that local control was achieved regularly by a limited resection when the tumor was a type for which effective chemotherapy and irradiation was available. However, tumor recurred in the same lobe in 50% of the others.[1] Therefore, when the metastatic nodule is likely to be unresponsive to chemotherapy and radiation, lobectomy is preferred for a single nodule (or multiple nodules in no more than 2 lobes), provided that resection will not compromise pulmonary function, extrapulmonary metastases are absent and the primary site of the tumor has been free from disease for more than 6 months.

REFERENCES

1. Ballantine, T. V. N., Wiseman, N. E., and Filler, R. M.: Assessment of pulmonary wedge resection for the treatment of lung metastases, J. Pediatr. Surg. 10:671, 1975.
2. Boyd, A. D., Spencer, F. C., and Lind, A.: Why has bronchial resection and anastomosis been reported infrequently for treatment of bronchial adenoma?, J. Thorac. Cardiovasc. Surg. 59: 359, 1970.
3. Cassady, J. R., et al.: Considerations in the radiation therapy of Wilms' tumor, Cancer 32:598, 1973.
4. Cayley, C. K., Caez, H. J., and Mersheimer, W.: Primary bronchogenic carcinoma of the lung in children, Am. J. Dis. Child. 82:49, 1951.
5. Dehner, L. P.: *Pediatric Surgical Pathology* (St. Louis: The C. V. Mosby Company, 1975).
6. Donahue, J. K., et al.: Bronchial adenoma, Ann. Surg. 167:873, 1965.
7. Dubilier, L. D., Bryant, L. R., and Danielson, G. K.: Histiocytoma (fibrous xanthoma) of the lung, Am. J. Surg. 115:420, 1968.
8. Gaitin-Gaitin, A., Rider, W. D., and Bush, R. S.: Carcinoid tumor—cure by irradiation, Int. J. Radiat. Oncol. Biol. Phys. 1:9, 1975.
9. Jaffe, N., et al.: Favorable response of metastatic osteogenic sarcoma to pulse high-dose methotrexate with citrovorum rescue and radiation therapy, Cancer 31:1367, 1973.
10. Jaffe, N., et al.: Multidisciplinary treatment for macrometastatic osteogenic sarcoma, Br. Med. J. 2:1039, 1976.
11. Kilman, J. W., et al.: Surgical resection for pulmonary metastases in children, Arch. Surg. 99:158, 1969.
12. Markel, S. F., et al.: Neoplasms of bronchus commonly designated as adenomas, Cancer 17:590, 1964.
13. Martini, N., et al.: Multiple pulmonary resections in the treatment of osteogenic sarcoma, Ann. Thorac. Surg. 12:271, 1971.
14. Niitu, Y., et al.: Lung cancer (squamous cell carcinoma) in adolescence, Am. J. Dis. Child. 127:108, 1974.
15. Postlethwait, R. W., Hogerty, R. F., and Trent, J. C.: Endobronchial polypoid hamartochondroma, Surgery 24:732, 1948.
16. Shermeta, D. W., Carter, D., and Haller, J. A., Jr.:Chondroma of the bronchus in childhood: A case report illustrating problems in diagnosis and management, J. Pediatr. Surg. 10:545, 1975.
17. Soutter, L.: Thirty-one-year hospital experience with bronchoscopic approach to bronchial adenoma, Ann. Otol. Rhinol. Laryngol. 63:509, 1954.
18. Verska, J. J., and Connolly, J. E.: Bronchial adenomas in children, J. Thorac. Cardiovasc. Surg. 55:411, 1968.
19. Wellons, H. A., Jr., et al.: Bronchial adenoma in childhood, Am. J. Dis. Child. 130:301, 1976.

49

Maurice Lev / Saroja Bharati

Embryology of the Heart and Pathogenesis of Congenital Malformations of the Heart

Embryology of the Heart

THE EMBRYOLOGY OF THE HEART will be presented as a synthesis of the views of Tandler,[1] Waterston,[2] Davis,[3] Pernkopf and Wirtinger,[4] Doerr,[5] Goerttler,[6, 7] Streeter,[8-10] Van Mierop,[11-13] Goor[14-16] and Anderson.[17] The development of the heart occurs from about 3 to 7 weeks after ovulation.

Stage I (Fig. 49–1)

At about 1 mm of fetal length (crown-rump) (1 somite – horizon 9–10), the heart begins to develop from paired angiogenic cell accumulations, which appear on both sides of the primitive pharynx in the splanchnic mesoderm. These cell accumulations form endocardial and myoepicardial tubes. These tubes are, at this stage, blind channels, which abut against but do not make connection with the primordial umbilico-vitelline channels. As the embryo lifts itself off the yolk sac, these tubes approach each other and fuse. During this period of migration, they become segmented from the cranial to the caudal aspect into aortic sac portions, bulbar portions and ventricular portions. Fusion of the two tubes (that is, both the endocardial tubes together and the myoepicardial tubes together) occurs at about 2 mm of fetal length (crown-rump) (7 somites – approximately 23 days after ovulation). Between the endocardial and myoepicardial tubes there is an amorphous, plastic and, in the beginning, noncellular gelatinous material called cardiac jelly. The cardiac tube now makes connection with the developing aortic arch system and the vitelline and umbilical veins. At this stage, the atria still are buried in the septum transversum. This may be called the first stage of the development of the heart.

Stage II (Fig. 49–2)

In the second stage, the atrio-ventriculo-bulbar loop is formed. This is due to the fact that the heart grows beyond its containing cavity, is fixed at its proximal and distal ends and the dorsal mesocardium disappears in the ventriculobulbar region. Thus, the bulboventricular part is affected first. This bends ventrally (anteriorly) and to the right. The direction of bending is related to lesser differential growth of the right side of the tube, as compared to the left. The bulboventricular loop so formed consists of a descending and an ascending limb. The descending limb may be called pro-ampulla. The ascending limb consists of meta-ampulla and bulbus, although some workers call the entire ascending limb bulbus. The bulbus is kinked on itself in the form of a bayonet. Its distal portion enters the truncus. Because of the difficulty in differentiating these parts, some workers call this the bulbotruncal area. In the formation of the bulboventricular loop, the mesocardial (dorsal) parts of the atrioventricular and bulboventricular regions are approximated. A deep indentation and associated spur (bulboventricular flange) is formed between the two limbs of the loop.

As the ventriculobulbar loop bends forward, the right and left sides of the atrium emerge out of the septum transversum, carrying along with it the right and left parts of the sinus venosus (11–20 somites – 2.5–3 mm). The bulbus falls into the groove between the developing right and left portions of the atrium. These portions develop from right and left anlagen, which retain their right and left sidedness vis-à-vis the position of the viscera. The sinus venosus is first connected to both sides of the atrium. However, it shifts to the right as the embryo favors the right side of the venous circuit with atrophy of the left. This is associated with a movement of the atrial canal to the left. Thus, in the formation of the atrio-ventriculo-bulbar loop, a bayonet-shaped structure is formed proximally in the sinoatrial region as well as distally in the bulbar region.

As judged by events in the chick embryo, it is during the stage of the development of the atrio-ventriculo-bulbar loop that contractions are thought to begin in the ventriculobulbar portion of the heart. The atrial portion of the heart and subsequently the sinus venosus portion as they develop take over the initiation of the beat. Thus, at 21–29 somites (3–4 mm – horizon 12), a distinct circulation has developed. Blood flows consecutively from the sinus venosus into the right atrium, into the left atrium, into the atrial canal present on the left side, into the descending limb of the bulboventricular loop, then into the ascending limb into the truncus. Thus, blood takes a markedly circuitous route through the heart.

Stage III (Fig. 49–3)

The next stage of the development of the heart has to do with the absorption of the bulbus and sinus venosus, the undoing of the twist of the sino-atrio-ventriculo-bulbar loop, the reorientation of the atrial canal to the bulbus and the development of septa, with the formation of a four-chambered heart. This occurs from about 4 mm to 17 mm of fetal length (crown-rump). The twist of the bulbus is undone by

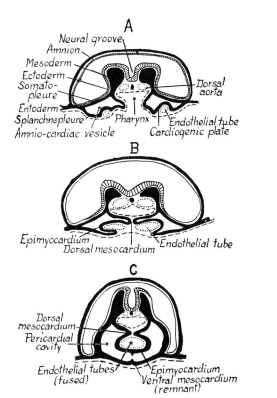

During this stage, the sinus venosus and the common pulmonary vein (which develops in part as an offshoot of the left atrium at about 5 mm) are also absorbed into the right and left atrium, respectively. The sinus venosus is divided into right, left and transverse portions. As stated above, the left horn early becomes smaller than the right and loses its connection with the left side, because of a shift of the venous blood from left to right. During the state of absorption of the bulbus, the sinus venosus lags behind the growth of the right atrium so that the right horn is absorbed into the latter. The transverse portion becomes the coronary sinus whereas the left horn becomes the vein of Marshall.

Septation

Associated with the above changes is the development of septation throughout the heart. Although these septa develop simultaneously, they will be dealt with separately for descriptive purposes.

Atrial Septum (Fig. 49–4)

At 4–5 mm of fetal length, the septum primum develops in the region of the indentation made by the bulbus. This septum grows downward from the dorsal wall of the atrium. Thus, a space is left between the septum primum and the developing endocardial cushions; this is called the ostium primum. This orifice eventually is closed by the endocardial cushions (10–12 mm). At about 7–8 mm, perforations occur in the septum primum that coalesce to form the ostium secundum. At about 17 mm, the septum secundum is formed by an infolding of the wall of the atrium to the right of the septum primum, joined by the septum spurium (formed by the junction of both valves of the sinus venosus) and by the left valve of the sinus venosus.[18] This produces the limbus overlying the ostium secundum. The eventual foramen ovale is thus the opening between the two septa. The further growth of these septa up to birth produces an approximation of their overlapping edges, so that blood can flow from the right atrium into the left due to the higher pressure of blood in the right atrium. At the same time, after birth, with the opening of the pulmonary circuit and the flow of blood into the left atrium, the overlapping of the septa produces a physiologic closure of the atrial septum at this point. Anatomic

Fig. 49–1.—Diagram of the first stage of the development of the heart. (From Jordan and Kindred, *Textbook of Embryology* [New York: Appleton-Century-Crofts, 1948].)

opposite torsions of the distal and proximal bulbar ostia. A telescoping of this chamber occurs, associated with ventral and to the left deviation of this chamber, and to a lesser extent the meta-ampulla. This is associated with a migration to the right of the atrial canal and the adjacent pro-ampulla. The bulbus is thus absorbed into the developing ventricles, the right side becoming the infundibulum of the right ventricle and the left side part of the vestibule of the left ventricle. Part of the pro-ampulla is given to the right side and a small part of the meta-ampulla to the left side.

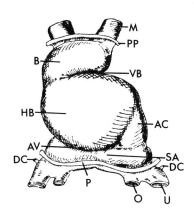

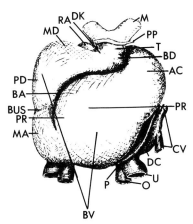

Fig. 49–2.—Second stage of the development of the heart (8–22 somites). *M*—mandibular arch; *B*—bulbus; *T*—truncus; *VB*—ventriculobulbar sulcus; *AV*—atrioventricular sulcus; *AC*—atrial canal; *O*—omphalomesenteric vein; *U*—umbilical veins; *DC*—duct of Cuvier; *P*—cut end of pericardium at venous entry; *PP*—cut end of pericardium at arterial origin; *RA*—right atrium; *DK*—

distal kink of bulbus; *MD*—middle portion of bulbus; *PD*—promixal portion of bulbus; *BA*—bulboauricular groove; *PR*—pro-ampulla; *MA*—meta-ampulla; *CV*—precardinal and postcardinal veins; *BV*—bulboventricular loop; *SA*—sinoatrial region; *HB*—cardiac tube bayonet; *BUS*—bulboventricular sulcus. (After Pernkopf, E., and Wirtinger, W., Z. Anat. 100:563, 1933.)

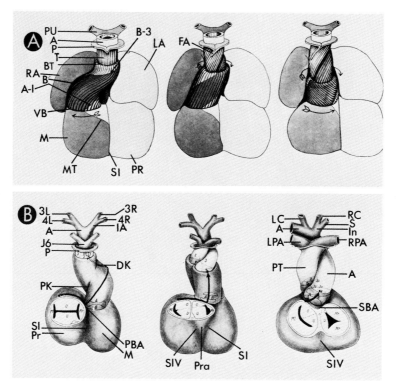

Fig. 49–3.—Third stage of the development of the heart, anterior **(A)** and posterior **(B)** views. *LA*—left atrium; *RA*—right atrium; *PR*—pro-ampulla; *M*—meta-ampulla; *B*—bulbus; *T*—truncus; *PU*—pulmonary trunk; *A*—aorta; *P*—pericardium; *BT*—bulbotruncal junction; *A-1*—bulbar ridge of A-1; *VB*—ventriculobulbar junction; *MT*—meta-ampullar portion of ventricular septal ridge; *SI*—interampullary sulcus; *B-3*—bulbar ridge B-3; *FA*—frenulum of aorta; *O*—anterior endocardial cushion; *U*—posterior endocardial cushion; *ML*—left lateral endocardial cushion; *MR*—right lateral endocardial cushion; *1–4*—bulbar swellings; *A, B*—proximal bulbar swellings; *3L*—3d left aortic arch; *3R*—3d right aortic arch; *4L*—4th left aortic arch; *4R*—4th right aortic arch; *J6*—junction of 6th aortic arch; *IA*—innominate artery; *PK*—proximal kinking groove; *PBA*—primary bulboauricular spur; *SBA*—secondary bulbo-ventricular spur; *DK*—distal kinking groove; *LC*—left cartoid; *RC*—right cartoid; *S*—subclavian; *LPA*—left pulmonary artery; *RPA*—right pulmonary artery; *Pra*—part of pro-ampulla that eventually will belong to the right ventricle; *SIV*—sulcus interventricularis. (According to Pernkopf, E., and Wirtinger, W., Z. Anat. 100:563, 1933.)

closure may take as long as a year. In about 25% of the cases, an oblique probe-patent foramen ovale remains.

Atrial Canal Cushions (Fig. 49–5)

At about 6 mm of fetal length, the superior (anterior, ventral) and inferior (posterior, dorsal) endocardial cushions make their appearance in the atrial canal. At about 9–10 mm, these cushions fuse, producing the mitral and tricuspid orifice. The small lateral cushions develop at about 11 mm. It must be recalled that while the cushions are developing, the atrial canal and its accompanying portion of the pro-ampulla are gradually moving toward the right, so that the tricuspid orifice first straddles the developing ventricular septum and then opens completely into the right ventricle.

Ventricular Septum (Fig. 49–6)

The ventricular septum is formed by the bulboventricular flange, the primordial main ventricular septum, the bulbar septum and the endocardial cushions. The earliest component to appear is the bulboventricular flange, which is developed during the formation of the bulboventricular loop. The main (posterior) interventricular septum develops as an infolding of the interampullary ring as the pro- and meta-ampulla expand. This begins at about 5–6 mm. The opening

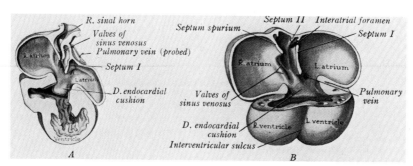

Fig. 49–4.—Development of the atrial septum. **A,** at 6.5 mm. **B,** at 9 mm. (From Arey, L. B., *Developmental Anatomy* [6th ed.; Philadelphia: W. B. Saunders Company, 1954].)

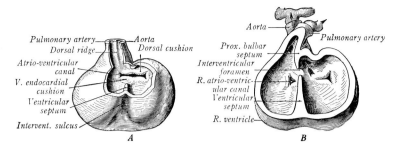

Fig. 49–5.—Formation of endocardial cushions and mitral and tricuspid valves. (From Arey, L. B., *Developmental Anatomy* [6th ed.; Philadelphia: W. B. Saunders Company, 1954].)

now between the developing right and left ventricles may be called the interventricular foramen. Those who call the entire ascending limb the bulbus call this opening the bulboventricular foramen. With the ventral and the left deviation of the bulbus and the dorsal and right deviation of the atrial canal, the posterior ventricular septum fuses with the dorsal endocardial cushion to the right of its midpoint (8–9 mm) and the bulboventricular flange fuses with the ventral endocardial cushion to the left of its midpoint.

Four cushions (called 1–4) are developed in the distal bulbus (also called truncus by some) and two cushions, A and B (sinistroventral and dextrodorsal, respectively), are developed in the proximal bulbus (also called conus by some). The truncus is considered a separate segment above the bulbus by others. We will so consider it here. Between the proximal and distal swellings stretch ridges 1A and 3B twisted about each other 270°. These first appear at about 4–5 mm. These ridges are accompanied by spur formation between the 4th and 6th arches. Septation spreads from downstream to upstream. Thus, the spurs between the 4th and 6th arches extend down to form truncal ridges that unite to form the proximal part of the aorta and pulmonary trunk. As the bulbus is absorbed into the ventricles, the bulbar ridges 1A and 3B are straightened out by the torsion and

countertorsion at the distal and proximal portions of the bulbus, and the ridges meet to form the bulbar septum. This septum is first at an angle to the main posterior ventricular septum. This leaves a four-way communication between the aorta, pulmonary trunk and the right and left ventricles. Recession of the bulboventricular flange brings the aortic portion of the proximal bulbus (conus) above the left ventricle so that it is continuous with the endocardial arch formed by the fused endocardial cushions. The superior endocardial cushion becomes attenuated in its midportion to accommodate the aortic root. The movement of the proximal bulbus to the left brings the proximal bulbar septum into alignment with the posterior ventricular septum and the shrunken bulboventricular flange. With the fusion of these components, an opening is left at the base between the two ventricles. The proximal bulbar septum is first endocardial and then becomes muscular.

The final separation of the right and left ventricles and the left ventricle from the right atrium is accomplished by the formation of atrioventricular septum and pars membranacea.[19] This occurs at about 16–17 mm—horizon 18. This is accomplished by the growth of the endocardial cushions, especially the posterior, perhaps aided by the bulbar cushions A and B. When formed, this segment is partly horizon-

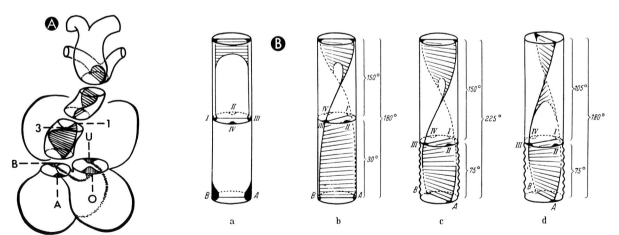

Fig. 49–6.—Formation of septation in ventricles, bulbus and truncus. **A,** the ventricles, the bulbus, the truncus, the large arterial trunks and the outline of the atria have been delineated in a transparent heart that is subdivided into portions at the ventriculobulbar and the bulbotruncal levels and at the origin of the 6th arches. In the AV orifice, the endocardial cushion O is in front and cushion U is in back. Ridges *(dotted)* start from these, i.e., a short ridge (OB) over the concavity and a long ridge (UA) over the convexity. A spiral septum (twisted more than 90°) formed from opposite ridges A-1 and B-3 extends from the ventriculobulbar ostium to the bulbotruncal ostium. From the bulbotruncal ostium, this septum connects with the aorticopul-

monary septum, which is twisted about 50°. (According to Goerttler.[6]) **B,** bulbotruncal septation according to Doerr. Diagrammatic sketches with the bulbotruncal area pictured as a straight tube. *(a)* Early stage. There are no bulbar ridges known to occur. However, truncal septation is shown developing. *(b)* After bulbotruncel torsion through 150°, the bulbotruncal septum is twisted through 180°. *(c)* At a later stage, torsion is increased, through 225°. *(d)* At the end of the second phase of development, slight reverse torsion at the aorticopulmonary division reduces the total torsion to 180°. (Doerr, W., Ergeb. Chir. Orthop. 36:1, 1950.)

tal, since the fusion of the endocardial cushions with the septum primum occurs somewhat to the left of the midpoint of the cushions, whereas the main ventricular septum joins to the posterior cushion considerably to the right of the midpoint, as stated above. Later, this portion becomes vertical and in line with the atrial and ventricular septa.

Atrioventricular and Semilunar Valve Apparatus

The atrioventricular valvular apparatus is fashioned from the endocardial cushions, the dextrodorsal bulbar cushion B and the connections of the endocardial cushions with the muscular trabeculae of the ventricular myocardium. This proceeds in three periods.[20] In the first period (11–23 mm), the various leaflets are first fashioned. The inferior leaflets of the mitral and tricuspid valves are formed from the lateral endocardial cushions, the aortic leaflet of the mitral valve from the fused anterior and posterior endocardial cushions, the anterior leaflet of the tricuspid from the fused anterior and posterior endocardial cushions and the dextrodorsal bulbar swelling B, and the septal cusp of the tricuspid from the posterior endocardial cushion, with perhaps a small part of the anterior. During this period, the leaflets consist of cushion material and muscular trabeculae. In the second period (23–61 mm), muscle gradually invades and replaces cushion material. Also during this period, as stated above, correlated with the changes in the pars membranacea, the developing tricuspid leaflets migrate to become more distal than the mitral leaflets. In the third period (85 mm to 4 mo), collagenous tissue invades and replaces muscle tissue.

The aortic and pulmonic valves are fashioned by an undermining process involving the distal bulbar cushions 1–4. This yields the aortic right and left anterior cusps (cushions 1 and 3), the posterior cusp (cushion 4), the pulmonic right and left posterior cusps (cushions 1 and 3) and the anterior cusp (cushion 2).

The Systemic Veins

At 3 mm there are three series of veins in the embryo: (1) the umbilical veins draining the chorion, (2) the vitelline veins draining the yolk sac and (3) the cardinal veins draining the embryo itself. The cardinals consist of the precardinals and the postcardinals uniting to form the common cardinals, which also drain the vitelline and the umbilical veins. Somewhat later, the subcardinals and the supracardinals develop, also draining the embryo.

The transformation of the vitelline and the umbilical veins is related to the development of the liver (4–9 mm). The growth of the liver breaks up the vitelline vessels into sinusoids with proximal and distal segments. At the same time, there is a shift of blood to the right horn of the sinus venosus, with atrophy of the left horn. The distal segments of the vitelline veins are converted into the portal vein, and the intermediate portions remain as the sinusoids, while the proximal portions become the hepatic veins, which at this stage drain into the right horn of the sinus venosus.

With the further growth of the liver, the developing umbilical veins are rerouted through the hepatic sinusoids. There now is a disappearance of the right and proximal part of the left umbilical vein, with the remainder of the left persisting. A diagonal passage now is dug out through the hepatic sinusoids to form the ductus venosus. Thus, at 9 mm, blood passes from the placenta through the umbilical vein through the ductus venosus into the sinus venosus.

The differentiation of the cardinal system and the development of the superior and the inferior venae cavae occur

from 4 to 22 mm. These changes are related to the development of the kidney. At 4 mm, the precardinal, the postcardinal and the subcardinal veins have developed. By 11 mm, the hepatic portion of the inferior vena cava develops from the vitelline veins and an anastomosis develops between the subcardinals. At 15 mm, the supracardinals develop and the postcardinal system begins to atrophy. By 22 mm, the inferior vena cava has developed from a fusion of various parts: the vitellines, the subcardinals and the supracardinals.

At about 20 mm, the superior vena cava is developed from the precardinal system as follows: At first, an oblique cross channel (left innominate) is formed, shunting blood from the left vein across to the right. This results in the loss of the communication of the left precardinal just caudal to the left common cardinal. The latter remains as the distal part of the vein of Marshall. The right common cardinal and the right precardinal become the superior vena cava. The azygos and the hemiazygos are developed from the supracardinals at about 22 mm.

The Pulmonary Vein

It is generally agreed that the pulmonary vein originates from two sources: (1) a presplanchnic source consisting of a channel formed from the confluence of the vascular plexuses of the lung, which extends to the middle part of the sinus venosus without opening into it, and (2) the main pulmonary stem being an outgrowth from the heart tube. However, there are differing opinions as to whether the latter originates from the sinus venosus or from the left atrium. The common vein is developed at 5 mm.

During the second phase of the development of the heart, concomitant with the absorption of the sinus venosus into the right atrium, the common pulmonary vein is absorbed into the left atrium. This is followed by the absorption of the right and the left pulmonary veins, so that, definitively, four separate pulmonary veins enter the left atrium.

The Aortic Arches (Fig. 49–7)

The aortic arches make their appearance as follows: first pair–1.3 mm, second–3 mm, third–4 mm, fourth–5–6 mm and sixth–6 mm. These arches form communications between the aortic sac and the two dorsal aortas. The first

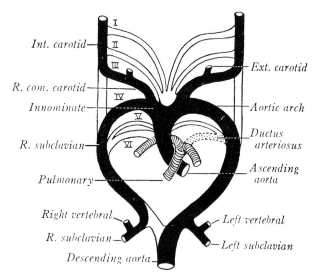

Fig. 49–7.–Transformation of the aortic arches. (From Arey, L. B., *Developmental Anatomy* [6th ed.; Philadelphia: W. B. Saunders Company, 1954].)

two pairs of arches disappear as the third pair of arches is forming. The dorsal aorta beyond the dorsal ends of the 3d arches persists as the internal carotid arteries. The 3d arches form the stems of the internal carotid arteries whereas the external carotid arteries are newly formed vessels on the 3d arches. The 3d arches between the external carotids and aortic sac form the common carotids. By 14 mm, the dorsal aorta between the 3d and the 4th arches atrophies. Between 14 and 16 mm, the right dorsal aorta between the subclavian and the common dorsal aorta likewise is lost. Thus, the 4th left arch and the common dorsal aorta now assume the topography of the definitive aorta and the right 4th remains as the proximal part of the right subclavian. Also at 14–16 mm, the right limb of the aortic sac elongates to form the innominate artery.

The distal portion of both subclavian arteries and the proximal part of the left develop from the 7th segmental arteries. Throughout their development, these derivatives undergo a constant cranial migration from their position low down on the 4th arches. Because of the difference in derivation of the two vessels, the left ascends more than the right. At about 16 mm, the left subclavian is just distal to the ductus arteriosus. Subsequently, it assumes its definitive position proximal to the isthmus. The right 6th aortic arch remains as the right pulmonary artery, and the left persists as the left pulmonary artery and the ductus arteriosus.

The Coronary Arteries

These vessels begin as thickenings of the aortic endothelium at 10–12 mm of fetal length. This is also the time the truncus septum is bisecting the larger pair of the distal bulbar swellings, which have fused in their centers. Both coronary arteries pass to the sides of the bulbus cordis, and the anterior descending coronary artery begins to be laid down. By 14 mm, both circumflexes are developed and by 20 mm, all larger branches are developed.

The Conduction System

There is a difference of opinion in regard to the method of development of the sinoatrial node. According to some (Walls[21]), it can be recognized at 7–10 mm and is derived from sinus venosus musculature. According to others (Shaner[22]), it appears as a new formation at 100 mm on the ventrolateral surface of the superior vena cava.

There is considerable controversy as to the development of the AV node, bundle of His and the right and left bundle branches. Mackenzie[23] believed that the AV node was derived from the sinus venosus and that the AV bundle arose from the atrial canal musculature. Koch[24] and Aschoff[25] thought that only the posterior part of the AV node arose from the sinus venosus and that the anterior part of the node and the bundle were derived from the atrial canal. Patten[26] suggested that the AV node is developed from the myocardium of the left sinus horn. Recently, Anderson[27] suggested that the proximal part of the AV node arises from the sinus venosus and the distal part comes from the atrial canal.

Most other authors,[28-32] however, believe that the AV node and bundle originate from the atrial canal musculature. According to these authors, they originate from the posterior part of the canal, which lies behind the posterior endocardial cushion at a time when the musculature of this canal still is unbroken. There is a difference of opinion as to whether both the AV node and bundle originate in situ[30, 31] or the bundle of His originates from a proliferation of AV nodal tissue.[21] There is also a difference of opinion as to whether the

bundle branches originate in situ[30, 31] from ventricular trabeculae or originate from a proliferation of the tissue of the bundle of His.[31] Anderson[27] recently has voiced the opinion that they originate in situ from the junction of the anterior and posterior (bulboventricular) part of the ventricular septum. Anderson[27] has also advanced the concept that the entire atrial part of the atrioventricular junction in the normal heart may be considered part of the conduction system.

The ideas of Wenink[32] deserve special mention. According to this author, the myocardium of the sinoatrial, atrioventricular, ventriculobulbar and bulbotruncal junctions or rings have morphologically specialized characteristics. The sinoatrial node develops from the sinoatrial ring, the AV node from both the sinoatrial and atrioventricular rings. The fusion of the bulboventricular and atrioventricular rings gives rise to the bundle of His, the bulboventricular ring to the right bundle branch and left bundle branch.

Whatever their origin, the AV node is seen at 8–9 mm, the bundle of His and the beginning of the left bundle branch at about 10–11 mm, the right bundle branch at 13 mm, and it can be traced to the moderator band at 22–25 mm.

Closure of the Ductus Arteriosus

The method of normal closure of the ductus is not clearly understood. It is in some way related to the onset of respiration. The latter results in a fall in pulmonary resistance and an increase in pulmonary flow. This is associated with an increase in left ventricular flow and in systemic pressure. Thus, blood is drawn away from the muscular ductus, which contracts and becomes nonfunctioning within hours after birth. Normally, it becomes anatomically closed by 3 months of age.

Possible Forces Operating in the Development of the Circulation

It has been shown by Goerttler[6] that in the early embryonic heart there are two currents swirling around each other with a line of stasis in between. The two currents are related to the vitelline-umbilical venous entry on both sides of the embryo. With the formation of the sino-atrio-ventriculo-bulbar loop, these two currents remain, albeit the venous return has been altered by changes in the veins. With the formation of the definitive heart, the two currents remain, with the superior vena cava feeding the right side and the inferior vena cava the left side. With the birth of the fetus, the two currents are appropriated by the pulmonary for the left side and the systemic for the right side. Thus, one might say that despite the various anatomic changes, a two-current circulation is present from the beginning.

Septation occurs at the line of stasis between the two currents. This septation is further enhanced by the various constrictive areas and by the difference in flow over convexities and concavities during the multiple curvatures and bayonet-like formations produced by the sino-atrio-ventriculo-bulbar loop. Furthermore, one might theorize that the increase in the volume of the two currents straightens the loop and telescopes the bulbus and sinus regions, which are absorbed into the ventricles. The hemodynamic principles involved in these changes are beyond the scope of the present work.

Pathogenesis of Congenital Malformations of the Heart

It is self evident that nothing is definitely known about the pathogenesis of congenital malformations of the heart;

hence, the various assumptions made by various investigators. However, conceptually it is useful to postulate the possible aberrancies that may occur in the pathogenesis of an individual anomaly. Only when abnormal embryos are studied by embryologists will it be possible to make more definitive statements.

Congenitally Abnormal Hearts in Pure Levocardia

In pure levocardia, the base-apex axis points to the left and there is normal position of chambers with concordance between atria and ventricles.

TETRALOGY OF FALLOT, DOUBLE OUTLET RIGHT VENTRICLE AND REGULAR COMPLETE (D) TRANSPOSITION.—These may be looked on as a group from the standpoint of pathogenesis. In all of these, one may postulate an abnormal absorption of the bulbotruncal area into the ventricles. This abnormality may be related to the abnormal formation of the bulbotruncal area in the formation of the bulboventricular loop and associated abnormal bulbotruncal ridge formation later. Or the bulbotruncal ridges may be abnormally formed primarily. Or there may be an abnormality in the process of absorption itself related to lack of resorption of the bulboventricular flange or some other unknown factor. Tetralogy of Fallot may be considered to be a mild form of such an anomaly and double outlet right ventricle with subaortic VSD a more severe form. In the case of double outlet right ventricle with subpulmonic VSD and in complete transposition, we may have partial or complete reversal of bulbus absorption into the ventricles.

The associated VSD, when present in these anomalies, represents an associated abnormality in the proximal bulbar septum. We do not know the pathogenesis of pulmonary stenosis in these anomalies.

TRUNCUS ARTERIOSUS COMMUNIS.—Here we are dealing with a lack of growth of the aorticopulmonary septum from the spurs between the 4th and 6th aortic arches, so that these spurs do not reach distal bulbar swellings 1 and 3. This is associated with abnormal incorporation of the bulbus into the ventricles and the lack of fusion of the distal bulbar swellings. It is possible that the lack of fusion of these swellings is related to the lack of approximation of the aorticopulmonary spurs to these swellings.

ISOLATED ATRIAL SEPTAL DEFECT.—In the *fossa ovalis or secundum type of ASD* there is either an abnormality in formation of the septum primum, whereby it becomes fragmented, or an abnormally wide formation of the septum secundum, whereby the two atrial septa cannot become properly approximated. We do not know whether abnormal currents from the sinus venosus or the inferior vena cava are related to this abnormality.

In *persistent ostium primum*, or the primum type of ASD, there apparently is an abnormality in either the formation or metamorphosis of the endocardial cushions. Here, one may postulate incomplete union of the anterior and posterior endocardial cushions on the left side reflected in the cleft of the aortic leaflet of the mitral valve. Since the septum primum meets the endocardial cushions to the left of its center, the endocardial cushions on the left side fail to close the ostium primum.

In the *sinus venosus type of atrial septal defect*, one must recall that the proximal (upstream) part of the atrial septum really is not a true septum but the infolding of the adjacent walls of the sinus venarum (coming from the sinus venosus) and the common pulmonary vein portion of the left atrium.

Defects in this region, therefore, may be related to an abnormality in either the common pulmonary vein or the sinus venosus—or both. Or there may be an abnormality in the absorption of these parts into the respective atria. This usually results in straddling or displaced superior vena cava, right pulmonary veins or inferior vena cava. Of course, one may postulate the reverse. That is, there may be primarily an abnormal entry of any of the above veins, resulting in a defect in the proximal (upstream) part of the atrial septum.

COMMON AV ORIFICE (CANAL)—COMPLETE AND INTERMEDIATE TYPES.—Here there is complete or almost complete lack of union of the anterior (superior) and posterior (inferior) endocardial cushions, thus producing one common opening for the tricuspid and mitral orifices. Because of the lack of union, no tissue is sent up from these cushions to close the foramen primum and none is sent down to close the interventricular foramen.

ISOLATED VENTRICULAR SEPTAL DEFECT.—Subaortic ventricular septal defects, which are located anterior to and sometimes involve the adjacent anterior part of the pars membranacea, may represent a lack of amalgamation of the main components of the ventricular septum—the posterior (inferior) main ventricular septum, the fused endocardial cushions and the proximal bulbar septum. Any one of these components may be defective, leading to such a lack of fusion. When the bulbar component is most defective, we have the usual type of ventricular septal defect. When the endocardial cushion component is defective, we may have a common AV canal type of ventricular septal defect or a defect within the pars membranacea or a left ventricular-right atrial type of ventricular septal defect. Where there is a defect within the upper part of the bulbar septum, we may have the high defect of Taussig with or without straddling of the pulmonary trunk. Where the straddling is marked there may be an incomplete double outlet left ventricle.

Since the junction of the bulbar septum and the main ventricular septum is wide, defects in the junction of these two septa may extend between the sinus and infundibulum of the ventricle from the anterior wall to the posterior wall.

Defects within the posterior septum itself may occur. There is no ready embryologic explanation of these defects. One may postulate that in the formation of this component of the ventricular septum by the infolding of the adjacent walls of the pro- and meta-ampulla, the loose trabecular arrangement of the left and right ventricles becomes confluent, producing a Swiss-cheese type of arrangement.

Where ventricular septal defects occur associated with other abnormalities, they may be hemodynamically produced.

ISOLATED AORTICOPULMONARY SEPTAL DEFECT.—Here we usually are dealing with a localized defective fusion of the spurs between the 4th and 6th arches, which form the aorticopulmonary septum. Where the defect is low there may be a lack of fusion of these spurs with the distal bulbar cushions.

ISOLATED PATENT DUCTUS ARTERIOSUS.—We do not know why the ductus remains patent in some cases. The various theories of this patency have been dealt with elsewhere.[33]

ISOLATED PULMONARY STENOSIS.—Where the stenosis is at the valve, the basic anomaly can be conceived to be in the formation of this valve from cushions 1, 2 and 3. We do not know whether there is a basic hemodynamic alteration that leads to both an abnormal valve and secondary stenosis or whether there is a structural abnormality with secondary hemodynamic stress.

In isolated infundibular stenosis we may be dealing with a faulty final incorporation of the bulbotruncal area into the right ventricle.

ISOLATED AORTIC STENOSIS. — In *stenosis at the valve ring*, the abnormally formed aortic valve is related to malformation of the aortic side of bulbar cushions 1 and 3 and of cushion 2, with secondary hemodynamic stresses. Thus, we may have a unicuspid, bicuspid or even an abnormally formed tricuspid valve. In *fibroelastic subaortic stenosis* there probably is faulty incorporation of the left side of the bulbus into the left ventricle. To what extent hemodynamic stresses are a part of this picture is not clear. In *idiopathic hypertrophic subaortic stenosis* there is also a strong possibility that the bulbar absorption is abnormal. One may postulate that the entire septal portion of the bulbus is absorbed in a bizarre way or in an aberrant angle, producng the thickened chaotic picture of the muscle in the basal part of the definitive septum. In *supravalvular aortic stenosis* there is an accentuation of the normal supravalvular ridge for reasons unknown to us. We do not know the cause of the rare form of supravalvular aortic stenosis above the sinus of Valsalva.

TRICUSPID STENOSIS AND ATRESIA. — To understand this entity embryologically, one must recall the vicissitudes of the tricuspid orifice during the various stages of development of the heart. After the junction of the anterior (superior) endocardial and posterior (inferior) endocardial cushions, the tricuspid and mitral orifices are formed. Since in the entity tricuspid stenosis and atresia the mitral orifice is more or less normally formed and there is a central fibrous body, this means that the anterior and posterior endocardial cushions must have fused. Thus, the explanation of the tricuspid stenosis and atresia must lie in the stage of the relatively dorsal and right migration of the atrial canal (during which the tricuspid orifice is forming) and the relatively ventral and leftward migration of the bulbotruncal area. During this migration, the tricuspid orifice fails to grow or becomes obliterated as it enters the right side. Thus, it may occur alone, without abnormalities in the bulbotruncal region (without transposition) or with this abnormality (with tetralogy, double outlet right ventricle or with complete transposition). Some consider tricuspid atresia complexes as a type of single ventricle (see below).

MITRAL STENOSIS AND ATRESIA. — Where these anomalies are associated with hypoplasia of the aortic tract complexes it is best to consider them as secondary hemodynamic consequences of lack of flow into the left side of the heart through the foramen ovale in fetal life. Similarly may be considered the aortic stenosis or atresia associated with these complexes. An alternative explanation might be that we are dealing with a true hypoplasia of part of the 4th arch system producing proximal (upstream) hemodynamic effects in the form of aortic stenosis or atresia with or without mitral stenosis or atresia. A third possibility exists—that there is an accentuated migration of the atrial canal posteriorly and to the right during the absorption of the bulbus. Of course, not to be forgotten is the possibility that we are dealing with fetal endocarditis of the aortic and mitral valves due to a virus.

COARCTATION OF THE AORTA. — Fetal (infantile, preductal) coarctation is fundamentally a hypoplasia of the left 4th arch derivatives. Where the isthmus alone is involved, this represents an exaggeration of the normal smallness of this part of the aorta related to lack of flow. The same factor may account for the more proximal extension of the narrowing. It is also possible to construct a pathogenesis based on the lack of blood flow to the left side of the heart in fetal life. In the latter case, this complex and hypoplasia of the aortic tract complex would represent variations of the same hemodynamic theme. The pathogenesis of paraductal (adult, segmental) type of coarctation is obscure. It may be related to the kind produced by the altered relationship of the ductus to the aorta, after birth, or even, in some cases, to the closure of the ductus after birth.

EBSTEIN'S DISEASE. — There are several possible explanations for this disease. One possibility is that Ebstein's disease represents an exaggeration of the normal slightly downward displacement of the tricuspid valve. Another pathogenesis can be constructed on the basis of the shift of the atrial canal and accompanying pro-ampulla to the right and dorsally. Thus, one might theorize that there is faulty fusion of the pro-ampullar component with the meta-ampullar component of the right ventricle, with resultant abnormality in the tricuspid valve and right ventricle.

SINGLE (PRIMITIVE) VENTRICLE. — This anomaly very likely is an abnormality in the shift of the atrial canal. The canal remains completely in the descending limb of the sino-atrio-ventriculo-bulbar loop. On the other hand, the bulbus is absorbed either relatively normally (Holmes heart) or abnormally (with d- or l-transposition, dependent on the loop) (see below).

PERSISTENT LEFT SUPERIOR VENA CAVA. — This results from the retention of the communication of the left precardinal vein with the left common cardinal vein.

ENTRY OF THE PULMONARY VEINS INTO THE SYSTEMIC CIRCUIT. — The following possibilities may occur: the presplanchnic channels in the lung regions, instead of uniting with an outgrowth from the cardiac tube, may effect a union with any of the following: (1) the precardinal veins (entry of the pulmonary veins into the right or the left superior vena cava), (2) the postcardinal, supracardinal or subcardinal veins (entry into the inferior vena cava or azygos), (3) the vitelline-umbilical venous system (entry into the portal vein), (4) the right horn of the sinus venosus (entry into the right atrium) or (5) the transverse horn of the sinus venosus (entry into the coronary sinus).

ABNORMAL AORTIC ARCHES AND BRACHIOCEPHALIC ARTERIES. — In *double aortic arch*, both 4th arches persist in their entirety, keeping their communication with the dorsal aorta. In *right aortic arch with a left diverticulum*, the right 4th arch persists as the aorta whereas the left 4th arch remains only in part as a diverticulum giving off the subclavian. In *right aortic arch with left descending aorta*, the right 4th arch persists and is pulled over by an aberrant left ductus or the left subclavian. Where the *right subclavian arises from the descending aorta* there is a persistence of the right dorsal aorta between the subclavian and the common dorsal aorta, accompanied by atrophy of its proximal portion. The various anomalies of the *left subclavian*, such as *origin from the ductus, from the pulmonary artery* or *from the aorta distal to the ductus,* are related to various stages in arrest in the proximal migration of the subclavian.

ORIGIN OF A CORONARY ARTERY FROM THE PULMONARY TRUNK. — Two possibilities present themselves: (1) either the primordial thickenings of the coronary arteries are laid down on the wrong side of the junction of the aorticopulmonary septum with the distal bulbar cushions or (2) the septum meets those ridges in an aberrant manner.

PREMATURE CLOSURE OR NARROWING OF FORAMEN OVALE. — It is not known whether this is an early, a progressive or a late anomaly in fetal life. In some cases, one may assume that the ostium secundum in the septum primum did not form or was fashioned very small. Here, secondary mitral atresias and ventricular septal defects would form related to altered hemodynamics. In other cases, a small ostium secundum might gradually become smaller and obliterated. This would produce a complex more typical of hypoplasia of the aortic tract complex.

MIXED (DISCORDANT) LEVOCARDIA. — In the usual type (atria normal, ventricles inverted), we are dealing with reversal of the bulboventricular loop. Normally, the bulboventricular loop forms anteriorly and to the right (d-loop). In the usual type of discordant levocardia it forms anteriorly and to the left (l-loop). With this, in the vast majority of cases there is inverted transposition (l-transposition) because the bulbus is absorbed in an aberrant manner. In the rarer type of mixed (discordant) levocardia (atria-situs inversus and ventricles normal), a d-loop is formed in situs inversus viscera. This usually is associated with regular (d-) transposition.

The cause of inverted (l-loops) in levocardia is not known.

Dextrocardia

We do not know the pathogenesis of dextroversion, mirror-image dextrocardia or discordant dextrocardia.

Mesocardia

In an early stage of the embryo (31 mm), the heart is in mesocardia.[34] Therefore, a definitive heart in mesocardia represents an early stage in the development of the heart whether in situs solitus or situs inversus viscera. At present, we do not know why the apex normally goes to the left or to the right.

REFERENCES

1. Tandler, J.: The Development of the Heart, in Keibel, F., and Mall, F. P. (eds.), *Manual of Human Embryology* (Philadelphia: J. B. Lippincott Company, 1912).
2. Waterston, D.: The development of the heart in man, Trans. R. Soc. Edinb., Part II, 52:257, 1918.
3. Davis, C. L.: Development of the human heart from its first appearance to the stage found in embryos of twenty paired somites, Contrib. Embryol. 19:245, 1927.
4. Pernkopf, E., and Wirtinger, W.: Die Transposition der Herzostien — ein Versuch der Erklärung dieser Erscheinung, Z. Anat. 100:563, 1933.
5. Doerr, W.: Morphogenese und Korrelation chirurgisch wichtiger angborener Herzfehler, Ergeb. Chir. Orthop. 36:1, 1950.
6. Goerttler, K.: Entwicklunggeschichte des Herzens, in Bargmann, W., and Doerr, W. (eds.), *Das Herz des Menschen* (Stuttgart: Georg Thieme, 1963).
7. Goerttler, K.: Normale und pathologische Entwicklung des menschlichen Herzens. Heftz, Zwanglose Abhandlungen aus dem Gebiet der Normalen und pathologischen Anatomie, in Bargmann, W., and Doerr, W. (eds.), *Das Herz des Menschen* (Stuttgart: Georg Thieme, 1958)
8. Streeter, G. L.: Developmental horizons in human embryos, Contrib. Embryol. 30:213, 1942.
9. Streeter, G. L.: Developmental horizons in human embryos, Contrib. Embryol. 31:29, 1945.
10. Streeter, G. L.: Developmental horizons in human embryos, Contrib. Embryol. 32:135, 1948.
11. Van Mierop, L. H. S., *et al.*: The anatomy and embryology of endocardial cushion defects, J. Thorac. Cardiovasc. Surg. 43:71, 1962.
12. Van Mierop, L. H. S.: Pathogenesis of transposition complexes. 1. Embryology of the ventricles and great arteries, Am. J. Cardiol. 12:216, 1963.
13. Van Mierop, L. H. S.: In Netter, F. H., The Ciba Collection of Medical Illustrations, Vol. 5, *Heart*, Section 3 (Embryology) (Summit, N. J.: Ciba Pharmaceutical Co., 1969).
14. Goor, D. A., *et al.*: The development of the interventricular septum of the human heart: Correlative morphogenetic study, Chest 58:453, 1970.
15. Goor, D. A., *et al.*: The construncus. 1. Its normal inversion and conus absorption, Circulation 46:375, 1972.
16. Goor, D. A., and Edwards, J. E.: The spectrum of transposition of the great arteries; with specific reference to developmental anatomy of the conus, Circulation 48:406, 1973.
17. Anderson, R. H., *et al.*: Morphogenesis of bulboventricular malformations. 1. Consideration of embryogenesis in the normal heart, Br. Heart J. 36:242, 1974.
18. Odgers, P. N. B.: The formation of the venous valves, the foramen secundum and the septum secundum in the human heart, J. Anat. 69:412, 1934 – 35.
19. Odgers, P. N. B.: The development of the pars membranacea septi in the human heart, J. Anat. 72:247, 1937 – 38.
20. Odgers, P. N. B.: The development of the atrioventricular valves in man, J. Anat. 73:643, 1938 – 39.
21. Walls, E. W.: The development of the specialized conducting tissue of the human heart, J. Anat. 81:93, 1947.
22. Shaner, R. F.: The development of the atrioventricular node, bundle of His, and sino-atrial node in the calf; with a description of a third embryonic node-like structure, Anat. Rec. 44:85, 1929 – 30.
23. Mackenzie, I.: The excitatory and connecting muscular system of the heart (a study in comparative anatomy), 17th Internat. Cong. Med. London, 1913. Section III, General Pathology and Pathologic Anatomy, Section I, Anatomy and Embryology, Discussion no. 1 (London: Oxford University Press).
24. Koch, W.: Über die Bedeutung der Reizbildungsstellen (kartiomotorischen Zentren) des rechten Vorhofes beim Saügetierherzen, Pfluegers Arch. 151:279, 1913. (Quoted by Eyster, J. A. E., and Meek, W. J., The origin and conduction of the heart-beat, Physiol. Rev. 1:1, 1921.)
25. Aschoff, L.: Bericht über die Verhandlungen der XIV. Tangung der Deutschen pathologischen Gesellschaft in Erfolgen Vom 4 – 6, April 10. (Quoted by Eyster, J. A. E., and Meek, W. J., The origin and conduction of the heartbeat, Physiol. Rev. 1:1, 1921.)
26. Patten, B. M.: Initiation and early changes in the character of the heart beat in vertebrate embryos, Physiol. Rev. 29:31, 1949.
27. Anderson, R. H., and Taylor, I. M.: Development of atrioventricular specialized tissue in human heart, Br. Heart J. 34:1205, 1972.
28. Mall, E. P.: On the development of the human heart, Am. J. Anat. 13:249, 1912.
29. Tandler, J.: *Anatomie des Herzens* (Jena: G. Fischer, 1913).
30. Sanabria, T.: Recherches sur la différenciation du tissu nodal et connecteur du coeur des mammifères, Arch. Biol. 47:1, 1936.
31. Field, E. J.: The development of the conducting system in the heart of sheep, Br. Heart J. 13:129, 1951.
32. Wenink, A. C. G.: Development of the human cardiac conduction system, J. Anat. 121:617, 1976.
33. Cassels, D. E.: *The Ductus Arteriosus* (Springfield, Ill.: Charles C Thomas, Publisher, 1973).
34. Licata, R. H.: The human embryonic heart in the ninth week, Am. J. Anat. 94:73, 1954.

50 LANGFORD KIDD / GEORGE A. TRUSLER

Methods of Diagnosis in Congenital Heart Disease

YOU HAVE THREE QUESTIONS TO ANSWER when you see a patient suspected of having congenital heart disease. Is heart disease present? Can you define the defect? How severe is it? These questions are the same whether you face a newborn, a growing child, an adolescent or an adult, for the answers dictate management, prognosis and family counseling. The classic methods of attacking these questions are the well-established tetrad of a careful history, a full and meticulous physical examination, a chest x-ray and a 12-lead electrocardiogram. In the majority of cases, the experienced cardiologist can arrive at an accurate diagnosis and prognosis with these methods alone.

He has available to him, however, a wide variety of tests, both noninvasive and invasive, to confirm, embellish and refine the original diagnosis. These newer tests, in turn, have enriched his skills so that newer clinical diagnoses such as a bicuspid aortic valve, or mitral valve prolapse, now can be made with confidence and accuracy. However, in other more complex lesions, very detailed and accurate anatomic and physiologic studies by cardiac catheterization are vital because of the advances in the ability of the cardiovascular surgeon to tackle these patients' problems.

Even in simple lesions, the diagnosis must be confirmed, severity assessed and other lesions excluded prior to operation. Also necessary is the serial study of patients, once diagnosed, for septal defects and ductuses may close spontaneously, obstructive lesions may develop or become more severe with time, and vascular disease, particularly in the pulmonary circulation, must be detected before it becomes irreversible. Finally, the more recent realization that many survivors of successful cardiac operations have residual problems has underlined the need for almost routine postoperative catheterizations.

Chest X-ray, Electrocardiography, Vectorcardiography

Although the skills of assessment, using these noninvasive techniques, have improved generally, there have been no major steps forward in this area. The Joint Study on the Natural History of Congenital Heart Defects has tested the correlation of many features of patients with aortic and pulmonic stenosis with the peak ventricular pressure measured at cardiac catheterization. Regression equations have been derived that are based only on the loudness of the murmur and simple electrocardiographic measurements and these have been found to be very reliable predictors of severity. The formula for aortic stenosis is LV-Ao gradient (mm Hg) = 13 (murmur score) + Rv6 − 6Qv6 − 9,[1] and for pulmonic stenosis the formula is RV-PA gradient = Rvl + 1.5Sv6 + 15 (murmur score) + mixed score − 30. The mixed score awards points for cyanosis (+25), P2 diminished (+15) or inaudible (+25), QRS axis to right (+10) and inverted T waves in AvF (+35) or vl (+15).[2]

Echocardiography

The use of ultrasound in cardiology is longstanding, with interest early on focused on mitral valve motion. However, echocardiography is of even greater value in congenital heart disease, particularly in identifying the disordered cardiac anatomy of the cyanotic newborn.[5] The technique has become well established and authoritative in some conditions so that, for instance, in hypoplastic left heart syndrome[3] cardiac catheterization no longer is necessary for definitive diagnosis.[7] Similarly, the echo picture is very typical in asymmetric septal hypertrophy.

The echocardiogram in the hands of the experienced pediatric cardiologist is of value in defining the hypoplastic right and left heart syndromes, endocardial cushion defects, tetralogy of Fallot, persistent truncus arteriosus and complete transposition of the great arteries. It can aid in assessing the size of the left-to-right shunt in atrial and ventricular septal defects and the shunt through a patent ductus. This last determination is especially valuable in the premature infant. In nearly all severely premature infants, the ductus is patent; however, when there is a large left-to-right shunt through the ductus, the left atrium dilates and the ratio between its anteroposterior diameter and that of the aorta increases, commonly exceeding 1.3:1. If the ductus closes spontaneously, this ratio quickly regresses to around 1:1.

A further enrichment of this investigative technique is the use of contrast echo techniques.[11] When a liquid is forcibly injected into the circulation, it produces microcavitations whether the fluid is indocyanine green dye, normal saline or the patient's own blood. These microcavitations show up as a dense cloud of echoes in the cardiac chambers in which they appear. Because they are filtered out in one passage of blood through the lungs, the finding of contrast echoes in the left heart following peripheral vein injection indicates right-to-left shunting, and focusing the transducer beam on the left atrium, ventricle or aorta will define at what level the shunt is occurring. We have also found this contrast echo technique to be of great value in the child after operation, to confirm or refute residual shunting.[12] Here, the injection can be alternatively through the central venous pressure line or the left atrial line to define right-to-left or left-to-right shunting, respectively.

Echocardiography can be used to scan the heart in two dimensions, either by using a rapidly oscillating transducer (the sector-scanner device) or by using an array of transducers (the multicrystal device). Both these developments allow the moving heart to be visualized in real time, in either the longitudinal or the transverse plane.

Cardiac Catheterization

Hemodynamic studies and angiocardiography remain the cornerstone of accurate diagnosis and the assessment of severity. Assessment of ventricular function and testing the integrity of the conducting system have become an integral part of routine pediatric cardiovascular diagnostic laboratory function.

In our laboratories, both the arterial and venous cardiac catheters are introduced percutaneously. This is a simple and quick procedure in children and infants down to 5 kg, and with practice and special miniaturized equipment it can be accomplished even in the newborn. Using this technique, loss of peripheral arterial pulses is much less frequent than with the cutdown technique, and subsequent catheterization using the same groin is not made more difficult.

Dye curves, using both forward flow, with venous injection and arterial sampling, and reverse flow, with injections in the left heart and sampling in the right, are used routinely as an estimate of the size of left-to-right or right-to-left shunts, or in purely obstructive lesions for the measurement of cardiac output. Oxygen saturations are routinely measured for Fick principle calculations of flows and shunts, and pressures are recorded from the pulmonary artery wedge position back to the cavae. The left heart can be entered fairly easily across the foramen ovale in infants and small children; if this·is not feasible, the arterial catheter is advanced across the aortic valve in the retrograde approach to the left ventricle. Swan-Ganz and Berman flow-guided balloon catheters have made catheter manipulation much easier in the complex malformed heart.

Pharmacologic Interventions

When there is an obstructive lesion such as aortic or pulmonic stenosis, measuring the gradient across the valve when the cardiac output has been raised, either by isoproterenol infusion or by exercise, frequently is valuable. In the investigation of suspected muscular subaortic stenosis, the gradient may be manipulated by making it either more severe with isoproterenol or less severe with propranolol. The other major pharmacologic procedure in most laboratories is the attempt to lower the raised pulmonary vascular resistance of the Eisenmenger syndrome with oxygen breathing or tolazoline hydrochloride; these two agents seem to have more effect at an altitude such as that in Denver.

Electrophysiology

Complex arrhythmias often can be elucidated by electrophysiologic studies and the recording of intracardiac electrograms. Multipolar catheters can help record the passage of the electrical impulse as it leaves the sinus node, arrives at the low right atrium, reaches the His bundle and enters the Purkinje system. With pacing and timed premature beats, we can study sinoatrial and atrioventricular node function and modify conduction with atropine or other agents. It is also possible to localize the accessory pathways in patients with Wolff-Parkinson-White syndrome. Noninvasively, the use of Holter monitors for 24-hour surveillance of cardiac conduction and ECG recording during exercise stress testing provide valuable supplementary data, and this information helps decide whether to use drugs to control dysrhythmias, to insert a pacemaker or to operate to divide accessory tracts.

Angiocardiography

Selective angiocardiography now is carried out in nearly every child undergoing cardiac catheterization. In most laboratories, filming, after the injection of 1 ml/kg of contrast material into the selected chamber, is done using biplane ciné techniques in the anteroposterior and lateral projections, although filming in right and left anterior obliques throws structures such as the ventricular septum and mitral valve into relief. With new equipment, the definition in these 60 frames per second films is excellent, and the dynamic picture of ventricular function allows one to compute ventricular end-diastolic volumes and ejection fractions. For fine detail, the large film changers at 6 or 12 frames per second are preferred. Special views, such as the head-up projection to see the pulmonary artery and its main branches clearly, may help.

Therapeutic Interventions

The example par excellence of a therapeutic measure as an addition to the diagnostic procedure is the Rashkind balloon atrial septostomy procedure. Since its introduction in 1966,[10] this has become a reliable palliative procedure, not only in complete transposition of the great arteries but in tricuspid and pulmonary atresia, in mitral atresia and in total anomalous pulmonary venous connection.

More recently, the closure of a patent ductus arteriosus and an atrial septal defect by mechanical devices introduced through the catheter have been described but still are in the experimental stage.[9]

The ductus arteriosus, however, has been proved to be amenable to pharmacologic manipulation in the newborn period. E-type prostaglandins infusion will maintain ductal patency for up to 24 hours in newborns with such lesions as pulmonary atresia where the ductus is life maintaining.[8] Conversely, inhibitors of prostaglandins synthesis, such as acetylsalicylic acid and indomethacin, have been demonstrated to close the ductus in newborn premature infants who are in congestive heart failure due to large left-to-right shunts through a patent ductus.[4, 6] These two new developments may be the beginning of new therapeutic fields for aiding the sick newborn with congenital heart disease.

REFERENCES

1. Ellison, R. C., *et al.:* Congenital valvular aortic stenosis: Clinical detection of small pressure gradient, Am. J. Cardiol. 37:757, 1976.
2. Ellison, R. C., *et al.:* Indirect assessment of severity in pulmonary stenosis, Circulation 56:1, 1977.
3. Farooki, Z. Q., *et al.:* Echocardiographic spectrum of the hypoplastic left heart syndrome, Am. J. Cardiol. 38:337, 1976.
4. Friedman, W. F., *et al.:* Pharmacologic closure of patent ductus arteriosus in the premature infant, N. Engl. J. Med. 295:526, 1976.
5. Godman, M. J., Tham, P. L., and Kidd, B. S. L.: Echocardiography in the evaluation of the cyanotic newborn infant, Br. Heart J. 36:154, 1974.
6. Heymann, M. A., *et al.:* Closure of the ductus arteriosus in premature infants by inhibition of prostaglandin synthesis, N. Engl. J. Med. 295:530, 1976.
7. Meyer, R. A.: Umbilical aortogram. Comment, Circulation 54: 347, 1976.
8. Olley, P. M., Coceani, F., and Bodach, E.: E-type prostaglandins: A new emergency therapy for certain cyanotic congenital heart malformations, Circulation 53:728, 1976.

9. Porstman, W., *et al.:* Catheter closure of the patent ductus arteriosus: 62 cases treated without thoracotomy, Radiol. Clin. North Am. 9:202, 1971.
10. Rashkind, W. J., and Miller, W. W.: Creation of an atrial septal defect without thoracotomy: A palliative approach to complete transposition of the great vessels, JAMA 196:991, 1966.
11. Valdez-Cruz, L. M., *et al.:* Echocardiographic detection of right-to-left shunts following peripheral vein injections, Circulation 54:558, 1976.
12. Valdez-Cruz, L. M., *et al.:* Recognition of residual postoperative shunts by contrast echocardiographic techniques, Circulation 55:148, 1977.

51 S. SUBRAMANIAN

Hypothermia and Circulatory Arrest

THE FEASIBILITY AND VALUE of early primary correction of congenital cardiac defects in infants are well established and the results of primary definitive correction reported from various centers[1-4] compare well with the results of staged procedures in the management of symptomatic infants with congenital cardiac defects.

The intraoperative management of the sick infant undergoing cardiac surgery has been greatly facilitated by the use of surface induced deep hypothermia and total cardiocirculatory arrest. In this chapter, I shall present our techniques of intraoperative management of infants undergoing cardiac operations and a brief summary of the results obtained using this method.

HISTORY. — "At Belle Isle in the beginning of the winter 1761–62 I conveyed worms and pieces of meat down the throats of lizards when they were going into winter quarters, keeping them afterwards in a cool place. On opening them at different periods I always found the substances which I had introduced, entire and free from any alteration; sometimes they were in the stomach, at other times they had passed into the intestine, and some of the lizards that were preserved alive voided them towards the spring with but very little alteration of their structure." Thus wrote John Hunter,[5, 6] the famous English surgeon, who first recognized the phenomenon of hibernation, which slows the life process of animals almost down to a halt. The first scientific application of hypothermia, however, was in 1797 by James Currie,[7] who lowered the body temperature of a patient with typhoid fever to 34° C.

The modern chapter on hypothermia as applied to cardiovascular surgery was opened by Bigelow,[8] who suggested the use of mild hypothermia as a means of reducing the metabolic rate during operations on infants with cyanotic cardiac disease. In animal experiments, Bigelow first demonstrated the feasibility of total circulatory arrest under hypothermia. He arrested the circulation completely for 15 minutes in a dog at 20–25° C and the animal fully recovered. In 1953, Lewis and Tauffic[9] first applied this method clinically for the correction of an atrial septal defect, and subsequently Swan[10] presented a series of successful corrections of various congenital cardiac lesions under hypothermia. The frequent occurrence of ventricular fibrillation during cooling, and the limited time (10–15 minutes) available for operation, restricted the use of such hypothermia to relatively simple cardiac defects. The successful application of the pump oxygenator systems developed by Gibbon[11] and others brought to an end the era of moderate total body hypothermia in cardiac surgery.

Extracorporeal cooling with the pump oxygenator and profound (20° C rectal) hypothermia and total circulatory arrest was reported by Sealy[12] in 1959 and, at the same time, Drew and Anderson[13] of England developed the technique of perfusion profound hypothermia, without a mechanical oxygenator, using the patient's own lung as an oxygenator. Despite these advances, problems continued to plague the technique of profound hypothermia—intravascular thrombosis,[14] central nervous system damage[15] and a higher mortality of the pump procedure in small infants. The problems seen in cardiopulmonary bypass were attributed by Morris *et al.*[16] to the nonpulsatile perfusion resulting in an alteration in metabolism, including release of catecholamines, serotonin and angiotensin, and depression in renal function.

In 1963, Horiuchi and associates[17] from Sendai in Japan reported good results with the repair of ventricular septal defects in babies less than 1 year of age using deep hypothermia by the surface cooling technique. Discouraged with the results of two-stage procedures in infants with congenital cardiac disease, the group at the University of Washington[18, 19] began to re-evaluate the technique of surface induced deep hypothermia and total circulatory arrest and achieved deep levels of hypothermia without ventricular fibrillation, providing safe circulatory arrest time of up to 50–60 minutes. The technique was modified by the Kyoto University group to include extracorporeal support during rewarming. The "Kyoto technique" has been used by numerous groups, including Barratt-Boyes,[3] Parenzan,[20] Binet,[21] Doty,[22] Mustard[23] and ourselves.[4] This is the technique that, with certain modifications, we have used at the Children's Hospital of Buffalo.

CLINICAL EXPERIENCE. — During the period from April, 1969 to November, 1976, 266 children with congenital heart defects were operated on at the Children's Hospital of Buffalo under profound hypothermia. The youngest was 7 days old and the oldest was 5 years; 170 were under the age of 1 year. Early in our experience, this technique was used in children for whom palliative operation was not available or had failed. Currently, we offer complete corrective operation for all operable congenital cardiac defects regardless of age or weight, and only occasionally perform palliative procedures.

INTRAOPERATIVE TECHNIQUES. — Cardiocirculatory support during intracardiac operations on infants can be obtained by the following methods: (a) conventional cardiopulmonary bypass—normothermic or hypothermic with or without local cardiac cooling; (b) surface induced hypothermia and surface induced rewarming and total cardiocirculatory arrest; (c) extracorporeal cooling total cardiocirculatory arrest and core rewarming; and (d) surface induced cooling, limited cardiopulmonary bypass, circulatory arrest and core rewarming.

Surface induced deep hypothermia with surface induced rewarming has been used extensively by the University of Washington group, but we have found this to be undesirable because the children then are exposed to a prolonged period of low cardiac output. In addition, the rate of rewarming is unpredictable and a long period of manual cardiac massage may be necessary to resuscitate the infant. Our experience with deep hypothermia and circulatory arrest has been limited to the use of surface cooling to 24° C, complete cardiocirculatory arrest for up to 60 minutes and core rewarming with the pump oxygenator.

The "bathtub" method was rapidly superseded by the technique of placing the child on a circulating water blanket, surrounded by crushed ice bags. This was the method used by us in the first 230 patients in our series. The disadvantages were the lack of visual assessment of the infant during cooling and the development of contact skin lesions, such as frostbite of the toes and ear lobes. This led us to develop a more suitable technique of cooling infants by circulating cool air around the exposed infant. The "hypothermia chamber" recently used by us[24] consists of two parts (Fig. 51–1). The lower half is a powerful refrigerating unit with a blower fan to circulate cold air into the transparent, plexiglass upper chamber surrounding the patient, who lies on a circulating water blanket to cool the back. The ambient temperature in the chamber is recorded on a chart paper and the esophageal and rectal temperatures are displayed on a console. The refrigerator is capable of lowering the ambient temperature down to −10° C. Usually, 0 to −5° C is adequate. The advantages of this chamber are self-evident. The chamber enables us to assess the child visually throughout the cooling phase; there are no bulky ice packs compressing the chest and abdomen of the child, and frostbite due to contact skin lesions does not occur. The time spent by paramedical personnel in preparing the child for hypothermia is appreciably shortened. An average 4-kg infant can be cooled from 37° to 25° C in 36 minutes with the chamber (45 sec/kg/1° C) compared to 60 minutes with the water bed (75 sec/kg/1° C). The chamber, therefore, reduces cooling time by nearly half.

ANESTHESIA. — We do not use any preoperative conditioning of the patients such as with fatty acids, advocated by the Kyoto group,[1] nor do we use deep ether anesthesia.[25] Induction is with halothane to 28° C, and anesthesia is maintained with halothane and the infant paralyzed with intermittent succinylcholine or pancuronium. Below 28°, it is not necessary to add any anesthetic to the gas mixture and the patient is maintained on normal ventilation with oxygen. Further use of paralyzing agents usually is unnecessary. The metabolism of curare at low temperatures is considerably delayed and these patients usually return to the ICU paralyzed and many require reversal.

No special adjuncts are used, normal ventilation is maintained, carbon dioxide is not added to the anesthetic mixture and the patient is not hyperventilated as recommended by Mohri.[18] Esophageal and rectal temperatures are monitored. The EEG was monitored in 44 infants and the EEG changes during hypothermia have been reported by us.[26] The hemodynamic effects of hypothermia have been well documented by other workers. These include decrease in cardiac output, decrease in heart rate and changes in ECG. Hemoconcentration occurs as a result of leakage of plasma into the tissues. It is important, therefore, to maintain adequate blood volume in these children to ensure an adequate cardiac output. Increased viscosity is prevented by administering plasma, plasma substitute or low molecular weight dextran, and this is especially relevant in the polycythemic infant. Metabolic acidosis is rare, and life-threatening arrhythmias are unusual. At an esophageal temperature of 25° C, the child is removed from the chamber and placed on the operating table. After thoracotomy, cardiopulmonary bypass is established with a single right atrial catheter and arterial return to the ascending aorta. Prior to total circulatory arrest, it is important to ligate a patent ductus arteriosus even if it is very small, because, during complete arrest, air may pass from the open right heart via the ductus into the aorta with fatal consequences. We use a Temptrol bubble oxygenator with total nonblood prime. The integral heat exchanger of this oxygenator has been found to be adequate for cooling and rewarming.

At about 18–20° C, the ascending aorta is cross-clamped proximal to the aortic cannula, perfusion is stopped and the

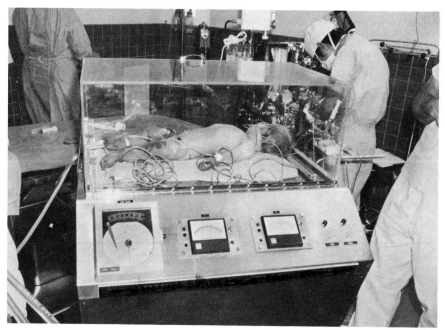

Fig. 51–1.—Hypothermia chamber. The lower half is a refrigerating unit with a blower fan that circulates cold air into the plexiglass chamber above. The patient lies on a circulating water blanket. The ambient temperature is recorded on the chart paper at the left; the esophageal and rectal temperatures are read from the other two dials.

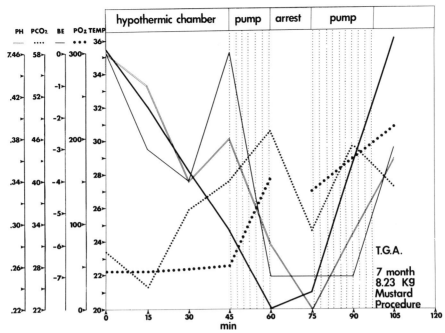

| | | | hypothermic chamber | pump | arrest | pump | |

Fig. 51-2.—Hypothermia and circulatory arrest. Intraoperative course of a child undergoing Mustard procedure for TGA.

patient exsanguinated through the venous cannula into the reservoir. The superior and inferior venae cavae then are occluded. The hemodiluted prime is discarded and replaced with platelet-free packed cells to raise the hematocrit to above 35%. Cardiac arrest is obtained by aortic cross-clamping only. On completion of the operation, the patient is transfused to the extent that he was exsanguinated, the right atrium cannulated again (left atrial appendage is cannulated in transposition) and rewarming is carried out with the pump oxygenator. At an esophageal temperature of 34° C, extracorporeal circulation is discontinued and protamine administered. At this point, fresh-frozen plasma is infused into the patient to compensate for coagulation factor deficiencies that may have occurred during cardiopulmonary bypass. Right and left atrial catheters are inserted for postoperative measurements and a thermodilution cardiac output catheter[27] is introduced via the right atrium through the tricuspid valve into the pulmonary artery (into the aorta in patients with transposition). Atrial and ventricular pacemaker wires are routinely implanted for postoperative management. Figure 51-2 illustrates the intraoperative course of an infant undergoing hypothermic arrest for transposition.

The postoperative care of these infants has been discussed by us extensively elsewhere.[28] This includes fluid restriction, careful and continuous monitoring of all hemodynamic variables (Fig. 51-3) (measurement of cardiac output is with the thermodilution cardiac output catheter and computer) and early administration of inotropic drugs before low cardiac output can become clinically evident. Postoperative pulmonary dysfunction after circulatory arrest has not been a major problem, and this may be attributed to hemodilution, maintenance of plasma protein levels, avoidance of platelets, use of filters in the pump oxygenator and in any postoperative transfusions and the free use of diuretics.

RESULTS.—Table 51-1 illustrates the results at the Buffalo Children's Hospital of intracardiac surgery using deep hypothermia. Of the 266 patients, only 15 were over 2 years

of age and 170 were under 1 year. The over-all mortality rate was 23%, and the mortality rate for those under 1 year of age was also 23%. The largest single group of lesions operated on was TGA, both simple and complex, which amounted to 46% of the total. The other large group of patients, listed as miscellaneous (18% of total), includes a variety of complex lesions, the operability of some being doubtful. Isolated ventricular septal defect, tetralogy of Fallot and total anomalous pulmonary venous drainage complete the list. Results in the simple TGA group have been uniformly good (10% mortality rate), and this seems to be a widespread experience. The complex TGA group, however, presents a different picture. When we carried out primary intracardiac correction in patients with TGA and VSD complicated by uncontrolled heart failure, the results were poor. The results in the same group, when the failure was controlled and operation done more electively by 6 months of age, are comparable to those in simple TGA. Similar results by others make us believe that perhaps in infants with TGA plus VSD and with failure, the two-stage approach in the very young infant (under 3 months of age) may provide a greater salvage. Results of banding of the pulmonary artery in TGA followed by debanding and correction are, however, not available. Our own experience of debanding of the pulmonary artery in TGA indicates that this is a relatively benign procedure. In the group of TGA complicated by left ventricular outflow tract obstruction, the results again fall in two groups. When the outflow tract obstruction is discrete, either at valvular or subvalvular level, primary intracardiac operation could be undertaken as in simple TGA with satisfactory results. When the outflow tract obstruction was caused by a long fibromuscular tunnel, the results were dismal, and we believe, therefore, that these patients should be offered a systemic to pulmonary artery shunt, followed by a Rastelli operation at 4 or 5 years of age. The results of operation for isolated VSD, as one would expect, have been very satisfactory. The cumulative death rate connected with the two-stage approach to VSD amounts to 25%. In view of the data presented here

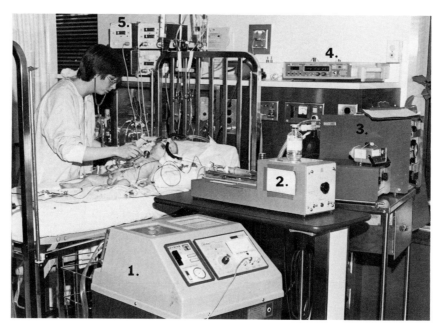

Fig. 51–3.—Postoperative intensive care monitoring of an infant after corrective surgery for tetralogy of Fallot. *1*, hypothermia machine. *2*, Harvard constant infusion syringe pump. *3*, Bourns ventilator. *4*, thermodilution cardiac output computer. *5*, three-channel monitor with alarm.

(5% mortality), we recommend primary intracardiac repair for VSD.

According to the mode of presentation at the hospital, these children are divided into four groups (Fig. 51–4): group A—emergency, failure of medical treatment; group B—elective, primary correction; group C—emergency, failure of palliation; group D—elective, after palliation.

It is clear from this figure that when operation was undertaken as an emergency measure on account of failure of medical treatment or failure of previous palliation, the mortality rate was consistently high and when undertaken electively to prevent the unfavorable natural history of the disease, the mortality rate was nearly nil.

CONCLUSIONS.—The enthusiasm generated by early reports of success with primary definitive intracardiac procedures in infants in heart failure from congenital cardiac disease has been sustained. The results obtained to date indicate that when operation is carried out in the extremely ill infant, the mortality rate is high but still superior to that of staged procedures. When operation is performed electively to prevent complications related to the natural history of the disease, the results of operation are excellent. There probably still is a place for two-stage procedures in selected lesions, complex TGA and a selected group of infants with te-

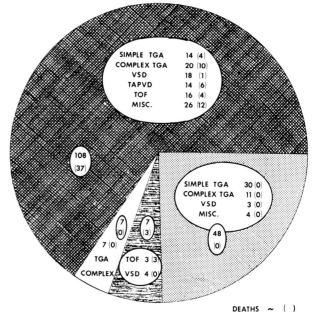

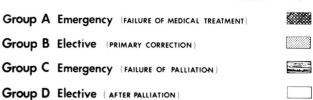

Group A Emergency (FAILURE OF MEDICAL TREATMENT)

Group B Elective (PRIMARY CORRECTION)

Group C Emergency (FAILURE OF PALLIATION)

Group D Elective (AFTER PALLIATION)

Fig. 51–4.—Open heart surgery in the first year of life—170 patients. Experience at Children's Hospital of Buffalo with cardiac surgery under hypothermia and circulatory arrest.

TABLE 51–1.—DEEP HYPOTHERMIA

	ALL AGES		<1 YEAR	
	Total	Deaths	Total	Deaths
TGA—simple	63	5	44	4
TGA—complex	59	19	38	10
Isolated VSD	40	2	25	1
Tetralogy	40	7	19	7
TAPVD	15	6	14	6
Miscellaneous	49	22	30	12
TOTALS	266	61	170	40

TGA = transposition of the great arteries; VSD = ventricular septal defect; TAPVD = total anomalous pulmonary venous drainage.

tralogy of Fallot. With the exception of these lesions, early one-stage correction of all operable symptomatic heart defects in infants is recommended.

Profound hypothermia with circulatory arrest greatly facilitated the operative manipulation and postoperative management. The experience at centers around the world with deep hypothermia and total circulatory arrest exceeds 1000 clinical cases. The advantages of this technique have been the availability of a clear bloodless field and absence of intracardiac cannulae, thus facilitating complete correction of difficult lesions and a completely relaxed heart. Total circulatory arrest with hypothermia also offers a myocardial protection that may be supplemented by local cooling and infusion of cardioplegic solutions into the root of the aorta. Most intracardiac procedures can be completed during the safe arrest period of 60 minutes, but the availability of the pump oxygenator permits more than one period of arrest. The early fears that brain damage might complicate total circulatory arrest have been dispelled. There have been no neurologic complications in the last 100 patients in this series. Our follow-up studies on an unselected group of patients[28] have shown clearly that when the technique was applied carefully with strict attention to detail, late neurologic and psychomotor complications were virtually nil. The IQ of these children falls within the normal distribution curve of a comparable group of children without heart disease. In view of these late follow-up findings, we believe that deep hypothermia and cardiocirculatory arrest is a safe technique for handling infants undergoing open intracardiac operations.

REFERENCES

1. Mori, A., Muraoka, R., *et al.*: Deep hypothermia combined with cardiopulmonary bypass for cardiac surgery in neonates and infants, J. Thorac. Cardiovasc. Surg. 64:422, 1972.
2. Hikasa, Y., Shirotani, H., *et al.*: Open heart surgery in infants with an aid of hypothermia anesthesia, Arch. Jpn. Chir. 36:495, 1967.
3. Barratt-Boyes, B. G., *et al.*: Intracardiac surgery in neonates and infants using deep hypothermia with surface cooling and limited cardiopulmonary bypass, Circulation 43 & 44 (Supp. I):25, 1971.
4. Venugopal, P., *et al.*: Early correction of congenital heart disease with surface induced deep hypothermia and circulatory arrest, J. Thorac. Cardiovasc. Surg. 66:375, 1973.
5. Gloyne, S. R.: *John Hunter* (Edinburgh: E. & S. Livingstone, Ltd., 1950).
6. Kobler, J.: *The Reluctant Surgeon—A Biography of John Hunter* (Garden City, N. Y.: Doubleday & Co., Inc., 1960).
7. Currie, J.: Medical reports on the effects of water, cold and warm as a remedy in fever and other diseases whether applied to the surface of the body or used internally. 1st ed., Cadell & Davis, 1797.
8. Bigelow, W. G., *et al.*: Hypothermia: Its possible role in cardiac surgery; an investigation of factors governing survival in dogs at low body temperatures, Ann. Surg. 132:849, 1950.
9. Lewis, F. J., and Tauffic, M.: Closure of atrial septal defects with aid of hypothermia: Experimental accomplishments and the report of one successful case, Surgery 33:52, 1953.
10. Swan, H., *et al.*: Hypothermia in surgery, analysis of 100 clinical cases, Ann. Surg. 142:382, 1955.
11. Gibbon, J. H., Jr.: Artificial maintenance of circulation during experimental occlusion of pulmonary artery, Arch. Surg. 34:1105, 1937.
12. Sealy, W. C., *et al.*: Hypothermia and extracorporeal circulation for open heart surgery. Its simplification with a heat exchanger for rapid cooling and rewarming, Ann. Surg. 150:627, 1959.
13. Drew, C. E., and Anderson, I. M.: Profound hypothermia in cardiac surgery. Report of three cases, Lancet 1:748, 1959.
14. Gelin, L.-E., and Lofstrom, B.: A preliminary study on peripheral circulation during deep hypothermia: Observations on decreased suspension stability of blood and its prevention, Acta Chir. Scand. 108:402, 1955.
15. Bjork, V. O.: An effective blood heat exchanger for deep hypothermia in association with extracorporeal circulation but excluding the oxygenator, J. Thorac. Cardiovasc. Surg. 40:237, 1960.
16. Morris, R. E., *et al.*: Nonpulsatile blood flow as a cause of metabolic changes in cardiopulmonary bypass (abstract), A.M.A. 117th Annual Convention, p. 17, 1968.
17. Horiuchi, T., *et al.*: Radical operation for ventricular septal defect in infancy, J. Thorac. Cardiovasc. Surg. 46:180, 1963.
18. Mohri, H., *et al.*: Use of rheomacrodex and hyperventilation in prolonged circulatory arrest under deep hypothermia induced by surface cooling. Method for open heart surgery in infants, Am. J. Surg. 112:241, 1966.
19. Dillard, D. H., *et al.*: Correction of total anomalous pulmonary venous drainage in infancy utilizing deep hypothermia with total circulatory arrest, Circulation 35 & 36 (Supp. I):I-105, 1967.
20. Parenzan, L.: Personal communication.
21. Weiss, M., *et al.*: A study of the electroencephalogram during surgery with deep hypothermia and circulatory arrest in infants, J. Thorac. Cardiovasc. Surg. 70:316, 1975.
22. Brunberg, J. A., *et al.*: Central nervous system consequences in infants of cardiac surgery using deep hypothermia and circulatory arrest, Circulation 49 & 50 (Supp. II):II-60, 1974.
23. Bailey, L. L., *et al.*: Surgical management of congenital cardiovascular anomalies with the use of profound hypothermia and circulatory arrest: Analysis of 180 consecutive cases, J. Thorac. Cardiovasc. Surg. 71:485, 1976.
24. Vidne, B. A., and Subramanian, S.: Surface induced profound hypothermia in infant cardiac operations: A new system, Ann. Thorac. Surg. 22:572, 1976.
25. Dillard, D. H., *et al.*: Correction of heart disease in infancy utilizing deep hypothermia and total circulatory arrest, J. Thorac. Cardiovasc. Surg. 61:64, 1971.
26. Olszowka, J., *et al.*: EEG and neurological correlates of deep hypothermia and circulatory arrest in infants, Ann. Thorac. Surg. (In press.)
27. Alfieri, O., *et al.*: Thermodilution cardiac output measurement in infants and small children following intracardiac surgery, J. Pediatr. Surg. 10:649, 1975.
28. Subramanian, S., *et al.*: Sequelae of Profound Hypothermia and Cardiocirculatory Arrest in Infants and Small Children, in Kidd, B. S. L., and Rowe, R. D. (eds.), *The Child with Congenital Heart Disease after Surgery* (Mount Kisco, N. Y.: Futura Publishing Company, Inc., 1976).

52 EOIN ABERDEEN

The Care of Infants and Children after Heart Operations

IN THE BEST of the congenital heart units over the past 15 years, more than 99% of children have survived the correction of certain uncomplicated intracardiac defects. These high survival rates have been achieved in an increasing number of centers in more recent years. The best survival rates following correction of the more complicated lesions such as Fallot's anomaly and transposition of the great arteries have also increased to 95% or better, and, in a few units, survival rates in infants having certain open heart operations have risen to better than 95%.

All good centers, perforce, have high standards of cardiology, of operative skills and of postoperative care. Usually, if the operation goes well, so goes the postoperative course, but success is not inevitable, so skilled and dedicated postoperative care should be available for every case. At least 1 nurse must be in attendance for every minute of the first 24 hours or longer (and that requires a staffing ratio of 5 nurses for 1 ICU bed) and at least 1 experienced resident physician must be available at any time around the clock (and that requires a team of at least 3 residents to ensure that 1 always will be instantly available to the ICU).

Preoperative Care

The emphasis of the 2 or 3 days in the hospital before operation is not only to complete all laboratory procedures required but to try to win the friendly confidence of the patient. Any apparatus or procedure that may intrude on the child's awareness after operation should be explained adequately before the day of operation. A careful explanation to the parents will not only help to allay their very reasonable fears but will also help them to explain more adequately to the child why an operation is necessary and what the child should expect.[128] Those counseling the parents of a child with a major congenital abnormality should be aware of the guilt feelings with which even the most rational of parents may be tormented.[108]

Postoperative Care

The care of children after heart operations has been steadily improved over more than 30 years, but two aspects of postoperative care have been the most important: one is the management of pulmonary insufficiency and the other is the management of low cardiac output. If the heart and the lungs perform well after operation, few other problems will prove insuperable.

The need for, and the techniques of, measuring cardiac output have been one of the special contributions of Dr. John Kirklin and his colleagues. A careful bedside clinical assessment of the patient is important, as important after major cardiac operations as it is after any other major operation, but the relationship of the clinical state to cardiac output has been slowly recognized, and only in recent years has it been possible to measure cardiac output frequently and reliably in infants and children.[81, 137]

Cardiac Output

The clinical estimate of cardiac output can be deceptive. Warm extremities of a good color and a good urine output in an alert, conscious patient strongly suggest that the circulatory volume is adequate. Systolic blood pressure is defended by the body almost to the bitter end; therefore, blood pressure is one of the least reliable indicators that blood volume and cardiac output are adequate. If the patient is pale and apprehensive or comatose, if the extremities are cold and urine output is low, cardiac output probably is inadequate and if hypotension should be present, the cardiac output may be dangerously low. If the cardiac output may be inadequate, it should be measured. The range of a normal cardiac output is about 2.5–4.4 l/m² of body surface/min, with a mean of about 3.5, and this "cardiac index" (CI) is the most widely used measurement for defining cardiac output, even though the use of surface area as a reference constant is not ideal in the early months and years of life. A cardiac index of 2.5 begins to be worrisome and a CI of 2.2 or 2.0 becomes a cause for concern.[16, 65, 68] If the CI is as low as 1.0 or less, survival becomes unlikely.[91] The cardiac index, however, is significantly less (about 20%) after operation in infants in the first months of life than it is in older children.[124]

Many attempts have been made to estimate both the cardiac output and the blood volume from bedside measurements. The criteria that have been used have been blood pressure, pulse rate, central venous pressure, changes in body weight, urine output, the arteriovenous oxygen saturation gradient across the systemic circulation, renal function and brain function, but none has been found to be sufficiently reliable, and if the question of low cardiac output arises there is no adequate substitute for its measurement, either by the use of dye dilution or thermodilution. The use of an electromagnetic flowmeter with a flexible head to measure cardiac output has not yet become clinically reliable.

If, after operation, a low cardiac output becomes a problem, the possible cause should be sought immediately and corrected. Usually the cardiac output is low because the heart is not contracting adequately. This basic problem may result from the heart failure present before operation, from the damage to myocardial function caused by the techniques of "myocardial preservation" used during operation or from the operation itself. Effective therapy to change the metabolic function of the myocardium is limited, but often much can be done to change the mechanical function.

The five principal cardiac factors that control cardiac output are:

1. Ventricular filling pressure (pre-load).
2. Chamber compliance or distensibility.
3. Myocardial contractility.
4. Heart rate.
5. Resistance to outflow (after-load).

After operation, we can readily control (1) ventricular filling pressure and (4) heart rate. We have some control over (5) resistance to outflow (after-load) and we can have some effect on (3) contractility, but we cannot affect (2) myocardial compliance.

A series of questions should be asked if low cardiac output is a problem.

1. *Blood volume.* Should blood, colloid or other fluids be given intravenously?

2. *Ventilation.* What are the blood gases?

3. *Acid-base balance.* What is the pH and base deficit or excess?

4. *Dysrhythmias.* Is the heart rate too slow or too fast? Is sinus conduction present?

5. *Tamponade.* Are the CI and arterial pressure falling? Are the atrial and venous pressures increasing?

6. *Other reasons* for low cardiac output, e.g., myocardial performance (including contractility and distensibility) and increased vascular resistance, either systemic or pulmonary.

Other decisions about treatment must be taken promptly once the cause has been considered, and three effective possibilities are available:

1. Are *positive inotropic* drugs needed?
2. Should the vascular resistance, systemic and/or pulmonary, be reduced?
3. Is mechanical cardiac assistance required?

1. Blood Volume and Transfusion

In the decade before open heart surgery, the need to replace blood loss had been increasingly appreciated, and techniques were developed to measure the amount of blood lost in the operating room,[22] but careful measurement of blood loss showed that it often was greatly underestimated[26] and led to the suggestion that part of the illness of trauma was, in fact, the illness of inadequate blood replacement.

Measurements of blood volume in children after cardiopulmonary bypass were reported by many centers[8, 13, 24, 27, 46, 65, 75] and, in these many hundreds of cases studied, almost every case was reported as having a postoperative blood volume less than the preoperative blood volume. Increasing the blood volume by transfusion had been shown, in many cases, to produce a dramatic increase in cardiac output of one-third or more.[11, 66, 69] The value of maintaining an adequate blood volume to achieve an adequate cardiac output has been emphasized repeatedly.

Simple measurement of the blood volume seemed to be the answer, but the variations in individuals of the same body weight and length are so wide as to make a single reading too inaccurate[24] and even when the blood volume was measured before operation, it was found that making the *post*operative blood volume equal to the *pre*operative blood volume sometimes produced unexpected pulmonary venous hypertension and pulmonary edema. Not only do the systemic vascular resistance and the pulmonary vascular resistance change during and after operation but venous tone increases,[104] the fluid compartments of the body may change in opposite directions and the metabolic rate may also change.[117]

If the blood volume is to be held at a level that will give the best cardiac output but will not cause pulmonary edema,

measuring the left atrial pressure is necessary. This pressure may be measured most accurately during and after operation via a cannula placed in the left atrium. It may also be measured by a balloon catheter placed in one pulmonary artery, or it may be assessed by measuring the right atrial pressure and guessing that the left atrial pressure bears a constant relationship to the right. However, the difference in pressure between the two atria does not remain constant even over a few hours. In low-risk patients having a good cardiac index postoperatively, the atrial pressures may be kept relatively low (about 7 torr) and then the gradient between them is unimportant. However, in higher-risk patients in whom the cardiac output might be a cause for concern after operation, measuring the pressure in each atrium becomes essential for optimal management. Knowledge of the difference in pressures that have been measured in various postoperative states may be of value. The clinical measurement of jugular venous pressures does not give an accurate enough assessment of central venous pressure,[35] and pressure in limb veins has even less relation to central venous pressure.

1.A. THE DIFFERENCE IN PRESSURE BETWEEN THE TWO ATRIA AFTER OPERATION.—As with so many other important measurements, Kirklin and his colleagues first recognized the need for monitoring pressures in both atria, and they published a vast amount of carefully recorded clinical data showing the relationship of right atrial to left atrial pressure after cardiac operations.

1.A.a. *Atrial septal defect.*—In all cases with a left-to-right shunt before operation, the left atrial pressure must be at least slightly higher than the right, and in one patient series,[94] the difference before operation was 3.5 torr (range 1–8) compared to the gradient between the two atria after operation, which was slightly higher at 4.2 torr (range increased to −1 to +18 torr). The higher gradients were associated with the higher cardiac outputs.[102] A further study[69] suggested that, in some patients, the right ventricle had better distensibility and so had a lower diastolic filling pressure, and perhaps these hearts had the larger pressure gradients between left and right atria after operation.

1.A.b. *Ventricular septal defect.*—After closure of a VSD, the atrial pressures will depend very much on the degree of pulmonary vascular obstructive disease.[12] In all patients having VSD closure, the left atrial pressure was higher than the right before operation, but in those with normal pulmonary vascular resistance, the left and right atrial pressures were very similar a few hours after operation. However, in those with moderate or severe pulmonary vascular obstructive disease, the right atrial pressure usually was greater than the left (range 1–6 torr). When using a transatrial incision, and avoiding a right ventriculotomy, the gradient, as expected, increased (range 3–8 torr).

1.A.c. *Fallot's anomaly.*—The left atrial pressure in most cases was higher than the right in one Mayo series (up to 9 torr) a few hours after operation, but the right atrial pressure was higher than the left (up to 2 torr) in a few cases; yet, 1 day after operation, the difference in the pressures was 3 torr or less.[120] In a further study, Kirklin and Theye[69] showed that there was little difference in the atrial pressure gradient between those having an RV outflow patch and those without, but the differences were over a wide range from −3 to +18 torr.

1.A.d. *Transposition of the great arteries (ventriculo-arterial discordance).*—When the intra-atrial flow has been rearranged by Mustard's operation, the systemic atrial pressure will be reduced if the patch has been so placed as to obstruct the systemic venous return. Presuming that suitable operative techniques can avoid this, the pliable patch would be expected to bulge inward if the pressure in the pulmonary venous atrium exceeded the pressure in the systemic venous atrium, but if the higher pressure were in the systemic venous atrium, the patch would simply balloon outward but still leave an adequate left atrial volume, and so the systemic venous atrial pressure could be higher than the pulmonary, but, in theory, the reverse should be unlikely. In practice, pulmonary atrial pressures a few torr higher than the systemic atrial pressure have been recorded,[92] partly explaining reduced cardiac outputs, but since the survival rate after Mustard's operation for patients with otherwise uncomplicated transposition of the great arteries has been so good, such pulmonary artery-systemic atrial pressure differences cannot be very significant. However, monitoring cannulae should be left in each atrium after operation in all cases, and the pulmonary atrial mean pressure should not exceed 12 torr in the early postoperative period. It is much better to increase the cardiac output with positive inotropes, such as dopamine, epinephrine or isoproterenol, than to push the pulmonary venous atrial pressure higher and so subject the patch to a higher pressure, which may impede systemic venous return (see Chap. 60).

1.A.e. *Total anomalous pulmonary venous drainage (TAPVD).* — This anomaly is as lethal as is TGA for untreated infants; that is, only 10–15% survive to their first birthday without intervention. Paar *et al.*,[95] in studying 9 infants having correction in the first 4 months of life, found that most required catecholamine and mechanical ventilatory support, during which time the LA pressure was kept between 11 and 14 torr ($\overline{13.1} \pm 2.2$) while the RA pressure was a mean of $\overline{8.7} \pm 1.6$ torr, that is, the LA mean pressure was $\overline{4.4}$ torr greater than the right atrial. Not only were the deaths in this series associated with low cardiac outputs (CI $\overline{2.32}$ in the survivors and $\overline{1.27}$ in nonsurvivors) and low mixed venous oxygen saturation (PO_2 $\overline{30.3}$ torr in all cases), but the stroke index was observed to be low (13.21 ml/m²), which is only about one-third the expected normal, but similar to measurements made in other infants after operation for congenital heart disease. Of special note was the observation that phasic pressures in the left atrium varied over a wide range, with a rapid Y descent in early diastole and a rapidly rising V wave in early systole, suggesting that the left atrium did not have an adequate volume to serve as the reservoir that converted continuous to intermittent flow. Even after operative enlargement of the left atrium, the same finding was observed. These data were not compared with preoperative pulmonary artery pressures, but severe pulmonary hypertension (pulmonary pressure 125–200% of the systemic pressure) has been shown to be associated with a much diminished survival in this condition.[9, 50] Perhaps true hypoplasia of the left atrium is associated with severe pulmonary hypertension and pulmonary vein obstruction,[9] but this has not been confirmed as yet.

1.B. REOPERATION FOR POSTOPERATIVE HEMORRHAGE. — Experience has taught that if postoperative bleeding is a problem it nearly always is better to return the patient to the operating room for a repeat thoracotomy — and the sooner the better. Blood drainage from the chest tubes is measured carefully, not as a precise indication of the amount of blood that should be replaced in the patient but so that the *rate* of blood loss can be estimated. Usually, if the amount of blood loss is steadily diminishing, it indicates that further observation is advisable and that bleeding will cease spontaneously.

Recording the blood loss on a graph chart helps to assess the rate of change. A blood loss of more than 10% of the blood volume in 1 hour, however, is exceeding a safe maximal rate of loss and is an indication to take the patient back to the operating room. Large amounts of blood within the chest are an added reason for reopening, to evacuate the clot.[95]

1.C. HEMATOCRIT LEVELS. — The hematocrit is best kept between 30 and 45. A hematocrit over 45 is associated with increased viscosity, which increases in an exponential manner (a power curve) with the increasing hematocrit, and so requires much more ventricular work.[100] A severely low hematocrit lowers the gas transport efficiency of the blood and also requires increased ventricular work,[51, 126] although the lower viscosity does allow increased flow.

1.D. RIGHT HEART FAILURE. — A residual obstruction of the pulmonary outflow tract would be expected to increase the right atrial pressure. Patients with an increased pulmonary vascular resistance or those who have had large right ventriculotomies, or still have some obstruction to the RV outflow, usually are transfused to a relatively high right atrial pressure (20–25 torr); however, the left atrial pressure should not be taken above 15 torr. This requires separate atrial monitoring lines for patients with pulmonary hypertension. Inserting the left atrial monitor line before the perfusion commences may also help in protecting the lung from unexpected venous hypertension.[41]

1.E. LEFT HEART FAILURE AND PULMONARY EDEMA. — Poor function of the left heart, or operations on the systemic side, should be followed after operation by special emphasis on avoiding pulmonary venous hypertension and alveolar pulmonary edema. Pulmonary edema can be life-threatening, so left-sided failure is much more dangerous than right-sided failure, which usually results only in liver enlargement or ascites or peripheral edema (see later discussion on colloid oncotic pressure).

Interstitial pulmonary edema may increase the extravascular lung water two- or threefold before causing clinical signs.[44] Chest x-rays, therefore, should be taken at least twice daily for at least 3 days after operation in these cases.

SUMMARY OF BLOOD REPLACEMENT. — The left atrial pressure is kept at over 7 torr in any complex case, with an upper limit preferably less than 12 and very rarely greater than 15, and left atrial pressures should be measured in any complex case. If a patient has a low cardiac output, or hypotension with a low left atrial pressure, a rapid transfusion of blood or colloid should be given promptly and it may require a surprisingly large amount (10–15% of the blood volume or more) before the cardiac output and arterial pressure respond adequately.

2. Ventilatory Support

Detail of techniques of ventilatory support is discussed by Downes and Raphaely in Chapter 2. They have themselves contributed much in the management of difficult cases after cardiac operations.

3. Acid-Base Changes and Management

3.A. METABOLIC ACIDOSIS. — Any prolonged period of poor tissue perfusion by the heart or the heart-lung machine may cause metabolic acidosis, but, with good perfusion, acidosis is avoidable[83, 85] even after 4 hours of cardiopulmonary bypass. A mild degree of acidosis (up to 3–4 mEq/l) usually is well tolerated and does not necessarily require correction. Severe degrees of acidosis require correction with a buffer, usually sodium bicarbonate, because severe degrees of acidosis depress cardiac output, reduce cerebral flow and increase pulmonary vascular resistance. The amount required may be calculated by measuring the base excess in the plasma (in mEq/l), multiplying this by the volume of the extracellular fluid, which normally is about 30% of body weight, but in newborns the ECF is 40% of body weight and falls progressively to 30% by age 6 months[119] (Fig. 52–1). A large deficit usually is best corrected in stages by giving half the calculated amount of buffer needed and then reassessing the position with further blood gas measurements.

3.B. METABOLIC ALKALOSIS.—This occurs more often after operation than is generally appreciated and in infants can be a major problem after open heart operations. It is in part the consequence of giving large amounts of buffer to correct the acidosis of bank blood used in the bypass machine. ACD blood has about 30 mEq/l of bicarbonate[53] and 1 blood volume of ACD blood given may produce a transfusion alkalosis.[77] Strongly acid urine precludes excretion of bicarbonate.[53] The postoperative response to injury with increased aldosterone secretion diminishes bicarbonate loss in urine.[86]

This degree of metabolic alkalosis not only decreases cardiac output but may also depress the serum potassium and increase the potassium loss in the urine, thus further increasing the metabolic alkalosis. For very young children, fresh blood taken into heparin without the use of ACD or CPD will avoid the problem of postoperative metabolic alkalosis.[37] The fresh heparinized blood is used for its biochemical rather than its hematologic advantages. If an infant's metabolic alkalosis exceeds +15 mEq/l after open heart surgery, survival is most unlikely. Direct infusion of 0.1 N hydrochloric acid may have a place in treating metabolic alkalosis.[55]

3.C. RESPIRATORY ALKALOSIS.—Overventilation of the patient often produces respiratory alkalosis. In early years, this was thought to be benign, and therefore overventilation was the routine practice to ensure good oxygenation. However, it now is appreciated that hypocarbia may:

a) Decrease cardiac output[98] and coronary flow.[25]

b) Diminish cerebral blood flow.

c) Shift the Hb–O_2 dissociation curve to the left, causing hemoglobin to retain oxygen (Bohr effect).

d) Increase urinary potassium excretion, so making digitalis toxicity more likely.[47]

If overventilation is continued until compensation develops, the buffer base is reduced, but this effect usually is small.[17, 49]

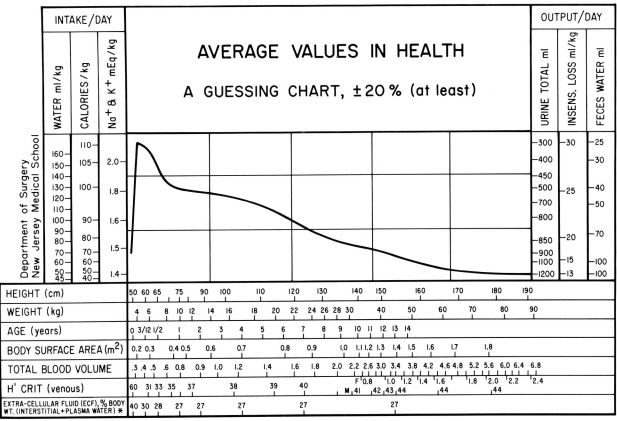

Fig. 52–1.—This chart correlates some of the important physiologic variables. The figures for daily intake, at the left in the chart, represent intake in health at rest. For IV therapy, the water intake is best reduced to 75% of the amount shown, and after major operations should be reduced to 33–40% for 2 days after operation. The daily output figures at the right include urine volume that would be expected when receiving 75% of the water intake shown. The chart is subtitled "Guessing Chart" to emphasize the variability of presumed normals. (Adapted from Aberdeen, E., Lancet 1:1024, 1961.)

3.D. RESPIRATORY ACIDOSIS.—Hypercarbia in lesser degrees (up to 50 torr) need not of itself be a cause for anxiety, and, in infants, a Pco_2 of up to 60 torr may be acceptable over a short period. Usually, a Pco_2 increasing above 50 torr is an indication for assisted ventilation of some type. The Pco_2 must be assessed in association with other data.

4. Dysrhythmias

Some changes in conduction after open heart operations are innocuous and common, but any dysrhythmia should be regarded as a warning signal.

4.A. SINUS TACHYCARDIA.—Sinus tachycardia should not be regarded as an abnormality that of itself may require specific treatment but rather as a clinical sign whose cause should be considered because the *cause* may need treatment. It is commonly caused by postoperative pain and anxiety or fever, but it may also be the first indication of a major complication such as low cardiac output, atelectasis or tamponade. Specific drug therapy rarely is required, but a very fast rate (greater than 160–170/min in a child or greater than 180–190/min in an infant) may reduce the cardiac output enough to cause hypotension.

4.B. JUNCTIONAL RHYTHM (NODAL RHYTHM).—Although not uncommon, and often of little significance in a good-risk patient, a junctional rhythm can mean not only that the ventricle is not having the benefit of a synchronized atrial contraction during the final phase of filling but may also be an early indication of digitalis intoxication, hypoxia, hypercalcemia or hyperkalemia. Slow junctional rhythm in infants early after operation may not be benign and pacing may be required.

4.C. BUNDLE-BRANCH BLOCK.—Right bundle-branch block is a common finding and is to be expected after right ventriculotomy[71] or even operations within the right ventricle that avoid a ventriculotomy.[40] The later development of RBBB may signify a severe ventricular strain. Left bundle-branch block is more serious than right and may be associated with the onset of left heart failure.

4.D. SUPRAVENTRICULAR TACHYCARDIA (PAROXYSMAL ATRIAL TACHYCARDIA, ATRIAL FLUTTER OR FIBRILLATION).—Mechanical stimulation of the vagi may effectively abort the tachycardia to a slower sinus rhythm. Pressure on the carotid sinus may be sufficient but pressure to the eyeballs with the thumb has caused damage to the eye and should be avoided. Atrial pacing may also have a place in some supraventricular tachycardias.[74, 129] Drug therapy usually is wise, and is essential if the tachycardia is producing heart failure. A vasopressor drug may stop the tachycardia promptly. Digoxin is the drug of first choice, but, if not effective, propranolol, diphenylhydantoin, lidocaine or verapamil may be used.

4.E. PREMATURE VENTRICULAR CONTRACTIONS.—Although seen often, premature ventricular contractions should be regarded with suspicion, as they may be the first sign of complications such as hypoxia, electrolyte imbalance or the onset of ventricular tachycardia or even fibrillation. The acid-base state should be checked, digoxin overdose should be considered and if catecholamines are being administered they should be reduced, if that is feasible. Lidocaine nearly always proves effective (1 mg/kg body weight). Propranolol, diphenylhydantoin or, rarely, procainamide may be required.

4.F. VENTRICULAR TACHYCARDIA.—See Section 4.E. The drug therapy is similar. A countershock may give prompt relief if hypotension develops.

4.G. BRADYCARDIA WITH OR WITHOUT HEART BLOCK.—Complete heart block always should raise the question of digitalis overdosage. Sinus bradycardia may be produced by overdosage with narcotics or sedatives or by hypothermia or hypoxia in infants.

4.G.a. *Heart block.*—First degree heart block (widening of P-R interval) is not usually a problem postoperatively. Slow His bundle or idioventricular bradycardia with complete heart block is a very serious abnormality. If the cardiac output remains satisfactory, no treatment may be necessary, especially if the QRS remains narrow (0.12 sec). If the heart rate increases with effort or atropine, it suggests a high level of the block, which is less dangerous.[87] However, a fixed rate of 45/min, or less, with a wide QRS suggests a trifascicular block, which will need permanent pacing. Any slow rate, even if self-limiting and in sinus rhythm and seemingly safe, nevertheless should be carefully observed. Electrical pacing of the heart should be commenced immediately if the cardiac output is low. Drugs that may be useful are atropine, isoproterenol and epinephrine.

4.G.b. *Electronic pacemaker.*—Pacemaker wires (atrial and ventricular) are routinely left in place after operation on all patients whose survival may be significantly at risk, or if any worrying dysrhythmia occurred during operation. Artificial pacing can be given a trial at any time should the cardiac output fall or the ventricular rate become slow. The presence of an atrial and ventricular wire also allows synchronized AV pacing, which may make a significant improvement in cardiac output.[56] Even if the heart is in sinus rhythm at a rate of 85, pacing the rate up to 100–120/min may increase the cardiac output. A demand pacemaker has obvious advantages. The temporary pacemaker wires are inserted into the epicardium and very rarely lead to complications.

5. Tamponade

Tamponade was a terror in the early days of open heart surgery because it could appear so rapidly in a patient who seemed to be doing well, and it could kill so quickly. It is much less common in recent years because of careful hemostasis at operation and perhaps because of the study of blood coagulation before operation, but it still is a complication to be feared in any patient, especially in those who were very cyanosed and had high hematocrits before operation. Even if the pericardium has been left widely open, blood in the mediastinum can surround and compress the venae cavae and pulmonary veins and especially the atria. This may give a widened mediastinal shadow on x-ray, but a wide mediastinum is not necessarily evidence of tamponade.

Compression of the atria restricts their filling and so ventricular output must be diminished severely even if the myocardium is capable of performing well. Tamponade may be suggested by a rapid increase in the central venous pressure or the right atrial pressure, especially if these pressures have been relatively low after operation, and tamponade is also suggested if an increasing pulse rate is accompanied by a falling arterial pressure. The pulmonary artery pressure will not be increased as is the central venous and right atrial pressure, and the finding of an increased right atrial pressure that is equal to the capillary wedge pressure may strongly suggest tamponade.[42, 131] The heart sounds may be poorly heard, an observation especially important if the heart sounds had been easily heard an hour or two before. The venous pressure may be higher in the superior than the inferior cava, causing a suffused appearance of the face and arms. The pulse pressure usually will show a so-called pulsus paradoxus change with respiration in tamponade; that is, a decrease in the systolic blood pressure greater than 10–15 torr with each inspiration.[101] (This is, in fact, an exaggeration of the normal relationship of blood pressure to ventilation, which gives a decrease in the systolic pressure of up to 10 torr with each inspiration.)

If tamponade is clinically apparent, the patient may be only moments from death. Treatment consists of rapid transfusion of blood, perhaps the infusion of catecholamine, but just as urgent is emergency reoperation for evacuation of the hematoma or blood. This reoperation should be performed within seconds or minutes and without procrastination for the full routine of "draping and prepping." The lower portion of the wound can be reopened and two fingers slipped under the sternum to the region of the heart. This may be enough to ease the immediate danger by evacuating the blood that is causing compression.[52, 122] This exploration should be done in the ICU if deterioration is rapid. An exploration that reveals no tamponade is relatively innocuous. The critical effect of tamponade usually is caused by the final 20–25 ml, which increases the pericardial pressure, or the area that a clot is compressing, and removing even a relatively small amount may be lifesaving, because it allows the atria to increase their effective capacity. The clot may not only cause a selective compression but may also make echocardiographic diagnosis more difficult.[109]

Exploration may be performed in the intensive care unit if the patient's deterioration is rapid. The hemothorax or hemopericardium that causes tamponade may also cause pulmonary insufficiency.

Lesser degrees of tamponade may persist for some days and can produce an otherwise unexplained sinus tachycardia. Tamponade may present as a later complication after open heart operation but this is quite rare in children.

6. Other Reasons for Low Cardiac Output

If the causes already discussed (headings 1–5) have been excluded or corrected, and output still is inadequate, it may be improved by positive inotropic drugs. The drugs should not be used to correct hypotension if the cause is hypovolemia or other correctable causes such as dysrhythmia, poor ventilation or tamponade. Cardiac output can be effectively increased by positive inotropes, but increased power requires increased energy and often the drug may have an associated and deleterious effect, either pharmacologically or mechanically, so only the minimal amount of drug necessary to achieve an increased output should be used. A bolus injection of a large amount of a positive inotrope should be used only in a last-ditch emergency. Drugs that raise the blood pressure by increasing peripheral vascular resistance (e.g., metaraminol, Neo-Synephrine and norepinephrine) usually have little place in treatment after cardiac operations.

6.A. CALCIUM.—Since calcium is so important in myocardial contractility, it is not surprising that ionized calcium is a strong inotrope. The citrate of ACD or CPD bank blood has a chelating effect on calcium, decreasing the available ionized portion.[63] Calcium chloride is a better source of ionized calcium than the gluconate or gluceptate salts and

is to be preferred,[132] but must not be given into a peripheral venous line, since its extravasation will cause tissue necrosis. The studies by Lappas et al.[73] suggest that calcium chloride (5 mg/kg) may increase the systemic vascular resistance more than myocardial contractility, especially in low-flow states, an undesirable effect of calcium.

6.B. CATECHOLAMINES.—The most commonly used catecholamines are epinephrine (Adrenalin), isoproterenol (Isoprenaline) and dopamine. Dobutamine, being used increasingly, still is regarded as an experimental drug. All catecholamines must be administered intravenously, into a central vein, to avoid the skin slough that may follow peripheral vein injection.

Catecholamine dosage in children must be expressed as micrograms per kilogram body weight per minute (μg/kg/min), since catecholamines are rapidly inactivated.

The administration of excess water should be prevented by calculating the concentration of the drug required to deliver enough drug but not too much water. Figure 52–2 has been compiled to help decide the concentration of the drug and the rate of administration.

The adrenergic receptor is the site of action of the catecholamines, both the natural amines (epinephrine and dopamine) and structurally related drugs (isoproterenol and dobutamine). The adrenergic receptors respond by (1) increased sinus heart rate, (2) increased force of myocardial contraction (positive inotropism), (3) increased rate of AV conduction, (4) vasoconstriction of most blood vessels and (5) vasodilatation of nutrient blood vessels.[3] The response of different circulations such as coronary, renal, splanchnic, cerebral, muscular and skin may vary one from the other.

Two different kinds of adrenergic receptors are recognized: alpha receptors, which cause vasoconstriction, and beta receptors, which cause cardiac stimulation and vasodilatation. Different catecholamines have different responses. Alpha stimulators such as phenylephrine (Neo-Synephrine), methoxamine and norepinephrine when administered simply increase the peripheral vascular resistance and thus have little place in the treatment of low output syndrome after open heart operations. These alpha stimulants do have a role in the high output failure of septic shock.

Epinephrine (Adrenalin) has both an alpha and a beta stimulant effect, but this varies with the dose, and in dogs it requires more than 1.0 μg/kg/min to increase the systemic vascular resistance.[28] Clinical experience would suggest a similar response in infants and children, in whom the drug has been widely used for its positive inotropic effect.[67] The adverse features of the drug are that it is moderately chronotropic and, in large doses, is a peripheral vasoconstrictor.

Isoproterenol has been widely used and, until recently, had been the drug of first choice for the low output state. It is the most potent beta stimulator of all the catecholamines[3] and has the advantage of dilating the peripheral vasculature. However, it is strongly chronotropic and may increase the heart rate to a degree that will cause hypoxic damage to the subendocardial portion of the left ventricle.[21] All catecholamines, and especially isoproterenol, should be given only in the minimal necessary dose, and often the smaller dose produces the maximal increase of cardiac output.

Dopamine is a naturally occurring precursor of epinephrine and norepinephrine, and has become the drug of first choice in the treatment of low output state in many centers. As a positive inotrope (a beta receptor stimulant), it is of the same level of effectiveness as isoproterenol[62] but does not

DRUGS USED IN LOW OUTPUT STATE - CALCULATION OF DOSE AND CONCENTRATION

TO CALCULATE TOTAL DOSE/MIN AND CONCENTRATION: MULTIPLY BODY WEIGHT (kg) x DESIRED DOSE IN µg/kg/min.
THIS → TOTAL DOSE/MIN — CHECK THIS ON VERTICAL AXIS AT LEFT — THEN LOOK RIGHT TO FIND DESIRED FLUID RATE. FLUID RATE IS
IN ml/hr ON UPPER HORIZONTAL SCALE AND IN ml/min ON LOWER HORIZONTAL SCALE. WHERE THE DESIRED DRUG DOSE AND FLUID
RATE INTERSECT WILL INDICATE THE AMOUNT OF STOCK MIXTURE OF DRUG TO BE MIXED WITH THE DILUENT AND MADE UP TO 100 ml
TO GIVE THE FINAL CONCENTRATION.

Epinephrine 1:1000 1 ml = 1000 µg
Dopamine 1:25 200 mg in 5 ml i.e, 1 ml = 40 mg = 40,000 µg
Isoproterenol 1:5000 1 ml = 0.2 mg = 200 µg
Na Nitroprusside 50 mg in 500 ml = 1:10,000 1 ml = 100 µg/ml

USUAL RANGE AND MAXIMAL DOSE

Epinephrine 0.1 - 0.5 - up to 1.0 or 1.5 µg/kg/min
Dopamine 1.0 - 10.0 - up to 30 µg/kg/min
Isoproterenol 0.01 - 0.2 - up to 0.5 µg/kg/min
Nitroprusside 0.5 - 4.0 - up to 8 µg/kg/min

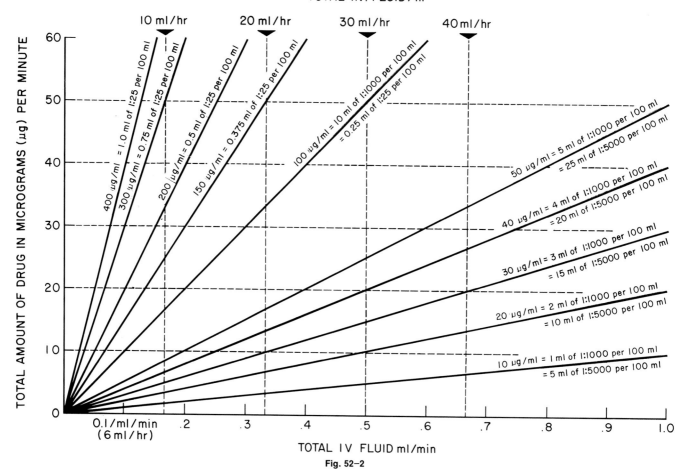

Fig. 52-2

increase heart rate. In the usual doses — up to 10 µg/kg/min — it lowers systemic vascular resistance, although in large doses it becomes a peripheral vasoconstrictor (an alpha stimulant). It acts on specific dopaminergic receptors, and has the great advantage of diminishing renal vascular resistance (in the usual doses), which increases renal blood flow and glomerular filtration rate, and it is the only catecholamine to do this.[105] One study suggests that the increase in renal flow is the only advantage of dopamine over epinephrine.[114]

An undesirable side-effect of catecholamines is the change in the pulmonary circulation as the lungs tend to clear the drug from the circulation, causing arteriovenous shunting in the lungs, which may result in arterial desatura-

tion.[14, 48] Infusion of the drugs into the left rather than the right atrium may help diminish this effect.[82]

A comparison of the positive inotropic effect of digitalis glucoside compared to catecholamines showed catecholamines to be 3 – 4 times more effective,[10] so that digoxin should not be used in the early postoperative phase to treat the low output state because digitalis toxicity can become a great problem at that time.

6.C. PERIPHERAL VASODILATORS. — It now is clear that reducing an increased peripheral vascular resistance does help increase cardiac output and survival after operation in patients who have an increased peripheral vascular resistance. From the early trials of a few years ago,[67] the data clearly establish the value of vasodilators after operation combined with careful control of atrial pressures.[70]

Several vasodilator drugs are available, but it seems that nitroprusside, which acts mainly at arteriolar levels, is the drug of choice at present and is near ideal.[96, 115] It has a rapid but short-lived action, which means that the vasodilator effect can be readily controlled, and it has few side-effects.

Benzing et al.[12] measured the effect in children with a cardiac index after operation of less than 2.0 l/min/m² and a systemic vascular resistance greater than 30 units and found the systemic resistance lowered by 54% and cardiac index increased by 77%, and they suggest that children are more able to change their resistance than are adults. They recommend a dose of nitroprusside between 0.5 and 8 µg/kg/min but not exceeding this level.

Appelbaum et al.[5] observed that only 3 of 21 patients aged 2 weeks to 17 months having intracardiac operations had normal blood pressures after operation, the other 18 having arterial hypertension and increased systemic vascular resistance (a mean of 48 ± 18 units in the study group, while their pulmonary vascular resistance was a mean of 8.6 units). Nitroprusside was given in sufficient amounts to bring the arterial pressure down to normal for that age, a fall of 27%, and this also lowered the pulmonary artery pressure and both atrial pressures by about one-fourth. The dose of nitroprusside was between 2.5 and 12 µg/kg/min and this was associated with a 17% increase in the cardiac index. The atrial pressures then were raised to their previous levels by expanding the blood volume, and the cardiac index increased to 141 ± 21% of the control level. The systemic resistance had fallen to 53% and the pulmonary vascular resistance to 38% of control values, changes that were highly desirable.

Side-effects that have been recorded include an increase in arteriovenous shunting in the lungs, which appeared to be dose related,[20] and the development of methemoglobinemia.[15]

Fluid Therapy

The optimal amount of water and electrolytes is simpler to calculate after cardiac operations than after general surgical operations because fewer choices are available for the patient having cardiopulmonary bypass.

After general operations, if heart function was normal before operation, one of several options can be chosen. These choices reflect the increasing knowledge of the illness of trauma gained over the past four decades.

Following the detailed analyses by Cuthbertson and by Moore and his colleagues, the principal changes in renal function were recognized to be the reduction in urine volume and the change in electrolyte excretion, especially the severe reduction in sodium and the increase in potassium. At the time that open heart operations were becoming routine, it was questioned whether the observed changes of the illness of trauma were desirable and were, in part at least, perhaps avoidable. Clarke and his colleagues[26] in England in the early 1950s measured blood volume and red cell mass changes after trauma and demonstrated that many of the severe changes (such as a urine Na/K ratio <1.0) were more the result of inadequate blood volume replacement than the effect of injury per se.[123] Studies by Hayes and colleagues[58] at New Haven in the later 1950s also demonstrated that part of the illness of trauma was the effect of fasting before operation, and that if water and sodium were given before and during operation, the postoperative severe reduction in urine sodium could be avoided. However, they found that giving extra sodium resulted in an over-all net gain of body sodium, even though urine sodium excretion was increased. When Shires and his colleagues[110] reported in 1961 and later that the measured sulfate space (i.e., extracellular fluid volume) was diminished by up to 28% during operation, this seemed to provide good reason for giving relatively large amounts of water and salt during operation. In one leading surgical center, the amount of water given during operations was increased fourfold, and the amount of sodium given intravenously increased elevenfold during this period,[106] but the development of pulmonary edema in some patients[64, 106] led to a reassessment of the technique of measurement of ECF and showed that the loss during operation was not nearly as large as had been assessed by Shires et al.[106, 111, 127] and, indeed, sometimes ECF was increased after noncardiac operations.[31, 36, 103, 106]

Measurements of ECF space after cardiac operations (open and closed) all showed an increase of ECF volume in the range of 5–33%[7, 8, 19, 27, 29, 89] and, as mentioned previously, the red cell mass and blood volume were consistently lowered.

Not only is the extracellular fluid volume increased after cardiac operations using cardiopulmonary bypass, but the kidney's ability to eliminate water and salt is severely limited because the kidney is forced into a nearly maximal concentration of solute load by the ADH and aldosterone response to such major operations and hemodynamic changes. The studies by Sturtz et al.[118] showed the solute concentration of urine after cardiac operations to be about 1 ml of urine per mOsm of solute (1000 mOsm/l), which is the same concentration that Hayes et al.[58] measured after major noncardiac operations. This leaves the patient unable to defend himself against excessive water or salt administration. In the early postoperative phase it is common to find some plasma hypo-osmolarity with hyponatremia developing over the first 2 or 3 days after operation,[118] even if water intake is severely restricted.[38] But measurement of total body sodium has shown total sodium to be increased,[19, 36, 88] so the hyponatremia is either dilutional or the result of intracellular sodium shift[34] rather than the result of a deficit of sodium. Thus, the management is not to give additional sodium but to allow or encourage water loss, and so increase plasma sodium and osmolar concentration. This is especially important in patients with heart failure who can be characterized as having an inability to excrete salt adequately.[18, 23, 90] Likewise, in infants whose ability to excrete salt is also less than a healthy adult's (because the infant kidney is so well suited to the infant's hypo-osmolar intake), it is an error to pour salt into the circulation simply because hyponatremia has been observed. If a hyperosmolar prime is used for the perfusion, the postoperative hypo-osmolarity may not occur[34] and a large amount of sodium may be transferred to the cell.[33]

The near shutdown of renal water and salt excretion (less than 10 mEq/l), the reduced urine volume and the near maximal concentration of solute (1 ml/mOsm) that occur after open heart operations in response to the increased ADH and aldosterone concentration can be overridden by a diuretic, either by a solute diuresis, such as is induced by mannitol or by glucose, or by a loop diuretic, such as furosemide or ethacrynic acid. Not only is urine volume increased but so is the concentration and the amount of sodium, so that a sodium deficit then may readily occur after an induced diuresis.

Sodium

A very small amount of sodium is required after operation on a patient with congestive heart failure, or after cardiopulmonary bypass, or after operation in the first months of life, unless sodium excretion has been excessively stimulated by diuretic therapy, which may happen frequently in adults with chronic heart failure but is uncommon in infants requiring heart operations. Even in health, a resting child requires a maximal maintenance intake of sodium of no more than 2 mEq/kg body weight, so, after operation, sodium intake should be less than 1 mEq/kg body weight, and for the first 24 hours after operation it usually is wise to give no sodium. This especially applies to an infant in the first months of life, who in health normally will have a very low sodium intake. Human breast milk is a low-sodium diet (about 7 mEq sodium/l, which is one-twentieth the concentration of sodium in "normal," 0.9%, saline), so a healthy infant taking 165 ml/kg/day of breast milk still is receiving only about 1.2 mEq Na/kg/day. After any major operation in an infant, the sodium intake should be low (no more than one-tenth "normal" saline), and if the infant has had heart failure (and is likely to have retained sodium chloride), a zero intake of sodium chloride is wise in the early postoperative period.

However, a severely premature infant (usually having had a patent ductus ligation) is an exception because the severely premature is not able to conserve sodium as effectively as a full-term newborn, and, without operation, requires about 3.5 mEq Na/kg/day for sodium balance.[4] Optimal management of the severely premature may require careful measurement of urine volume and daily weighing in addition to measurement of sodium levels in the urine and plasma every 8 hours.[133]

Potassium

Potassium loss is increased by the renal response after cardiopulmonary bypass, and therefore it is wise to add potassium to the IV fluid soon after the operation. The usual concentration is 40 mEq K/l, which is safe provided that the urine volume is above oliguric levels (0.5 ml/kg/hr in infants, 0.4 ml/kg/hr in children and 0.3 ml/kg/hr in adolescents) and also provided that the plasma potassium stays below 5.0 mEq/l. Plasma potassium levels should be measured frequently, and the general rule of keeping plasma potassium above 3.5 mEq/l is a reasonable approach, but it should be recognized that plasma potassium levels between 3.0 and 3.5 are found quite often in children with a low risk after cardiopulmonary bypass, and the low potassium levels can be an indication of good cardiovascular function in these children. High potassium levels may be found in the newborn, and the plasma potassium up to 7 mEq/l may be acceptable in the early days of life.

Dextrose

The calories supplied by 5% dextrose in water (D_5W) are the minimum required to produce the desired reduction of solute load that glucose produces in the fasting state.[49] In the newborn, an increased need for calories is better met by 10% dextrose in water ($D_{10}W$), but this hypertonic concentration of dextrose may cause thrombophlebitis if delivered into a peripheral vein and can cause skin necrosis if extravasated into the subcutaneous tissue, so $D_{10}W$ usually should be delivered through a cannula.

Water

The rate at which water should be administered can be calculated with some accuracy, because the patient really has no options at this time. If the kidney is locked into a maximal concentration phase, insensible loss via skin and respiratory tract are the only other variables to be considered, because usually the water lost in feces and the water gained by oxidizing metabolites are both small amounts and are about equal, so they cancel each other and can be omitted from calculations.

The normal water intake varies greatly, from the relatively high intake of the newborn after the first week of life to the near-adult needs of late adolescence. Various techniques have been tried to give a common reference scale that can be applied at any age, such as referring to a presumed surface area or a presumed calorie intake, but none gives an acceptable constant, so it becomes easier, and is just as accurate, to calculate fluids on a basis of body weight (kg), but still allowing for the difference of age. A healthy newborn takes an average of about 165 ml/kg body wt/day (24 hr). By the age of 1 year, this is down to about 125 ml/kg/day, falling to 100 ml/kg/day at 5 years of age and about 75 ml/kg/day at 10 years and reaches the adult level of 45 ml/kg/day in late adolescence. This water is lost half in urine and half by insensible loss. In infants, the insensible loss is a little greater than the urine loss, but by the adult age the reverse is usual.

For a patient receiving parenteral fluids, the amount should be reduced to three-fourths of these values, but early after a major operation the amount should be only about one-third for the first day, increasing to about 40% for the next 2 days. Sturtz *et al.*[118] made careful measurements in children from 3 to 14 years of age and concluded that water intake should be limited after cardiopulmonary bypass operations to 500 ml/m² for the first 24 hours and 750 ml/m² for 24 hours for the next 2 days. This regimen has been quite widely used. However, in infants, the over-all requirements may be higher.

The insensible loss from the respiratory tract varies with the humidity of the inspired air, and this can cover a wide range in different climates. On a winter day, if the air is at the freezing point, only 5 mg/L of H_2O vapor fully saturates the air whereas at body temperature of 37° C the air requires 44 mg of water vapor for saturation. But the human upper airway functions as a superbly efficient humidifying system and can also retain about 25% of water vapor by cooling the exhaled air to about 32° C.[130] An adolescent breathing a minute volume of about 5L in a severe winter can lose almost 200 mg H_2O/min (about 250 gm H_2O/24 hr) from the respiratory tract whereas the same person on a very humid, hot summer day may lose very little water from the respiratory tract. Likewise, a patient connected to a mechanical ventilator with a good humidifier (and any patient connected to artificial ventilation should be inhaling air that is well humidified at body temperature) will have little insensible loss by the respiratory route.

Insensible loss from skin and lungs normally varies quite widely in individuals of similar age and size[59] and will be increased by fever (and, of course, by sweating), but an additional calculation must be reckoned in a newborn being nursed under a radiant heat shield after PDA ligation.

Williams and Oh[134] measured the insensible loss in full-term newborns and found the insensible loss to be only 0.53 ml/kg/hr (12.7 ml/kg/24 hr) when infants were nursed in an incubator, but the loss doubled in amount to 1.08 ml/kg/hr (26 ml/kg/24 hr) when nursed under a radiant heat warmer.

Wu and Hodgman[135] measured the increased insensible water loss in the severely premature and found that prematures weighing less than 1500 gm lost 3.49 ml/kg/hr (84 ml/kg/24 hr) under an infrared radiant warmer compared with 1.56 ml/kg/hr when nursed in an incubator. Those weighing between 1500 and 2000 gm lost 2.15 ml/kg/hr under radiant heating compared with 0.7 ml/kg/hr (17 ml/kg/24 hr) when nursed in an incubator. This wide difference in insensible loss, between 12.7 ml/kg/24 hr and 84 ml/kg/24 hr, again emphasizes how haphazard any single rule-of-thumb calculation may be. Any calculations must be recognized as starting estimates that must be reviewed and modified, every few hours if need be.

Renal Output

Acute renal failure has been associated with a mortality rate greater than 50% after open heart operations, despite dialysis and other expert treatment.[72] Postoperative renal failure became much less frequent with the use of a diluted bypass prime, which resulted in large urine volumes during and early after bypass.[84] A reduced incidence of renal problems after operations on the abdominal aorta, and in the management of traumatic shock, also emphasized the need to correct oliguria early, before irreversible tubular cortical necrosis occurred.

Powers and colleagues[97] had demonstrated on a dog model that a degree of trauma that led to severe renal damage in almost all control experiments could be made much less damaging by stimulating renal flow with IV mannitol (an osmotic diuretic) soon after the onset of oliguria but could be avoided if the mannitol was used prophylactically and preceded the trauma. Other studies[116] supported the conclusions of Powers on the prevention of renal failure with prophylactic diuresis, and many units have included mannitol in the prime to stimulate urine flow. However, the amount of mannitol should be limited, so that plasma osmolarity is kept close to a normal range (see later). Mannitol, as with other colloid blood volume expanders, will constantly leak from the vascular system and may contribute to pulmonary edema if given in excessive amounts, so loop diuretics such as furosemide (1–2 mg/kg body wt) or ethacrynic acid are used, especially in infants,[76] if urine volume is falling dangerously low, and loop diuretics have also been shown to lower the incidence of postoperative renal failure.[112] Diuretics should not be used if the cardiac output is low, until the usual measures, such as increasing the blood volume, have been taken to increase cardiac output.

The early signs of acute renal failure are an inability of the kidney to excrete both a solute load and water and a failure to retain sodium. The ability to handle solutes can best be judged by comparing urine and plasma osmolarities, and these should be measured every few hours if renal function seems to be a problem. Perhaps the best index of impending renal failure is measured as a reduction in free water clearance, which should be a negative volume.[6, 72] (Free water clearance [C_{H_2O}] in ml/hr is simply a statement of how much plasma has been cleared of solutes and is calculated by subtracting osmolar clearance [C_{osm}] in ml/hr from the urine volume [UV].) ($C_{H_2O} = UV - C_{osm}$.) Osmolar clearance (C_{osm}) is derived from the equation $\dfrac{\text{urine osmolarity}}{\text{plasma osmolarity}} \times UV$, so if the kidney was excreting isosmotic fluid, the free water clearance would be zero, but since the kidney is concentrating the solute load, the free water clearance is a negative number in patients with good renal function after operation.

Falling urine volume is the first danger sign and a urine volume >1.0 ml/kg/hr is desirable. A volume of <0.5 ml/kg/hr in an infant (or <0.4 ml/kg/hr in a child or <0.3 ml/kg/hr in an adolescent) may be reasonably regarded as a significant oliguria and, if continued for more than 2–3 hours despite diuretic therapy, raises concern about renal failure. If the urine osmolarity is >450 mOsm/l (2.5 ml/mOsm) and plasma osmolarity is near normal, a free water clearance of an adequate amount (more negative than −0.3 ml/kg/hr) must be occurring. Other indications of adequate renal performance are $\dfrac{\text{urine osmolarity}}{\text{plasma osmolarity}}$ ratio >1.2 and a urine sodium <10 mEq/l whereas a urine sodium >40 mEq/l suggests a failing renal function.

Established renal failure may be defined in terms of an increasing blood urea nitrogen (>5 times the control value) and an increasing blood creatinine (>2 times the control value),[72] and before this has been reached, consultation should have been had with a nephrologist for consideration of renal dialysis. Dialysis may also greatly help pulmonary failure if pulmonary congestion or edema is partly the result of escaped colloid. As soon as oliguria has been observed for 3 hours despite diuretics, water intake should be recalculated and limited to the insensible water loss plus the measured urine volume. Electrolytes should be limited, potassium usually completely avoided and antibiotic dosage should be reviewed. An IV fluid containing amino acids and hypertonic glucose may be of value,[1] but each detail of treatment should be coordinated with the nephrologist.

Colloid Oncotic Pressure

The Starling equation of capillary function summarizes an essential principle, namely that the balance of hydrostatic pressure and oncotic pressure within and without the capillary determines capillary function, but it is an oversimplification if it does not take into account other factors such as capillary permeability and leakage of colloids, as well as lymphatic flow. Colloid oncotic pressure now can be measured readily, and Weil's group recommend that a regular measurement should be made of the difference between colloid osmotic pressure and pulmonary wedge or left atrial pressure. A gradient of less than 9 torr indicates a significant risk of pulmonary edema.[32]

Changes in colloid oncotic pressure during and after bypass depend largely on the priming solution used in the heart-lung machine. English et al.,[41] using a mixed prime with a hematocrit of 30, found that colloid osmotic pressure fell from a preoperative mean of 29.5 torr to almost 18 torr 30 minutes after bypass had begun, and emphasized that the early fall in colloid osmotic pressure accented the need to avoid episodes of left atrial hypertension, especially at the beginning of the perfusion. The colloid osmotic pressure returned toward normal an hour after bypass but still was only 90% of normal 24 hours after bypass. Marty et al.[80] confirmed a similar range of changes in colloid oncotic pressure, and recorded a linear relationship of colloid oncotic pressure to total plasma protein, but demonstrated no change in postoperative lung function when salt-poor albumin was administered to increase the oncotic pressure. Attempts to manipulate the colloid osmotic pressure should be used with caution, especially in infants. Marty[79] reviewed the dangers of hyperoncotic albumin therapy and, recognizing that the amount of albumin escaping from the circulation varies from 5% per hour in adults to 18% per hour in newborns and that the rate of escape could be tripled by administering concentrated albumin, concluded that "excessive albumin therapy may aggravate rather than aid patients with pulmonary insufficiency."

Hesse *et al.*[60] studied the rate of transcapillary escape of albumin in patients with heart failure and found an increased rate of 8.3 ± 1.6%, but the escape of albumin could be reduced to near the normal 5% by water and sodium restriction, which also reduced the right atrial pressure. So, concentrated albumin probably should not be used, especially in infants and/or patients with heart failure.

Hyperosmolarity

Pediatricians have recognized for the past 10 years that a sudden increase in osmolar concentration (crystalloid concentration) can result in brain damage, which includes cerebral hemorrhage and subarachnoid and subdural hemorrhage. Finberg[43] suggested that the maximal safe rate of change may be no more than 25 mOsm/l over a period of 4 hours. However, changes greater than this must be induced suddenly when bypass is commenced with a hyperosmolar prime. Several centers have reported using a bypass prime with an osmolarity as high as 390 mOsm/l, and seemingly without observed brain damage. So brain damage from hyperosmolarity is an undetermined risk, but perhaps one we should take more note of.

Normal serum osmolarity is 285 ± 8 mOsm/l for adults[78] but is slightly lower in infants, at 278 ± 7 mOsm/l.[107] A dangerous level of hyperosmolarity can be unwittingly reached quite readily by adding various solutes, so osmolarity should be checked every few hours in the early postoperative phase.

Some Important Osmolarities

Sodium chloride 0.9% ("normal")	= 296 mOsm/l.
Dextrose 5% in water (D_5W)	= 266 mOsm/l.
Dextrose 5% in 0.23% saline (D_4 ¼ S)	= 335 mOsm/l.
Ringer's lactate	= 256 mOsm/l.
Ringer's lactate in 5% dextrose	= 528 mOsm/l.

50% dextrose has 27.5 mOsm in 10 ml.

20% mannitol has 12 mOsm in 10 ml, so an infusion of 1 gm/kg body wt of mannitol will increase the serum osmolarity by 24 mOsm/l if given quickly.

Sodium bicarbonate given at 3 mEq/kg body wt will increase the osmolarity by 7.5 mOsm/l, so perhaps 3 such infusions over a 4-hour period may be maximal.

Plasma osmolarity can be calculated by the Mansberger formula[78]:

$$\text{Osmolarity} = \text{Na}(1.86) + \frac{\text{BUN}}{2.8} + \frac{\text{Glucose}}{18} + 5\,\text{mOsm/l}$$

which emphasizes the importance of sodium in controlling plasma osmolarity.

Some Special Features of the Physiology of Infants

Hemoglobin and *hematocrit* levels vary greatly during the first year of life. At birth, the infant has a high hemoglobin (18 gm/dl), the result of the preceding weeks of desaturation. This level falls during the next 3 months to an average of 11 gm (lower if the infant has been prematurely born) but rises back to 13 gm/dl by the age of 1 year and to 14 gm/dl by 10 years of age (see Fig. 52–1). Many infants of 3 months with hemoglobin within a normal range are transfused unneces-

sarily because the decision maker ignores this detail of natural history.

Blood glucose levels are low in the newborn. The definition of hypoglycemia in a newborn is a blood glucose of less than 30 mg/dl and in a premature less than 20 mg/dl.[30]

Renal function. The glomerular filtration rate (GFR) is low at birth, in one series $\overline{10.8}$ ml/min/m² at age 0–4 days and doubled to 20 ml/min/m² by 14 days old.[54] GFR was not related to gestational age in newborns older than 32 weeks' gestation. The renal threshold for bicarbonate in infants is 21.5–22.5 mmol/l compared to 26–28 in adults. The neonate can concentrate urine to only 700 mOsm/l compared to 1200 mOsm/l in the older child and adult. This is mainly because there is so little urea to excrete.[39] The expected urine solute load of infants fed on breast milk is 79 mOsm/l,[137] so the use of free water clearance is inappropriate as a guide to incipient renal failure in neonates because it is normally a positive value. The diuretic response to water load develops after 3–4 days.[39] However, adults subjected to a water load of 100 ml/kg/day for 48 hours had their maximal renal concentration fall from 1209 to 851 mOsm/l,[125] which is, in fact, close to the neonate's maximal concentrating power.

High protein intakes are advocated by some neonatologists for prematures, but a study by Räihä *et al.*[99] showed that prematures fed between 3 and 8 gm protein/kg/day gained weight adequately and those fed more than 9 gm protein/kg/day had an early extra weight gain associated with a higher blood ammonia and more frequent metabolic acidosis, but when assessed over a longer term had growth patterns identical to prematures fed human milk.

Ambient temperature is especially important for the naked newborn. Oxygen consumption is much affected by skin temperature, more so than core temperature. Oxygen consumption is minimal for the naked newborn when ambient temperature is 32–34° C, which gives a skin temperature of 36.1–36.5° C and a rectal temperature of 37° C. An ambient temperature of 30° C may double oxygen consumption, and cold may cause some systemic desaturation.[113] Total heat loss ranges between a minimum and a maximum of 5–10 kcal/kg/hr and is lost in approximately equal amounts by evaporation, convection and radiation. Conduction heat loss is slight.[61] The newborn has an ability to produce heat by a nonshivering thermogenesis, which uses stores of a special brown fat, and this heat production is more efficient than shivering. Thermal neutrality for a lightly clothed adult is about 23° C, too cold for most newborns, so some method of warming is needed.

Despite all efforts, the long-term results in surviving prematures leave cause for much concern. Fitzhardinge *et al.*[45] reviewed 73 patients whose birth weights had been less than 1500 gm and who required intensive care, including ventilation. After 2 years, major neurologic defects were recognized in 28%.

Summary

The changes occurring after heart operations in infants and children are complex, and the younger the age of the patient the more valuable is knowledge of the physiology of the infant, normal and abnormal. The changes following operation place the infant at the mercy of the physician controlling the intensive care, and the infant has good reason to hope that that physician is aware of the changes that follow major operations in general and heart operations in particular, and is also familiar with the differences that distinguish the infant from a scaled-down version of an adult. Given this level of postoperative care, the results of cardiac operations, even in a severely stressed newborn with complex lesions, can be very rewarding. It no longer is acceptable to claim that small infants are fragile creatures. Given postoperative management guided by available knowledge, infants have proved to be robust surgical specimens.

REFERENCES

1. Abel, R. M., Beck, C. H., Jr., Abbott, W. M., Ryan, J. A., Jr., Barnett, G. O., and Fischer, J. E.: Improved survival from acute renal failure after treatment with intravenous essential L-amino acids and glucose, N. Engl. J. Med. 288:695, 1973.
2. Aberdeen, E.: Average fluid values and electrolyte needs, Lancet 1:1024, 1961.
3. Ahlquist, R. P.: Present state of alpha- and beta-adrenergic drugs. 1. The adrenergic receptor, Am. Heart J. 92:661, 1976.
4. Aperia, A., Broberger, O., Thodenius, K., and Zetterström, R.: Renal control of sodium and fluid balance in newborn infants during intravenous maintenance therapy, Acta Paediatr. Scand. 64:725, 1975.
5. Appelbaum, A., Blackstone, E. H., Kouchoukos, N. T., and Kirklin, J. W.: Afterload reduction and cardiac output in infants early after intracardiac surgery, Am. J. Cardiol. 39:445, 1977.
6. Baek, S., Makabali, G. G., Brown, R. S., and Shoemaker, W. C.: Free-water clearance patterns as predictors and therapeutic guides in acute renal failure, Surgery 77:632, 1975.
7. Beall, A. C., Jr., Johnson, P. C., Shirkey, A. L., Crosthwait, R. W., Cooley, D. A., and DeBakey, M. E.: Effects of temporary cardiopulmonary bypass on extracellular fluid volume and total body water in man, Circulation 29:59, 1964.
8. Beattie, H. W., Evans, G., Garnett, E. S., and Webber, C. E.: Sustained hypovolemia and extracellular fluid volume expansion following cardiopulmonary bypass, Surgery 71:891, 1972.
9. Behrendt, D. M., Aberdeen, E., Waterston, D. J., and Bonham-Carter, R. E.: Total anomalous pulmonary venous drainage in infants. 1. Clinical and hemodynamic findings, methods, and results of operation in 37 cases, Circulation 46:347, 1972.
10. Beiser, G. D., Epstein, S. E., Goldstein, R. E., Stampfer, M., and Braunwald, E.: Comparison of the peak inotropic effects of a catecholamine and a digitalis glycoside in the intact canine heart, Circulation 42:805, 1970.
11. Benzing, G., III, Helmsworth, J., Schreiber, J. T., and Kaplan, S.: Cardiac performance and oxygen consumption during intracardiac operations in children, Ann. Thorac. Surg. 22:176, 1976.
12. Benzing, G., III, Helmsworth, J. A., Schreiber, J. T., Loggie, J., and Kaplan, S.: Nitroprusside after open-heart surgery, Circulation 54:467, 1976.
13. Berger, R. L., Polanzak, M. L., and Ryan, T. J.: Central venous pressure and blood volume pattern following open-heart surgery, Ann. Thorac. Surg. 6:57, 1968.
14. Berk, J. L., Hagen, J. F., Koo, R., Beyer, W., Dochat, G. R., Rupright, M., and Nomoto, S.: Pulmonary insufficiency caused by epinephrine, Ann. Surg. 178:423, 1973.
15. Bower, P. J., and Peterson, J. N.: Methemoglobinemia after sodium nitroprusside therapy, N. Engl. J. Med. 293:865, 1975.
16. Boyd, A. D., Tremblay, R. E., Spencer, F. C., and Bahnson, H. T.: Estimation of cardiac output soon after intracardiac surgery with cardiopulmonary bypass, Ann. Surg. 150:613, 1959.
17. Brandfonbrener, M., and Whang, R.: Effect of respiratory alkalosis on survival in hemorrhagic shock, Circ. Res. 21:461, 1967.
18. Braunwald, E., Plauth, W. H., Jr., and Morrow, A. G.: A method for the detection and quantification of impaired sodium excretion. Results of an oral sodium tolerance test in normal subjects and in patients with heart disease, Circulation 32:223, 1965.
19. Breckenridge, I. M., Digerness, S. B., and Kirklin, J. W.: Increased extracellular fluid after open intracardiac operation, Surg. Gynecol. Obstet. 131:53, 1970.
20. Brodie, T. S., Gray, R., Swan, H. J. C., and Matloff, J. M.: Effect of nitroprusside on arterial oxygenation, intrapulmonic shunts and oxygen delivery (abstract), Am. J. Cardiol. 37:123, 1976.
21. Buckberg, G. D., and Ross, G.: Effects of isoprenaline on coronary blood flow: Its distribution and myocardial performance, Cardiovasc. Res. 7:429, 1973.
22. Bull, J. P.: Historical landmarks in the study and treatment of blood loss, Br. J. Clin. Pract. 10:743, 1956.
23. Cannon, P. J.: The kidney in heart failure, N. Engl. J. Med. 296:26, 1977.
24. Cartmill, T. B., Ricks, R. K., Garrett, H. E., Williams, J. A., and DeBakey, M. E.: Blood volume measurements in cardiovascular surgical patients, Surg. Gynecol. Obstet. 121:1269, 1965.
25. Case, R. B., Greenberg, H., and Moskowitz, R.: Alterations in coronary sinus pO_2 and O_2 saturation resulting from pCO_2 changes, Cardiovasc. Res. 9:167, 1975.
26. Clarke, R., and Fisher, M. R.: Assessment of blood loss following injury, Br. J. Clin. Pract. 10:745, 1956.
27. Cleland, J., Pluth, J. R., Tauxe, W. N., and Kirklin, J. W.: Blood volume and body fluid compartment changes soon after closed and open intracardiac surgery, J. Thorac. Cardiovasc. Surg. 52:698, 1966.
28. Coffin, L. H., Ankeney, J. L., and Beheler, E. M.: Experimental study and clinical use of epinephrine for treatment of low cardiac output syndrome, Circulation 33–34 (supp.):78, 1966.
29. Cohn, L. H., Angell, W. W., and Shumway, N. E.: Body fluid shifts after cardiopulmonary bypass. I. Effects of congestive heart failure and hemodilution, J. Thorac. Cardiovasc. Surg. 62:423, 1971.
30. Cornblath, M.: Unique metabolic adaptation in the fetus and newborn, N. Engl. J. Med. 285:631, 1971.
31. Cornell, G. N., Gilder, H., Filippone, A., Fuller, F. W., and Beal, J. M.: Changes in body compartments following operation, Surgery 44:125, 1958.
32. daLuz, P. L., Shubin, H., Weil, M. H., Jacobson, E., and Stein, L.: Pulmonary edema related to changes in colloid osmotic and pulmonary artery wedge pressure in patients after acute myocardial infarction, Circulation 51:350, 1975.
33. Das, J. B., Eraklis, A. J., and Gross, R. E.: Water and cation content of red blood cells and muscle tissue before and after the cardiopulmonary bypass. The effects of the osmolarity of the perfusion prime, J. Thorac. Cardiovasc. Surg. 57:824, 1969.
34. Das, J. B., Eraklis, A. J., and Jones, J. E.: Water and solute excretion following cardiopulmonary bypass with hemodilution. The effects of the osmolarity of the perfusion prime, J. Thorac. Cardiovasc. Surg. 58:789, 1969.
35. Davison, R., and Cannon, R.: Estimation of central venous pressure by examination of jugular veins, Am. Heart J. 87:279, 1974.
36. DeCosse, J. J., Randall, H. T., Habif, D. V., and Roberts, K. E.: The mechanism of hyponatremia and hypotonicity after surgical trauma, Surgery 40:27, 1956.
37. Deverall, P. B.: Non-respiratory alkalosis following open-heart surgery, Proc. Assoc. Eur. Paediatr. Cardiol. 9:21, 1973.
38. Deverall, P. B., Muss, D. C., Macartney, F. J., and Settle, J. D.: Osmolal balance after open intracardiac operations in children, Thorax 28:756, 1973.
39. Edelmann, C. M., Jr., and Spitzer, A.: The maturing kidney. A modern view of well-balanced infants with imbalanced nephrons, J. Pediatr. 75:509, 1969.
40. Edmunds, L. H., Saxena, N. C., Friedman, S., Rashkind, W. J., and Dodd, P. F.: Transatrial repair of tetralogy of Fallot, Surgery 80:681, 1976.
41. English, T. A. H., Digerness, S., and Kirklin, J. W.: Changes in colloid osmotic pressure during and shortly after open intracardiac operation, J. Thorac. Cardiovasc. Surg. 61:338, 1971.
42. Field, J., Shiroff, R. A., Zelis, R., and Babb, J. D.: Limitations in the use of the pulmonary capillary wedge pressure. Cardiac tamponade, Chest 70:451, 1976.
43. Finberg, L.: Dangers to infants caused by changes in osmolal concentration, Pediatrics 40:1031, 1967.
44. Fishman, A. P.: Pulmonary edema. The water-exchanging function of the lung, Circulation 46:390, 1972.
45. Fitzhardinge, P. M., Pape, K., Arstikaitis, M., Boyle, M., Ashby, S., Rowley, A., Netley, C., and Swyer, P. R.: Mechanical ventilation of infants of less than 1,501 gm birth weight: Health, growth, and neurologic sequelae, J. Pediatr. 88:531, 1976.
46. Flanagan, J. P., Steinmetz, G. P., Jr., Crawford, E. W., and Merendino, K. A.: Observations on blood volume with special attention to loss and replacement in cardiac surgery, Surgery 56:925, 1964.
47. Flemma, R. J., and Young, W. G., Jr.: The metabolic effects of mechanical ventilation and respiratory alkalosis in postoperative patients, Surgery 56:36, 1964.
48. Fordham, R. M. M., and Resnekov, L.: Arterial hypoxaemia. A side-effect of intravenous isoprenaline used after cardiac surgery, Thorax 23:19, 1968.
49. Gamble, J. L.: *Chemical Anatomy, Physiology and Pathology of Extracellular Fluid.* A lecture syllabus (6th ed.; Cambridge, Mass.: Harvard University Press, 1954).
50. Gathman, G. E., and Nadas, A. S.: Total anomalous venous connection: Clinical and physiologic observations of 75 pediatric patients, Circulation 42:143, 1970.

51. Geha, A. S.: Coronary and cardiovascular dynamics and oxygen availability during acute normovolemic anemia, Surgery 80: 47, 1976.

52. Gengos, D. C., Celermajer, J. M., and Morgan, W. W., Jr.: A simplified method of internal cardiac compression and open pericardial drainage in the infant, J. Pediatr. 72:543, 1968.

53. Grigor, K. C.: Metabolic alkalosis and acid urine following open-heart surgery with cardiopulmonary bypass, Br. J. Anaesth. 40:943, 1968.

54. Guignard, J. P., Torrado, A., DaCunha, O., and Gautier, E.: Glomerular filtration rate in the first three weeks of life, J. Pediatr. 87:268, 1975.

55. Harken, A. H., Gabel, R. A., Fencl, V., and Moore, F. D.: Hydrochloric acid in the correction of metabolic alkalosis, Arch. Surg. 110:819, 1975.

56. Hartzler, G. O., Maloney, J. D., Curtis, J. J., and Barnhorst, D. A.: Hemodynamic benefits of atrioventricular sequential pacing after cardiac surgery, Am. J. Cardiol. 40:232, 1977.

57. Hayes, M. A., Byrnes, W. P., Goldenberg, I. S., Greene, N. M., and Tuthill, E.: Water and electrolyte exchanges during operation and convalescence, Surgery 46:123, 1959.

58. Hayes, M. A., Williamson, R. J., and Heidenreich, W. F.: Endocrine mechanisms involved in water and sodium metabolism during operation and convalescence, Surgery 41:353, 1957.

59. Heeley, A. M., and Talbot, N. E.: Insensible water losses per day by hospitalized infants and children, Am. J. Dis. Child. 90: 251, 1955.

60. Hesse, B., Parving, H., Lund-Jacobsen, H., and Noer, I.: Transcapillary escape rate of albumin and right atrial pressure in chronic congestive heart failure before and after treatment, Circ. Res. 39:358, 1976.

61. Hey, E. N., and Mount, L. E.: Heat losses from babies in incubators, Arch. Dis. Child. 42:75, 1967.

62. Holloway, E. L., Stinson, E. B., Derby, G. C., and Harrison, D. C.: Action of drugs in patients early after cardiac surgery. I. Comparison of isoproterenol and dopamine, Am. J. Cardiol. 35:656, 1975.

63. Howland, W. S., Schweizer, O., Jascott, D., and Ragasa, J.: Factors influencing the ionization of calcium during major surgical procedures, Surg. Gynecol. Obstet. 143:895, 1976.

64. Hutchin, P., Terzi, R. G., Hollandsworth, L. C., Johnson, G., Jr., and Peters, R. M.: The influence of intravenous fluid administration on postoperative urinary water and electrolyte excretion in thoracic surgical patients, Ann. Surg. 170:813, 1969.

65. Kaplan, S., Edwards, F. K., Helmsworth, J. A., and Clark, L. C.: Blood volume during and after total extracorporeal circulation, Arch. Surg. 80:39, 1961.

66. Kerr, A. R., and Kirklin, J. W.: Effect of rapid increase of blood volume on atrial pressures and pulmonary blood volume: An experimental study, Ann. Surg. 272:278, 1970.

67. Kirklin, J. W., and Archie, J. P., Jr.: The cardiovascular subsystem in surgical patients, Surg. Gynecol. Obstet. 139:17, 1974.

68. Kirklin, J. W., and Rastelli, G. C.: Low cardiac output after open intracardiac operations, Prog. Cardiovasc. Dis. 10:117, 1967.

69. Kirklin, J. W., and Theye, R. A.: Cardiac performance after open intracardiac surgery, Circulation 28:1061, 1963.

70. Kouchoukos, N. T., and Karp, R. B.: Management of the postoperative cardiovascular surgical patient, Am. Heart J. 92:513, 1976.

71. Krongrad, E., Hefler, S. E., Bowman, F. O., Jr., Malm, J. R., and Hoffman, B. F.: Further observations on the etiology of the right bundle branch block pattern following right ventriculotomy, Circulation 50:1105, 1974.

72. Landes, R. G., Lillehei, R. C., Lindsay, W. G., and Nicoloff, D. M.: Free-water clearance and the early recognition of acute renal insufficiency after cardiopulmonary bypass, Ann. Thorac. Surg. 22:41, 1976.

73. Lappas, D. G., Drop, L. J., Buckley, M. J., Mundth, E. D., and Laver, M. B.: Hemodynamic response to calcium chloride during coronary artery surgery, Surg. Forum 26:234, 1975.

74. Lister, J. W., Gosselin, A. J., Nathan, D. A., and Barold, S. S.: Rapid atrial stimulation in the treatment of supraventricular tachycardia, Chest 63:995, 1973.

75. Litwak, R. S., Gilson, A. J., Slonim, R., McCune, C. C., Kiem, I., and Gadboys, H. L.: Alterations in blood volume during "normovolemic" total body perfusion, J. Thorac. Cardiovasc. Surg. 42:477, 1961.

76. Loggie, J. M. H., Kleinman, L. I., and Van Maanen, E. F.: Renal function and diuretic therapy in infants and children. Part III, J. Pediatr. 86:825, 1975.

77. Lyons, J. H., and Moore, F. D.: Posttraumatic alkalosis: Incidence and pathophysiology of alkalosis in surgery, Surgery 60: 93, 1966.

78. Mansberger, A. B., Boyd, D. R., Cowley, R. A., and Buxton, R. W.: Refractometry and osmometry in clinical surgery, Ann. Surg. 196:672, 1969.

79. Marty, A. T.: Hyperoncotic albumin therapy, Surg. Gynecol. Obstet. 139:105, 1974.

80. Marty, A. T., Prather, J., Matloff, J. M., and Schauble, J.: Oncotic effects of dilutional bypass, albumin, and diuretics, Arch. Surg. 107:21, 1973.

81. Mathur, M., Harris, E. A., Yarrow, S., and Barratt-Boyes, B. G.: Measurement of cardiac output by thermodilution in infants and children after open-heart operations, J. Thorac. Cardiovasc. Surg. 72:221, 1976.

82. McEnany, M. T., Morgan, R. J., Mundth, E. D., and Austen, W. G.: Circumvention of detrimental pulmonary vasoactivity of exogenous catecholamines in cardiac resuscitation, Surg. Forum 26:98, 1975.

83. McGoon, D. C., Moffitt, E. A., Theye, R. A., and Kirklin, J. W.: Physiologic studies during high flow, normothermic, whole body perfusion, J. Thorac. Cardiovasc. Surg. 39:275, 1960.

84. Mielke, J. E., Hunt, J. C., Maher, F. T., and Kirklin, J. W.: Renal performance during clinical cardiopulmonary bypass with and without hemodilution, J. Thorac. Cardiovasc. Surg. 51: 229, 1966.

85. Moffitt, E. A., Kirklin, J. W., and Theye, R. A.: Physiologic studies during whole-body perfusion in tetralogy of Fallot, J. Thorac. Cardiovasc. Surg. 44:180, 1962.

86. Moore, F. D.: Convalescence: The Metabolic Sequence after Injury, in Kinney, J. M., *et al.* (eds.), *Manual of Preoperative and Postoperative Care* (2d ed.; Philadelphia: W. B. Saunders Company, 1971), p. 19.

87. Narula, O. S., Scherlag, B. J., Javier, R. P., Hildner, F. J., and Samet, P.: Analysis of the A-V conduction defect in complete heart block utilizing His bundle electrograms, Circulation 41: 437, 1970.

88. Pacifico, A. D., Digerness, S., and Kirklin, J. W.: Acute alterations of body composition after open intracardiac operations, Circulation 41:331, 1970.

89. Pacifico, A. D., Digerness, S., and Kirklin, J. W.: Regression of body compositional abnormalities of heart failure after intracardiac operations, Circulation 42:999, 1970.

90. Pacifico, A. D., Digerness, S., and Kirklin, J. W.: Sodium-excreting ability before and after intracardiac surgery, Circulation 41 – 42 (supp.):142, 1970.

91. Parr, G. V. S., Blackstone, E. H., and Kirklin, J. W.: Cardiac performance and mortality early after intracardiac surgery in infants and young children, Circulation 51:867, 1975.

92. Parr, G. V. S., Blackstone, E. H., Kirklin, J. W., Pacifico, A. D., and Lauridsen, P.: Cardiac performance early after interatrial transposition of venous return in infants and small children, Circulation 49 – 50 (supp.): 2, 1974.

93. Parr, G. V. S., Kirklin, J. W., Pacifico, A. D., Blackstone, E. H., and Lauridsen, P.: Cardiac performance in infants after repair of total anomalous pulmonary venous connection, Ann. Thorac. Surg. 17:561, 1974.

94. Pemberton, A. H., Kirklin, J. W., and Wood, E. H.: Interatrial pressure relationships after closure of atrial septal defects in man, Circulation 15:568, 1957.

95. Pillsbury, R. C., Dong, E., Jr., Lower, R. R., Hurley, E. J., and Shumway, N. E.: Emergency reoperation following open-heart surgery, Ann. Thorac. Surg. 1:50, 1965.

96. Poole-Wilson, P. A., Lewis, G., Angerpointer, T., Malcolm, A. D., and Williams, B. T.: Haemodynamic effects of salbutamol and nitroprusside after cardiac surgery, Br. Heart J. 39:721, 1977.

97. Powers, S. R., Jr., Boba, A., Hostnik, W., and Stein, A.: Prevention of postoperative acute renal failure with mannitol in 100 cases, Surgery 55:15, 1964.

98. Prys-Roberts, C., Kelman, G. R., Greenbaum, R., Kain, M. L., and Bay, J.: Hemodynamics and alveolar-arterial Po$_2$ differences at varying Paco$_2$ in anesthetized man, J. Appl. Physiol. 25:80, 1968.

99. Räihä, N. C. R., Heinonen, K., Rassin, D. K., and Gaull, G. E.: Milk protein quantity and quality in low-birthweight infants: I. Metabolic responses and effects on growth, Pediatrics 57:659, 1976.

100. Reemtsma, K., and Creech, O., Jr.: Viscosity studies of blood,

plasma, and plasma substitutes, J. Thorac. Cardiovasc. Surg. 44:674, 1962.

101. Reeve, R., Reeve, F. J. S., and Lin, T. K.: Paradoxical pulse revisited, Am. Heart J. 92:120, 1976.

102. Rehder, K., Kirklin, J. W., and Theye, R. A.: Physiologic studies following surgical correction of atrial septal defect and similar lesions, Circulation 24:1302, 1962.

103. Reid, D. J.: The body fluid compartments during surgery, Ann. R. Coll. Surg. Engl. 44:88, 1969.

104. Reid, D. J., Digerness, S. B., and Kirklin, J. W.: Changes in whole body venous tone and distribution of blood after open intracardiac surgery, Am. J. Cardiol. 22:621, 1968.

105. Rosenblum, R.: Physiologic basis for the therapeutic use of catecholamines, Am. Heart J. 87:527, 1974.

106. Roth, E., Lax, L. C., and Maloney, J. V., Jr.: Ringer's lactate solution and extracellular fluid volume in the surgical patient: A critical analysis, Ann. Surg. 169:149, 1969.

107. Rowe, M. I.: The role of serum osmolality measurement in the management of the neonatal surgical patient, Surg. Gynecol. Obstet. 133:93, 1971.

108. Rozansky, G. I., and Linde, L. M.: Psychiatric study of parents of children with cyanotic congenital heart disease, Pediatrics 48:450, 1971.

109. Schiller, N. B., and Botvinick, E. H.: Right ventricular compression as a sign of cardiac tamponade. An analysis of echocardiographic ventricular dimensions and their clinical implications, Circulation 56:774, 1977.

110. Shires, T., Williams, J., and Brown, F.: Acute change in extracellular fluids associated with major surgical procedures, Ann. Surg. 154:803, 1961.

111. Shizgal, H. M., Solomon, S., and Gutelius, J. R.: Body water distribution after operation, Surg. Gynecol. Obstet. 144:35, 1977.

112. Stahl, W. M., and Stone, A. M.: Prophylactic diuresis with ethacrynic acid for prevention of postoperative renal failure, Ann. Surg. 172:361, 1970.

113. Stephenson, J. M., and Oliver, T. K.: The effect of cooling on blood gas tensions in newborn infants, J. Pediatr. 76:848, 1970.

114. Stephenson, L. W., Blackstone, E. H., and Kouchoukos, N. T.: Dopamine vs epinephrine in patients following cardiac surgery: Randomized study, Surg. Forum 27:272, 1976.

115. Stinson, E. B., Holloway, E. L., Derby, G., Oyer, P. E., Hollingsworth, J., Griepp, R. B., and Harrison, D. C.: Comparative hemodynamic responses to chlorpromazine, nitroprusside, nitroglycerin, and trimethaphan immediately after open-heart operations, Circulation 51–52 (supp.): 26, 1975.

116. Stone, A. M., and Stahl, W. M.: Renal effects of hemorrhage in normal man, Ann. Surg. 172:825, 1970.

117. Sturridge, M. F., Theye, R. A., Fowler, W. S., and Kirklin, J. W.: Basal metabolic rate after cardiovascular surgery, J. Thorac. Cardiovasc. Surg. 47:298, 1964.

118. Sturtz, G. S., Kirklin, J. W., Burke, E. C., and Power, M. H.: Water metabolism after cardiac operations involving a Gibbon-type pump-oxygenator. 1. Daily water metabolism, obligatory water losses, and requirements, Circulation 16:988, 1957.

119. Talbot, N. B., Richie, R. H., and Crawford, J. D.: *Metabolic Homeostasis.* A syllabus for those concerned with the care of patients (Cambridge, Mass.: Harvard University Press, 1959).

120. Theye, R. A., and Kirklin, J. W.: Physiologic studies early after repair of tetralogy of Fallot, Circulation 28:42, 1963.

121. Theye, R. A., and Kirklin, J. W.: Physiologic studies following surgical correction of ventricular septal defect, Circulation 27: 530, 1963.

122. Thomas, T. V.: Emergency evacuation of acute pericardial tamponade, Ann. Thorac. Surg. 10:566, 1970.

123. Topley, E., and Fisher, M. R.: The illness of trauma, Br. J. Clin. Pract. 10:768, 1956.

124. Truccone, N. J., Spotnitz, H. M., Gersony, W. M., Dell, R., Bowman, F. O., Jr., and Malm, J. R.: Cardiac output in infants and children after open-heart surgery, J. Thorac. Cardiovasc. Surg. 71:410, 1976.

125. Vaamonde, C. A., Presser, J. I., and Clapp, W.: Effect of high fluid intake on the renal concentrating mechanism of normal man, J. Appl. Physiol. 36:434, 1974.

126. Varat, M. A., Adolph, R. J., and Fowler, N. O.: Cardiovascular effects of anemia, Am. Heart J. 83:415, 1972.

127. Virtue, R. W., LeVine, D. S., and Aikawa, J. K.: Fluid shifts during the surgical period: RISA and S[35] determinations following glucose, saline or lactate infusion, Ann. Surg. 163:523, 1966.

128. Visintainer, M. A., and Wolfer, J. A.: Psychological preparation for surgical pediatric patients: The effect on children's and parents' stress responses and adjustment, Pediatrics 56:187, 1975.

129. Waldo, A. L., MacLean, W. A. H., Karp, R. B., Kouchoukos, N. T., and James, T. N.: Entrainment and interruption of atrial flutter with atrial pacing. Studies in man following open heart surgery, Circulation 56:737, 1977.

130. Walker, J. E. C., and Wells, R. E., Jr.: Heat and water exchange in the respiratory tract, Am. J. Med. 30:259, 1961.

131. Weeks, K. R., Chatterjee, K., Block, S., Matloff, J. M., and Swan, H. J. C.: Bedside hemodynamic monitoring. Its value in the diagnosis of tamponade complicating cardiac surgery, J. Thorac. Cardiovasc. Surg. 71:250, 1976.

132. White, R. D., Goldsmith, R. S., Rodriguez, R., Moffitt, E. A., and Pluth, J. R.: Plasma ionic calcium levels following injection of chloride, gluconate, and gluceptate salts of calcium, J. Thorac. Cardiovasc. Surg. 71:609, 1976.

133. Wilkening, R. B.: Etiology of hyponatremia, J. Pediatr. 91: 1026, 1977.

134. Williams, P. R., and Oh, W.: Effects of radiant warmer on insensible water loss in newborn infants, Am. J. Dis. Child. 128: 511, 1974.

135. Wu, P. Y. K., and Hodgman, J. E.: Insensible water loss in preterm infants: Changes with postnatal development and nonionizing radiant energy, Pediatrics 54:704, 1974.

136. Wyse, S. D., Pfitzner, J., Rees, A., Lincoln, J. C. R., and Branthwaite, M. A.: Measurement of cardiac output by thermal dilution in infants and children, Thorax 30:262, 1975.

137. Ziegler, E. E., and Fomon, S. J.: Fluid intake, renal solute load, and water balance in infancy, J. Pediatr. 78:561, 1971.

53 EOIN ABERDEEN
Palliative Cardiac Procedures

THE RADICAL CORRECTION of congenital heart lesions during the first year of life has been reported in increasing numbers since the first successful intracardiac operations from 1955 onward by Kirklin[14] and his colleagues at the Mayo Clinic and in 1957 by Sloan[24] and his colleagues in Ann Arbor. When radical correction can be performed, be it anatomic correction or only physiologic or functional correction, at a low risk in the first year of life, the advantages are compelling. Correction limits the underlying risks of the lesion itself, as well as avoiding the risks of palliative surgery. Correction also relieves the parents and family of the pressures, psychologic and financial, that a major illness forces into the home environment. Palliative surgery, even though it may involve a very small early risk, may also include long-term complications of the palliative operation itself and the possibility that patients may be lost to further treatment or follow-up examination because the palliative operation has seemed so successful. To be acceptable, a palliative operation needs to offer a survival chance at least 10% better than the risk of the corrective procedure performed on *that* patient at *that* time. Therefore, any corrective procedure that has a survival rate better than 90% probably is to be preferred to a palliative operation at any age. The accurate assessment of the risk involved can be made only after the anomaly has been completely diagnosed (which usually requires cardiac catheterization and angiocardiography), and then the natural history of the condition must be known so that an assessment of risks can be made. This includes detailed knowledge of the achievements of the surgical team in the center where operation is being considered, in addition to an accurate assessment of the patient.

"Correction" can be defined in several ways, and pedantic distinctions have been made. Corrective operations imply that physiologic correction is achieved, but it is recognized that almost no heart with a congenital lesion can be converted to a heart that is normal physiologically and anatomically in every macroscopic and microscopic detail. "Correction" almost never means "perfection," and very few children with congenital heart disease are "completely cured" by operation if complete cure implies no myocardial hypertrophy, no valve prolapse or regurgitation, no incomplete bundle-branch block, no persisting systemic or pulmonary hypertension. At times, physiologic correction is achieved using external conduits of Dacron and heterograft valves, sometimes of a size that will require replacement before adult life, or the heart is left with the right ventricle as the systemic ventricle, as after Mustard's operation for transposed great arteries. These cases must be considered in one sense "palliative" or, at least, a palliative form of physiologic correction. Often there is no sharp distinction between a palliative and a corrective procedure.

Some conditions are incorrectable at any age, such as:
1. Severe hypoplasia of the left heart or the right heart and/or their outflows.

2. Atresia of the mitral or aortic valves.
3. Some forms of tricuspid atresia with or without pulmonary valve atresia.
4. Some forms of Ebstein's anomaly.
5. Some forms of single ventricle.

For these, a purely palliative operation is the only help that can be offered. The palliative operation will add yet one more abnormality, but may lead to a survival in worthwhile status for many years or even decades. These conditions will not be discussed further here.

For some conditions, corrective operation is the only effective therapy to be considered. For example:
1. Severe pulmonary valve stenosis with an intact ventricular septum.
2. Some forms of severe aortic valve stenosis.
3. Coarctation of the aorta and/or
4. Patent ductus arteriosus.
5. Cardiac tumors.
6. Atrial septal defect (rarely).
7. Perhaps an anomalous left coronary artery (see p. 656).

These conditions will not be considered further here.

The conditions most worth discussion are a few that have, in the past, been treated with varying success by purely palliative operations, but now may be treated by primary corrective operation in the first year of life. As cardiac surgery progresses, it will surely become possible to correct more and more lesions at the first operation in infancy. During the past decade especially, the proportion of patients requiring palliative cardiac operations has become less and the proportion having corrective intracardiac operation in infancy has increased, but we have not yet reached the desired stage where there is no place for any palliative operation in these potentially correctable lesions. The anomalies to be considered further include ventricular septal defects, valve stenoses, especially the combination that presents in Fallot's anomaly, and transposition of the great arteries, especially in its complex forms.

Four palliative operations warrant further consideration.
1. Pulmonary artery constriction (banding).
2. Systemic to pulmonary artery anastomoses (shunts).
3. Palliative valvotomy.
4. Atrial septectomy.

Pulmonary Artery Constriction (Banding)

Because the natural history of Fallot's anomaly is so much better in infants than is the natural history of a large VSD without any pulmonary outflow tract obstruction, it was logical that constriction of the pulmonary artery was tried as a means of helping infants with large ventricular septal defects and heart failure to recover from the effects of the huge left-to-right shunt. Pulmonary artery constriction was first performed by Muller and Dammann[18] in 1951 and simple banding of the pulmonary artery was first reported by Albert

TABLE 53–1.—PULMONARY ARTERY CONSTRICTION (BANDING)°

DEFECT	NO. OF REPORTS ANALYZED	NO. OF CASES	NO. OF HOSPITAL DEATHS	% MORTALITY RATE
VSD – isolated and single Some ± PDA	34	413	35	8.5%
VSD – multiple	Not identifiable from the literature reports			
VSD + ASD	15	83	30	36%
VSD + coarctation	14	95	38	40%
Single ventricle	10	73	21	28%
VSD + AV canal	20	140	45	32%
No VSD ostium primum	6	10	9	90%
VSD – DORV	5	22	6	27%
VSD + TGA (complete)	18	225	71	32%
VSD + congenitally corrected TGA	7	21	5	24%
VSD + truncus arteriosus	20	99	52	53%
VSD + mitral valve anomaly	5	8	4	50%
VSD + miscellaneous	11	179	94	52%

°Analysis from available literature, 1953–1977.

et al. in 1958,[1] and was applied to an increasing number of cases during the next 10 years. However, banding has been required much less in recent years as open heart operations in the first year of life have become safer. The experience gained emphasized the need to look carefully at the varieties of VSDs treated, and of their natural history. Ventricular septal defects are not just holes in the ventricular septum but may vary greatly in size, in their position in the septum, may be single or multiple, may be isolated or associated with other congenital heart defects. The effect of the VSD or VSDs will also depend on whether the pulmonary outflow tract is obstructed and whether the great arteries are transposed or normally related.

Most series that have reported the treatment by pulmonary artery banding of ventricular septal defect causing failure in the first year of life have revealed mortality rates varying from 2% to 11% if the VSD was uncomplicated, but much higher mortality rates, often more than 50%, when the VSD was complicated by other lesions. The report that most emphasizes this variation in prognosis was from the Hospital for Sick Children, London, covering the years 1957–1966.[25] In a consecutive series of 146 patients, only one-third had a ventricular septal defect without additional lesions, and these cases of isolated single VSD rarely required operation in the first 6 weeks of life. Of the infants in this series requiring banding in the first 6 weeks of life, only 2 of 22 had a ventricular septal defect without other intracardiac lesions whereas of those operated on between the ages of 3 and 6 months, 20 of 49 had a ventricular septal defect without other intracardiac lesions. Not only was there a contrast in the age at presentation of infants with a large isolated VSD but even more in the survival rate. Of 44 children in this series who had pulmonary artery banding for VSD alone, only 1 (2%) died whereas the mortality rate of those with ventricular septal defect and additional lesions such as a large patent ductus, coarctation of the aorta or atrial septal defect was between 54% and 77%—an extraordinary contrast. Similar results had been reported in a number of other series of children treated by pulmonary artery banding, and although it may be thought that the addition of an atrial septal defect would not alter the outlook greatly for a child with a large ventricular septal defect, in most series it increased the risk of dying after banding by 4 times or more (Table 53–1).

When these children came to corrective operation, a further unusual aspect of the natural history was revealed. In the series from Great Ormond Street, of the first 22 patients having intracardiac correction after pulmonary artery banding, 8 of 22 had multiple VSDs and 12 of 22 had defects that were very large or huge (such as 40 × 20 mm, or 35 × 25 mm, or an absence of almost half the septum). This was in sharp contrast to the type of ventricular septal defect treated in the routine correction of VSD in older children, and strongly suggested that the operation of pulmonary artery banding interfered with natural selection and salvaged patients with very large or multiple defects who otherwise would have died in infancy. Debanding of the pulmonary artery and closure of the VSD when the VSD was single and no larger than the usual Fallot's anomaly VSD did not result in any deaths. So it would seem that a single VSD of moderate size rarely causes severe heart failure in the first 6 weeks of life, the patients rarely die at pulmonary artery banding and rarely die at later VSD closure and unbanding—but however low the risk of PA banding for a single VSD, banding should not now be used because the risk of primary correction in many centers is so low.

Likewise, the high mortality rates reported after pulmonary artery banding in such lesions as VSD + ASD or VSD + a large PDA or VSD + coarctation of the aorta argue strongly for primary correction, because the excellent results of VSD closure in infants have included many with ASDs or patent ductus.

Personal analysis° of the literature has identified at least 17 centers reporting mortality rates of less than 10% for infants under 1 year of age having primary correction of a single VSD (a total of 406 patients, with 21 deaths—a 5.2% mortality rate), some of these having VSD + ASD or VSD + PDA, which compares with the mortality rate of 8.5% (35 deaths in 413 cases) in 16 reports of pulmonary artery banding in infants with isolated VSD. Of 83 patients identified in 15 reports as having PA banding for VSD + ASD (nearly all being in the first year of life), the mortality rate was 36% (30 patients died). For patients with VSD and associated coarctation of the aorta, 14 reports identified 95 patients having PA banding with a mortality rate of 40% (38 patients died), but there is a wide variation among the small groups reported.

The surprisingly high mortality rate reported after repair

—————

°The large number of publications analyzed has made it impractical to present an all-inclusive bibliography for this chapter.

of multiple VSDs was reviewed recently by Blackstone *et al.,*[4] who observed that among 11 centers reporting their results, the lowest mortality rate was 30%, many reporting mortality rates of 50% or higher. (The risk of pulmonary artery banding for multiple VSDs cannot be identified from the literature, but presumably it is not higher than the risk associated with banding for a single ventricle, which was 28% in 9 reports—20 of 71 patients operated on died, most in the first year of life.) An acceptable explanation of this high mortality rate has not yet been provided. Before any series of results of VSD operations can be fully assessed, the incidence of multiple VSD and the size of the VSD must be known.

Early primary correction of atrioventricular canal is also suggested by the high risk of banding (45 (32%) of 140 patients died). Acceptable results of primary correction in infants are being reported with increasing frequency, but, again, this provides an example of natural selection, and infants with atrioventricular canal presenting with uncontrollable heart failure in the first 4 months of life may prove to be much more difficult to correct than those presenting after 6 months of age, because the worst deformity presents earliest.

Pulmonary artery banding still would seem to have a place in the management of an infant with TGA and a VSD large enough to elevate the pulmonary artery pressure to systemic levels. If not operated on, such an infant assuredly will develop severe pulmonary vascular disease during the first 12 months of life. Since correction of TGA by Mustard's operation and VSD closure in the first months of life has carried a high mortality rate, PA banding in the first months of life still is used for these cases. Perhaps as methods of myocardial preservation improve, PA banding will have less use in these cases.

Truncus arteriosus is a lesion for which PA banding has been very unsatisfactory. Over-all, a 53% mortality rate has been recorded in infants, mostly in the early months of life, having PA banding (52 deaths in 99 cases identified in 20 reports). Selection of patients for banding would favor the form of truncus with a common pulmonary artery, although some cases in which the right and left pulmonary arteries were banded separately are included. Not only was the hospital survival rate so poor, but the later survival and quality of life of the infants were even more discouraging, partly as a result of technical problems when the short length of pulmonary artery available for banding caused the band to occlude the branch pulmonary arteries asymmetrically, and also because of the inherent problems of the lesion. The data indicate that pulmonary artery banding, by conventional methods, has been well tried in truncus arteriosus and has failed. Therefore, an alternative operation is essential. Primary "correction," using a valve-containing external conduit, may prove to be satisfactory, or preferable to PA banding, at least in the early survival rates and the later quality of life.

A recently suggested palliative operation, not yet given an effective trial, is operative creation of stenosis of the orifice of the pulmonary artery, performed from inside the aorta under a brief period of bypass support.[17] This could allow regulation of the pulmonary flow as effectively as a carefully measured Waterston shunt, and perhaps also allow for some growth, without producing a pulmonary flow so excessive as to cause pulmonary vascular disease. Should the operation have a high salvage rate and allow the infant to grow to a size permitting a corrective operation at a reasonably low risk, it would become yet one more among the many major contributions to surgery associated with the names Varco and Minneapolis.

One other important observation in truncus arteriosus is the function of the common truncal valve. If severe aortic regurgitation is occurring, both the prognosis and the management will be greatly altered, and again the natural history for each case must be assessed before comparing the results of treatment in different case series.

Systemic to Pulmonary Artery Anastomoses (Shunts)

Palliative surgery for Fallot's anomaly still is the subject of controversy. Primary correction is obviously desirable for the general advantages already stated, and for the additional reasons that there is good evidence that much of the obstruction to right ventricular outflow is acquired during the early years of life, and early primary correction avoids that complication. Complete closure (atresia) of the stenosed pulmonary valve may develop after successful shunting, although this may not be a very significant complication. Some data suggest that the lower diastolic pressure and the wider systemic pulse pressure that may be produced by a good systemic to pulmonary artery shunt can contribute to increased hypoxia of the right ventricular myocardium when right ventricular hypertension is present.[6] Therefore, the initial case reports of successful primary correction in the first year of life by Ross in 1960,[3] McMillan in 1962[16] and of 4 cases without a death by Baffes[2] in the mid-1960s were important contributions and have been followed by several recent reports of correction in the first year of life with mortality rates of less than 10% (5 reports can be identified covering 152 children less than 2 years of age having primary correction, with only 12 hospital deaths—a 7.9% mortality rate). This would suggest that palliative operations for Fallot's anomaly now may have no place. However, the reports from some of the other leading centers of infant heart surgery producing excellent results in other types of heart disease requiring primary correction record mortality rates of 20%, 21%, 27%, 37% and even 60% in relatively small groups of patients, so that all the problems in primary correction in the infant with Fallot's anomaly have not yet been identified.

Most centers reporting good results from Fallot correction in the first year of life have reported a high proportion of cases having right ventricular outflow patches, at first considered a possible disadvantage of early correction. However, a recent study by Pacifico *et al.*[20] indicated that when precise measurement and a standardized protocol were used to ensure an adequate right ventricular outflow, the proportion of 55 patients of all ages having outflow tract patches was 44%, which was a higher proportion than the same surgeons had found necessary previously. The concern about inserting outflow patches has diminished as many patients with known postoperative pulmonary valve regurgitation have been followed for more than 15 years and nearly all have good heart function.

Fortunately, in the past few years, at the same time that the early primary correction of Fallot's anomaly has been more widely applied, it has also become evident that systemic to pulmonary artery shunts can be performed at low risk even in the first days of life. The literature identifies at least 8 reports describing 82 infants having Blalock-Taussig shunts, with 2 hospital deaths. My personal experience of the past 6 years includes 16 patients under 1 year of age, 5 in the first week of life, with no deaths and no later shunt closures. The improved results follow several changes of technique, the most important being extensive dissection of the right carotid artery well into the neck, to allow the subclavian-carotid bifurcation to be brought closer to the right pulmonary artery, so that the right subclavian can be divided at the site of the first branch and anastomosed without undue tension. The diameter of the anastomosis usually is 3.0–3.5 mm, which permits a large flow. The use of fine 7-0 monofilament suture and optical magnification have also helped greatly.

Waterston's anastomosis can easily be made too large, and many centers have reported high mortality rates, as high as 40%, in the first months of life, but precise measurement of the aortic incision,[9] limiting its length to exactly 3 mm in patients in the first months of life, has resulted in several reports of survival rates of 90% or better after Waterston's anastomosis for Fallot's anomaly. One factor affecting selection should be recognized. If severe hypoplasia of the branch pulmonary arteries is present, it is more likely that a Waterston shunt will be attempted rather than a Blalock-Taussig, so the latter should be expected to have a better survival rate both early and late.

The results of correction of Fallot's anomaly have been reported from many centers in the past 15 years, and all who use Blalock-Taussig shunts have, without exception, shown an interesting feature—the survival of patients having primary correction without any palliative operation either has not been as good (only half as good in two large series) or has been the same as the survival of patients who have been corrected following a single classic Blalock-Taussig shunt. Since the shunt group is biased toward the more severe forms of Fallot's anomaly, because it is their severe desaturation that leads to the shunt, and these severe forms would be expected to have a higher mortality rate, especially as additional operative time is required to close the palliative shunt, the reasons for equal survival rates are interesting. Since a successful shunt usually lowers the hemoglobin level, one factor may be the better survival rate of patients with a hemoglobin level below 16 gm/dl compared to those over 16 gm/dl.

An important study by Jarmakani and colleagues[13] compared right ventricular function in 25 Fallot's anomaly without any operation and 18 patients after palliative shunts. The RV end-diastolic volume and RV ejection fraction were decreased in Fallot's anomaly (but not in other patients with isolated pulmonary valve stenosis). The authors suggest that this may be the result of the myocardial hypoxia that occurs with severe Fallot's anomaly. RV output increased, as did LV output, in patients with effective palliative shunts, and this was coincident with increased RV and LV volumes. Hypoplasia of the left ventricle in Fallot's anomaly has been discussed for many years. It has been measured recently,[11] and it is suggested that an LV end-diastolic volume of less than 55% of the predicted normal perhaps is an indication for a palliative shunt, with radical correction to follow in a year or more, after the LV volume has increased to near normal.

Two other recent studies have measured a better postoperative cardiac function in patients having radical correction of Fallot's anomaly after an initial palliative shunt, compared to patients having primary correction without any palliative operation.[21, 22]

The problem of the patients with Fallot's anomaly and severe hypoplasia of the pulmonary arterial tree cannot be answered adequately with the experience so far reported. Small arteries of 2 mm diameter or less make palliative shunting an unsatisfactory operation and also have been the main cause of failure of the corrective operation in at least one center's experience with radical correction of infants.[26] Perhaps the best answer will prove to be enlargement of the pulmonary outflow tract under cardiopulmonary bypass, leaving the VSD untouched, to be closed later when the pulmonary arteries have enlarged enough to allow left-to-right shunting. Occasional cases have been mentioned in the literature, and Gerbode and Carr[10] reported a follow-up of 5 patients treated with this two-stage plan. Three had successful second-stage VSD closure. Two had not yet developed a left-to-right shunt, so the VSD closure had not yet been performed. A larger experience will be needed to confirm these encouraging results.

In summary, it is clear that the problems of Fallot's anomaly, especially those in the first year of life, have not yet been solved, but the results of operative treatment are most encouraging. Early primary correction in infants has been reported from a few centers with mortality rates less than 10%, and so suggest that the ideal treatment is becoming feasible. However, other centers of proved expertise and experience in infant cardiac surgery have reported discouragingly high mortality rates after primary correction in infants. The reason for these differences is not clear. Further observation will demand precise assessment of the size of the RV outflow tract and of pulmonary arteries, and perhaps careful assessment of ventricular volumes and function. The arguments for primary correction are compelling, stand on their own merits and do not need to be supported by comparing the results with some of the poorer shunt survival rates reported one or two decades ago. Should palliation be used, the results of shunting (especially the Blalock-Taussig operation) have been excellent in some centers in recent years—mortality rates of less than 5%, even in the first week of life, have been reported—and the subsequent results of the corrective operation have been as good as with primary correction, or better. For the rare cases with severe hypoplasia of the branch pulmonary arteries, perhaps a two-stage approach is advisable, with relief from the outflow tract obstruction under cardiopulmonary bypass as a first procedure, and later VSD closure if and when a left-to-right shunt has developed.

Pulmonary Valve Atresia with Intact Ventricular Septum

This anomaly is rare, fortunately, because results of treatment are not yet satisfactory. At first, pulmonary valve atresia and severe pulmonary valve stenosis were thought to be similar variations of a single problem, but results of treatment have revealed an enormous difference in the patients' ability to survive operation. Severe pulmonary stenosis has had a good survival rate after valvotomy, whether direct via the pulmonary artery or indirect via the infundibulum (Brock operation), with survival rates about 90%. With pulmonary valve atresia, the same operations have yielded survival rates of less than 50% and as low as 20%. The results have been better in the uncommon cases with a large right ventricle.

A survey of 1963–1977 publications on pulmonary valve atresia with intact ventricular septum reveals the results after operations performed on infants in the first month of life (Table 53–2).

These summarized results perhaps oversimplify the conclusions, because one of the best series reported has been of pulmonary valvotomy done at the same initial procedure as the systemic pulmonary arterial shunt (14 cases, with 3 deaths) whereas another center reporting superb results for

TABLE 53–2.—PULMONARY VALVE ATRESIA WITH INTACT VENTRICULAR
SEPTUM—RESULTS OF OPERATIONS°

OPERATION	NO. OF REPORTS ANALYZED	NO. OF PATIENTS OPERATED ON	HOSPITAL DEATHS
Valvotomy only (direct—via PA)	10	87	64 (74%)
Valvotomy only (indirect—Brock operation)	8	39	20 (51%)
Systemic to pulmonary artery shunt only	9	81	48 (59%)
Glenn anastomosis	4	5	4 (80%)
Systemic to pulmonary artery shunt + valvotomy	7	32	17 (53%)
Shunt + atrial septostomy or septectomy	8	48	10 (21%)

°Analysis from available literature, 1963–1977.

other conditions treated operatively in newborns reports an 83% mortality (10 deaths in 12 cases) with combined valvotomy and shunt. Although the best survivals have come from balloon septostomy and shunt, the patients faced further risks. If no valvotomy was done, deaths occurred from the age of 3 months—in some series less than half survived the first year of life without valvotomy. On the other hand, risks of later valvotomy (performed weeks or months after the shunt) are difficult to define because insufficient experience is reported and most reports are of one or two cases only. It seems that some children have died at closed valvotomy done within days or weeks of the shunt operation, but the degree of risk cannot be defined. Likewise, the risk of open heart correction in the first few years of life is not clear, but the risks of not surviving may be significant. Ideally, correction of the pulmonary valve atresia by open heart correction in the first hours of life is desirable, and again data are not available. Some who advocated open correction at any age now are advising balloon septostomy and shunting in the first months of life, which implies that their, unpublished, results are not encouraging.

One problem of lung function that should be considered further is the response of the pulmonary vasculature to severe hypoxia and acidosis. A sixfold increase in pulmonary vascular resistance has been recorded in fetal lambs when the pH has been lowered to 7.2 and the P_{O_2} to 25.[23] Yet, in newborn humans with pulmonary valve atresia, the pH may be as low as 6.8 and the P_{O_2} as low as 14 torr. My own experience has included two such cases in the first day of life, in one of which the Blalock-Taussig anastomosis seemed to be flowing from right to left when studied by aortography. Effective management of such cases will require a successful method of reducing the pulmonary vascular resistance in newborns with a pH below 7.0 and a P_{O_2} below 20 torr, before any operative method can have a chance to succeed. If drug therapy cannot achieve this, perhaps membrane oxygenator support will be required.

Clearly the best method of treating pulmonary valve atresia with intact septum has not been conclusively determined. Future reports should define the anatomy of the heart more precisely, not only as to the size of the right ventricle and the competence of the tricuspid valve but whether the more frequently occurring small ventricle has a conus or not,[8] whether sinusoids are prominent and whether they drain blood retrograde into the coronary system; and whether abnormal coronary vessel connections are present. When the results of operation are assessed with these factors taken into consideration, a clearer answer may emerge.

Atrial Septostomy and Septectomy

Surgical methods of producing an atrial septal defect are discussed in Chapter 60.

External Conduits and Dacron Grafts

Artificial conduits are discussed in Chapter 56. The definition of palliation again may be raised. Several reports of long-term failure of Dacron grafts in the systemic arteries[5, 7, 12, 15, 19] suggest that patients having Dacron grafts inserted during childhood may require reoperation for aneurysm formation or graft failure in their adult years. The degree of risk would, at present, seem to be very small, but the next decade may reveal more complications. If so, the advantage of using natural artery tissue will again be made clear; for example, such as can be achieved by direct anastomosis of the aorta or even of an inlay graft of the subclavian for coarctation of the aorta. For severe obstruction of the hypoplastic aortic annulus, enlargement of the aortic ring and insertion of an adequately sized aortic valve heterograft or allograft may prove to be preferable to placing a valve-bearing Dacron conduit between the apex of the LV and the descending aorta. Some years of observation may be required before sufficient information is available to make an adequate assessment.

REFERENCES

1. Albert, H. M., Atik, M., and Fowler, R.: Production and release of pulmonary stenosis in dogs, Surgery 44:904, 1958.
2. Baffes, T. G.: Total body perfusion in infants and small children for open heart surgery, Pediatr. Surg. 3:551, 1968.
3. Benson, P. F., Joseph, M. C., and Ross, D. N.: Total surgical correction of Fallot's tetralogy in the first year of life, Lancet 2: 326, 1962.
4. Blackstone, E. H., Kirklin, J. W., Bradley, E. L., DuShane, J. W., and Appelbaum, A.: Optimal age and results in repair of large ventricular septal defects, J. Thorac. Cardiovasc. Surg. 72:661, 1976.
5. Cooke, P. A., Nobis, P. A., and Stoney, R. J.: Dacron aortic graft failure, Arch. Surg. 108:101, 1974.
6. Cooper, N., Brazier, J., and Buckberg, G.: Effects of systemic-pulmonary shunts on regional myocardial blood flow in experimental pulmonary stenosis, J. Thorac. Cardiovasc. Surg. 70:166, 1975.
7. Deterling, R. A., Jr.: Failure of Dacron arterial prostheses, Arch. Surg. 108:13, 1974.
8. Dobell, A. R. C., and Grignon, A.: Early and late results in pulmonary atresia, Ann. Thorac. Surg. 24:264, 1977.
9. Donahoo, J. A., and Aberdeen, E.: A new instrument for measurements in cardiovascular surgery, Ann. Thorac. Surg. 22:494, 1976.
10. Gerbode, F., and Carr, I.: Surgery of Congenital Lesions of the

Heart and Great Vessels, in *Practice of Surgery* (Hagerstown, Md.: Harper & Row, Publishers, 1974), Chap. 21.

11. Graham, T. P., Jr., Faulkner, S., Bender, H., Jr., and Wender, C. M.: Hypoplasia of the left ventricle: Rare cause of postoperative mortality in tetralogy of Fallot, Am. J. Cardiol. 40:454, 1977.
12. Hussey, H. H.: Arterial replacement: Failure of synthetic prostheses, JAMA 235:848, 1976.
13. Jarmakani, J. M., Nakazawa, M., Isabel-Jones, J., and Marks, R. A.: Right ventricular function in children with tetralogy of Fallot before and after aortic-to-pulmonary shunt, Circulation 53:555, 1976.
14. Kirklin, J. W., and DuShane, J. W.: Repair of ventricular septal defect in infants, Coll. Papers Mayo Clin. 52:286, 1960.
15. Kirsh, M. M., Perry, B., and Spooner, E.: Management of pseudoaneurysm following patch grafting for coarctation of the aorta, J. Thorac. Cardiovasc. Surg. 74:636, 1977.
16. McMillan, K. R., Johnson, A. M., and Machell, E. S.: Total correction of tetralogy of Fallot in young children, Br. Med. J. 1: 348, 1965.
17. Mistrot, J. J., Varco, R. L., and Nicoloff, D. M.: Palliation of infants with truncus arteriosus through creation of a pulmonary artery ostial stenosis, Ann. Thorac. Surg. 22:495, 1976.
18. Muller, W. H., Jr., and Dammann, J. F., Jr.: The treatment of certain congenital malformations of the heart by the creation of pulmonic stenosis to reduce pulmonary hypertension and ex-

cessive pulmonary blood flow. A preliminary report, Surg. Gynecol. Obstet. 95:213, 1952.
19. Olsson, P., Söderlund, W., Dubiel, W. T., and Ovenfors, C-O.: Patch grafts or tubular grafts in the repair of coarctation of the aorta. A follow-up study, Scand. J. Thorac. Cardiovasc. Surg. 10: 139, 1976.
20. Pacifico, A. D., Kirklin, J. W., and Blackstone, E. H.: Surgical managment of pulmonary stenosis in tetralogy of Fallot, J. Thorac. Cardiovasc. Surg. 74:382, 1977.
21. Pouleur, H., Goenen, M., Jaumin, P. M., Vliers, A. C., Charlier, A. A., and Trémouroux, J.: Cardiac function early after repair of tetralogy of Fallot, J. Thorac. Cardiovasc. Surg. 70:24, 1975.
22. Richardson, J. P., and Clarke, C. P.: Tetralogy of Fallot risk factors associated with complete repair, Br. Heart J. 38:926, 1976.
23. Rudolph, A. M., and Yuan, S.: Response of the pulmonary vasculature to hypoxia and H+ ion concentration changes, J. Clin. Invest. 45:399, 1966.
24. Sloan, H., Mackenzie, J., Morris, J. D., Stern, A., and Sigmann, J.: Open-heart surgery in infancy, J. Thorac. Cardiovasc. Surg. 44:459, 1962.
25. Stark, J., Aberdeen, E., Waterston, D. J., Bonham-Carter, R. E., and Tynan, M.: Pulmonary artery constriction (banding): A report of 146 cases, Surgery 65:808, 1969.
26. Venugopal, P., and Subramanian, S.: Intracardiac repair of tetralogy of Fallot in patients under 5 years of age, Ann. Thorac. Surg. 18:228, 1974.

54 John H. Foster / Richard H. Dean

Surgically Correctable Hypertension in Children*

ONE TO TWO PER CENT of children and up to 11% of adolescents have high blood pressure.[23] This frequency is similar to that of congenital heart disease; yet, although physicians routinely listen for murmurs and look for signs of congenital heart disease in children, they do not routinely measure blood pressure. In most cases, children are not recognized to be hypertensive until they develop a complication: heart failure, seizure, stroke or other central nervous system signs. Table 54–1 lists causes of hypertension in children. This presentation will be limited to the surgically correctable causes: adrenal or renal tumors, coarctation of the aorta, unilateral renal disease and renovascular hypertension. Renovascular hypertension is more common than all of the other causes combined, except for coarctation of the aorta (Fig. 54–1).

Over the past 14 years, our multidisciplinary group evaluated 107 hypertensive children in the hospital. During the same period, more than 2000 adults with hypertension were studied. The work-up in children included the usual history, physical examination, laboratory studies, chest x-ray and cardiogram; in the history and physical examination, special attention is given to a history of urinary infections, abdomi-

nal trauma, a family history of hypertension and signs or symptoms of an abdominal mass or of one of the adrenal causes of hypertension.

In the vast majority of children, the next steps are the rapid-sequence IVP and renal arteriography. If the renal arteries are normal, peripheral renin activity is determined to screen for aldosteronism.

Table 54–2 shows the diagnosis in the 107 children. Adrenal and renal tumors were not seen among these patients referred to the hypertension clinic for evaluation, because these diagnoses usually are made or suspected by the referring physician and the patients sent directly for operative therapy. Sixty per cent had essential hypertension.

Adrenal Causes of Hypertension

Pheochromocytoma

Pheochromocytoma is an uncommon cause of hypertension (0.3–5% of the hypertensive population,[34] of which 5% are children). In 1960, Stackpole et al.[39] collected the reports of 100 children with pheochromocytoma; boys predominated 2:1. It is a catecholamine-secreting tumor of the chromaffin cells found in the adrenal medulla, sympathetic chain, organ of Zuckerkandl, bladder, neck or thorax: 24% are bilateral, 23% extrarenal, 8% both adrenal and extra-adrenal and 4% of patients have 3 or more tumors. Ten per cent of the

*Supported in part by NHLBI Grant #HL-14192 and USPHS Grant #5M01RR00095. From the Department of Surgery and the Specialized Center of Research in Hypertension, Vanderbilt University School of Medicine, Nashville, Tennessee.

TABLE 54-1.—CAUSES OF HYPERTENSION IN CHILDREN°

I. RENAL
    A. Acute and chronic glomerulonephritis
    B. Pyelonephritis—*unilateral*
    C. Polycystic kidney
    D. *Hypoplastic* or *atrophic kidney*
    E. Tumors: *Wilms' neuroblastoma*
    F. Misc.: *Radiation nephritis*, periarteritis
    G. Aneurysms
    H. Trauma
II. CENTRAL NERVOUS SYSTEM
    A. Poliomyelitis, encephalitis
    B. Expanding intracranial mass: tumor, hemorrhage, trauma
    C. Misc.: Dysautonomia, polyneuritis
III. CARDIOVASCULAR
    A. *Coarctation: thoracic* or *abdominal aorta*
    B. *Takayasu's arteritis*
    C. *Renovascular occlusive lesions*
IV. ADRENAL
    A. *Pheochromocytoma*
    B. *Cushing's syndrome*
    C. *Primary aldosteronism*
    D. *Adrenogenital syndrome*
V. POISONINGS—lead, mercury, licorice
VI. IATROGENIC HYPERTENSION—glucosteroids, oral contraceptives
VII. ESSENTIAL HYPERTENSION

°Surgically correctable causes in italics.

TABLE 54-2.—CAUSE OF HYPERTENSION IN 107 CHILDREN REFERRED TO HYPERTENSION CLINIC AT VANDERBILT

	NO.	%
Coarctation of the aorta		
Thoracic	3	
Abdominal	4	5
Renal parenchymal disease		
Bilateral	8	
Unilateral	4	12
Renovascular hypertension	25	24
Essential hypertension	63	60

definitive evidence of metastasis to a nonchromaffin tissue. Five per cent of childhood pheochromocytomas are malignant.[20]

CLINICAL MANIFESTATIONS.—In adults with pheochromocytoma, hypertension may be paroxysmal (65%), sustained (30%) or absent (5%) whereas, in children, 92% have sustained hypertension and only 8% are paroxysmal. The most frequent manifestations in children are: headache, sweating, nausea, weight loss and visual changes, including retinopathy.

DIAGNOSIS.—Most pheochromocytomas secrete norepinephrine and about half secrete epinephrine as well; in children, the tumor is primarily norepinephrine secreting. The finding of an elevated 24-hour urinary output of catecholamines (>130 mg/24 hr), establishes the diagnosis.° An IVP may localize the tumor, especially one located in the adrenal medulla. Pheochromocytomas are extremely vascular and often are opacified on angiography (Fig. 54–2). *Before undertaking arteriography, provision must be made for an immediate infusion to control blood pressure should a hypo- or hypertensive crisis occur.*

OPERATIVE TREATMENT.—Pheochromocytoma results in a blood volume deficit in most patients. An adrenergic blockade with oral phenoxybenzamine or IV phentolamine to control the blood pressure may be required preoperative-

cases are familial, inherited as an autosomal dominant trait; the tumors frequently are multiple and may be associated with neurofibromatosis, medullary carcinoma of the thyroid, parathyroid adenoma or hyperplasia (Sipple's syndrome). The tumor may vary from a tiny nodule to a mass of 100 gm or more. Histologically, most pheochromocytomas appear malignant, but the only acceptable criterion of malignancy is

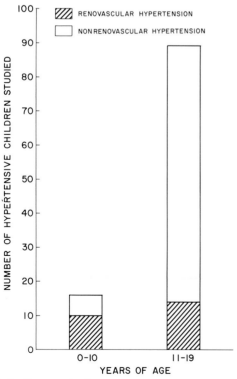

Fig. 54–1.—Renovascular hypertension versus nonrenovascular hypertension in children.

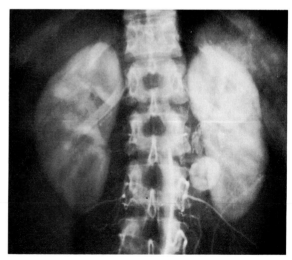

Fig. 54–2.—Pheochromocytoma located just below and adherent to the left renal artery demonstrated by aortography.

°N.B.: Normal values given here and elsewhere are for our endocrine laboratory. Diet, medication and other factors can influence results as well.

ly. The anesthesiologist has a critical role to play in successful operative treatment. Again, provisions must be made for immediate infusion of phentolamine to control hypertension, norepinephrine and blood to counteract hypotension and propranolol to control arrhythmias. We prefer a generous incision, which allows minimal manipulation when removing the tumor.[35] A thorough exploration is performed looking for bilateral or multiple tumors. Earlier, operative mortality was high (13–45%); today, with better knowledge of the problems and pharmacologic control of the blood pressure, the operative mortality is low. The Vanderbilt series now totals 20 patients without an operative death. Two were children; 1 had bilateral tumors. After removal of a tumor, the vast majority (90–95%) of patients are cured.

Cushing's Syndrome

In 1932, Cushing described a syndrome of truncal obesity, hypertension, hirsutism, abdominal striae, polydipsia, polycythemia and susceptibility to infection. Four of his 8 patients had, at autopsy, a basophil adenoma of the pituitary, to which he attributed the syndrome. Today, it is known that the cause is hypersecretion of cortisol by the adrenal. Excluding cases secondary to steroid hormone therapy, hypercortisolism occurs most commonly from three causes: (1) bilateral adrenocortical hyperplasia secondary to the stimulatory effect of increased secretion of ACTH by the pituitary, which may or may not contain an adenoma; (2) bilateral adrenocortical hyperplasia secondary to the stimulus of ectopic ACTH from a nonendocrine tumor (e.g., oat cell carcinoma of the lung); or (3) an adrenocortical tumor. Of 85 patients with Cushing's syndrome due to pituitary and adrenal causes observed at Vanderbilt since 1952, 16 were 19 years

of age or younger.[29] Seven had adrenal tumors (adenoma in 3 and carcinoma in 4) and 9 had bilateral hyperplasia (Fig. 54–3).[33, 36] Up to 1969, 93 cases of Cushing's syndrome were reported in children under 15 years of age—61 had carcinoma, 14 had adenomas and 18 had hyperplasia.[14, 24] Twenty-seven of the children were under 1 year of age—11 of them had carcinoma, 10 had adenoma and 6 had hyperplasia. Associated congenital anomalies were common in infants.

CLINICAL MANIFESTATIONS.—Females predominate; under the age of 1 year, the ratio is 5:1. The signs and symptoms are: obesity, hypertension, failure to thrive, osteoporosis and cessation of linear growth. Most have an abnormal glucose tolerance test.

DIAGNOSIS.—The diagnosis is established by first measuring the 24-hour urinary output of 17-hydroxycorticosteroids (17-OHCS); patients with Cushing's syndrome excrete more than 12 mg/day. Then, dexamethasone is given orally (0.5 mg q6h); in normal subjects this causes a decrease in urinary secretion of 17-OHCS to less than 2.5 mg/day within 48 hours. Patients with Cushing's syndrome show resistance to suppression with this small dose of dexamethasone.

TREATMENT.—The IVP and arteriography usually will localize the site of a tumor. Removal of the tumor is followed by permanent remission, except in patients with malignant adrenocortical tumors, in whom recurrence of the tumor is associated with recurrence of symptoms.[33] Patients with Cushing's disease secondary to hyperplasia usually are treated first by pituitary irradiation; the remission rate was 60% in the 69 patients so treated by Liddle's group at Vanderbilt. In the 8 of these who were children there was an excellent remission in 5.[29] If pituitary radiation therapy fails,

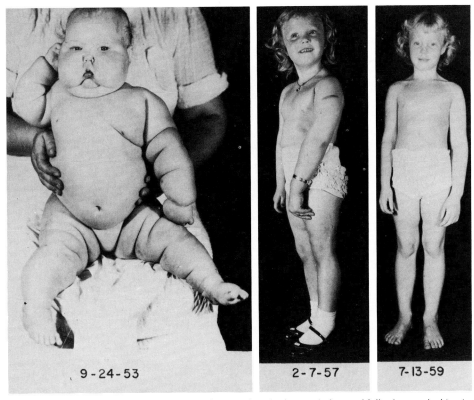

9 - 24 - 53   2 - 7 - 57   7 - 13 - 59

Fig. 54–3.—Child with Cushing's syndrome secondary to adrenal adenoma before and following surgical treatment. (From Weidener, M. G., and Towery, B. T., Surgery 39:492, 1956.)

we resort to bilateral total adrenalectomy via simultaneous bilateral, posterior incisions. (For anterior approach, see Chap. 128.) Four children so treated during the past 20 years were cured.[36] These patients require lifelong glucocorticoid and mineralocorticoid replacement therapy.

Primary Aldosteronism

Primary aldosteronism is an uncommon cause of hypertension (<0.5% of the hypertensive population) characterized by excess adrenal production of the mineralocorticoid aldosterone; in adults, it usually is secondary to a solitary small adrenal adenoma (90%); the other 10% have bilateral hyperplasia or adenoma or carcinoma. In children, 4 cases with an adenoma and more than 10 with hyperplasia have been reported.[17, 20, 28] The tumors have ranged in weight from 0.5 gm to 13 gm.

CLINICAL MANIFESTATIONS.—Females predominated 3:1, ranging in age from infancy to 12 years. Signs and symptoms included severe hypertension (160/120–300/180 mm Hg), visual disturbances, polyuria, polydipsia, retinopathy and hypokalemic alkalosis. Muscle weakness, growth retardation, tetany or intermittent paralysis may occur.

DIAGNOSIS.—Serum K is low (<3 mEq/1), CO_2 and Na usually are elevated. Urinary K is high and urinary aldosterone excretion is elevated (>3–17 mg/day). Plasma renin activity is low. An elevated aldosterone secretion rate (ASR > 40–180 mg/day) is considered diagnostic. Angiography rarely will localize the tumor; it may be difficult to find at operation. However, secondary aldosteronism (including renovascular hypertension) must be ruled out. Thus, it is important to do renal arteriography. Adrenal vein catheterization and determination of aldosterone levels allow localization of the tumor;[9, 26] in cases of hyperplasia, the levels are elevated bilaterally.

TREATMENT.—Preoperatively, the patient is given a low Na, high K diet. If the site of the tumor has been localized, a unilateral approach is used. In cases of hyperplasia, bilateral total adrenalectomy by a one-stage posterior approach is advocated. Obviously, glucocorticoid and mineralocorticoid therapy then are required postoperatively. Operative mortality is low and the patient usually is cured.

Adrenogenital Syndrome

The adrenogenital syndrome may be due to congenital adrenal hyperplasia or secondary to a virilizing adrenocortical tumor (adenoma or carcinoma); both may have associated hypertension.[8] Congenital hyperplasia is treated medically.

DIAGNOSIS AND TREATMENT.—Clinical manifestations include masculinization in the female and pseudoprecocious puberty in the male, hypertension is common, manifestations of Cushing's syndrome may be present and associated congenital defects are common. Urinary 17-ketosteroid (17-KS) excretion is increased (>0.3–15 mg/day depending on age and sex). Congenital adrenal hyperplasia can be differentiated from a tumor by administering cortisone; urinary excretion of 17-KS is reduced to normal in hyperplasia but not in the virilizing tumor. X-ray studies will localize a tumor that is calcified or that displaces the kidney on pyelography or whose tumor vessels are revealed arteriographically. The treatment is removal of the tumor. Many of these neoplasms are highly malignant, but cure may be expected following removal of an adenoma or in some of the encapsulated less malignant tumors.[8] Temporary adrenal insufficiency postoperatively may require glucocorticoid therapy.

Neuroblastoma

Neuroblastomas usually (50%) arise in the adrenal medulla from tissue derived from the neural crest but may also arise from the sympathetic chain or paraganglia. Some neuroblastomas secrete large amounts of catecholamines and the children have elevated urinary catecholamines and VMA; 10–15% of these children are hypertensive. Neuroblastoma is discussed in detail in Chapter 99.

Renal Tumors

Wilms' Tumor

Ten per cent to 15% of children with Wilms' tumor are hypertensive, often severely so (pressure 190/155). The hypertension usually is attributed to compression or kinking of the renal artery by the tumor. Renin-angiotensin studies showing elevated activity have been reported. Wilms' tumor is discussed in detail in Chapter 99.

Coarctation of the Aorta

Coarctation of the aorta may be divided into two general categories: *isthmic*, those involving the thoracic aorta isthmus, and *subisthmic*, those arising below the isthmus and usually involving the abdominal aorta.

Coarctation of the Thoracic Aorta (Isthmic)

Coarctation of the thoracic aorta is a congenital anomaly that is found in 10–15% of patients with congenital heart disease. Hypertension above the coarctation is the almost invariable result. Coarctation of the thoracic aorta is presented in detail in Chapter 56.

Coarctation of the Abdominal Aorta (Subisthmic)

About 2% of coarctations of the aorta are subisthmic.

HISTORICAL DATA.—Subisthmic coarctation was first described by Schlesinger[32] in 1835. Bjork and Intonti[2] and DeBakey *et al.*[7] have published reports describing 26 cases. The first successful repair was done by Beattie in 1951, using an aortic homograft to bypass the lesion.[1] In 1952, Glenn anastomosed the distal splenic artery to the thoracic aorta to bypass a focal supraceliac coarctation.[15]

PATHOLOGIC ANATOMY.—Robicsek's classification of subisthmic coarctations as either suprarenal, juxtarenal or subrenal is useful because of the differing clinical presentations.[31] These lesions may be focal (63%) or elongated (37%).

PATHOPHYSIOLOGY.—As the child grows older, collateral circulation around the site of aortic constriction increases. Degenerative changes and subsequent fibrosis and thickening occur early in the course of thoracic coarctation and similar changes occur in the subisthmic lesions. Abdominal coarctation has a natural history similar to that of thoracic coarctation, with a life expectancy of 30–40 years; 25% of the patients die from each of the following causes: heart failure, ruptured intracranial aneurysm, rupture of the aorta or bacterial endocarditis. Senning and Johansson[37] reviewed 32 patients with abdominal coarctation, of whom 10 died before the age of 34 due to cerebral hemorrhage or cardiac failure. Renal failure, which rarely occurs in thoracic coarctation, is a not infrequent problem in juxtarenal coarctation.

CLINICAL MANIFESTATIONS AND DIAGNOSIS.—The signs and symptoms are related to the location: suprarenal coarctations produce findings like thoracic coarctations, with hypertension as a predominant sign, juxtarenal coarctation results in hypertension, may cause impaired renal function, and infrarenal coarctation causes symptoms in the lower extremities without hypertension. An abdominal bruit often is audible and femoral pulses usually are impaired. Blood pressure in the legs is decreased. Cardiomegaly is frequent; rib notching is limited to the lower rib cage. Aortography visualizing both the thoracic and abdominal aorta establishes both diagnosis and location; some coarctations are multiple. Oblique views may be necessary to visualize the renal arteries well.

TREATMENT. — Several techniques of revascularization have been used in abdominal coarctations. The appropriate technique depends on the location and extent of coarctation. Suprarenal coarctations may be confined to the lower thoracic aorta but commonly extend to the celiac axis. If the coarctation involves both the thoracic and proximal abdominal aorta, a combined left thoracotomy and midline abdominal incision is made. Short subisthmic thoracic coarctations are replaced with a Dacron graft. For elongated coarctations, one inserts a Dacron bypass. A partial occluding clamp usually can be used for the proximal anastomosis. Lesions extending to the celiac axis are best bypassed to the infrarenal aorta; the graft is brought through the left retroperitoneal space.

Coarctation with Renal Artery Stenosis

The majority of these coarctations arise close to the celiac axis and extend to the inferior mesenteric artery; stenosis usually is limited to the orifice of the renal artery but may be more extensive. Unilateral renal artery stenosis has been seen; bilateral involvement is the rule. Split renal function studies (SRFS) and renal vein renin assays (RVRA) are done preoperatively.

Bypass grafting from the thoracic aorta to the distal abdominal aorta through a left thoracic and midline abdominal incision is the preferred treatment. The decision to perform unilateral or bilateral renal artery reconstruction is complex. Bilateral renal artery reconstruction is necessary in patients with severe bilateral renal artery stenosis. If the preoperative RVRA and SRFS point to a predominantly unilateral lesion, only that side may require revascularization. The decision must be on the basis of the findings in the individual case. Autogenous saphenous vein, splenic or hypogastric artery or a Dacron graft can be used. Either a secondary bypass graft from the Dacron aorta—aorta graft to the renal arteries—or a patch angioplasty is done. Other approaches can be used in particular cases; e.g., a splenorenal arterial anastomosis can be used to bypass a left renal artery stenosis.

Results of Treatment

The results with abdominal coarctations without renal artery stenosis have been excellent; 90–95% of the patients become normotensive. The postoperative course is similar to that of patients with thoracic lesions. Occasionally, paradoxic hypertension and bowel ischemia may occur in the early postoperative period.

Following operation for juxtarenal coarctations, the results have also been good. The risk of operation is greater because the procedure is more extensive; nevertheless, DeBakey had no early or late deaths in 16 patients and all remained normotensive 5 years or more following operation.[7] During the past 8 years, 4 cases of abdominal aortic coarctation have been treated at Vanderbilt.

There were 3 boys and 1 girl; ages at the time of recognition were 3 months, 4, 9 and 18 years. The abdominal aorta was hypoplastic in all 4. At the time of operation, in the 9-year-old and the 18-year-old, the renal arteries originated from the hypoplastic segment. The main renal arteries were stenotic bilaterally in the 9-year-old and only on the right in the 18-year-old. Blood pressures ranged from 240/140 to 160/100 mm Hg. Differential renal renin assays identified a unilateral lesion in 3 patients and were nonlateralizing in the 9-year-old with bilaterally severe stenosis. In the 4-year-old, a Dacron bypass from the thoracic to the infrarenal abdominal aorta resulted in normal blood pressure (Fig. 54–4). A left nephrectomy was done in the 3-month-old. He is markedly improved but requires antihypertensive medication and may have right renal stenosis; this will be studied subsequently. The 9-year-old with coarctation and stenotic renal arteries had a patch angioplasty, using autologous splenic artery, of the aorta and the main renal arteries, which resulted in marked improvement and is easily controlled with small amounts of medication. He also had small bilateral accessory renal arteries, one of which was seen to be occluded on the preoperative arteriogram. A recent follow-up aortogram shows widely patent main renal arteries, but now both accessory arteries are occluded. Eventually, he may require segmental resections. The fourth patient, an 18-year-old girl, was admitted to the hospital in 1968 following a seizure. There was a history of repeated urinary infections. The BP was 210/160 mm Hg and she had grade IV hypertensive retinopathy. IVP showed a small left kidney with clubbing of the calyces and dilatation of the distal left ureter, which drained into the urethra. Aortogram showed hypoplasia of the abdominal aorta from just below the celiac axis to the aortic bifurcation. The left renal artery and kidney were small but otherwise normal. There were two right renal arteries with stenotic occlusion of the one to the upper pole. The BUN was 38 mg/100 ml, urine culture grew out Aerobacter and Klebsiella. Following these studies, the patient developed severe renal failure, refractory hypertension, congestive failure and uremic pneumonitis and died, despite peritoneal dialyses. Late recognition in this last patient and the ultimate result sharply contrasts with the 9-year-old boy with abdominal coarctation and bilateral renal artery stenosis.

Renovascular Hypertension

Renovascular hypertension (RVH) is the second most common cause of surgically remediable hypertension. Only coarctation of the aorta is more frequent. It is being recognized with increasing frequency, especially in centers interested in the problem.[13, 19, 25, 45] Prior to 1962, RVH in a child had not been recognized at Vanderbilt; since that time, 24 children with RVH have been identified and treated surgically, with an excellent result in 23 of the children.

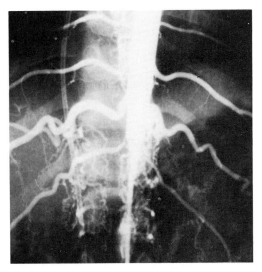

Fig. 54–4. — Retrograde catheter aortogram in a 4-year-old white boy with abdominal coarctation who was cured following Dacron graft from the thoracic aorta to the infrarenal aorta. Note the prominent and enlarged intercostal arteries and collaterals. A roentgenogram in a later phase of the aortogram showed a small aorta below the superior mesenteric artery; renal arteries appeared normal, although the right one was not optimally demonstrated.

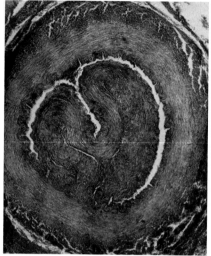 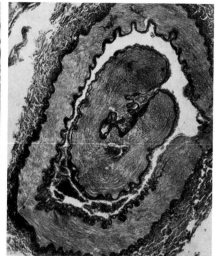

Fig. 54–5.—Photomicrographs of right renal artery of a 5-year-old black boy with RVH due to fibromuscular dysplasia of artery to an ectopic right kidney. A fibromuscular plug almost occluded the artery. First documented case of RVH and of FMD of renal artery. Compare with Figure 54–12. (From Leadbetter, W. F., and Burkland, C. E., J. Urol. 39:611, 1938.)

Renovascular hypertension may be defined as main or branch renal artery occlusive disease of sufficient severity to activate the renal pressor mechanism.

HISTORICAL DATA.—In 1934, Goldblatt *et al.*[16] reported the experimental production of hypertension in the dog by constricting both renal arteries. The first case of renovascular hypertension was documented in 1938 by Leadbetter and Burkland,[21] who reported a 5-year-old black boy with hypertension (240/140 mm Hg) and a nonfunctioning, ectopic right kidney, who was treated by nephrectomy and cured of his hypertension. Figure 54–5 shows photomicrographs of the fibromuscular lesion that almost completely occluded the right renal artery in the patient. This was also the first reported case of fibromuscular dysplasia of the renal artery.

INCIDENCE.—As in adults, the incidence of RVH is not known. Using Loggie's[23] estimate of incidence of hypertension in children as 1–2% of those under 12 and 11% in adolescence, a reasonable estimate can be made; in hypertensive children under 12, 50% probably have RVH; over 12 years of age, the incidence probably is over 5%, just as in hypertensive adults.

ETIOLOGY AND PATHOLOGIC ANATOMY.—The etiology and pathologic anatomy of the occlusive lesions are classified and listed in Table 54–3. By far the most common etiology is fibromuscular dysplasia[13] (Figs. 54–6 and 54–7) (over 90% of the reported cases), bilateral in 10–15%. The etiology of fibromuscular dysplasia is not known, and it involves other arteries as well. The youngest reported patient (recognized at autopsy) was 10 days of age;[22] our youngest surgically treated patient was 4 months of age.[12]

PATHOPHYSIOLOGY.—The mechanism whereby renal artery stenosis causes hypertension remains somewhat uncertain. It is commonly believed that renal artery stenosis re-

TABLE 54–3.—ETIOLOGY OF RENOVASCULAR
HYPERTENSION IN CHILDREN

I. EXTERNAL COMPRESSION OF THE RENAL ARTERY
   A. Renal, adrenal and para-aortic tumors
   B. Crus of diaphragm
   C. Ligature
II. INTRALUMINAL OBSTRUCTION OF RENAL ARTERY
   A. Embolus
   B. Thrombosis
III. LESIONS OF THE RENAL ARTERY
   A. Trauma—blunt or penetrating
   B. Fibromuscular dysplasia—intimal, medial or adventitial
   C. Neurofibromatosis
   D. Arteritis—Takayasu's arteritis
   E. Aneurysms—congenital, idiopathic, arteriovenous
IV. COARCTATION OF THE ABDOMINAL AORTA

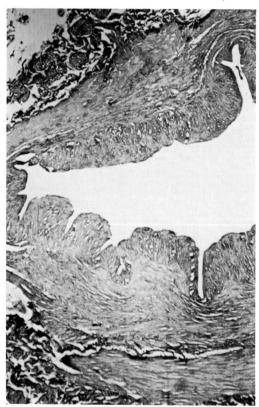

Fig. 54–6.—Medial fibromuscular dysplasia of the renal artery, the most common cause of RVH in children.

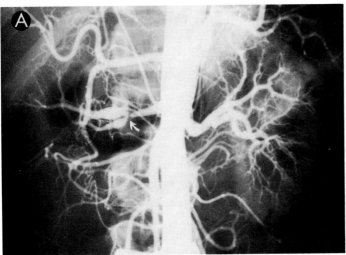

Fig. 54–7.—A, hypertension due to renal artery stenosis from fibrodys-
plasia in a 17-year-old girl whose first manifestation of hypertension was a
stroke. (From Foster, J. H., in Dale, W. A. [ed.], *Management of Arterial Occlu-* *sive Disease* [Chicago: Year Book Medical Publishers, Inc., 1971], p. 275.)
B, operative photograph of the right renal artery *(RRA)* stenosis.

duces renal blood flow or diminishes the pulse pressure, which, in turn, causes the juxtaglomerular apparatus to release renin, which is converted to angiotensin—a powerful vasoconstrictor (Fig. 54–8).

The deleterious effects of sustained diastolic hypertension are reflected in the susceptible target organs: the heart, brain and kidneys, especially in the arteries and arterioles of these organs. Left ventricular hypertrophy, encephalopathy, retinopathy, cerebral vasculitis, intracranial hemorrhage and arteriolar nephrosclerosis occur singly or in various combinations. The end result may include congestive heart failure, stroke and/or renal failure. In the adult, hypertension accelerates the course of arteriosclerosis and atherosclerosis throughout the body. How early in life this process begins is not certain. Secondary aldosteronism is not an uncommon accompaniment of severe renovascular hypertension.

CLINICAL MANIFESTATIONS.—The signs and symptoms of hypertension rarely are attributable to the elevated blood pressure per se but rather are due to the effects on the target organs. Early in the disease there are few or no signs or symptoms. There is little in the history, physical examination or routine laboratory examinations that will help to differentiate RVH from essential hypertension (EH) in children. Under 12 years of age, a renovascular cause becomes much more likely. A history of abdominal or flank trauma may be important in the etiology of RVH. A family history of hypertension and hypertension of recent onset occur equally frequently in RVH and EH. Cardiomegaly and retinopathy are helpful only in gauging the severity of the hypertension. The vast majority of children with RVH are symptomatic, and markedly so, at the time of the recognition of the hypertension.[15] In our series, central nervous system signs and symptoms (headache, extreme irritability, seizures, stroke, severe retinopathy), congestive heart failure and cardiomegaly were the common modes of presentation. Half of the children had malignant hypertension when their high blood pressure was recognized.

DIAGNOSIS.—Prior to beginning the diagnostic studies, the blood pressure is brought under control with drugs. This may require several days. The screening tests that we use

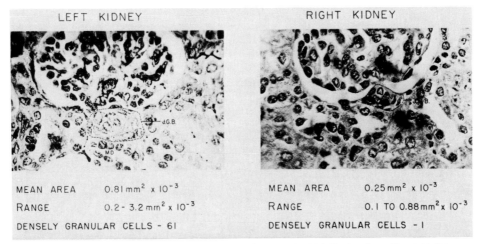

Fig. 54–8.—Photomicrographs of juxtaglomerular apparatus (JGA) in kidneys of a 4-month-old child with malignant RVH due to FMD of left renal artery, showing hypertrophy of the JGA and an increase in granular cells (source of renin). Nephrectomy (the right kidney was biopsied) resulted in cure.

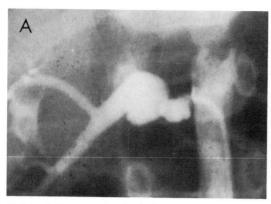

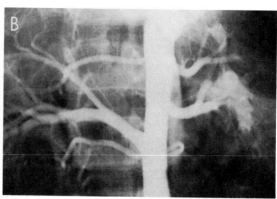

Fig. 54–9.—Unilateral fibromuscular dysplasia and aneurysm of right renal artery before **(A)** and after **(B)** Dacron aortorenal graft in a 7-year-old white boy, who now has been normotensive for 3 years. He was first seen at the age of 3 and received drug therapy for 4 years before the revascularization.

are the rapid-sequence excretory urogram (IV) and renal arteriography. The arteriogram is our major screening test. We obtain AP and oblique aortographic and selective renal arteriographic views. If renal artery stenosis or a hypoplastic kidney is found, we do split renal function studies and renal venous renin assays to determine the functional significance of the lesions. In children under 6–8 years of age, we reluctantly omit the split renal function studies because of the problems with ureteral catheterization in small children. We say "reluctantly" because we know that about 10% of the time one radiographic test or the other will be falsely normal in cases of RVH. Our criteria for interpreting the functional tests have been described previously.[6]

If either the split renal function studies or differential renin assays are positive, we consider the diagnosis of RVH established and usually recommend operative treatment.

OPERATIVE TREATMENT.—About 30% of patients with RVH will have a blood volume deficit, markedly so in severe cases. Drug therapy (usually Aldomet) is continued up to the time of operation *if necessary* to keep the diastolic pressure under 100 mm Hg.

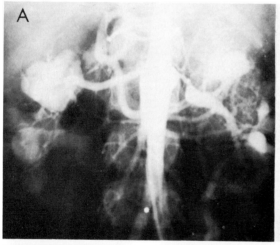

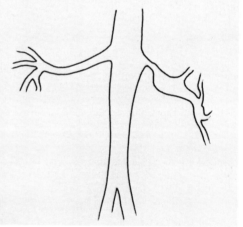

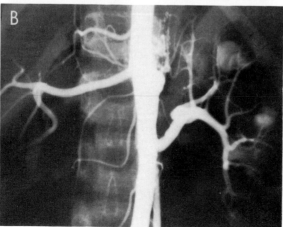

Fig. 54–10.—**A,** aortogram in an 8-year-old white boy with Takayasu's arteritis causing left renal artery stenosis. Celiac, superior mesenteric and right subclavian arteries were also involved. Caliceal clubbing and ureteral dilatation bilaterally 2° reflux is present but renal function was normal. Tracing at the right depicts aorta and renal arteries more clearly. **B,** postoperative study, showing patent aortorenal bypass graft; left hypogastric artery was utilized as graft material. He has been normotensive for 6 years.

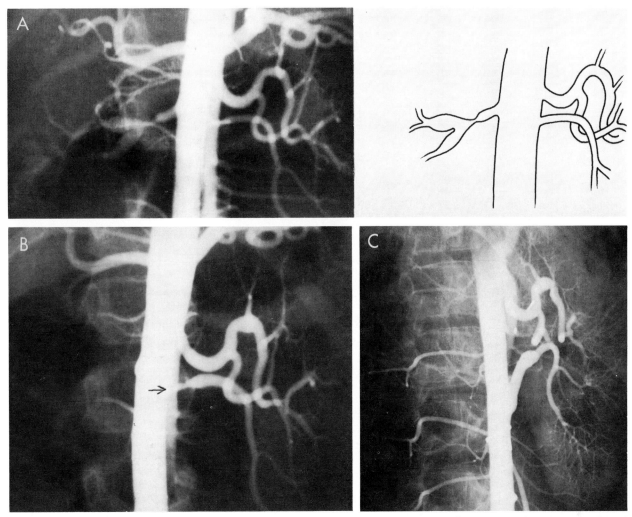

Fig. 54–11.—A, aortogram showing FMD of right renal artery in a 2-year-old white boy treated by right nephrectomy after thrombosis of a vein patch angioplasty. Tracing at the right depicts aorta and renal arteries more clearly. B, hypertension recurred (after 4 years of normotension) secondary to left inferior renal artery stenosis. C, saphenous vein, aortorenal graft resulted in normotension for the past 3 years. End-to-end anastomosis to renal artery was done. After hypertension recurred, he was followed on drug therapy for 5 years before the bypass was done.

Our basic operation has been the aortorenal bypass graft utilizing the saphenous vein as the graft. Dacron grafts and autologous hypogastric artery have also been used. In anastomosing the graft to the renal artery. We have used both the end-to-side and the end-to-end techniques, depending on the anatomic configuration. Monofilament polypropylene sutures (4.0 or 5.0) are used. Mannitol is administered intravenously about 15 minutes before the renal artery is occluded and intravenous heparin is given just prior to clamping.

In our 24 children (2 patients with abdominal coarctation are included) (Figs. 54–9, 54–10, 54–13 and 54–14), an aortorenal bypass was done in 12 (bilateral in 2), a vein patch angioplasty was done in 4, primary nephrectomy was done in 5 and a single segment of the kidney was resected in 3 (Fig. 54–12). Two of the patch angioplasties (done in 1962–1963) thrombosed and required nephrectomy. There were no operative deaths, but in a 4-year-old boy treated by nephrectomy in 1965 who then was normotensive for 4 months, the hypertension recurred and he was found to have severe stenosing lesions of the branch renal arteries in his contralateral kidney (Fig. 54–15). He died 8 months postoperatively with malignant hypertension and renal failure. A second patient treated by nephrectomy in 1963 remained

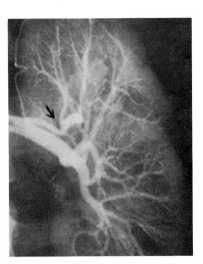

Fig. 54–12.—Fibromuscular stenosis of a segmental branch artery (arrow). Hypertension in this 16-year-old girl has been relieved for the 4 years since segmental nephrectomy.

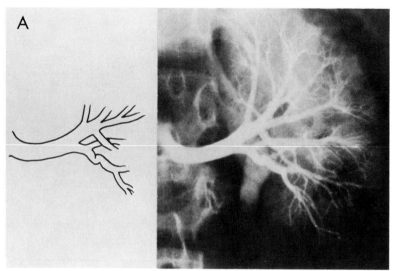

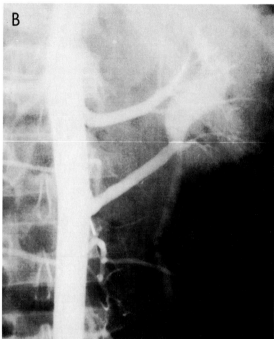

Fig. 54–13.—FMD in a segmental branch of the left renal artery in an 8-year-old boy with hypertension. **A,** arteriogram and accompanying outline drawing showing the affected vessel to the lower pole. **B,** postoperative study showing aortorenal saphenous vein graft (an end-to-end anastomosis was made to the segmental renal artery).

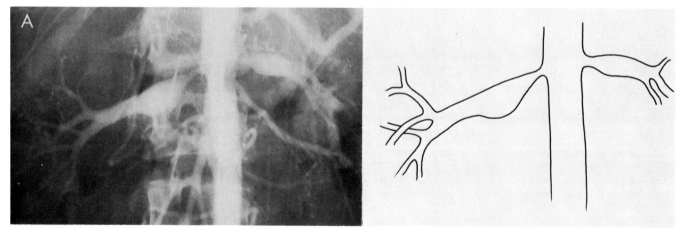

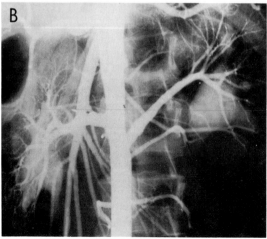

Fig. 54–14.—Bilateral FMD renal artery stenosis in a 12-year-old girl. **A,** aortogram and sketch show the juxta-aortic stenoses and poststenotic dilatation. **B,** postoperative study, 1 year later, showing relief of the obstruction and patent bilateral Dacron aortorenal grafts. She has been normotensive for the past 2½ years.

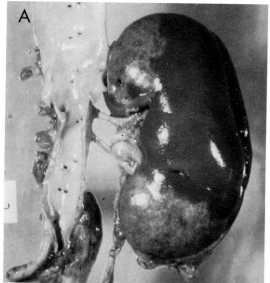 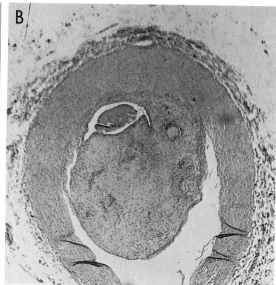

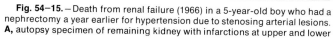

Fig. 54–15.—Death from renal failure (1966) in a 5-year-old boy who had a nephrectomy a year earlier for hypertension due to stenosing arterial lesions. **A,** autopsy specimen of remaining kidney with infarctions at upper and lower pole. **B,** photomicrograph showing organized thrombosis in a renal artery. Note similarity to Fig. 54–5. We have since avoided nephrectomy in apparently unilateral fibromuscular disease.

normotensive for 4 years only to become hypertensive again (Fig. 54–11). Contralateral renal artery stenosis had developed in the interim. He subsequently had a successful renal artery bypass and has been normotensive for the past 3 years. The development of contralateral renal artery stenosis in these 2 patients has made us reluctant ever again to perform a nephrectomy for RVH in childhood, if it possibly can be avoided. If the child is too small to allow a successful reconstruction, we will treat the child with drugs until sufficient size is reached (Figs. 54–9 and 54–11).

The postoperative course in these children has been largely uneventful as contrasted to more frequent morbidity in the adult RVH patients. Most of the children were normotensive prior to discharge from the hospital or shortly thereafter.

Twenty-three of the 24 children are living and well. They have had follow-up studies, including renal arteriography, at 1–2-year intervals; follow-up ranges from 6 months to 14 years (mean 4.6 years). Nineteen are normotensive and require no medication. Four patients are clearly improved but require mild antihypertensive medication. In the 2 from the abdominal coarctation group, the reasons for their residual RVH already has been explained, a third has developed a new segmental renal artery stenosis and the final patient had bilateral bypasses for longstanding hypertension (<10 years). A similar series of childhood RVH has been reported by Fry *et al.*[13] with equally good results; they, too, use the saphenous vein as a graft. Smaller series have been reported by Kaufman *et al.*[19] and by Wylie and Stoney.[25, 40] The latter prefer to use the autologous hypogastric artery for the aorto-renal graft.

Unilateral Renal Parenchymal Disease

An occasional case of severe unilateral renal parenchymal disease results in hypertension that can be relieved by nephrectomy.[43] These usually are cases of pyelonephritis with a small, largely destroyed kidney on one side. Radiation nephritis accounts for some of the cases. If such a patient has lateralizing renal venous renin assays, a favorable blood

pressure response may be expected following nephrectomy. The hypertension should be severe (diastolic pressures of 100 mm Hg or greater) to justify removing one kidney and the function of the uninvolved kidney should be normal. We have treated 4 such children ranging in age from 7 to 16 years with a beneficial response in each; 2 are cured and 2 clearly improved 1–12 years following nephrectomy.

REFERENCES

1. Beattie, E. J., Jr., Cooke, F. N., Paul, J. S., and Orbison, J. A.: Coarctation of aorta at level of diaphragm treated successfully with preserved human blood vessel graft, J. Thorac. Surg. 21: 506, 1951.
2. Bjork, V. O., and Intonti, F.: Coarctation of abdominal aorta with right renal artery stenosis, Ann. Surg. 160:54, 1964.
3. Conn, J. W., Cohen, E. L., and Rovner, D. R.: Suppression of plasma renin activity in primary aldosteronism, JAMA 190:125, 1964.
4. Conn, J. W., Cohen, E. L., Rovner, D. R., and Nesbit, R. M.: Special communication: Normokalemic primary aldosteronism, JAMA 193:100, 1965.
5. Conn, J. W., Knopf, R. F., and Nesbit, R. M.: Primary Aldosteronism: Present Evaluation of Its Clinical Characteristics and the Results of Surgery, in Baulieu, E. E., and Robel, R., *Aldosterone* (Oxford: Blackwell Scientific Publications, 1964).
6. Dean, R. H., and Foster, J. H.: Criteria for the diagnosis of renovascular hypertension, Surgery 74:926, 1973.
7. DeBakey, M. E., Garrett, H. E., Howell, J. F., and Morris, G. C., Jr.: Coarctation of the abdominal aorta with renal arterial stenosis: Surgical considerations, Ann. Surg. 165:830, 1967.
8. diGeorge, A.: Disorders of the Adrenal Glands, in Vaughan, V. C., and McKay, R. J. (eds.), *Nelson's Textbook of Pediatrics* (10th ed.; Philadelphia: W. B. Saunders Company, 1969), p. 1327.
9. Egdahl, R. H., Kahn, P. C., and Melby, J. C.: Unilateral adrenalectomy for aldosteronomas localized preoperatively by differential adrenal vein catheterization, Surgery 64:117, 1968.
10. Fishman, L. M., Kuchel, O., Liddle, G. W., Michelakis, A. M., Gordon, R. D., and Chick, W. T.: Incidence of primary aldosteronism in uncomplicated "essential" hypertension, JAMA 205: 497, 1968.
11. Foster, J. H.: Surgically Correctible Hypertension, in Schwartz, S. I. (ed.), *Principles of Surgery* (New York: McGraw-Hill Book Company, Inc., 1974), p. 939.
12. Foster, J. H., Pettinger, W. A., Oates, J. A., *et al.*: Malignant hypertension secondary to renal artery stenosis in children, Ann. Surg. 164:700, 1966.

13. Fry, W. J., Ernst, C. B., Stanley, J. C., and Brink, B.: Renovascular hypertension in the pediatric patient, Arch. Surg. 107:692, 1973.
14. Gilbert, M. G., and Cleveland, W. W.: Cushing's syndrome in infancy, Pediatrics 46:217, 1970.
15. Glenn, F., Keefer, E. B. C., Speer, D. S., and Dotter, C. T.: Coarctation of the lower thoracic and abdominal aorta immediately proximal to the celiac axis, Surg. Gynecol. Obstet. 94:561, 1952.
16. Goldblatt, H., Lynch, J., Hanzal, R. F., and Summerville, W. W.: Studies on experimental hypertension. I. The production of persistent elevation of systolic blood pressure by means of renal ischemia, J. Exp. Med. 59:347, 1934.
17. Grim, C. E., McBryde, A. C., Glenn, J. F., and Gunnels, J. C., Jr.: Childhood primary aldosteronism with bilateral adrenocortical hyperplasia: Plasma renin activity as an aid to diagnosis, Pediatrics 71:377, 1967.
18. Hume, D. M., and Harrison, T. S.: Pituitary and Adrenals, in Schwartz, S. I. (ed.), *Principles of Surgery* (New York: McGraw-Hill Book Company, Inc., 1974), p. 363.
19. Kaufman, J. J., Goodwin, W. E., Waisman, J., and Gyepes, M. T.: Renovascular hypertension in children: Report of seven cases treated surgically including two cases of renal autotransplantation, Am. J. Surg. 124:149, 1972.
20. Kelly, V. C., and Limbeck, G. A.: The Adrenal Glands, in Brenneman, J., and Kelly, V. C. (eds.), *Practice of Pediatrics* (Hagerstown, Md.: Harper & Row, Publishers, 1971), Vol. 1, Part 2, p. 235.
21. Leadbetter, W. F., and Burkland, C. E.: Hypertension in unilateral renal disease, J. Urol. 39:611, 1938.
22. Ljungquist, A., and Wallgren, G.: Unilateral renal artery stenosis and fatal arterial hypertension in a newborn infant, Acta Paediatr. 51:575, 1962.
23. Loggie, J. M. H.: Hypertension in children and adolescents, Hosp. prac., p. 81, June, 1975.
24. Loridan, L., and Senior, B.: Cushing's syndrome in infancy, J. Pediatr. 75:349, 1969.
25. Lye, C. S., String, T., Wylie, E. J., and Stoney, R. J.: Aortorenal arterial autografts: Late observations.
26. Melby, J. C., Spark, R. F., Dale, S. L., Egdahl, R. H., and Kahn, P. C.: Diagnosis and localization of aldosterone-producing adenomas by adrenal-vein catheterization, N. Engl. J. Med. 277:1050, 1967.
27. Morris, G. C., Jr., DeBakey, M. E., Cooley, D. A., and Crawford, E. S.: Subisthmic aortic stenosis and occlusive disease, Arch. Surg. 80:87, 1960.
28. New, M. I., and Peterson, R. E.: Aldosterone in Childhood, in Levine, S. Z. (ed.), *Advances in Pediatrics* (Chicago: Year Book Medical Publishers, Inc., 1968), Vol. 15, p. 111.
29. Orth, D. N., and Liddle, G. W.: Results of treatment in 108 patients with Cushing's syndrome, N. Engl. J. Med. 285:243, 1971.
30. Pyorala, K., Heinoney, O., Doskelo, P., and Keikel, P. E.: Coarctation of the abdominal aorta. Review of twenty-seven cases, Am. J. Cardiol. 6:650, 1960.
31. Robicsek, F., Sanger, P. W., and Daugherty, H. K.: Coarctation of the abdominal aorta diagnosed by aortography: Report of three cases, Ann. Surg. 162:227, 1965.
32. Schlesinger: Merkwurdige Verschliessung der Aorta, Wochenschr. Heilk., No. 31, p. 489, 1835.
33. Scott, H. W., Jr.: Tumors of the Endocrine Glands: Tumors of the Adrenal Cortex and Cushing's Syndrome. Seventh National Cancer Conference Proceedings, p. 513, 1973.
34. Scott, H. W., Jr., and Foster, J. H.: Surgical Considerations in Hypertension, in *Current Problems in Surgery* (Chicago: Year Book Medical Publishers, Inc., July, 1964).
35. Scott, H. W., Jr., Liddle, G. W., Mulherin, J. L., Jr., et al.: Surgical experience with Cushing's disease, Ann. Surg. (In press.)
36. Scott, H. W., Jr., Riddell, D. H., and Brockman, S. K.: Surgical management of pheochromocytoma, Surg. Gynecol. Obstet. 120:707, 1965.
37. Senning, A., and Johansson, L.: Coarctation of the abdominal aorta, J. Thorac. Cardiovasc. Surg. 40:517, 1960.
38. Silen, W., Biglieri, E. G., Slaton, P., and Galante, M.: Management of primary aldosteronism, Ann. Surg. 164:600, 1966.
39. Stackpole, R. H., Melicow, M. M., and Uson, A. C.: Pheochromocytoma in children, J. Pediatr. 63:314, 1963.
40. Stoney, R. J., and Wylie, E. J.: Arterial autografts, Surgery 67:18, 1970.
41. Tanaka, N., Kubota, S., and Kamimae, A.: An autopsy case of aldosteronism accompanied by unilateral renovascular hypertension in a young child and the demonstration of juxtaglomerular granules, Acta Pathol. Jpn. 15 (1):21, 1965.
42. Van Way, C. W., III, Michelakis, A. M., Alper, B. J., Hutcheson, J. K., Rhamy, R. K., and Scott, H. W., Jr.: Renal vein renin studies in a patient with renal hilar pheochromocytoma and renal artery stenosis, Ann. Surg. 172:212, 1970.
43. Vaughan, E. D., Jr., Buhler, F. R., Laragh, J. H., Sealey, J. E., Gavras, H., and Baer, L.: Hypertension and unilateral parenchymal renal disease: Evidence for abnormal vasoconstriction-volume interaction, JAMA 233:1177, 1975.
44. Vermeulen, F., Stas, F., Delegher, C., Buyssens, N., et al.: Surgical correction of renovascular hypertension in children, J. Cardiovasc. Surg. 16:21, 1975.
45. Wylie, E. J., Perloff, D., and Stoney, R. J.: Autogenous tissue revascularization techniques in surgery for renovascular hypertension, Ann. Surg. 170:416, 1969.

Arterial Anomalies

55 Henry T. Bahnson

Patent Ductus Arteriosus

HISTORICAL PERSPECTIVE.—Although in 1888 Munro knew that the patent ductus arteriosus should be closed, and in 1907 suggested an operation for its interruption, this was not attempted until Strieder in 1937 operated on a patient with subacute bacterial endocarditis and ligated the ductus; the patient died 4 days later of acute gastric dilatation. Unaware of this attempt, Gross in 1938 operated electively on a patient with a patent ductus, obliterating it by ligation, and thus placed the first entering wedge into the surgical treatment of congenital heart disease. Early surgical treatment was by ligation of the ductus, later followed by the theoretically more effective approach of division. Safe division of a short, broad ductus was not possible, however, until the development of improved instruments, most of which involved the multitoothed principle developed by Potts.

Treatment of the patent ductus arteriosus has reflected the rapid advances made in cardiovascular surgery in the past four decades. Initially one of the very few operations on the heart and great vessels and performed by only a few surgeons, interruption by ligation or division now is done by most thoracic surgeons, is one of the simpler operations and often is performed almost incidentally as part of the open repair of intracardiac defects or as one of several treatments, as in the care of the infant with respiratory distress syndrome.

Anatomy and Physiology

The ductus arteriosus is the distal portion of the left 6th aortic arch of the embryo and in fetal life conducts blood flow from the pulmonary artery to the aorta, away from the unused lungs. At birth, as ventilation begins, pulmonary vascular resistance drops abruptly and flow reverses in the ductus. The increased oxygen level of arterial blood and drop of pulmonary resistance are associated with contraction of the ductus,[10] followed by firm closure. In 558 infants studied anatomically by Christie,[2] the ductus was open 2 weeks after birth in 65%, but this number rapidly decreased with age and only 2% were open after 32 weeks and 1% at 1 year. Many of these openings were small and functionally unimportant.

When patent, the ductus commonly is the only cardiovascular abnormality, but it also is a common accompaniment of other malformations within the heart itself or of the aorta. It joins the main, or left, pulmonary artery with the lesser curvature of the aortic arch just distal to the left subclavian artery and thus conducts an aortic-pulmonary left-to-right shunt of blood. It may vary in diameter from 1 mm to around 2 cm and is also variable in length. Some of the large ductus may be nearly flush aortic-pulmonary connections. The ductus may exist in aberrant positions, but these are rare and it almost always is on the left even in the presence of a right aortic arch, in which case it often connects the pulmonary artery and the distal portion of the left innominate artery.

In most cases, the increased pulmonary blood flow is tolerated with few secondary changes; but, in some patients, pulmonary hypertension develops, associated with marked intimal proliferation of the medium and small pulmonary arteries, muscular hypertrophy of these vessels and organizing thrombi in the pulmonary arteries.[4] Some of these arterial changes are noted in the lung of normal infants, the lung during fetal life being subjected to the same pressure as that of the systemic circulation, but these features normally regress rapidly after birth with lowering of the pulmonary arterial pressure.[6] In patients with pulmonary hypertension there may be some failure of regression of these changes with, in time, progression associated with the increased flow and pressure in the pulmonary circulation. Those patients in whom these changes occur, however, represent the minority, and in most patients measurable changes occur only in pulmonary blood flow.

The ductus may be protective in patients with diminished pulmonary circulation, as in the tetralogy of Fallot. In such patients, the use of prostaglandin E, a potent vasodilator, may serve to keep the ductus open.[16] Conversely, inhibitors of prostaglandin have been used to encourage closure.[9]

Clinical Features

Patent ductus arteriosus occurs in about 1 in 4000 of the general population. About 70% are female.[7] Patency is part of the rubella syndrome of infants, stemming from rubella during the first trimester of pregnancy, and epidemics of rubella have resulted in a sporadic increased incidence.

Symptoms attributable to patent ductus arteriosus vary greatly from none to severe cardiac failure, depending on age, the size of the aortic-pulmonary shunt and undetermined factors. Some patients grow normally, have no limitation of activity and no detectable abnormality except for the murmur. Some children, however, will have frequent respiratory distress and be retarded in physical growth, sometimes strikingly. The added burden on the heart may be made apparent in older children by loss of energy, shortness of breath and fatigue. Cardiac failure from the overload of a large patent ductus is rare in the absence of pulmonary hypertension, which, in turn, may be aggravated by an elevated left atrial pressure.

Subacute bacterial endarteritis at the site of the ductus has not been commonly seen since the common use of antibiotics began, but the disease and prevention of it were common indications for operation in early experience. Endarteritis occurs most commonly in young adults and rather infrequently in children and is manifested by the signs similar to those of endocarditis—fever, weight loss, anemia and positive blood cultures.

Although the condition is compatible with a long life and little or no disability, this is not usually the case. As reported by Keys and Shapiro,[13] those patients alive at 17 years of age with a patent ductus arteriosus have a subsequent life expectancy about one-half that of the normal population. From Campbell's[1] own large experience and that reported by others, he concluded that by age 45, 42% of patients with a patent ductus arteriosus will have died. Although he found that spontaneous closure of the ductus may occur even later in life, this occurs too infrequently to rely on. Data such as these related to the untreated natural course of the abnormality no longer can be obtained, since operation is commonly recommended for prophylactic reasons.

The heart usually is normal in size or only minimally enlarged. It may be overactive in the presence of a large shunt. Commonly there is a normal systolic blood pressure with a low diastolic level because of the runoff into the pulmonary circuit, and in the advanced stage there may be peripheral signs similar to those of aortic insufficiency. The murmur is a characteristic one and the condition can be accurately diagnosed by it in the vast majority of cases. Typically, it is a continuous murmur, often rumbling in systole, sometimes obscuring the pulmonary second sound, heard most prominently in the right second to third intercostal spaces and often associated with a thrill. The pulmonary second sound may be accentuated. The rumbling systolic phase, banging second sound and continuous murmur give the impression of running machinery, the term usually applied to it. The murmur can be transmitted over the chest, the extent depending mainly on its intensity. Only the systolic component may be heard in the presence of a small ductus although the flow and turbulence probably are continuous. When the shunt of blood to the ductus is extremely large there may be a rumbling diastolic murmur at the apex of the heart suggestive of relative mitral stenosis. Systolic murmurs may be heard due to the large flow through the active heart. The murmur may be obscured or altered when heart failure occurs with pulmonary hypertension.

When the heart is enlarged, roentgenography may demonstrate that the enlargement is predominantly of the left atrium and left ventricle. The region of the left pulmonary artery often is full and the lung fields may show increased vascularity, sometimes leading to a hilar dance, although this is not so striking with the ductus as with an atrial septal defect. Ventricular septal defect may also cause enlargement of the left-sided chambers, but the ascending aorta characteristically is larger with a patent ductus, because of the flow through it, than with ventricular septal defect. Enlargement of the left atrium may be demonstrated by echocardiography, the size of the left atrium being compared with that of the aortic root to detect an increase in the former.[18] This study has been helpful, especially in the newborn.

In recent years it has become evident that the ductus may be patent and be an important aggravating element in the respiratory distress syndrome of the newborn, especially when this occurs in premature infants. Probably because of the immaturity of the tissue in the wall of the ductus, it commonly remains patent in premature infants.[15] Hypoxia, which occurs with the respiratory distress syndrome, probably contributes to patency inasmuch as the rapid rise in arterial oxygen with ventilation is one factor that favors closure at birth.[10] In the newborn infant with respiratory distress, the usual signs of an appropriate murmur, bounding femoral pulses, unusual pulmonary vascularity and increased left atrial size as indicated by echocardiography suggest that the ductus plays a significant role in the respiratory distress syndrome. This should indicate the need for diagnostic cardiac catheterization and operation if a large shunt is found. Ductal tissue in these infants may be responsive to irritation during catheterization and in some instances the ductus has closed as a result of catheterization. Although operative closure of the ductus is well tolerated in these small sick infants, it is only one of many important elements in their sophisticated care.

It has been shown that prostaglandins E_1 and E_2 have a powerful vasodilating action. Inhibition of prostaglandin synthesis produces constriction of the ductus arteriosus in normal fetal lambs in utero. Based on this experimental evidence, indomethacin, a potent inhibitor of prostaglandin synthetase, has been administered in an effort to cause constriction and closure of the patent ductus. The drug has been effective in premature infants with the respiratory distress syndrome, but has been much less effective in older children. The role of this form of treatment in anyone other than a neonate remains obscure.[9, 11]

The typical picture may not be present when significant pulmonary hypertension exists. This may be the case in infants soon after birth with an otherwise ordinary ductus because, at birth, the pulmonary artery pressure is elevated, normally falling rapidly in the first few months. Because of a lower gradient between aorta and pulmonary artery, blood may not flow continuously and only a systolic or even no murmur may be heard. As the child grows older, the typical continuous murmur appears.

There is also a group of patients, most commonly infants or young children, who have pulmonary hypertension and a large ductus who may be severely distressed. The murmur usually is a systolic one with only a short diastolic component, sometimes separated by a pause, and the pulmonary second sound is unusually loud, all indicating severe pulmonary hypertension. The heart usually is enlarged and the lung fields are vascular, due to both increased flow and congestion. The principal concern in this atypical condition is the increased pulmonary vascular resistance. If this is not present in the infant or young child, it will surely develop unless the abnormal communication is corrected.[21] By the time adult years are reached, the pulmonary hypertension is unlikely to be reversible, and in its extreme form there is a reversed flow through the ductus from pulmonary artery to aorta, giving rise to cyanosis of the toes in contrast to more normal color of the fingers. Such a late and irreversible stage is not often seen in children, and in adults it usually is associated with a large ductus. Uncertainty about the development of pulmonary hypertension, however, is another reason for elective interruption of the ductus in childhood.

The diagnosis can be made in most instances simply on the basis of the characteristic murmur with other clinical features that are consistent with the diagnosis. A venous hum may simulate the patent ductus arteriosus, but the hum usually varies with the position of the patient or with occlusion of the jugular veins in the neck. Several shunts between the pulmonary and systemic circuits may give continuous murmurs such as a ruptured sinus of Valsalva and coronary or pulmonary arteriovenous fistula, but these usually can be detected by other findings. The most difficult and important differential diagnosis may be from an aortic-pulmonary window located near the origins of the great arteries and otherwise similar to a patent ductus. Such communications usually are large, produce atypical findings and can be diagnosed by catheterization and cineangiogram.

Operation often may be undertaken with a diagnosis supported only by the noninvasive studies, but if there is doubt, the ductus should be demonstrated by cardiac catheterization and cineangiogram made by injection into the aorta near the ductus. Catheterization and assessment of the hemodynamic state should be undertaken in all cases of atypical patent ductus and in those with cardiac defects.

Selection of Patients for Operation

Once the diagnosis is established in a child or young adult there is sufficient indication for operative interruption of the patent ductus arteriosus, the risk of operation being very low. It was pointed out by Clatworthy and McDonald[3] that operative morbidity in infants and young children is no greater than that in older children; they advocated operation forthwith in all symptomatic patients, and in asymptomatic patients before the age of 5. There may be psychological advantages to operation before the age of 2, as recommended by Trusler et al.[19] In premature infants with respiratory distress syndrome, interruption of the ductus should be done urgently if there are signs of increased pulmonary blood flow and embarrassment from this. The clinical course has been strikingly changed in some infants weighing even less than a kilogram.[12]

Patients with severe pulmonary hypertension may present a perplexing problem. In young children there rarely is sufficient pulmonary vascular obstructive disease to contraindicate operation and there is good reason to believe that interruption of the increased pulmonary blood flow will allow regression of anatomic pulmonary vascular changes as the child grows. On the other hand, when pulmonary vascular obstructive disease is severe and there is evidence of reversal of flow with cyanosis of the toes, the patient may not tolerate the stresses of operation nor will there be a significant hemodynamic improvement with interruption. A good analysis of the problem has been presented by Ellis et al.,[8] who proposed that if the shunt is predominantly left to right but nearly equal, operation probably is indicated but involves significant risk. There are clear indications for operation when the shunt is only left to right without right-to-left components even in the presence of severe pulmonary hypertension, since several studies have shown a decrease in pulmonary artery pressure and vascular resistance after interruption of the ductus under these circumstances.

Deductions can be drawn from a study by DuShane and Kirklin[5] and their follow-up of 68 patients after closure of ventricular septal defects with pulmonary hypertension and severely elevated pulmonary vascular resistance. Half of those over the age of 2 had persistence of high pulmonary vascular resistance whereas of those operated on before age 2, more than 90% had a favorable result. There seems little question that elevated pulmonary vascular resistance may become a limiting factor when there is any one of the several types of left-to-right shunt and that this should be prevented by early operation when possible.

Operative Technique

Exposure from either an anterolateral or posterolateral incision may be adequate and the choice depends on personal preference. The adjacent aorta may be mobilized more easily from laterally and behind, and this approach may be especially useful when the pulmonary artery is unusually large. Good exposure can be obtained, however, more easily and with less disturbance of ventilation from the front and anterolateral incision, and this has been my preference. The incision is made through the third interspace, going well below the breast in females. The incision should extend well around laterally to the edge of the latissimus dorsi and well up into the axilla. Good exposure of the pulmonary artery, ductus and adjacent aorta must be obtained. The pleura is incised over the pulmonary artery between and parallel to the vagus and phrenic nerves. The ductus often can be seen and identified but if it is not, the recurrent nerve from the vagus should be traced in its course around the ductus and aorta. The nerve is displaced posteriorly from the anterolateral approach. A small lappet of pericardium invariably overlies the ductus and this should be dissected up and the ductus freed of adventitia and adjacent attachments. The entire area around the ductus, adjacent pulmonary artery and aorta should be freed by sharp dissection. Once the ductus is mobilized and the aorta and pulmonary artery cleared

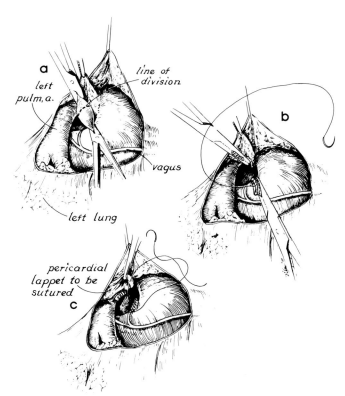

Fig. 55–2.—The author's usual method of interruption of the ductus arteriosus by division. Exposure is as in Figure 55–1. Ductus clamps are placed at either end. Once divided, the clamps are pushed toward the pulmonary artery and aorta, which increases exposure and reduces the likelihood of slippage of the clamps. The usual closure is a continuous mattress suture down and an over-and-over suture back.

of adventitia, a right-angle clamp may be passed around the ductus and a tape passed for gentle traction.

How the ductus is interrupted probably is not critical. Theoretically, closure of any large artery can best be accomplished by division, but in actual practice multiple suture ligature of the ductus with occlusion over a 3–5-mm distance has given excellent results.[17] Blalock championed ligation with multiple transfixion sutures when division was associated with considerable risk. The method is satisfactory even though the differential of safety is not as great now as previously. When ligation is used, pursestring sutures should be placed at the aortic and pulmonary ends and tied down snugly, nearly or completely interrupting flow. Mattress sutures then should be placed between the two pursestrings and the ductus obliterated over a distance of 8–10 mm (Fig. 55–1).

The risk of division of a ductus has decreased as increasing experience has been gained with handling of the great vessels and especially with the development of finer instruments for occluding them. Division probably is more widely practiced now than ligation and is my preference under most circumstances. After the ductus is fully mobilized, fine vascular clamps, such as the Potts multitoothed ductus clamps, are placed at the aortic and pulmonary ends and the ductus is divided between them (Fig. 55–2). At this time, pressure of each clamp against the adjacent great vessel will give better exposure and also diminish the chance of the clamp being pulled off. Although a single-layer closure may be satisfactory, my preference is for a continuous mattress suture adjacent to the clamp with a single over-and-over whipstitch

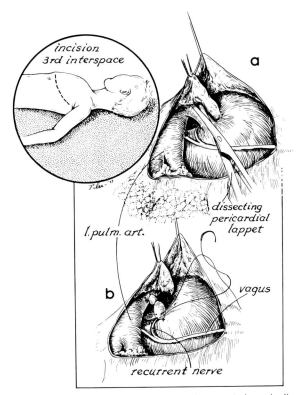

Fig. 55–1.—Operative treatment of patent ductus arteriosus by ligation. Incision is through the third interspace anteriorly with wide exposure laterally into the axilla. The incision goes below the breast in females. Identified by tracing the recurrent nerve around it, the ductus is exposed by dissecting off the pericardial lappet. Nonpenetrating pursestring sutures are placed at either end and perforating mattress sutures are placed between to obliterate the ductus over a distance of 8–10 mm.

on the free edge. This usually will suffice, but occasionally an additional suture is required after the occluding clamps are removed. The lappet of pericardium then is sutured over the pulmonary end to adventitia lying posterior to the pulmonary artery in order further to separate the two suture lines.

Simple ligation of the ductus is not advised when the structure is unusually large because of the danger of tearing through the wall, and division is advocated in such patients. When the ductus is extremely short and large, additional security can be obtained by clamping the ductus at the pulmonary end and then cross-clamping the aorta proximal and distal to the ductus. Sufficient cuff can be left on the pulmonary end for satisfactory closure, and the opening in the aorta can be closed while the aorta is collapsed. Although the safe aortic occlusion time is not known,[7] 10 minutes probably is safe and this should be ample to allow closure.

Operative Results

Results of operation for patent ductus arteriosus are among the most gratifying in the treatment of congenital heart disease. There is immediate reduction in the work of the heart and convalescence usually is smooth. In a collective review of 3986 cases, operative mortality was 2% with ligation and 2.1% with division in children and 4.3% and 5.2% respectively in adults.[20] In 689 cases of all types at the Johns Hopkins Hospital, including those with pulmonary hypertension, cardiac failure and additional defects, the mortality rate was 2.6%.

Studies by Lueker *et al.*[14] have demonstrated evidence of residual pulmonary vascular hyperactivity with exercise, and hypoxia, after interruption of a patent ductus arteriosus. This is in keeping with other studies, including those of DuShane and Kirklin referred to above, which show that increased pulmonary vascular resistance diminishes little after interruption of a left-to-right shunt even though pressure may fall significantly with the decrease in pulmonary blood flow. Long-term results, however, show that most patients are normal, and hence, in view of the low risk, operative interruption of the ductus is indicated in children and young adults, including those who are asymptomatic.

REFERENCES

1. Campbell, M.: Natural history of patent ductus arteriosus, Br. Heart J. 30:4, 1968.
2. Christie, A.: Normal closing time of the foramen ovale and the ductus arteriosus: Anatomical and statistical study, Am. J. Dis. Child. 40:323, 1930.
3. Clatworthy, H. W., Jr., and McDonald, V. G., Jr.: Optimum age for surgical closure of patent ductus arteriosus, JAMA 167:444, 1958.
4. Dammann, J. F., Jr., and Sell, C. G. R.: Patent ductus arteriosus in the absence of a continuous murmur, Circulation 6:110, 1952.
5. DuShane, J. W., and Kirklin, J. W.: Late Results of the Repair of Ventricular Septal Defect on Pulmonary Vascular Disease, in Kirklin, J. W. (ed.), *Advances in Cardiovascular Surgery* (New York: Grune & Stratton, 1973), pp. 9–16.
6. Edwards, J. E.: Structural changes of the pulmonary vascular bed and their functional significance in congenital cardiac disease, Proc. Inst. Med. Chic. 18:134, 1950.
7. Ekstrom, G.: The surgical treatment of patent ductus arteriosus. A clinical study of 290 cases, Acta Chir. Scand., Supp. 169, 1952.
8. Ellis, F. H., Jr., *et al.*: Patent ductus with pulmonary hypertension, J. Thorac. Surg. 31:268, 1956.
9. Friedman, W. F., *et al.*: Pharmacologic closure of patent ductus arteriosus in the premature infant, N. Engl. J. Med. 295:526, 1976.
10. Heymann, M. A., and Rudolph, A. M.: Control of the ductus arteriosus, Physiol. Rev. 55:62, 1975.
11. Heymann, M. A., Rudolph, A. M., and Silverman, N. H.: Closure of the ductus arteriosus in premature infants by inhibition of prostaglandin synthesis, N. Engl. J. Med. 295:530, 1976.
12. Horsley, B. L., *et al.*: Respiratory distress from patent ductus arteriosus in the premature newborn, Ann. Surg. 177:806, 1973.
13. Keys, A., and Shapiro, M. J.: Patency of the ductus arteriosus in adults, Am. Heart J. 25:158, 1943.
14. Lueker, R. D., Vogel, J. N. K., and Blount, S. G., Jr.: Cardiovascular abnormality following surgery for left to right shunts. Observations in atrial septal defect, ventricular septal defect and patent ductus arteriosus, Circulation 40:783, 1969.
15. McMurphy, D., *et al.*: Developmental changes in constriction of the ductus arteriosus: Responses to oxygen and vasoactive agents in the isolated ductus arteriosus of the fetal lamb, Pediatr. Res. 6:231, 1972.
16. Olley, P. M., Coceani, F., and Bodach, E.: E-type prostaglandins. A new emergency therapy for certain cyanotic congenital heart malformations, Circulation 53:728, 1976.
17. Scott, H. W., Jr.: Closure of patent ductus by suture ligation technique, Surg. Gynecol. Obstet. 90:91, 1950.
18. Silverman, N. H., *et al.*: Echocardiographic assessment of ductus arteriosus shunt in premature infants, Circulation 50:821, 1974.
19. Trusler, G. A., Arayangkoon, P., and Mustard, W. T.: Operative closure of isolated patent ductus arteriosus in the first two years of life, Can. Med. Assoc. J. 99:879, 1968.
20. Waterman, D. H., Samson, P. C., and Bailey, C. P.: The surgery of patent ductus arteriosus. A report of the Section on Cardiovascular Surgery, Dis. Chest 29:102, 1956.
21. Ziegler, R. F.: The importance of patent ductus arteriosus in infants, Am. Heart J. 43:553, 1952.

56 Clarence S. Weldon

Congenital Obstruction to Left Ventricular Outflow, Including Coarctation of the Aorta

OBSTRUCTION to the outflow of blood from the left ventricular cavity occurs in many forms and at multiple levels. Major categories include coarctation of the aorta, interruption of the aortic arch, supravalvar aortic stenosis, valvar aortic stenosis, subvalvar aortic stenosis and intraventricular obstructions resulting from hypertrophic cardiomyopathy. Surgical techniques now have been developed for relief from these obstructions in all forms and at all levels.

Coarctation of the Aorta

Coarctation of the aorta is a narrowing or an obliteration of the aortic lumen that occurs in proximity to the ductus arteriosus or ligamentum arteriosum. There is much evidence to suggest that this condition is indeed not a primary malformation but a secondary defect resulting from a maldistribution of blood flow during the fetal development of the central circulation. The first precise description of the condition was provided by Paris.[95] Originally, it was assumed that the malformation resulted from a maldevelopment of aortic arches and that the involution of the 4th aortic arch during the cephalad migration of the left subclavian artery was the principal cause for coarctation. An analysis of the timed events of aortic arch development does not fit the development of coarctation of the aorta in its usual locations.[7, 97] Craigie[31] and, later, Skoda[117] proposed that coarctation of the aorta resulted from ectopic ductal tissue extending into the aorta. This theory, once widely accepted, has been abandoned because of a failure to find such tissue in coarctation sites.[39, 61] Coarctation is recognized to be a curtain-like infolding of the aortic media.[39, 103] The aortic wall at the attachment of the ligamentum arteriosum or ductus arteriosus does not participate in the constriction. The "coarctation curtain" points toward the ductus or ligamentum in all cases.[19, 131] Coarctation may be located opposite the ductus arteriosus, proximal to it or distal to it. The left subclavian artery has its usual relationship to the great arteries in coarctation that is situated proximal to the ductus (preductal coarctation) but is shifted distally in coarctation that is juxtaductal or distal to the ductus arteriosus (postductal coarctation).[61, 108] In infants, the involved portion of the aorta frequently includes the entire isthmus (that portion located between the left subclavian artery and the ductus arteriosus). In older children and adults, an intimal hyperplasia is observed over the curtain of medial infolding. This is thought to be a secondary postnatal phenomenon.[32] The constriction of the aortic lumen may vary from mere indentation of the aorta to complete luminal obliteration. Although coarctation of the aorta occurs as an isolated abnormality, it is recognized that in newborns and infants with symptomatic coarctation, associated congenital heart abnormalities are the rule rather than the exception.[8, 24, 41, 43, 55, 65, 116, 120] Most reported series document that patent ductus arteriosus, ventricular septal defect, left ventricular outflow obstructing lesions,[66] left ventricular inflow obstructing lesions[37] and transposition of the great arteries are seen in that order of frequency.[41, 43, 55, 65, 120] Rudolph[108] was the first to suggest that coarctation was the result of altered fetal hemodynamics and proposed that a preductal coarctation was an exaggeration of the normally small aortic isthmus that resulted from a reduced isthmic flow during fetal life. Hutchins[61] advanced a second hemodynamic theory, proposing that excessive ductal flow during fetal life would produce retrograde flow through the isthmus of the aorta and create a branch point opposite the ductus and streamlining of the left subclavian artery toward the ductus. Thus, with ductal closure, there would be produced a juxtaductal coarctation of the aorta. These two hemodynamic theories now may be amalgamated into a unified theory of coarctation development, and such a theory is strongly supported by the following facts: (1) The malformations associated with coarctation, namely, patent ductus arteriosus, ventricular septal defects, aortic valve abnormalities, aortic arch hypoplasia and vascular malformations in the cerebral circulation, would all produce a diminution of blood flow across the isthmus during fetal life and, with the exception of cerebral AV malformations, an augmentation of ductal flow. (2) Coarctation of the aorta has never been observed in conditions in which aortic blood flow exceeds ductal flow during fetal life. Such conditions include tricuspid atresia, pulmonary stenosis and the tetralogy of Fallot malformation. (3) In the absence of other malformations, a smaller or deformed mitral valve has been demonstrated in 75% of patients with coarctation.[41, 105] (4) Angiographic measurements performed in infants with isolated coarctation and heart failure have demonstrated that the left ventricular volume is abnormally small.[47] (5) Infants with isolated coarctation always have right ventricular electrocardiographic preponderance, never left ventricular electrocardiographic preponderance.[55]

The Theory of Hemodynamic Molding of the Fetal Descending Thoracic Aorta

A statement concerning this unified hemodynamic theory for the development of coarctation of the aorta follows: The fetal circulation[32, 107] involves a system of three shunts that permit the distribution of oxygen-poor blood (Fig. 56–1). Placental vein blood with a PO_2 of 30 mm Hg is diverted for the most part away from the liver through the ductus venosus. Entering the heart, this blood is directed by the crista dividens across the foramen ovale into the left side of the heart and, preferentially, to the fetal brain. *In its course, it molds the development of the left side of the heart, determining size by volume and shaping configuration with a flow*

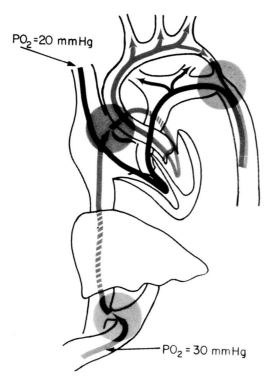

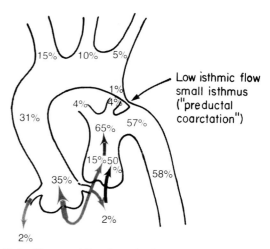

Fig. 56–3. — Diagram of the effect of reducing fetal left ventricular output down to 30% of total blood flow and augmenting fetal ductal flow. The aortic isthmus conducts greatly reduced flow and remains a diminutive vessel (preductal coarctation).

Fig. 56–1. — Diagram of the fetal circulation. A system of three shunts permitting the hypoxemic fetus to distribute blood flow.

profile. Should the foramen ovale fail altogether as a fetal shunt, this blood is diverted into the right side of the heart and the left side of the heart fails to develop properly, producing a so-called hypoplastic left heart syndrome.[73] Meanwhile, blood from the superior vena cava with a Po_2 of 20 mm Hg courses through the right side of the heart and, on its way, molds its development. Pulmonic blood flow is diverted, for the most part, away from the lungs, through the ductus arteriosus to the distal part of the body and the umbilical arteries. There is evidence that the outputs of the right and left ventricles during fetal life are approximately equal. Experimental measurements of peripheral fetal flow have permitted a composite of the distribution of blood flow in a normal fetus to be constructed[1, 108, 113] (Fig. 56–2). Of 50% of the total flow that crosses the aortic valve, 4% enters the coronary circulation, 15% the innominate artery, 10% the left

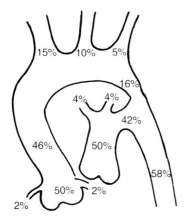

Fig. 56–2. — Diagram of the distribution of blood flow in a normal fetus. The size of vessels is determined by the volume they carry.

carotid artery and 5% the left subclavian artery, leaving 16% for distal flow through the isthmic portion of the aorta, which is located between the left subclavian artery and the ductus arteriosus. At this point, it joins the 42% of blood flow flowing through the ductus to provide the 58% entering the distal aorta. Isthmic flow is small and therefore the size of the vessel is small. The size of blood vessels is determined, as they develop, by the volume they carry and their configuration is determined by the pressure and flow profile of the blood passing through them. The isthmic portion of the aorta is normally small at birth and this has been shown angiographically and by autopsy studies.[38, 108, 116] At birth, the isthmus of the aorta is forced to carry 66% of total cardiac output and quickly enlarges proportionally. A variety of cardiac abnormalities, however, reduce the proportion of blood flow that crosses the aortic valve. These abnormalities include (1) obstruction to left ventricular outflow, such as aortic valve stenosis and aortic arch hypoplasia, (2) obstruction to the left ventricular inflow, which results whenever a small foramen ovale provides obstruction to flow and favors distribution of inferior caval flow through the right side of the heart or whenever there is obstruction at the mitral valve, (3) a runoff from the left ventricle to the right ventricle, as occurs with a ventricular septal defect. In the presence of any of these abnormalities, if the aortic blood flow is reduced down to 35% of total blood flow and ductal flow is augmented by 15%, the effect is to reduce the amount of blood flow that goes across the isthmic portion of the aorta to nearly nothing. A vessel that does not carry blood flow during fetal life does not develop and remains very small indeed. This condition of an underdeveloped isthmic portion of the aorta results in a preductal coarctation of the aorta (Fig. 56–3). A still further decrease in blood flow across the aortic valve, in combination with an augmentation of ductal flow, results in the ductal flow supplying not only the descending aorta but also portions of the brachiocephalic circulation. Isthmic flow then is retrograde. The molding effect of such flow is to streamline the developing left subclavian toward the ductus and to create opposite the ductus a bifurcating vessel (Fig. 56–4). The effect of ductal closure opposite this bifurcation point produces an infolding of the media of the aorta opposite the ductus or ligamentum, the so-called coarctation curtain, tipped toward the ductus. Such an arrangement is what

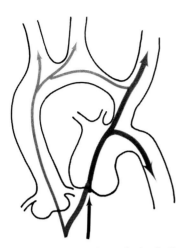

Fig. 56–4.—Diagram of the effect of a marked reduction in fetal ventricular outflow. Ductal flow provides flow to both the descending aorta and the brachiocephalic circulation, creating, by hemodynamic molding, a bifurcation opposite the ductus and a malposition of the left subclavian artery.

is known as a juxtaductal or postductal coarctation of the aorta (Fig. 56–5).

Coarctation of the aorta, therefore, no longer is regarded as a primary malformation of the central circulation but is seen to be a consequence of abnormal blood flow distribution during fetal development. The most common cause probably is an inadequate shunt at the foramen ovale, which limits left ventricular flow and favors right ventricular or ductal flow. The eventual location of a coarctation is dependent on both the volume and the direction of fetal isthmic flow.

Pathophysiology of Coarctation in Infancy

The natural history of coarctation from the time of birth is variable. On one hand, many coarctations later discovered to be total interruptions of aortic continuity produce little or no signs in the neonatal period. On the other hand, infants with less severe coarctations experience early-onset left ventricular failure and death. Because of the high incidence of association, intracardiac defects have been assumed to be the cause of this early failure and death with infantile coarctation of the aorta.[120] Although associated malformations occur with 70–90% of such reported cases,[61, 103, 108, 113] this assumption leaves unexplained the remaining 10–30% of cases that are not associated with cardiac malformations. It

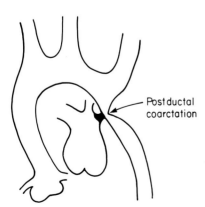

Fig. 56–5.—Diagram of the effect of ductal closure opposite a bifurcation point. An infolding (lipping) of the aortic wall points toward the ductus (postductal coarctation).

has further been suggested that the cause of this variable natural history is the development or lack of development of collaterals prior to the events of birth. There, of course, is no reason for collaterals to develop prior to birth, provided that the ductus carries its ordinary 42% of fetal blood flow, and, indeed, collaterals at the time of birth around a coarctation site are extremely rare.[65, 79, 122] The heart failure that complicates infantile coarctation is relatively unresponsive to medical management. It *is* left ventricular failure. However, the determinants of this left ventricular failure are multiple. A doubling of blood flow across the aortic valve occurs at birth. Whenever this occurs against an obstructed aorta there is an enormous increase in the after-load against which the left ventricle must eject. Such an after-load is well tolerated by a normal left ventricle. It will not, however, be tolerated by a left ventricle that already is excessively after-loaded, pre-loaded or hypoplastic to a degree that renders it incompetent. In those instances in which the cause of coarctation was a reduction of inflow into the developing left ventricle, the neonatal left ventricle will be to a degree hypoplastic and incompetent. In those cases in which the developmental abnormality responsible for the coarctation was obstruction to left ventricular outflow, excessive after-loads at birth become additive, and in those cases in which the causative factor for the coarctation was a runoff of left ventricular volume through a ventricular septal defect, the events of birth produce an excessive pulmonary blood flow, which adds to the after-loaded left ventricle and excessive volume pre-load. Similarly, ductus closure produces a sudden and excessive volume loading of a stressed and incompetent left ventricle. Thus, the presence or absence of heart failure in infants with coarctation is dependent on the balance of left ventricular competence and the multiple loads placed on the left ventricle at birth or in the neonatal period.

Diagnosis of Coarctation in Infancy

The diagnosis of coarctation in infancy should be suspected whenever severe heart failure occurs within the first 3 months of life. Differential pressures between the upper and lower extremities often can be demonstrated, but this sign frequently is destroyed by the presence of severe left ventricular failure or by an associated ventricular septal defect and a persistently patent ductus arteriosus. The electrocardiogram demonstrates right ventricular hypertrophy but is influenced by associated anomalies. The diagnosis is established by cardiac catheterization and selective angiocardiography. Precise diagnosis of the coarctation is most easily established by selective aortography. This can be performed by catheterization of the ductus when it is persistently patent, by catheterization of the aorta through the umbilical artery or by retrograde brachial artery catheterization.

Treatment of Coarctation in Infancy

The superiority of early surgical therapy over medical management, although controversial for some time, now has been established beyond doubt. Following the demonstration by Crafoord and Nylin[30] in 1945 that coarctation could be corrected by resection of the coarctate segment and end-to-end aortic anastomosis, and confirmation of this by Gross and Hufnagel[49] in 1945, Kirklin and his associates[69] in 1952, showed that the operation was feasible in infants less than 1 year of age. The view that all infants with proved coarctation of the aorta who present initially in heart failure should be managed by surgical resection of the coarctation is amplified when the results of medical and surgical therapy are com-

TABLE 56–1.—Comparative Reported Results of Medical and Surgical Therapy in Infants Less than 6 Months of Age with Congestive Heart Failure and Coarctation of the Aorta

	THERAPY	COMPOSITE REPORTS[†] NO. LIVING/NO. CASES	TOTAL EXPERIENCE ST. LOUIS CHILDREN'S HOSPITAL NO. LIVING/NO. CASES	TOTAL CASES NO. LIVING/NO. CASES (% SURVIVAL)
Isolated coarctation	Medical[°]	37/42	1/1	38/43 (88)
	Surgical	46/51	11/12	57/63 (90)
Coarctation with	Medical	12/33		12/33 (36)
persistently patent ductus arteriosus	Surgical	100/126	8/8	108/134(81)
Coarctation with VSD	Medical	6/31	2/3	8/34 (23)
with and without persistently patent ductus arteriosus	Surgical	45/80	7/8	52/88 (59)
Coarctation with ASD	Medical	0/9	0/1	0/10 (0)
with and without persistently patent ductus arteriosus	Surgical	6/7	3/8	9/15 (60)
Coarctation with	Medical	5/38	2/10	7/48 (15)
severe defects[‡]	Surgical	54/161	8/20	62/181(34)

[°]Medical therapy includes digitalis derivatives, diuretics, oxygen and sedatives.
[†]References: 2, 20, 41, 43, 45, 50, 53, 55, 69, 71, 75, 85, 110, 120, 127.
[‡]Aortic stenosis or atresia, mitral stenosis or atresia, atrioventricular canal, single ventricle, transposition of great arteries.

pared. Table 56–1 is a comprehensive review of the literature concerning the mortality rates of infants with coarctation of the aorta in heart failure reported between 1945 and the present. Salvage rates with surgical intervention are higher in all categories in which coarctation is associated with another defect, as well as when it is an isolated abnormality. The most significant postnatal event influencing the natural history of coarctation of the aorta is closure of the ductus arteriosus. It is this event that actually produces the postductal or juxtaductal coarctation. In preductal coarctation, ductal closure produces an augmentation of pulmonary blood flow with diastolic overload of the left ventricle, an event that aggravates the function of the already overloaded left ventricle. It is now recognized that an important part of the treatment of infantile coarctation is maintenance of ductal patency until surgical correction can be performed. This can usually be accomplished by infusing exogenous prostaglandin E-1 while preparations are being made for surgery. Digitalis and diuretics are usually also given to improve the function of the failing left ventricle. The maneuvers essential for correcting an infant coarctation, namely, clamping the aorta above and below the coarctation and ligating a ductus arteriosus when it is persistently patent, throw an additional load on the failing left ventricle. The effect of ductal ligation is to force more blood through the pulmonary circulation and into the left ventricle, thereby providing an acute left ventricular volume overload (preload). The effect of cross-clamping the aorta (frequently proximal to the left subclavian artery) produces an increased after-load on the failing left ventricle. In the presence of a ventricular septal defect, this cross-clamping maneuver redistributes the relative resistances in the two circuits, forcing more blood through the pulmonary circulation, again producing an acute volume load on the failing left ventricle. It therefore is of extreme importance that during the repair of infant coarctation, efforts be made to reduce the severity of acute volume overloading. Fishman and associates[40] recently have demonstrated that the simple expedient of substituting a rapid ductal ligation just prior to coarctectomy for the more leisurely division and oversewing of the ductus has improved their surgical mortality. Connors and associates,[27] in an effort to minimize the acute volume overloading of the left ventricle that occurs with aortic cross-clamping and ductal ligation, proposed the technique of prebanding the pulmonary artery in the presence of a ventricular septal defect before either ligating the ductus or cross-clamping the aorta. Whenever the preoperative catheterization demonstrated that there was no gradient between the ventricular pressures, the band was left in place after correction of the coarctation, but in those instances in which there still was some gradient between the left ventricular pressure and right ventricular pressure, the band was removed following the repair of coarctation. Using this technique since 1969, 24 patients under 1 year of age, of whom 18 were under 1 month of age, have been operated on at St. Louis Children's Hospital. Pulmonary artery bandings were done in 7 instances. In 3 patients, a temporary band was placed prior to ductal ligation and excision of the coarctation, and then removed. There was no intraoperative mortality in this series, although among 5 (21%) patients with severe associated cardiac abnormalities there were 3 early and 2 late deaths. In recent years, techniques have become available for performing extensive intraoperative corrections in infants. This, therefore, raises the possibility of combining resection of the coarctation with the immediate subsequent repair of intracardiac defects, such as ventricular septal defects. Efforts are being made to explore this approach.[106] However, up to the present, no one has produced a sizable series of patients in which infantile coarctation repair and the correction of intracardiac anomalies have been combined in the same procedure. The superiority of total correction over coarctation repair with later correction of other anomalies has yet to be demonstrated.

The Problem of Recoarctation Following Repair in Infancy

The technique of end-to-end aortic anastomosis performed in infants for relief from coarctation of the aorta now is recognized to produce a rather high incidence of anastomotic stenosis, which is noted later in childhood. Reports have indicated that this anastomotic stenosis may occur in as high as 25% of infants who survive such repairs performed during the first year of life.[54, 67] This stenosis at the anastomosis has been variously attributed to a failure to make a proper-size anastomosis,[96] to a failure to resect so-called coarctate tissue,[88] to a failure of the anastomosis to grow[86] and, finally, to suture granulomata in the region of the anastomosis.[67] The occurrence of stenosis at the anastomosis recreates precisely the pathophysiology of coarctation of the aorta allowing for hypertension in the brachiocephalic circulation and for the development of systemic collaterals to the lower part of the body (Fig. 56–6). Unfortunately, the situation presents a particularly hazardous state of affairs for surgical treatment. This is so because the stenotic site has been displaced proximally and, in many cases, now is in the transverse aortic arch. It is so because the enlarged intercostal vessels that function as collaterals have been displaced closer to the site of stenosis and because the previous dissection of the aorta now has resulted in a more friable aortic tissue. In addition, the previously operated-on aorta must be freed from surrounding fibrosis, which is variably intense

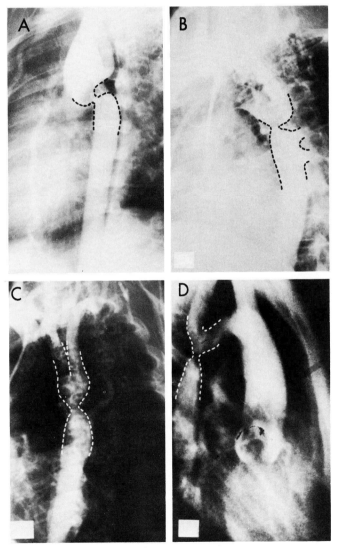

Fig. 56–6.—Aortograms obtained in 4 children with recurrent coarctation (anastomotic stenosis). The site of narrowing has been moved proximally. Intercostal arteries are closer to the "coarctation site." Well-formed collateral arteries are evident. (From Weldon, C. S., Hartmann, A. F., Jr., Steinhoff, N. G., and Morrissey, J. D., Ann. Thorac. Surg. 15:510, 1973.)

and which involves the vagus nerve and its recurrent laryngeal branch. In 1973, Weldon and his associates[129] reported a technique that makes the correction of these recurrent coarctations quite simple, safe and rapid. They used a very short and sharply beveled bypass graft inserted around the area of the anastomotic stenosis (Fig. 56–7). Side-biting clamps were used on the aorta above and below the stenosis. Eight patients with severe anastomotic stenosis producing recoarctation of the aorta now have been operated on at St. Louis Children's Hospital. Of these, 3 had a resection of the previous anastomosis with a second end-to-end aortic anastomosis and 5 were treated by the insertion of a short bypass graft. There was no mortality in this series and there was 100% relief from upper extremity hypertension and a restoration of pulses in the lower extremities. The condition of an anastomotic stenosis producing recurrent coarctation, however, is one that begs less for treatment than for prevention. Examination of the anastomoses that were resected from 3 patients indicates that in all 3 an extensive suture granuloma was the cause of the stenosis. The introduction of fine nonreactive suture material for the performance of infantile coarctation resection may prove beneficial in preventing the complication of anastomotic stenosis.

In 1957, Vosschulte[126] described a procedure that he termed "isthmusplastik." This procedure involves incision of the aorta longitudinally across an aortic coarctation and insertion of a diamond-shaped patch. Moor and his associates[83] reported a rather extensive experience using this technique in 19 patients, some of whom were infants. They used primarily prosthetic materials and, in one instance, an opened mammary artery. Follow-up data are not available. In 1966, Waldhausen and Nahrwold[127a] reported repair of coarctation using a subclavian-flap technique. They recommended division of the left subclavian artery at the apex of the chest, followed by longitudinal incision through the left subclavian arterial stump, the origin of the left subclavian artery and the descending thoracic aorta through the coarctate segment into the normal descending thoracic aorta. This procedure creates a flap of subclavian tissue that can be folded down and sewn into the incision in the descending thoracic aorta with a U-shaped suture line. The technique provides adequate enlargement of the coarctate segment and avoids a transverse aortic incision. Pierce and associates[96a] have recently reviewed a series of patients for whom such repairs were done. Anastomotic stenosis was not a complication in this group of patients. There is growing enthusiasm for the use of this technique to avoid the complications of recurrent coarctation of the aorta. At St. Louis Children's Hospital, we have, during the past year, abandoned the use of end-to-end aortic anastomoses in favor of the subclavian-flap technique whenever an operation is indicated in an infant less than 1 month of age.

Pathophysiology of Coarctation of the Aorta in the Older Child

Children between the ages of 1 and 15 years with coarctation of the aorta usually are asymptomatic. Nonetheless, upper extremity hypertension usually is present. Surgical repair of the coarctation is recommended during childhood because of the recognized complications of this hypertensive disease. The prognosis of untreated coarctation of the aorta was demonstrated by Campbell.[21] His study showed that approximately 20% of people with coarctation of the aorta die before the first or second decade of life and that approximately 80% die before the age of 50. Death in un-

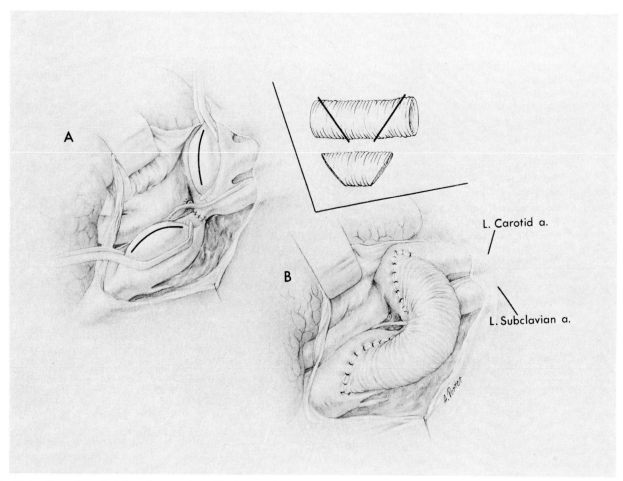

L. Carotid a.

L. Subclavian a.

Fig. 56–7.—The author's technique for managing difficult cases of recurrent coarctation. Side-biting arterial clamps are placed above and below the stenotic anastomosis. A short segment of sharply beveled prosthetic artery is used to bypass the stenosis. (From Weldon, C. S., Hartmann, A. F., Jr., Steinhoff, N. G., and Morrissey, J. D., Ann. Thorac. Surg. 15:510, 1973.)

treated coarctation of the aorta results from cerebrovascular hemorrhage, aortic dissection or rupture, chronic congestive heart failure and subacute bacterial endocarditis. The nature and natural history of the hypertensive disease that complicates coarctation of the aorta has produced controversy. Blumgart and co-workers[14] suggested that hypertension in the brachiocephalic circulation was a simple consequence of mechanical blockade. This hypothesis was supported by the work of Gupta and Wiggers,[51] who performed animal experiments demonstrating that a 50% constriction of the aortic lumen produced an immediate systolic pressure elevation above the constriction and a fall below it. Following the demonstration by Goldblatt and his associates[44] that constriction of the aorta just above the renal arteries produced hypertension in the dog, Page[94] suggested that a renal factor was responsible for the hypertension in coarctation of the aorta. An ingenious experiment performed by Scott and Bahnson[111] supported this hypothesis. They transplanted one kidney to the neck of a dog, then produced experimental coarctation, with resulting brachiocephalic hypertension. Subsequently, they relieved this hypertension by excising the remaining kidney from below the diaphragm. Kirkendall and associates[68] studied renal hemodynamics in patients with coarctation and found no evidence for renal hypertension. More recently, renin assays[13, 130] performed in patients

with coarctation have provided conflicting evidence for a renal factor in the hypertension associated with coarctation of the aorta. Furthermore, Sealy[112] pointed out a third feature of the hypertensive disease, namely, a postoperative augmentation or persistence of systemic hypertension. Sealy demonstrated that following adequate surgical relief from the coarctation, certain patients had an initial drop and then a rise in blood pressure within the first 36 hours postoperatively. A second type of hypertension also noted by Sealy was longer lasting and more delayed, usually subsiding in from 2 to 3 weeks. Sealy suggested that this phenomenon was the consequence of abnormal baroreception in the aortic arch, which persisted after the relief from the obstruction. Srouji and Trusler[119] suggested that hyperactive adrenal glands or a vascular spasm might be causative factors. Postoperative follow-up studies[77, 98] in patients with coarctation of the aorta have been reported and have shown that from 5% to 10% of the patients had persistent hypertension despite an adequate aortic lumen at the anastomotic site. Maron and his associates[77] have shown in a 20-year postoperative follow-up of patients with coarctation of the aorta that prolonged preoperative hypertension, with operation after 25 years of age, is associated with an increased risk of postoperative hypertension and premature cardiovascular death. It appears, at present, that the hypertensive disease that complicates coarctation of the aorta and is responsible for the early death of patients is complex, multifactorial and variable.

Diagnosis of Coarctation in the Older Child

Diagnosis of coarctation of the aorta in the older child is made by the finding of weak or absent pulses in the lower extremity in combination with upper extremity hypertension. There usually is a short systolic murmur and evidences of collateral development, which include palpable pulsations along the anterior borders of the latissimus dorsi and along the scapulae. Electrocardiographic findings are variable. Roentgenographic changes usually are pronounced. Abnormalities of the aortic arch and descending aorta are the most useful findings. Traction by the ligamentum arteriosum frequently causes a notch or impression on the left lateral border of the aorta in the frontal view. This finding in combination with an ectatic left subclavian origin above and poststenotic dilatation below the coarctate segment gives the appearance of the so-called double aortic knob or "figure 3 sign" to the left aortic border. Furthermore, the medial and anterior borders of the aortic arch can be visualized by their impression on a barium-filled esophagus. Important radiographic indicators of increased collateral flow around the coarctate aortic segment include notching of the posterior ribs from enlarged intercostal vessels and a prominent retrosternal internal mammary vessel seen in the true lateral film of the chest. Diagnosis is proved by selective aortography.

Treatment of the Older Child with Coarctation of the Aorta

Surgical correction is indicated whenever a patient has significant hypertension in the upper extremities or a pressure gradient of at least 50 mm Hg between the upper and lower extremities, or evidence of a well-developed collateral circulation. The technique for surgical repair was developed by Gross.[48] The approach is through the fourth intercostal interspace posterolaterally on the left. The aorta above and below the coarctation and the ligamentum arteriosum is mobilized. The ligamentum arteriosum or the ductus arteriosus is ligated. The coarctate segment is isolated between specially designed aortic clamps. It is wise to avoid ligation of intercostal arteries. However, when these are situated close to the coarctation, ligation sometimes is necessary to secure adequate mobilization of the coarctate segment. Resection of the coarctation is followed by end-to-end aortic anastomosis. This usually can be accomplished within a period of approximately 15 minutes of aortic clamping. On occasion, the coarctate segment is long, or the aorta cannot be adequately mobilized. It then is necessary to insert a portion of prosthetic aorta. Some confusion continues about the optimal age for surgical correction. The recommended age varies from 3 years to 20 years.[64, 90, 92, 98, 104, 114] Confusion arises because of concern about the growth of the anastomosis site. Moss and his associates[86] have shown with angiocardiography that by the age of 3 years, the cross-sectional area of the aorta at the level of the diaphragm has achieved 52% of the cross-sectional area of the adult aorta. Since restriction to flow is not achieved until there is at least a 50% constriction of the aorta, surgical anastomosis performed between the ages of 4 and 8 years should not be complicated by a recurrent coarctation of the aorta in adulthood. A current recommendation is that elective surgical correction of uncomplicated coarctations be performed between the ages of 4

and 8 years. If there is marked hypertension or cardiomegaly demonstrated by roentgenography and electrocardiography, operation should be at an even younger age.

Results of Coarctation Repair in the Older Child

Surgical resection of coarctation in children over 1 year of age has, in my experience, not been associated with any perioperative mortality or with the development of paraplegia. Mustard of Toronto had only 2 deaths in more than 300 children operated on. At St. Louis Children's Hospital, 76 patients between the ages of 1 and 15 years with coarctation of the aorta have been studied. Of these, 66 have been treated by surgical resection. The average age at the time of operation was 8.9 years, with a range of 2.75–14.75 years. Primary anastomosis was performed in 61 patients. In 4 patients, a short Dacron prosthesis was inserted and in 1 patient, a patch was used to enlarge the coarctate segment. Among the 66 patients undergoing correction there was 1 perioperative death, and that resulted from an operation performed elsewhere and followed infection of an inserted prosthetic graft. Of the 10 patients not operated on, 8 had a coarctation mild to a degree that operation was not required. One patient in the series had a large associated ventricular septal defect and pulmonary vascular obstructive disease, which contraindicated operation. Five patients had a coexisting ventricular septal defect, 3 had a persistently patent ductus arteriosus and 1 had an atrial septal defect. Although it once was assumed that successful repair of coarctation of the aorta would provide normal life expectancy, long-term assessment of patients operated on[115] has indicated that there remains a high incidence of deaths after operation as a consequence of coexistent cardiac disease, cerebrovascular malformation or residual hypertension.

Complications of Surgical Resection of Coarctation in the Older Child

Paraplegia is a recognized complication of coarctation. In a collaborative report by Brewer and his associates,[17] the incidence was 0.4% of patients operated on.

Acute arteritis involving vessels of medium and small size below the anastomosis was first reported by Sealy and co-workers.[112] This complication may lead to thrombosis, aneurysm formation or bowel infarction. In an effort to prevent this complication, Ho and Moss[56] recommended the administration of parenteral reserpine to patients who had severe hypertension and complained of abdominal pain in the postoperative period. It has been our practice to regulate paradoxic hypertension in the postoperative period with antihypertension agents, bringing the pressure into a normal range. The complication of mesenteric arteritis has not been observed in our series of patients.

Interruption of the Aortic Arch

Interruption of the aortic arch is a condition in which there is actual discontinuity of the aorta. It is generally held that this condition is a consequence of maldevelopment of the fetal aortic arch system. However, the invariable incidence of severe intracardiac anomalies, especially left heart hypoplasia, suggests that this may, indeed, also be a consequence of hemodynamic molding. Aortic arch interruption is uncommon. Approximately 250 such cases have been recorded in the literature,[111] but this probably does not represent a true incidence. The natural history is bleak. In excess of 90% of patients with interrupted aortic arch die in very early infancy.[82, 124] Only 20 cases of successful surgical management have been reported in the literature. Whenever patients with an interrupted aortic arch survive to childhood or adult life, this has been achieved by spontaneous slow closure of the ductus arteriosus and the development of marked collaterals. The repair of aortic arch interruption in children or adults is quite simple and can be done by interposing a prosthetic graft between the ascending aorta and the descending aorta. A number of such cases have been reported.[63, 72, 135] Interruption of the aortic arch is divided into three types, lettered "A," "B" and "C," depending on the site of arch interruption. Type A refers to an interruption distal to the left subclavian artery, Type B to an interruption between the left carotid and the left subclavian artery and Type C to an interruption between the innominate and the carotid arteries. Each of these has two variants, one occurring with the right subclavian artery arising from the distal aorta and another with the right subclavian artery arising from the right pulmonary artery. Several palliative procedures have been recommended for these conditions and include the proposal of Hairston[52] for bilateral banding of the pulmonary arteries to control pulmonary blood flow while still permitting perfusion of the distal aorta through the patent ductus. Another proposal has been made recently by Fishman and associates[40] to formalinize the periductal area in an effort to maintain ductal patency while performing bilateral banding of the pulmonary arteries. A still further variation was recommended by Van Praagh.[124] He suggested interposition of a prosthetic graft between the pulmonary artery and the distal aorta to bypass a closing ductus, adding to this a banding of each pulmonary artery. Efforts at repair ordinarily have involved attempts to reconstruct the aortic arch with the use of the arch branches. The major problem has been that, in small infants, these branches provide only very small conduits and the operation fails because there is inadequate relief from the aortic obstruction. Considering Type A aortic arch interruption, which resembles preductal coarctation, the usual technique is to sacrifice the left subclavian artery, turning it down to make an anastomosis into the distal aorta, or, whenever it is possible, to bring together the ends of the aorta and suture the distal aorta to the lateral aspect of the subclavian artery at its origin. Fishman and associates[40] have reported success with both of these techniques. More recently, Barratt-Boyes[4] has performed a corrective operation in an 8-day-old infant during which a prosthetic graft was interposed between the ascending aorta and the descending aorta at the ductus level. This was combined with an intracardiac repair of a ventricular septal defect and anomalous pulmonary venous drainage. Concerning Type B, the usual technique has been to attempt to reconstruct the arch by sacrificing the left carotid artery, which can be turned down and sewn to the distal aorta. In certain instances it has been possible to bring the descending aorta to the level of the base of the left carotid. Fishman and associates[40] have reported success using this technique. More recently, repair of the arch has been combined with intracardiac repairs using deep hypothermia and circulatory arrest. Murphy and co-workers[89] have reported the repair of a Type B interruption using a saphenous vein allograft obtained from the father of their patient and interposing this between the ascending aorta and the descending aorta, and then combining the repair of the interruption with the intracardiac repair of a ventricular septal defect. Trusler and Izukawa[123] have demonstrated that through a median sternotomy it is possible to free the descending aorta so that it can be brought into approximation with the ascending aorta and

a direct anastomosis done with these structures. They combined such a repair of a Type B arch interruption with the intracardiac repair of a ventricular septal defect. Bowman[15] subsequently has reported on the successful management of 3 patients using Trusler's technique. No one has yet reported a successful repair of Type C malformation in an infant but this malformation is extremely rare. It would appear at present that Trusler's technique has much to recommend it, as there have been many and repeated failures when an effort is made to construct an aortic arch from the available branch vessels.

Supravalvar Aortic Stenosis

Constriction of the aorta just distal to the aortic valve was first described by Chevers[26] in 1842. In 1930, Mencarelli[81] introduced the term supravalvular aortic stenosis. Nuffield and his associates[93] classified supravalvar aortic stenosis according to three anatomic types, which included a localized diaphragm-like obstruction in the ascending aorta, a localized narrowing of the ascending aorta and diffuse narrowing of the entire ascending aorta. Williams and his associates[133] reported a syndrome characterized by supravalvar aortic stenosis, mental deficiency and typical facies. Black and Bonham-Carter[12] suggested that hypercalcemia may be an etiologic factor in the syndrome. Garcia and his co-workers[42] demonstrated an association of this defect with high blood calcium levels in early life. The syndrome described by Williams now is classified as clinical Type A supravalvar aortic stenosis. Williams and his associates[133] also identified a small group of patients who have supravalvar aortic stenosis in the absence of mental deficiency and facial or dental characteristics, but in which there is a familial association. This has been called Type B supravalvar aortic stenosis. A third type (Type C) occurs sporadically in the absence of any familial characteristics, or in the absence of mental deficiency or association with facial and dental changes. The clinical findings in all cases include a systolic murmur resulting from the obstruction to left ventricular outflow and a varying degree of left ventricular hypertrophy that depends on the degree of obstruction. At left heart catheterization, it is possible to demonstrate gradients across the obstruction and to demonstrate by aortography the abnormal anatomy of the ascending aorta. In 1961, McGoon and his associates[80] provided surgical relief for this condition by incising across the narrowed segment of the aorta and inserting a prosthetic diamond-shaped patch. DeBakey and Beall[33] have reported their success with McGoon's technique. At St. Louis Children's Hospital, 9 patients between the ages of 3 and 15 years with supravalvar aortic stenosis have been studied and operated on. Prosthetic patch angioplasty has been performed in all cases. None of our patients fits the familial pattern. Three patients had the full hypercalcemic syndrome and a fourth had unusual facies but normal growth and development. The clinical findings in all of these cases were indistinguishable from those of valvar or subvalvar obstruction, and, indeed, 4 of the patients had gradients across the aortic valve and 3 had a gradient within the left ventricle in addition to the gradient recorded in the ascending aorta. The technique used to correct the defects in our patients was slightly modified from that originally reported by McGoon, in that the incision across the narrowed segment was carried down to the aortic annulus, enlarging the posterior sinus of Valsalva. A very generous, nearly rectangle-shaped patch was inserted, purposefully separating the commissural attachments of the posterior aor-

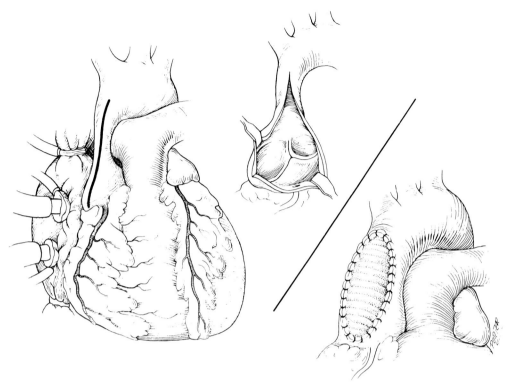

Fig. 56–8.—The technique for repair of supravalvar aortic stenosis. The aorta is incised through the stenosis all the way to the aortic annulus. The commissures supporting the noncoronary cusp of the aortic valve are sepa- rated by inserting an oval (nearly rectangular) patch of polyester cloth. (From Weisz, D., Hartmann, A. F., Jr., and Weldon, C. S., Am. J. Cardiol. 37:75, 1976.)

tic valve leaflet (Fig. 56–8). In several cases, the patch extended all the way to the origin of the innominate artery. In 1975, 6 of the 9 patients who had been operated on were evaluated by repeat cardiac catheterization and angiography 7–14 months after the operation. This study[128] demonstrated that preoperative systolic gradients, which ranged from 40 to 90 mm Hg (average 70), had been reduced postoperatively to gradients ranging from 0 to 20 mm Hg. The average gradient was 11 mm Hg. The postoperative appearance of the ascending aorta as demonstrated by aortography was near normal in all 6 patients. The results of the operation for supravalvar aortic stenosis are judged to be excellent (Fig. 56–9). Doty and associates[36a] recently have reported a technique for the repair of supra-aortic stenosis that permits enlargement of two of the three sinuses of Valsalva. An incision is made through the stenotic area into the posterior sinus of Valsalva. A connecting incision is made into the right sinus of Valsalva. The aortic incision, which is in the form of an inverted "Y," is enlarged by the insertion of a prosthetic patch in the form of a Roman arch with broad plinths. The published description of this technique reported 8 successful cases.

Valvar Aortic Stenosis

Valvar aortic stenosis occurs rarely in the form of hypoplasia of the annulus of the aortic valve[101] and commonly in the form of abnormal formation of the valve leaflets. The incidence of aortic stenosis—which includes supravalvar aortic stenosis, valvar aortic stenosis and subvalvar aortic stenosis—usually is stated to be 3% of congenital heart disease.[22] However, the precise incidence probably has not been accurately determined. Recent information has shown that a large percentage of calcific aortic stenosis, which becomes apparent in the adult, has as its basis congenital malformations of the aortic valve not previously recognized in childhood.[102] The abnormalities of the leaflet tissue that produce obstruction at the aortic valve cover a wide spectrum that extends from a tricuspid semilunar valve with mild commissural fusion to a valve that is represented only by verrucous tissue without evidence of sinus or commissural development. The most common arrangement is a basically bicuspid valve in which the third commissure is represented only by a raphe or thickening in one of the two leaflets.[118] As with coarctation of the aorta, two distinct clinical syndromes have been recognized.

The Clinical Syndromes of Valvar Aortic Stenosis in Infancy and in Childhood

The first syndrome is characterized by severe left ventricular failure during the first year of life. The second syndrome is characterized by a milder degree of left ventricular failure appearing in late childhood or early adolescence and is associated with a recognized risk of sudden death.[57, 78, 91, 134] It is characteristic for aortic valve stenosis not to produce symptoms between the ages of 1 and 5 years. Congenital aortic valve stenosis frequently is associated with preductal coarctation of the aorta, endocardial fibroelastosis and abnormalities of the mitral valve (see above). In the infantile syndrome of fatal congestive heart failure with aortic stenosis, the mortality usually is associated with combined defects that result from either the addition to the afterload of the heart, as in coarctation and aortic stenosis, or with a combination of ventricular incompetence and excessive after-load, as occurs with aortic stenosis in combination with

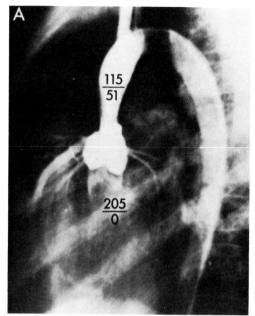 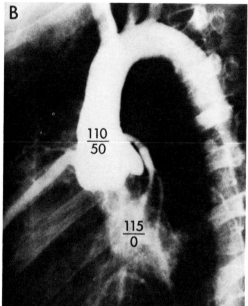

Fig. 56–9.—Supravalvar aortic stenosis. **A,** preoperative aortogram obtained on a child with severe supravalvar aortic stenosis. **B,** postoperative aortogram on the same child. The appearance of the aorta is near normal.

(From Weisz, D., Hartmann, A. F., Jr., and Weldon, C. S., Am. J. Cardiol. 37:75, 1976.)

endocardial fibroelastosis or mitral valve abnormalities.[76] The infantile syndrome is also recognized in patients with isolated aortic stenosis. It occurs in those patients with the most severe forms of aortic stenosis and those whose valves lack all sinus and commissural development. The childhood syndrome, which is characterized by the development of dyspnea, syncope, exercise intolerance and chest pain in late childhood or early adolescence, occurs in only about 10% of patients with recognized aortic stenosis. Indeed, of 300 patients with recognized congenital aortic stenosis, followed at The Hospital for Sick Children and the Toronto General Hospital in Toronto,[64] only 8% developed evidence of left ventricular failure prior to the age of 30, and most of those who developed left ventricular failure did so during the first year of life. The recognized risk of sudden death rather than the problem of uncontrollable left ventricular failure now is frequently accepted as the indication for surgical correction of valvar aortic stenosis in childhood.

Diagnosis of Valvar Aortic Stenosis

The condition usually is suspected by the presence of a characteristic systolic murmur heard in the aortic area. In 80% of cases this is accompanied by a thrill.[74] The presence of a systolic ejection click is said to differentiate valve stenosis from subvalvar stenosis,[125] but this distinction is not absolute. Roentgenographic findings include evidence of left ventricular enlargement and aortic enlargement. Calcification of the aortic valve is extremely rare in children. Catheterization of the left ventricle, usually via the aorta, establishes the diagnosis when pressure gradients across the valve area are measured during systole. Angiography and cineangiography provide a reliable method for distinguishing between valvar, supravalvar and subvalvar aortic stenosis. The electrocardiogram, which frequently demonstrates evidence of left ventricular hypertrophy or a strain pattern,

has both diagnostic and prognostic significance. Hugenholtz and Gamboa[59] demonstrated that by using the vectorcardiogram and measuring the sum of selected spatial vectors, one could obtain an excellent correlation with the left ventricular peak pressure. Thus, the electrocardiogram became a useful indicator of the need for further investigation of patients or indeed for operation. Furthermore, Hugenholtz and co-workers[60] demonstrated that although there is no change in the maximal spatial vector over the years of growth in a normal heart there is a remarkable linear increase in the maximal spatial vector once an elevated resting diastolic pressure is produced in either the right or left ventricle. This finding demonstrated that the vectorcardiogram reflects accurately the average peak pressure developed by either ventricle.

Management of Valvar Aortic Stenosis

Asymptomatic aortic stenosis in the infant or child with a measured gradient of less than 50 mm Hg does not require operation. In more severe forms of the disease, operation is indicated by the appearance of symptoms or by the rapidity of the rate of change of electrocardiographic or radiologic findings. The operation for congenital aortic stenosis is aortic valve commissurotomy. The extent of the commissurotomy depends on the type of valvar stenosis. In infants with unrecognizable commissures, short anterior and posterior incisions usually are made. In monocusp valves, only a single incision is made. Concerning valves with recognizable sinus and commissural development, we have established and followed a rule that the extent of the commissurotomy should be related to the height of the developed commissure and to the depth of the developed adjacent sinuses. Thus, if a commissure, although fused, is normally high, the commissure may be opened to the aortic valve annulus. If, however, the commissural and sinus development is only 50% of normal, the valve should be opened only halfway from the

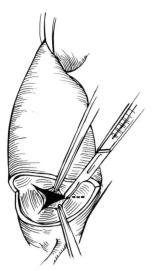

Fig. 56–10.—The proper technique for performing an aortic valve commissurotomy for relief from congenital aortic valve stenosis. Adjacent leaflets are supported while the commissure is incised with a knife directly in the middle of the fusion. Scissors should be avoided.

central orifice to the aortic valve annulus. If there is only rudimentary sinus development and no height to the commissure (the commissure being represented by a raphe), no incision should be made. While using this rule since 1969, in a consecutive series of 14 patients, commissurotomy always has provided relief from the aortic gradient, reducing it to below 50 mm Hg, and has never resulted in significant aortic regurgitation. A second rule is that commissurotomy always should be performed with a knife and not with scissors. Scissors blades have a tendency to slip off the thickened commissure onto the valve leaflet, cutting the valve leaflet and rendering the valve insufficient. A proper technique is to support the valve leaflet on either side of the commissure with surgical forceps and, with a fine knife and using a sawing motion, to divide the commissure precisely in the middle (Fig. 56–10). In infants under 1 year of age with left ventricular failure, the operation has been accomplished with the aid of cardiopulmonary bypass with an inflow occlusion technique, sometimes in conjunction with hyperbaric oxygenation and, more recently, with the technique of deep hypothermia using surface cooling followed by cardiopulmonary bypass with cooling to 18° or 20° C.[6] This permits a period of circulatory arrest during which the commissurotomy may be performed with excellent visualization of the valve. Rewarming then is accomplished on cardiopulmonary bypass to 32° C, followed by additional surface rewarming. In older children, the operation is accomplished on standard cardiopulmonary bypass with moderate hypothermia and, in more recent years, with selective cardiac hypothermia by infusion of cold saline over the myocardium during a period of aortic cross-clamping. Following aortotomy, a suction catheter is introduced through the stenotic valve and, with the heart arrested, cooled and decompressed, excellent visualization of the valve is obtained. A precise commissurotomy then can be performed.

Results of Operation

The most comprehensive review of the results of operation for congenital aortic stenosis was provided in a follow-up study reported by Bernhard and his associates[9] from Bos-

ton Children's Hospital. Their report involved 140 patients undergoing operation for valvar stenosis. All patients were followed, and cardiac catheterization was repeated in 106 patients. Twenty-four infants under 1 year of age were operated on by various methods. Sixteen surviving patients operated on in infancy were followed for from 6 months to 9½ years. Four of this group have required reoperation. The repeat catheterization in 9 of the group revealed that residual gradients ranged from 17 to 90 mm Hg. Most reported series of patients operated on using deep hypothermia techniques have included a few patients with congenital valvar aortic stenosis, but no sizable series of such patients with this technique has as yet been reported.

The results of operation performed for relief from aortic stenosis in childhood or adolescence have been more encouraging. The report by Bernhard and associates included 116 patients operated on between 1956 and 1972. Three died at operation and 7 later. Survivors were followed for from 1 to 15 years and 68 patients were restudied by repeat catheterization. A second operation was carried out for severe calcification in 4 patients at 4, 8 and 12 years after the initial operation. Among the 106 survivors, 60 had no significant aortic regurgitation. Of these 60 patients, 39 have been followed for from 4 to 15 years and 27 had one or more cardiac catheterizations. In 18 of the restudied patients, a residual gradient was found to be less than 50 mm Hg, in 3, to be between 50 and 100 mm Hg and in 3, to exceed 100 mm Hg. Among the remaining 33 of the 60 patients without aortic regurgitation, the results were judged to be satisfactory on clinical grounds. Forty-six of the 106 patients had significant postoperative aortic regurgitation. The degree of incompetence was judged to be mild in 27, moderate in 13 and severe in 6. It was noted, however, that 13 of the 19 patients with moderate or severe aortic regurgitation were operated on before 1961.

Considering results from a more recent era. Since 1969, at St. Louis Children's Hospital, 31 children with a diagnosis of congenital aortic stenosis have been operated on. Of these, 14 (45%) had valvar aortic stenosis, 10 (33%) had supravalvar aortic stenosis and 7 (22%) had subvalvar aortic stenosis. No deaths have occurred during or after operation in the entire group. Six of the 10 patients with supravalvar aortic stenosis have been studied by repeat catheterization and those data are presented above. The largest gradient recorded at operation following repair of supravalvar stenosis was 30 mm Hg. Among the patients with valvar aortic stenosis, only 1 was operated on during the first year of life and that child was operated on at the age of 2 months for severe congestive heart failure. A commissurotomy was performed on a bicuspid valve with the aid of deep hypothermia and circulatory arrest. The child has survived, with normal growth and development and without symptoms for 8 years after operation. One patient had a commissurotomy performed in an earlier era and was reoperated on for recurrent aortic stenosis at 14 years of age and required a valve replacement. Commissurotomy was performed in all the remaining patients with valvar aortic stenosis. Aortic regurgitation has not been recognized in any patient following a commissurotomy. Intraoperative measurement of the peak systolic gradients between the left ventricle and the radial artery were made following all commissurotomies and in no instance was a gradient greater than 40 mm Hg recorded. In 7 patients with subvalvar aortic stenosis, resection of the fibrous membrane was performed with total relief from the gradient in 3 patients, with reduction of the gradient to between 5 mm Hg and 30 mm Hg in 3 patients and with reduction of the systolic gradient to 50 mm Hg in 1 patient.

Subvalvar Aortic Stenosis

Subaortic stenosis usually exists in the form of a discrete ring of fibrous tissue encircling the outflow tract of the left ventricle. The abnormality was first described by Chevers[26] in 1842. As with valvar stenosis, the obstruction leads to left ventricular hypertrophy, heart failure and, in certain instances, sudden death.[132] A more severe form of subaortic stenosis has been described as the left ventricular outflow tract tunnel syndrome,[99] in which the fibrous tissue exists as a cylinder rather than as a ring and occupies most of the left ventricular outflow tract. Subvalvar aortic stenosis is extremely difficult to distinguish from valvar aortic stenosis in the clinical setting. Although the absence of a systolic click or splitting of the second heart sound in the pulmonic area leads to the suspicion of the proper diagnosis, the differential diagnosis usually is made with cineangiography, which clearly demonstrates the appearance of the fibrous ring situated below a normal valve. Ordinarily, portions of this fibrous ring are attached to the anterior leaflet of the mitral valve, and much has been made of the hazards of surgical resection of the fibrous ring because of reported instances of injury to the anterior leaflet of the mitral valve.[11] This complication has been totally avoided by using the simple technique of placing sutures in the fibrous ring to put traction on it and thereby delineate the relationship of fibrous ring to adjacent structures (Fig. 56–11). With the patient on cardiopulmonary bypass and with the heart cold, arrested and decompressed, the aortic valve can be retracted and traction placed on the fibrous ring with the sutures that have been placed in it. This brings the fibrous ring into sharp relief and it can be precisely and accurately resected from the left ventricular septum and from the anterior leaflet of the aortic valve without producing injury to either of these structures. Relief from discrete fibrous stenosis in the outflow tract portion of the left ventricle nearly always is complete.

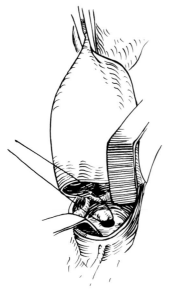

Fig. 56–11.—A simple technique that permits precise resection of a subvalvar membrane (subvalvar aortic stenosis). Sutures are placed in the membrane. Traction on the suture throws the margins of the membrane into relief, allowing the membrane to be excised with accuracy from the interventricular septum and the anterior leaflet of the mitral valve.

Aortic Valve Atresia

Aortic valve atresia, which ordinarily exists in combination with hypoplasia of the left ventricle and the ascending aorta (hypoplastic left heart syndrome), is an untreatable and lethal form of obstruction to left ventricular outflow.

Muscular Subaortic Stenosis

Muscular subaortic stenosis, also known as idiopathic hypertrophic subaortic stenosis (IHSS), hypertrophic obstructive cardiomyopathy (HOCM) and asymmetric septal hypertrophy (ASH), is a familial disorder in which abnormal myocardium produces a hypertrophic bulging of the interventricular septum. The abnormal septum impinges on the mitral valve apparatus during systole and thus produces obstruction to the outflow from the left ventricle. Although the average age of patients reported in the literature is between 20 and 30 years, approximately 50% of patients with this disorder are first identified in childhood.[16] This condition, which produces outflow tract obstruction, results in secondary muscular hypertrophy of the left ventricle and, consequently, left ventricular failure. Fortunately, the symptoms of left ventricular failure rarely develop in children. However, in the most severe forms of the disease, biventricular outflow tract obstruction is produced and may progress rapidly even in infancy. Symptoms include breathlessness and exercise intolerance. Angina, dizziness and palpitations, which are frequent symptoms in the adult condition, are rare in childhood. Physical findings include a double impulse on palpation of the apex of the heart and a systolic murmur. The electrocardiogram generally demonstrates an abnormal hypertrophic pattern. Roentgenography usually shows enlargement of the left ventricle. The definitive diagnosis is made by left ventricular angiography. The left ventricular cavity is small. The left ventricular wall is thickened. The outflow tract of the ventricle as defined by selective angiography has an abnormal configuration. A diagnostic sign obtained at the time of cardiac catheterization is the postextrasystolic accentuation of the arterial pulse.[18] Considerable success has been obtained with the use of beta blockade as a pharmacologic technique for manipulating the force of left ventricular contraction and thereby the severity of the obstruction produced by the hypertrophic myocardium.[46] A variety of operations have been developed for surgical relief from the obstruction. These include transaortic myotomy or resection of the hypertrophy,[84] resection of the hypertrophic septum by way of the right ventricular outflow tract,[70] trans left ventricular resection of the hypertrophy[5] and prosthetic replacement of the mitral valve.[28] None of these operations, however, is ideally performed in infancy and childhood. The reasons are that the child's aorta is too small to give proper visualization of the left ventricular outflow tract, the left ventricular approach has been associated with aneurysm formation and prosthetic replacement of the mitral valve in infants and small children probably carries a prognosis more dire than does the disease itself. Development of methods for the creation of a new unobstructed left ventricular outflow tract[34] (see below) recently have provided a new and acceptable technique for managing patients with muscular subaortic stenosis in childhood.

Bypass of Uncorrectable Lesions Producing Obstruction to Left Ventricular Outflow

Theoretically, whenever obstruction to left ventricular outflow at any level cannot adequately be relieved, it can be

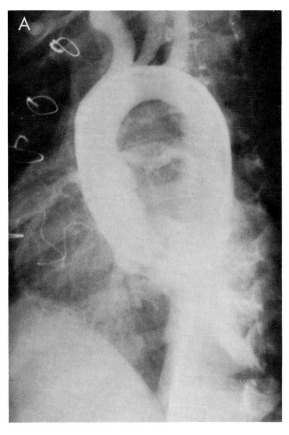
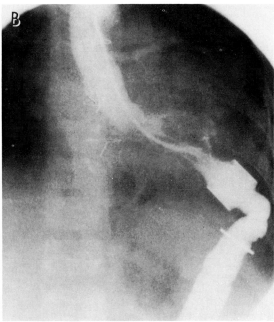

Fig. 56–12.—Subaortic stenosis. **A,** preoperative left ventriculogram of a child with severe intraventricular obstruction from cardiomyopathy. **B,** postoperative left ventriculogram obtained following the construction of an apical-aortic shunt as a new left ventricular outflow tract to bypass the unresectable obstruction. (From Dembitsky, W. P., and Weldon, C. S., Ann. Surg. 184:317, 1976.)

bypassed by constructing a second and new left ventricular outflow tract between the left ventricle and the aorta distal to the level of obstruction. Recently, it has been shown that such a bypass can be accomplished by the insertion of a valve-bearing conduit between the apex of the left ventricle and the descending aorta. The modern effort, which is based on older experimental findings, became feasible with the development of a polyester prosthesis into which a preserved tissue valve had been inserted. In 1910, Carrel[23] recorded his efforts using paraffin rubber tubes and jugular vein to create a bypass from the left ventricular cavity to the descending aorta. In 1923, Jeger[62] improved on these experiments by inserting a valve-bearing conduit and kept alive, over a 4-day period, an experimental animal. In 1950, Bailey and his associates[3] described a technique to treat aortic valve stenosis using ventricular aortic shunts composed of canine aortic homografts. In 1951, Hufnagel[58] reported similar experiments. In 1954, Donovan and Sarnoff[36] described aortic apical anastomosis used in acute animal experiments and, by 1955, Sarnoff and his co-workers[109] reported on 7 long-term dog survivors with valve-bearing conduits inserted between the apex of the left ventricle and the aorta. The technique was applied clinically in the 1960s by Templeton,[121] who inserted rigid Hufnagel-type prostheses into 5 patients with aortic stenosis, interposing the prosthesis between the apex of the left ventricle and the thoracic aorta. One of these patients survived for 13 years. In 1975, Bernhard[10] inserted a rigid apical aortic conduit into a 22-year-old man for the treatment of a hypoplastic aortic annulus. The prosthesis was manufactured from a stainless steel tube covered with flocked Dacron fibrils. A porcine xenograft glutaraldehyde-treated tissue valve was mounted into a polyester sleeve and interposed between the rigid conduit,

which had been inserted into the left ventricle and the thoracic aorta. Later in the same year, Cooley[29] attached a Hancock prosthesis designed for the construction of a new right ventricular outflow tract directly onto the left ventricle and led it to the suprarenal abdominal aorta. His patient had a hypoplastic aortic valve annulus. In 1976, Dembitsky and Weldon[34] reported results in 2 children with unresectable intraventricular obstruction. One of these children had severe hypertrophic obstructive cardiomyopathy (Fig. 56–12) and the other had a combination of supra-aortic stenosis, aortic stenosis and fibrous tunnel obstruction of the left ventricular outflow tract (Fig. 56–13). A commercially available Hancock prosthesis was fastened to a rigid cloth-covered metal cylinder, which was inserted directly into the left ventricular cavity by way of the left ventricular apex. The distal end of the valve-bearing conduit was sewn to the infrarenal abdominal aorta. Subsequently, Cooley has used the technique for relief from valvar, supravalvar and intraventricular obstruction as well as recurrent coarctation of the aorta.[100] With the development of this procedure, severe obstructions to left ventricular outflow, which were not previously correctable by standard operations, can be managed effectively. Such conditions include coarctation in a calcified aorta, certain recurrent coarctations, interruption of the aortic arch, tubular hypoplasia of the ascending aorta, annular hypoplasia of the aortic valve, monocusp aortic valve, fibrous tunnel obstruction of the left ventricular outflow tract and severe hypertrophic obstructive cardiomyopathy. Indeed, the success of this procedure has suggested that whenever relief from outflow tract obstruction in an infant or child involves replacement of the aortic valve, it may be better to leave the obstructed valve in situ and to perform a bypass from the left ventricle to the aorta so that the valve will be easily accessi-

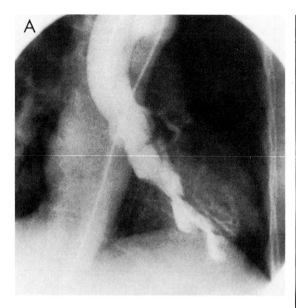

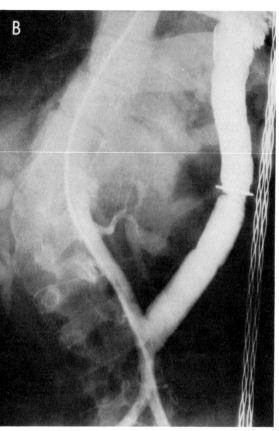

Fig. 56–13.—Relief from left ventricular outflow obstruction by valve-bearing left ventricle-to-aorta shunt. **A,** preoperative left ventriculogram of a child with combined valvar, subvalvar and intraventricular obstruction. **B,** postoperative left ventriculogram following the construction of an apical aortic shunt. The prosthetic aortic valve is in the abdomen. (From Dembitsky, W. P., and Weldon, C. S., Ann. Surg. 184:317, 1976.)

ble for re-replacement when this becomes necessary. The technique for constructing a new left ventricular outflow tract is quite simple. My technique[34] (Fig. 56–14) utilizes a commercially available prosthesis designed for right ventricular outflow tract reconstruction. This prosthesis is modified by covering a stainless steel cylinder with polyester cloth and then suturing this cloth-covered cylinder to the end of the prosthesis. With the patient supported on cardio-

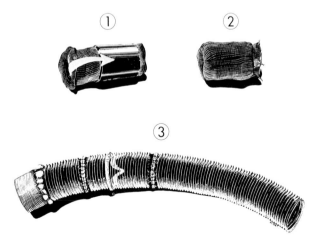

Fig. 56–14.—Technique for modifying a commercially available valve-bearing arterial prosthesis for use as an apical aortic shunt. *1,* a metal cylinder is drawn over a cloth cylinder. *2,* the cloth is doubled over the metal cylinder and sewn to itself, thus enclosing the metal cylinder in porous polyester cloth. *3,* the cloth-covered cylinder is sewn to the prosthesis and a ring of felt is used to cover the junction. (From Dembitsky, W. P., and Weldon, C. S., Ann. Surg. 184:317, 1976.)

pulmonary bypass, the apex of the left ventricle is exposed. A conical section of left ventricular myocardium is removed and the modified prosthesis is inserted directly into the heart so that the rigid end of the prosthesis projects at least 0.5 cm into the left ventricular cavity. The prosthesis is sutured to the epicardial surface of the left ventricle. A defect is created in the diaphragm adjacent to the left ventricular apex. The valve-bearing conduit is led through the diaphragmatic defect and placed retroperitoneally or transperitoneally and sutured into the infrarenal abdominal aorta. In this position, the valve is readily available for re-replacement. Postoperative studies of patients with a second left ventricular outflow tract bypassing an obstructive lesion have demonstrated that the distribution of blood flow between the obstructed and the unobstructed new left ventricular outflow tract is dependent on the degree of obstruction in the naturally occurring outflow tract. So long as the newly created outflow tract remains widely patent, all obstruction, regardless of the level or of the severity, is relieved. I have made an effort to adapt this procedure to the neonate, using a parental saphenous vein oriented so that the venous valve would prevent regurgitation into the ventricle. A single clinical trial in a 1-month-old infant with severe obstructive cardiomyopathy was unsuccessful.

REFERENCES

1. Assali, N. S., Kirschman, T. H., and Dilts, P. V.: Effects of hyperbaric oxygen on uteroplacental and fetal circulation, Circ. Res. 22:573, 1968.
2. Bahn, R. C., Edwards, J. E., and DuShane, J. W.: Coarctation of the aorta as a cause of death in early infancy, Pediatrics 8:192, 1951.
3. Bailey, C. P., Glover, R. P., O'Neill, T. J., and Ramirez, H. P.:

Experiences with the experimental surgical relief of aortic stenosis, J. Thorac. Surg. 20:516, 1950.

4. Barratt-Boyes, B. G., Nicholls, T. T., Brandt, P. W. T., and Neutze, J. M.: Aortic arch interruption associated with patent ductus arteriosus, ventricular septal defect and total anomalous pulmonary venous connection, J. Thorac. Cardiovasc. Surg. 63:367, 1972.

5. Barratt-Boyes, B. G., and O'Brien, K. P.: Surgical Treatment of Idiopathic Hypertrophic Subaortic Stenosis Using a Combined Left Ventricular-Aortic Approach in Hypertrophic Obstructive Cardiomyopathy, in Wolstenholme, G. E. W., and O'Connor, M. (eds.), *Hypertrophic Obstructive Cardiomyopathy* (London: J. & A. Churchill, Ltd., 1971), pp. 150–159.

6. Barratt-Boyes, B. G., Simpson, M. B., and Neutze, J. M.: Intracardiac surgery in neonates and infants using deep hypothermia with surface cooling and limited cardiopulmonary bypass, Circulation 43(Supp. I):25, 1971.

7. Barry, A.: The aortic arch derivatives in the human adult, Anat. Rec. 111:221, 1951.

8. Becker, A. E., Becker, M. J., and Edwards, J. E.: Anomalies associated with coarctation of the aorta, Circulation 41:1067, 1970.

9. Bernhard, W. F., Keane, J. F., Fellows, K. E., Litwin, S. B., and Gross, R. E.: Progress and problems in the surgical management of congenital aortic stenosis, J. Thorac. Cardiovasc. Surg. 66:44, 1973.

10. Bernhard, W. F., Poirier, V., and LaFarge, G. C.: Relief of congenital obstruction to left ventricular outflow with a ventricular-aortic prosthesis, J. Thorac. Cardiovasc. Surg. 69:223, 1975.

11. Bjork, V. D., Holtquist, G., and Lodin, H.: Subaortic stenosis produced by abnormally placed anterior mitral leaflet, J. Thorac. Cardiovasc. Surg. 41:659, 1961.

12. Black, J. A., and Bonham-Carter, R. E.: Association between aortic stenosis and facies of severe infantile hypercalcemia, Lancet 2:745, 1963.

13. Blaine, E. H., and Davis, J. O.: Evidence for a renal vascular mechanism in renin release: New observations with graded stimulation by aortic constriction, Circ. Res. 28–29 (Supp. II): 118, 1971.

14. Blumgart, H. L., Lawrence, J. S., and Ernstene, A. C.: The dynamics of the circulation in coarctation (stenosis of the isthmus) of the aorta of the adult type, relation to essential hypertension, Arch. Intern. Med. 47:806, 1931.

15. Bowman, F. O., in discussion of Fishman, N. H., Bronstein, M. H., Berman, W., Jr., Roe, B. B., Edmunds, L. H., Jr., Robinson, S. J., and Rudolph, A. M.: Surgical management of severe aortic coarctation and interrupted aortic arch in neonates, J. Thorac. Cardiovasc. Surg. 71:35, 1976.

16. Braunwald, E., and Morrow, A. G.: Obstruction to left ventricular outflow: Current criteria for the selection of patients for operation, Am. J. Cardiol. 12:53, 1963.

17. Brewer, L. A., Fosburg, R. G., Mulder, G. A., and Veroka, J. J.: Spinal cord complications following surgery for coarctation of the aorta, J. Thorac. Cardiovasc. Surg. 64:368, 1972.

18. Brockenbrough, E. C., Braunwald, E., and Morrow, A. G.: A hemodynamic technique for the detection of hypertrophic subaortic stenosis, Circulation 23:189, 1961.

19. Brom, A. G.: Narrowing of the aortic isthmus and enlargement of the mind, J. Thorac. Cardiovasc. Surg. 50:166, 1965.

20. Calodney, M. D., and Carson, M. J.: Coarctation of the aorta in early infancy, J. Pediatr. 37:46, 1950.

21. Campbell, M.: Natural history of coarctation of the aorta, Br. Heart J. 32:63, 1970.

22. Campbell, M., and Kauntze, R.: Congenital aortic valve stenosis, Br. Heart J. 48:485, 1954.

23. Carrel, A.: Experimental surgery of the aorta and heart, Ann. Surg. 52:83, 1910.

24. Chang, J. H. T., and Burrington, J. D.: Coarctation of the aorta in infants and children, J. Pediatr. Surg. 7:127, 1972.

25. Chevers, N.: A collection of facts illustrative of the morbid conditions of the pulmonary artery as bearing on the treatment of cardiac and pulmonary disease, Lond. Med. Gaz. 38, 1846.

26. Chevers, N.: Observation on the diseases of the orifices and valves of the aorta, Guy's Hosp. Rep., p. 387, 1842.

27. Connors, J. P., Hartmann, A. F., Jr., and Weldon, C. S.: Considerations in the surgical management of infantile coarctation of the aorta, Am. J. Cardiol. 36:489, 1975.

28. Cooley, D. A., Leachman, R. D., and Wukasch, D. C.: Diffuse muscular subaortic stenosis: Surgical treatment, Am. J. Cardiol. 31:1, 1973.

29. Cooley, D. A., Norman, J. C., Mullins, C. E., and Randall, G.: Left ventricle to abdominal aortic conduit for relief of aortic stenosis, Cardiovasc. Dis. 2:376, 1975.

30. Crafoord, C., and Nylin, G.: Congenital coarctation of the aorta and its surgical treatment, J. Thorac. Surg. 14:347, 1945.

31. Craigie, D.: Instance of the obliteration of the aorta beyond the arch, illustrated by similar cases and observations, Edinb. Med. Surg. J. 56:427, 1841.

32. Dawes, G. S.: Changes in the circulation at birth, Br. Med. J. 17:148, 1961.

33. DeBakey, M. E., and Beall, A. C., Jr.: Successful surgical correction of supravalvular aortic stenosis, Circulation 27:858, 1963.

34. Dembitsky, W. P., and Weldon, C. S.: Clinical experience with the use of a valve-bearing conduit to construct a second left ventricular outflow tract in cases of unresectable intraventricular obstruction, Ann. Surg. 184:317, 1976.

35. Dische, M. R., Tsai, M., and Baltaxe, H. A.: Solitary interruption of the arch of the aorta, Am. J. Cardiol. 35:271, 1975.

36. Donovan, T. J., and Sarnoff, S. J.: Apical-aortic anastomosis for the relief of aortic stenosis, Circ. Res. 11:381, 1954.

36a. Doty, D. B., Polansky, D. B., and Conrad, B.: Supravalvular aortic stenosis—repair by extended aortoplasty, J. Thorac. Cardiovasc. Surg. 74:362, 1977.

37. Easthope, R. N., Tawes, R. L., Bonham-Carter, R. E., Aberdeen, E., and Waterston, D. J.: Congenital mitral valve disease associated with coarctation, Am. Heart J. 77:743, 1969.

38. Edmunds, L. H., McClenathan, J. E., and Hufnagel, C. A.: Subclinical coarctation of the aorta, Ann. Surg. 156:180, 1962.

39. Edwards, J. E., Christensen, N. A., Clagett, O. T., and MacDonald, J. R.: Pathologic considerations in coarctation of the aorta, Proc. Staff Meet. Mayo Clin. 23:324, 1948.

40. Fishman, N. H., Bronstein, M. H., Berman, W., Jr., Roe, B. B., Edmunds, L. H., Jr., Robinson, S. J., and Rudolph, A. M.: Surgical management of severe aortic coarctation and interrupted aortic arch in neonates, J. Thorac. Cardiovasc. Surg. 71: 35, 1976.

41. Freundlich, E., Engle, M. A., and Goldberg, H. P.: Coarctation of the aorta in infancy, Pediatrics 27:427, 1961.

42. Garcia, R.-G., Friedman, W. F., Kaback, M. M., and Rowe, R. D.: Idiopathic hypercalcemia and supravalvular aortic stenosis, documentation of a new syndrome, N. Engl. J. Med. 271: 117, 1964.

43. Glass, I. H., Mustard, W. T., and Keith, J. D.: Coarctation of the aorta in infants, Pediatrics 26:109, 1960.

44. Goldblatt, H., Kahn, J. R., and Hanzal, R. F.: IX. The effect on blood pressure of constriction of the abdominal aorta above and below the site of origin of both main renal arteries, J. Exp. Med. 69:649, 1939.

45. Goldring, D., Padilla, H., Ferguson, T. B., Behrer, M. R., Hartmann, A. F., Jr., Zwirn, B., and Kraus, F. T.: Coarctation of the aorta and associated patent ductus arteriosus. Part I. Experimental studies in dogs, J. Pediatr. 56:11, 1960.

46. Goodwill, J. F.: Clarification of the cardiomyopathies, Mod. Concepts Cardiovasc. Dis. 41:41, 1972.

47. Graham, T., Atwood, G., Boerth, R., Bouchek, R., Dykes, C., and Smith, C.: Right and left heart size and function in infants with symptomatic coarctation (abstract), Circulation 54(Supp. II):227, 1976.

48. Gross, R. E.: Coarctation of the aorta: Surgical treatment of 100 cases, Circulation 1:41, 1950.

49. Gross, R. E., and Hufnagel, C. A.: Coarctation of the aorta: Experimental studies regarding its surgical correction, N. Engl. J. Med. 233:287, 1945.

50. Groves, L. K., and Effler, D. B.: Problems in the surgical management of coarctation of the aorta, J. Thorac. Cardiovasc. Surg. 39:60, 1960.

51. Gupta, T. C., and Wiggers, C. J.: Basic hemodynamic changes produced by aortic coarctation of different degrees, Circulation 3:17, 1951.

52. Hairston, P., Webb, H., and Lee, W. H., Jr.: Aortic arch interruption: Treatment with pulmonary artery banding, J. Thorac. Cardiovasc. Surg. 54:60, 1967.

53. Hallman, G. L., Yashar, J. J., Bloodwell, R. D., and Cooley, D. A.: Surgical correction of coarctation of the aorta in the first year of life, Ann. Thorac. Surg. 4:106, 1967.

54. Hartmann, A. F., Jr., Goldring, D., Hernandez, A., Behrer, M. R., Schad, N., Ferguson, T. B., and Burford, T. H.: Recurrent coarctation of the aorta after successful repair in infancy, Am. J. Cardiol. 25:405, 1970.

55. Hartmann, A. F., Jr., Goldring, D., and Staple, T. W.: Coarctation of the aorta in infancy: Hemodynamic studies, J. Pediatr. 70:95, 1967.

56. Ho, E. C. K., and Moss, A. J.: The syndrome of mesenteric arteritis following surgical repair of aortic coarctation, Pediatrics 49:40, 1972.

57. Hohn, A. P., Van Praagh, S., Moore, D., Vlad, P., and Lambert, E. C.: Aortic stenosis, Circulation 32:1114, 1965.

58. Hufnagel, C. A.: Aortic plastic valvular prosthesis, Bull. Georgetown Univ. Med. Center 4:128, 1951.

59. Hugenholtz, P. G., and Gamboa, R.: Effect of chronically increased ventricular pressure on the electrical forces of the heart, Circulation 30:511, 1964.

60. Hugenholtz, P. G., Lees, M. M., and Nadas, A. S.: The scalar electrocardiogram, vectorcardiogram, and exercise electrocardiogram in the assessment of congenital aortic stenosis, Circulation 26:79, 1962.

61. Hutchins, G. M.: Coarctation of the aorta explained as a branch-point of the ductus arteriosus, Am. J. Pathol. 63:203, 1971.

62. Jeger, cited by Kuttner, H.: *Chirurgische operationslehre* (5th ed.; Leipzig: Barth, 1923), Vol. 2.

63. Kauff, M. K., Bloch, J., and Baltaxe, H. A.: Complete interruption of the aortic arch in adults, Radiology 106:53, 1973.

64. Keith, J. D., Rowe, R. D., and Vlad, P.: Coarctation of the Aorta, in *Heart Disease in Infancy and Childhood* (2d ed.; New York: The Macmillan Company, 1967), p. 226.

65. Kelminson, L. L.: Coarctation of the aorta in infancy, Adv. Cardiol. 11:43, 1974.

66. Kerber, R. E., Greene, R. A., Cohn, L. H., Nexler, L., Kriss, J. P., and Harrison, D. C.: Multiple left ventricular outflow obstruction, J. Thorac. Cardiovasc. Surg. 63:374, 1972.

67. Khoury, G. H., and Hawes, C. R.: Recurrent coarctation of the aorta in infancy and childhood, J. Pediatr. 72:801, 1968.

68. Kirkendall, W. M., Culbertson, J. W., and Eckstein, J. W.: Renal hemodynamics in patients with coarctation of the aorta, J. Lab. Clin. Med. 53:6, 1959.

69. Kirklin, J. W., Burchell, H. B., Pugh, D. G., Purke, E. C., and Mills, S. D.: Surgical treatment of coarctation of the aorta in a ten-week-old infant: Report of a case, Circulation 6:411, 1952.

70. Kirklin, J. W., and Ellis, S. H.: Surgical relief of diffuse subvalvular aortic stenosis, Circulation 26:739, 1961.

71. Lang, H. T., Jr., and Nadas, A. S.: Coarctation of the aorta with congestive heart failure in infancy—medical treatment, Pediatrics 17:45, 1956.

72. LePage, J. R., Viamonte, M., and Jude, J. R.: Complete interruption of the arch of the aorta: An enigma?, J. Can. Assoc. Radiol. 22:60, 1971.

73. Lev, M., Arcilla, R., Rimoldi, H. J. A., Licata, R. H., and Gasul, B. M.: Premature narrowing or closure of the foramen ovale, Am. Heart J. 65:638, 1963.

74. Levine, S., and Harvey, W. P.: *Clinical Auscultation of the Heart* (Philadelphia: W. B. Saunders Company, 1949).

75. Malm, J. R., Blumenthal, S., Jameson, A. G., and Humphreys, G. H., II: Observations on coarctation of the aorta in infants, Arch. Surg. 86:110, 1963.

76. Manning, J. A., Sellers, F. J., Bynum, R. S., and Keith, J. D.: The medical management of endocardial fibroelastosis, Circulation 17:359, 1958.

77. Maron, B. J., Humphries, J. O., Rowe, R. D., and Mellits, E. D.: Prognosis of surgically corrected coarctation of the aorta, Circulation 47:119, 1973.

78. Marquis, R. M., and Logan, A.: Congenital aortic stenosis and its surgical treatment, Br. Heart J. 17:373, 1955.

79. Mathew, R., Simon, G., and Joseph, M.: Collateral circulation in coarctation of aorta in infancy and childhood, Arch. Dis. Child. 47:950, 1972.

80. McGoon, D. C., Mankin, H. T., Vlad, P., and Kirklin, J. W.: The surgical treatment of supravalvular aortic stenosis, J. Thorac. Cardiovasc. Surg. 41:125, 1961.

81. Mencarelli, L.: Stenosi sopravalvolare aortica ad anello, Arch. Ital. Anat. Istol. Patol. 1:829, 1930.

82. Moller, J. H., and Edwards, J. E.: Interruption of aortic arch: Anatomic patterns and associated cardiac malformations, Am. J. Roentgenol. 95:557, 1965.

83. Moor, G. F., Ionescu, M. I., and Ross, D. N.: Surgical repair of coarctation of the aorta by patch grafting, Ann. Thorac. Surg. 14:626, 1972.

84. Morrow, A. G., and Brockenbrough, E. C.: Surgical treatment of idiopathic hypertrophic stenosis: Technique and hemodynamic results of subaortic ventriculomyotomy, Ann. Surg. 154:181, 1961.

85. Mortensen, J. D., Cutler, P. R., Rumel, W. R., and Veasy, L. G.: Management of coarctation of the aorta in infancy, J. Thorac. Surg. 37:502, 1959.

86. Moss, A. J., Adams, F. H., O'Loughlin, B. J., and Dixon, W. J.: The growth of the normal aorta and of the anastomotic site in infants following surgical resection of coarctation of the aorta, Circulation 19:338, 1959.

87. Moss, A. J., Emmanouilides, G. C., Adams, F. H., and Chuang, K.: Response of ductus arteriosus and pulmonary and systemic arterial pressure to changes in oxygen environment in newborn infants, Pediatrics 33:937, 1964.

88. Mulder, D. G., and Linde, L. M.: Recurrent coarctation of the aorta in infancy, Am. Surg. 25:908, 1959.

89. Murphy, D. A., Lemire, G. G., Tessler, I., and Dunn, G. L.: Correction of type B aortic arch interruption with ventricular and atrial septal defects in a three-day-old infant, J. Thorac. Cardiovasc. Surg. 65:882, 1973.

90. Nadas, A. S., and Fyler, D. C.: *Pediatric Cardiology* (3d ed.; Philadelphia: W. B. Saunders Company, 1972), p. 460.

91. Nadas, A. S. Hauwaert, L. V., Hauck, A. J., and Gross, R. E.: Combined aortic and pulmonic stenosis, Circulation 25:346, 1962.

92. Nelson, W. E., Vaughan, V. C., III, and McKay, R. J.: *Textbook of Pediatrics* (9th ed.; Philadelphia: W. B. Saunders Company, 1969), p. 1004.

93. Nuffield, H. N., Wagenvoort, C. A., Omgley, P. A., and Edwards, J. E.: Hypoplasia of ascending aorta, an unusual form of supravalvular aortic stenosis with special reference to localized coronary arterial hypertension, Am. J. Cardiol. 10:746, 1962.

94. Page, I. H.: The effect of chronic constriction of the aorta on arterial blood pressure in dogs: An attempt to produce coarctation of the aorta, Am. Heart J. 19:218, 1940.

95. Paris, M.: Considerable stenosis of the thoracic aorta, observed at the Hôtel-Dieu of Paris, J. Chirurg. 2:107, 1791. Cited by Jarcho, S., Am. J. Cardiol. 7:844, 1961.

96. Parsons, C. G., and Astley, R.: Recurrence of aortic coarctation after operation in childhood, Br. Med. J. 1:573, 1966.

96a. Pierce, W. S., Waldhausen, J. A., Berman, W., Jr., and Whitman, V.: Late results of the subclavian flap procedure in infants with coarctation of the thoracic aorta, Circulation 56:103, 1977.

97. Pillsbury, R. C., Lower, R. R., and Shumway, N. E.: Atresia of the aortic arch, Circulation 30:749, 1964.

98. Rathi, L., and Keith, J. D.: Postoperative blood pressure in coarctation of the aorta, Br. Heart J. 26:671, 1964.

99. Reis, R. L., Peterson, L. M., Mason, D. T., Simon, A. L., and Morrow, A. G.: Congenital fixed subvalvular aortic stenosis: An anatomical classification and correlations with operative results, Circulation 43–44 (Supp. I):11, 1971.

100. Reul, G. J., Nihill, M. R., Norman, J. C., and Cooley, D. A.: Surgical treatment of left ventricular outflow tract obstruction with apicoaortic valved conduit, Surgery 80:674, 1976.

101. Richter, G. W.: Co-existing congenital stenosis of aortic and pulmonic ostia: Report of a case, Arch. Pathol. 56:392, 1953.

102. Roberts, W. C.: Anatomically isolated aortic valvular disease: The case against its being of rheumatic etiology, Am. J. Med. 49:151, 1970.

103. Rosenberg, H. S.: Coarctation of the aorta: Morphology and pathologic considerations, Perspect. Pediatr. Pathol. 1:339, 1973.

104. Rosenberg, H. S., Klima, T., Henderson, S. R., and McNamara, D. G.: Maturation of the aortic isthmus, Cardiovasc. Res. 47, Oct.–Dec., 1971.

105. Rosenquist, G. C.: Congenital mitral valve disease associated with coarctation of the aorta, Circulation 49:985, 1974.

106. Rowe, R. D., and Vlad, P.: Diagnostic Problems in the Newborn: Origins of Mortality in Congenital Cardiac Malformation, in Barratt-Boyes, B. G., Neutze, J. M., and Harris, E. A. (eds.), *Heart Disease in Infancy* (Baltimore: The Williams & Wilkins Company, 1973), p. 3.

107. Rudolph, A. M.: The changes in the circulation after birth, Circulation 41:343, 1970.

108. Rudolph, A. M., Heyman, M. A., and Spitznas, U.: Hemodynamic considerations in the development of narrowing of the aorta, Am. J. Cardiol. 30:514, 1972.

109. Sarnoff, S. J., Donovan, T. J., and Case, R. B.: The surgical relief of aortic stenosis by means of apical-aortic valvular anastomosis, Circulation 11:564, 1955.

110. Schuster, S. R., and Gross, R. E.: Surgery for coarctation of the aorta: A review of 500 cases, J. Cardiovasc. Surg. 43:54, 1962.

111. Scott, H. W., Jr., and Bahnson, H. T.: Evidence for a renal factor in the hypertension of experimental coarctation of the aorta, Surgery 30:206, 1951.

112. Sealy, W. C.: Indications for surgical treatment of coarctation of the aorta, Surg. Gynecol. Obstet. 97:301, 1953.

113. Shinebourne, E. A., and Elseed, A. M.: Relation between fetal flow patterns, coarctation of the aorta, and pulmonary blood flow, Br. Heart J. 36:492, 1974.

114. Shumacker, H. B., Jr., Nahrwold, D. L., King, H., and Waldhau-

sen, J. A.: Coarctation of the Aorta, in *Current Problems in Surgery* (Chicago: Year Book Medical Publishers, Inc., February, 1968).

115. Simon, A. B., and Zloto, A. E.: Coarctation of the aorta: Longitudinal assessment of operated patients, Circulation 50:456, 1974.

116. Sinha, S. N., Kardatzke, M. L., Cole, R. B., Muster, A. J., Wessel, H. V., and Paul, M. H.: Coarctation of the aorta in infancy, Circulation 40:385, 1969.

117. Skoda, J.: Protokoll der sections—Sitzung fur physiologie und pathologie, WBL Z. Aerzte Wien. 1:720, 1855.

118. Spencer, F. C., Neil, C. A., and Bahnson, H. T.: Forty-six patients with congenital aortic stenosis, Am. Surg. 26:204, 1960.

119. Srouji, M. N., and Trusler, G. A.: Paradoxical hypertension and the abdominal pain syndrome following resection of coarctation of the aorta, Can. Med. Assoc. J. 92:412, 1965.

120. Tawes, R. L., Jr., Aberdeen, E., Waterston, D. J., and Bonham-Carter, R. E.: Coarctation of the aorta in infants and children: A review of 333 operative cases including 179 infants, Circulation 39(Supp. I):173, 1969.

121. Templeton, J. Y., III: Personal communication.

122. Thomas, H. M., Groves, B. M., Treasure, R. L., *et al.*: Coarctation of the aorta with complete luminal obstruction, Am. J. Med. Sci. 266:59, 1974.

123. Trusler, G. A., and Izukawa, T.: Interrupted aortic arch and ventricular septal defect: Direct repair through a median sternotomy incision in a 13-day-old infant, J. Thorac. Cardiovasc. Surg. 69:126, 1975.

124. Van Praagh, R., Bernhard, W. F., Rosenthal, A., Parisi, L. F., and Fyler, D. C.: Interrupted aortic arch: Surgical treatment, Am. J. Cardiol. 27:200, 1971.

125. Vogel, J. H., and Blount, S. G., Jr.: Clinical evaluation in localizing level of obstruction to outflow from the left ventricle:

Importance of early ejection click, Am. J. Cardiol. 15:782, 1965.

126. Vosschulte, K.: Isthmusplastik zur behandlung der aortem isthmusstenose, Thoraxchirurgie 4:443, 1957.

127. Waldhausen, J. A., King, H., Nahrwold, D. L., Lurie, P. R., and Shumacker, H. B, Jr.: Management of coarctation in infancy, JAMA 187:116, 1964.

127a. Waldhausen, J. A., and Nahrwold, D. L.: Repair of coarctation of the aorta with subclavian flap, J. Thorac. Cardiovasc. Surg. 51:532, 1966.

128. Weisz, D., Hartmann, A. F., Jr., and Weldon, C. S.: Results of surgery for congenital supravalvular aortic stenosis, Am. J. Cardiol. 37:75, 1976.

129. Weldon, C. S., Hartmann, A. F., Jr., Steinhoff, N. G., and Morrissey, J. D.: A simple, safe, and rapid technique for the management of recurrent coarctation of the aorta, Ann. Thorac. Surg. 15:510, 1973.

130. Werning, C., Schonbeck, M., Weidmann, P., Baumann, K., Gysling, E., Wirz, P., and Siegenthaler, W.: Plasma renin activity in patients with coarctation of the aorta, Circulation 40:731, 1969.

131. Wielenga, G., and Dankmelzer, J.: Coarctation of the aorta, J. Pathol. Bacteriol. 95:265, 1968.

132. Wiglesworth, F. W.: A case of subaortic stenosis with acute aortic endocarditis, J. Tech. Methods 17:102, 1937.

133. Williams, J. C., Barratt-Boyes, B. G., and Lowe, J. B.: Supravalvular aortic stenosis, Circulation 24:1311, 1961.

134. Wood, P.: *Diseases of the Heart and Circulation* (London: Eyre and Spottiswoods, Ltd., 1956).

135. Zetterqvist, P.: Atypical coarctation of the aorta with bilateral vertebral-subclavian pathway, Scand. J. Thorac. Cardiovasc. Surg. 1:68, 1967.

57   EDUARDO ARCINIEGAS

Vascular Anomalies Compressing the Trachea and Esophagus

HISTORY.—Double aortic arch was first described in 1737 by Hommel,[4] and a case of retroesophageal right subclavian artery was reported in 1794 by Bayford.[2] In 1932, Abbott[1] described 5 cases of double aortic arch and noted their surgical importance, but it was Gross,[3] in 1945, who first successfully divided a vascular ring. Numerous additional reports[7, 8, 12, 13] have been published subsequently.

Incidence

Vascular rings are rare lesions. They comprise less than 1% of all congenital cardiac malformations.[5] The related embryology is discussed in Chapter 49.

Types

The term "vascular ring" has been loosely applied to a group of congenital malformations that result from faulty embryonic development of the aortic arch and cause compression of the esophagus and/or trachea. Since some of these vascular developmental abnormalities form only partially encircling rings and are less frequently the source of obstructive symptoms, it may be clinically useful to consider vascular rings as either "complete" or "incomplete."

COMPLETE VASCULAR RINGS.—In order of frequency, the most common are: (a) double aortic arch, (b) right aortic arch with retroesophageal left subclavian artery and left ligamentum arteriosum and (c) right aortic arch with mirror-image branching and left ligamentum arteriosum. A left aortic arch with right descent and right ligamentum arteriosum may be encountered occasionally.

INCOMPLETE RINGS.—The most frequent are: (a) retroesophageal right subclavian artery and (b) anomalous left pulmonary artery (pulmonary artery sling).

OTHER VASCULAR LESIONS CAUSING TRACHEOBRONCHIAL COMPRESSION.—These are: (a) anomalous innominate artery and (b) pulmonary artery aneurysms in patients with tetralogy of Fallot and absent pulmonary valve.

Double aortic arch (Fig. 57–1).—This is caused by persistence of the right 4th aortic arch and right dorsal aorta. The ascending aorta divides into two arches, which pass on either side of the trachea and esophagus and join posteriorly to form the descending aorta and create an almost always tight ring. The right or posterior arch is larger in about 80% of

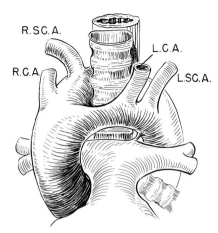

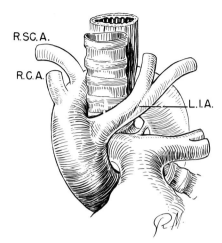

Fig. 57–1.—Double aortic arch. The right, or posterior, arch is the larger in 80% of the cases. Both are usually patent. Atresia is more likely to occur in the anterior arch at its junction with the descending aorta, where in other cases a narrowing makes it the site of choice for operative division.

Fig. 57–3.—Right aortic arch with mirror-image branching and left ligamentum arteriosum. As in all rings with a right aortic arch, the ductus or ligament must be divided.

cases and gives origin to the right carotid and right subclavian arteries. Both arches usually are patent. When atretic, the occluded segment most frequently is located in the anterior arch, at or near the posterior junction of the two arches. It is the most common type and comprised 27 of 36 vascular rings in our experience.

Right aortic arch with retroesophageal left subclavian artery and left ligamentum arteriosum (Fig. 57–2).—This is produced by persistence of the right aortic arch and absence of the left arch between the left carotid and left subclavian arteries. The left subclavian artery arises from the descending aorta, often from a diverticulum, and passes to the left behind the esophagus. The left ligamentum completes the ring. It is the second most frequent type.

Right aortic arch with mirror-image branching and left ligamentum arteriosum (Fig. 57–3).—This results from persistence of the right aortic arch and disappearance of the left arch between the left subclavian artery and the left ligamen-

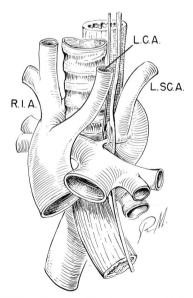

Fig. 57–2.—Right aortic arch with retroesophageal left subclavian artery and left ligamentum arteriosum. It is the ligament of the ductus that completes the ring, and division of the ligament is the operative treatment.

tum arteriosum. The latter originates from the descending aorta and connects with the left pulmonary artery to complete the ring. It is a rare anomaly. More commonly, in cases of right aortic arch with mirror-image branching, the ligamentum takes origin anteriorly, from the left subclavian artery, and there is no ring at all, an arrangement that is found in about 20% of patients with tetralogy of Fallot.

Left aortic arch with right descent and right ligamentum arteriosum.—In this anomaly the aortic arch courses to the left of the trachea and esophagus, turns sharply to the right behind the esophagus and gives origin to the right subclavian artery. The left ligamentum arteriosum disappears but the right ligamentum persists and connects the right descending aorta with the right pulmonary artery and completes the ring. It is a very uncommon lesion, often associated with intracardiac defects.[9]

Retroesophageal right subclavian artery.—This is caused by disappearance of the right aortic arch between the right carotid and right subclavian arteries. The right subclavian artery arises from the descending aorta and passes to the right chest behind the esophagus. The right ligamentum arteriosum is absent and, consequently, there is no ring. It is a frequent anomaly and a common radiographic finding but it rarely, if ever, is symptomatic, despite the old name dysphagia lusoria.

Anomalous innominate artery.—The innominate artery occasionally may originate more distally and to the left in the aortic arch than normally. When this happens, the artery, as it passes to the right, may compress the trachea anteriorly and cause obstructive symptoms. It probably is a very rare lesion. Only 1 of our 36 vascular ring patients had clearly demonstrable innominate artery-induced tracheal obstruction.

Anomalous left pulmonary artery (Fig. 57–4).—The left pulmonary artery originates from the right pulmonary artery and compresses the right bronchus and lower trachea as it passes to the left between the trachea and the esophagus, causing obstructive emphysema and/or atelectasis of the right lung (and occasionally of the left). Hypoplasia and cartilaginous abnormalities of the distal trachea and right bronchus occur frequently and contribute greatly to worsening of the ventilatory obstruction. The esophagus is indented anteriorly but not obstructed. Associated congenital cardiovascular anomalies are found in more than half of the cases. Also

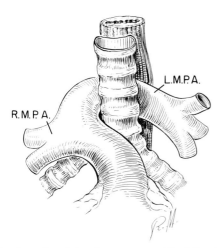

Fig. 57–4.—Anomalous left pulmonary artery. The left main pulmonary artery must be divided, and anastomosed to the pulmonary artery trunk anterior to the trachea (see Fig. 46–14).

called "pulmonary artery sling," it is a rare and unfavorable lesion due to the associated obstructive tracheobronchial anomalies.[10]

Pulmonary artery aneurysm in association with tetralogy of Fallot and absent pulmonary valve.—This is another uncommon but very important cause of tracheobronchial obstruction in infancy. As in other types of Fallot's complex there is a ventricular septal defect with varying degrees of aortic dextroposition. The pulmonary valve ring is small and stenotic but the pulmonary valve is virtually absent, consisting of several small and gelatinous nodular remnants. The pulmonary artery trunk and both main pulmonary arteries develop severe aneurysmal dilatation and compress the distal trachea and main bronchi. The aneurysmal process involves the right pulmonary artery more frequently and with greater severity, causing hyperinflation and/or atelectasis of the right lung.[6]

Clinical Features

Vascular rings sometimes cause little or no tracheoesophageal compression and may be asymptomatic. Respiratory distress and/or dysphagia develop as the severity of the obstruction increases. Dyspnea, apneic episodes, intermittent cyanosis, stridor, brassy cough, wheezing and noisy breathing in various combinations are the most common symptoms, and tend to be either provoked or aggravated by feedings. The head may be held hyperextended by the infant to relieve dyspnea. Dysphagia is less common and, when present, often is episodic. Symptoms appear earlier and are more severe in cases of double aortic arch. Most patients require operation within the first weeks or months of life.

Diagnosis

A history of recurrent respiratory and/or feeding problems always should raise the possibility that a vascular ring is present. Diagnostic delays may result in preventable deaths or additional airway damage.

Plain chest roentgenograms usually are not helpful but occasionally may show tracheal narrowing and, in patients with pulmonary artery sling, hyperinflation of either lung, more commonly the right. A barium esophagogram, diagnostic in all cases, is the single most important study needed. The impressions produced on the barium-filled esophagus by the anomalous aortic arch and/or branches often are quite characteristic for each lesion and may allow diagnosis of the specific ring type present. Bilateral and posterior indentations are present in double aortic arch, the right-sided indentation usually being higher (Fig. 57–5, A); the posterior impression frequently courses down and to the left (Fig. 57–5, B). Retroesophageal subclavian arteries cause typically slanted posterior filling defects. An anterior esophageal indentation at the level of the tracheal bifurcation is characteristic of "pulmonary artery sling" (Fig. 57–6). Bronchoscopy, esophagoscopy and tracheograms are not only unnecessary but may be harmful in these often critically ill babies. Angiography adds little except in doubtful cases and in

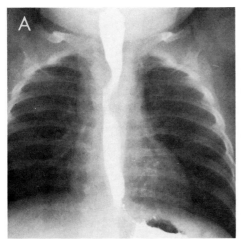
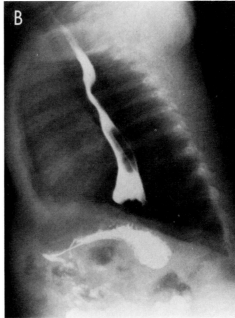

Fig. 57–5.—Double aortic arch. Esophagograms showing bilateral **(A)** and posterior **(B)** esophageal indentations typical of double aortic arch. As in this instance, the typical double indentation in the barium-filled esophagus seen in the PA view is higher on the right. Barium swallow is usually the only study required in diagnosis of vascular rings.

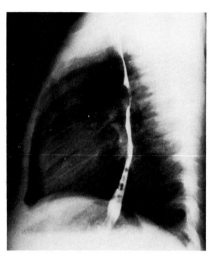

Fig. 57-6.—Anomalous left pulmonary artery producing an anterior esophageal filling defect.

those with either pulmonary artery sling or aneurysm of the pulmonary arteries (Fig. 57-7).

Surgical Considerations

Operation is indicated in all symptomatic patients. A left posterolateral thoracotomy provides excellent exposure in most cases. Thorough dissection of all vascular components is required. In double aortic arch, the smaller arch is the one to be divided, usually near the posterior junction of the arches and always at a point that avoids compromise of any major aortic arch branch. The ligamentum should also be divided. Suspension of the anterior arch is not required. Division of the ligamentum arteriosum opens the ring in all right aortic arch types. Division of the retroesophageal left subclavian artery is unnecessary and may lead to late development of subclavian steal syndrome. The trachea and esophagus should be thoroughly freed above and below the level of the ring in all cases. The left recurrent laryngeal nerve should be carefully protected from injury.

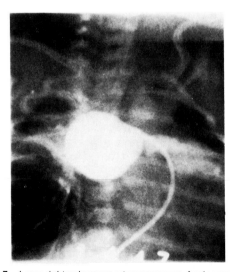

Fig. 57-7.—Large right pulmonary artery aneurysm. Angiogram in a 7-day-old infant with tetralogy of Fallot and absent pulmonary valve. The right ventricular outflow tract lies rather horizontally and to the left. The left pulmonary artery is absent.

Suspension of the ascending aorta and innominate artery to the anterior chest wall as described by Gross dramatically relieved the tracheal obstruction in our single case of anomalous innominate artery. In cases of pulmonary artery sling, the anomalous left pulmonary artery should be divided at its origin from the right pulmonary artery and reimplanted into the main pulmonary artery trunk. Plication or partial excision of the involved arteries should be considered in symptomatic infants with aneurysm of the pulmonary artery in association with tetralogy of Fallot and absent pulmonary valve.

Postoperative Care

Additional airway trauma should be carefully avoided. Humidified oxygen, thorough aspiration of tracheobronchial secretions and antibiotic treatment of any associated pneumonitis are essential. Tracheostomy rarely is needed and is best avoided.

Results

Two of our 36 patients with vascular rings died early after operation. Both deaths occurred early in our experience, in patients with double aortic arch, and were related to postoperative airway problems. In 2 patients with double aortic arch who were referred late to us, prolonged endotracheal intubation was responsible for erosion of the esophagus and posterior aortic arch and sudden, massive upper gastrointestinal hemorrhage, which was fatal in 1 of them. There have been no late deaths. Similar results have been reported by others.[7, 8, 12, 13] Noisy breathing and some stridor may persist for several months, but long-term relief from the tracheoesophageal compression symptoms following operation should be excellent in most patients. Operative mortality is higher and late results less satisfactory in cases of pulmonary artery sling and aneurysms involving the pulmonary arteries.

REFERENCES

1. Abbott, M. E.: Congenital Heart Disease, in *Nelson's Loose-Leaf Medicine* (New York: Thomas Nelson & Sons, 1932), Vol. 4, p. 155.
2. Bayford, D.: An account of a singular case of deglutition, Mem. Med. Soc. Lond. 2:275, 1794.
3. Gross, R. E.: Surgical relief for tracheal obstruction from a vascular ring, N. Engl. J. Med. 233:586, 1945.
4. Hommel: Cited by Turner, W.: On irregularities of the pulmonary artery, arch of the aorta and the primary branches of the arch with an attempt to illustrate their mode of origin by a reference to development, Br. Foreign Med.-Chirurg. Rev. 30:173; 461, 1962.
5. Keith, J. D., Rowe, R. D., and Vlad, P.: *Heart Disease in Infancy and Childhood* (2d ed.; New York: The Macmillan Company, 1967).
6. Lakier, J. B., et al.: Tetralogy of Fallot with absent pulmonary valve, Circulation 50:167, 1974.
7. Lincoln, J. C. R., et al.: Vascular anomalies compressing the esophagus and trachea, Thorax 24:295, 1969.
8. Nikaidoh, H., Riker, W. L., and Idriss, F. S.: Surgical management of vascular rings, Arch. Surg. 105:327, 1972.
9. Park, S. C., *et al.*: Left aortic arch with right descending aorta and right ligamentum arteriosum, J. Thorac. Cardiovasc. Surg. 71:779, 1976.
10. Saade, R. M., *et al.*: Pulmonary artery sling, J. Thorac. Cardiovasc. Surg. 69:333, 1975.
11. Shuford, W. H., and Sybers, R. G. L.: *The Aortic Arch and Its Malformations* (Springfield, Ill.: Charles C Thomas, Publisher, 1974).
12. Tucker, B., et al.: Congenital aortic vascular ring, Arch. Surg. 99:521, 1969.
13. Wychulis, A. R., et al.: Congenital vascular ring: Surgical considerations and results of operation, Mayo Clin. Proc. 46:182, 1971.

58 EOIN ABERDEEN

Anomalies of the Aortic Root

Aortic Sinus Fistulas

Definition and History

A COMMUNICATION between the aortic sinus (of Valsalva) and one of the cardiac chambers must be of hemodynamic significance, because the large difference of pressure ensures a big flow. A fistula may follow the rupture of an aneurysm of the sinus of Valsalva, and most of the reported cases have been observed in adults. However, a fistula may be found from an aortic sinus to a cardiac chamber without there being an aneurysm of the sinus. Such cases present at an earlier age than those with sinus aneurysm. As well, an aneurysm of the sinus may be found without a fistula being present.

The first report of an aortic sinus fistula was by Hope[6] in 1839, and the first successful correction was by Lillehei et al.[9] using cardiopulmonary bypass on May 2, 1956, a year in which at least 3 other centers also achieved successful correction of the lesion.

Pathology

The essential lesion in congenital aortic sinus aneurysm, as demonstrated by Edwards and Burchell,[5] is separation of the media of the aortic wall from the valve ring tissue. Whether a fistulous tract without an aneurysmal sinus has a similar defect is not clear.

About two-thirds of the reported fistulas have arisen from the right coronary sinus, about one-fourth from the noncoronary sinus and the remaining 8% from the left coronary sinus. The chamber of termination is shown in Figure 58–1, which is taken from a recent review of the literature by Nowicki et al.[12] The most common fistula is from the right sinus to the right ventricle and the next most common is from the noncoronary sinus to the right atrium, and then the right sinus to the right atrium. Other varieties are rare, but a fistula from each sinus to each cardiac cavity has been described, except for a right sinus to left atrial fistula, and that seems anatomically impossible.

Associated cardiac defects were found in slightly more than half of the reported cases, with a ventricular septal defect occurring in one-third, an aortic valve anomaly being next most common in 8% and a pulmonary valve lesion in 5%. It is of interest that of 35 patients described as having a ventricular septal defect in combination with an aortic sinus fistula, the fistula arose from the right aortic sinus in all but 1 case.

A fibrous tissue tube or sac from the sinus was described in 76% of patients. In the others, the fistula was simply a tract. Bacterial endocarditis had occurred in 8% of cases.

Signs and Symptoms

The presenting symptoms were either dyspnea or dyspnea and pain in the chest, a few having pain without dys-

pnea. About one-sixth of patients had no symptoms. Of those who had symptoms, slightly more than half had a gradual onset and slightly less than half had a sudden onset. When the onset was sudden, the symptoms usually were severe and sometimes death occurred within days. The ages of the patients ranged from 6 weeks to 79 years (mean 31 years).

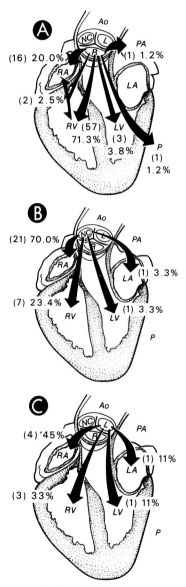

Fig. 58–1.—The chamber of termination for fistulas arising from the right sinus (80 patients) (A), noncoronary sinus (30 patients) (B) and left sinus (9 patients) (C). Ao = aorta; NC = noncoronary sinus; L = left coronary sinus; R = right coronary sinus; RA = right atrium; PA = pulmonary artery; LA = left atrium; RV = right ventricle; LV = left ventricle; P = pericardium. (From Nowicki, E. R., et al.[12])

653

Only 18 cases have been recorded in the first decade of life. The average age at onset for those without symptoms was 21 years as against 34 years for those who had a gradual onset of symptoms and 32 years for those in whom the onset was sudden.

A precordial thrill was palpated in about three-fourths of patients and a collapsing or bounding pulse was felt in about 80%. A continuous murmur was recorded in 94% and clinical signs of heart failure were apparent in 60%. Chest x-ray showed increased vascular markings in three-fourths and increased heart size in 90%. Abnormal ECG patterns were observed in 80%, with most showing left ventricular hypertrophy or a strain pattern. Pulmonary blood flow usually increased to about twice the systemic flow and the pulmonary artery pressure usually was increased (mean 42 torr systolic). The correct diagnosis was made after angiocardiography in 84% of patients having this investigation. More than 10% of patients had had an operation for a presumed patent ductus arteriosus, which was not present.

The subject has been well reviewed over the past 3 decades.[7, 8, 13, 14]

Diagnosis

Young children are not likely to present with a history of a sudden appearance of symptoms, but the diagnosis may be suspected from the clinical finding of a continuous murmur, and the diagnosis will be confirmed by aortography, provided that the aortic root is filled with the radiopaque injection.

Differential Diagnosis

The differential diagnosis usually rests with other causes of a continuous murmur, of which patent ductus arteriosus is the most frequent, but other forms of fistulous communication between the systemic arteries and systemic veins, cardiac chambers or pulmonary circulation may cause a continuous murmur.

Treatment

The only effective treatment is operation, and cardiopulmonary bypass now is essential. Earlier reports describe techniques for closure of the fistula using hypothermia and inflow occlusion.[11] At first, the closure of the fistula was made from its distal end, in the chamber to which it drained, and this was done either through an atrial well or with surface hypothermia and inflow occlusion, or with cardiopulmonary bypass. Repair has also been done from the pulmonary artery through fistulas of the outflow tract to the left ventricle. Experience now has made clear that the preferable method of treatment is from the aorta using an aortotomy. This allows a direct attack on the prime defect, which is the absence of continuity between the media of the aortic wall and the aortic valve ring.[15, 16] The defect can be closed either by direct suture or by a patch. Cross-clamping of the aorta is essential before the aortotomy is performed and, in the past, the heart has been protected by topical hypothermia or by coronary perfusion; in the future, it seems more likely that cardioplegic hypothermic arrest will be chosen. The aortic approach allows excision of the aneurysmal sac and accurate placement of sutures in the aortic wall and the valve ring without danger of injuring a coronary artery or the aortic valve cusps.

If a ventricular septal defect requires closure, the defect nearly always is associated with a right sinus fistula and the defect itself usually is supracristal. It may well be possible to close it through the aortic approach. If not, the right

ventricle can be opened and the VSD repaired through a right ventriculotomy. Several reviews of the results of operation have been published.[1-4, 10]

Prognosis

In the cases so far recorded, the surgical mortality was 12.7%, with failure to close the fistula in 1.6%. Most deaths were associated with additional cardiac lesions and with failure to close the fistula (which occurred only in cases in which aortotomy was not used). At present, in a case with an isolated fistula and using an aortic approach, the chance of survival is about 95% or perhaps better. The long-term outlook should be good but, of course, observation for 50 years or more is required before this can be stated with assurance. Certainly the risks of operation are sufficiently low as to recommend operative correction for all cases, in the younger age group at least.

REFERENCES

1. Bloor, K., Douglas, W. K., and Riddell, A. G.: Successful repair of an aneurysm of the aortic sinus, Thorax 17:146, 1962.
2. Bonfils-Roberts, E. A., DuShane, J. W., McGoon, D. C., and Danielson, G. K.: Aortic sinus fistula—surgical considerations and results of operation, Ann. Thorac. Surg. 12:492, 1971.
3. DeBakey, M. E., Diethrich, E. B., Liddicoat, J. E., Kinard, S. A., and Garrett, H. E.: Abnormalities of the sinuses of Valsalva. Experience with 35 patients, J. Thorac. Cardiovasc. Surg. 54:312, 1967.
4. Dubost, C. H., Blondeau, P. H., and Piwnica, A.: Right aorta-atrial fistulas resulting from a rupture of the sinus of Valsalva, J. Thorac. Cardiovasc. Surg. 43:421, 1962.
5. Edwards, J. E., and Burchell, H. B.: Specimen exhibiting the essential lesion in aneurysm of the aortic sinus, Proc. Staff Meet. Mayo Clin. 31:407, 1956.
6. Hope, J.: Case of an Aneurismal Pouch of the Aorta Bursting into the Right Ventricle, in *Diseases of the Heart & Great Vessels* (London: J. Churchill, 1839).
7. Jones, A. M., and Langley, F. A.: Aortic sinus aneurysms, Br. Heart J. 11:325, 1949.
8. Kieffer, S. A., and Winchell, P.: Congenital aneurysms of the aortic sinuses with cardioaortic fistula, Dis. Chest 38:49, 1960.
9. Lillehei, C. W., Stanley, P., and Varco, R. L.: Surgical treatment of ruptured aneurysms of the sinus of Valsalva, Ann. Surg. 146:459, 1957.
10. Meyer, J., Wukasch, D. C., Hallman, G. I., and Cooley, D. A.: Aneurysm and fistula of the sinus of Valsalva. Clinical considerations and surgical treatment in 45 patients, Ann. Thorac. Surg. 19:170, 1975.
11. Morrow, A. G., Baker, R. R., Hanson, H. E., and Mattingly, T. W.: Successful surgical repair of a ruptured aneurysm of the sinus of Valsalva, Circulation 16:533, 1957.
12. Nowicki, E. R., Aberdeen, E., Friedman, S., and Rashkind, W. J.: Congenital left aortic sinus-left ventricle fistula and review of aortocardiac fistulas, Ann. Thorac. Surg. 23:378, 1977.
13. Onat, A., Ersanli, O., Kanuni, A., and Aykan, T. B.: Congenital aortic sinus aneurysms, Am. Heart J. 72:158, 1966.
14. Sakakibara, S., and Konno, S.: Congenital aneurysm of the sinus of Valsalva associated with ventricular septal defect, Am. Heart J. 75:595, 1968.
15. Shumacker, H. B., Jr., and Judson, W. E.: Rupture of aneurysm of sinus of Valsalva into left ventricle and its operative repair, J. Thorac. Cardiovasc. Surg. 45:650, 1963.
16. Spencer, F. C., Blake, H. A., and Bahnson, H. T.: Surgical repair of ruptured aneurysm of sinus of Valsalva in two patients, Ann. Surg. 152:963, 1960.

Aortic-Pulmonary Septal Defect

Definition and History

AN AORTIC-PULMONARY (aortopulmonary) septal defect or aorticopulmonary window is a congenital communication between the ascending aorta and the main trunk of the pulmonary artery. The first case report was by Elliottson[6] in 1830. The first case to be diagnosed clinically was that by Gasul et al.,[7] although the first patient to be successfully treated by operation was operated on May 22, 1948 by Dr. Robert Gross, the case having been diagnosed as a patent ductus arteriosus. The first patient to be diagnosed preoperatively and operated on was reported by Scott and Sabiston,[13] and the first correction using cardiopulmonary bypass was by Cooley et al.[4]

Pathology

The defect usually is large, although it may vary in size from a few millimeters in diameter to more than 2 centimeters. The lower margin of the defect usually is separated from the aortic valve ring by at least a few millimeters of aorta but sometimes the lower margin may be absent.[11] When this occurs, although the defect is similar to a persistent truncus arteriosus, the separate valve rings of the aortic and pulmonary valves distinguish the lesion from the truncus, in which there is a common aortic-pulmonary valve. The ductus and ligamentum may be absent in this lesion, but the presence of a ductus by no means excludes an aorticopulmonary window and the combination of the two has been described quite frequently. Additional lesions such as ventricular septal defect or Fallot's anomaly or atrial septal defect have been observed in about half the cases described.[2, 14] The pulmonary vasculature may be affected by the increased pressure and flow quite early, and pulmonary vascular disease may develop after several years.

A case with two aortopulmonary defects has been reported.[1]

Signs, Symptoms and Natural History

Although the statement often has been made that aorticopulmonary window presents in a manner identical to the presentation of patent ductus arteriosus, this is true only in a general sense. Pulmonary hypertension is more frequent and more severe in aorticopulmonary window, because the defect is larger than a ductus.[15] The increased pulmonary resistance results in a diminished flow in diastole, so the clinical findings frequently are those of a systolic murmur, perhaps with a diastolic murmur, whereas a continuous ductus-like machinery murmur is found in only about one-tenth of cases.[10] Two patients lived beyond 30 years of age.[9]

Diagnosis and Special Tests

If a murmur has been heard, and if an accented pulmonary second sound suggests pulmonary hypertension and especially if heart failure has developed, a complete cardiac catheterization and angiocardiographic examination are advisable. The murmur is maximally heard rather lower along the left sternal border than the characteristic ductus murmur. Diagnosis is confirmed by the passage of the catheter from the pulmonary artery into the ascending aorta and then into one of the proximal branches of the ascending aorta, such as the innominate or the left or right common carotid. This x-ray picture of the catheter through an aorticopulmonary septal defect is in contrast to that seen when the catheter is passed through a patent ductus into the descending aorta and down toward the abdominal aorta. The second special test is roentgenography with injection of radiopaque material into the proximal aortic root. This will outline the aortic root and the pulmonary artery if an aorticopulmonary win-

dow is present, but aortography, which does not fill the aorta proximally as far as the aortic valve, may fail to demonstrate an aortic-pulmonary septal defect. Dye dilution curves may also help to localize the shunt in the proximal aorta.

Differential Diagnosis

Many of the reported cases have been mistaken for patent ductus arteriosus or ventricular septal defect. A patent ductus usually presents with a continuous machinery murmur, although the atypical patent ductus with pulmonary hypertension may not have more than a systolic murmur with some diastolic component, but this is heard at the level of the second interspace, that is, it is higher than the maximal intensity area of the aorticopulmonary window murmur. Passage of the catheter, as mentioned, may also be diagnostic of a ductus rather than an aorticopulmonary window. Roentgenography may also show other causes of continuous murmur in this region, such as an aortic sinus of Valsalva fistula, and coronary arteriography may demonstrate coronary artery fistulas or an anomalous left coronary artery.

Treatment

The only effective treatment is operative correction. The early cases were treated by simple ligation, but this was shown to be associated with a high recurrence rate, or incomplete closure, and major bleeding occurred not infrequently during dissection of this region. Division and suture was the next technique to be tried,[12] but, again, bleeding from the posterior aspect of the window during dissection caused major problems on occasion. The use of cardiopulmonary bypass gave much greater safety to the technical aspects of the operation, and since it was first used by Cooley et al.,[4] has been the usual method of cardiac support during operation, although it may be combined with hypothermic circulatory arrest, or, indeed, hypothermic circulatory arrest may be used without bypass.

Various operative techniques have been used in association with cardiopulmonary bypass. Simple division of the fistula and suture-closure of the aorta and pulmonary artery have been used, sometimes placing a patch in the pulmonary artery, which allows a generous closure of the aorta to be made without narrowing the pulmonary artery, because insufficient tissue is left on the pulmonary side. Another suggested technique was opening the pulmonary artery and closure of the defect from within the pulmonary artery. The rather posterior position of the defect can make definition and dissection difficult.[16] The simplest and safest approach has proved to be through the aorta anteriorly, closing the defect by suturing a Dacron patch in place.[3] This has the added advantage of allowing the surgeon to see exactly where the right coronary artery arises, and to be sure that the patch is placed on the pulmonary side of the orifice of this artery. This operative technique for managing aorticopulmonary window was introduced by David Waterston in London in 1965[5] and is another of the major contributions to pediatric surgery made by this most gifted surgeon.

Prognosis and Results of Treatment

The results of treatment in the past do not reflect the current risk because Waterston's method of closing the defect is much safer than the techniques used earlier. The problem of increased pulmonary vascular resistance is a major concern. If the defect is closed in the first year of life, the pulmonary resistance is unlikely to be much increased, and, in infants, the technique of surface induced hypothermia and circulatory arrest with rewarming by cardiopulmonary bypass is quite adequate, as is cardiopulmonary bypass with hypothermia. In older children, if the pulmonary vascular resistance is increased, the risk of operation is also considerably increased and, as with other forms of left-to-right shunt, operative correction should be avoided if the pulmonary resistance is three-fourths or more of systemic or if it exceeds 12 or perhaps even 10 units. For uncomplicated cases, most of which are not in the first year of life, the survival rate should be over 90%. Twenty-five infants, less than 1 year of age, have been reported in 17 publications (identified in a personal review of the English-language literature); 8 were operated on without bypass or hypothermia in the earlier years, with 1 death; 16 were operated on using cardiopulmonary bypass or hypothermic arrest, with 2 deaths (1 survivor could not be further identified).

Without treatment, the outlook is limited by the development of severe pulmonary vascular disease. This is the common complication, since the defect usually is a large one. Survival beyond the third or fourth decade is very unlikely in an untreated patient, but if closure of the defect has been achieved before the pulmonary vascular resistance is increased, the outlook should be very good. Nearly all associated anomalies, which are found in about half the cases, can be dealt with at the same operation and will, of course, affect the prognosis.

REFERENCES

1. Baronofsky, I. D., Gordon, A. J., Grishman, A., Steinfeld, L., and Kreel, I: Aorticopulmonary septal defect. Diagnosis and report of case successfully treated, Am. J. Cardiol. 5:273, 1960.
2. Blieden, L. C., and Moller, J. H.: Aorticopulmonary septal defect. An experience with 17 patients, Br. Heart J. 36:630, 1974.
3. Clarke, C. P., and Richardson, J. P.: The management of aortopulmonary window. Advantages of transaortic closure with a Dacron patch, J. Thorac. Cardiovasc. Surg. 72:48, 1976.
4. Cooley, D. A., McNamara, D. G., and Latson, J. R.: Aorticopulmonary septal defect: Diagnosis and surgical treatment, Surgery 42:101, 1957.
5. Deverall, P. B., Aberdeen, E., Bonham-Carter, R. E., and Waterston, D. J.: Aortopulmonary window, J. Thorac. Cardiovasc. Surg. 57:479, 1969.
6. Elliottson, J.: Malformation of the heart, Lancet 1:247, 1830.
7. Gasul, B. M., Fell, E. H., and Casa, R.: The diagnosis of aortic septal defect by retrograde aortography. Report of a case, Circulation 4:251, 1951.
8. Gross, R. E.: Surgical closure of an aortic septal defect, Circulation 5:858, 1952.
9. Meisner, H., Schmidt-Habelmann, P., Sebening, F., and Klinner, W.: Surgical correction of aorto-pulmonary septal defects. A review of the literature and report of eight cases, Dis. Chest 53: 450, 1968.
10. Morrow, A. G., Greenfield, L. J., and Braunwald, E.: Congenital aortopulmonary septal defect. Clinical and hemodynamic findings, surgical technic, and results of operative correction, Circulation 25:463, 1962.
11. Neufeld, H. N., Lester, R. G., Adams, P., Jr., Anderson, R. C., Lillehei, C. W., and Edwards, J. F.: Aorticopulmonary septal defect, Am. J. Cardiol. 9:12, 1962.
12. Putnam, T. C., and Gross, R. E.: Surgical management of aortopulmonary fenestration, Surgery 59:727, 1966.
13. Scott, H. W., Jr., and Sabiston, D. C., Jr.: Surgical treatment for congenital aorticopulmonary fistula. Experimental and clinical aspects, J. Thorac. Surg. 25:26, 1953.
14. Tandon, R., da Silva, C. L., Moller, J. H., and Edwards, J. E.: Aorticopulmonary septal defect coexisting with ventricular septal defect, Circulation 50:188, 1974.
15. Wertheimer, M., Moller, J. H., and Castaneda, A. R.: Pulmonary hypertension and congenital heart disease, Ann. Thorac. Surg. 16:416, 1973.
16. Wright, J. S., Freeman, R., and Johnston, J. B.: Aorto-pulmonary fenestration, J. Thorac. Cardiovasc. Surg. 55:280, 1968.

Anomalous Left Coronary Artery

ORIGIN of the left coronary artery from the pulmonary artery is a very rare congenital anomaly, which perhaps explains why the natural history of this condition has unfolded so gradually. Although the first description of a case (at autopsy) was by Konstantinowitsch[14] in 1906, it was not until 1933 that the typical clinical presentation in infants was described by Bland, White and Garland.[3] Mustard attempted (unsuccessfully) an anastomosis of the left carotid artery to the anomalous left coronary artery in 1953.[2]

The development of myocardial infarction, observed in most cases, has been regarded as the major pathologic complication. However, excessive left ventricular hypertrophy has been recorded in all cases, and I advance the hypothesis that the development of very severe myocardial hypertrophy is the major pathologic complication of this anomaly, and that infarction is not necessarily important, and may on occasion be a red herring. If this hypothesis is correct, it follows that we should change our emphasis in treating this condition. Every effort should be made to prevent the development of severe ventricular hypertrophy, and that can be achieved only by early diagnosis (in the first weeks and months of life), followed promptly by an anastomosis of a systemic artery to the left coronary artery. Enough information is available from the literature to reconstruct the true natural history of this condition (personal analysis of 154 reports).

Natural History of Anomalous Left Coronary Artery (ALCA)

A sequence of problems afflicts the left ventricle starting soon after birth when a child is born with a left coronary artery arising from the pulmonary artery. The anomalous artery is at first perfused by venous blood at or about systemic pressure, but by the second week of life, as the pulmonary vascular resistance falls, the left coronary artery is perfused with blood at low pressure and still with the low oxygen content of mixed venous blood. However, although myocardial hypoxia must be severe, the risk of dying from this anomaly does not begin until near the end of the second month of life. By then, severe hypertrophy of the left ventricle and ventricular septum is present and increases. This age also corresponds with the development of the "normal anemia" of infants, when the hemoglobin level falls from 18 gm/dl (the average level at birth) to the nadir of 11 gm/dl (the average normal hemoglobin of 3 months of age). During the remainder of the first year of life, gross hypertrophy in the left ventricle increases, as does fibrosis of the hypertrophic myocardium, especially in the subendocardial region and papillary muscles. The mortality rate remains high during the first 12 months of life. By the end of the first year of life, the average heart weight of those who died had increased to 4 times or more that of the normal, and death had claimed about 70% of reported patients. The average heart weight of those dying at 9 months of age was equal to the average heart weight of a normal 13-year-old child. Myocardial infarction at the apex of the left ventricle occurred frequently but not invariably and sometimes was not extensive. The typical ECG changes sometimes were found in the absence of an infarct, but severe hypertrophy of the left ventricle always was present. Once a child had survived the second year of life, the risk of dying became much less, and data are not available to estimate average heart weights at these and later ages.

During the first year of life, the anastomoses between the right and left coronary artery systems enlarge, allowing the right artery to perfuse the left arterial area so that the direction of flow is reversed in the left coronary artery, which now delivers arterial blood into the pulmonary artery. Fibrotic replacement of the inner third of the left ventricular myocardium has been described in a number of cases reported over the past 30 years.[16, 23] This condition demonstrates, more than any other, the mechanical problems that the hypertrophied left ventricle faces in supplying an adequate circulation to the inner layers of myocardium. The cause of the gross hypertrophy is of great interest, since the hypertrophy of the heart is so severe but is confined to the left ventricle and the septum. An additional factor is that the left ventricle does not face an increased after-load, and yet this very severe hypertrophy develops in that portion of the heart supplied by venous blood at a low pressure; that is, hypoxia is combined with poor perfusion.[8] This severe hypertrophy is in marked contrast to the heart of a child with transposed great arteries, when venous blood perfuses the coronary circulation but at a normal pressure, and hypertrophy does not occur disproportionately in either ventricle.

One other feature that could be important is the dominance of a left or right coronary artery in supplying the myocardium.[22] Perhaps in future years, as coronary arteriography is done more frequently and interpreted more expertly, it may be possible to assess whether a child who has a dominant coronary right artery may better survive with an anomalous left coronary artery than a child who has a dominant left coronary artery.

Almost 200 patients have been reported in the literature, about half having had some form of corrective operation. Of those reported as not having had operation, nearly all were reported after death, and about 70% were in the first year of life. Those reported after the first year of life were nearly all in the first two decades, but 1 patient was reported in the sixth and 1 in the seventh decade.

Diagnosis

An infant may present with a history that is almost diagnostic, as first described in 1933 in a model of medical reporting by Bland, White and Garland,[3] after whom the syndrome has been named. The characteristic presentation is of an infant with "paroxysmal attacks of acute discomfort precipitated by the exertion of nursing." There may be "short inspiratory grunts, followed immediately by marked pallor and cold sweat." The state seems like that of severe shock and there may be "transient loss of consciousness." The attack may last 5–10 minutes and the infant then may feed normally for several days. The onset of these signs usually is between the fourth and sixteenth weeks, but in a few cases the signs have appeared in the second and third weeks of life. Death has not occurred until near the end of the second month of life (with the exception of 2 cases).

In older children and adults, the lesion may be uncovered during examination of a patient who may have no symptoms or may have the symptoms of developing heart failure. Wesselhoeft et al.[23] reviewed the literature in 1968 in one of the finest examples of scholarly review in the cardiologic literature.

They recognized 4 types of presentation, the *first* being the infant with the Bland-White-Garland syndrome suggesting angina, which accounted for three-fourths of the cases. The *second* presentation is that of mitral insufficiency of undetermined etiology, which may present in infants or older children and adults. The *third* presentation is that of the continuous murmur syndrome, which appears only in older children and adults. The *fourth* type of presentation is sudden death in adults who usually had no previous symptoms, although some had a history of exercising at the time of sudden death. The last three groups accounted for the other one-fourth of the cases in about equal proportion.

Wesselhoeft et al. also emphasized the ECG changes. All patients had evidence of left ventricle hypertrophy and 80% of the infants had a Q-T pattern, that is, with an enlarged Q-wave (more than 4 mm) and inversion of the T-wave in aVL or in left precordial leads V_4-V_6. Almost every patient showed T-wave inversion in one or more leads.

The diagnosis is confirmed at cardiac catheterization. Angiographic dye injected into the aortic root in almost all children who have survived the early period of infancy will demonstrate the enlarged right coronary artery flowing through a large anastomosis to a left coronary artery, which drains into the pulmonary artery. In all cases, the left coronary artery, if it is visualized, does not arise from the aorta.

Echocardiography of the aortic valve in these patients may show dominance of the right coronary cusp and posterior dislocation of the aortic valve, in addition to dilatation of the left ventricle and poor posterior wall movement.[12]

Routine lung scan after IV injection of radioactive macroaggregates of human serum albumin suggested the diagnosis of ALCA in a 2-month-old patient when the myocardium was unexpectedly visualized.[21]

Differential Diagnosis

In an infant, the other causes of cardiac enlargement and cardiomyopathy must be considered, and when mitral regurgitation is the presenting problem, other causes of mitral valve disease must be considered. At a later age, if the child presents with a continuous murmur, other causes of a continuous murmur must be excluded, such as patent ductus arteriosus, ventricular septal defect with aortic valve regurgitation, aortic sinus fistula, coronary artery fistula or AV fistula of the lung or chest wall.

Treatment

The only effective treatment is operation. In the past, operation often has been postponed if the patient seemed to be doing well, but the natural history of this lesion now is sufficiently defined that nonoperative management is known to be inadvisable.

The first successful operation, ligation of the anomalous artery at its origin from the pulmonary artery, was performed by Jahnke at the suggestion of Morrow and reported by Case et al.[5] The performing of this procedure, in fact, had been preceded by a gradual recognition over many years of the natural history of the condition. In 1927, Abbott first suggested that the flow in the anomalous left coronary artery was from the heart into the pulmonary artery. (In 1886, Brooks[4] had first described reversed flow in an anomalous coronary artery but careful reading of this paper suggests that it was an anomalous conus [3d coronary] artery and not an anomalous left coronary artery.) The first suggestion that ligation of the anomalous artery would be physiologically advantageous was made by Edwards[10] in 1954. The actual observation of the reversed flow was reported by Apley et al.[2] in 1957 and the following year came the report of the first successful ligation by Jahnke.

Since that report, more than 60 patients have been described as having had ligation of the anomalous coronary. Of those operated on over the age of 18 months, all have survived to leave the hospital. Of those operated on under the age of 18 months, only about half have survived and this has not been much influenced by the age at operation, from the second month of life on to 1½ years of age. Since more than two-thirds of the patients with ligation fell in the group of less than 18 months, ligation clearly is not an adequate answer.

Cooley *et al.*[7] reported the first connection of the anomalous coronary artery to the systemic circuit using a graft. The first successful direct anastomosis of a systemic artery to the anomalous coronary was reported by Meyer *et al.*,[17] so achieving the physiologic correction first attempted by Mustard in 1953 when he sutured the carotid artery to the anomalous coronary. A number of reports subsequently have described the use of autologous vein grafts to connect the anomalous coronary to the aorta, but since the patency of these grafts over a 2-year period rarely is more than 80% in adult coronary surgery, it is not surprising that graft failure occurred in children,[11] and this has been reported associated with sudden death in 2 patients, 10 months or more after operation. It cannot be assumed that failure of a graft is simply the same as ligating the anomalous artery. In one case of postoperative occlusion of the vein graft, the entire left coronary system was found to be thrombosed at the postmortem study.[1] It seems desirable, therefore, that the anomalous artery should be directly anastomosed to a systemic artery either by using the left subclavian, as Meyer *et al.* suggested, or, as described by Neches *et al.*[18] in 1974 (and also successfully applied by Grace *et al.*[13]), detaching the ALCA with a surrounding cuff of pulmonary artery wall and anastomosing this to the aortic root, after completely dividing the pulmonary artery to improve the exposure, an operation requiring heart-lung bypass.

Further experience is required to determine which operative technique is the most suitable. A left subclavian artery can be attached to the anomalous coronary through a left thoracotomy without using cardiopulmonary bypass. A successful case has been reported by Senderoff *et al.*[20] and I have used this technique in the last 2 of 4 children operated on. In a 3-month-old child, the subclavian artery gradually occluded over the next 6 months, seemingly because it was acutely kinked at its origin from the aorta, although the anastomosis and the attached portion of the subclavian artery remained patent. The child continued to do well. A second child operated on at 3 years of age had follow-up studies 2 years later that showed full patency of the graft and coronary system.

Pinsky *et al.*[19] reported angiographic studies 3 years and 5 years after direct anastomosis of the subclavian to the anomalous left coronary artery in 2 patients, 1 aged 8 months and the other 4 months at the time of operation. Both children were in good health. The anastomosis had closed in the infant operated on at 8 months but was widely patent in the other, with marked improvement in the ECG.

Perhaps a form of subclavian arterioplasty as described by Laks and Cataneda[15] may help.

Summary

Enough evidence is at hand now to recognize that this rare lesion was lethal in at least three-fourths of the recognized cases, and death usually occurred in infancy. Ligation of the anomalous left coronary artery in the first 18 months of life has been attempted in an adequate enough number of cases to know that the mortality is at least 50%, which is unacceptable. The evidence strongly suggests that the lethal factor is gross hypertrophy of the left ventricle, not myocardial infarction. Since the hypertrophy is a result of perfusion at low pressure with desaturated blood, the only effective way to prevent the hypertrophy and the fibrotic replacement of the subendocardium is to perfuse the anomalous artery from a systemic artery. If this is to be done early enough to prevent severe hypertrophy, the condition must be recognized as early as possible and the child operated on as soon as the diagnosis has been made. If this can be achieved in the first 3 months of life, perhaps much of the damage to the heart can be averted. The conventional expectant approach of simply observing patients in relatively good health no longer is justified. The alternative, that is, connecting the anomalous left coronary artery to the systemic arterial circuit as early as possible, has not yet been done sufficiently often for its full value to be assessed.

REFERENCES

1. Anthony, C. L., Jr., McAllister, H. A., Jr., and Cheitlin, M. D.: Spontaneous graft closure in anomalous origin of the left coronary, Chest 68:586, 1975.
2. Apley, J., Horton, R. E., and Wilson, M. G.: The possible role of surgery in the treatment of anomalous left coronary artery, Thorax 12:28, 1957.
3. Bland, E. F., White, P. D., and Garland, J.: Congenital anomalies of the coronary arteries: Report of an unusual case associated with cardiac hypertrophy, Am. Heart J. 8:787, 1933.
4. Brooks, H. S. J.: Two cases of an abnormal coronary artery of the heart arising from the pulmonary artery: With some remarks upon the effect of this anomaly in producing cirsoid dilatation of the vessels, J. Anat. Physiol. 20:26, 1886.
5. Case, R. B., Morrow, A. G., Stainsby, W., and Nestor, J. O.: Anomalous origin of the left coronary artery. The physiologic defect and suggested surgical treatment, Circulation 17:1062, 1958.
6. Chiariello, L., Meyer, J., Reul, G. J., Jr., Hallman, G. L., and Cooley, D. A.: Surgical treatment for anomalous origin of left coronary artery from pulmonary artery, Ann. Thorac. Surg. 19: 443, 1975.
7. Cooley, D. A., Hallman, G. L., and Bloodwell, R. D.: Definitive surgical treatment of anomalous origin of left coronary artery from pulmonary artery: Indications and results, J. Thorac. Cardiovasc. Surg. 52:798, 1966.
8. Deckelbaum, L., Green, R., III, Mueller, M., Hood, W. B., Jr., and Apstein, C. S.: Acute hypoxic heart failure: Comparison of hypoxemia and ischemia, Am. J. Cardiol. 35:131, 1975.
9. Edwards, J. E.: Anomalous coronary arteries with special reference to arteriovenous-like communications, Circulation 17: 1001, 1958.
10. Edwards, J. E.: Functional pathology of congenital cardiac disease, Pediatr. Clin. North Am. 1:13, 1954.
11. El-Said, G. M., Ruzyllo, W., Williams, R. L., Mullins, C. E., Hallman, G. L., Cooley, D. A., and McNamara, D. G.: Early and late result of saphenous vein graft for anomalous origin of left coronary artery from pulmonary artery, Circulation 47–48(supp. 3):2, 1973.
12. Glaser, J., Bharati, S., Whitman, V., and Liebman, J.: Echocardiographic (EG) findings in patients (PTS) with anomalous origin of the left coronary artery (ALCA), Circulation 47–48 (supp. 4):63, 1973.
13. Grace, R. R., Angelini, P., and Cooley, D. A.: Aortic implantation of anomalous left coronary artery arising from pulmonary artery, Am. J. Cardiol. 39:608, 1977.
14. Konstantinowitsch, W. V.: Ein seltener Fall von Herzmissbildung. (Cor biloculare, atresia ostii aortae.) (In German.), Prag. Med. Wochenschr. 31:657, 1906.
15. Laks, H., and Cataneda, A. R.: Subclavian arterioplasty for the ipsilateral Blalock-Taussig shunt, Ann. Thorac. Surg. 19:319, 1975.
16. Lyon, R. A., Johansmann, R. J., and Dodd, K.: Anomalous origin of the left coronary artery, Am. J. Dis. Child. 72:675, 1946.
17. Meyer, B. W., Stefanik, G., Stiles, Q. R., Lindesmith, G. G., and Jones, J. C.: A method of definitive surgical treatment of anomalous origin of left coronary artery, J. Thorac. Cardiovasc. Surg. 56:104, 1968.
18. Neches, W. H., Mathews, R. A., Park, S. C., Lenox, C. C., Zuber-

buhler, J. R., Siewers, R. D., and Bahnson, H. T.: Anomalous origin of the left coronary artery from the pulmonary artery. A new method of surgical repair, Circulation 50:582, 1974.

19. Pinsky, W. W., Fagan, L. R., Mudd, J. F. G., and Willman, V. L.: Subclavian-coronary artery anastomosis in infancy for the Bland-White-Garland syndrome. A three-year and five-year follow-up, J. Thorac. Cardiovasc. Surg. 72:15, 1976.

20. Senderoff, E., Slovis, A. J., Moallem, A., and Kahn, R. E.: Subclavian-coronary artery anastomosis. A technique for definitive correction of anomalous origin of left coronary artery, J. Thorac. Cardiovasc. Surg. 71:142, 1976.

21. Sfakianakis, G. N., Damoulaki-Sfakianaki, E., McClead, R. E., and Craenen, J.: Anomalous origin of left coronary artery diagnosed by a lung scan, N. Engl. J. Med. 296:675, 1977.

22. Vasko, J. S., Gutelius, J., and Sabiston, D. C., Jr.: A study of predominance of human coronary arteries determined by arteriographic and perfusion technics, Am. J. Cardiol. 8:379, 1961.

23. Wesselhoeft, H., Fawcett, J. S., and Johnson, A. L.: Anomalous origin of the left coronary artery from the pulmonary trunk. Its clinical spectrum, pathology, and pathophysiology, based on a review of 140 cases with seven further cases, Circulation 38:403, 1968.

Bulbus Cordis Anomalies

59

Denton A. Cooley / Don C. Wukasch

Anomalous Pulmonary Venous Return

HISTORY. – Anomalous communication between the pulmonary and systemic venous systems was first described more than two centuries ago in 1739 by Winslow.[63] In 1798, a case of total pulmonary venous drainage into the right side of the heart was described by Wilson,[62] and Friedlowsky[30] (1868) subsequently described this pathologic entity in more detail. In 1942, Brody[10] focused attention on anomalous pulmonary venous drainage in a collective review of reported cases, with consideration of the types and location of such anomalies. As recently as 1947, operative correction of these lesions had not been accomplished, when Brantigan[9] suggested that resection of the portion of lung thus drained would palliate the partial anomalous drainage. For complete anomalous drainage of the entire pulmonary circulation, he speculated that removal of the interatrial septum might be performed or a major pulmonary vein could be anastomosed to the left atrium.

In 1951, Muller[46] reported successful side-to-side anastomosis of an anomalous pulmonary vein into the left atrium, and in 1954 Gerbode[32] reported a similar case. Successful repair of partial anomalous drainage involving both left and right lungs subsequently was reported by Kirklin,[43] Neptune et al.,[49] Bailey et al.[3] and Cooley and Mahaffey.[19] Correction of total anomalous pulmonary venous drainage presented a more difficult technical problem, which ultimately was solved with development of the pump-oxygenator for temporary cardiopulmonary bypass. Repair of total anomalous drainage of the type directly into the right atrium was reported by Gott et al.,[35] who referred to the work of Lewis and Varco, who had used hypothermia and cardiac inflow occlusion. Burroughs and Kirklin[12] also were successful in repair of this type of defect using an atrial-well technique.

The first successful open correction of total anomalous drainage of the supracardiac type was reported by Cooley and Ochsner[21] in 1957. Subsequently, various techniques for repair have been described.[2, 8, 34, 55, 56] In 1962, Mustard and co-workers[47] described a two-stage repair in critically ill infants. During the first procedure for the supracardiac type of total anomalous pulmonary venous return (TAPVR), a posterior anastomosis between the common pulmonary venous trunk and left atrium was performed using cardiopulmonary bypass; ligation of the vertical vein and closure of the atrial septal defect were postponed until several years later. More recent advances in technique and postoperative management have allowed complete one-stage repair even in young infants. In 1971, Gersony et al.[33] reported successful repair in 7 of 10 infants under the age of 5 months, demonstrating the feasibility of early correction in young infants. Using deep hypothermia by surface cooling and only limited cardiopulmonary bypass, Barratt-Boyes et al.[7] performed successful correction in 4 of 6 infants, the youngest survivor being only 9 days old.

Embryology

The primordia of the lungs, larynx and tracheobronchial tree are derived by division of the foregut, with which the lungs initially share a common blood supply. The splanchnic plexus drains into the neighboring veins, which are the systemic precardinal and postcardinal veins and the visceral veins of the abdomen, i.e., the umbilicovitelline vessels and associated hepatic sinusoids. Thus, initial drainage of the lungs is into the superior vena cava, coronary sinus, innominate veins, portal system, ductus venosus and inferior vena cava and without direct communication with the heart. The developing left atrium must make connection with that portion of the splanchnic bed that is draining the primordial lungs. It does this by developing a "common pulmonary vein" that extends into the dorsal mesocardium.[1] As this junction is taking place, separation of the primary venous connections with the cardinal and umbilicovitelline venous system occurs. According to Edwards,[26] the underlying cause for anomalous connection is (1) failure of the atrial portion of the heart to connect with the pulmonary portion of the splanchnic plexus or (2) a secondary obliteration of normally developed communications between the atrial portion of the heart and the pulmonary portion of the splanchnic plexus. This does not provide an adequate explanation for those cases in which the drainage of one or both lungs is directly into the right atrium. An abnormality in development of the atrial septum probably accounts for the formation of the sinus venosus type of anomaly. If the septum develops farther than normal to the left, the site of the outpouching of the left atrium (sinoatrial region), which joins the primitive pulmonary veins, may lie to the right of the septum, thus creating a connection with the right atrium. If the atrial septum occupies a position midway between the normal and the extreme left position, the sinoatrial pouch may be divided so that the left lung drains into the left atrium normally and the right lung into the right atrium.

Anatomy and Pathophysiology

PARTIAL ANOMALOUS DRAINAGE.—The venous system within the lung is normal in this condition, but wide variation occurs in the anatomic site to which the anomalous veins drain. Partial anomalous drainage of the right lung into the right atrium or venae cavae is several times more common than for the left lung. Only rarely do both lungs have partial anomalous drainage into the systemic circulation.[40] The site of partial drainage from the right lung is, in order of frequency, to the superior vena cava, to the right atrium or to the inferior vena cava.[39] On the left side, the veins usually empty into a persistent left superior vena cava (persistent cardinal vein) or into the innominate vein and, rarely, enter the coronary sinus posteriorly. In most cases, the partial drainage is accompanied by a patent foramen ovale or a true atrial septal defect. In some instances with a large-volume left-to-right shunt via the pulmonary veins, a septal defect may be a factor in preventing overload of the right heart and provides for adequate left ventricular filling. Occasionally the lung itself is abnormal, and we have demonstrated abnormal lobulation and pleural reflection in a right lung where all of the drainage was into the inferior vena cava below the diaphragm. Anomalous venous drainage of the entire right lung with normal left pulmonary drainage occurs in the absence of a patent foramen ovale, with drainage of the right pulmonary veins to the inferior vena cava via a common vein. This condition has been termed the "scimitar deformity." The fanciful name for this anomaly results from the curved, sword-like appearance, on chest films, of the large anomalous pulmonary vein draining the blood from the right lung (Fig. 59–1). The anomaly occurs only in the right lung.

SINUS VENOSUS DEFECT.—This anomaly is a combination of a high interatrial septal defect and anomalous pulmonary venous drainage of the right upper and sometimes middle lobe veins. Although this lesion was described first in 1868,[61] the term sinus venosus defect was coined in 1956 by Ross.[51] Characteristically, the sinus venosus defect is located adjacent to the orifice of the superior vena cava, and no superior margin of the atrial septum is present.[16] The septal defect is located cephalad to the fossa ovalis, which usually is intact. The point of entry of anomalous veins is at the atriocaval junction or higher, directly into the superior vena cava. In many instances, one or more segmental veins empty separately into the superior vena cava.

TOTAL ANOMALOUS DRAINAGE.—Although an atrial septal defect is present in most instances of partial anomalous pulmonary venous drainage, an interatrial communication must be present in total anomalous drainage in order for the patient to survive. All of the blood normally destined for the

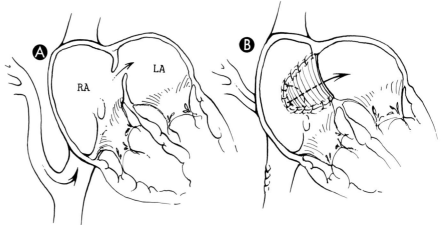

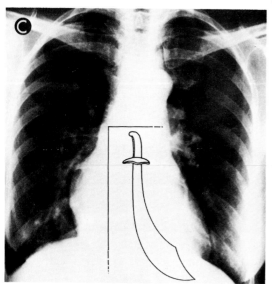

Fig. 59–1.—"Scimitar deformity." **A,** drainage of common pulmonary venous trunk into inferior vena cava below the diaphragm. **B,** method of repair consisting of anastomosis of the pulmonary venous trunk into the right atrium, enlargement of the foramen ovale and creation of a Dacron tunnel to direct blood into the left atrium. (For complete technique see Fig. 59–5.) **C,** roentgenogram of the chest of a patient with anomalous venous return of entire right lung into the inferior vena cava demonstrating the typical "scimitar-shaped" right paracardial shadow. The heart is moderately shifted to the right.

left atrium enters the right atrium, where it mixes freely with unoxygenated venous blood. Whereas most of this blood enters the right ventricle, some of the mixed pulmonary and systemic venous blood is shunted right to left to enter the left ventricle and is pumped out into the body, producing cyanosis. Mild cyanosis may or may not be apparent early in life but always will appear later as the right-to-left shunt increases. Usually the diameter of the pulmonary artery is twice that of the ascending aorta. The left atrium and ventricle are small in comparison to the right side of the heart; but since the left ventricle still is adequate to provide for complete cardiac outflow, surgical correction usually is possible in a one-stage operation.

Total anomalous drainage of pulmonary venous blood occurs in several anatomic forms. Darling *et al.*[22] have described anatomic classification of the types of total anomalous drainage based on the location or level at which the communication of the veins enters the systemic veins or right side of the heart. Thus, either supracardiac, cardiac, infracardiac or mixed types occur (Fig. 59–2).

SUPRACARDIAC TYPE.—The common pulmonary venous trunk usually drains to the left innominate vein through an anomalous vertical vein. This is the most frequent type.[64] A connection to the dorsal aspect of the right superior vena cava is less common. Survival of infants born with this anomaly depends on the absence of pulmonary venous obstruction and the presence of an atrial septal defect; the larger the defect the better the prognosis. In patients with this anomaly, all of the pulmonary venous blood from the right and left lungs enters a common vein behind the heart and passes through a persistent left vertical vein into the left innominate vein (see Fig. 59–6, A).

CARDIAC TYPE.—Venous return occurs either directly into the posterior aspect of the right atrium or through a connection to the coronary sinus (Fig. 59–2, B). Communication with the left atrium is through a foramen ovale or atrial septal defect.

INFRACARDIAC TYPE.—The blood of both lungs passes below the diaphragm through a descending vein that drains into the inferior vena cava, hepatic veins, portal vein or ductus venosus (Fig. 59–2, C). Of all types of total anomalous venous return, this type (see Fig. 59–8, A) produces the greatest early mortality, probably because of the frequent presence of obstruction to the pulmonary veins below the diaphragm.[64] With few exceptions, these patients die during infancy unless operation is performed within the first few days or weeks of life. Since no effective palliative treatment is available, operation must be performed early despite the high surgical risk.

MIXED TYPE.—The pulmonary venous blood drains into the right side of the heart by a combination of the routes described above.

Incidence

Among patients with cyanotic congenital cardiac defects who require operation during the first year of life, TAPVR ranks fourth in frequency at the Texas Heart Institute, following transposition of the great arteries, tetralogy of Fallot and tricuspid atresia.[64]

The exact incidence of partial anomalous pulmonary venous drainage is difficult to determine, since instances obviously will escape detection by the usual autopsy technique, which involves separating the heart and lungs without studying them as a unit. Healey[39] found 1 (0.4%) case among 251 cadavers, and Hughes and Rumore[40] found 2 (0.7%) in 280 postmortem subjects. One should recognize that anomalous drainage of the partial type is relatively common and frequently accompanies atrial septal defect. In a survey of 147 cases of anomalous drainage, Healey[39] reported 61 complete or total and 86 partial anomalies. In the instances of total anomalous drainage, approximately 39% connected with the superior caval system, usually in the region of the innominate vein.

In our own experience with 154 patients who underwent surgical treatment for TAPVR, 92 patients (60%) demonstrated the supracardiac type, among whom 20 (22%) had drainage to the right superior vena cava and 72 (78%) had drainage into an anomalous vertical vein. The cardiac type of drainage was seen in 41 patients (27%), among whom drainage was to the body of the right atrium in 18 (44%) and into the coronary sinus in 23 (56%). The infracardiac type was observed in 11 patients (7%), in whom drainage was to the portal vein in 6 (55%), the inferior vena cava in 3 (27%) and into the hepatic veins in 2 (18%). Ten patients (6%) demonstrated a mixed type of anomaly.

Symptoms and Findings on Examination

Partial anomalous pulmonary drainage of the right lung into the right atrium produces minimal symptoms and findings.[60] Since the vascular shunt is left to right, no cyanosis is evident. Usually right atrial and ventricular enlargement is present, but often no murmur is heard. In the presence of an associated atrial septal defect of significant size, symptoms of a large-volume left-to-right shunt are evident. The patient

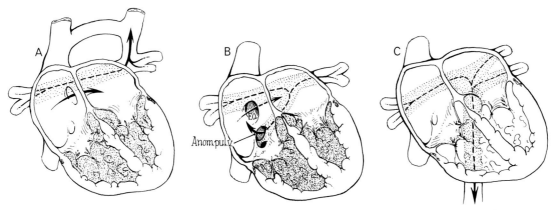

Fig. 59–2.—The three anatomic types of total anomalous pulmonary venous return. **A,** supracardiac. **B,** cardiac. **C,** infracardiac.

has dyspnea on exertion, palpitation and occasional pre-cordial fullness or discomfort. A frail or so-called gracile habitus may be noted, depending on the volume of the shunt and the degree of vascular resistance.

Total anomalous pulmonary venous drainage usually causes severe symptoms, primarily of pulmonary congestion and heart failure, and striking physical findings. Infants demonstrate severe right-sided failure, with cardiomegaly, hepatomegaly and variable cyanosis, depending on the size of the interatrial communication. Pulmonary congestion is common because of the excessive pulmonary blood flow. As the heart enlarges, compression of the left lower lobe may occur and be mistaken for pneumonia. A left-sided chest deformity develops at an early age because of the tremen-dous load placed on the right side of the heart and conse-quent enlargement. The findings on physical examination are determined by whether there is obstruction to the pul-monary venous return to the right side of the heart, which may result from either stenosis of the vertical anomalous vein in the supracardiac type,[38] or resistance of an organ, such as the liver, on the infracardiac drainage into the portal vein.[37] If obstruction is present, the heart usually is not en-larged or overactive on physical examination, and murmurs frequently are absent. The pulse usually is of small volume during infancy and blood pressure is low. Patients without obstruction and, consequently, with large left-to-right shunts have evidence of increased cardiac activity on inspection and palpation of the precordium. A systolic ejection murmur frequently is present over the area of the pulmonary valve, but infants may not have an appreciable murmur.

The clinical picture of the patient who has survived infan-cy and childhood is similar to that of patients with other forms of mild cyanotic heart disease. In general, these pa-tients have an interatrial communication of sufficient size to vent the right atrial overload into the left atrium. Often, symptoms in these patients are surprisingly mild, and in 1 of our patients who was 36 years of age, the symptoms were not disabling and cyanosis was barely evident. The number of anatomic variations in the anomalous drainage results in a wide variation in the degree of incapacity.

ELECTROCARDIOGRAPHY, RADIOGRAPHY, ECHOCARDIOG-RAPHY AND CARDIAC CATHETERIZATION. — Electrocardio-grams demonstrate evidence of right axis deviation and right ventricular hypertrophy. The P waves are unusually tall and may be peaked. According to Keith and associates,[42] the most striking feature about the electrocardiogram in pa-tients with TAPVR is the presence of a Q wave in the right precordial leads. But if the anomalous pulmonary drainage represents only a small segment of the lung, the electrocar-diographic changes may be undetectable. In instances of total anomalous drainage, an impressive degree of right atri-al enlargement is present.

Roentgenograms of the chest in patients with partial anomalous pulmonary venous drainage reveal right atrial and right ventricular enlargement with dilatation of the main pulmonary artery. Pulmonary vessels in the periphery of the lung fields often are prominent, depending on the volume of pulmonary overload. In the sinus venosus type of anomaly, the diagnosis may be suggested by a right hilar bulge at the atriocaval junction. Tomography and selective angiography may aid in this diagnosis.[25]

Roentgenograms of the chest in patients with total anoma-lous pulmonary venous return also vary, depending on the presence or absence of obstruction to pulmonary venous return. Patients without obstruction usually have increased

pulmonary vascularity with a prominent main pulmonary artery segment,[37] over-all cardiac size is increased and there is no enlargement of the left atrium according to the normal path of the barium-filled esophagus in the right anterior oblique view. The right atrium is enlarged. The roentgeno-graphic appearance of total anomalous pulmonary venous return into the left innominate vein in children reveals an almost pathognomonic cardiac silhouette (Fig. 59–3). These findings were clearly described by Snellen and Albers,[58] who reported a figure-of-eight configuration of the mediasti-num. The upper half of the eight is formed by the ascending or vertical anomalous pulmonary vein on the left and the prominence of the distended right superior vena cava. This same configuration also has been referred to as the "snow-man" and "cottage loaf" appearance, the latter being the shape of a particular bread loaf in Great Britain. A hilar dance usually is demonstrable in the pulmonary vessels on fluoroscopy. The above pattern is typical of the total anom-aly in children and adults but usually is not characteristic in infants. In infants, cardiac enlargement involving the right ventricle and engorgement of the pulmonary vessels reveal the presence of a large left-to-right shunt. The superior me-diastinal shadow may be widened, with a box-like appear-ance of the heart caused by a somewhat horizontal left bor-der of the heart at its junction with the aortic arch.[35]

Echocardiography recently has been reported to aid in the diagnosis of TAPVR. Recent work by Paquet *et al.*[50] and Sasse *et al.*[53, 54] in 10 patients with TAPVR at Texas Children's Hospital has demonstrated a characteristic echo-free space posterior to the left atrial wall. The significance of their finding is that apparently TAPVR can be differentiated from primary pulmonary disease in the critically ill newborn infant before cardiac catheterization.

Cardiac catheterization is necessary to make the diagnosis and should be performed whenever the condition is sus-pected. The objective of cardiac catheterization is not only to make or confirm the diagnosis but to delineate the precise anatomy of the pulmonary veins and assess the physiologic disturbance.[52] The presence of frequently occurring pul-monary venous obstruction must be determined and its ex-act location demonstrated. Because the degree of elevation of the pulmonary vascular resistance is one of the major fac-tors determining the mortality in surgical treatment,[64] its careful assessment is imperative. Although the significance of hypoplasia of the left ventricle on the prognosis following operation has not been established,[52] the size of the left atrium and ventricle should be noted. The coexistence of associated lesions, notably ventricular septal defect and pa-tent ductus arteriosus, obviously must be determined. In general, it is preferable to use a saphenous or femoral vein approach rather than one through the upper limb, to facili-tate passage of the catheter across the atrial opening into the left atrium and ventricle as well as to provide easier access to the entrance of the pulmonary veins.[52]

Cardiac catheterization in all patients with anomalous venous return reveals an increased oxygen saturation of right atrial blood when compared to systemic venous blood. These findings are of little value, however, in differentiating partial anomalous drainage from an atrial septal defect. Usu-ally, the volume of left-to-right shunt in the anomalous veins is smaller than with atrial septal defect, in which the shunt may be 2 or 3 times the systemic flow.

In total anomalous drainage of pulmonary veins, the blood oxygen saturation in the right side of the heart is similar or equal to the saturation in the systemic arteries and is consid-ered almost diagnostic. Exploration of the superior caval sys-

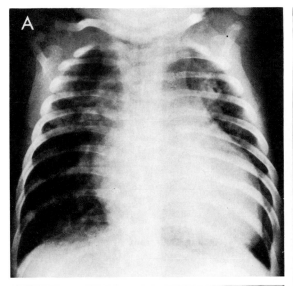

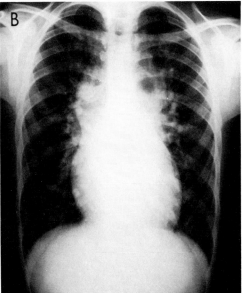

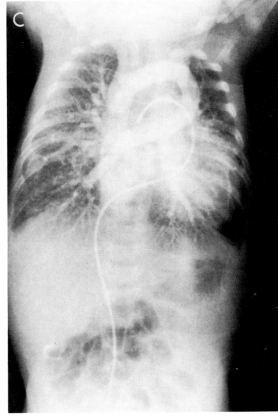

Fig. 59–3.—Total anomalous venous return into left innominate vein: roentgenographic features in various age groups. **A,** posteroanterior roentgenogram of chest of a 3-month-old male with TAVR of the supracardiac type with a left "vertical anomalous vein." Note cardiac enlargement and increased pulmonary vascular markings. Vascular engorgement in superior mediastinum results in "snowman appearance." **B,** roentgenogram of chest of a 14-year-old male showing enlarged left superior vena cava and right superior vena cava producing the mediastinal configuration referred to as "snowman deformity." **C,** anteroposterior angiocardiogram of 4-month-old male with TAVR, supracardiac type. Contrast material injected via catheter in right pulmonary artery. Pulmonary veins from each lung unite in a common retrocardiac trunk. From the left side of this vein there ascends the vertical anomalous vein ("persistent left superior vena cava") to join the innominate vein. Engorged veins in superior mediastinum give "snowman appearance" to the heart.

tem with the catheter introduced through the left antecubital vein may reveal the connection of the pulmonary venous trunk with the left innominate vein. Passage of the catheter through the anomalous channel into both lungs occasionally is possible. The pressure within the right side of the heart and pulmonary artery is elevated, frequently to a striking degree. Entry of the catheter into the left atrium from the superior vena cava usually is more difficult than from the inferior vena cava because of the preferential flow of blood through the foramen from below.

In general, indicator dye dilution curves do not add great-ly in establishing the diagnosis of anomalous pulmonary venous return but when done from the left atrium or left ventricle may detect associated anomalies, such as ventricular septal defect or patent ductus arteriosus. Dye dilution studies do reveal a shorter appearance time from the atrium than from the right ventricle or pulmonary artery. Dye dilution studies are extremely useful for precisely locating the anomalous drainage and estimating the volume of the shunt. Comparison of right atrial dilution curves is made following injection of indicator solution into the right and left pulmonary veins.[62] This reveals the volume of blood being recirculated but does not differentiate, in every case, the possible sites where this occurs. Often it is difficult to distinguish anomalous pulmonary venous drainage from an atrial septal defect, since in large atrial defects, because of the preferential flow, dilution curves frequently demonstrate a greater degree of venous drainage to the right atrium from the right lung than from the left lung. Exploration of the anomalous veins with the catheter, together with combinations of various injection sites and sampling sites, usually provides adequate diagnostic data.

Differential Diagnosis

The problems of differential diagnosis have been clearly described by Rudolph[52] to fall in three separate categories, depending on the presenting clinical picture and age of the patient.

NEWBORN INFANT WITH RESPIRATORY DISTRESS.—The diagnosis of TAPVR must be considered in any newborn infant with respiratory distress, cyanosis, weak pulses, mottling of the extremities or pallor. Primary pulmonary disease is the most frequent etiology of this syndrome and, formerly, cardiac catheterization often was necessary to differentiate this condition from TAPVR. However, recent use of echocardiography in our institution has indicated the feasibility of excluding possible TAPVR by this noninvasive technique, thus avoiding unnecessary cardiac catheterization in critically ill infants with primary pulmonary disease.[50, 53, 54] Aortic or mitral valve atresia, cor triatriatum and congenital mitral stenosis can produce a clinical picture identical to TAPVR. Differential diagnosis must be made with the aid of cardiac catheterization and angiocardiography.

OLDER INFANTS WITH CARDIAC FAILURE.—The possibility of TAPVR must be considered in any infant who develops cardiac failure within the first few months of life, especially if mild cyanosis is present. According to Rudolph,[52] the most frequent congenital cardiac lesions that must be differentiated by cardiac catheterization are Ebstein's anomaly, common atrium, endocardial cushion defect, double-outlet right ventricle and single ventricle.

OLDER CHILDREN WITH LARGE-VOLUME OVERLOAD OF RIGHT HEART.—The clinical picture of older children with a hyperactive right ventricle, diastolic murmur, mild cyanosis, cardiomegaly and increased pulmonary vascular markings may also be produced by atrial septal defect with or without partial anomalous venous return, common atrium or Ebstein's anomaly. Definitive diagnosis of TAPVR is made by cardiac catheterization and angiocardiography.

Prognosis

Prognosis usually is good in *partial anomalous pulmonary connection*, and patients frequently have no outward signs of disability. In Brody's series,[10] 76% of patients reached maturity, and Dean and Fox[23] described a patient who lived to be 86 years of age. Under ordinary circumstances, a single anomalous pulmonary vein without associated atrial septal defect does not cause symptoms during childhood. The appearance of symptoms early in life usually indicates the presence of a large associated atrial septal defect or anomalous drainage of an entire lung. According to Brody,[10] if less than half of the blood from the pulmonary parenchyma is drained anomalously, the patients exhibit little disability. When more than half of the pulmonary circulation enters the right side of the heart, evidence of right-sided failure becomes evident, often interferes with development and shortens the life span.

In contrast to partial anomalous drainage, the prognosis in *total anomalous pulmonary venous connection* is poor. In a review of reported cases, Healey[39] observed the average age at death to be 1.8 years, and most patients did not survive infancy.[11, 22] The interatrial communication in the usual instance of the malformation is small and often is of the "probe patent" type. Since the presence of the interatrial defect is vital to survival, the size of the defect is critical, and those patients surviving infancy and early childhood have a sizable interatrial opening that permits right-to-left shunting.

In order to improve the survival rate, cardiac catheterization should be performed immediately to delineate specific features of the malformation. The infant in critical condition may be improved by atrial septostomy, and especially is this required if the atrial septal defect is so small as to leave a pressure gradient between left and right atria,[28, 57] but if pulmonary hypertension persists, if there is a known obstruction in the anomalous veins[50] or if congestive heart failure develops, operation is required.[17] In patients who have obstruction to pulmonary venous return especially, e.g., from external compression or intrinsic stenosis,[27, 35, 36] no attempt should be made to manage the infant by medication alone on a long-term basis because death may occur suddenly and operation for these patients is an emergency procedure, as Gathman and Nadas[31] advised. Older children and adults may be operated on but with less urgency when the diagnosis is established.[17]

The nature of the anatomic defect sometimes strongly influences the outcome. For example, in our experience, the mortality rate in patients with the supracardiac type with drainage into the right superior vena cava is twice that of the more commonly found connection to the left innominate vein.[64]

Operative Treatment

Repair of anomalous pulmonary venous drainage is recommended in all patients if the volume of shunt is significant and the anatomic arrangements permit complete correction. Repair requires redirection of the pulmonary venous blood into the left atrium.

Patients are operated on using cardiopulmonary bypass with a disposable bubble oxygenator.[15, 18, 21] If the patient weighs more than 14 kg, the extracorporeal circuit is primed with 5% dextrose in distilled water. In small infants, freshly drawn blood preserved in heparin is used to prime the system. Since 1963 we have utilized a midline sternotomy and elevated the heart by traction on the apex to permit creation of the largest possible anastomosis between the common pulmonary venous trunk and the left atrium. The anomalous vertical vein or the connection to the superior or inferior vena caval system is ligated. The patent foramen ovale usually is closed with several interrupted sutures through a right atriotomy. If the entire left lung is draining into the superior vena cava, it may be corrected by transferring the communicating trunk into the left auricular appendage.[19, 45]

PARTIAL ANOMALOUS PULMONARY VENOUS RETURN WITH ASSOCIATED ATRIAL SEPTAL DEFECT.—Since most of the right pulmonary lesions are associated with an atrial septal defect, such redirection usually is accomplished by closing the septal defect laterally and anteriorly to the rim of the anomalous veins. The coronary sinus and pulmonary venous orifices are identified in the right atrial chamber (Fig. 59–4, A). Repair usually consists of diverting the blood

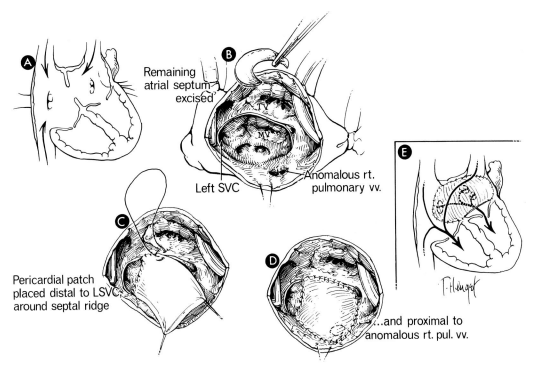

Fig. 59–4.—Partial anomalous pulmonary venous return. Technique of correction of atrial septal defect. **A,** diagram of atrial septal defect and anomalous right pulmonary veins. **B,** anomalous right pulmonary veins are identified and remaining atrial septum excised. **C,** pericardial patch placed distal to left superior vena cava around septal ridge. **D,** suture line continued proximal to anomalous right pulmonary veins. **E,** pattern of flow after completion of repair.

from the right lung to the left atrium (Fig. 59–4, *E*). Portions of the interatrial septum may be excised if there is interference or obstruction to flow into the left atrium (Fig. 59–4, *B*).

Direct repair with a double row of continuous sutures occasionally is satisfactory but may produce tension on the suture line, with possible distortion and obstruction of the pulmonary veins. Therefore, we usually use a Dacron or pericardial patch (Fig. 59–4, *C* and *D*). The direction of the suture line should be planned carefully so that the patch will not be redundant or become folded. The coronary sinus should be identified and not included in the suture line.

ANOMALOUS PULMONARY VENOUS RETURN WITH ASSOCIATED REPAIR OF PARTIAL SINUS VENOSUS DEFECT. — Sinus venosus defects are associated with a persistent left superior vena cava in about 10% of the patients. In all such defects, the extra cava should be suspected and, if present, taped before cardiotomy. The cannulations are performed in the usual manner. A superior caval catheter smaller than the inferior catheter may be selected to facilitate accurate suturing at the superior atriocaval junction, which can be difficult. The lateral surface of the superior vena cava should be exposed to identify the anomalous veins, which are common in this defect. Efforts should be made to divert all of the pulmonary venous return into the left atrium.

Single small segmental branches of the pulmonary venous system, however, may be simply ligated without serious consequences. The superior caval tourniquet should be passed above the entry of all pulmonary veins. The azygos vein may require separate control or ligation to allow proper placement of the tourniquet at a position more cephalad than usual.

SCIMITAR DEFORMITY (TOTAL ANOMALOUS VENOUS RETURN FROM THE RIGHT LUNG TO THE INFERIOR VENA CAVA). — Repair of the defect (Fig. 59–5, *A*) requires the use of temporary cardiopulmonary bypass. The lower end of the anomalous vein is dissected free at its juncture with the inferior vena cava just above the point where the hepatic veins enter but usually below the caval hiatus in the diaphragm (Fig. 59–5, *B* and *C*). The usual cannulations are performed, the vena cava occluded and the pulmonary vein clamped and divided (Fig. 59–5, *D*). The caval end is sutured (Fig. 59–5, *E*). The vein will not reach the left atrium, which is located farther to the left than usual and does not present normally along the right cardiac border; thus, a special technique is necessary to divert the blood into the left atrium. The right atrium is opened, exposing the interatrial septum. Usually the septum has either no defect or a small patent foramen ovale. An incision is made in the lateral wall of the right atrium and the vein is anastomosed to the atrium (Fig. 59–5, *F* and *G*). A small segment of atrial tissue may be excised to prevent obstruction of the anastomosis or subsequent stenosis.

The foramen ovale is enlarged to the fullest extent (Fig. 59–5, *H*). An oblong patch of knitted Dacron fabric is fashioned, which will create a tunnel for blood from the veno-atrial anastomosis to enter the foramen ovale (Fig. 59–5, *I*). This technique has never failed to provide satisfactory results. We have used a similar technique for diverting large pulmonary veins entering the superior vena cava at the atrio-caval junction into the left atrium. First, an atrial septal defect is created and a patch graft is used to divert blood from the anomalous veins into the left atrium.

TAPVR, SUPRACARDIAC TYPE. — Repair of the anomaly requires temporary cardiopulmonary bypass. The approach

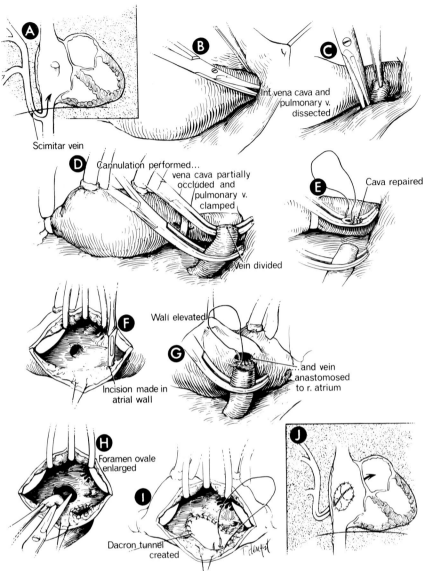

Fig. 59–5.—Total anomalous venous return from right lung to inferior vena cava. **A,** diagram showing common venous trunk entering inferior vena cava below diaphragm. **B,** inferior vena cava and pulmonary vein dissected. **C,** cannulation performed and vena cava partially occluded. **D,** pulmonary vein is clamped and divided. **E,** inferior vena cava is repaired. **F,** an incision is made in right atrial wall. **G,** right atrial wall is elevated and common pulmonary vein anastomosed to right atrium. **H,** foramen ovale is enlarged. **I,** a Dacron tunnel is created to direct right pulmonary venous blood into left atrium. **J,** pattern of flow after completion of repair.

is through a median sternotomy. With the heart and lungs bypassed, the apex of the heart is lifted upward, exposing the common venous trunk posteriorly (Fig. 59–6, *B*). The vertical vein is either temporarily occluded with a tape snare or ligated. This always should be done outside the pericardium and in the superior mediastinum to avoid compromising additional veins, which may be entering from the left lung.

After an incision is made in the long axis of the retrocardiac vein, an incision is made in the left atrium (Fig. 59–6, *C*). The anastomosis between these two structures then is completed using a continuous running technique with a 4-0 monofilament polypropylene suture (Fig. 59–6, *D*). A separate right atriotomy is made to expose the atrial septal defect. This may be closed with a running suture; or, if the left atrium appears to be compromised, by direct suture; a small patch of knitted Dacron fabric may be used (Fig. 59–6, *E*). After the atriotomy is closed, the repair is completed by ligating the vertical vein (Fig. 59–6, *F*).

We have seen several cases in which the common venous trunk drained into the right superior vena cava posteriorly.

No left vertical vein was present. In those instances, the repair was done in a similar manner, closing the caval communication by ligature or intracardiac patch and anastomosing the vein to the posterior wall of the left atrium.[20]

TAPVR, CARDIAC TYPE. — In this anomaly, the pulmonary veins from the right and left lungs empty directly into the posterior aspect of the right atrium. Repair is performed during temporary cardiopulmonary bypass after opening the right atrium in the standard manner to expose the septum and pulmonary venous orifices located posteriorly. The coronary sinus ostium is identified and separated from the pulmonary venous ostia. The remainder of the interatrial septum is excised. A patch of knitted Dacron fabric is used to cover the pulmonary orifices and divert the venous blood into the left atrium while closing the interatrial defect. The final results are shown in Figure 59–7, with blood from the pulmonary veins draining normally to the left atrium.

TAPVR, PARACARDIAC TYPE DRAINING INTO THE CORONARY SINUS. — Anatomically, this anomaly is very similar to the type in which the pulmonary venous drainage is directly

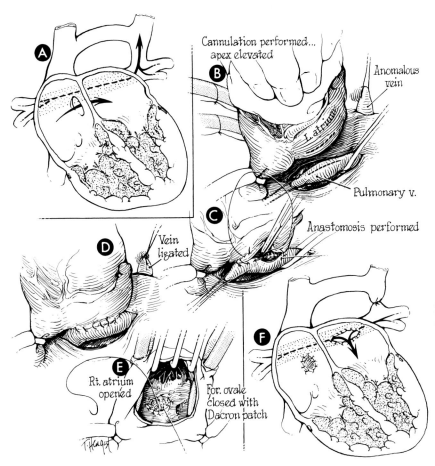

Fig. 59–6.—Total anomalous venous drainage, *supracardiac type* with vertical anomalous pulmonary vein ("persistent left superior vena cava"). **A,** pattern of venous connections. **B,** cannulation done, the ascending aorta clamped and the heart retracted anteriorly with gauze square or traction suture. Retrocardiac transverse pulmonary venous trunk is dissected and taped. Location of incision in left atrium and pulmonary vein indicated by dotted line. **C,** anastomosis performed. **D,** "persistent" left superior vena cava is ligated. **E,** right atrium is opened and foramen ovale is closed with a Dacron patch. **F,** pattern of flow after completion of repair.

into the right atrium (Fig. 59–7, *A*). Repair is nearly identical, with the exception that the coronary sinus is dilated and a membrane or partition representing the superior wall of the dilated coronary sinus exists (Fig. 59–7, *B*). This partition must be excised and the remaining intra-atrial septal tissue removed as described for the other paracardiac type (Fig. 59–7, *C*). The resulting defect is closed with a patch of knitted Dacron material diverting the pulmonary venous blood into the left atrium (Fig. 59–7, *D*). Usually individual coronary veins in the floor of the coronary sinus may be identified, and the patch is placed so that these veins enter the right atrium in a normal manner. On completion of repair, the pulmonary veins drain fully into the left atrium (Fig. 59–7, *E*).

TAPVR, INFRACARDIAC TYPE.—Repair of the infracardiac type of drainage is performed through a median sternotomy. With the patient on cardiopulmonary bypass, with or without hypothermia, the apex of the heart is elevated, exposing the retrocardiac vein, which runs in a vertical direction (Fig. 59–8, *B*). The common trunk is occluded at the diaphragm. A transverse incision is made in the posterior left atrium, and the anastomosis is performed using a continuous running suture of 4-0 or 5-0 monofilament polypropylene (Fig. 59–8, *C*). The descending vertical vein is ligated at the diaphragm (Fig. 59–8, *D*) and the foramen ovale is closed through a right atriotomy. At completion of the anastomosis, free flow of blood from the venous trunk into the left atrium is present (Fig. 59–8, *E*).

TAPVR, MIXED TYPE.—Since patients in this category have a variety of venous connections, no single technique is applicable. Often a vertical anomalous vein drains only the left lung or the left upper lobe. In this instance, side-to-side anastomosis to the left atrium or left atrial appendage is used. The right lung usually drains into the right atrium or the coronary sinus, and repair must be accomplished by the techniques already described for these anomalies. Because of the complicated nature of the anomaly in most patients in this group, successful complete anatomic repair is accomplished less frequently than in the other types.

Results of Operation

Between 1955 and November 30, 1976 at the Texas Heart Institute, 329 patients underwent operation for anomalous pulmonary venous return; 154 patients had correction of TAPVR and 175 patients had correction of partial anomalous pulmonary venous return (PAPVR). In patients with PAPVR, early death occurred in 12 (6.9%). Early death in all types of TAPVR occurred in 52 patients (33.8%). Analysis of these 154 patients operated on for TAPVR demonstrated that age at the time of the operative procedure significantly influenced mortality, which was highest in patients requiring operation during the first year of life (Table 59–1). Of 76 infants less than 1 year of age, 40 (53%) died. With increasing age, the mortality rate decreased significantly. Of 22 patients between the ages of 13 and 24 months, 4 (27%) died and of 41 patients between 2 and 10 years of age only 6 (15%) died. All 14 patients over 10 years of age survived. The oldest patient in the series was 55 years of age.

A total of 92 patients had the supracardiac type of anomaly (Table 59–2); in 80%, drainage was through an anomalous

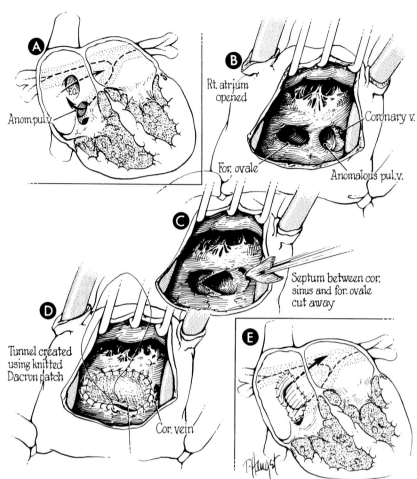

Fig. 59–7.—Total anomalous venous return, *cardiac type,* in which pulmonary veins drain into the coronary sinus. **A,** pattern of venous connection. **B,** right atrium is opened and the anomalous pulmonary vein visualized. **C,** the septum between the coronary sinus and foramen ovale is excised. **D,** a tunnel is created using a Dacron patch, preserving the entrance of the coronary vein into the right atrium. **E,** pattern of flow after repair is completed.

vertical vein connecting with the left innominate vein and in 20% was through a connection directly to the right superior vena cava. Among 41 patients with the cardiac type, direct drainage into the body of the right atrium occurred in 45% and drainage through the coronary sinus occurred in 55%. Mortality was 30% in the supracardiac type and 27% in the cardiac type. Of 11 patients with infracardiac defect, 7 (64%) died. Three patients had drainage into the inferior vena cava and all survived. Drainage was into the hepatic veins in 2 patients, both of whom died, and 6 patients had drainage into the portal vein, 5 of whom died.

Of the 10 patients with mixed venous drainage, 6 died, a mortality rate of 60% (Table 59–3). Drainage to the innominate veins and coronary sinus was observed in 4 patients, 2 of whom died. In a 40-year-old patient, all the pulmonary venous blood gained access to the systemic venous system through both the coronary sinus ostium into the right atrium and a vertical vein to the left innominate vein. Connections of the back of the right atrium and through a vertical anomalous vein were observed in 3 patients, 2 of whom died. One patient who had drainage into the right superior vena cava and inferior vena cava also died.

Among the 52 patients who died, pulmonary edema was the most common cause of death, occurring in 26 patients. Other causes were severe postoperative pulmonary hypertension (6 patients), sudden cardiac arrest (6), heart block (3), respiratory insufficiency (3), portal vein thrombosis (2), renal failure (2), cerebral edema (1) and a technical perfu-

sion problem in 1. An anomaly in which the right and left lung drained individually into the dorsal aspect of the right superior vena cava was observed in a 4-day-old infant who died a few hours after exploratory thoracotomy. Nonfatal complications included postoperative pneumonia (3 patients), heart block (3), postcardiotomy syndrome (2), atelectasis (2), pericardial effusion (1), pulmonary edema (1) and melena (1).

The influence of pulmonary venous return on the outcome of surgical treatment of patients with TAPVR remains a matter of debate. Keith and colleagues[42] pointed out that increased pulmonary venous return may be a limiting factor in the survival of patients with TAPVR. In contrast, McNamara and associates did not agree with this concept in an analysis of 35 patients.[28] In order to evaluate its influence on surgical mortality, the pulmonary venous return was obtained by plotting the ratio of pulmonary-to-systemic pressure in 91 patients whose complete physiologic data were available.[64] The 91 patients were divided into two groups by age: those older than 1 year and those less than 1 year. The distribution of patients older than 1 year who had a normal pulmonary venous return and those whose pulmonary venous return was greater than normal was almost equal (28 and 22 patients, respectively). The operative mortality in the group with increased pulmonary venous return exceeded that in the group with normal pulmonary venous return (27 and 11, respectively) (see Table 59–3). In patients less than 1 year of age, again it was apparent that the outcome was more suc-

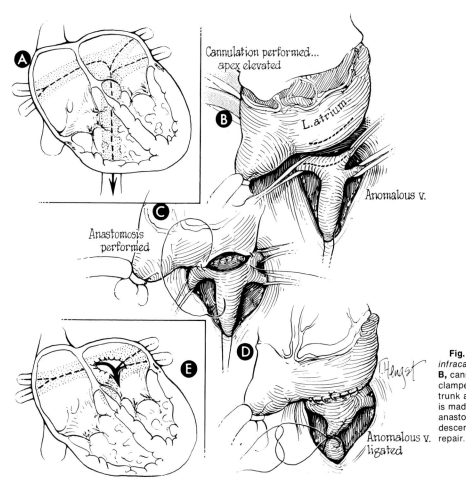

Fig. 59-8.—Total anomalous venous return, *infracardiac type.* **A,** pattern of venous connection. **B,** cannulation is performed, the ascending aorta clamped and the heart is elevated. The retrocardiac trunk and descending vein are dissected. An incision is made in the vein and left atrium (dotted lines). **C,** anastomosis is performed. **D,** the anomalous descending vein is ligated. **E,** pattern of flow after repair.

TABLE 59-1.—RELATIONSHIP OF AGE AND MORTALITY IN 154 PATIENTS UNDERGOING CORRECTION OF TAPVR

AGE GROUPS	NO. PATIENTS	NO. DEATHS	MORTALITY(%)
0-12 months	76	40	52.6
13-24 months	22	6	27.0
2-10 years	41	6	14.6
11-20 years	9	0	0.0
21 years or older	6	0	0.0
TOTAL	154	52	33.8

cessful if pulmonary venous return was not increased. Of 9 infants with normal pulmonary venous return, 4 (44%) died whereas of 32 infants with increased pulmonary venous return, 24 (75%) died after surgical intervention (see Table 59-3). In addition, it is noteworthy that 32 (78%) of 41 patients less than 1 year of age had increased pulmonary venous return.

The over-all mortality of 34% in our present series compares favorably with that of other large reported series, both for infants less than 1 year and over 1 year of age. Comparison of other collected series is shown in Table 59-4.

Debate continues regarding the theoretic advantages of utilizing profound hypothermia with circulatory arrest.[4, 6, 24, 29] Barratt-Boyes[5] has presented a well-documented report suggesting that profound hypothermia and circulatory arrest as used in a small series can result in a 70% survival rate in infants with TAPVR presenting in the first year of life, with little difference in the mortality rate of those operated

on during the first and second 6 months of life. However, a comparison of results from a collected group of a large number of patients reported from major centers using profound hypothermia and circulatory arrest with those utilizing conventional perfusion techniques demonstrates no significant difference in the results with either technique (Table 59-5). Therefore, at present, we concur with Malm[33] and prefer conventional perfusion techniques, with careful attention to cannulation and to maintenance of optimal flow rate and oxygenation.

TABLE 59-2.—INFLUENCE OF ANATOMIC TYPE OF TAPVR ON MORTALITY

TYPE	NO. PATIENTS	NO. DEATHS	MORTALITY (%)
Supracardiac	92	28	30
RSVC	(20)	(9)	(45)
Anomalous vertical vein	(72)	(19)	(26)
Cardiac	41	11	27
Body of right atrium	(18)	(4)	(22)
Coronary sinus	(23)	(7)	(30)
Infracardiac	11	7	63
IVC	(3)	(0)	(0)
Portal vein	(6)	(5)	(83)
Hepatic vein	(2)	(2)	(100)
Mixed	10	6	60
TOTAL	154	52	33

TABLE 59–3.—PULMONIC-TO-SYSTEMIC RESISTANCE RATIO AND
SURGICAL MORTALITY IN TAPVR

AGE	PULMONIC-TO-SYSTEMIC RESISTANCE RATIO	NO. PATIENTS	NO. DEATHS	SURGICAL MORTALITY(%)
More than 1 yr	>0.2	22	6	27
	<0.2	28	3	11
Less than 1 yr	>0.2	32	24	75
	<0.2	9	4	44
TOTAL		91	37	41

TABLE 59–4.—RESULTS OF SURGERY FOR TAPVR

AUTHOR	INSTITUTION	TOTAL NO. PATIENTS OPERATED ON	MORTALITY	PATIENTS BELOW AGE 1 YR	MORTALITY
Gomez et al.[34]	Mayo Clinic	59	10 (17%)	15	7 (47%)
Mustard et al.[47]	The Hospital for Sick Children, Toronto	71	45 (63%)	37	31 (84%)
Behrendt et al.[8]	The Hospital for Sick Children, London	56	33 (59%)	37	26 (70%)
Present series	Texas Heart Institute	154	52 (33.8%)	76	40 (53%)

TABLE 59–5.—COMPARISON OF SURGICAL RESULTS OF TAPVR REPAIR DURING FIRST
YEAR OF LIFE USING PROFOUND HYPOTHERMIA AND CIRCULATORY ARREST
WITH CONVENTIONAL PERFUSION TECHNIQUES

PROFOUND HYPOTHERMIA AND CIRCULATORY ARREST			CONVENTIONAL PERFUSION TECHNIQUES		
AUTHOR	TOTAL PATIENTS	DEATHS MORTALITY(%)	AUTHOR	TOTAL PATIENTS	DEATHS MORTALITY(%)
Subramanian et al.[59]	7	4 (57)	Wukasch et al.[64]	63	36 (57)
Clarke[14]	7	3 (43)	McGoon[34]	15	7 (47)
Cartmill et al.[13]	6	2 (33)	Behrendt et al.[8]	37	26 (70)
Kirklin[44]	4	1 (25)	Present series (1973–1976)	13	4 (31)
Barratt-Boyes[6]	9	2 (22)			
Mustard et al.[48]	25	13 (52)			

REFERENCES

1. Auer, J.: The development of the human pulmonary vein and its major variations, Anat. Rec. 101:581, 1948.
2. Bahnson, H. T., Spencer, F. C., and Neill, C. A.: Surgical treatment of 35 cases of drainage of pulmonary veins to the right side of the heart, J. Thorac. Surg. 36:777, 1958.
3. Bailey, C. P., et al.: Surgical treatment of 46 interatrial septal defects by atrioseptopexy, Ann. Surg. 140:805, 1954.
4. Bailey, L. L., et al.: Surgical management of congenital cardiovascular anomalies with the use of profound hypothermia and circulatory arrest: Analysis of 180 consecutive cases, J. Thorac. Cardiovasc. Surg. 71:485, 1976.
5. Barratt-Boyes, B. G.: Primary Definitive Intracardiac Operations in Infants: Total Anomalous Pulmonary Venous Connection, in Kirklin, J. W. (ed.), *Advances in Cardiovascular Surgery* (New York: Grune & Stratton, 1973), pp. 127–139.
6. Barratt-Boyes, B. G., Neutze, J. M., and Harris, E. A. (eds.), *Heart Disease in Infancy. Diagnosis and Surgical Treatment* (London: Churchill Livingstone, 1973).
7. Barratt-Boyes, B. G., Simpson, M., and Neutze, J. M.: Intracardiac surgery in neonates and infants using deep hypothermia with surface cooling and limited cardiopulmonary bypass, Circulation 43–44(Supp.):25, 1971.
8. Behrendt, D. M., et al.: Total anomalous pulmonary venous drainage in infants, Circulation 46:347, 1972.
9. Brantigan, O. C.: Anomalies of the pulmonary veins, Surg. Gynecol. Obstet. 84:63, 1947.
10. Brody, H.: Drainage of the pulmonary veins into the right side of the heart, Arch. Pathol. 33:221, 1942.
11. Burroughs, J. T., and Edwards, J. E.: Total anomalous pulmonary venous connection, Am. Heart J. 59:913, 1960.
12. Burroughs, J. T., and Kirklin, J. W.: Complete surgical correction of total anomalous pulmonary venous connection: Report of 3 cases, Proc. Staff Meet. Mayo Clin. 31:182, 1956.
13. Cartmill, T. B., Overton, J. H., and Celermajer, J. M.: Deep Hypothermia and Perfusion in Infancy, in Barratt-Boyes, B. G., Neutze, J. M., and Harris, E. A. (eds.), *Heart Disease in Infancy. Diagnosis and Surgical Treatment* (London: Churchill Livingstone, 1973), p. 45.
14. Clarke, C. P.: Discussion, in Barratt-Boyes, B. G., Neutze, J. M., and Harris, E. A. (eds.), *Heart Disease in Infancy. Diagnosis and Surgical Treatment* (London: Churchill Livingstone, 1973), p. 64.
15. Cooley, D. A., and Collins, H. A.: Anomalous drainage of entire pulmonary venous system into left innominate vein: Clinical and surgical considerations, Circulation 19:486, 1959.
16. Cooley, D. A., Ellis, P. R., Jr., and Bellizzi, M. D.: Atrial septal defects of the sinus venosus type: Surgical considerations, Dis. Chest 39:185, 1961.
17. Cooley, D. A., and Hallman, G. L.: Criteria for recommending surgery in total anomalous pulmonary venous drainage, Am. J. Cardiol. 12:98, 1963.
18. Cooley, D. A., Hallman, G. L., and Leachman, R. D.: Total anomalous pulmonary venous drainage: Correction with the use of cardiopulmonary bypass in 62 cases, J. Thorac. Cardiovasc. Surg. 51:88, 1966.
19. Cooley, D. A., and Mahaffey, D. E.: Anomalous pulmonary venous drainage of entire left lung: Report of case with surgical correction, Ann. Surg. 142:986, 1955.

20. Cooley, D. A., and Norman, J. C.: *Techniques in Cardiac Surgery* (Houston: Texas Medical Press, 1975), p. 119.
21. Cooley, D. A., and Ochsner, A., Jr.: Correction of total anomalous pulmonary venous drainage, Surgery 42:1014, 1957.
22. Darling, R. C., Rothney, W. B., and Craig, J. M.: Total pulmonary venous drainage into the right side of the heart: Report of 17 autopsied cases not associated with other major cardiovascular anomalies, Lab. Invest. 6:44, 1957.
23. Dean, J. C., and Fox, G. W.: A left pulmonary vein emptying into the left innominate, Wis. Med. J. 27:120, 1928.
24. Dillard, D. H., *et al.*: Correction of total anomalous pulmonary venous drainage in infancy utilizing deep hypothermia with total circulatory arrest, Circulation 35–36(Supp. 1):105, 1967.
25. Dotter, C. T., Hardisty, N. M., and Steinberg, I.: Anomalous right pulmonary vein entering the inferior vena cava: 2 cases diagnosed during life by angiocardiography and cardiac catheterization, Am. J. Med. Sci. 218:31, 1949.
26. Edwards, J. E.: Pathologic and developmental considerations in anomalous pulmonary venous connections, Proc. Staff Meet. Mayo Clin. 28:441, 1953.
27. Elliott, L. P., and Edwards, J. E.: The problem of pulmonary venous obstruction in total anomalous pulmonary venous connection to the left innominate vein, Circulation 25:913, 1962.
28. El-Said, G., Mullins, C. E., and McNamara, D. G.: Management of total anomalous pulmonary venous return, Circulation 45:1240, 1972.
29. Engle, M. A.: Total anomalous pulmonary venous drainage: Success story at last, Circulation 46:209, 1972.
30. Friedlowsky: Cited by Brody.[10]
31. Gathman, G. E., and Nadas, A. S.: Total anomalous pulmonary venous connection, Circulation 42:143, 1970.
32. Gerbode, F. L.: In discussion of Scannell, J. G., and Shaw, R. S.: Surgical reconstruction of the superior vena cava, J. Thorac. Surg. 28:163, 1954.
33. Gersony, W. M., *et al.*: Management of total anomalous pulmonary venous drainage in early infancy, Circulation 43–44(Supp. 1):19, 1971.
34. Gomez, M. M., *et al.*: Total anomalous pulmonary venous connection: Surgical considerations and result of operations, J. Thorac. Cardiovasc. Surg. 59:748, 1970.
35. Gott, V. L., Lester, R. G., Lillehei, C. W., and Varco, R. L.: Total anomalous pulmonary venous return: An analysis of 30 cases, Circulation 13:543, 1956.
36. Guntheroth, W. G., Nadas, A. S., and Gross, R. E.: Transposition of the pulmonary veins, Circulation 18:117, 1958.
37. Hallman, G. L., and Cooley, D. A. (eds.): Total Anomalous Pulmonary Venous Return, in *Surgical Treatment of Congenital Heart Disease* (Philadelphia: Lea & Febiger, 1975), p. 133.
38. Hastreiter, A. R., *et al.*: Total anomalous pulmonary venous connection with severe pulmonary venous obstruction. A clinical entity, Circulation 25:916, 1962.
39. Healey, J. E., Jr.: An anatomic survey of anomalous pulmonary veins: Their clinical significance, J. Thorac. Surg. 23:433, 1952.
40. Hughes, C. W., and Rumore, P. C.: Anomalous pulmonary veins, Arch. Pathol. 37:364, 1944.
41. Keith, J. D., *et al.*: Complete anomalous pulmonary venous drainage, Am. J. Med. 16:23, 1954.
42. Keith, J. D., Rowe, R. D., and Vlad, P.: *Heart Disease in Infancy and Childhood* (New York: The Macmillan Company, 1958), p. 341.
43. Kirklin, J. W.: Surgical treatment of anomalous pulmonary venous connection, Proc. Staff Meet. Mayo Clin. 28:476, 1953.
44. Kirklin, J. W.: Surgical Treatment of Total Anomalous Pulmonary Venous Return in Infancy, in Barratt-Boyes, B. G., Neutze, J. M., and Harris, E. A. (eds.), *Heart Disease in Infancy, Diagnosis and Surgical Treatment* (London: Churchill Livingstone, 1973), p. 89.
45. Kirklin, J. W., Ellis, F. H., and Wood, E. H.: Treatment of anomalous pulmonary venous connections in association with interatrial communications, Surgery 39:389, 1956.
46. Muller, W. H., Jr.: The surgical treatment of transposition of the pulmonary veins, Ann. Surg. 134:683, 1951.
47. Mustard, W. T., Keith, J. D., and Trusler, G. A.: Two stage correction for total anomalous pulmonary venous drainage in childhood, J. Thorac. Cardiovasc. Surg. 44:477, 1962.
48. Mustard, W. T., Keon, W. J., and Trusler, G. A.: Transposition of great arteries and transposition of lesser veins, Prog. Cardiovasc. Dis. 11:145, 1968.
49. Neptune, W. B., Bailey, C. P., and Goldberg, H.: Surgical correction of atrial septal defects associated with transposition of pulmonary veins, J. Thorac. Surg. 25:623, 1953.
50. Paquet, M., and Gutgesell, H.: Echocardiographic features of total anomalous pulmonary venous connection, Circulation 51:599, 1975.
51. Ross, D. N.: Atrial septal defect: Surgical anatomy and technique, Guy's Hosp. Rep. 105:376, 1956.
52. Rudolph, A. M. (ed.): Total Anomalous Pulmonary Venous Drainage, in *Congenital Diseases of the Heart* (Chicago: Year Book Medical Publishers, Inc., 1974), p. 581.
53. Sasse, L.: Letter: Echo recordings in TAPVC, Circulation 52:527, 1975.
54. Sasse, L., Bozio, A., and Davignon, A.: Letter: Interpreting the echocardiogram in TAPVC, Circulation 53:1041, 1976.
55. Senning, A.: Complete correction of total anomalous pulmonary venous return, Ann. Surg. 148:99, 1958.
56. Serrato, M., Bucheleres, H. G., and Bicoff, P.: Palliative balloon atriostomy for total anomalous pulmonary venous connection in infancy, J. Pediatr. 73:734, 1968.
57. Silove, E. D., *et al.*: Total anomalous pulmonary venous drainage. II. Spontaneous functional closure of interatrial communication after surgical correction in infancy, Circulation 46:351, 1972.
58. Snellen, H. A., and Albers, F. H.: The clinical significance of anomalous pulmonary venous drainage, Circulation 6:6, 1952.
59. Subramanian, S., *et al.*: Experiences with Deep Hypothermia in Infancy using Surface Cooling, in Barratt-Boyes, B. G., Neutze, J. M., and Harris, E. A. (eds.), *Heart Disease in Infancy. Diagnosis and Surgical Treatment* (London: Churchill Livingstone, 1973), p. 37.
60. Taussig, H.: *Congenital Malformations of the Heart* (New York: The Commonwealth Fund, 1947).
61. Wagstaffe, W. W.: Two cases of free communication between the auricle by deficiency of the upper part of the septum auricularum, Trans. Pathol. Soc. Lond. 19:96, 1868.
62. Wilson, J.: A description of a very unusual formation of the human heart, Philos. Trans. R. Soc. Lond. Pt. 1, 88:346, 1798.
63. Winslow: Cited by Brody.[10]
64. Wukasch, D. C., *et al.*: Total anomalous pulmonary venous return: Review of 125 patients treated surgically, Ann. Thorac. Surg. 19:622, 1975.

Transposition of the Great Arteries (Ventriculo-Arterial Discordance)

Natural History

Transposition of the great arteries is one of the most frequently occurring forms of severe congenital heart disease. Earlier studies clearly underestimated both the incidence of congenital heart disease and the proportion of these patients who had transposition. It now is apparent that about 1% of live-born infants have congenital heart disease. The reports of the New England Regional Infant Cardiac Program[131] showed that 10.8% of 1564 infants studied with congenital heart disease had TGA. Transposition is the most common form of fatal cyanotic heart disease in the first year of life. The majority of the children are males, as with most other forms of congenital heart disease, and in TGA the ratio is about 2 males to 1 female.[103] Birth weights are in the normal range or slightly higher than normal.[159]

Severe cyanosis is present from birth and the hypoxia threatens survival from the day of birth. In the short term, a large communication between the pulmonary and systemic circulations is beneficial because it allows better mixing of the two circulations. In general, about half the hearts described have had an intact ventricular septum and have owed their initial survival to an atrial septal defect or a patent foramen ovale. About a quarter of the patients have had a ventricular septal defect as an additional lesion, and in about another eighth of cases left ventricular outflow tract obstruction (LVOTO) has been present either with or without a ventricular septal defect. Slightly less than an eighth of the patients described have had more complex additional lesions together with transposition of the great arteries. Patent ductus arteriosus has been recognized in about half of the cases studied[103]; however, the proportion has varied in other series.[159]

Development of the Operative Treatment

Transposition of the great arteries is the grossest derangement of the connections of the heart occurring in congenital heart disease, and yet the heart has four good chambers and four good valves. Inevitably, surgeons have been looking for the operative key to this most provoking challenge. Despite the progress in the past quarter century, we have yet to reach our only acceptable goal—to be able to offer almost all of the children born with this anomaly the prospect of a normal existence for a normal life span. Survival without operation is possible only if additional anomalies allow mixing of the pulmonary and systemic circulations, and even then survival usually is short.

Matthew Baillie[14] gave the first precise description of the abnormal anatomy of transposition in 1797. Effective palliative treatment first began at Johns Hopkins. Hanlon and Blalock's description of a method of creating an atrial septal defect in 1948 [70] was followed by their application of it to the human in 1950.[21]

The principle of rearrangement of venous flow within the atria was introduced by Albert[4] in 1955. This brilliant contribution was the forerunner of a number of different methods of rerouting the atrial flow paths.[37, 39, 120] The first successful corrective operation on a human was by Senning in 1958,[84] who redirected the venous return within the atria by an ingenious technique that made the atria into inner and outer tubes by repositioning the atrial septum and the atrial walls. Kirklin,[91] using the Senning operation, reported in 1961 a series of 11 cases. Many of the anomalies were complex, and 7 patients died. It is only with later experience that one can look back at this series and recognize that it was a superb achievement in a group of cases that even now would be mostly regarded as high risk. Occasional reports of a single successful application of the Senning operation appeared in the next few years.

When Mustard,[127] in 1964, published his method of redirecting the venous flow within the atria using pericardium for the partition, the prospect for children with transposition of the great arteries seemed suddenly transformed and, as this technique was adopted around the world, successful physiologic corrections of transposition were reported in increasing numbers.[3, 33, 68, 202] Its successful application to younger children led to the routine application in the first year of life beginning in 1967.[1]

The success of the intra-atrial operation was followed by the development at the Mayo Clinic[145, 146] of a technique, the Rastelli operation, that connected the left ventricle to the aorta by a patch placed in the upper portion of the right ventricle, so that the ventricular septal defect was connected to the aortic ring and thus directed the output of the left ventricle to the aorta, while the output of the right ventricle was conducted to the pulmonary artery by an external conduit that contained a semilunar valve.

The complete correction of transposed great arteries by rearrangement of the flow within the ventricles was first reported by McGoon[118] in 1972. A very large ventricular septal defect was found so placed as to allow the left ventricle to be connected to the aorta by a patch that funneled the LV contents from the VSD to the aortic root yet allowed the RV contents to be ejected directly into the pulmonary valve and artery, thus restoring the normal relationships of ventricles to great arteries for the first time in complete TGA.

Lindesmith et al.[106] introduced the concept of a "palliative" Mustard operation for patients with TGA + VSD + PVOD in 1972. They performed the Mustard operation without closing the ventricular septal defect, so that the septal defect could act as a vent should pulmonary vascular resistance suddenly increase. The same concept has been applied to patients with transposition of the great arteries with an intact ventricular septum and severe pulmonary vascular obstructive disease, by creating a ventricular septal defect in the apical part of the interventricular septum in addition to the Mustard operation.[176]

In patients with severe LVOTO and an intact interventricular septum, either the Mustard operation with a left ventricle to pulmonary artery conduit can be used[171] or the principle of biventricular conduits is applicable.[119]

The long-sought goal of arterial correction of TGA was achieved in São Paulo in 1975 by Jatene et al.[82, 83] A modified Baffes procedure[12] was successfully used in a 40-day-old infant with TGA + VSD. Several additional successes have been reported,[95, 112, 116, 153, 207] but it seems that the overall mortality rate of this operation is high (about 70%) at present.

An alternative technique for arterial correction has been described independently by Damus,[41] by Kaye[86] and by Stansel.[174] The pulmonary artery is transected proximal to the bifurcation and the proximal pulmonary artery is anastomosed to the ascending aorta end to side. The right ventricle then is connected to the distal pulmonary artery with a valved conduit, an operation not well suited to the small infant.

Definition and Classification

The heart of a child with a typical transposition of the great arteries is simple to describe, but categorizing the variants of transpositions has proved to be very difficult and, so far, no generally accepted classification has emerged, despite much discussion and debate.

A desirable classification uses terms that describe congenital heart disease accurately and without ambiguity. The terms should be as valid for use at operation or autopsy as during diagnostic investigations. A classification based on morphogenetic concepts is speculative, and each time a new morphogenetic theory is accepted, changes in nomenclature would be required, which is undesirable. The classification should be suitable for modern medical recording purposes and it is helpful if it is easy to remember.

The nomenclature proposed by a European group in 1977[190] approaches these desirable criteria. Their nomenclature is based on the connection of cardiac segments to reflect the route of the circulation, and that is fundamental to the abnormal physiology of congenital heart disease. The following steps are required in this descriptive classification.

1. Define the atrial situs (solitus, inversus, ambiguus).
2. State the type of atrioventricular connection (concordant, discordant, ambiguus, double inlet, absence of right or left atrioventricular connection).
3. State the mode of atrioventricular connection, i.e., one or two patent atrioventricular valves, etc.
4. State the ventriculo-arterial connections (concordant, discordant, double outlet of ventricle, single outlet of the heart).
5. State the anatomic relationship of the great arteries, e.g., the aortic valve ring anterior or anterior to the right, etc., of the pulmonary valve ring.
6. List all additional anomalies.
7. Describe any abnormal morphology, e.g., primitive ventricle etc.

Chamber Definition

Before defining the connections, the heart segments must be defined. Definition of the atrial chambers is generally accepted.[45, 100, 165, 195]

Definition of the ventricular chambers is more difficult. Tynan et al.[190] suggest that a chamber possessing an inlet portion and a trabecular portion be described as a ventricle whereas chambers that do not possess inlet portions are described as rudimentary chambers, of left or right ventricular type, depending on the nature of their

trabecular portions. Two variants of rudimentary chamber are recognized—outlet chambers possess both trabecular and outlet portions whereas trabeculated pouches have only the trabeculated portion. If either or both the inlet or outlet components straddle or override the septum that separates the trabeculated portions, the overriding valve is assigned to the ventricle supporting more than half of its circumference. This concept, suggested by Kirklin[90] in 1973 for the classification of arterial valves, can readily be applied to an atrioventricular valve as well. A chamber receiving less than half of an atrioventricular valve is termed a rudimentary chamber, not a ventricle.

Connection of the Cardiac Chambers

ATRIAL SITUS.—Three possibilities exist—solitus, inversus and ambiguus.[194] Atrial situs reflects visceral situs almost without exception, provided that the visceral situs is clearly solitus or inversus, so the visceral situs (readily determined from a plain x-ray) establishes the atrial situs. In doubtful situations such as situs ambiguus (visceral heterotaxia), the bronchial anatomy is the most reliable guide to the atrial situs.[141]

ATRIOVENTRICULAR CONNECTION (THE CHAMBERS ARE REFERRED TO AS MORPHOLOGICALLY LEFT OR RIGHT, NOT ANATOMICALLY LEFT OR RIGHT).—A concordant connection is present when the right atrium connects to the right ventricle and the left atrium connects to the left ventricle. In a discordant connection, conversely, the left atrium connects to the right ventricle and the right atrium to the left ventricle. If the two atria cannot be differentiated one from the other, the term "ambiguus" is used for the connection with the ventricles. When both atria do not connect directly with separate chambers in the ventricular mass, double inlet ventricle or absence of the right or left atrioventricular connection is present. Distinguishing between the mitral and tricuspid valves sometimes is difficult, so the nonspecific term "left" and "right" atrioventricular valve is preferred.[11]

VENTRICULO-ARTERIAL CONNECTIONS.—Ventricles connect to the arteries in one of four ways. In concordant connection, the aorta arises from the left ventricle or an outlet chamber of the left ventricular type and the pulmonary artery arises from the right ventricle or an outlet chamber of the right ventricular type. Discordant connection exists when the aorta arises from the right ventricle or an outlet chamber of the right ventricular type and the pulmonary artery from the left ventricle or an outlet chamber of the left ventricular type. Thus, discordant ventriculo-arterial connection is an alternative description for complete transposition of the great arteries. As already mentioned, the 50% rule for the aortic and pulmonary valve overriding applies here.[90]

A double outlet ventricle or chamber exists when one, and more than half of the other, aortic valve and pulmonic valve arise from one ventricle or chamber. In a single outlet heart, the chambers in the ventricular mass possess only one patent outlet (aorta, pulmonary artery or persistent truncus arteriosus).

ANATOMIC RELATIONS.—A description of the anatomic relations of the cardiac structures, one to another, is important for planning and performing operations. Relations in both the frontal and sagittal planes must be described. The position of the heart within the thorax is described as apex to the left, to the right or a centrally placed heart. The relationship of the ventricles or rudimentary chambers and the great arteries is described, one to the other, within this frame of reference.

ADDITIONAL CARDIAC ANOMALIES.—These are described in as much detail as the investigation defines. They include stenosis or incompetence of valves, septal defects, anomalies of venous return, etc.

This nomenclature avoids using terms such as D- or L-transposition, malposition of the great arteries, etc. Classic or complete transposition of the great arteries is described as solitus, atrioventricular concordance, ventriculo-arterial discordance, and the relationship of the aortic valve to the pulmonic valve is specified, e.g., aorta anterior or aorta anterior and to the right, etc. Eight positions give sufficient accuracy to describe the aortic-pulmonic valve relationship—aorta posterior (i.e., posterior to the pulmonic valve), posterior to the left, to the left, anterior to the left, anterior, anterior to the right, to the right and posterior to the right (of the pulmonic valve). In situs inversus, typical transposition is described as inversus, concordant, discordant. "Congenitally corrected transposition" is termed solitus, discordant, discordant or, in the mirror image, inversus, discordant, discordant. Relationship of the ventricles, one to the other, then is added; for example, right ventricle to the left or right of, and superior or inferior to, the left ventricle.

The Abnormal Physiology of Transposed Great Arteries

Transposition of the great arteries results in a pattern of circulation that will not permit survival unless there are some additional anomalies. The normal circulation consists of a pulmonary and a systemic circulation, which are linked in series to make one continuous flow path, and the volume flowing through one circuit must be identical to the volume flowing through the other circuit because each is the source of blood for the other. In TGA, however, the circuits are completely separate and independent. Not only are they not in series, they are not even in parallel [104] (Fig. 60–1).

Each circuit, therefore, can flow quite independently of the other. The pulmonary circuit, with a low resistance and a powerful pump, has a rapid rate of circulation; the systemic circulation, with a higher resistance, has a slower circulation. Output on the pulmonary side has been shown to be 3 times or more greater than on the systemic side.

The complete separation of the circulations has one result that is not always recognized; there can be no *unidirectional flow*, from one circulation to the other, for more than a very brief period. In the normal heart, because the circulations are in series, there can be a preferential shunt from left to right or from right to left, and the circulations *must* adjust to this alteration. With transposition, however, a *one-way shunt* necessarily would empty one circulation into the other if continued for more than a brief period. The communication between the pulmonary and systemic circulations, necessary to allow life to continue, is at atrial level in most cases. To-and-fro flow, from left to right at the beginning of the cardiac cycle and then right to left, was demonstrated by Jonson *et al.*[84] in 1959 and by Carr (quoted by Lev *et al.*[102]).

We prefer to describe this to-and-fro flow as "mixing" and to reserve the use of the word "shunt" to indicate a unidirectional flow. As explained, this cannot occur in TGA, but must be balanced by an equal and opposite flow at that site or elsewhere in the two circulations.

The increase of flow through the pulmonary circulation

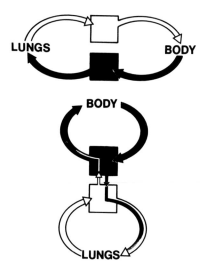

Fig. 60–1. — The relationship of the systemic and pulmonary circulations. The normal circulations *(top)* are in series. In ventriculo-arterial discordance (TGA) *(bottom)*, the circulations are not in series, not even in parallel. They are completely separate, hence the importance of interatrial communication.

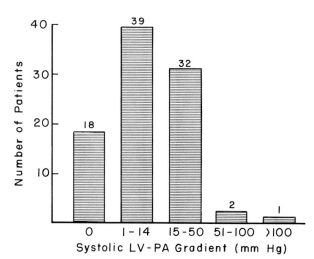

Fig. 60–2. — The pressure gradient measured between the left ventricle and the pulmonary artery in 92 patients with simple TGA (Hospital for Sick Children, Great Ormond Street, London).

can produce changes in pressure that may be mistakenly thought to indicate pulmonary stenosis. The anatomy of the left ventricular outflow tract does become changed in transposition, and gradients of over 70 torr may be measured in the left ventricular outflow tract. Yet, the obstructive element must be slight if the pulmonary flow is about 3 times faster than the systemic (Fig. 60–2).

Rarely, a transposition may present with a slower flow in the pulmonary circuit, which may mask a significant obstruction. If the pulmonary circulation is only half the output of the systemic, the pulmonary artery pressure may be deceivingly low, and an increased pulmonary vascular resistance may not be recognized. Flows in the systemic and pulmonary circulations must be known before the significance of difference between pressures can be accurately assessed. Direct measurement of flows now is recognized as more accurate than simple calculation of resistance ratios.[108]

The combination of transposed great arteries and a large ventricular septal defect presents another interesting variation in physiology. The pressures in the two circulations may reach equilibrium but a unidirectional shunt is not possible in TGA. The VSD allows the two ventricles to balance their pressures and so moves the left ventricular output more to the right on the Frank-Starling curve as the filling pressure increases, and thus increases stroke volume.[62] In this way, the pulmonary circulation is increased by a ventricular septal defect that does not act as a unidirectional shunt.

Another rare variation of this abnormal physiology is found in a few infants who have a large atrial septal defect but present with a low systemic arterial saturation of less than 30%. This indicates that there must be poor mixing across the atrial septal defect. Presumably this results when the compliance in each ventricle is so similar that there is little difference in atrial pressures, especially in the diastolic phase of the cardiac cycle, and thus there is little physical reason for mixing to occur in the atria, whatever the size of the atrial defect.

An additional reason for desaturation in some infants with TGA may be a difference in flow between the left and the right lungs. A flow through the left lung of only about one-third of the flow through the right lung has been demonstrated by Muster *et al.*[129] and by Vidne *et al.*[197]

Symptoms and Signs

Transposition has no diagnostic clinical symptoms or signs. The cyanosis occurring in all these infants usually is observed in the day or two after birth, and most babies have heart failure by the end of the second week of life. Respiratory infections are common. Cyanotic spells may occur, usually in infants with left ventricular outflow tract obstruction.

Physical examination may show tachypnea, dyspnea and tachycardia in a severely cyanosed infant with a very large liver. Auscultation may not demonstrate any murmur, although the second heart sound is loud and often single because the aortic valve is anterior. If an associated anomaly is present, the murmur from that lesion may be dominant. Cyanosis usually is severe and the arterial saturation in the range of 50–60%. In one series, it ranged from 12% to 82%.[135] Hemoglobin levels and hematocrits usually are raised, varying with the age and the degree of palliation provided by the additional defects.

Spontaneous closure of both VSD and PDA has been well shown.[142] Sudden deterioration in infants having spontaneous closure of a large ductus in the first 3 weeks of life has been described by Waldman *et al.*[203]

Complications

HEART FAILURE, HYPOXIA AND ACIDEMIA. – Blood pH is close to normal in children with transposition who do not have heart failure, but heart failure is associated with acidemia[161] and the arterial oxygen may fall to 20 torr or even as low as 10 torr in infants with TGA and heart failure.

PULMONARY VASCULAR OBSTRUCTIVE DISEASE (PVOD). – Obstructive change in the lung arterioles is a major problem for those surviving with TGA and becomes a special problem if a large VSD is present. With TGA and a large VSD, almost every factor known to cause PVOD is combined in one patient – pulmonary arterial flow is high, pulmonary arterial pressure is high, pulmonary arterial oxygen saturation is high,[36] the hematocrit is high and the systemic arterial oxygen saturation is low.[130] Inevitably, an infant with this combination of changes will develop severe pulmonary vascular disease during the first year of life.

Ferencz[57] and Wagenvoort *et al.*[201] emphasized the very high incidence of PVOD in patients with transposition and VSD. The protective effect of true pulmonary valve stenosis (rare) was recognized. Studies from the Mayo Clinic[200] and from Children's Memorial Hospital in Chicago[134] confirmed the high incidence of severe PVOD in the first year of life. Studies from the Hospital for Sick Children, Great Ormond Street, London[180] demonstrated not only the high incidence of pulmonary vascular disease in children with TGA and VSD who had survived beyond the first year of life but also demonstrated that the pulmonary resistance was not reduced to acceptable levels by pulmonary artery banding performed after the first year of life whereas pulmonary artery banding performed earlier – in the first year – subsequently was associated with a near to normal pulmonary resistance.

The studies by Clarkson *et al.*[35] of the hearts of 35 children dying with TGA showed that 15–20% had developed evidence of severe PVOD by 3–11 months of age even when the ventricular septum was intact and the ductus was closed. Lakier *et al.*[98] found that 5 of 29 patients with TGA and intact ventricular septum had developed increased pulmonary vascular resistance (3.6–12.9 units) between 7 and 30 months of age.

PULMONARY OUTFLOW TRACT OBSTRUCTION. – The response of the left ventricular outflow tract perhaps is the least well understood feature of transposition. Since only 1 case of supravalvar pulmonary artery stenosis has been described,[73] it is reasonable to describe pulmonary outflow tract obstruction by the more anatomically precise term of left ventricular outflow tract obstruction (LVOTO). Apart from the change in shape of the heart that occurs as the right ventricle becomes the dominant, systemic ventricle and occupies a greater portion of the outflow area, a variety of types of obstruction afflict the left ventricular outflow tract. These are:

1. Subvalvar pulmonary stenosis of the LV outflow tract.
   a) Fibrous tunnel between VSD and pulmonary ring.[162]
   b) Fibrous diaphragm.[162]
   c) Hypertrophied septum.[191]
   d) Abnormal systolic anterior movement of anterior mitral leaflet.[133]
   e) Abnormal insertion of mitral valve anterior leaflet, chordae or papillary muscles.[152, 168]
   f) Accessory fibrous tissue associated with mitral valve.[166]
   g) Aneurysm of membranous ventricular septum or tricuspid tissue, with or without VSD.[148, 199]
2. Valvar pulmonic stenosis and/or hypoplasia of the pulmonary valve ring.

Subvalvar stenosis often may occur without valvar stenosis, and has been observed to develop during infancy.[191] The different types of outflow stenosis should be recognized before operation because their operative management varies. The cylindrical fibrous tunnel of that portion of the LV outflow tract immediately below the pulmonary valve is relatively long, usually 1 cm or more in length, and may or may not be associated with a VSD, which, if present, usually is of moderate or large size. The left circumflex coronary artery often lies anterior to the LV outflow tract in this region.[164]

Subvalvar obstructions from hypertrophy of the septum and from accessory tissue associated with the mitral valve would seem to be acquired lesions, like the narrowing of the LV outflow tract caused by muscular hypertrophy of the septum (presumably the result of the right ventricle becoming the systemic ventricle). This narrowed outflow tract may be readily obstructed by further additions, such as insertion of the anterolateral papillary muscle or the mitral valve anteriorly.[133] Functional obstruction of the left ventricular outflow tract can be suspected from pressure measurements or from angiocardiographic appearances or from inspection of the heart, but dynamic measurements of flow are required to confirm finally that the lesion is acting as an effective obstruction; otherwise, the wrong operation may be performed, with serious consequences.

The relative frequency with which the different forms of LVOTO occur still is being assessed. Some of the earlier studies made from autopsy material overemphasize the effect of valvar obstruction.[164] Three more recent studies, made by diagnostic investigations during life or from a review of hearts in an autopsy collection but assessed in the light of recent hemodynamic experience, are shown in Table 60–1. The London and Buffalo analyses were based on diagnostic studies and that from Minneapolis on an autopsy collection. The relative infrequency of pulmonary valve stenosis is seen.

TABLE 60-1.—MAIN CAUSE OF LVOTO (16 PATIENTS AT GREAT ORMOND STREET, LONDON AND 2 SERIES PREVIOUSLY REPORTED)

	LONDON, GREAT ORMOND STREET	MINNEAPOLIS, SHRIVASTAVA et al.[166]	BUFFALO, CHIARIELLO et al.[30]
Subpulmonary fibrous membrane or shelf	6	9 (+5)	
Anomalous attachment of mitral valve	6	5 (+2)	
Accessory tissue of mitral valve		1 (+4)	
Fibromuscular tunnel	3		17
Aneurysm, membranous septum or tricuspid valve tissue	2	2 (+3)	3
Pulmonary valve stenosis	1	1 (+2)	3
Acquired pulmonary valve atresia	1		
TOTAL	19	18	23

Numbers in parentheses in the Minneapolis series are lesions that occurred in combination with each other.

Acquired obstruction of the LV outflow tract seems to occur very rarely after the Mustard operation. Possibly the lower flow and lower blood hematocrit after operation are both significant. Muster et al.[128] studied 50 children after the Mustard operation and found no case with progression of LV outflow tract stenosis.

An aneurysm of a membranous portion of the ventricular septum, either with or without a VSD, may balloon into the pulmonary outflow tract, and Vidne et al.[199] reported 8 cases.

Diagnostic Techniques

Chest Roentgenogram

Overfilled lung fields, an enlarged heart and a narrow vascular pedicle may be very suggestive of TGA on the plain AP roentgenogram. The appearance has been likened to "an egg on its side." The heart usually is not enlarged in the first days of life. The wide variety of roentgenographic findings in transposition has been emphasized by Noonan et al.[135]

Electrocardiogram

TGA does not give a diagnostic ECG. RVH is the principal change if the communication between the two circulations is primarily at atrial level, and biventricular hypertrophy in patients with a significant VSD or PDA.

Echocardiogram

Dillon et al.[48] demonstrated superimposition of the great arteries without an intervening crista in all patients with TGA and nearly all gave a simultaneous recording of echoes from the semilunar valves. Such findings were not observed in other forms of congenital heart disease. Echocardiography has also given useful diagnostic information about subpulmonic obstruction[133] and aneurysm of the membranous septum.[158]

Cardiac Catheterization and Angiocardiography

Any infant with central cyanosis should be referred for investigation to a center where efficient angiocardiography is done, to establish the diagnosis of transposition and to exclude severe additional lesions. Investigation expeditious enough to avoid causing deterioration in the patient allows the Rashkind[144] balloon atrial septostomy to be performed as soon as possible.

Mair et al.[110] emphasized the variability of Rp/Rs ratios and preferred to calculate pulmonary and systemic flows separately so that they then could calculate the "effective pulmonary flow" from the formula:

Effective pulmonary flow =
$$\frac{\text{Oxygen consumption}}{\text{Pulmonary venous } O_2 \text{ content} - \text{systemic venous } O_2 \text{ content}}$$

They also suggested that pulmonary vascular resistance was best determined by the difference in the oxygen content between the arterial and venous blood in the pulmonary circuit, and that patients whose difference in oxygen content is greater than 2.6 vol/100 ml are likely to have a pulmonary vascular resistance of more than 10 units/m² and so be unsuitable for total correction whereas those with a gradient of less than 2.3 vol/100 ml are likely to have a resistance of less than 10 units/m² and so would be good candidates for correction, although they preferred patients with an oxygen difference of less than 2.0 vol/100 ml. Newfeld et al.[134] found that oxygen differences of less than 2.0 vol/100 ml were necessary to exclude severe pulmonary vascular obstructive disease. Recent experience suggests that a measured pulmonary resistance of less than 8 or even 6 units is required if VSD closure is to be performed at the time of correction.

For the future, surgeons should require the direct measurement of pulmonary flow by one or more of the several methods available.

Differential Diagnosis

The likely other causes of severe cyanosis in infants are Fallot's anomaly and tricuspid atresia. In both, lung fields are underfilled on the plain chest roentgenogram and in tricuspid atresia, the ECG shows severe left ventricular hypertrophy. In total anomalous pulmonary venous drainage, cyanosis usually is mild, as also in persistent truncus arteriosus.

Operative Treatment

Palliative Operations

The survival of infants with TGA depends, in the short term at least, on the presence of a sufficiently large defect in the atrial septum to allow adequate mixing in the two circulations. A naturally occurring atrial septal defect usually is not of sufficient size and larger defects must be created. The indirect technique, balloon septostomy, introduced by Rashkind and Miller,[144] has proved to be one of the major contributions to the management of infants with TGA. It is especially applicable to infants in the first 3 months of life. After that age, the septum does not yield so readily and does not tear adequately with traction on the balloon. The direct operative techniques have proved to have very effective results and good survival rates in infants over the age of 3 months. If the result of a Rashkind balloon septostomy is not adequate after the first few months of infancy, the septal defect can be enlarged by an operative method. Survival rates after operation in patients over the age of 3 months should be of the order of 95%.[46]

We have had a large experience with the Blalock-Hanlon operation for creating an atrial septal defect and prefer it. A number of other operative techniques have been described using caval inflow occlusion or excising a portion of the atrial septum with a rongeur or a specially designed punch introduced through the right atrium. The Edwards operation[51] is not recommended. The technique of the Blalock-Hanlon operation is outlined in Figure 60–3.

If transposition of the great arteries is complicated by se-

vere pulmonary stenosis with a ventricular septal defect, systemic desaturation may be severe. Systemic-pulmonary artery shunting continues to have a place in the treatment of such cases and survival rates have been surprisingly good for the past two decades. Stark *et al.*[178] reported 58 children over 3 months of age having palliative shunts between the years 1953 and 1968, with a 93% survival rate. The Blalock-Taussig anastomosis is preferred. Using microtechniques and extensive mobilization of the innominate and carotid arteries, the operation can be reliably performed even on the first day of life. If the subclavian artery arising from the innominate artery is hypoplastic, the Waterston anastomosis is a useful alternative, and safe if the incision made in the aorta for the anastomosis is a measured 3 mm in an infant in the early months of life.

Recent experience has encouraged our use of the "Gore-

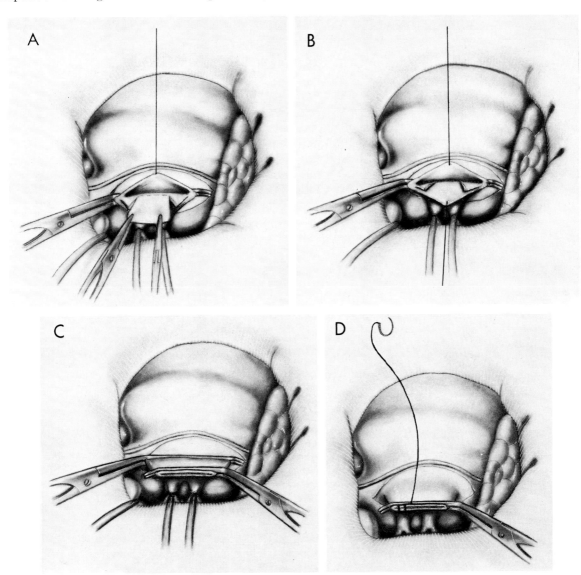

Fig. 60–3.—The Blalock-Hanlon operation for atrial septectomy. Through a right lateral thoracotomy, 5th interspace, snares are placed around the right pulmonary artery and the right pulmonary veins. **A,** a partial occlusion clamp is placed with one jaw posterior to the pulmonary veins, the other anterior, so that, when closed, portions of the right and left atria are included. Parallel incisions are made in the right and left atria, the intervening atrial septum grasped with hemostats. A segment 12–15 mm wide is isolated with scissor cuts, then an extra portion of the atrial septum withdrawn from the heart, while the operator momentarily releases the partial occlusion clamp enough to pull the septum through it. **B,** the flap of atrial septum then is excised. **C,** the edges of the atrial incision are approximated with a small partial occlusion clamp and the larger occlusion clamp and snares released. **D,** the atrial incision then can be closed at leisure. Total clamping time usually is 3–4 minutes. (From Aberdeen, E., Blalock-Hanlon Operation and Rashkind Procedure, in Rob, C., and Smith, R., *Operative Surgery* [2d ed.; London: Butterworths, 1968] Vol. 2, pp. 193–199.)

Tex" prosthetic graft. The tube prosthesis is anastomosed end to side to both the pulmonary and subclavian arteries. A 5 or 6 mm diameter graft can be inserted, because the flow still is controlled by the size of the subclavian artery, and flow can increase as the artery grows with the child. Prosthetic grafts with a diameter of 4 mm or less have a higher incidence of thrombosis than the larger-diameter grafts. A useful technical contribution to an old operation was made by Laks and Castaneda[99] when they described a form of arterioplasty to be used when the subclavian artery arises directly from the aorta, and which moves the origin of the subclavian more anterior on the aorta, so the kinking of the artery on the aorta no longer becomes an obstruction. This technique can be very difficult in small infants. The Glenn anastomosis is not used now in TGA.

Constriction (Banding) of the Pulmonary Artery

Pulmonary artery banding has been largely abandoned in the management of ventricular septal defect in children with ventricular arterial concordance (normal great artery connections), because primary VSD repair in early infancy has proved to be so reliable. Unfortunately, this stage has not yet been reached in the management of TGA with VSD (see Table 60–4), in which the mortality rate of primary repair in most centers with experience has been between 25% and 50%. Therefore, in TGA with VSD, pulmonary artery banding has continued to have a place, with a mortality rate of about 12%.[180] It is not yet demonstrated whether it is best to reoperate before the end of the first year to remove the band, perform a Mustard operation and close the ventricular septal defect or to wait until later for a Rastelli operation, with the placement of an external conduit. As with the treatment of other forms of congenital heart disease, total correction of the lesion at a first operation in infancy has obvious advantages for the child and for the family. Perhaps a more effective method of cardiac preservation during operation, or of cardiac support after operation, will allow the application of corrective techniques in early infancy so that palliative procedures can be almost totally avoided.

Rearrangement of Flow within the Atria

Mustard Operation

The Mustard operation is used commonly at this time to correct the abnormal physiology of transposed great arteries. Experience gained in many centers since the first successful operation in 1964 has shown the initial design to be sound. Various minor modifications have been introduced, mainly to facilitate the operation and to minimize the incidence of complications, namely, obstructions of systemic or pulmonary venous return, and atrial dysrhythmias. The following is a description of the Mustard operation as being currently used at the Hospital for Sick Children, Great Ormond Street. The technique evolved over a period of 12 years, during which time 460 Mustard operations have been performed. In most children with TGA and an intact ventricular septum, balloon septostomy provides adequate palliation so that the Mustard operation can be delayed. At present, an age of 8–12 months is considered optimal.[1, 15, 177, 181] Should balloon septostomy fail or the child deteriorate earlier, the Mustard operation can be carried out even in the first week of life.[170] Patients with transposition and ventricular septal defects should be operated on before the age of 6 months, or even earlier, because they may develop pulmonary vascular disease early. Similar criteria apply to infants with TGA and a large patent ductus arteriosus.

Operation

ANESTHESIA. — Premedication and anesthesia are as in other open heart operations in infants and children.[71]

MONITORING. — An arterial cannula is inserted percutaneously into a radial artery. Alternatively, a brachial artery can be exposed and a cannula inserted under direct vision. Two venous cannulae, esophageal and nasopharyngeal temperature probes, ECG electrodes and a urinary catheter are inserted.

PERFUSION. — For most Mustard operations we use standard cardiopulmonary bypass with hemodilution, moderate hypothermia (25° C) and one period of ischemic cardiac arrest. More recently we have used the cardioplegic solution described by Jynge et al.[85] to improve myocardial protection. The technique of cardiopulmonary bypass combined with hypothermia and cardioplegia enables us to use periods of low flow or even short periods of circulatory arrest should the venous return be excessive. For infants under the age of 3–6 months and under certain special circumstances we use the Kyoto technique of hypothermia and circulatory arrest.[16, 72] We use surface cooling in all sick infants, whether we plan to operate under cardiopulmonary bypass or to use deep hypothermia and circulatory arrest.

INCISION. — Through a midline sternotomy, the pericardium is cleaned of adventitia between the phrenic nerves and the intact pleura pushed to both sides. The pericardium is incised on the right side parallel to the phrenic nerve and 20 mm anterior to it (Fig. 60–4, A). An adequate pocket of pericardium is left around the apex of the heart so that it does not dislocate anteriorly. If the pericardium is not suitable for the patch, we use a Dacron patch.[173] Dacron patches were used regularly at Great Ormond Street in 1971 and 1972 but resulted in too many obstructions to venous (both pulmonary and systemic) return.[179] Others have used Dacron in older children with satisfactory long-term and short-term results. Animal experiments have shown that autogenous pericardial grafts in the atrial septum become surrounded by fibrous tissue on each side but acquire a vascular supply in the middle portion.[126] Pericardial autografts in the atrial wall of growing pigs have been observed to increase in size by 2½ times.[42] Studies of free grafts of human pericardium 1–3 years after the Mustard operation show that the tissue is well vascularized.

Currently, we use a pericardial patch that is cut into the trouser shape suggested by Brom[24, 179] (Fig. 60–4, B). When the pericardium contracts in the next few months, the atrial wall should form at least 50% of the circumference of the pathway (Fig. 60–4, C). The shape of each atrium is slightly different, so we do not hesitate to adjust the size of the patch during the operation. The measurements are only an approximate guide.

CANNULATION. — A left atrial line is inserted through a purse string on the left upper pulmonary vein. The IVC is cannulated at the junction of the right atrium with the IVC. The SVC is cannulated directly through the SVC at least 1½ cm above the SVC-RA junction (Fig. 60–4, D). This avoids damage to the sinoatrial node and sinus node artery. Right-angled cannulae with semirigid tips facilitate the caval cannulation (Fig. 60–4, E). The arterial return is via a cannula to the ascending aorta. We vent the uppermost part of the

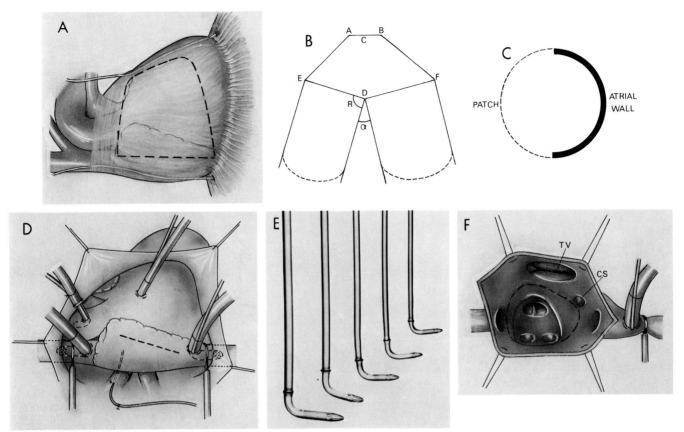

Fig. 60–4. — The Mustard operation. **A,** the extent of resection of the pericardium is indicated by a dotted line. **B,** Brom patch for Mustard operation. *A–B* is the distance from the left upper to the left lower pulmonary vein, *E–D* twice the flat diameter of the SVC, *D–F* twice the flat diameter of the IVC. *C–D* equals *E–D + D–F* divided by 2. *R* is 90° angle. Alpha is 30° angle. **C,** newly formed pathway consists of at least 50% of the circumference of the atrial wall. **D,** arterial, SVC and IVC cannulae. Right ventricular vent and left atrial monitoring line in place. **E,** various sizes and different lengths of tips of the Rygg cannulae for venous cannulation. **F,** line of the excision of the interatrial septum is shown, as well as the traction sutures in the atrial wall.

(continued)

right ventricle with a small vent. In infants, a metal coronary artery cannula tip connected to a feeding tube is used for this vent.

The right atrium is opened from the base of the right atrial appendage inferiorly and parallel to the AV groove. In small infants, we prefer to enlarge the pulmonary venous atrium, and therefore the incision is made transversely across the crista terminalis and between the AV groove to between the right upper and lower pulmonary veins. This incision slows the conduction from the SA node to the AV node[204] and could, in theory at least, increase the incidence of atrial dysrhythmias, so that we do not use it routinely on all patients.

Traction sutures are placed anteriorly, close to the tricuspid valve ring and on the right side near the crista terminalis. Excellent exposure is thus obtained without use of intraatrial retractors. The atrial septum is excised (Fig. 60–4, *F*) and the edges of the raw area sutured together. Whether the coronary sinus orifice should be enlarged by a cutback remains controversial. Electrophysiologic studies by Wittig *et al.*[204] showed that such an incision slowed the conduction from SA node to AV node. Clinical experience, however, has not demonstrated an increased incidence of dysrhythmias in patients in whom the coronary sinus cutback was used.[32] In small infants, we often use coronary sinus cutback because it widely opens the IVC pathway.

A continuous mattress suture through the wall of the atrium prevents tunnels behind the atrial trabeculations that may cause atrial shunts later. It is important that the lower and upper suture lines diverge to avoid a constricting ring that may obstruct pulmonary venous return (Fig. 60–4, *H*). The placement of the completed patch is shown in Figure 60–4, *I*. Should the pulmonary venous atrium need enlargement, we separate the upper and lower pulmonary veins with an inlay patch (Fig. 60–4, *J*).

TERMINATION OF PERFUSION. — Perfusion is terminated as with other intracardiac procedures. The initial placement of the catheter in the pulmonary venous atrium was mentioned. The monitoring cannula to the systemic venous atrium can be readily placed through the IVC cannulation site. Temporary atrial and ventricular pacemaker wires are inserted.

Postoperative Care

All patients are intubated with a nasotracheal tube and ventilated with a volume-cycled ventilator for a few hours at least. They then are weaned from the ventilator and either placed directly in an oxygen tent or the continuous positive airway pressure (CPAP) system is used. If the cardiac output is inadequate, the usual methods are used to increase it.[140] Pre-load is increased by transfusion of blood or plasma, depending on the child's hematocrit. The left atrial pressure is

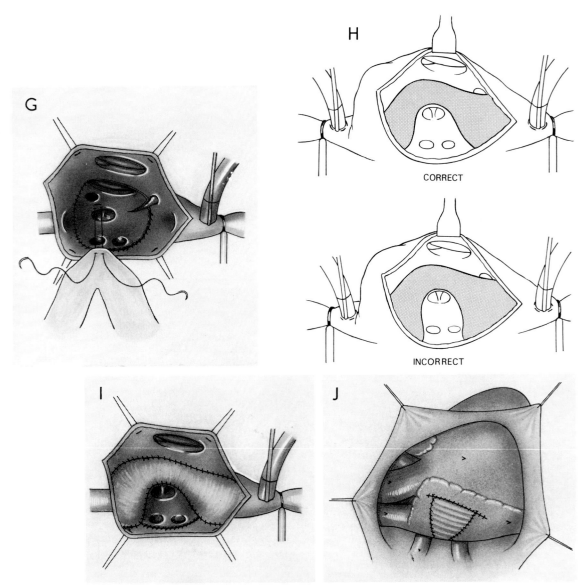

Fig. 60–4. (cont.).–**G,** the raw area after the excision of the interatrial septum is sutured over. The coronary sinus is cut back, still a controversial point. The first stitch anchoring the patch is placed between the orifice of the left atrial appendage and left pulmonary veins. A double-armed 5–0 suture is used to insert the patch, starting on the patch at point *C* (see **B**), which is thus attached to the left atrial wall between the orifice of the left pulmonary vein and the left atrial appendage. **H,** the correct and incorrect placement of the interatrial patch on the lateral atrial wall is illustrated. It is important that the lower and upper suture lines diverge to avoid constriction that may ob- struct pulmonary venous return. **I,** completed patch. The pericardial patch diverts caval and coronary sinus return to the left atrium. The pulmonary veins now drain into the right atrium and the venous drainage thus has been transposed. **J,** Dacron patch separating the right upper and lower pulmonary veins, frequently used to secure the necessary enlargement of the pulmonary venous (right) atrium. (From Stark, J., Transposition of the Great Arteries. Mustard Operation, in Rob, C., and Smith, R., *Operative Surgery* [3d ed.; London: Butterworths. In press].)

not raised above 12 torr. If the systemic vascular resistance is high, chlorpromazine, nitroprusside or phentolamine may be used. For positive inotropic support we prefer dopamine, isoproterenol and epinephrine – in that order.

Surgical Technique in the Presence of Associated Cardiac Lesions

PATENT DUCTUS ARTERIOSUS. — If the child with TGA + PDA remains in severe congestive heart failure despite intensive medi- cation, interruption of the ductus may be required in early infancy. Improvement in heart failure often is dramatic but hypoxemia may increase so that the adequacy of interatrial communication must be established before the duct is ligated. Occasionally, hy- poxemia becomes so severe that a Mustard operation may be ur- gently required.[203]

A PDA that does not cause intractable heart failure may be left to be dealt with at the time of the Mustard operation. Double liga- tion from the midline sternotomy,[55] as in other congenital heart defects, remains our technique of choice.

VENTRICULAR SEPTAL DEFECT. — The localization of ven- tricular septal defects was studied in 86 autopsied hearts by Idriss *et al.*[73] The majority of the defects are of the malalignment type and are located high in the interventricular septum. These defects are readily accessible through the retracted but not detached tricuspid valve. The atrioventricular conduction bundle in TGA usually is in the normal position, i.e., on the left side of the septum, and passes close to the posteroinferior margin of the VSD.[19] Its position in an AV canal type of VSD or midseptal VSD does not differ from such defects in normally related great arteries, so we do not hesitate to use cardioplegic arrest with hypothermia.[85]

If the VSD is easily accessible, it is closed with a Dacron patch

TABLE 60-2.—THE MUSTARD OPERATION FOR SIMPLE TGA WITH INTACT SEPTUM—
CHILDREN OF ALL AGES

AUTHOR AND YEAR OF REPORT	NO. OF PATIENTS	HOSPITAL DEATHS	MORTALITY RATE
Clarkson et al., 1972[33]	45	7	15.5%
Danielson et al., 1972[44]	25	3	12%
Ebert et al., 1974[50]	54	3	5.5%
Kilman et al., 1973[87]	15	0	0%
Lindesmith et al., 1972[106]	31	2	6%
Oelert and Borst, 1977[136]	60	0	0%
Parr et al., 1974[140]	24	3	12.5%
Shumway et al., 1975[167]	32	2	6%
Sørland et al., 1976[172]	32	3	9%
Subramanian and Wagner, 1973–1974[181]	34	3	9%
Stark et al., 1977*	292	25	9%
Trusler and Mustard, 1974[187]	97	11	11.3%
Waldhausen et al., 1971[202]	18	0	0%

*These are the most recent data available from Great Ormond Street.

and a continuous suture of 4-0 Prolene. If access is difficult, single mattress sutures may be preferred. Occasionally, the VSD may have to be closed through a left ventriculotomy, or even through a right ventriculotomy. A right ventriculotomy should be short and high under the aortic valve ring to minimize the impairment of right ventricular function after operation.

LEFT VENTRICULAR OUTFLOW TRACT OBSTRUCTION.— Causes of LVOTO are described on page 675. Pulmonary valve stenosis is rare (see Table 60-1) and usually can be visualized without difficulty from the pulmonary artery. An anterior incision in the pulmonary artery from the left side of the aorta should be used with caution if previous operations have left adhesions, because the left coronary artery may be hidden in the adhesions and may be unexpectedly injured. The subvalvar area can be inspected through the pulmonary valve from above, using a nasal speculum,[17] through a ventricular septal defect or through a left ventriculotomy. Direct relief from the obstruction is difficult in some patients and may even be impossible (for example, a long fibromuscular tunnel or an abnormal attachment of the mitral valve). Alternative techniques for bypassing the obstruction are described later.

TGA + VSD + PREVIOUS PULMONARY ARTERY BANDING. —The band may be divided by incision in the long axis of the pulmonary artery and a patch (pericardial) inserted, the banded segment of the pulmonary artery may be resected and the artery anastomosed end to end or a Rastelli operation performed using a valved conduit.

JUXTAPOSITION OF THE ATRIAL APPENDAGES.—Usually this variation can be managed without serious problems.[192, 198] In our experience the right atrium is small in all patients with TGA and juxtaposed atrial appendages. We therefore enlarge the pulmonary venous atrium with a generous patch in all such patients.

COARCTATION OF THE AORTA.—Resection of the coarctation or arterioplasty is used as in patients with normally related great arteries (ventriculo-arterial concordance). The combination of TGA + VSD + coarctation of the aorta has proved to have a high mortality rate in most reported series.

TRICUSPID VALVE REGURGITATION.— Severe tricuspid regurgitation may, occasionally, be present. We have replaced the tricuspid valve with a bio-prosthesis (Hancock heterograft no. 23) in a 3¼-year-old child at the time of the Mustard operation. The valve deteriorated badly after 3 years and required replacement.

Results of the Mustard Operation

The hospital mortality rate after the Mustard operation for TGA + intact ventricular septum (IVS) as reported from various centers is shown in Table 60-2. A 90–95% survival rate of patients with uncomplicated TGA has been achieved in recent years. Interestingly, the risks of the Mustard operation during the first year of life are not greater, and may even be less than later (Table 60-3). The best treatment for a sick infant with TGA + IVS in the first few weeks of life who has had a balloon septostomy but has not improved, or has deteriorated soon afterward, is controversial. Surgical septectomy may be performed without improving mixing at atrial level,[177] presumably because the pressure difference between the two atria is too small to encourage bidirectional flow. The risk of an emergency Mustard operation in these sick infants is high in our experience and that of others.[5, 181]

TABLE 60-3.—SIMPLE TGA WITH INTACT VENTRICULAR SEPTUM:
THE MUSTARD OPERATION IN THE FIRST YEAR OF LIFE

AUTHOR AND YEAR OF REPORT	NO. OF PATIENTS	HOSPITAL DEATHS	MORTALITY RATE	TECHNIQUE OF CARDIOPULMONARY SUPPORT
Alfieri et al., 1977[5]	28 (< 7 mo)	5	18%	Hypothermic arrest
Bailey et al., 1976[13]	27	0	0%	Hypothermic arrest
Barratt-Boyes, 1973[15]	17	2	12%	Hypothermic arrest
Ebert et al., 1974[50]	14	0	0%	Hypothermic arrest
Kilman et al., 1973[87]	8	0	0%	Cardiopulmonary bypass— normothermia
Oelert and Borst, 1977[136]	26	0	0%	
Parr et al., 1975[139]	10	2	20%	Hypothermia and low flow
Rittenhouse et al., 1974[149]	8 (< 7 mo)	1	13%	Hypothermic arrest
Stark et al., 1977	80	5	6%	Cardiopulmonary bypass and hypothermia
Zavanella and Subramanian[208]	44	4	8.5%	Hypothermic arrest

TABLE 60-4.—TGA AND VSD: THE MUSTARD OPERATION AND VSD CLOSURE—ALL AGES

AUTHOR AND YEAR OF REPORT	NO. OF PATIENTS	HOSPITAL DEATHS	MORTALITY RATE
Castaneda *et al.*, 1976[27]	25	2	8%
Champsaur *et al.*, 1973[29]	22	10	45%
Danielson *et al.*, 1972[44]	29	16	55%
Ebert *et al.*, 1974[50]	13	1	8%
Kilman *et al.*, 1973[87]	6	1	17%
Mori *et al.*, 1976[126]	23	9	39%
Oelert and Borst, 1977[136]	13	0	0%
Stark *et al.*, 1977	52	13	25%

Additional cardiac lesions are associated with an increased hospital mortality rate for the Mustard operation. The results for correction of TGA + VSD are shown in Table 60-4. The risk depends partly on the position of the VSD and its relationship to the tricuspid and mitral valves, and also on the degree of pulmonary vascular obstructive disease (PVOD). The operative mortality rate for TGA + VSD in the first year of life is even higher (Table 60-5) than later. Some surgeons therefore advocate pulmonary artery banding in the first month of life and debanding, closure of the VSD and the Mustard operation at about 1 year of age.[25]

Results of the Mustard operation in children with TGA + intact ventricular septum (IVS) and left ventricular outflow tract obstruction (LVOTO) depend very much on the anatomy of the obstruction. A fibrous shelf can easily be relieved and satisfactory results achieved. Between 1971 and 1977, we corrected 15 such patients, with 2 deaths (13% mortality rate). When effective relief from the obstruction within the ventricle is not possible, alternative operations are available.

Complications of the Mustard Operation

Several complications have been widely reported after the Mustard operation. Vena caval pathway obstruction, usually the superior vena cava, has been reported frequently.[31, 34, 55, 63, 67, 117, 125, 179, 196] In our own experience, vena caval pathway obstruction was much more common when Dacron was used for the patch (30%) than when pericardium was used (5%).[179] In patients who required reoperation after the use of the Dacron partition, Dacron was found to be folded on itself like a concertina and surrounded by thick scar tissue[2, 175] (Fig. 60-5). Obstruction of the inferior vena cava, very unusual, especially if pericardium has been used for the atrial partition,[2] has not occurred at all in some series. It has been reported to lead to a protein-losing enteropathy,[124] as has SVC obstruction.[96]

Obstruction to pulmonary venous return has been reported less frequently than caval pathway obstruction.[17a, 34, 67, 136, 179, 202] The obstruction may occur either at the suture line, if this has been placed so that the superior and inferior suture lines come too close to each other on the right pulmonary vein opening (see Fig. 60-4, *H*), or in the midportion of a too voluminous patch. Pulmonary venous obstruction is more serious than caval pathway obstruction and more often fatal. For these reasons, if the distance between the SVC and IVC suture lines seems to be too short, we extend the atriotomy incision posteriorly to between the right upper and lower pulmonary vein orifices and insert a large patch to enlarge the pulmonary venous atrium, as described by Replogle and Lin[147] and Ebert *et al.*[50] We use this technique routinely in all infants under the age of 6 months.

More recent changes in surgical technique have decreased the incidence of obstructive complications. During 1974–1976, we used pericardium cut into the trouser-shaped patch described by Brom[24, 177] and we encountered only 2 SVC obstructions and 2 pulmonary venous obstructions among 115 survivors of the Mustard operation. In one of these patients who developed obstruction, a Dacron patch had been used because pericardium was not available. Clarkson *et al.*[34] reported 3 severe and 4 mild obstructions to the SVC and 2 severe and 6 mild obstructions to the pulmonary venous outflow in a group of 49 survivors of the Mustard operation. In the Toronto series, no caval obstructions were observed in 97 cases.[29]

Obstruction of the pulmonary venous return can be disastrous. It is an acquired lesion, hemodynamically similar to a triatrial heart. Patients with symptoms should have a corrective operation performed without delay.

We prefer the right thoracotomy approach through the fifth interspace for operative revision for systemic or pulmonary vein obstruction, tricuspid valve incompetence or residual ventricular septal defect. The sternum can be transected to improve the approach. Cannulation of the inferior and superior venae cavae is easier and dissection of adhesions (and bleeding) less extensive than with repeat sternotomy. The right coronary arteries and the right phrenic nerve are more likely to be spared.[184] Access to intracardiac pathways and to the tricuspid valve is better from the right side than from the front when the right ventricle is trapped in adhesions.

DYSRHYTHMIAS.—Conduction disturbances and dysrhythmias have been recorded after operation in all of the large

TABLE 60-5.—TGA AND VSD: THE MUSTARD OPERATION AND VSD REPAIR
IN THE FIRST YEAR OF LIFE

AUTHOR AND YEAR OF REPORT	NO. OF PATIENTS	HOSPITAL DEATHS	MORTALITY RATE
Alfieri *et al.*, 1977[5]	5 (< 7 mos)	3	60%
Barratt-Boyes, 1973[15]	9	5	55%
Castaneda *et al.*, 1976[27]	9	2	22%
Oelert and Borst, 1977[136]	7	0	0%
Stark *et al.*, 1977	15	4	27%

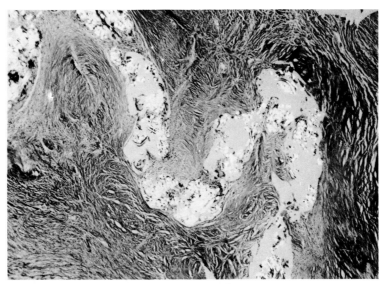

Fig. 60–5.—Transverse section through Dacron patch showing late stage of contraction caused by heavy deposition of fibrous tissue, which has crinkled the Dacron during the phase of fibrous tissue contraction and so caused obstruction to venous flow.

series.[53] Among 14 patients who died after the Mustard operation at the Mayo Clinic,[75] none was in sinus rhythm. The Houston group[52] observed 128 survivors of the Mustard operation, with an incidence of sinus rhythm in less than 40% of their earlier cases, increasing to about 70% in their most recent years. A high incidence of atrial flutter and complete AV dissociation was reported previously from Great Ormond Street.[23]

Modifications in operative technique were introduced by many surgeons in order to reduce dysrhythmias after operation. The three main aims were: (1) To avoid trauma to the AV node and bundle of His caused by coronary sinus suction techniques or by suture lines crossing the bundle or running close to it. (2) To avoid injury to the sinus node, the sinus node artery and its nerve supply. (3) To avoid interruption of the so-called internodal pathways.[70, 121] A reduced incidence of dysrhythmias has been recorded in several published series.[32, 52] In our own experience of 84 consecutive survivors of the Mustard operation during 1974 and 1975, only 9 dysrhythmias were observed (5 had transient junctional rhythm, 3 had permanent junctional rhythm, 1 had transient supraventricular tachycardia). Insufficient data are available to confirm the exact reason for the improvement or to determine what other steps could be taken to decrease further the incidence of dysrhythmias. Direct damage to the AV node or the sinus node obviously should be avoided. Careful use of intracardiac suction, especially around the coronary sinus, and placement of the SVC cannula well away from the SA node are recommended. Injury to the sinus node artery should also be avoided. Excision of the atrial septum, plus cutback of the coronary sinus, in addition to a long transverse atriotomy does not leave much atrial wall intact for conduction. Careful further study is required to assess the importance of the technical points, so that changes intended to *decrease* the incidence of obstruction to blood flow do not *increase* the incidence of dysrhythmias or vice versa.

TRICUSPID VALVE REGURGITATION.—Tricuspid valve regurgitation was reported by Tynan *et al.*[189] in 17 of 173 patients surviving the Mustard operation, but it was severe in only 3, and 2 of these had abnormal valve cusps with myxomatous degeneration. Hagler *et al.*[67] reported mild tricuspid regurgitation in 7 patients and moderate to severe regurgitation in 6 patients of a series of 44 studied late after the Mustard operation at the Mayo Clinic. Champsaur *et al.*[29] did not observe tricuspid regurgitation in any of 97 patients in the Toronto series, nor did Muster *et al.*[128] when studying 50 patients in the Chicago postoperative series. A later study by the Toronto group showed mild tricuspid incompetence in only 2 of 14 patients studied in detail,[60] so function of the tricuspid valve late after the Mustard operation does not yet seem to be a cause for great concern.

INTERATRIAL SHUNTS.—Leaks between the atria or through the ventricular septum have been recorded when careful studies have been made after the operation. The first report of atrial leaks came from Toronto,[160] and they introduced the method of releasing the caval snares after the patch was placed and before the atrium was closed so that the patch can be checked for leaks. We have found that clamping the caval line for a few seconds makes a leak much easier to recognize. In our experience, a right-to-left shunt is significant only if there also is obstruction of the caval pathway downstream from the leak.

RIGHT VENTRICULAR FUNCTION.—A decrease in right ventricular function has been measured in some patients after the Mustard operation. Jarmakani and Canent[81] measured a diminished right ventricular ejection fraction in patients after the Mustard operation. It still is difficult to assess whether this is a problem of the right ventricle, which now carries the systemic load and eventually may fail, or whether it is more a consequence of inadequate myocardial protection during operation, especially as the techniques used in the earlier years perhaps were less effective in preserving full myocardial function.

DIMINISHED SIZE OF THE RIGHT ATRIUM.—The atrial capacity is of critical importance in regulating cardiac output. Studies by Trusler *et al.*[186] showed that, in dogs, reduction of atrial volume by up to 50% had little effect on the resting cardiac output but reduction of atrial size beyond this reduced the output significantly. Suga,[182] using an ana-

TABLE 60–6.—LONG-TERM FOLLOW-UP AFTER THE MUSTARD OPERATION

AUTHOR AND YEAR OF REPORT	NO. OF PATIENTS SURVIVING THE MUSTARD OPERATION	LATE DEATHS NO.	%	PERIOD OF FOLLOW-UP
Champsaur et al., 1973[29]	97	12	12	From May 1963
Clarkson et al., 1976[34]	49	5	10	From 1964
Mair et al., 1974[107]	49	10	20	From 1964
Stark et al., 1977	164	25	15	From 1965
Sunderland et al., 1975[183]	18	2	11	From 1970

log model, showed the importance of atrial compliance in transforming the continuous venous return into the intermittent filling flow. The importance of venous return in the regulation of cardiac output has been emphasized for many years by Guyton.[66] Perhaps an atrial capacity that is adequate at rest is inadequate for high cardiac outputs. A careful study of cardiac performance soon after the Mustard operation by Parr et al.[140] showed large pressure fluctuations in the systemic venous atrium, suggesting that the systemic atrium may not have been adequate as a reservoir and thus may have impaired the cardiac output. Studies by Silove and Taylor[169] showed evidence of somewhat reduced compliance of the systemic venous atrium. The pulmonary atrium seemed affected to a lesser degree.

CHYLOTHORAX.—Chylothorax developing after the Mustard operation should be accepted as presumptive evidence of SVC obstruction.

Long-Term Results

Although the Mustard operation has dramatically improved the survival rate of children born with TGA, and many of them lead normal lives, the long-term observations have some disquieting features (Table 60–6). Mair et al.[107] studied 49 of 54 children surviving the Mustard operation at the Mayo Clinic, 4–10 years after operation. Ten had died (20%), including 2 with pulmonary vascular obstructive disease, 3 with dysrhythmias, 2 who required reoperation and 1 with pulmonary venous obstruction. The Toronto group reported 12 late deaths in a series of 97 survivors.[29] Four were the result of heart failure, 3 from possible dysrhythmias and 3 from pulmonary venous obstruction. The late results from the Great Ormond Street Hospital for Sick Children, reviewed in 1976, showed that there were 25 late deaths (15%) in a group of 164 patients surviving operation in 1965–1971. Fifty-six of the survivors attended normal schools and participated in sporting activities. A further 46 led unrestricted lives, but with some complications (e.g., dysrhythmias or tricuspid incompetence). Twenty-one patients were restricted by severe dysrhythmias. Severe neurologic deficit was present in 7 survivors, but this deficit was present in some patients before the operation. Eight patients known to be alive were not assessed in detail because they were living abroad.

Senning Operation

The first successful correction of a human with TGA was achieved by Senning in Stockholm on June 10, 1958 on a 9-year-old boy.[84] The practical value of this extraordinary achievement was only slowly appreciated and some of the advantages of the operation still are being recognized almost 20 years later. The operation applied the principle of rearrangement of venous flow within the atria, as first proposed by Albert.[4] Senning's technique made the atria into two concentric tubes, by rearranging the atrial septum and walls so that the inner tube carried the desaturated systemic venous blood to the mitral valve and the outer tube carried the saturated pulmonary venous blood to the tricuspid valve.

Successful results of the Senning operation were recorded by four surgeons in the next few years,[2] and others tried the operation without success.

Senning[157] reported 4 cases, 1 an infant of 6 weeks, the others 6–10 years of age, 2 having VSDs—so only one of his 4 patients was a good-risk case, and this was his only survivor. Kirklin[91] likewise operated on what now is recognized as a series with many high-risk cases. Of 11 patients, 5 were infants, of whom 4 were less than 6 months of age, 9 were in intractable heart failure and only 2 of the 11 had an intact septum and several had severe pulmonary vascular disease. Of the 4 survivors in this series, the youngest was 3 months of age. At this time, these results were considered good evidence that TGA was a very difficult condition to treat. In fact, reviewing the information recorded then with our present knowledge of TGA makes it clear that the natural history of the disease was not considered, and the assessment of the risks of the Senning operation made then were not correct. The few patients who did survive these early attempts did well; so well, in fact, that Brom of Leyden[143] was sufficiently impressed with the results in 2 patients seen 6 and 7 years after operation that he returned to using the Senning operation, as have several other surgeons. Senning used modifications of his original technique, one using a Dacron patch and another fashioning a flap from the atrial wall,[156] and, although the results were excellent for the simple TGA (3 deaths of 41 patients) and the complex cases (5 deaths of 25 patients), Senning has returned to using his original technique, one advantage of which is that only viable cardiac tissue is used for the repair, so presumably atrial contraction is more effective than with other techniques. The relatively low incidence of dysrhythmias after the Senning operation now has been achieved after the Mustard operation. Perhaps a longer period of observation will provide enough evidence to decide which method of rearrangement of atrial flow provides the best cardiac function.

Intraventricular Correction

Rearrangement of flow within the ventricles is possible only in the rare event that a large and high VSD is present. A large patch is sutured to the lower edge of the VSD and then to the wall of the right ventricle and finally around the aortic valve annulus. The shape and placement of the patch is critical to avoid obstruction to flow. Since the first successful case reported by McGoon[118] on a 2-year-old child operated on in 1969, reported successes have been those of Taguchi et al.,[185] an 11-year-old patient, and Cooley et al. in a 13-year-old.[38]

Great Artery Reversal for TGA

When Jatene and his colleagues[82, 83] achieved in 1975 the first successful survival by great artery reversal, they modified a technique that had been described by Baffes et al.[12] in 1961. Baffes excised the coronary arteries from the aorta, with a small cuff of aortic wall still attached, transected the great arteries and then reanastomosed them in their physiologically correct position, transferring the coronary arteries. Jatene's technique differed from Baffes' in that the great arteries were divided well distal to the semilunar valves, the pulmonary artery at a point near the bifurcation and the aorta a similar distance distal from the heart. Each of the stomas left in the aortic sinuses following excision of the coronary arteries was closed with a patch and the coronary arteries transferred to the pulmonary artery root. The aorta and pulmonary arteries then were transferred, with the necessary tailoring of the enlarged pulmonary artery to make a matching diameter at the anastomosis. Jatene et al.[83] reported 8 patients, with 2 surviving. The second successful case had the pulmonary artery lengthened by a Dacron tube graft.

Lower[116] reported the first instance of an infant with TGA and an intact ventricular septum surviving arterial rearrangement, followed by Yacoub.[207]

Although several additional successes with great artery reversal have been reported,[95, 112, 153, 206] it seems that, overall, patients dying after arterial rearrangement outnumber the survivors by perhaps 3 or 4 to 1. Before this technique, so desirable in theory, can prove to be acceptable in regular practice, a survival rate of about 90% should be expected for uncomplicated transpositions, since the survival rate now is better than 90% for intra-atrial rearrangement of flow. If this survival rate is to be achieved for great artery reversal, it seems that some extra factor will be required—either a better means of myocardial preservation during operation and/or a better support method after operation, perhaps mechanical left heart assistance.

Another technique for arterial correction is described during the discussion of external conduits.

Operations Using External Conduits

Rastelli Operation

The relief from left ventricular outflow tract obstruction (LVOTO) in children with TGA may be difficult (such as with a long fibromuscular tunnel) or impossible (such as with abnormal attachment of the mitral valve). The difficulty in relieving the LVOTO without causing damage to important adjacent structures such as the bundle of His or the mitral valve has resulted in a high mortality rate of correction of TGA with VSD and LVOTO in the past[23, 44] (Table 60-7).

The prognosis for patients with this combination of lesions has improved greatly since Rastelli[146] described his innovative technique for anatomic correction. The principle of the operation is illustrated in Figure 60-6, A-C. The ventricular septal defect is not closed but is used to connect the left ventricle to the aorta by a large patch. The pulmonary artery is either ligated or divided and the pulmonary end oversewn. Continuity between the right ventricle and the pulmonary artery is re-established with an external valve conduit. Kirklin[94] first introduced this principle of correction using a conduit without a valve. Rastelli initially proposed an aortic homograft for the conduit such as had been used in the repair of pulmonary atresia by Ross.[153] A Dacron conduit containing a porcine heterograft[22] is another alternative that is widely used at present.

Currently, we prefer the Rastelli operation for patients with TGA + VSD + LVOTO. It is possible to use the operation in patients with TGA + VSD whether or not there has been previous pulmonary artery banding. We prefer to defer the operation until the age of 4 or 5 years, because the survival rate has proved to be better in older children[114] and because a larger conduit can be placed at this age, although conduit of a size sufficient for an adult can be used even at the age of 2–3 years. Should a child require operation before the age of 4, a systemic-to-pulmonary artery shunt (Blalock-Taussig) is our treatment of choice.

The Rastelli operation has also been used successfully in children with TGA, VSD and PS who previously had had a Glenn anastomosis. The SVC was reanastomosed to the right atrium, the right pulmonary artery reconnected to the main pulmonary artery by a Dacron tube graft and the Rastelli procedure then performed.[115, 151]

OPERATIVE TECHNIQUE (Fig. 60-6).—Currently, we use hypothermia to 22–25° C, combined with cold cardioplegic cardiac arrest.[85] When the desired body temperature is reached, the aorta is crossclamped and the right atrium opened (Fig. 60-6, A). An ASD or patent foramen ovale is closed. The ventricular anatomy then is assessed from the right atrium via the tricuspid valve, to establish whether the positions of the VSD and the papillary muscles are suitable for the Rastelli operation. This approach also allows the right ventriculotomy incision to be safely placed after inspection from inside the right ventricle. The incision points in the direction of the pulmonary artery, and that usually is to the left. A button of right ventricular myocardium is not excised, but occasionally the edges of the incision are thinned. The VSD is enlarged if its diameter is smaller than that of the aortic valve ring (Fig. 60-6, B), to ensure a wide outflow from the left ventricle to the aorta. Through the VSD, the pulmonary valve is sutured closed and the pulmonary artery doubly ligated above the valve (Fig. 60-6, C).

TABLE 60-7.—TGA AND VSD AND LVOTO*: THE MUSTARD OPERATION, VSD CLOSURE AND OUTFLOW TRACT CORRECTION—ALL AGES

AUTHOR AND YEAR OF REPORT	NO. OF PATIENTS	HOSPITAL DEATHS	MORTALITY RATE
Chiariello et al., 1975[30]	17	10	59%
Danielson et al., 1971[43]	14	5	36%
Ebert et al., 1974[50]	14	2	14%
Idriss et al., 1974[73]	8	0	0%
Rastelli et al., 1969[146]	7	0	0%
Stark et al., 1973–1977	15	2	13%
Trusler and Mustard, 1974[187]	9	3	33%

*Left ventricular outflow tract obstruction.

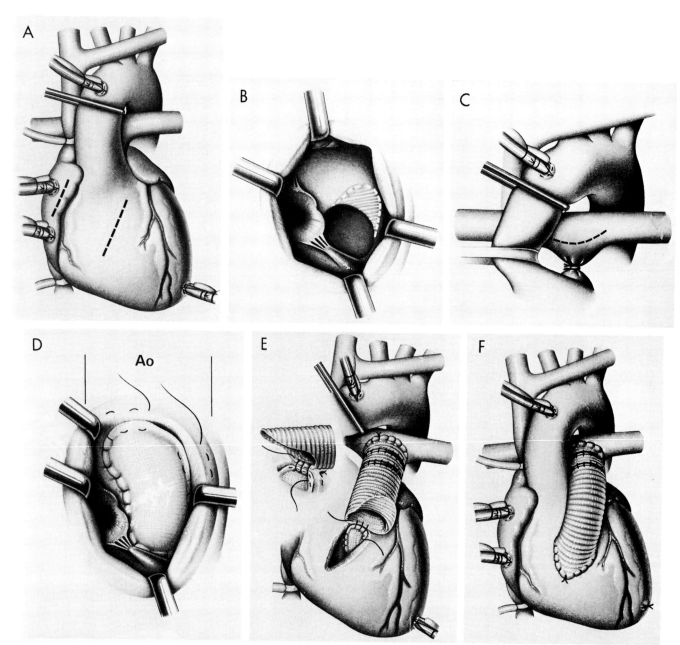

Fig. 60–6. — The Rastelli operation. **A,** ventriculotomy and atriotomy indicated by dotted lines. The atriotomy is performed first, the interior of the ventricle inspected through the tricuspid valve, the anatomy assessed and the appropriate ventriculotomy performed. **B,** cross-hatched area of septum is excised if need be to enlarge defect to diameter of aortic valve ring. **C,** the pulmonary artery is doubly ligated above the valve. Incision in the pulmonary artery is indicated by a dotted line. The pulmonary valve has been sutured closed through the VSD. **D,** left ventricle is connected to aorta using a large Dacron patch. **E,** anastomosis of the conduit to the pulmonary artery has been completed. Proximal end of the conduit is trimmed obliquely *(inset)* and then sutured to the right ventriculotomy. In the upper corner of the ventriculotomy, the conduit is attached to the ventricular patch. **F,** Rastelli operation completed. (From Stark, J., Transposition of the Great Arteries. Rastelli Operation, in Rob, C., and Smith, R., *Operative Surgery* [3d ed.; London: Butterworth. In press].)

This is preferred to transection of the pulmonary artery because the suture line of the proximal pulmonary artery may be difficult to reach after the conduit has been placed, and bleeding from this area can be troublesome.

A large patch of Dacron velour is sutured around the VSD to connect the LV to the aorta (Fig. 60–6, *D*). The pulmonary artery is opened widely at the bifurcation so that a large anastomosis with the conduit can be performed. We presently use a fresh aortic homograft, which has been preserved in an antibiotic solution. The area between the anterior valve ring and the right ventricle is closed with a patch of woven Dacron tube. An alternative to the fresh aortic homograft is a Dacron conduit containing a porcine heterograft. The advantages and disadvantages are summarized in Table 60–8. The proximal end of the Dacron conduit is trimmed obliquely to achieve a wide anastomosis with the RV (Fig. 60–6, *E*). Gradients at the proximal anastomosis[150] seemingly can be avoided. Figure 60–6, *F* shows the completed conduit.

The conduit must be placed so as not to cross the midline, in order to avoid compression by the sternum. If compres-

TABLE 60–8.—THE CHOICE OF A VALVED CONDUIT FOR THE RASTELLI OPERATION

	PRO	CON
Aorta with homograft valve in situ	Cheap Larger size can be inserted Easier distal anastomosis	Irradiated and frozen grafts calcify readily Not readily available
Heterograft valve in Dacron tube	Readily available Quality control simpler	Expensive Bulky in infants Gradients with small sizes

sion of the conduit is conceivable, the pericardium and pleura can be opened widely on the left, behind and parallel to the left phrenic nerve. The heart thus can rotate to the left, moving the conduit farther away from the midline. This incision of the pericardium and pleura on the left is a preferred routine in all conduit operations performed on infants.

TERMINATION OF PERFUSION AND POSTOPERATIVE CARE.—Evacuation of air and control of bleeding are even more meticulous than usual. Preclotting of the conduit is helpful, because bleeding from the porous Dacron may be a problem. Normal or near-normal intracardiac pressures may be recorded after the repair if the intraoperative myocardial protection has been adequate, and no special measures are required to discontinue bypass. Mechanical ventilation for at least 12 hours after operation is preferred in all these patients.

RESULTS.—Between 1971 and 1975, we operated on 23 patients, with 2 hospital deaths (8%) and 2 late deaths (8%) (Table 60–9). The largest series has been published from the Mayo Clinic,[115] and their hospital mortality decreased from 26% of 34 children operated on between 1968 and 1972 to only 8% in 25 patients operated on during 1972–1975.

COMPLICATIONS.—Several complications following the Rastelli operation have been described.[76, 114, 138, 150] Residual defects of the ventricular septum have been frequent and probably result from the use of the very large ventricular patch. Aneurysm of the right ventricle, obstruction of the conduit, obstruction of the newly constructed left ventricular outflow tract and compression of the conduit by the sternum have all been described. Poor results may be caused by the unfavorable anatomy. These problems are related to the position of the ventricular septal defect and its relationship to the tricuspid valve attachments. Papillary muscle reimplantation was used in 1 of our patients and replacement of the tricuspid valve in another, but both died. Others[113] have described an increased mortality rate after the Rastelli operation for patients with TGA + VSD + pulmonary valve atre-

sia and suggested that the increased risk was mainly because of hypoplasia of the pulmonary arteries. Many of their patients had residual right ventricular hypertension following repair, and of 13 operated on in this group, 4 died.

The Left Ventricle to Pulmonary Artery Conduits

If a patient has TGA + LVOTO and an intact ventricular septum, alternative techniques are available for correction. If the obstruction can be resected adequately, resection is combined with either a Mustard operation or possibly with reversal of the great arteries. However, if the obstruction cannot be relieved, the Mustard operation can be done and the obstruction bypassed by a valved conduit from the left ventricle to the pulmonary artery. Only a few patients treated by such a technique have been reported[119, 171] and, so far, the mortality rate has been high. A left ventricle to pulmonary artery conduit can be considered if the preoperative angiocardiogram suggests that the LVOTO cannot be resected. The LVOTO bypass may also be used in patients in whom the LV pressure after "correction" is found to be at systemic levels, but with the PA pressure below normal, or the LV pressure is found to be suprasystemic even if the PA pressure is normal.

Biventricular Conduits

This technique, introduced by McGoon[119] in 1976, provides external conduits to bypass the outflow tracts of both ventricles. Rarely required, it provides an opportunity for correction in some unusual situations that otherwise may be impossible to correct.

Arterial Correction by Pulmonary Aortic Anastomosis and External Conduit

This method of great artery reversal was described independently by Damus,[41] by Stansel[174] and by Kaye.[86] The technique includes transection of the main pulmonary artery close to the bifurcation. The proximal end of the pulmonary artery is anastomosed end to side to the ascending aorta, the VSD is closed and continuity of the RV to the pulmonary artery is established by a valved conduit from the RV to the distal end of the pulmonary artery at the bifurcation. The aortic valve was not closed in the early cases, because it was presumed that the aortic pressure would remain higher than the PA and RV pressure and therefore keep the aortic valve closed, but one surviving patient had to be reoperated on for closure of the aortic orifice because of the persistent ejection through the aortic valve. Two of 4 patients operated on at the Mayo Clinic have survived and are doing well. This technique has the obvious advantage that variations of coronary artery anatomy do not prevent this form of great artery correction as they do not transfer the coronary artery ostia.

TABLE 60–9.—TGA WITH VSD AND LVOTO: THE RASTELLI OPERATION–ALL AGES

AUTHOR AND YEAR OF REPORT	NO. OF PATIENTS	HOSPITAL DEATHS	MORTALITY RATE
Daenen et al., 1976[40]	23	2+2 late death	8%
Griepp, 1974[64]	9	3	33%
Imamura et al., 1977[74]	8	3	38%
Marcelletti et al., 1976[113]	13 c̄ pulmonary atresia	4+1 late death	31%
Marcelletti et al., 1976[114]	59	11	19%
	9 < 5 mo	5	56%
	50 > 5 mo	6	12%
	Dacron conduit (1972–75) 25	2	8%

TABLE 60-10.—PALLIATIVE MUSTARD OPERATION FOR TGA WITH SEVERE PVOD ± VSD

AUTHOR AND YEAR OF REPORT	NO. OF PATIENTS	HOSPITAL DEATHS	MORTALITY RATE
Bernhard *et al.*, 1976[18]	3	0	0%
Lindesmith *et al.*, 1975[105]	10	0	0%
Mair *et al.*, 1976[109]	8	0	0%
Oelert and Borst, 1977[136]	8	1	12%
Stark *et al.*, 1977	34	2	6%
	(incl. 4 VSD created for IVS)		

Variations of coronary anatomy are quite common in TGA,[155] and one study suggests perhaps as many as one-third (47 of 149) being unsuited for transplantation.[163] The obvious disadvantage is that a conduit inserted in the first year of life probably will require a larger replacement before growth of the child is complete.

Operation for Transposition of the Great Arteries in the Presence of Pulmonary Vascular Obstructive Disease

Pulmonary vascular obstructive disease (PVOD) can develop early in patients with transposition of the great arteries (TGA),[57, 98, 134, 200, 201] almost inevitably during the first year of life in patients with TGA and an associated large VSD and/or PDA and occasionally in infants with TGA and an intact ventricular septum. Children with a severely elevated pulmonary arteriolar resistance (Rp) either have incurred a high operative mortality after the Mustard operation and closure of the VSD or have been refused operation.[110] Even after survival from the Mustard operation, the PVOD may progress and cause death.[109]

In 1972, Lindesmith *et al.*[106] reported the concept of the palliative Mustard operation for patients with TGA and VSD and severe PVOD. The venous inflow is redirected within the atria in the usual way but no attempt is made to close the ventricular septal defect. Presumably the VSD "decompresses" the left ventricle if the pulmonary vascular resistance increases. Whatever the functional explanation, the results have been astonishingly good (Table 60-10). Not only has the hospital mortality been low but the improvement in most cases has been striking. Of 23 patients operated on at Great Ormond Street between 1973 and January of 1977, the arterial oxygen saturation ranged between 45% and 79% (mean 65%), hemoglobin 13-23 gm/dl (mean 19) and pulmonary arterial resistance 6.4-35 units/m^2 (mean 17) before operation. All these patients survived and improved. After operation, the arterial O$_2$ saturation was 75-96% (mean 89) (p<0.001) (Table 60-11).

Stark *et al.*[176] extended this principle to children with TGA, intact ventricular septum and PVOD by adding creation of an apical VSD to the standard Mustard procedure.

Our present policy in patients with TGA and PVOD is: if the Rp is over 8 units/m^2, a palliative Mustard operation is performed (if there is no VSD, a VSD is created). If the Rp is less than 6 units/m^2, the Mustard operation is performed and the VSD is closed. Patients with an Rp in the mid-range of 6-8 units/m^2 are assessed carefully on an individual basis. The appearance of the pulmonary vessels on angiocardiography, the age of the patient and perhaps a study of a lung biopsy may affect the decision as to whether to close the VSD or leave it open, but the Mustard operation is done in any case.

Summary

Although so much has been achieved to help patients with ventriculo-arterial discordance (transposed great arteries), we still are not able to provide these children with the prospect of a normal existence for a normal life span, and anything less must be unacceptable when a heart has near-normal valves and myocardium. Careful long-term observations must be made, and some may be discouraging, such as the observation that right ventricular function is reduced after the Mustard operation,[61] but the reason for this is not yet defined. From the first attempted correction of TGA, arterial correction seemed to be the obvious procedure because it has the advantage of utilizing the left ventricle as the systemic ventricle. After more than 20 years of repeated failures, arterial correction now has been performed successfully, but, as yet, the risks of this highly desirable procedure are too high for it to be acceptable for routine use. The coming years no doubt will reveal better methods of myocardial preservation at operation and perhaps more effective methods of cardiac assistance for the first few days after operation, so that survival rates after arterial correction will improve greatly, but until that acceptable survival rate is clearly established, it seems prudent to continue operations that reverse the venous inflow, the Mustard and Senning operations, as the routine corrective operations for ventriculo-arterial discordance (TGA).

TABLE 60-11.—PALLIATIVE MUSTARD OPERATION (Preoperative and Postoperative Arterial Oxygen Saturation [SaO$_2$] and Serum Hemoglobin [Hb])

	PREOPERATIVE		POSTOPERATIVE		
Art. O$_2$ sat. %	45-79	$\overline{65}$	75-96	$\overline{89}$	p < 0.001
Hb gm/dl	13-25	$\overline{19}$	11-18	$\overline{14}$	p < 0.05

REFERENCES

1. Aberdeen, E.: Correction of uncomplicated cases of transposition of the great arteries, Br. Heart J. 33(Supp. 6):66, 1971.
2. Aberdeen, E.: Transposition of the Great Arteries, in Sabiston, D. C., and Spencer, F. C. (eds.), *Gibbon's Surgery of the Chest* (Philadelphia: W. B. Saunders Company, 1976), Chap. 41.
3. Aberdeen, E., Waterston, D. J., Carr, I., Graham, G., Bonham-Carter, R. E., and Subramanian, S.: Successful "correction" of transposed great arteries by Mustard's operation, Lancet 1: 1233, 1965.
4. Albert, H. M.: Surgical correction of transposition of great vessels, Surg. Forum 5:74, 1955.
5. Alfieri, O., Bianchi, T., Locatelli, G., Vanini, V., and Parenzan, L.: Open heart surgery in the first six months of life, J. Pediatr. Surg. 12:113, 1977.
6. Alfieri, O., and Subramanian, S.: A new instrument for surgical exposure of subaortic and subpulmonic stenosis, Ann. Thorac. Surg. 19:589, 1975.
7. Anderson, R. H., Arnold, R., and Jones, R. S.: D-bulboventricular loop with L-transposition in situs inversus, Circulation 46:173, 1972.

8. Anderson, R. H., Arnold, R., and Wilkinson, J. L.: The conducting system in congenitally corrected transposition, Lancet 1: 1286, 1973.

9. Anderson, R. H., Becker, A. E., Arnold, R., and Wilkinson, J. L.: The conducting tissues in congenitally corrected transposition, Circulation 50:911, 1974.

10. Anderson, R. H., Stark, J., de Leval, M., Aberdeen, E., Taylor, J. F. N., and Urban, A. E.: An autopsy study of hearts from patients with transposition of the great arteries after Mustard's operation, Am. J. Cardiol. 37:117, 1976.

11. Anderson, R. H., Wilkinson, J. L., Gerlis, L. M., Smith, A., and Becker, A. E.: Atresia of the right atrioventricular orifice, Br. Heart J. 39:414, 1977.

12. Baffes, T. G., Ketola, F. H., and Tatooles, C. J.: Transfer of coronary ostia by "triangulation" in transposition of the great vessels and anomalous coronary arteries: A preliminary report, Dis. Chest 39:648, 1961.

13. Bailey, L. L., Takeuchi, Y., Williams, W. G., Trusler, G. A., and Mustard W. T.: Surgical management of congenital cardiovascular anomalies with the use of profound hypothermia and circulatory arrest. Analysis of 180 consecutive cases, J. Thorac. Cardiovasc. Surg. 71:485, 1976.

14. Baillie, M.: *The Morbid Anatomy of Some of the Most Important Parts of the Human Body* (London: Johnson and Nicol, 1797), p. 38.

15. Barratt-Boyes, B. G.: Complete Correction of Cardiovascular Malformation in the First Two Years of Life Using Profound Hypothermia, in Barratt-Boyes, B. G., Neutze, J. H., and Harris, E. A. (eds.), *Heart Disease in Infancy. Diagnosis and Surgical Treatment* (London: Churchill Livingstone, 1973), pp. 25–36.

16. Barratt-Boyes, B. G., Simpson, M., and Neutze, J. M.: Intracardiac surgery in neonates and infants using deep hypothermia with surface cooling and limited cardiopulmonary bypass, Circulation 43 (Supp. 1):25, 1971.

17. Bentall, H. H.: The place of surgery in hypertrophic obstructive cardiomyopathy (idiopathic hypertrophic subaortic stenosis), J. Thorac. Cardiovasc. Surg. 51:49, 1966.

17a. Berman, M. A., Talner, N. S., and Stansel, H. C., Jr.: Experience with Mustard's operation in infants less than one year of age: Emphasis on late complications including patch stenosis, Surgery 73:133, 1973.

18. Bernhard, W. F., Dick, M., II, Sloss, L. J., Castaneda, A. R., and Nadas, A. S.: The palliative Mustard operation for double outlet right ventricle or transposition of the great arteries associated with ventricular septal defect, pulmonary arterial hypertension, and pulmonary vascular obstructive disease. A report of eight patients, Circulation 54:810, 1976.

19. Bharati, S., and Lev, M.: The conduction system in simple, regular (d-), complete transposition with ventricular septal defect, J. Thorac. Cardiovasc. Surg. 72:194, 1976.

20. Billette, J. Elharrar, V., Porlier, G., and Nadeau, R. A.: Sinus slowing produced by experimental ischemia of the sinus node in dogs, Am. J. Cardiol. 31:331, 1973.

21. Blalock, A., and Hanlon, C. R.: The surgical treatment of complete transposition of the aorta and the pulmonary artery, Surg. Gynecol. Obstet. 90:1, 1950.

22. Bowman, F. O., Hancock, W. D., and Malm, J. R.: A valve-containing Dacron prosthesis. Its use in restoring pulmonary artery-right ventricular continuity, Arch. Surg. 107:724, 1973.

23. Breckenridge, I. M., Stark, J., Bonham-Carter, R. E., Oelert, H., Graham, G. R., and Waterston, D. J.: Mustard's operation for transposition of the great arteries. Review of 200 cases, Lancet 1:1140, 1972.

24. Brom, G. A.: Technique of Mustard Operation, in Hahn, C. (ed.), *Thorax Chirurgie, Leiden 1950–1975* (Leiden: Netherlands Drukkerij Bedrijf B. V., 1975).

25. Carpena, C., and Subramanian, S.: Management of the ventricular septal defect in transposition, Am. J. Cardiol. 33:130, 1974.

26. Carpentier, A., Deloche, A., Hanania, G., Forman, J., Sellier, Ph., Piwnica, A., and Dubost, Ch.: Surgical management of acquired tricuspid valve disease, J. Thorac. Cardiovasc. Surg. 67:53, 1974.

27. Castaneda, A. R., Metras, D., and Buckley, L. P.: Transposition of the great arteries with ventricular septal defect: Surgical experience with the Mustard operation and closure of the ventricular septal defect, Proc. 7th Eur. Congr. Cardiol., Amsterdam, June, 1976, p. 566.

28. Castaneda, A. R., Norwood, W. I., Williams, R., and Nadas, A.: Deep hypothermia and circulatory arrest technique for repair of congenital heart defects in infancy, Proc. 7th Eur. Congr. Cardiol., Amsterdam, June, 1976, p. 409.

29. Champsaur, G. L., Sokol, D. M., Trusler, G. A., and Mustard, W. T.: Repair of transposition of the great arteries in 123 pediatric patients: Early and long-term results, Circulation 47: 1032, 1973.

30. Chiariello, L., Agosti, J., Vlad, P., and Subramanian, S.: Management of left ventricular outflow tract obstruction in complex transposition: A critical review of our experience, Circulation 51–52(Supp. 2):169, 1975.

31. Clarke, C. P., Bath, S. T., Curtis, K., and Brown, T. C. K.: A simple method of perfusion for refashioning the intra-atrial baffle after physiological correction of transposition of the great vessels, Aust. N.Z. J. Surg. 42:238, 1973.

32. Clarkson, P. M., Barratt-Boyes, B. G., and Neutze, J. M.: Late dysrhythmias and disturbances of conduction following Mustard operation for complete transposition of the great arteries, Circulation 53:519, 1976.

33. Clarkson, P. M., Barratt-Boyes, B. G., Neutze, J. M., and Lowe, J. R.: Results over a ten-year period of palliation followed by corrective surgery for complete transposition of the great arteries, Circulation 45:1251, 1972.

34. Clarkson, P. M., Neutze, J. M., Barratt-Boyes, B. G., and Brandt, P. W. T.: Late postoperative hemodynamic results and cineangiocardiographic findings after Mustard atrial baffle repair for transposition of the great arteries, Circulation 53:525, 1976.

35. Clarkson, P. M., Neutze, J. M., Wardill, J. C., and Barratt-Boyes, B. G.: The pulmonary vascular bed in patients with complete transposition of the great arteries, Circulation 53: 539, 1976.

36. Cohn, L. H., Kosek, J. C., and Angell, W. W.: Pulmonary arteriosclerosis produced by hyperoxemic normotensive perfusion, Surgery 70:723, 1971.

37. Cooley, D. A.: Personal communication, August, 1972.

38. Cooley, D. A., Angelini, P., Leachman, R. D., and Kyger, E. R., III: Intraventricular repair of transposition complexes with ventricular septal defect, J. Thorac. Cardiovasc. Surg. 71:461, 1976.

39. Creech, O., Jr., Mahaffey, D. E., Sayegh, S. F., and Sailors, E. L.: Complete transposition of the great vessels: A technique for intracardiac correction, Surgery 43:349, 1958.

40. Daenen, W., de Leval, M., and Stark, J.: Transposition of great arteries, ventricular septal defect, and left ventricular outflow tract obstruction: Results of 23 Rastelli operations, Br. Heart J. 38:878, 1976.

41. Damus, P. S.: Letter to the Editor, Ann. Thorac. Surg. 20:724, 1975.

42. Danielson, G. K., Cooper, E., Talwar, J., Ifuku, M., and Bryant, L. R.: Cardiac growth following atrial replacement with prosthetic materials, J. Thorac. Cardiovasc. Surg. 55:842, 1968.

43. Danielson, G. K., Mair, D. D., Ongley, P. A., Wallace, R. B., and McGoon, D. C.: Repair of transposition of the great arteries by transposition of venous return, J. Thorac. Cardiovasc. Surg. 61:96, 1971.

44. Danielson, G. K., Ritter, D. G., Coleman, H. N., III, and DuShane, J. W.: Successful repair of double-outlet right ventricle with transposition of the great arteries (aorta anterior and to the left), pulmonary stenosis, and subaortic ventricular septal defect, J. Thorac. Cardiovasc. Surg. 63:741, 1972.

45. de la Cruz, M. V., Berrazueta, J. R., Arteaga, M., Attie, F., and Soni, J.: Rules for diagnosis of arterioventricular discordances and spatial identification of ventricles. Crossed great arteries and transposition of the great arteries, Br. Heart J. 38:341, 1976.

46. Deverall, P. B., Tynan, M. J., Carr, I., Panagopoulos, P., Aberdeen, E., Bonham-Carter, R. E., and Waterston, D. J.: Palliative surgery in children with transposition of the great arteries, J. Thorac. Cardiovasc. Surg. 58:721, 1969.

47. Dick, M., II, Van Praagh, R., Rudd, M., Folkerth, T., and Castaneda, A. R.: Electrophysiologic delineation of the specialized atrioventricular conduction system in two patients with corrected transposition of the great arteries in situs inversus (I,D,D), Circulation 55:896, 1977.

48. Dillon, J. C., Feigenbaum, H., Konecke, L. L., Keutel, J., Hurwitz, R. A., Davis, R. H., and Chang, S.: Echocardiographic manifestations of d-transposition of the great vessels, Am. J. Cardiol. 32:74, 1973.

49. Duran, C. G., and Ubago, J. L. M.: Clinical and hemodynamic performance of a totally flexible prosthetic ring for atrioventricular valve reconstruction, Ann. Thorac. Surg. 22:458, 1976.

50. Ebert, P. A., Gay, W. A., Jr., and Engle, M. A.: Correction of transposition of the great arteries: Relationship of the coronary sinus and postoperative arrhythmias, Ann. Surg. 180:433, 1974.

51. Edwards, W. S., Bargeron, L. M., Jr., and Lyons, C.: Reposition

of right pulmonary veins in transposition of great vessels, JAMA 188:522, 1964.

52. El-Said, G. M., Gillette, P. C., Cooley, D. A., Mullins, C. E., and McNamara, D. G.: Protection of the sinus node in Mustard's operation, Circulation 53:788, 1976.

53. El-Said, G. M., Gillette, P. C., Mullins, C. E., Nihill, M. R., and McNamara, D. G.: Significance of pacemaker recovery time after the Mustard operation for transposition of the great arteries, Am. J. Cardiol. 38:448, 1976.

54. El-Said, G. M., Mullins, C. E., Gillette, P. C., Cooley, D. A., and McNamara, D. G.: Effect of modifications to protect the S-A node on dysrhythmias after Mustard operation for transposition of the great arteries, Circulation 52(Supp. 2):178, 1975.

55. El-Said, G., Mullins, C. E., Nihill, M. R., Hallman, G. L., Cooley, D. A., and McNamara, D. G.: Hemodynamic changes after Mustard's operation for transposition of the great arteries, Am. J. Cardiol. 31:129, 1973.

56. Engel, T. R., Meister, S. G., Feitosa, G. S., Fischer, H. A., and Frankl, W. S.: Appraisal of sinus node artery disease, Circulation 52:286, 1975.

57. Ferencz, C.: Transposition of the great vessels: Pathophysiologic considerations based upon a study of the lungs, Circulation 33:232, 1966.

58. Fox, L. S., Kirklin, J. W., Pacifico, A. D., Waldo, A. L., and Bargeron, L. M., Jr.: Intracardiac repair of cardiac malformations with atrioventricular discordance, Circulation 54:123, 1976.

59. Friedberg, D. Z., and Nadas, A. S.: Clinical profile of patients with congenital corrected transposition of the great arteries. A study of 60 cases, N. Engl. J. Med. 282:1053, 1970.

60. Godman, M. J., Friedli, B., Pasternac, A., Kidd, B. S. L., Trusler, G. A., and Mustard, W. T.: Hemodynamic studies in children four to ten years after Mustard operation for transposition of the great arteries, Circulation 53:532, 1976.

61. Graham, T. P., Jr., Atwood, G. F., Boucek, R. J., Jr., Boerth, R. C., and Bender, H. W., Jr.: Abnormalities of right ventricular function following Mustard's operation for transposition of the great arteries, Circulation 52:678, 1975.

62. Graham, T. P., Jr., Jarmakani, J. M., Canent, R. V., Jr., and Jewett, P. H.: Quantification of left heart volume and systolic output in transposition of the great arteries, Circulation 44:899, 1971.

63. Grehl, T. M., and Shumway, N. E.: Transposition of the great arteries: Reoperation for dysfunctional intra-atrial baffle, J. Thorac. Cardiovasc. Surg. 67:863, 1974.

64. Griepp, R.: In discussion of Idriss, F. S., *et al.*: Transposition of the great vessels with ventricular septal defect: Surgical and anatomic considerations, J. Thorac. Cardiovasc. Surg. 68:732, 1974.

65. Grondin, P., Meere, C., Limet, R., Lopez-Bescos, L., Delcan, J-L., and Rivera, R.: Carpentier's annulus and De Vega's annuloplasty. The end of the tricuspid challenge, J. Thorac. Cardiovasc. Surg. 70:852, 1975.

66. Guyton, A. C., Jones, C. E., and Coleman, T. G.: *Circulatory Physiology: Cardiac Output and Its Regulation* (Philadelphia: W. B. Saunders Company, 1973).

67. Hagler, D. J., Ritter, D. G., and Mair, D. D.: Hemodynamic assessment of the Mustard procedure for complete transposition of the great arteries, Am. J. Cardiol. 39:295, 1977.

68. Haller, J. A., Crisler, C., Brawley, R., Cameron, J., and Rowe, R. D.: Operative correction and postoperative management of transposition of the great vessels in nine children, Ann. Thorac. Surg. 7:212, 1969.

69. Hallman, G. L., Gill, S. S., Bloodwell, R. D., McNamara, D. G., Latson, J. R., Leachman, R. D., and Cooley, D. A.: Surgical treatment of cardiac defects associated with corrected transposition of the great vessels, Circulation 35–36(Supp. 1):133, 1967.

70. Hanlon, C. R., and Blalock, A.: Complete transposition of the aorta and the pulmonary artery: Experimental observations on venous shunts as corrective procedures, Ann. Surg. 127:385, 1948.

71. Hatch, D. J.: Cardiac Surgery in the First Year of Life, in Branthwaite, M. A. (ed.), *Anaesthesia for Cardiosurgery* (Oxford: Blackwell Scientific Publications, 1977), Chap. 9, pp. 151–181.

72. Hikasa, Y., Shirotani, H., Satomura, K., Muraoka, R., Abe, K., Tsushimi, K., Yokota, Y., Miki, S., Kawai, J., Mori, A., Okamoto, Y., Koie, H., Ban, T., Kanzaki, Y., and Yokota, M.: Open heart surgery in infants with an aid of hypothermic anesthesia, Arch. Jpn. Chir. 36:495, 1967.

73. Idriss, F. S., Aubert, J., Paul, M., Nikaidoh, J., Lev, M., and Newfeld, E. A.: Transposition of the great vessels with ventric-

74. Imamura, E., Morikawa, T., Tatsuno, K., Okamoto, K., Imai, Y., and Konno, S.: Conduit repairs of transposition complexes. A report of 14 cases, J. Thorac. Cardiovasc. Surg. 73:570, 1977.

75. Isaacson, R., Titus, J. L., Merideth, J., Feldt, R. H., and McGoon, D. C.: Apparent interruption of atrial conduction pathways after surgical repair of transposition of great arteries, Am. J. Cardiol. 30:533, 1972.

76. Jacobs, T., de Leval, M., and Stark, J.: False aneurysm of right ventricle after Rastelli operation for transposition of great arteries, ventricular septal defect, and pulmonary stenosis, J. Thorac. Cardiovasc. Surg. 67:543, 1974.

77. James, T. N.: The connecting pathways between the sinus node and A-V node and between the right and the left atrium in the human heart, Am. Heart J. 66:498, 1963.

78. James, T. N., and Hershey, E. A., Jr.: Experimental studies on the pathogenesis of atrial arrhythmias in myocardial infarction, Am. Heart J. 63:196, 1962.

79. James, T. N., and Reemtsma, K.: The response of sinus node function to ligation of the sinus node artery, Henry Ford Hosp. Med. Bull. 8:129, 1960.

80. Janse, M. J., and Anderson, R. H.: Specialized internodal atrial pathways—fact or fiction? Eur. J. Cardiol. 2:117, 1974.

81. Jarmakani, J. M. M., and Canent, R. V., Jr.: Preoperative and postoperative right ventricular function in children with transposition of the great vessels, Circulation 49–50(Supp. 2):39, 1974.

82. Jatene, A. D., Fontes, V. F., Paulista, P. P., Souza, L. C. B., Neger, F., Galantier, M., and Souza, J. E. M. R.: Successful anatomic correction of transposition of the great vessels. A preliminary report, Arq. Bras. Cardiol. 28:461, 1975.

83. Jatene, A. D., Fontes, V. F., Paulista, P. P., Souza, L. C. B., Neger, F., Galantier, M., and Souza, J. E. M. R.: Anatomic correction of transposition of the great vessels, J. Thorac. Cardiovasc. Surg. 72:364, 1976.

84. Jonsson, B., Ovenfors, C., and Senning, A.: Surgically corrected case of transposition of the great vessels, Acta Chir. Scand. 245(Supp.):297, 1959.

85. Jynge, P., Hearse, D-J., and Braimbridge, M. V.: Myocardial protection during ischemic cardiac arrest. A possible hazard with calcium-free cardioplegic infusates, J. Thorac. Cardiovasc. Surg. 73:848, 1977.

86. Kaye, M. P.: Anatomic correction of transposition of great arteries, Mayo Clin. Proc. 50:638, 1975.

87. Kilman, J. W., Williams, T. E., Jr., Kakos, G. S., Craenen, J., and Hosier, D. M.: Surgical correction of the transposition complex in infancy, J. Thorac. Cardiovasc. Surg. 66:387, 1973.

88. Kinsley, R. H., McGoon, D. C., and Danielson, G. K.: Corrected transposition of the great arteries, Circulation 49:574, 1974.

89. Kinsley, R. H., Ritter, D. G., and McGoon, D. C.: The surgical repair of positional anomalies of the conotruncus, J. Thorac. Cardiovasc. Surg. 67:395, 1974.

90. Kirklin, J. W.: Surgery for Transposition of the Great Arteries and Other Types of Malposition of the Great Arteries, in Barratt-Boyes, B. G., Neutze, J. M., and Harris, E. A. (eds.), *Heart Disease In Infancy. Diagnosis and Surgical Treatment* (London: Churchill Livingstone, 1973).

91. Kirklin, J. W., Devloo, R. A., and Weidman, W. H.: Open intracardiac repair for transposition of the great vessels: 11 cases, Surgery 50:58, 1961.

92. Kirklin, J. W., Pacifico, A. D., Bargeron, L. M., Jr., and Soto, B.: Cardiac repair in anatomically corrected malposition of the great arteries, Circulation 48:153, 1973.

93. Kirklin, J. W., and Silver, A. W.: Technic of exposing the ductus arteriosus prior to establishing extracorporeal circulation, Proc. Staff Meet. Mayo Clin. 33:423, 1958.

94. Kiser, J. C., Ongley, P. A., Kirklin, J. W., Clarkson, P. M., and McGoon, D. C.: Surgical treatment of dextrocardia with inversion of ventricles and double-outlet right ventricle, J. Thorac. Cardiovasc. Surg. 55:6, 1968.

95. Kreutzer, G., Neirotti, R., Galindez, E., Coronel, A. R., and Kreutzer, E.: Anatomic correction of transposition of the great arteries, J. Thorac. Cardiovasc. Surg. 73:538, 1977.

96. Krueger, S. K., Burney, D. W., and Ferlic, R. M.: Protein-losing enteropathy complicating the Mustard procedure, Surgery 81:305, 1977.

97. Kupersmith, J., Krongrad, E., Gersony, W. M., and Bowman, F. O., Jr.: Electrophysiologic identification of the specialized conduction system in corrected transposition of the great arteries, Circulation 50:795, 1974.

98. Lakier, J. B., Stanger, P., Heymann, M. A., Hoffman, J. I. E.,

and Rudolph, A. M.: Early onset of pulmonary vascular obstruction in patients with aortopulmonary transposition and intact ventricular septum, Circulation 51:875, 1975.

99. Laks, H., and Castaneda, A. R.: Subclavian arterioplasty for the ipsilateral Blalock-Taussig shunt, Ann. Thorac. Surg. 19:319, 1975.
100. Lev, M.: Pathologic diagnosis of positional variations in cardiac chambers in congenital heart disease, Lab. Invest. 3:71, 1954.
101. Lev, M., Fielding, R. T., and Zaeske, D.: Mixed levocardia with ventricular inversion (corrected transposition) with complete atrioventricular block. A histopathologic study of the conduction system, Am. J. Cardiol. 12:875, 1963.
102. Lev, M., Rimoldi, H. J. A., Paiva, R., and Arcilla, R. A.: The quantitative anatomy of simple complete transposition, Am. J. Cardiol. 23:409, 1969.
103. Liebman, J., Cullum, L., and Belloc, N. B.: Natural history of transposition of the great arteries: Anatomy and birth and death characteristics, Circulation 40:237, 1969.
104. Lillehei, C. W., and Varco, R. L.: Certain physiologic, pathologic, and surgical features of complete transposition of the great vessels, Surgery 34:376, 1953.
105. Lindesmith, G. G., Stanton, R. E., Lurie, P. R., Takahashi, M., Tucker, B. L., Stiles, Q. R., and Meyer, B. W.: An assessment of Mustard's operation as a palliative procedure for transposition of the great vessels, Ann. Thorac. Surg. 19:514, 1975.
106. Lindesmith, G. G., Stiles, Q. R., Tucker, B. L., Gallaher, M. E., Stanton, R. E., and Meyer, B. W.: The Mustard operation as a palliative procedure, J. Thorac. Cardiovasc. Surg. 63:75, 1972.
107. Mair, D. D., Danielson, G. K., Wallace, R. B., and McGoon, D. C.: Long-term follow-up of Mustard operation survivors, Circulation 49–50(Supp. 2):46, 1974.
108. Mair, D. D., and Ritter, D. G.: Factors influencing intercirculatory mixing in patients with complete transposition of the great arteries, Am. J. Cardiol. 30:653, 1972.
109. Mair, D. D., Ritter, D. G., Danielson, G. K., Wallace, R. B., and McGoon, D. C.: The palliative Mustard operation: Rationale and results, Am. J. Cardiol. 37:762, 1976.
110. Mair, D. D., Ritter, D. G., Ongley, P. A., and Helmholz, H. F., Jr.: Hemodynamics and evaluation for surgery of patients with complete transposition of the great arteries and ventricular septal defect, Am. J. Cardiol. 28:632, 1971.
111. Maloney, J. D., Fiddler, G. I., Danielson, G. K., McGoon, D. C., Wallace, R. B., and Ritter, D. G.: Intraoperative identification of the conduction system in congenital heart disease with atrioventricular discordance (ventricular inversion), Circulation 55–56(Supp. 3):105, 1977.
112. Mamiya, R. T., Moreno-Cabral, R. J., Nakamura, F. T., and Sprague, A. Y.: Retransposition of the great vessels for transposition with ventricular septal defect and pulmonary hypertension, J. Thorac. Cardiovasc. Surg. 73:340, 1977.
113. Marcelletti, C., Mair, D. D., McGoon, D. C., Wallace, R. B., and Danielson, G. K.: Complete repair of transposition of the great arteries with pulmonary atresia, J. Thorac. Cardiovasc. Surg. 72:215, 1976b.
114. Marcelletti, C., Mair, D. D., McGoon, D. C., Wallace, R. B., and Danielson, G. K.: The Rastelli operation for transposition of the great arteries. Early and late results, J. Thorac. Cardiovasc. Surg. 72:427, 1976a.
115. Marcelletti, C., Wallace, R. B., and Ritter, D. G.: Reconstruction of superior vena cava-right atrial continuity and "anatomic" repair of transposition of great arteries with ventricular septal defect. Report of case, Mayo Clin. Proc. 51:163, 1976.
116. Mauck, H. P., Robertson, L. W., Parr, E. L., and Lower, R. R.: Anatomic correction of transposition of the great arteries without significant ventricular septal defect or patent ductus arteriosus, J. Thorac. Cardiovasc. Surg. 74:631, 1977.
117. Mazzei, E. A., and Mulder, D. G.: Superior vena cava syndrome following complete correction (Mustard repair) of transposition of the great vessels, Ann. Thorac. Surg. 11:243, 1971.
118. McGoon, D. C.: Intraventricular repair of transposition of the great arteries, J. Thorac. Cardiovasc. Surg. 64:430, 1972.
119. McGoon, D. C.: Left ventricular and biventricular extracardiac conduits, J. Thorac. Cardiovasc. Surg. 72:7, 1976.
120. Merendino, K. A., Jesseph, J. E., Herron, P. W., Thomas, G. I., and Vetto, R. R.: Interatrial venous transposition. A one-stage intracardiac operation for the conversion of complete transposition of the aorta and pulmonary artery to corrected transposition: Theory and clinical experience, Surgery 42:898, 1957.
121. Merideth, J., and Titus, J. L.: The anatomic atrial connections between sinus and A-V node, Circulation 37:566, 1968.

122. Miller, B. L., Posner, P., and Daicoff, G. R.: Early detection of dysrhythmias following repair of transposition of the great arteries, Circulation 52(Supp. 2):217, 1975.
123. Mohri, H., Barnes, R. W., Rittenhouse, E. A., Reichenbach, D. D., Dillard, D. H., and Merendino, K. A.: Fate of autologous pericardium and Dacron fabric used as substitutes for total atrial septum in growing animals, J. Thorac. Cardiovasc. Surg. 59:501, 1970.
124. Moodie, D. S., Feldt, R. H., and Wallace, R. B.: Transient protein-losing enteropathy secondary to elevated caval pressures and caval obstruction after the Mustard procedure, J. Thorac. Cardiovasc. Surg. 72:379, 1976.
125. Morgan, J. R., Miller, B. L., Daicoff, G. R., and Andrews, E. J.: Hemodynamic and angiocardiographic evaluation after Mustard procedure for transposition of the great arteries, J. Thorac. Cardiovasc. Surg. 64:878, 1972.
126. Mori, A., Ando, F., Setsuie, N., Yamaguehi, K., Oku, H., Kanzaki, Y., Kawai, J., Shirotani, H., Makino, S., and Yokoyama, T.: Operative indication for corrective surgery in cases of complete transposition of the great arteries associated with large ventricular septal defect, J. Thorac. Cardiovasc. Surg. 71:750, 1976.
127. Mustard, W. T.: Successful two-stage correction of transposition of the great vessels, Surgery 55:469, 1964.
128. Muster, A. J., Paul, M. H., and Idriss, F. S.: Hemodynamics and angiography after the Mustard operation, Am. J. Cardiol. 37:159, 1976.
129. Muster, A., Paul, M., Levin, D., Conway, J., and Newfeld, E.: Diminished left pulmonary blood flow in transposition of the great arteries, Am. J. Cardiol. 31:150, 1973.
130. Nadas, A. S., and Fyler, D. C.: Corrected Transposition of the Great Arteries, in Nadas, A. S., and Fyler, D. C., *Pediatric Cardiology* (Philadelphia: W. B. Saunders Company, 1972), pp. 629–638.
131. Nadas, A. S., Fyler, D. C., and Castaneda, A. R.: The critically ill infant with congenital heart disease, Mod. Concepts Cardiovasc. Dis. 42:53, 1973.
132. Nagai, I., Kawashima, Y., Fujita, T., Mori, T., and Manabe, H.: Successful closure of ventricular septal defect through a left-sided ventriculotomy in corrected transposition of the great vessels, Ann. Thorac. Surg. 21:492, 1976.
133. Nanda, N. C., Gramiak, R., Manning, J. A., and Lipchik, E. O.: Echocardiographic features of subpulmonic obstruction in dextro-transposition of the great vessels, Circulation 51:515, 1975.
134. Newfeld, E. A., Paul, M. H., Muster, A. J., and Idriss, F. S.: Pulmonary vascular disease in complete transposition of the great arteries: A study of 200 patients, Am. J. Cardiol. 34:75, 1974.
135. Noonan, J. A., Nadas, A. S., Rudolph, A. M., and Harris, G. B. C.: Transposition of the great arteries: A correlation of clinical, physiologic, and autopsy data, N. Engl. J. Med. 263:592, 1960.
136. Oelert, H., and Borst, H.: Atrial Inversion for Transposition of the Great Arteries Using an Intra-atrial Dacron Baffle. Surgical Technique and Results, in Longmore, D. B. (ed.), *Modern Cardiac Surgery* (London: Medical Technical Press, 1977).
137. Okamura, K., and Konno, S.: Two types of ventricular septal defect in corrected transposition of the great arteries: Reference to surgical approaches, Am. Heart J. 85:483, 1973.
138. Park, S. C., Neches, W. H., Lenox, C. C., Zuberbuhler, J. R., and Bahnson, H. T.: Massive calcification and obstruction in a homograft after the Rastelli procedure for transposition of great arteries, Am. J. Cardiol. 32:860, 1973.
139. Parr, G. V. S., Blackstone, E. H., and Kirklin, J. W.: Cardiac performance and mortality early after intracardiac surgery in infants and young children, Circulation 51:867, 1975.
140. Parr, G. V. S., Blackstone, E. H., Kirklin, J. W., Pacifico, A. D., and Lauridsen, P.: Cardiac performance early after interatrial transposition of venous return in infants and small children, Circulation 49–50(Supp. 2):2, 1974.
141. Partridge, J. B., Scott, O., Deverall, P. B., and Macartney, F. J.: Visualization and measurement of the main bronchi by tomography as an objective indicator of thoracic situs in congenital heart disease, Circulation 51:188, 1975.
142. Plauth, W. H., Jr., Nadas, A. S., Bernhard, W. F., and Fyler, D. C.: Changing hemodynamics in patients with transposition of the great arteries, Circulation 42:131, 1970.
143. Quaegebeur, J. M., Rohmer, J., Brom, A. G., and Tinkleberg, J.: Revival of the Senning operation in the treatment of transposition of the great arteries, Thorax 32:517, 1977.
144. Rashkind, W. J., and Miller, W. W.: Creation of an atrial septal

defect without thoracotomy: A palliative approach to complete transposition of the great arteries, JAMA 196:173, 1966.

145. Rastelli, G. C., McGoon, D. C., and Wallace, R. B.: Anatomic correction of transposition of the great arteries with ventricular septal defect and subpulmonary stenosis, J. Thorac. Cardiovasc. Surg. 58:545, 1969.

146. Rastelli, G. C., Wallace, R. B., and Ongley, P. A.: Complete repair of transposition of the great arteries with pulmonary stenosis. A review and report of a case corrected by using a new surgical technique, Circulation 39:83, 1969.

147. Replogle, R. L., and Lin, C.: Surgical correction of transposition of the great vessels, J. Thorac. Cardiovasc. Surg. 63:196, 1972.

148. Riemenschneider, T. A., Goldberg, S. J., Ruttenberg, H. D., and Gyepes, M. T.: Subpulmonic obstruction in complete (d) transposition produced by redundant tricuspid tissue, Circulation 39:603, 1969.

149. Rittenhouse, E. A., Mohri, H., Dillard, D. H., and Merendino, K. A.: Deep hypothermia in cardiovascular surgery, Ann. Thorac. Surg. 17:63, 1974.

150. Rocchini, A. P., Rosenthal, A., Castaneda, A. R., Keane, J. F., and Jeresaty, R.: Subaortic obstruction after the use of an intracardiac baffle to tunnel the left ventricle to the aorta, Circulation 54:957, 1976.

151. Rohmer, J., Quaegebeur, J. M., and Brom, A. G.: Takedown and reconstruction of cavopulmonary anastomosis, Ann. Thorac. Surg. 23:129, 1977.

152. Rosenquist, G. C., Stark, J., and Taylor, J. F. N.: Congenital mitral valve disease in transposition of the great arteries, Circulation 51:731, 1975.

153. Ross, D., Rickards, A., and Somerville, J.: Transposition of the great arteries: Logical anatomical arterial correction, Br. Med. J. 1:1109, 1976.

154. Ross, D. N., and Somerville, J.: Correction of pulmonary atresia with a homograft aortic valve, Lancet 2:1446, 1966.

155. Rowlatt, U. F.: Coronary artery distribution in complete transposition, JAMA 149:269, 1962.

156. Senning, A.: Correction of the transposition of the great arteries, Ann. Surg. 182:287, 1975.

157. Senning, A.: Surgical correction of transposition of the great vessels, Surgery 45:966, 1959.

158. Seward, J. B., Tajik, A. J., Giuliani, E. R., and Mair, D. D.: Aneurysm of the membranous ventricular septum in TGA: Echo features, Circulation 54:161, 1976.

159. Shaher, R. M.: *Complete Transposition of the Great Arteries* (New York: Academic Press, 1973).

160. Shaher, R. M., Keith, J. D., and Mustard, W. T.: Necropsy findings eight months after total correction of complete transposition of the great vessels by the interatrial baffle technique, Can. Med. Assoc. J. 94:1127, 1966.

161. Shaher, R. M., and Kidd, L.: Acid-base balance in complete transposition of the great vessels, Br. Heart J. 29:207, 1967.

162. Shaher, R. M., Moes, C. A. F., and Khoury, G.: Radiologic and angiocardiographic findings in complete transposition of the great vessels with left ventricular outflow tract obstruction, Radiology 88:1092, 1967.

163. Shaher, R. M., and Puddu, G. C.: Coronary arterial anatomy in complete transposition of the great vessels, Am. J. Cardiol. 17:355, 1966.

164. Shaher, R. M., Puddu, G. C., Khoury, G., Moes, C. A. F., and Mustard W. T.: Complete transposition of the great vessels with anatomic obstruction of the outflow tract of the left ventricle: Surgical implications of anatomic findings, Am. J. Cardiol. 19:658, 1967.

165. Shinebourne, E. A., Macartney, F. J., and Anderson, R. H.: Sequential chamber localization—logical approach to diagnosis in congenital heart disease, Br. Heart J. 38:327, 1976.

166. Shrivastava, S., Tadavarthy, S. M., Fukuda, T., and Edwards, J. E.: Anatomic causes of pulmonary stenosis in complete transposition, Circulation 54:154, 1976.

167. Shumway, N. E., Griepp, R. B., and Stinson, E. B.: Surgical management of transposition of the great arteries, Am. J. Surg. 130:233, 1975.

168. Silove, E. D., and Taylor, J. F. N.: Angiographic and anatomical features of subvalvar left ventricular outflow obstruction in transposition of the great arteries: The possible role of the anterior mitral valve leaflet, Pediatr. Radiol. 1:87, 1973.

169. Silove, E. D., and Taylor, J. F. N.: Haemodynamics after Mustard's operation for transposition of the great arteries, Br. Heart J. 38:1037, 1976.

170. Singh, A. K., Dillon, M., and Stark, J.: Mustard operation for TGA in a 3-day-old infant, complicated by acute renal failure, J. Thorac. Cardiovasc. Surg. 18:387, 1977.

171. Singh, A. K., Stark, J., and Taylor, J. F. N.: Left ventricle to pulmonary artery conduit in treatment of transposition of great arteries, restrictive ventricular septal defect, and acquired pulmonary atresia, Br. Heart J. 38:1213, 1976.

172. Sørland, S. J., Tjønneland, S., and Hall, K. V.: Transposition of great arteries. Early results of Mustard's operation in paediatric patients, Br. Heart J. 38:584, 1976.

173. Stafford, E. G., and McGoon, D. C.: The Mustard operation: Use of an elastic knitted Dacron patch, Mayo Clin. Proc. 48:119, 1973.

174. Stansel, H. C., Jr.: A new operation for d-loop transposition of the great vessels, Ann. Thorac. Surg. 19:565, 1975.

175. Stark, J.: Operation results for transposition of the great arteries, Adv. Cardiol. 17:20, 1976.

176. Stark, J., de Leval, M. R., and Taylor, J. F. N.: Mustard operation and creation of ventricular septal defect in two patients with transposition of the great arteries, intact ventricular septum and pulmonary vascular disease, Am. J. Cardiol. 38:524, 1976.

177. Stark, J., de Leval, M. R., Waterston, D. J., Graham, G. R., and Bonham-Carter, R. E.: Corrective surgery of transposition of the great arteries in the first year of life: Results in 63 infants, J. Thorac. Cardiovasc. Surg. 67:673, 1974.

178. Stark, J., Hucin, B., Aberdeen, E., and Waterston, D. J.: Cardiac surgery in the first year of life: Experience with 1,049 operations, Surgery 69:483, 1971.

179. Stark, J., Silove, E. D., Taylor, J. F. N., and Graham, G. R.: Obstruction to systemic venous return following the Mustard operation for transposition of the great arteries, J. Thorac. Cardiovasc. Surg. 68:742, 1974.

180. Stark, J., Tynan, M., Tatooles, C. J., Aberdeen, E., and Waterston, D. J.: Banding of the pulmonary artery for transposition of the great arteries and ventricular septal defect, Circulation 41–42(Supp. 2):116, 1970.

181. Subramanian, S., and Wagner, H.: Correction of transposition of the great arteries in infants under surface-induced deep hypothermia, Ann. Thorac. Surg. 16:391, 1973.

182. Suga, H.: Importance of atrial compliance in cardiac performance, Circ. Res. 35:39, 1974.

183. Sunderland, C. O., Henken, D. P., Nichols, G. M., Dhindsa, D. S., Bonchek, L. I., Menashe, V. D., Rahimtoola, S. H., Starr, A., and Less, M. H.: Postoperative hemodynamic and electrophysiologic evaluation of the interatrial baffle procedure, Am. J. Cardiol. 35:660, 1975.

184. Szarnicki, R. J., Stark, J., and de Leval, M.: Reoperation for complications following inflow correction for transposition of the great arteries, Ann. Thorac. Surg. 25:150, 1978.

185. Taguchi, K., Matsumura, H., Hirao, M., Kato, K., and Itano, M.: A new approach to total repair of transposition of the great vessels. A technique for atrial autotransplantation, J. Thorac. Cardiovasc. Surg. 70:282, 1975.

186. Trusler, G. A., Bull, R. C., Hoeksema, T., and Mustard, W. T.: The effect on cardiac output of a reduction in atrial volume, J. Thorac. Cardiovasc. Surg. 46:109, 1963.

187. Trusler, G. A., and Mustard, W. T.: Palliative and reparative procedures for transposition of the great arteries, Ann. Thorac. Surg. 17:410, 1974.

188. Tynan, M.: Transposition of the great arteries: Changes in the circulation after birth, Circulation 46:809, 1972.

189. Tynan, M., Aberdeen, E., and Stark, J.: Tricuspid incompetence after the Mustard operation for transposition of the great arteries, Circulation 45–46(Supp. 1): 111, 1972.

190. Tynan, M. J., Becker, A. E., Macartney, F. J., Quero-Jimenez, M., Shinebourne, E. A., and Anderson, R. H.: The nomenclature of congenital cardiac malformation (In press.)

191. Tynan, M., Carr, K., Graham, G., and Bonham-Carter, R. E.: Subvalvar pulmonary obstruction complicating the postoperative course in balloon atrial septostomy in transposition of the great arteries, Circulation 39–40(Supp. 1):223, 1969.

192. Urban, A. E., Stark, J., and Waterston, D. J.: Mustard's operation for transposition of the great arteries complicated by juxtaposition of the atrial appendages, Ann. Thorac. Surg. 21:304, 1976.

193. Utley, J. R., Todd, E. P., Noonan, J. A., and Achtel, R. A.: Aortopulmonary anastomosis for complex congenital heart disease: Greater mortality with l-transposition, Circulation 52(Supp. 2):252, 1975.

194. Van Mierop, L. H. S., Eisen, S., and Schiebler, G. L.: The radiographic appearance of the tracheobronchial tree as an indicator of visceral situs, Am. J. Cardiol. 26:432, 1970.

195. Van Praagh, R., Ongley, P. A., and Swan, H. J. C.: Anatomic types of single or common ventricle in man. Morphologic and geometric aspects of 60 necropsied cases, Am. J. Cardiol. 13: 367, 1964.

196. Venables, A. W., Edis, B., and Clarke, C. P.: Vena caval obstruction complicating the Mustard operation for complete transposition of the great arteries, Eur. J. Cardiol. 1/4:401, 1974.

197. Vidne, B., Duszynski, D., and Subramanian, S.: Pulmonary flow distribution in transposition of the great arteries, Am. J. Cardiol. 37:178, 1976a.

198. Vidne, B. A., and Subramanian, S.: Complete correction of transposition of the great arteries with left juxtaposition of the atrial appendages, Thorax 31:178, 1976.

199. Vidne, B. A., Subramanian, S., and Wagner, H. R.: Aneurysm of the membranous ventricular septum in transposition of the great arteries, Circulation 53:157, 1976b.

200. Viles, P. H., Ongley, P. A., and Titus, J. L.: The spectrum of pulmonary vascular disease in transposition of the great arteries, Circulation 40:31, 1969.

201. Wagenvoort, C. A., Nauta, J., van der Schaar, P. J., Weeds, H. W. H., and Wagenvoort, N.: The pulmonary vasculature in complete transposition of the great vessels, judged from lung biopsies, Circulation 38:746, 1968.

202. Waldhausen, J. A., Pierce, W. S., Park, C. D., Rashkind, W. J., and Friedman, S.: Physiologic correction of transposition of the great arteries: Indications for and results of operation in 32 patients, Circulation 43:738, 1971.

203. Waldman, J. D., Paul, M. H., Newfeld, E. A., Muster, A. J., and Idriss, F. S.: Transposition of the great arteries with intact ventricular septum and patent ductus arteriosus, Am. J. Cardiol. 35:175, 1975.

204. Wittig, J. H., de Leval, M. R., and Stark, J.: Intraoperative mapping of atrial activation before, during, and after the Mustard operation, J. Thorac. Cardiovasc. Surg. 73:1, 1977.

205. Yacoub, M., and Radley-Smith, R.: Functional anatomy and correction of mitral regurgitation in infants and children, Circulation 51–52(Supp. 2):259, 1973.

206. Yacoub, M. H., Radley-Smith, R., and Hilton, C. J.: Anatomical correction of complete transposition of the great arteries and ventricular septal defect in infancy, Br. Med. J. 1:1112, 1976.

207. Yacoub, M. H., Radley-Smith, R., and Maclaurin, R.: Two-stage operation for anatomical correction of transposition of the great arteries with intact interventricular septum, Lancet 1: 1275, 1977.

208. Zavanella, C., and Subramanian, S.: Surgery for transposition of the great arteries in the first year of life, Ann. Surg. 187:143, 1978.

61 Dwight C. McGoon

Double-Outlet Right Ventricle

A CONTINUUM that defies sharp demarcation exists between various categories of conotruncal anatomy.[1] Double-outlet right ventricle (DORV) is a condition representing only a portion of this spectrum, and it blends imperceptibly with adjacent anomalies.[2] DORV sometimes has been defined as a condition in which both great arteries originate from the right ventricle, with circumferential myocardium present proximal to both semilunar valves and, hence, separation of each atrioventricular valve from both semilunar valves. At the opposite extreme, DORV is defined as any condition in which one great artery and at least one-half of the other originates from the right ventricle. In the latter instance, many patients previously designated as having tetralogy of Fallot would be included in the group with DORV. The problem would not exist if it were not for the ventricular septal defect that invariably is associated with DORV, since, in the spectrum of DORV, one or the other great artery can override the ventricular septal defect and, hence, originate in complementary proportion from each ventricle.

This problem of definition is not significantly relevant to the surgical management of an individual patient but becomes important when patients are grouped for the purpose of analyzing their characteristics, prognosis and results of management. For the individual patient, surgical repair involves one consideration that transcends these various definitions, namely, to route the blood from the cavae to the pulmonary artery and from the pulmonary veins to the aorta via the appropriate ventricle. However, since some position must be taken with respect to this dilemma of classification, our group includes as DORV only those conditions in which both semilunar valves originate essentially entirely from the right ventricle. Thus, when the aorta overrides the ventricular septal defect, the deformity is classified as severe tetralogy if pulmonary stenosis is associated—or, if not, as ventricular septal defect with overriding aorta. When the aorta originates from the right ventricle and the pulmonary artery overrides the ventricular septal defect, the deformity is classified as a variant of transposition of the great arteries.

Sixteen possible variations of DORV with regard to the interrelationships of the great arteries and to the location of the ventricular septal defect have been described.[3] These do not include the variants related to situs inversus and ventricular inversion. For practical purposes, and especially from the standpoint of surgical intervention, there are four types, and each of the four may or may not be associated with pulmonary stenosis (Fig. 61–1). These four types result from the two basic great arterial relationships (aorta to right of pulmonary artery—usually side by side or aorta slightly posterior or anterior—or aorta anterior or to the left of the pulmonary artery) and two basic locations of the ventricular septal defect (posterior or anterior in the septum). Sridaromont and associates[3] studied 60 hearts and found that the aorta was to the right in 56 and to the left in 4. Of the 56 with the aorta to the right, 39 had a subaortic (posterior) ventricular septal defect (Fig. 61–1, A), 2 had a subaortic and subpulmonary ventricular septal defect and 5 had a remote (malalignment of ventricular septum or muscular defect) ventricular septal defect; in 10 hearts, the ventricular septal defect was subpulmonary (anterior) (Fig. 61–1, B). Of the 4 hearts with aorta to the left, 3 had a subpulmonary ventricular septal defect (Fig. 61–1, C) and 1 had a subaortic ventric-

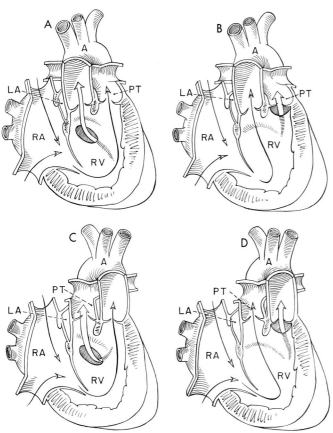

Fig. 61–1.—Four basic types of DORV. **A** and **B,** aorta to right. **A,** ventricular septal defect, subaortic (posterior). **B,** ventricular septal defect, subpulmonary (posterior). **C** and **D,** aorta anterior and to left. **C,** ventricular septal defect, subpulmonary (posterior). **D,** ventricular septal defect, subaortic (anterior). *A,* aorta; *PT,* pulmonary trunk; *LA,* left atrium; *RA,* right atrium; *RV,* right ventricle. (From Sridaromont, S., *et al.:* Double outlet right ventricle: Hemodynamic and anatomic correlations, Am. J. Cardiol. 38:85, 1976. By permission of Dun-Donnelley Publishing Corporation.)

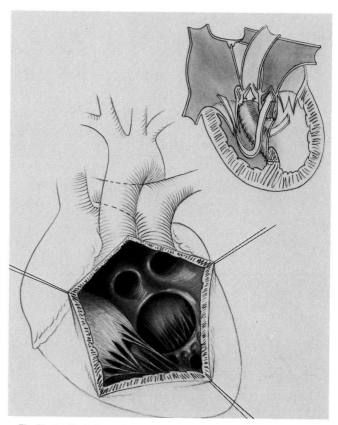

Fig. 61–2.—Technique of repair of DORV with aorta to right and subaortic (posterior) ventricular septal defect. Tunnel directs blood from left ventricle to aorta. (From Kinsley, R. H., Ritter, D. G., and McGoon, D. C.: The surgical repair of positional anomalies of the conotruncus, J. Thorac. Cardiovasc. Surg. 67:395, 1974. By permission of C. V. Mosby Company.)

ular septal defect (Fig. 61–1, *D*). Thus, the most common type of DORV is with the aorta to the right of the pulmonary artery and the ventricular septal defect is subpulmonary (posterior). This was the type first described and first encountered surgically and, hence, often called "classic" DORV. Kirklin first repaired this anomaly in 1957.[4, 5] As experience and knowledge regarding DORV advanced, the concept of four basic surgical types emerged in 1968.[6]

The surgeon has at least six techniques that allow correction of the various types of DORV. These include four methods for the correction of the four basic types of DORV, plus two that may be required for relief from associated pulmonary stenosis. These latter two are standard; the first is outflow-tract patch-graft reconstruction when the pulmonary outflow tract is to the left and the left coronary branches pass posteriorly to it, and the second is insertion of an extracardiac conduit from the right ventricle to the pulmonary artery when patch reconstruction is not feasible (outflow tract overlain by major coronary arteries).

Repair for the classic and most common type (Fig. 61–1, *A*) is shown in Figure 61–2, and this is really an extension of the classic repair for tetralogy, since, in effect, there is a 100% "dextrorotation" of the aorta. The left ventricular blood is simply directed by a tunnel created with a patch on the "floor" and rightward aspect of the right ventricular outflow tract through the ventricular septal defect and out the aorta.

When the aorta remains to the right but the ventricular septal defect is anterior and, hence, subpulmonary (Fig. 61–1, *B*), the accepted repair has been to close the ventricular septal defect so that the left ventricle drains to the pulmonary artery, thus creating transposition of the great arteries. The repair is completed by performing intra-atrial transposition of venous return (Mustard operation).[7] One must assess the possibility, even for this type of DORV, of creating a tunnel from ventricular septal defect to aorta as in the previous type, since success with this method has been reported.[8] Also, in this type of DORV there is the potential for newer methods other than the Mustard operation that are being explored for correction of transposition of the great arteries.

In the spectrum of interrelationships among the great arteries in DORV, when the aorta becomes situated more and more anteriorly, a point is reached where it no longer is feasible to extend a tunnel from a posterior ventricular septal defect along the "floor" and right wall of the outflow tract to reach the aorta. Beyond that point, the aortic annulus lies anteriorly or leftward from the pulmonic annulus (Fig. 61–1, *C*). For the repair of this anomaly, the tunnel must be placed along the "roof" and left wall of the outflow tract in order to reach the aorta (Fig. 61–3.)[6]

The most favorable anatomy, and rarest, is the leftward

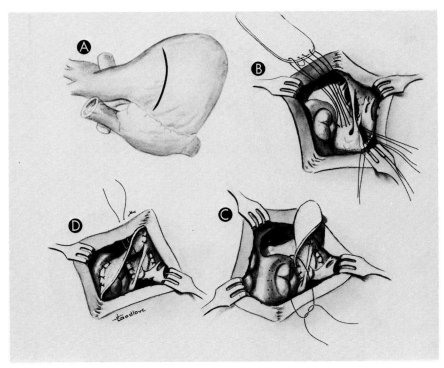

Fig. 61–3.—Technique of repair of DORV with aorta anterior or to left and subpulmonary (posterior) ventricular septal defect. Semilunar valve seen in **B, C** and **D** is the pulmonary valve, which lies posteriorly and to the right. (From Patrick, D. L., and McGoon, D. C.: An operation for double-outlet right ventricle with transposition of the great arteries, J. Cardiovasc. Surg. (Torino) 9:537, 1968. By permission of Edizioni Minerva Medica.)

position of the aorta, with respect to the pulmonary artery, and a subaortic (anterior) ventricular septal defect (Fig. 61–1, D). In this variant, the ventricular septal defect is closed so as to direct the left ventricular blood behind it to the aorta.[9] In a sense, this repair is similar to that for the previous type, except it is simplified because the ventricular septal defect and aortic annulus are more closely approximated.

These descriptions and discussions are confined to hearts with situs solitus and concordant atrioventricular relationships. With respect to situs inversus of the atria and viscera, it seems simpler to retain the same anatomic descriptions and surgical concepts as described but to recognize them as being mirror image rather than to invoke different terminology.[10] With respect to DORV in the presence of ventricular inversion (discordant atrioventricular relationships, which embryologically oriented classifications refer to as L-loop) there currently is only one appropriate surgical repair, which replaces the intracardiac repair originally described.[11] Thus, from the surgeon's standpoint, subclassification in the presence of inverted ventricles is not a practical exercise. The repair for this condition consists of a left ventriculotomy (that is, an incision in the right-sided "pulmonic" ventricle), closure of the ventricular septal defect to the right of both semilunar valves, division of the pulmonary trunk, closure of its proximal stump and, finally, insertion of an extracardiac valved conduit from the ventriculotomy to the distal end of the pulmonary trunk.

Since the simplification of classification and concept is desirable, if nothing is lost in validity and practicality, a surgical classification of DORV that is believed to be comprehensive and oriented toward technique of repair is presented in Table 61–1. It is a modification of many preceding contributions.[2, 12 14]

Angiocardiography remains the key to correct preoperative diagnosis. Principles of patient management are basical-

TABLE 61–1.—SURGICAL CLASSIFICATION OF DOUBLE-OUTLET RIGHT VENTRICLE°

TYPE	REPAIR
Atrioventricular Concordance	
Situs solitus	
Aorta to right, subaortic VSD	Tunnel RV "floor" (LV to aorta)
Aorta to right, subpulmonary VSD	Tunnel RV "roof" (LV to PT) plus Mustard operation
Aorta anterior or to left, subpulmonary VSD	Tunnel RV "roof" (LV to aorta)
Aorta anterior or to left, subaortic VSD	Tunnel RV "roof" (LV to aorta)
Situs inversus	
Same as above, except anatomy and repair in mirror image	
Atrioventricular Discordance	
Situs solitus or situs inversus	
Aorta anterior (pulmonary artery is posterior, either directly or to right or left of aorta)	Ventriculotomy in morphologic LV; closure VSD; extracardiac conduit

°Each type may or may not be associated with pulmonary stenosis. VSD, ventricular septal defect; RV, right ventricular; LV, left ventricle; PT, pulmonary trunk.

ly similar to those used in the management after repair of ventricular septal defect or tetralogy of Fallot. However, the risks of operation for the more complex repairs are higher than for simple ventricular septal defect or tetralogy repair.[5, 15, 16] Nevertheless, the risk of corrective operation is sufficiently low in current practice to make this the clearly indicated approach for the child with DORV. For infants, however, in whom continued medical management is inappropriate because of congestive heart failure (large pulmonary blood flow), progressive pulmonary vascular obstructive disease or severe cyanosis or hypoxic spells, there is a stronger reason to do the palliative operation (banding the pulmonary trunk or a systemic-to-pulmonary artery shunt, respectively) than exists for simple ventricular septal defect or tetralogy. This decision must be made on the basis of local factors and individual experience.

REFERENCES

1. Kinsley, R. H., Ritter, D. G., and McGoon, D. C.: The surgical repair of positional anomalies of the conotruncus, J. Thorac. Cardiovasc. Surg. 67:395, 1974.
2. Lev, M., *et al.:* A concept of double-outlet right ventricle, J. Thorac. Cardiovasc. Surg. 64:271, 1972.
3. Sridaromont, S., *et al.:* Double outlet right ventricle: Hemodynamic and anatomic correlations, Am. J. Cardiol. 38:85, 1976.
4. McGoon, D. C.: Origin of both great vessels from the right ventricle, Surg. Clin. North Am. 41:1113, 1961.
5. Kirklin, J. W., Harp, R. A., and McGoon, D. C.: Surgical treatment of origin of both vessels from right ventricle, including cases of pulmonary stenosis, J. Thorac. Cardiovasc. Surg. 48: 1026, 1964.
6. Patrick, D. L., and McGoon, D. C.: An operation for double-outlet right ventricle with transposition of the great arteries, J. Cardiovasc. Surg. (Torino) 9:537, 1968.
7. Hightower, B. M., *et al.:* Double-outlet right ventricle with transposed great arteries and subpulmonary ventricular septal defect: The Taussig-Bing malformation, Circulation 39(Supp. 1): 207, 1969.
8. Kawashima, Y., *et al.:* Intraventricular rerouting of blood for the correction of Taussig-Bing malformation, J. Thorac. Cardiovasc. Surg. 62:825, 1971.
9. Danielson, G. K., *et al.:* Successful repair of double-outlet right ventricle with transposition of the great arteries (aorta anterior and to the left), pulmonary stenosis, and subaortic ventricular septal defect, J. Thorac. Cardiovasc. Surg. 63:741, 1972.
10. Stewart, S., *et al.:* Complete correction of double-outlet right ventricle with situs inversus, l-loop, and l-malposition (I, L,L) with subaortic VSD and pulmonary stenosis, J. Thorac. Cardiovasc. Surg. 71:129, 1976.
11. Kiser, J. C., *et al.:* Surgical treatment of dextrocardia with inversion of ventricles and double-outlet right ventricle, J. Thorac. Cardiovasc. Surg. 55:6, 1968.
12. Pacifico, A. D., Kirklin, J. W., and Bargeron, L. M., Jr.: Complex Congenital Malformations: Surgical Treatment of Double-Outlet Right Ventricle and Double-Outlet Left Ventricle, in Kirklin, J. W. (ed.), *Advances in Cardiovascular Surgery* (New York: Grune & Stratton, 1973).
13. Van Praagh, R., *et al.:* Double outlet right ventricle (S,D,L) with subaortic ventricular septal defect and pulmonary stenosis: Report of six cases, Am. J. Cardiol. 35:42, 1975.
14. Stewart, S.: Double-outlet right ventricle: A collective review with a surgical viewpoint, J. Thorac. Cardiovasc. Surg. 71:355, 1976.
15. Gomes, M. M. R., *et al.:* Double-outlet right ventricle without pulmonic stenosis: Surgical considerations and results of operation, Circulation 43 (Supp. 1):31, 1971.
16. Gomes, M. M. R., *et al.:* Double-outlet right ventricle with pulmonic stenosis: Surgical considerations and results of operation, Circulation 43:889, 1971.

62 DWIGHT C. McGOON

Truncus Arteriosus and Pulmonary Atresia with Ventricular Septal Defect

A GROUP OF congenital cardiac defects shares the characteristic of discontinuity between the heart and the pulmonary artery. In such hearts, the proximal pulmonary trunk is absent and, in some, additional portions of the normal pulmonary arterial tree may be atretic. The three segments of the normal pulmonary arteries have separate embryonic origins: (1) the main pulmonary artery, or pulmonary trunk, from the truncus arteriosus, (2) right and left main pulmonary arteries from the sixth aortic arches and (3) intraparenchymal pulmonary arteries from the lung buds. Many combinations of absence or defective development of these segments may occur. Modifications of several prior classifications have led to the one presented in Table 62–1. The basic types of discontinuity between the heart and pulmonary artery are shown in Figures 62–1–62–6.

In a retrospective study,[1] two-thirds of the patients had pulmonary arteries present, one-fourth had them absent and one-twelfth had them absent in one lung. However, present techniques utilizing aortography and selective angiocardiographic contrast injections often reveal pulmonary arteries, sometimes of diminutive size, in patients who formerly were dismissed as having none.

If the pulmonary arteries originate from the ascending aorta, the condition is called "persistent truncus arteriosus" and if pulmonary blood flow is via some other source, the condition is called "pulmonary atresia."

Truncus Arteriosus

Persistent truncus arteriosus is an uncommon congenital cardiac malformation comprising about 1–4% of congenital cardiac defects in autopsy studies. The malformation results from a failure of the embryonic truncus and conus to partition during the first few weeks of fetal development. Thus, a single arterial vessel guarded by a single valve receives blood from both ventricles through a high ventricular septal defect, and this artery supplies blood to the coronary arteries, the pulmonary arteries and the thoracic aorta.

Several lesions are commonly associated with truncus arteriosus. The truncal valve usually has three cusps, but about one-third of hearts show two to four or even five or six cusps. The valve cusps often are thickened and deformed, resulting in significant truncal valve regurgitation in about one-fourth of patients. Truncal valve stenosis is seen occasionally, but rarely beyond infancy. The truncus frequently is dilated, probably secondary to the large blood flow. There are frequent anomalies of location of the coronary ostia, but usually with normal coronary arterial distribution. A right

TABLE 62-1.—CLASSIFICATION OF ABSENCE OF ANATOMIC ORIGIN FROM HEART OF PULMONARY ARTERIAL SUPPLY

I. Pulmonary arteries present
  A. Confluence of right and left pulmonary arteries
    1. Atresia of pulmonary trunk
      a. Proximal
      b. Diffuse
    2. Persistent truncus arteriosus (types 1 and 2)
  B. Nonconfluence of right and left pulmonary arteries
    1. Independent ductal origins
    2. Independent bronchial arterial origins
II. Pulmonary arteries absent (agenesis or atresia)
III. Mixed type
  One pulmonary artery and pulmonary trunk absent, flow to present pulmonary artery via:
  A. Ascending aorta (truncus arteriosus)
  B. Patent ductus arteriosus
  C. Potts' shunt
  D. Blalock-Taussig shunt
  E. Bronchial collateral arteries only

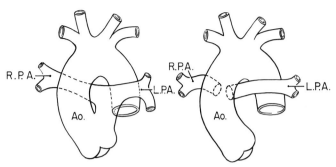

Fig. 62–3.—Truncus arteriosus, pulmonary arteries present. Confluence of right (R.P.A.) and left (L.P.A.) pulmonary arteries, plus persistent truncus arteriosus. *Left*, type 1. *Right*, type 2. *Ao.*, aorta. (From Berry, B. E., *et al.*: Absence of anatomic origin from heart of pulmonary arterial supply: Clinical application of classification, J. Thorac. Cardiovasc. Surg. 68:119, 1974. By permission of C. V. Mosby Company.)

aortic arch is encountered in at least 30% of patients. Complete interruption of the aortic arch was found in 6% of a surgical series of patients with truncus arteriosus,[2] and in each of these patients, the interruption was in the left aortic arch between the left common carotid and the left subclavian artery; a large patent ductus arteriosus provided the blood supply to the left subclavian artery and descending aorta. Sixteen per cent (11 patients) of a group of patients with truncus arteriosus who were studied by cardiac catheterization[3] had unilateral complete absence of a pulmonary artery. Seven of the 11 patients had absence of the left pulmonary artery and 4 had absence of the right pulmonary artery. Interestingly, 9 of the 11 had absence of the pulmonary artery on the same side as the aortic arch.

Truncus arteriosus originally was classified into four types by Collett and Edwards,[4] but Table 62-1 shows that only types 1 and 2 are now recognized. Type 1 is characterized by the presence of a short segment of pulmonary trunk from which the right and left pulmonary arteries bifurcate. Type 2 is characterized by the absence of a true pulmonary trunk with adjacent origin of the right and left pulmonary arteries from the posterolateral aspect of the truncus arteriosus. Since there seldom is significant separation of the origin of the right pulmonary artery from the truncus itself, it is difficult to subclassify most patients into type 1 or 2. The previously identified type 3 truncus seems to be only a slightly wider separation of the origins of the right and left pulmonary arteries from the posterolateral aspect of the truncus arteriosus, so that this rare variant can be readily absorbed into the type 2 classification. The original type 4 truncus arteriosus and the so-called pseudotruncus are conditions that are more clearly designated as types of pulmonary atresia.

Infants born with truncus arteriosus usually manifest symptoms of congestive heart failure early in infancy. During the first few weeks of life, as pulmonary resistance gradually decreases and flow through the lungs increases, congestive heart failure may commence. The failure is further aggravated by the presence of truncal valvular regurgitation. Most infants in whom congestive heart failure develops die within the first year of life.[5] Those who survive are subject to the early onset of severe pulmonary vascular obstructive disease.

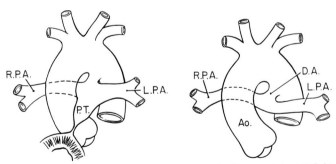

Fig. 62–1 (left).—Pulmonary arteries present. Confluence of right (R.P.A.) and left (L.P.A.) pulmonary arteries, plus atresia of proximal pulmonary trunk (P.T.) (cord-like remnant of atretic segment of pulmonary trunk present in this case). Ductus arteriosus present. (From Berry, B. E., *et al.*: Absence of anatomic origin from heart of pulmonary arterial supply: Clinical application of classification, J. Thorac. Cardiovasc. Surg. 68:119, 1974. By permission of C. V. Mosby Company.)

Fig. 62–2. (right).—Truncus arteriosus, pulmonary arteries present. Confluence of right (R.P.A.) and left (L.P.A.) pulmonary arteries, plus diffuse atresia of pulmonary trunk (no remnant of atretic pulmonary trunk in this case). Ductus arteriosus (D.A.) present. *Ao.*, aorta. (From Berry, B. E., *et al.*: Absence of anatomic origin from heart of pulmonary arterial supply: Clinical application of classification, J. Thorac. Cardiovasc. Surg. 68:119, 1974. By permission of C. V. Mosby Company.)

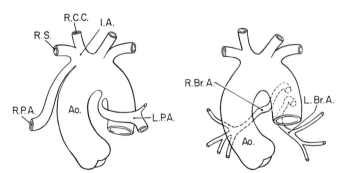

Fig. 62–4 (left).—Truncus arteriosus, pulmonary arteries present. Nonconfluence of right (R.P.A.) and left (L.P.A.) pulmonary arteries, which have independent ductal origins. R.S., right subclavian artery. R.C.C., right common carotid artery. I.A., innominate artery. Ao., aorta. (From Berry, B. E., *et al.*: Absence of anatomic origin from heart of pulmonary arterial supply: Clinical application of classification, J. Thorac. Cardiovasc. Surg. 68:119, 1974. By permission of C. V. Mosby Company.)

Fig. 62–5 (right).—Truncus arteriosus, pulmonary arteries absent with arterial supply to lungs via bronchial collateral (R.Br.A. and L.Br.A.) arteries only. Ao., aorta. (From Berry, B. E., *et al.*: Absence of anatomic origin from heart of pulmonary arterial supply: Clinical application of classification, J. Thorac. Cardiovasc. Surg. 68:119, 1974. By permission of C. V. Mosby Company.)

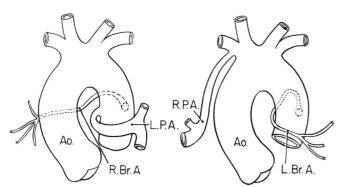

Fig. 62–6.—Truncus arteriosus, mixed type. *Left,* right pulmonary artery and main pulmonary artery absent, with ductal origin of left pulmonary *(L.P.A.)* artery. Small bronchial *(R.Br.A.)* artery nourishes right lung. *Right,* left pulmonary artery and main pulmonary artery absent, with ductal origin of right pulmonary *(R.P.A.)* artery. Small bronchial *(L.Br.A.)* artery nourishes left lung. *Ao.,* aorta. (From Berry, B. E., et al.: Absence of anatomic origin from heart of pulmonary arterial supply: Clinical application of classification, J. Thorac. Cardiovasc. Surg. 68:119, 1974. By permission of C. V. Mosby Company.)

The clinical findings are not unlike those of a patient with a large ventricular septal defect or a large patent ductus arteriosus and are related to the increased volume of pulmonary blood flow plus the presence or absence of truncal valve regurgitation. Because of the large "runoff" from the aorta through the lungs, the peripheral pulses are accentuated or even bounding in character, with a corresponding increase in pulse pressure. Definitive diagnosis depends on cardiac catheterization and angiocardiography. Study should include the careful assessment of pulmonary resistance, which can be calculated from the determination of pulmonary blood flow and pressure. As with other patients having increased pulmonary blood flow, a level of pulmonary resistance at about 10 units m² represents the demarcation between operability (at levels lower than 10 units) and inoperability.

Surgical correction was attempted sporadically, beginning in the early 1960s, and was successfully accomplished in 1967.[6, 7] The basic steps of the operative repair as originally described remain essentially unchanged: (1) separation of the pulmonary artery (or arteries) from the truncus and closure of the resulting truncal defect (Fig. 62–7, *A*); (2) longitudinal right ventriculotomy and patch closure of the ventricular septal defect (Fig. 62–7, *A* and *B*); and (3) establishment of continuity between the right ventricle and the pulmonary artery using a Dacron conduit containing a porcine valve (Fig. 62–7, *C* and *D*).

Ninety-two operations for truncus arteriosus recently were reviewed with respect to early and late results.[8] The mortality rate in the earlier years of the experience when a homograft aorta was used as a conduit was 34% whereas since 1972, when the Dacron conduit with porcine valve was used, the mortality rate had decreased to 9%. Other factors probably contributing to the improved mortality rate were better selection of patients and increased experience. In this series,[8] exactly half of the patients had normal anatomy of the right and left pulmonary arteries. The remainder had various abnormalities, including bilateral hypoplasia, absence or hypoplasia of one or the other pulmonary arteries and stenosis of the right, left or both pulmonary arteries, either of natural cause or resulting from previous operative banding of the pulmonary artery.

Fifty-one of the 92 patients had some truncal valve regur-

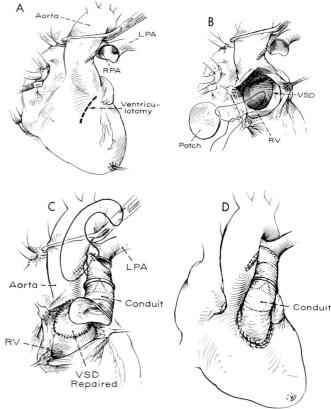

Fig. 62–7.—Repair of truncus arteriosus. **A,** pulmonary artery transected at high level from its origin in truncus, and closure of truncus, which now becomes the aorta. Longitudinal ventriculotomy is made in anticipated direction of extracardiac conduit. **B,** ventricular septal defect (VSD) is closed with patch. (From Parker, R. K., et al.: Repair of truncus arteriosus in patients with prior banding of the pulmonary artery, Surgery 78:761, 1975. By permission of C. V. Mosby Company.) **C** and **D,** extracardiac Dacron conduit containing porcine valve is anastomosed distally to pulmonary artery and proximally to the ventriculotomy. (From Wallace, R. B.: Truncus Arteriosus, in Sabiston, D. C., Jr., and Spencer, F. C. (eds.), *Gibbon's Surgery of the Chest* [3d ed.; Philadelphia: W. B. Saunders Company, 1976]. By permission.)

gitation, but it was so mild as to be insignificant in 28 of these. In the remaining 23 patients, the regurgitation was severe enough to require attention during operation.[9] Experience and extended follow-up studies have demonstrated that an increasingly radical approach to the treatment of truncal valve regurgitation is indicated, meaning that replacement of the valve is indicated in most patients whose regurgitation is more than mild. Otherwise, persistence of left ventricular overwork and progressive left ventricular failure are to be expected. However, truncal valve replacement in infants may not be a feasible solution, a fact that contributes significantly to the complexity of management of patients in this age group.

Twenty-nine per cent of patients[10] had previously undergone banding of the pulmonary artery or arteries. Usually, the origins of the right and left pulmonary arteries are involved in the banded zone, whether or not the band was placed about the pulmonary trunk or about each of the pulmonary arteries. A special technique for repair in previously banded patients has evolved (Fig. 62–8).

No statistically significant relationship was found[8] between the risk of early mortality and the sex of the patient, the anatomic type of truncus arteriosus, the anatomy of the pulmonary blood supply, the presence of truncal valve re-

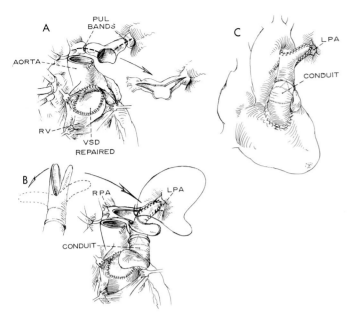

Fig. 62–8.—Repair of truncus in presence of bilateral pulmonary arterial bands. **A,** pulmonary artery is opened through banded sites. **B,** trimmed conduit is anastomosed to pulmonary artery. **C,** completed repair. (From Parker, R. K., *et al.*: Repair of truncus arteriosus in patients with prior banding of the pulmonary artery, Surgery 78:761, 1975. By permission of C. V. Mosby Company.)

gurgitation or the presence of associated cardiovascular anomalies or previous operation. However, a significantly higher operative mortality was found for repairs performed on infants when the need for surgical therapy is most important. Only recently have significant successes been reported during infancy.[11, 12] It remains a moot point whether or not to attempt complete repair for the infant with truncus arteriosus or whether to perform banding of the pulmonary trunk or separate bandings of the right and left pulmonary arteries. The significant risk of repair and the necessity for use of a small-sized conduit, which would require later replacement, are detractions from the corrective approach. Likewise, banding of the pulmonary artery has resulted in a high risk[13] and somewhat complicates the subsequent corrective procedure. With further refinements of management and techniques, the corrective approach during infancy may prove to be the better choice.

After a median follow-up period of 36 months, ranging from 4 to 92 months, 5 of 69 patients surviving repair of truncus arteriosus had died of complications related to their condition or operation.[8] Fifty-nine per cent of surviving patients were in functional Class I, with all but 1 of the remainder in Class II. The clinical status of patients having significant truncal valve regurgitation preoperatively was suggestively worse than for patients having no or only mild truncal valve regurgitation.

In summary, truncus arteriosus remains a complex problem for the cardiac surgeon, but salvage of many patients has been made possible by corrective operation. The challenge for the future is the achievement of an increasingly successful approach to the management of the infant with truncus arteriosus.

Pulmonary Atresia with Ventricular Septal Defect

A portion of the pulmonary arterial tree has failed to develop in this condition, and an almost endlessly variable pat-

TABLE 62–2.—LEVELS OF PULMONARY ATRESIA°

LEVEL	NO. OF PATIENTS
Right ventricular outflow tract	11
Pulmonary valve	44
Proximal pulmonary trunk	16
Pulmonary trunk	21
Proximal branch arteries (nonconfluence)	11
TOTAL	103

°Most downstream level.

tern of pulmonary arterial development may be encountered. When there is total absence of the pulmonary arterial tree, no corrective operative procedure can be done. Lung transplantation may be the only corrective approach to total agenesis of the pulmonary arterial tree. At the opposite extreme, only the proximal portion of the pulmonary arterial trunk may be deficient, leaving a well-developed arterial tree beyond this. Correction in this situation consists of closure of the ventricular septal defect and re-establishment of continuity between the right ventricle and the intact arterial tree. Between these two extremes exists a borderline between operability and inoperability. Currently, the minimal requirement for operability is the presence of a well-developed pulmonary arterial branch in an accessible location at the hilus of one lung.

In a surgical series,[14] various levels of pulmonary atresia were noted (Table 62–2). When the atretic zone included the pulmonary valve, pulmonary trunk and proximal portions of the right and left pulmonary arteries, separate origin or nonconfluence of the right and left pulmonary arteries necessarily resulted.

In addition to this incidence of nonconfluence of the branch pulmonary arteries, additional anomalies of the right and left pulmonary arteries were encountered in 30 of the 103 patients. These included severe hypoplasia of one or both pulmonary arteries in 13, absence or atresia of one pulmonary artery in 10 and segmental stenosis of one or both pulmonary arteries in 7. Additional associated cardiovascular anomalies were encountered frequently, including atrial septal defect in 15%, persistent left superior vena cava in 7%, tricuspid regurgitation in 7%, anomalous origin of the right coronary artery in 6% and other less common associated anomalies.

In pulmonary atresia, because there is absence of origin

TABLE 62–3.—SOURCES° OF PULMONARY BLOOD SUPPLY IN PULMONARY ATRESIA

	NO. OF PATIENTS	
SOURCE	Total	With Single Source
Patent ductus arteriosus	37	5
Large bronchial collateral arteries	35	18
Blalock-Taussig shunt (or shunts)	31	20
Potts' anastomosis	18	13
Waterston shunt	8	5
Left coronary-pulmonary artery fistula	4	1
Aorta-pulmonary artery shunt	2	1
Aorta-pulmonary artery communication†	1	0
Glenn shunt	1	0

°Many patients had two or more significant sources.
†Possibly a fistula from an accessory right coronary artery to the proximal pulmonary trunk.

of the pulmonary artery from the right ventricle, some source of pulmonary blood flow other than the usual invariably must be present. The sources of pulmonary blood supply encountered in one surgical series[14] are listed in Table 62–3. In most patients, the original natural source of pulmonary blood flow was inadequate so that a supplemental surgical shunt had been established which, in many, was the sole remaining significant source of pulmonary blood flow.

Perhaps the single most important feature of the management of this group of patients is the accurate and precise preoperative angiographic definition of the existing portion of the pulmonary arterial tree and of every significant source of pulmonary blood flow.

The operative management of patients with pulmonary atresia consists of (1) control of the source of pulmonary blood flow, (2) closure of the ventricular septal defect in the standard manner, (3) correction of associated anomalies and (4) establishment of continuity between the right ventricle and the distal patent pulmonary arterial tree.

The technique for control of the source of pulmonary blood supply varies according to the type present. If a small patent ductus exists, it often can be isolated before the onset of bypass, after which it can be ligated as soon as perfusion is instituted. In instances in which the ductus is large and thin-walled or otherwise inaccessible, the pulmonary orifice of the ductus can be sutured while working through an incision in the distal pulmonary trunk and proximal left pulmonary artery during an interval of circulatory arrest under conditions of profound hypothermia, a technique identical to the Kirklin-Devloo[15] method for control of the Potts anastomosis. The various other surgical anastomoses are controlled in the standard fashion.[16, 17] The large bronchial collateral arteries are preferably exposed for ligation[18] by working through the median sternotomy and dissecting through the posterior pericardium or via the pleural space into the perihilar mediastinum. Lacking accessibility by this approach, a complementing lateral thoracotomy can be performed on the side of the descending aorta. With respect to the rarely encountered fistula that provides communication between the left coronary artery and the proximal pulmonary trunk,[19] the ascending aorta can be cross-clamped after institution of extracorporeal circulation and the fistula can be closed by direct suture, working through a pulmonary arteriotomy overlying the fistula; in this way, injury to peripheral continuation of the left coronary artery can be avoided.

Continuity between the right ventricle and the distal pulmonary arterial tree can be established either by patch graft reconstruction of the outflow tract of the right ventricle, similar to that utilized in tetralogy with severe pulmonary stenosis, or by extracardiac valved conduit reconstruction. Although a functional pulmonary valve at the completion of repair may be preferable, whether such surgically inserted valves will provide an improvement in the long-term result is not certain. Therefore, new pulmonary valves probably should not be used when a more conservative approach, such as patch graft reconstruction of the outflow tract, is feasible because of the short length of the atretic zone and of the adequate size of the distal pulmonary arterial tree. However, where the "runoff" into the lungs is restricted by ab-

sence of one pulmonary artery, hypoplasia of one or both pulmonary arteries or the presence of pulmonary vascular obstructive disease or peripheral stenoses, the advantage of a functioning pulmonary valve would be greatest and the practice of inserting such a valve in these patients is justified.

The early death rate was 11% after operation for pulmonary atresia and ventricular septal defect in a surgical series,[13] with the principal causes of death being inability to relieve right ventricular hypertension because of restricted pulmonary arterial outflow and low cardiac output after repairs for associated complex anomalies. The late results of the operation seem to be equally as good as those after tetralogy of Fallot procedures. The poor results are related to persistent right ventricular hypertension and acute right ventricular failure resulting from inadequacy of the peripheral pulmonary arterial tree.

REFERENCES

1. Berry, B. E., et al.: Absence of anatomic origin from heart of pulmonary arterial supply: Clinical application of classification, J. Thorac. Cardiovasc. Surg. 68:119, 1974.
2. Gomes, M. M. R., and McGoon, D. C.: Truncus arteriosus with interruption of the aortic arch: Report of a case successfully repaired, Mayo Clin. Proc. 46:40, 1971.
3. Mair, D. D., et al.: Selection of patients with truncus arteriosus for surgical correction: Anatomic and hemodynamic considerations, Circulation 49:144, 1974.
4. Collett, R. W., and Edwards, J. E.: Persistent truncus arteriosus: A classification according to anatomic types, Surg. Clin. North Am. 29:1245, 1949.
5. Marcelletti, C., McGoon, D. C., and Mair, D. D.: The natural history of truncus arteriosus, Circulation 54:108, 1976.
6. McGoon, D. C., Rastelli, G. C., and Ongley, P. A.: An operation for the correction of truncus arteriosus, JAMA 205:69, 1968.
7. Weldon, C. S., and Cameron, J. L.: Correction of persistent truncus arteriosus, J. Cardiovasc. Surg. 9:463, 1968.
8. Marcelletti, C., et al.: The natural history of truncus arteriosus, Circulation 54:108, 1976.
9. DeLeval, M. R., et al.: Management of truncal valvular regurgitation, Ann. Surg. 180:427, 1974.
10. Parker, R. K., et al.: Repair of truncus arteriosus in patients with prior banding of the pulmonary artery, Surgery 78:761, 1975.
11. Ebert, P. A., et al.: Pulmonary artery conduits in infants younger than six months of age, J. Thorac. Cardiovasc. Surg. 72:351, 1976.
12. Sullivan, H., et al.: Surgical correction of truncus arteriosus in infancy, Am. J. Cardiol. 38:113, 1976.
13. Singh, A. K., et al.: Pulmonary artery banding for truncus arteriosus in the first year of life, Circulation 54(Supp. 3): 17, 1976.
14. Olin, C. L., et al.: Pulmonary atresia: Surgical considerations and results in 103 patients undergoing definitive repair, Circulation 54(Supp. 3):35, 1976.
15. Kirklin, J. W., and Devloo, R. A.: Hypothermic perfusion and circulatory arrest for surgical correction of tetralogy of Fallot with previously constructed Potts' anastomosis, Dis. Chest 39: 87, 1961.
16. Kirklin, J. W., and Payne, W. S.: Surgical treatment for tetralogy of Fallot after previous anastomosis of systemic to pulmonary artery, Surg. Gynecol. Obstet. 110:707, 1960.
17. Ebert, P. A., Gay, W. A., Jr., and Oldham, H. N.: Management of aorta-right pulmonary artery anastomosis during total correction of tetralogy of Fallot, Surgery 71:231, 1972.
18. McGoon, D. C., Baird, D. K., and Davis, G. D.: Surgical management of large bronchial collateral arteries with pulmonary stenosis or atresia, Circulation 52:109, 1975.
19. Krongrad, E., et al.: Pulmonary atresia or severe stenosis and coronary artery-to-pulmonary artery fistula, Circulation 46:1005, 1972.

63 GEORGE A. TRUSLER

Pulmonary Atresia and Pulmonic Stenosis with Normal Aortic Root

Pulmonary Atresia

THIS COMPLEX ANOMALY comprises less than 1% of all congenital heart disease.[13] The atresia usually is at the pulmonary valve, with three small ridges marking the vestigial commissures between three partially formed valve leaflets. The pulmonary artery, although underdeveloped to a variable extent, frequently is close to normal in size and rarely small. The interventricular septum is intact. Usually there is gross hypertrophy of the right ventricular myocardium, with a diminutive right ventricular chamber, a narrow infundibular channel and a small tricuspid valve (Fig. 63–1). An interatrial communication, most often a small patent foramen ovale, always is present, with dilatation of the right atrium and hypertrophy of its wall. All blood entering the right atrium must cross the interatrial communication into the left atrium to reach the systemic circulation. Pulmonary circulation, and life, are maintained by flow through the patent ductus arteriosus. In 10–15% of cases,[7] the right ventricle has a larger lumen and is less hypertrophied, often with severe tricuspid valve incompetence.

Clinical Features

Usually the patent ductus arteriosus is small and the infant is severely cyanotic shortly after birth. There are no cardiac murmurs except those originating in the patent ductus arteriosus or a blowing murmur of tricuspid insufficiency. Radiographic examination shows decreased pulmonary vascular markings and a heart that usually is large but may be small. A left ventricular overloading pattern in the electrocardiogram distinguishes this lesion from tetralogy of Fallot with characteristic right ventricular hypertrophy. In both pulmonary atresia and severe pulmonary stenosis, the venous angiocardiogram shows a filling sequence similar to that in tricuspid atresia, and it may be difficult to differentiate these conditions.

The demonstration of pure left ventricular hypertrophy with a QRS axis of less than 130 in the frontal plane of the electrocardiogram, but not frank left axis deviation, suggests that the right ventricle is small.[24] If a cardiac catheter can be positioned in the right ventricle, selective angiocardiography will clearly show the size of the ventricle with complete occlusion of its outflow tract.

Treatment

Without treatment, the prognosis is exceedingly poor. Keith et al.[13] found that one-quarter of the infants died in the first week of life and 78% were dead by 6 months. Frequently death coincided with closure of the ductus arteriosus.

At operation, one must avoid misjudging the size of the right ventricle, for the thickness of its wall makes it look large in contrast to the actual volume of the chamber. One should suspect a small right ventricular chamber if its wall feels thick and firm with an appearance of poor contractility, if there is a dimple over the lower interventricular sulcus or an anomalous coronary vessel communicating with the right ventricular chamber.

When the right ventricular lumen is normal or large, the right ventricular outflow tract should be reconstructed to eliminate all obstruction. This is done with either cardiopulmonary bypass or deep hypothermia and circulatory arrest. Often outflow patch enlargement of the pulmonary valve ring and infundibulum will be required in addition to pulmonary valvotomy. If there is severe tricuspid incompetence, the tricuspid valve should be repaired or replaced. If good right heart function is achieved, the atrial septal defect should be closed.

In most cases, the right ventricle has a small or diminutive lumen and it is advisable to perform a systemic-pulmonary shunt and pulmonary valvotomy. A balloon atrial septostomy will have been done previously at cardiac catheterization. Bowman et al.[2] have obtained good results combining a Waterston shunt with a transventricular pulmonary valvotomy. We prefer a left-sided incision and combine a Potts anastomosis with a transarterial valvotomy. If the patent ductus arteriosus is large, it may be ligated following the anastomosis.

In 23 infants with pulmonary atresia we have used this approach, with 4 early deaths.[27] Two children died during a second pulmonary valvotomy. Seventeen children survive. Subsequently, in 1 child, the RV enlarged sufficiently that a formal repair was possible. However, further experience is needed to determine how often this will occur. Some infants have such a small hypoplastic tricuspid valve that complete repair will never be possible. When more help is needed, a Glenn cavopulmonary anastomosis through the right chest is an easy alternative, an advantage of the original left-sided incision.

The separation into small and large right ventricular types is not strict. There are many cases in which there are ventricles of intermediate size, which, in part, may account for the few good long-term results following pulmonary valvotomy alone.

Pulmonic Stenosis with Normal Aortic Root

In 1888, Fallot separated this malformation from that associated with an interventricular septal defect, and in 1951 Abrahams and Wood[1] introduced the term pulmonic stenosis with normal aortic root. Sellors[23] in 1947 and Brock[4] in 1948 independently performed the first successful valvotomies by a transventricular approach, Brock using a specially designed valvotome. Swan and Zeavin[25] introduced the transarterial approach with inflow occlusion and hypothermia in 1954. The open transarterial technique with cardiopulmonary bypass using the artificial heart-lung apparatus now is

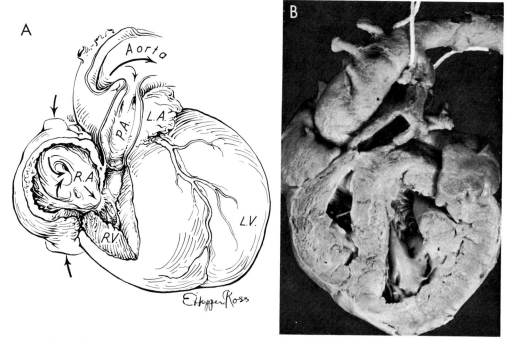

Fig. 63–1.—Pulmonary atresia with normal aortic root. The drawing **(A)** of the specimen **(B)** demonstrates the small right ventricular chamber that almost prohibits surgical correction.

widely used and, more recently, deep hypothermia with circulatory arrest has been useful in infants.

Incidence and Pathologic Anatomy

The incidence of pulmonic stenosis appears to be 10% of all congenital heart disease.[13] In all severe forms of pulmonic stenosis, the pulmonary artery is the site of poststenotic dilatation and low pressure. On palpation of the vessel, the valve can be felt projecting into the lumen of the artery like a cervix with a forceful jet of blood, which can be eliminated by digital occlusion of the valvar orifice. On inspection, the commissures may be found to be completely fused to the edge of an orifice measuring 2 or 3 mm in diameter. In more moderate pulmonary stenosis, the commissural fusion is less marked, resulting in a larger opening measuring 4–8 mm in diameter. Occasionally, the valve is bicuspid and presents a "fishmouth" appearance. In some cases there is no actual commissural fusion but a thickening of valve tissue with shortening of its free margin creating a relatively small orifice. There may be some narrowing of the pulmonary artery at the free margin of the valve.

In a small number of children, the pulmonary valve is dysplastic, with thick fleshy leaflets, poorly formed commissures and shallow sinuses.[14] This type of valve is seen commonly in children with the Noonan syndrome.[19]

Not infrequently, valve stenosis is combined with some degree of infundibular stenosis. Pure infundibular stenosis is uncommon.[6, 26] The stenosis in these cases is muscular and located approximately 1 cm below the valve. Our experience with childhood lesions leads us to believe that most infundibular stenosis probably is a physiologic hypertrophy of the infundibular area in the presence of a valvar stenosis.[9, 10, 21] However, Danielson *et al.*[6] believe that the incidence of combined infundibular and valvar stenosis is the same at all ages. Regardless of the type of stenosis, right atrial and right ventricular hypertrophy are present and the fora-

men ovale often is patent. In approximately 15% of our cases, a secundum type of atrial septal defect accompanied the pulmonic stenosis. Isolated supravalvar pulmonary stenosis also may occur but it usually is mild.[20]

Hemodynamics

In severe stenosis, the right ventricular pressure may be as high as 260 mm Hg. If a patent foramen ovale or atrial septal defect is present, there may be some degree of cyanosis when the pressure is high. Usually with moderate stenosis, right ventricular pressure from 70 to 110 mm Hg, the shunt across an atrial septal defect is from left to right and the patient is not cyanotic.

Diagnosis

The signs usually are most dramatic in the first year of life. Figure 63–2 illustrates the clinical signs in 26 infants operated on when under 1 year of age at The Hospital for Sick Children, Toronto.

Invariably, a systolic murmur is present over the pulmonary area, usually accompanied by a thrill in severe and in some instances of moderately severe stenosis. In severe cases, the second heart sound is reduced and there is a precordial heave. In moderate stenosis, the electrocardiogram may be normal, but in the more severe forms, the electrocardiogram shows right axis deviation with a tall R in V₁ (Fig. 63–3). In severe cases, on the plain chest roentgenogram, hilar shadows are either normal or reduced; depending on the presence of a right-to-left shunt, the right atrium and right ventricle may be enlarged. There nearly always is a poststenotic pulmonary artery bulge regardless of the severity of the stenosis. The heart with only moderate stenosis is not enlarged. Echocardiography may indicate the presence of a small right ventricle and is particularly useful in differentiating tetralogy of Fallot from pulmonary stenosis.

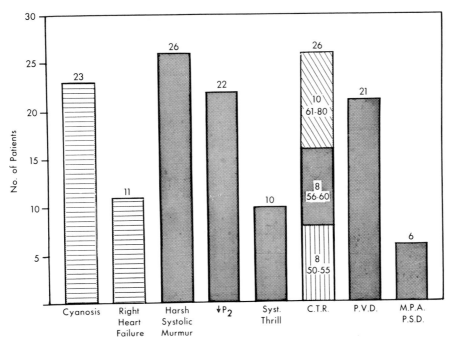

Fig. 63–2.—Pulmonic stenosis with normal aortic root. Clinical and radiographic features in 26 infants in the first year of life. ↓ P_2, pulmonary second sound reduced; *C.T.R.*, cardiothoracic ratio; *P.V.D.*, pulmonary vasculature diminished; *M.P.A.*, *P.S.D.*, main pulmonary artery, poststenotic dilatation.

Cardiac catheterization (Fig. 63–4) confirms the diagnosis and the severity of the stenosis. Selective angiocardiography demonstrates the size and function of the right ventricle in severe forms of stenosis as well as the thickness of the valve leaflets and degree of obstruction. In young infants with severe stenosis, tricuspid insufficiency is common. Angiocardiography is particularly important to identify a small right ventricle or a dysplastic pulmonary valve.[12] (Figs. 63–5 and 63–6).

Differential Diagnosis

In the infant, mild to moderately severe pulmonic stenosis with normal aortic root may be difficult to distinguish from aortic stenosis. The cyanotic infant without a murmur or with a continuous murmur due to a ductus and with left ventricular hypertrophy may have pulmonary atresia. Transposition of the great vessels with pulmonic stenosis may be diagnosed by selective angiocardiography to demonstrate the anteriorly placed aorta. Associated Ebstein malformation is rare and diagnosed by selective angiocardiography.

Natural History

Since operative relief from pulmonary stenosis now is widely available, the natural nonoperative history of the condition no longer is observed.[5] The outlook in pulmonary stenosis is related to the severity of the stenosis. Most mild cases remain mild. Children with moderate or severe stenosis eventually require operation. Without operation, death in the first year of life is not uncommon; of 14 deaths in the first

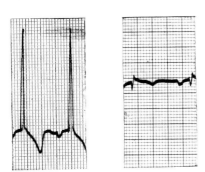

Fig. 63–3.—Pulmonic stenosis with normal aortic root. Height of the R wave in the ECG may be as significant as the pressure recorded in the right ventricle. In this 6-year-old patient, division of the pulmonic valve under direct vision led to dramatic reduction of the R wave 4 years later.

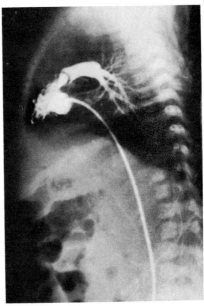

Fig. 63–4.—Pulmonic stenosis with normal aortic root. Angiocardiogram, lateral view, of a 6-week-old infant, demonstrates the size of the right ventricle, outline of the stenosed valve and the large pulmonary artery. Selective angiocardiography may aid in diagnosis of severe pulmonic stenosis in infancy.

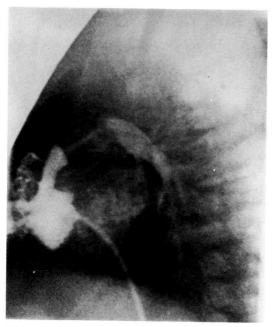

Fig. 63–5.–Small right ventricle. Lateral angiocardiogram in an infant with pulmonic stenosis.

6 years of life reported by Keith,[13] 9 were in the first year. Mody[17] suggested that when pulmonary stenosis was identified in infancy, even though mild, it was likely to progress.

Indications for Operation

As with most congenital defects, the indications for operation become more clearly defined as experience is gained by both cardiologist and surgeon. The severity of the lesion must be weighed against the morbidity and mortality of operative intervention. With a mortality of less than 1% and very little morbidity, we operate in cases of moderate stenosis when the pressure gradient across the valve is 50 mm Hg or over. In severe cases, particularly in infancy, operation

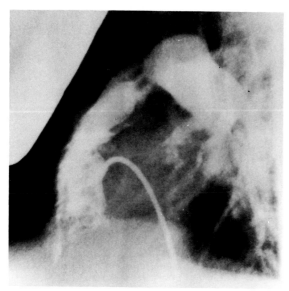

Fig. 63–6.–Noonan syndrome and thickened dysplastic pulmonary valve leaflets. Lateral angiocardiogram.

should be undertaken when the diagnosis has been established. The infant in severe distress may present a surgical emergency.

Operative Technique

Valvotomy through the right ventricle, introduced by Sellors and by Brock, still is performed in some centers. Perhaps the most effective transventricular technique has been with the Himmelstein valvulotome.[11] We prefer to divide the valve under direct vision to obtain an adequate opening with minimal valve incompetence. Lam and Taber[15] reported division of the valve with inflow occlusion at normothermic temperatures. Many surgeons have used hypothermia with inflow occlusion to provide more time, as advocated by Swan. Almost all now prefer cardiopulmonary bypass. In infants, the addition of moderate to deep hypothermia and a period of circulatory arrest improves exposure and facilitates the repair.

The chest is opened with a median sternotomy incision. When using hypothermia and inflow occlusion, the venae cavae are taped intrapericardially and the pulmonary artery is opened just distal to the valve. The valve is grasped with two forceps, delivered into the incision and inspected to assess the amount of stenosis present and the position of the commissures. In severe forms, where the commissures are fused to a significant degree, simple commissurotomy is effective. Sometimes, the commissures are short, so that division of the commissures would not produce an adequate opening of the stenosed valve. Occasionally there is no commissural fusion but rather a shortening of the free margin of the valve. In such cases, two or three commissures are cut free from the pulmonary artery wall for an appropriate distance so that the point of attachment of the commissure now is deeper in the pulmonary valve sinus, where the diameter is wider[3] (Fig. 63–7). The extended commissure then is split to the pulmonary artery wall. After valvotomy, a sound is passed through the lumen to determine the size of the orifice and the presence of infundibular stenosis or other right ventricular obstruction. In older children, a finger may be inserted. In a relaxed flaccid heart, it is difficult to assess physiologic muscular infundibular hypertrophy, which is present only in systole. However, significant isolated infundibular stenosis in the presence of an intact ventricular septum usually is quite obvious and prevents passage of a large sound or a finger.

Following valvotomy and closure of the pulmonary artery, when the child is hemodynamically stable, a pullback pressure recording should be made to identify any residual ob-

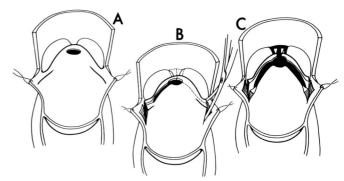

Fig. 63–7.–Technique of pulmonary valvotomy when valve commissures are short and commissurotomy alone will not create an adequate orifice. The commissures are extended by partial detachment from the pulmonary artery wall and then split.

struction. In older children, the drop in pressure at operation may be surprisingly small, and, in some, the pressure in the right ventricle is elevated following division of the valve, likely due to a temporary hyperdynamic state following bypass or inflow stasis. True anatomic infundibular stenosis, although relatively uncommon, should be excised. If this is inadequate, the outflow tract is reconstructed.

Postoperative Care

Generally these children have an excellent postoperative course. Particularly gratifying are results in the children with severe stenosis, whose improvement over the preoperative state is striking. The need for oxygen therapy is brief. After removal of chest drains, older children usually are up within a few days of operation. Complications are exceedingly rare beyond the usual ones involved in a simple thoracotomy or median sternotomy incision. On the other hand, infants with critical pulmonary stenosis may be in a low output state with some degree of right-to-left atrial shunting. Inotropic cardiac support may be necessary and if there is persistent severe cyanosis, a shunt or some other form of therapy may be required.

Results of Operation

Beyond infancy, results are excellent. From 1956 to 1976 inclusive, we performed primary pulmonary valvotomy in 162 children over 1 year of age, using inflow stasis in early cases but cardiopulmonary bypass in the most recent cases. There were no deaths. An associated atrial septal defect was closed in 25 children. In only 2 children was infundibular stenosis resected whereas some evidence of infundibular stenosis was recorded in another 17 children and there was angiographic evidence of a hypercontractile infundibulum in others. Three children had mild to moderate stenosis of the pulmonary artery at the free margin of the valve leaflets, treated by either arterioplasty or patch graft. Five children had tricuspid incompetence, 1 requiring annuloplasty. Three children had an aortic valvotomy carried out at the same operation and 2 had resection of a subvalvar aortic diaphragm. A patent ductus arteriosus was ligated in 3 children.

Pulmonic stenosis in infants under 1 year of age is a more complex problem and often urgent.[18] From 1956 to 1976 inclusive, we operated on 80 such infants. Eight of the 80 infants had obvious infundibular narrowing but we enlarged this with an outflow patch in only 2. One other infant had moderate supravalvar stenosis, which required patching. Many infants had a patent foramen ovale and in 9 there was an atrial septal defect. In 1 infant, this was closed at the time of valvotomy and in 2 others it was closed several years later because of persisting right-to-left shunt. A patent ductus arteriosus was ligated in 2 infants and 9 infants had secondary tricuspid incompetence.

These infants may be critically ill and need careful support during operation. Eighteen of the 80 infants died. Eight deaths occurred in the operating room, either before or soon after the valvotomy. The other 10 deaths were due to cardiac failure, either of low output type or with cyanosis from continued right-to-left atrial shunting, suggesting inadequate blood flow through the right ventricle and pulmonary artery. Five of these 10 infants had either a dysplastic pulmonary valve or a small right ventricle or both.

The dysplastic pulmonary valve is a special problem seen chiefly in the infant group. We have encountered this in 2 children over 1 year of age and in 9 of the 80 infants under 1 year. Schieken et al.[22] and others[16] advise either excision of the valve or patch reconstruction of the outflow tract rather than valvotomy. Our experience tends to support this view. Four of 8 infants who had only pulmonary valvotomy died from inadequate right heart function, Later, 2 of the 4 survivors required patch reconstruction of the right ventricular outflow tract. We now prefer to use deep hypothermia and circulatory arrest, and if a good 10–12-mm channel cannot be achieved by pulmonary valvotomy, the narrow part of the outflow tract is enlarged by a patch of pericardium. The valve leaflets are excised only when they show no possibility of useful function.

The presence of a small or diminutive right ventricle is another special problem usually seen early in the first year of life in critically ill infants cyanotic with right-to-left shunting. When the right ventricular volume is reasonable and there is no infundibular stenosis, good results can be expected from pulmonary valvotomy.[8] However, when there is a diminutive right ventricular chamber and a narrow infundibular channel, similar to pulmonary atresia, pulmonary valvotomy alone is inadequate and should be accompanied by a systemic-pulmonary shunt to increase pulmonary blood flow and reduce hypoxemia, allowing the right ventricle to grow with the passage of time. Nine of our 80 infants had a diminutive right ventricle. Only 2 of 6 survived pulmonary valvotomy alone. In the other 3 infants, the pulmonary valvotomy was combined with a systemic-pulmonary shunt and all survived.

Most children have a good long-term result following pulmonary valvotomy.[16] However, a few will need repeat valvotomy, particularly when the initial operation was carried out in infancy. Five of the 62 infant survivors in our series required either a second valvotomy or right ventricular outflow tract reconstruction 10 months to 15 years later. Some degree of pulmonary incompetence is common after pulmonary valvotomy but appears to be well tolerated in almost all cases.

REFERENCES

1. Abrahams, D. G., and Wood, P. H.: Pulmonary stenosis with normal aortic root, Br. Heart J. 13:519, 1951.
2. Bowman, F. O., Jr., et al.: Pulmonary atresia with intact ventricular septum, J. Thorac. Cardiovasc. Surg. 61:85, 1971.
3. Braimbridge, M. V., et al.: Pulmonary valve stenosis without ventricular septal defect; results of surgery, Thorax 21:164, 1966.
4. Brock, R. C.: Pulmonary valvotomy for the relief of congenital pulmonary stenosis; report of 3 cases, Br. Med. J. 1:1121, 1948.
5. Campbell, M.: Simple pulmonary stenosis; pulmonary valvular stenosis with a closed ventricular septum, Br. Heart J. 16:273, 1954.
6. Danielson, G. K., et al.: Pulmonic stenosis with intact ventricular septum; surgical considerations and results of operation, J. Thorac. Cardiovasc. Surg. 61:228, 1971.
7. Davignon, A. L., et al.: Congenital pulmonary atresia with intact ventricular septum; clinicopathologic correlation of two anatomic types, Am. Heart J. 62:591, 1961.
8. Freed, M. D., et al.: Critical pulmonary stenosis with a diminutive right ventricle in neonates, Circulation 48:875, 1973.
9. Hardy, J. D., et al.: Isolated pulmonic stenosis; surgical results in 26 cases, Surgery 60:980, 1966.
10. Hessel, E. A., II, et al.: Surgical treatment of pulmonic stenosis with intact ventricular septum with the use of cardiopulmonary bypass, J. Thorac. Cardiovasc. Surg. 49:796, 1965.
11. Himmelstein, A., et al.: Closed transventricular valvulotomy for pulmonic stenosis; description of a new valvulotome and results based on pressures during operation, Surgery 42:121, 1957.
12. Jeffrey, R. F., Moller, J. H., and Amplatz, K.: The dysplastic pulmonary valve; a new roentgenographic entity; with a discussion of the anatomy and radiology of other types of valvular pulmonary stenosis, Am. J. Roentgenol. 114:322, 1972.
13. Keith, J. D., Rowe, R. D., and Vlad, P.: Heart Disease in Infancy and Childhood (2d ed.; New York: The Macmillan Company, 1967).

14. Koretzky, E. D., *et al.*: Congenital pulmonary stenosis resulting from dysplasia of valve, Circulation 40:43, 1969.
15. Lam, C. R., and Taber, R. E.: Simplified technique for direct vision pulmonary valvotomy, J. Thorac. Surg. 38:309, 1959.
16. Mistrot, J., *et al.*: Pulmonary valvulotomy under inflow stasis for isolated pulmonary stenosis, Ann. Thorac. Surg. 21:30, 1976.
17. Mody, M. R.: The natural history of uncomplicated valvular pulmonic stenosis, Am. Heart J. 90:317, 1975.
18. Mustard, W. T., Jain, S. C., and Trusler, G. A.: Pulmonary stenosis in the first year of life, Br. Heart J. 30:255, 1968.
19. Noonan, J. A., and Ehmke, D. A.: Associated noncardiac malformations in children with congenital heart disease, J. Pediatr. 63:468, 1963.
20. Roberts, N., and Moes, C. A. F.: Supravalvular pulmonary stenosis, J. Pediatr. 82:838, 1973.
21. Rowe, R. D., *et al.*: Severe valvular pulmonary stenosis with a normal root; immediate results of transarterial valvotomy, with notes on the clinical assessment of patients before and after operation, Can. Med. Assoc. J. 78:311, 1958.
22. Schieken, R. M., Friedman, S., and Pierce, W. S.: Severe congenital pulmonary stenosis with pulmonary valvular dysplasia syndrome, Ann. Thorac. Surg. 15:570, 1973.
23. Sellors, T. H.: Surgery of pulmonic stenosis; a case in which the pulmonary valve was successfully divided, Lancet 1:988, 1948.
24. Shams, A., *et al.*: Pulmonary atresia with intact ventricular septum; report of 50 cases, Pediatrics 47:370, 1971.
25. Swan, H., and Zeavin, I.: Cessation of circulation in general hypothermia. III: Technics of intracardiac surgery under direct vision, Ann. Surg. 139:385, 1954.
26. Swan, H., *et al.*: The surgical treatment of isolated infundibular stenosis, J. Thorac. Cardiovasc. Surg. 38:319, 1959.
27. Trusler, G. A., *et al.*: Surgical treatment of pulmonary atresia with intact ventricular septum, Br. Heart J. 38:957, 1976.

64 John W. Kirklin / Albert D. Pacifico

Tetralogy of Fallot

HISTORY. — Although Stensen described the syndrome in 1672,[21] Fallot's[9] report published in 1888 gave the entity of the tetralogy of Fallot its name. The palliative operation of subclavian-pulmonary artery anastomosis, developed and described by Blalock and Taussig,[6] brought practical importance to the identification of this defect in cyanotic children. Lillehei and associates[15] first achieved complete intracardiac repair of the malformation. Through the observations, experiments and vision of many workers, the patient who has tetralogy of Fallot no longer faces progressing invalidism and death but has a high probability of surviving a corrective intracardiac operation.

Anatomic Features

The tetralogy of Fallot is a specific and unique combination of defects.[20] These include a large ventricular septal defect (VSD), which is immediately beneath the aortic valve. The defect usually is rather posterior and extends to the annulus of the tricuspid valve. In some patients it is somewhat anterior to this position, with a bar of septal muscle between the defect and the tricuspid valve. This small difference in location is important because, in the former, the bundle of His lies along the rim of the defect on the left ventricular side.[14] When the defect is somewhat more anterior, the bundle of His is rather far removed from the edges of the defect, and stitches used to make the repair may be placed along the rim of the defect. The ventricular septal defect is subpulmonary in 2–5% of patients. In about 1% of patients, the VSD is the ventricular component of a large complete atrioventricular canal.[10] Table 64–1 indicates the spectrum of patients with tetralogy of Fallot who come to operation.

The aorta is dextroposed and arises to a variable degree from the right as well as the left ventricle. The infundibulum of the right ventricle is underdeveloped to a variable degree, resulting in infundibular, at times valvar and at times supravalvar pulmonary stenosis. There may be stenosis of the ostium infundibulum, which alone or associated with additional narrowing downstream to this area offers sufficient resistance to blood flow to result in essentially equal peak systolic pressures in the two ventricles.

The *ostium infundibulum* is produced by hypertrophy and anterior displacement of the crista supraventricularis. The parietal band and the septal band usually are hypertrophied and produce additional narrowing at and/or just upstream to the ostium infundibulum. Between the ostium infundibulum and the pulmonary valve is the variably sized but always to some degree underdeveloped *infundibular chamber* (Fig. 64–1). The *orifice of the pulmonary valve*, which may or may not be narrowed, is a little downstream to the attachment of the base of the cusps of this valve to the junctional area between the artery and right ventricle. The level of basal attachment of the cusps is termed the *pulmonary valve ring*. The cusps are also attached at their commissures to the wall of the pulmonary artery. A localized *stenosis* of this area of the main *pulmonary artery* may result from shortening of the free edge of these cusps. Uncommonly, there is stenosis at the origin of the left and right pulmonary arteries, which complicates considerably the repair of the tetralogy of Fallot.

In *tetralogy of Fallot with congenital pulmonary atresia*, no luminal connection exists between the right ventricle and the pulmonary artery. Usually the pulmonary artery is present but narrow and the right and left pulmonary arteries are confluent. The malformation may be even more extreme, in which case the pulmonary artery is absent. In the most extreme form of this variant of the tetralogy of Fallot there is no confluence between the right and left pulmonary arteries. Pulmonary valve atresia may develop later in life in some patients with tetralogy of Fallot who have had anastomotic operations.

Patients with tetralogy of Fallot have varying degrees of cyanosis because of differences in the severity of the pulmonary stenosis. Neither the location of the ventricular septal defect nor the degree of dextroposition of the aorta apparently has any direct effect on the degree of cyanosis.

TABLE 64-1.—Spectrum of Patients Operated on for
Tetralogy of Fallot, University of Alabama Medical
Center, 1967-1977

CATEGORY	NUMBER OF PATIENTS
Classic tetralogy of Fallot	429
Tetralogy of Fallot with congenital pulmonary atresia	41
Tetralogy of Fallot with acquired pulmonary atresia	18
Tetralogy of Fallot with subpulmonary VSD	14
Tetralogy of Fallot with complete AV canal	4
Tetralogy of Fallot with pulmonary valve incompetence	8
Tetralogy of Fallot with aorto-pulmonary window	1
Total	515

Diagnosis*

CLINICAL FEATURES.—Cyanosis occurs at or soon after birth in about a third of the patients, before the first year of life in a third and at any time during the next several years in the remaining third. Since the degree of cyanosis depends on the total amount of unsaturated hemoglobin rather than on the arterial oxygen saturation, cyanosis increases as polycythemia develops. Dyspnea depends on the severity of the disease and is increased by exertion or emotional stress. Clubbing of the fingers rarely is noted before 2 years of age and is proportional to the degree of cyanosis. Squatting following exertion is common in younger children when the condition is severe; however, social consciousness makes older children live within their tolerance for exercise, and the need for squatting lessens.

Infants, most often those under 1 year of age, may suffer from attacks of severe anoxia resulting in episodes of unconsciousness that may end fatally. Polycythemia develops as a

---

*This discussion was prepared originally by Dr. P. A. Ongley, then of the Section of Pediatrics of the Mayo Clinic.

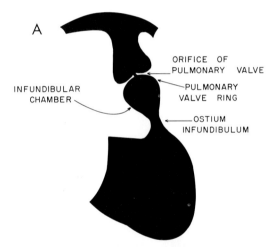

INFUNDIBULAR CHAMBER

ORIFICE OF PULMONARY VALVE

PULMONARY VALVE RING

OSTIUM INFUNDIBULUM

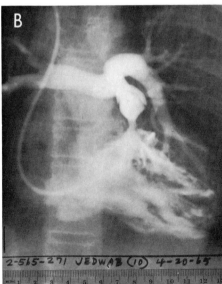 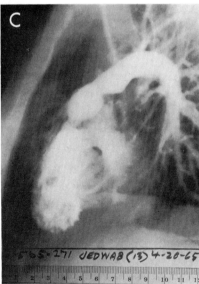

Fig. 64–1.—Tetralogy of Fallot. **A,** schematic representation of the right ventricle and pulmonary artery. **B,** anteroposterior and **C,** lateral angiocardiograms after right ventricular injection of dye. In **C,** dye is seen passing from the right ventricle through the ventricular septal defect into the left ventricle. The infundibulum is underdeveloped (small). There is severe infundibular pulmonary stenosis and a moderate-sized infundibular chamber. The thickened, stenotic pulmonary valve can be seen in profile.

response to the anoxic state and leads to congestive changes in the viscera, with the occasional appearance of epistaxis or hemoptysis. Cerebrovascular thrombosis with deficits of the central nervous system may occur and cerebral abscesses may develop. Mild albuminuria is common.

PHYSICAL EXAMINATION.—Over-all enlargement of the heart is unusual. The cardiac impulse is dominantly right ventricular in type, with a systolic thrill at the mid-left sternal border in most cases. The first heart sound is normal and is loudest at the apex or lower left sternal border. The second sound almost always is single; it is diminished at the upper left sternal border and is loudest at the middle and lower portions of the left sternal border. This clear single sound almost certainly represents closure of the aortic valve. If a clear-cut splitting of the second sound is noted in a cyanotic patient considered to have tetralogy of Fallot, the accuracy of the diagnosis should be seriously questioned.

The characteristic murmur is systolic in timing and is of variable intensity, depending on the severity of the stenosis, being loudest with moderate stenosis and least apparent with severe stenosis. The murmur ends before aortic closure and rarely is more than grade 3 in intensity; occasionally, when the condition is severe, it is no greater than grade 1. During an episode of anoxia, a murmur that usually is grade 2 or 3 may become greatly diminished or even inaudible. Because the pulmonary stenosis commonly is infundibular, the murmur is loudest at the mid-left sternal border, but when valvar stenosis also is present, the murmur may be heard best at the upper left sternal border. Pulmonic diastolic murmurs are rare and, if present, may be associated with congenital hypoplasia of the cusps of the pulmonary valve.

ELECTROCARDIOGRAPHY.—The findings on electrocardiography are dominated by evidence of overwork of the right ventricle. The findings are those of right ventricular systolic overload; this is not so pronounced as that seen in severe pulmonary stenosis with an intact septum but it is perhaps more consistent for a large group of patients. Right atrial hypertrophy is less common and less severe than it is in pulmonary stenosis with an intact septum, but P waves 5 or 6 mm or more in height sometimes are encountered.

ROENTGENOLOGIC ASPECTS.—The majority of patients display a typical contour, the so-called coeur en sabot. The heart is normal or even small in size in the posteroanterior projection, with elevation of the apex giving a right ventricular contour. A concavity is present in the region of the right ventricular outflow tract and the main pulmonary artery. The main pulmonary artery and the hilar vessels are diminished in size and the peripheral vascular shadows in the lungs are less prominent than usual. Moderate enlargement of the right atrium and the aorta is frequent. A right aortic arch occurs in 20–25% of cases whereas such an anomaly is virtually never present in pulmonary stenosis with an intact septum. Right ventricular hypertrophy is best evaluated in the lateral view, in which it is noted as a forward bulging of the anterior surface of the cardiac silhouette toward the posterior surface of the sternum. When the condition is mild, an infundibular chamber of considerable size may be present and may project as a prominence in the expected region of the main pulmonary artery, thus confusing the picture. The true size of the pulmonary artery is not always obvious from routine studies, and angiocardiography may show a pulmonary artery of reasonable size in cases in which the presence of extreme hypoplasia might be suspected from the usual views and from fluoroscopic observations.

ANGIOCARDIOGRAPHY.—Cardiac catheterization and biplane angiocardiography provide the most precise information concerning diagnosis and anatomy. Not only the classic views should be used but special views must be made to profile the ventricular septum and identify the number and location of the ventricular septal defects.[1, 8] Special views of the bifurcation of the pulmonary artery are also required, in order to identify, if present, stenoses at the origins of the right and/or left pulmonary artery.

Course without Treatment

Patients with the tetralogy of Fallot who are not treated surgically have an unfavorable life history. Only about 70% of them live to 6 months of age, about 50% to 2 years of age, 40% to 5 years of age and 20% to 10 years of age (Fig. 64–2). Patients with the tetralogy of Fallot and congenital pulmonary atresia have an even worse prognosis, only about 40% of them being alive at the age of 2 years.

The usual cause of death in infants who die from the tetralogy of Fallot is severe hypoxia. The tendency of patients with this malformation to severe hypoxia increases with age. Also, in patients with the severe form of tetralogy of Fallot a group of complications begins to develop if the patient survives the early months of life. These include polycythemia, thrombotic pulmonary vascular disease, cerebral thrombosis and the development of an aorto-pulmonary collateral circulation. Individuals who die after the age of about 10 years generally do so as a result of these complications. Thus, hemoptysis may develop and cause death. Cerebral thrombosis and abscesses may complicate the life history of these patients and cause death.

Congestive heart failure is uncommon as a complication of the tetralogy of Fallot, except in those patients who live into the fourth and fifth decades of life. These rare individuals may die as a result of chronic congestive heart failure, which, in part, is the result of the effects of chronic hypoxia on myocardial function.

Surgical Treatment

INTRACARDIAC REPAIR.—The operation for tetralogy of Fallot has evolved over a period of more than 20 years. The

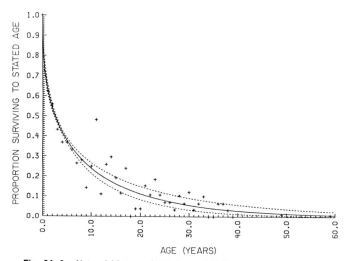

Fig. 64–2.—Natural history of tetralogy of Fallot estimated from Danish population study.[19] (From Bertranou, Blackstone and Kirklin, unpublished data). Pluses (+) represent actual data points from the Danish study. These data have been statistically smoothed (solid line with its 70% confidence interval enclosed by the dashed lines).

TABLE 64–2.—The Need for Patch-Graft Enlargement Across the Pulmonary Valve Ring

BODY SURFACE AREA (m²)	PROBABILITY°					
	15% (MEAN NORMAL)†	35% (< NORMAL BUT WITHIN 50% CL)	50% (< NORMAL BUT WITHIN 72.5%CL)	75% (< NORMAL BUT WITHIN 95% CL)	90% SMALL (< THAN 95% CL)	HIGHEST VALUE WITHIN 95% CL°°°
0.15	5.9	5.1	4.6	3.6	< 3.6	8.1
0.20	7.3	6.5	6.1	5.1	< 5.1	9.6
0.25	8.4	7.6	7.2	6.2	< 6.2	10.7
0.30	9.3	8.5	8.1	7.1	< 7.1	11.6
0.35	10.1	9.3	8.8	7.8	< 7.8	12.3
0.40	10.7	10.0	9.5	8.5	< 8.5	13.0
0.45	11.3	10.6	10.1	9.1	< 9.1	13.6
0.50	11.9	11.1	10.6	9.6	< 9.6	14.1
0.55	12.3	11.6	11.1	10.1	<10.1	14.6
0.60	12.8	12.0	11.5	10.5	<10.5	15.0
0.65	13.2	12.4	11.9	10.9	<10.9	15.4
0.70	13.5	12.7	12.3	11.3	<11.3	15.8
0.75	13.9	13.1	12.6	11.6	<11.6	16.1
0.80	14.2	13.4	12.9	11.9	<11.9	16.4
0.90	14.8	14.0	13.5	12.5	<12.5	17.0
1.0	15.3	14.5	14.0	13.0	<13.0	17.6
1.2	16.2	15.4	14.9	13.9	<13.9	18.5
1.4	17.0	16.2	15.7	14.7	<14.7	19.2
1.6	17.6	16.8	16.4	15.4	<15.4	19.9
1.8	18.2	17.4	16.9	15.9	<15.9	20.5
2.0	18.7	18.0	17.5	16.5	<16.5	21.0

CL = confidence limits.
The probability (°) that patch-graft enlargement is necessary is indicated as a percentage above each of the columns. The phrases within parentheses (†) describe the size of the pulmonary valve ring relative to the patient's body surface area with reference to the data of Rowlatt, Rimoldi and Lev.[18] The numbers under each of these columns are the measured internal diameter of the pulmonary valve ring (mm) after valvotomy in the individual patient. The column to the right indicates a valve above which the pulmonary valve ring is abnormally large (°°°). This is an appropriate size for the woven Dacron tube from which the patch-graft is cut. (From Pacifico, Kirklin and Blackstone.[16])

present practices at the University of Alabama Medical Center are presented, and are representative of those of most surgeons.

After the patient has been anesthetized and appropriate recording devices inserted, a primary median sternotomy incision is made. The various anatomic features of the tetralogy of Fallot are identified after opening the pericardium. Since nearly all patients have a woven Dacron patch inserted either into the right ventriculotomy incision or across the pulmonary valve ring, a woven Dacron tube of appropriate size is selected and preclotted twice. (Pericardium is used as the outflow patch material by many surgeons.) A table has been developed (Table 64–2) relating the size of the patient's pulmonary valve ring to the mean normal values developed by Rowlatt, Rimoldi and Lev.[18] The Dacron tube selected is about as large as the highest normal value within the 95% confidence limits of Lev's mean normal value. Practically, the patient's body surface area is determined, this value determined from the right-hand column of Table 64–2, and the next largest woven Dacron tube is selected. As is seen later, the tube is cut in half longitudinally and one half used for the patch. In a basically similar manner, the proper size of a pericardial patch can be determined.

Cardiopulmonary bypass is established using two venous cannulas (except in infants less than about 3 months of age, in whom a single venous cannula and the Barratt-Boyes Kyoto method[2, 3] are used). Arterial cannulation is into the ascending aorta. With the perfusate, the patient's body temperature is gradually lowered to 22° C (measured in the nasopharynx). The heart, of course, is cooled as well during this procedure. During the cooling, the right atrium is opened, the foramen ovale is closed with two rows of fine monofilament sutures and the right atrium closed. When the patient's body temperature reaches 22° C, the aorta is cross-clamped and a cold (7° C) cardioplegic solution containing 20–30 mEq/l of potassium is injected. This produces electromechanical quiescence and keeps the myocardial temperature between 10° and 20° C. In small infants, total circulatory arrest then is established at a body temperature of 20° C and can be maintained safely up to 45 minutes. In patients over about 3 months of age, total circulatory arrest usually is not necessary and the flow is reduced to 0.5 l/min/m² for about 30 minutes and then to 1.6 l/min/m² as long as it is required while the perfusate temperature is maintained at 20° C. Prior to opening the heart, measurements are made of the length of the proposed ventriculotomy incision and the length should the incision have to be extended across the pulmonary valve ring to the bifurcation of the pulmonary artery (Fig. 64–3, A). Then a short vertical incision is made in the infundibulum of the right ventricle (Fig. 64–3, B). The pulmonary valve, if stenotic, is opened as much as is possible by direct incision of its commissures. The markedly hypertrophied parietal band is identified on the right side of the infundibular chamber and excised. Any obstructing septal bands on the left side are excised and the free wall of the right ventricle is mobilized. The ventricular septal defect is repaired in a manner similar to that for an isolated ventricular septal defect. A Dacron velour patch is used, which is sutured into place with continuous fine monofilament sutures. As indicated earlier, when the defect is in the typical position back up against the tricuspid valve, the sutures must be kept on the right ventricular side and well away

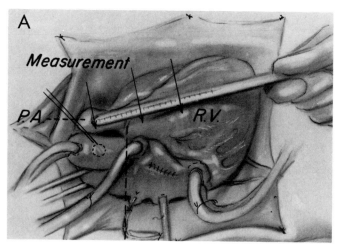

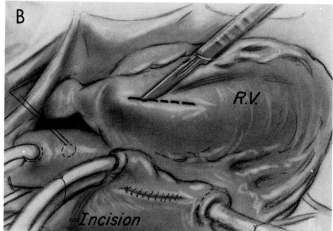

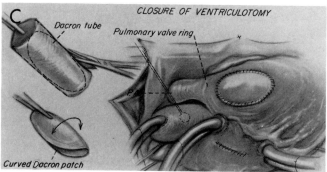

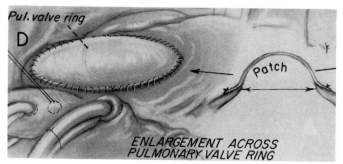

Fig. 64–3.—Repair of tetralogy of Fallot. **A,** prior to cardiotomy, measurements are made of the length of the incision if it is to be limited to the ventricle and its length if it is to be carried to the end of the pulmonary artery. When angiocardiography has showed some narrowing at the origin of the left pulmonary artery, the incision is carried onto the left pulmonary artery. **B,** a short vertical incision is made in the infundibulum of the right ventricle. **C,** after excising the infundibular elements, mobilizing the free wall of the right ventricle, opening the pulmonary valve and repairing the ventricular septal defect, the twice preclotted Dacron tube has been trimmed and sutured into the ventriculotomy incision. **D,** when the ventriculotomy incision has been extended across the pulmonary valve ring to the bifurcation of the pulmonary artery, a longer patch-graft is sutured into the entire area. Note that in both **C** and **D** the patch-graft has a convex contour both longitudinally and transversely to provide the largest possible pathway.

from the edge of the defect posteriorly and inferiorly. Defects that are more anterior, with a bar of muscle between the defect and the tricuspid valve, can be closed by suturing the patch into place with stitches that are along the very edge of the defect just along the right ventricular side.

Now the difficult decision must be made as to whether patch-graft enlargement across the pulmonary valve ring is to be done. We believe that this should be done if the ratio of the peak pressure in the right ventricle to that in the left ($P_{RV/LV}$) will be greater than about 0.65 without it. There is a relationship between the size of the pulmonary valve ring measured with Hegar dilators and this ratio after repair without patch-graft enlargement across the pulmonary valve ring[16] (Fig. 64–4). Although one may decide about patch-graft enlargement across the pulmonary valve ring by "eyeballing" the situation, or may routinely avoid patch-graft enlargement across the pulmonary valve ring unless pressure measurements immediately after repair indicate its need, we believe that a more rational approach is to use the available data and measurements in an attempt to refine the indication for this. Thus, we measure the pulmonary valve diameter with Hegar dilators and refer again to Table 64–2. If the measured pulmonary valve ring is either normal (far left column) or smaller than normal but within the 50% confidence limits of normal, we do not extend the incision across the pulmonary valve ring primarily. (The chance that patch-graft enlargement across the ring is necessary is 15%

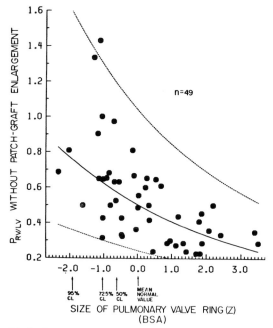

Fig. 64–4.—Relationship of $P_{RV/LV}$ and size of the pulmonary valve ring (expressed for each patient as Z). The mean normal value of the valve ring was calculated from each patient's body surface area.[16]

and 35%, respectively, according to the table.) Instead, the ventriculotomy incision is closed with a patch of woven Dacron (Fig. 64–3, C). In the uncommon circumstance in which $P_{RV/LV}$ immediately after repair is greater than about 0.65, usually cardiopulmonary bypass is re-established for patch-graft enlargement across the pulmonary valve ring. If the measured pulmonary valve ring is abnormally small, that is, less than the lower 95% confidence limits of Lev's normal data, or is within the normal range but outside the lower 72.5% confidence limits, then, according to the table, a 75–90% chance exists of an unacceptably high right ventricular pressure without patch-graft enlargement across the pulmonary valve ring. Under these circumstances, the incision is promptly carried across the pulmonary valve ring to the end of the main pulmonary artery and, if necessary, onto the origin of the left pulmonary artery. The outflow patch, trimmed from the preclotted woven Dacron tube, is sewn into place through this entire area (Fig. 64–3, D).

After discontinuing cardiopulmonary bypass and before closing the chest, fine recording catheters are placed in the left atrium through the right superior pulmonary vein and in the right atrium. These are used for pressure monitoring and for injecting indocyanine green for measurement of cardiac output postoperatively. Hemostasis is carefully secured, two drainage tubes are left within the pericardium, fine steel wire is used to reapproximate the sternum and the remainder of the wound is closed as usual.

Palliative Operations

The palliative operation of choice in most circumstances is the Blalock-Taussig operation made on the side opposite that of the ascending aorta (Fig. 64–5). This end-to-side left subclavian-left pulmonary artery anastomosis is constructed through a lateral incision entering the chest usually through the top of the bed of nonresected fifth rib. After dissecting out the structures, and using, when necessary, optical magnification and interrupted 7–0 monofilament sutures, the anastomosis is constructed in the classic manner.[5, 12]

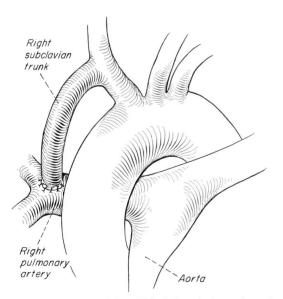

Right subclavian trunk

Right pulmonary artery

Aorta

Fig. 64–5.—Tetralogy of Fallot: Blalock-Taussig type of anastomosis (end-to-side junction of subclavian artery to pulmonary artery). An anterolateral incision through the bed of the nonresected right fourth rib is used. The subclavian artery arising from the innominate artery is utilized in making this shunt between the systemic and the pulmonary circulation. When a right aortic arch is present, the anastomosis is made on the left side.

Side-to-side anastomosis of the ascending aorta to the right pulmonary artery, the so-called Waterston anastomosis, is preferred by some, particularly in very small infants. It is easier and therefore quicker to perform, an advantage in the critically ill, very small infant. The size of the stoma is difficult to control, and if it is too large, congestive heart failure occurs promptly in the early postoperative period, and hypertensive pulmonary vascular disease develops later. Its use, therefore, probably should be restricted to the critically ill, very small infant.

Postoperative Management

Management of infants and children, as well as adults, who have undergone open intracardiac repair for the tetralogy of Fallot is similar to that of other patients undergoing intracardiac operations.

Primary consideration is given to management of the cardiovascular system. Either by clinical criteria or the use of indicator-dilution curves, the cardiac output is estimated. If it is adequate, that is, above about 2.0 l/min/m², no special pharmacologic intervention is indicated. The higher of the two atrial pressures is kept at 10–12 mm Hg by the infusion of blood or, if the hematocrit is high, of an albumin solution, unless cardiac performance is optimal at lower atrial pressures. When a patch has been placed across the pulmonary valve ring and cardiac performance is not optimal, the patient is digitalized intravenously with the use of digoxin. (The estimated digitalizing dose of this drug is 0.9 mg/m² of body surface area, usually given over a period of 24 hours in divided doses.)

A nasotracheal tube is placed at the end of the operation, and the patient is ventilated by the technique of intermittent mandatory ventilation. A positive end-expiratory pressure of about 4–8 mm Hg is desirable. The rate of intermittent mandatory ventilation is gradually decreased, and it usually can be as low as 5 per minute within 20–24 hours of operation. If the patient's spontaneous breathing is adequate and gas exchange is good at this point, extubation is performed.

The performance of the renal system usually is adequate following operation. However, if urine flow falls below about 25 ml/m²/hr, a powerful diuretic agent such as furosemide is given.

An important consideration in patients operated on for the tetralogy of Fallot is that of the indications for return to the operating room for the control of continuing bleeding. Many of these patients are polycythemic and some have had previous anastomotic operations, both contributing at times to excessive chest drainage. We have found the use of a table (Table 64–3) indicating the need for reoperation on the basis of the quantity of chest drainage to be extremely useful in this regard. Whenever the chest drainage exceeds the criteria indicated, the patient is returned to the operating room. Usually, only diffuse bleeding is found, but the re-entry with additional electrocoagulation of bleeding points nearly always stops further bleeding.

Hospital Mortality

The hospital mortality for primary complete repair of the classic type of tetralogy of Fallot is primarily related to the age of the patient at the time of operation. Thus, in our own experience since 1972, there have been no deaths in patients over the age of 4 years at the time of repair (Table 64–4). In younger patients, the risk of the operation has been higher, and under the age of 12 months our own mortality is 18%. Barratt-Boyes[3] has reported superior results in

TABLE 64–3.—LEVELS OF CHEST DRAINAGE ABOVE
WHICH REOPERATION IS INDICATED

PREOP WEIGHT (kg)	CHEST DRAINAGE INDICATING REOPERATION					
	Ml/hr No. of Hr in Succession			Total ml Hour Number		
	1	2	3	4th	5th	6th
≤5.0	70	60	50	120	130	140
6.0	70	60	50	130	155	NA
7.0	70	61	50	152	181	NA
8.0	90	69	52	174	207	NA
9.0	90	78	59	195	233	NA
10.0	108	87	65	217	259	NA
12.0	130	104	78	260	311	NA
14.0	152	122	91	304	363	NA
16.0	174	139	104	347	414	NA
18.0	195	156	117	391	466	NA
20.0	217	174	130	434	518	NA
25.0	271	217	163	542	647	NA
30.0	325	260	195	651	777	NA
35.0	380	304	228	759	906	NA
40.0	434	347	260	868	1036	NA
45.0	488	391	293	976	1165	NA
≥50.0	500	400	300	1000	1200	NA

NOTE: The columns headed "No. of Hr in Succession" indicate the drainage in any 1 hour above which re-entry is indicated, the drainage per hour in any 2 successive hours above which re-entry is indicated and the drainage per hour in any 3 successive hours above which re-entry is indicated. The columns headed "Total ml" refer to the cumulative drainage in any 4-hour period above which re-entry is indicated and for any 5- or 6-hour period.

infants in the first 2 years of life, as has Castaneda[7] (Table 64–5). Whether we and others can duplicate the superb results in very small infants shown in Table 64–5 remains to be seen.

The hospital mortality in our experience is somewhat higher (9%, 70% confidence limits 5–15%) when a patch-graft across the pulmonary valve ring is required than when it is not (4%, 70% confidence limits 2–9%). The risk of complete repair has been very low, 3.4%, in patients requiring repair after a single Blalock-Taussig anastomosis (Table 64–6). The mortality has been slightly higher in patients coming to complete repair after a single Waterston anastomosis (Table 64–7).

Few institutions have, in recent years, systematically performed anastomotic operations for infants with the tetralogy of Fallot because of the impression that the risk of these op-

TABLE 64–4.—RESULTS OF PRIMARY REPAIR
OF THE TETRALOGY OF FALLOT ACCORDING
TO AGE, EXCLUSIVE OF PATIENTS WITH
MULTIPLE VSD, UNIVERSITY OF ALABAMA
MEDICAL CENTER, 1972–1977

AGE (MONTHS)	NO.	HOSPITAL DEATHS		
		No.	%	70% CL
<12	34	6	18	11–27%
≥12 < 24	27	2	7	2–17%
≥24 < 48	29	4	14	7–24%
≥48	61	0	0	0–3%
TOTAL	151	12	7.9	5.7–10.9%

CL = confidence limits.
NOTE: In this and subsequent tables, the 70% confidence limits of all proportions are given to aid in the interpretation of the data.[4]

TABLE 64–5.—CURRENT MORTALITY (1973–1977) FOR
PRIMARY INTRACARDIAC REPAIR OF THE TETRALOGY OF
FALLOT AT BOSTON CHILDREN'S HOSPITAL[°]

AGE (MONTHS)		TOTAL NO.	HOSPITAL DEATHS		
			No.	%	70% CL
<3		12	2	16.7	5.6–35.1%
≥3 < 6	0% to {	12	0	0	0–14.8%
≥6 < 12	7.2% {	14	0	0	0–12.8%
TOTAL		38	2	5.3	1.7–12.1%

CL = confidence limits.
[°] Modified from Castaneda *et al.*[7]

TABLE 64–6.—RESULTS ACCORDING TO AGE AT
REPAIR OF THE CLASSIC TYPE OF TETRALOGY OF
FALLOT IN PATIENTS WHO PREVIOUSLY HAD HAD
A SINGLE BLALOCK-TAUSSIG ANASTOMOSIS,
EXCLUSIVE OF PATIENTS WITH MULTIPLE VSD,
UNIVERSITY OF ALABAMA MEDICAL CENTER,
1967–1977

AGE (MONTHS)	TOTAL NO.	HOSPITAL DEATHS		
		No.	%	70% CL
<12				
≥12 < 24	1	0	0	0–86%
≥24 < 48	2	0	0	0–61%
≥48 < 72	26	2	8	3–17%
≥ 6 < 12 yr	48	1	2	0.3–7%
≥12 < 18 yr	13	0	0	0–14%
≥18 < 30 yr	15	0	0	0–12%
≥30 < 45 yr	10	1	10	1–30%
≥45 yr	2	0	0	0–61%
TOTAL	117	4	3.4	1.7–6.1%

CL = confidence limits.

TABLE 64–7.—RESULTS ACCORDING TO AGE AT
REPAIR OF THE CLASSIC TYPE OF TETRALOGY OF
FALLOT IN PATIENTS WHO PREVIOUSLY HAD HAD
A SINGLE WATERSTON ANASTOMOSIS, EXCLUSIVE
OF PATIENTS WITH MULTIPLE VSD, UNIVERSITY
OF ALABAMA MEDICAL CENTER, 1967–1977

AGE (MONTHS)	TOTAL NO.	HOSPITAL DEATHS		
		No.	%	70% CL
<6	–			
≥ 6 < 12	1	1	100	14–100%
≥12 < 24	1	0	0	0–86%
≥24 < 48	7	0	0	0–24%
≥48 < 72	14	1	7	1–22%
≥ 6 < 12 yr	7	1	14	2–41%
≥12 < 18 yr	1	0	0	0–86%
≥18 < 30 yr	–			
≥30 < 45 yr	–			
≥45 yr	–			
TOTAL	31	3	10	4–19%

CL = confidence limits.

erations in small infants is high. Arciniegas has systematically performed anastomotic operations for all patients with the tetralogy of Fallot less than 5 years of age over the past 5 years (personal communication). His results are superb, with a hospital mortality of 8% in infants under the age of 1

TABLE 64-8.—RESULTS OF ANASTOMOTIC OPERATIONS°

AGE (MONTHS)	BLALOCK-TAUSSIG			WATERSTON			TOTAL			
	No.	Early Deaths	70% CL	No.	Early Deaths	70% CL	No.	Early Deaths	70% CL	
≤1	5	0(0%)	0-32%	8	1(12.5%)	2-36%	13	1(8%)	1-24%	
>1 ≤ 3	4	0(0%)	0-38%	3	0(0%)	0-47%	7	0(0%)	0-24%	2%
>3 ≤ 6	2	0(0%)	0-61%	2	0(0%)	0-61%	4	0(0%)	0-38%	0.3-8%
>6 ≤ 12	12	0(0%)	0-15%	8	0(0%)	0-21%	20	0(0%)	0-9%	
>12 ≤ 60	25	1(4%)	0.5-13%	19	0(0%)	0-10%	44	1(2%)	0.3-8%	
TOTAL	48	1(2%)	0.3-7%	40	1(2.5%)	0.3-8%	88	2(3%)	1-5%	

CL = confidence limits.
°These are the results of anastomotic operations in a center in which these are routinely done for patients with the tetralogy of Fallot requiring surgical intervention before the age of 5 years: 72 patients had classic tetralogy of Fallot and 16 patients tetralogy of Fallot with congenital pulmonary atresia. There is no significant difference in proportion of early deaths in the two groups. (Data from Arciniegas, personal communication, 1977.)

month, and with essentially no deaths in infants over this age (Table 64-8). This experience indicates clearly that the risk of anastomotic operations in infants, with modern techniques of anesthesia and postoperative care, is extremely low.

All of the above data concerning the hospital mortality of intracardiac repair pertain to patients operated on without the modality of cold cardioplegic arrest as it now is practiced by most cardiac surgeons. Since three-fourths of the hospital deaths after repair of the tetralogy of Fallot in our experience have been from low cardiac output, improved myocardial preservation can be expected to reduce hospital mortality rates still further.

Late Results

A number of studies have documented the superb late results that follow the repair of tetralogy of Fallot in most patients. An example is the report from the Mayo Clinic of late results in patients operated on between 1964 and 1971[17] (Table 64-9). More than 80% of the patients have an excellent long-term result and only 4% have a poor result or late death related to the disease. Except in those patients who had severe pulmonary vascular disease as a result of earlier aorto-pulmonary anastomoses, most of the late deaths were sudden, and probably were a result of rhythm disturbances.

The late functional and occupational results of the tetralogy of Fallot are well illustrated in the report by Gersony et al.[11] (Table 64-10). Their study again shows the very high proportion of patients obtaining an excellent long-term result, and most of these are completing their education or are gainfully employed.

TABLE 64-9.—LATE RESULTS OF THE REPAIR OF TETRALOGY OF FALLOT°

CATEGORY	NO.	%	70% CL
Excellent result	236	83	80-85%
Fair result	26	9	7-11%
Poor result	4	1	0.7-2.6%
Late death related to disease	9†	3	2-5%
Late death unrelated to disease	4	1	0.7-2.6%
No late follow-up	6	2	1-3%

CL = confidence limits.
°These are the late results of the repair of tetralogy of Fallot, as modified from Poirier, McGoon et al.[17] The study refers only to patients who survive the first 30 postoperative days. Three of the 9 late deaths (†) were sudden and unexpected, and occurred 1, 3 and 4 years postoperatively. Three other deaths were from severe pulmonary vascular disease in patients who had undergone preliminary Potts anastomoses.

TABLE 64-10.—OCCUPATIONAL STATUS IN A GROUP OF PATIENTS 5-10 YEARS AFTER COMPLETE REPAIR OF THE TETRALOGY OF FALLOT°

	NO.
Full-time student	21
Housewife	13
Clerical worker	11
Registered nurse	4
Secretary	4
Teacher	1
Farmer	1
Naval officer	1
Unemployed	1

°Data from Gersony et al.[11]

The repair of the tetralogy of Fallot, then, clearly is an operation with decreasing hospital mortality rates and superb long-term results.

Present Indications and Timing for Operation

The patient with mild cyanosis, mild polycythemia and mild disability can have his operation safely deferred until the age of about 4 years. The data presented above indicate that the risk of the operation under these circumstances is very low, less than 3%.

Frequently, however, infants and small children present with either severe and progressing cyanosis and polycythemia or recurrent severe hypoxic spells. In this situation, one good choice is a preliminary anastomotic operation, which has been shown by Arciniegas to have a very low mortality, and later complete repair, which we and others have shown can be safely accomplished after the preliminary anastomotic operation. Since very few children die between the time of the anastomotic operation and later complete repair, the combined mortality of this surgical approach is no more than 5%. Another good choice is the performance of primary intracardiac repair at whatever age urgent symptoms develop. Data from many centers indicate that the risk of this approach in general is 15-20% when the operation is required in the first 3 months of life, 5-15% when it is required within 3 and 12 months of age and less than 5% when it is required between 12 and 48 months. Because we believe that these risks are steadily being reduced, we continue to practice primary intracardiac repair for all infants needing operation for the tetralogy of Fallot.

REFERENCES

1. Bargeron, L. M., Jr., Elliott, L. P., Soto, B., Beam, P. R., and Curry, G. C.: Axial cineangiography in congenital heart disease. Section 1, Circulation 56:1075, 1977.
2. Barratt-Boyes, B. G.: Primary Definitive Intracardiac Operations in Infants: Tetralogy of Fallot, in Kirklin, J. W. (ed.), *Advances in Cardiovascular Surgery* (New York: Grune & Stratton, 1973), p. 155.
3. Barratt-Boyes, B. G., and Neutze, J. W.: Primary repair of tetralogy of Fallot in infancy using profound hypothermia with circulatory arrest and limited cardiopulmonary bypass: A comparison with conventional two stage management, Ann. Surg. 178:406, 1973.
4. Blackstone, E. H., Kirklin, J. W., Bradley, E. L., DuShane, J. W., and Appelbaum, A.: Optimal age and results in repair of large ventricular septal defects, J. Thorac. Cardiovasc. Surg. 72:661, 1976.
5. Blalock, A.: Surgical procedures employed and anatomic variations encountered in the treatment of congenital pulmonic stenosis, Surg. Gynecol. Obstet. 87:385, 1948.
6. Blalock, A., and Taussig, H. B.: The surgical treatment of malformations of the heart in which there is pulmonary stenosis or pulmonary atresia, JAMA 128:189, 1945.
7. Castaneda, A. R., Freed, M. D., Williams, R. G., and Norwood, W. I.: Repair of tetralogy of Fallot in infancy: Early and late results, J. Thorac. Cardiovasc. Surg. 74:372, 1977.
8. Elliott, L. P., Bargeron, L. M., Jr., Beam, P. R., Soto, B., and Curry, G. C.: Axial cineangiography in congenital heart disease. Specific lesions. Section II, Circulation 56:1084, 1977.
9. Fallot, A.: Contribution a l'anatomie pathologique de la maladie bleue (cyanose cardiaque), Marseille-méd. 25:77, 138, 207, 341 and 403, 1888.
10. Fisher, R. D., Bone, D. K., Rowe, R. D., and Gott, V. L.: Complete atrioventricular canal associated with tetralogy of Fallot. Clinical experience and operative methods, J. Thorac. Cardiovasc. Surg. 70:265, 1975.
11. Gersony, W. M., Batthany, S., Bowman, F. O., Jr., and Malm, J. R.: Late follow-up of patients evaluated hemodynamically after total correction of tetralogy of Fallot, J. Thorac. Cardiovasc. Surg. 66:209, 1973.
12. Kirklin, J. W., and Karp, R. B.: *The Tetralogy of Fallot from a Surgical Viewpoint* (Philadelphia: W. B. Saunders Company, 1970).
13. Kirklin, J. W., and Payne, W. S.: Surgical treatment for tetralogy of Fallot after previous anastomosis of systemic artery to pulmonary artery, Surg. Gynecol. Obstet. 110:707, 1960.
14. Lev, M.: The architecture of the conduction system in congenital heart disease. II. Tetralogy of Fallot, A.M.A. Arch. Pathol. 67:572, 1959.
15. Lillehei, C. W., *et al.*: Direct vision intracardiac surgical correction of the tetralogy of Fallot, pentalogy of Fallot, and pulmonary atresia defects: Report of first 10 cases, Ann. Surg. 142:418, 1955.
16. Pacifico, A. D., Kirklin, J. W., and Blackstone, E. H.: Surgical management of the pulmonary stenosis in the tetralogy of Fallot, J. Thorac. Cardiovasc. Surg. 74:382, 1977.
17. Poirier, R. A., McGoon, D. C., Danielson, G. K., Wallace, R. B., Ritter, D. G., Moodie, D. S., and Wiltse, C. G.: Late results after repair of tetralogy of Fallot, J. Thorac. Cardiovasc. Surg. 73:900, 1977.
18. Rowlatt, U. F., Rimoldi, H. J. A., and Lev, M.: The quantitative anatomy of the normal child's heart, Pediatr. Clin. North Am. 10:499, 1963.
19. Rygg, I. H., Bertelsen, S., Borgeskov, S., Fabricius, J., Hansen, P. F., Hasner, E., Lauridsen, P., Melchior, J., and Sandoe, E.: The palliative surgical treatment of tetralogy of Fallot, Dan. Med. Bull. 18:59, 1971.
20. Van Mierop, L. H. S., and Wiglesworth, F. W.: Pathogenesis of transposition complexes, Am. J. Cardiol. 12:216, 1963.
21. Willius, F. A.: An unusually early description of the so-called tetralogy of Fallot, Proc. Staff Meet. Mayo Clin. 23:316, 1948.

Defects of Septal Closure

65 George G. Lindesmith

Secundum Type Atrial Septal Defects

Atrial septal defects of the ostium secundum variety are one of the most common congenital heart defects and were submitted to operative repair early in the history of cardiac surgery. This occurred because of the frequency of these lesions among congenital heart defects and because repair could be carried out quickly and without involving the ventricular chambers. Several techniques were developed allowing correction of secundum type atrial septal defects without direct visualization of the lesion. These included the use of an atrial well in the open atrium by Gross[1] and indirect techniques, the heart unopened, described by several authors.[2-5] Closure of atrial septal defects under direct vision was made possible by the technique of using hypothermia with inflow occlusion.[6, 7] All of these earlier techniques either placed severe time constraints on the operating surgeon or prevented adequate visualization of the defect. Because of such limitations, these techniques not infrequently led to inadequate closure of the defect or inappropriate positioning of the pulmonary or systemic veins as they entered the atria. By the first half of the 1960s, the techniques of cardiopulmonary bypass had become standardized and the use of extracorporeal circulation had become safe enough so that the use of the heart-lung machine became the accepted technique to allow surgical repair of all intracardiac defects.

Since secundum type atrial septal defects constitute approximately 10% of congenital heart lesions,[8] the frequency of this lesion has allowed some assessment of its hereditary epidemiology. The apparent familial incidence of this defect is well known to all cardiac surgeons. Studies have shown that the genetic influence on the occurrence of this defect is on a multifactorial basis.[9-11] Therefore, some assessment of the risk to the newborn can be obtained by a careful analysis of the family members, the risk increasing with the number of involved relatives.

Anatomy

Defects of the septum secundum can be grouped easily into three categories, based entirely on the anatomic location of the defect in the septum.

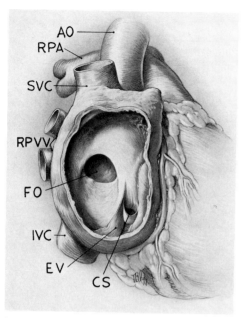

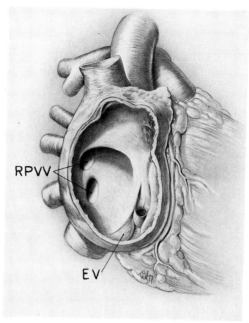

Fig. 65–1.—Patent foramen ovale. A sizable foramen is seen in the central portion of the atrial septum. A prominent eustachian valve *(EV)* is shown in this and subsequent drawings, because of the importance of the structure in the closure of atrial septal defects. *AO* = aorta, *RPA* = right pulmonary artery, *SVC* = superior vena cava, *RPVV* = right pulmonary veins, *FO* = foramen ovale, *IVC* = inferior vena cava, *EV* = eustachian valve, *CS* = coronary sinus.

Fig. 65–2.—Ostium secundum type of atrial septal defect. The usual arrangement is shown, with the openings of the right pulmonary veins clearly visible at the lateral margin of the defect. *RPVV* = right pulmonary veins, *EV* = eustachian valve.

PATENT FORAMEN OVALE.—The most commonly encountered defect in the septum secundum is simple patency of the foramen ovale (Fig. 65–1). This defect is seen frequently in combination with other intracardiac defects. The size of the opening varies from mere probe patency to a defect encompassing the bulk of the area of the foramen ovale. In defects of this type, a portion of the valve of the foramen ovale always is present as the inferior rim of the defect. In the absence of accompanying defects, a small patent foramen ovale usually remains unsuspected and is reported only as an incidental finding at autopsy.

OSTIUM SECUNDUM DEFECT.—This defect is the secundum type atrial septal defect most commonly encountered surgically as an isolated lesion. The area of the septum involved includes, most frequently, the area of the foramen ovale and the septal tissue lateral and inferior to it (Fig. 65–2). Usually the defect has no inferior or lateral rim. On occasion, a portion or all of the valve of the foramen ovale persists in its inferior or lateral rim. If remnants of the valve of the foramen ovale are present, they usually contain multiple fenestrations (Fig. 65–3). The openings of the right pulmonary veins usually can be seen clearly through this type of defect. If a eustachian valve is present, its location is such that it may appear to be the inferior margin of the defect. This anatomic relationship must be clearly understood or the inferior vena cava will be transposed to the left atrium during closure of the defect.

SINUS VENOSUS DEFECT.—The sinus venosus secundum type ASD occurs in the superior portion of the atrial septum immediately subjacent to the superior vena cava (Fig. 65–4). The relationship of sinus venosus defects to the superior vena cava is such that there is no clear-cut superior rim to the opening. There also is no lateral rim, this portion of the

opening being occupied by one or more of the right pulmonary veins. This type of defect is regularly accompanied by anatomic drainage of a portion of the right pulmonary veins into either the right atrium or the superior vena cava (Fig. 65–5). The anomalous location of the right superior pulmonary veins can be detected at operation by external examination of the heart and the nature of the septal defect anticipated.

Anomalous drainage of either systemic or pulmonary

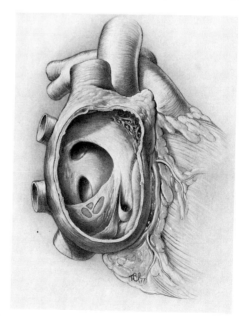

Fig. 65–3.—Ostium secundum type of atrial septal defect. A fenestrated residual valve of the foramen ovale persists as a portion of the anterior and inferior rim of the defect.

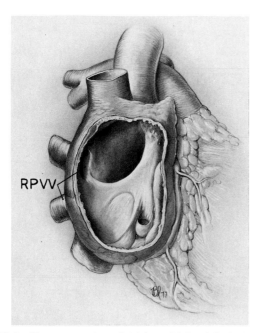

Fig. 65–4.—Sinus venosus type of atrial septal defect. It lies in the superior portion of the atrial septum. The superior right pulmonary vein can be seen entering the atrial chamber in the lateral margin of this defect. The defect has no clear superior rim. *RPVV* = right pulmonary veins.

veins occurs often enough in conjunction with secundum type atrial septal defects that the presence of these anomalies of pulmonary venous drainage always should be borne in mind when these defects are being repaired.

The size of sinus venosus defects, of course, varies considerably. Even with openings that are quite small (1–2 cm in diameter) there may be left-to-right shunting of significant magnitude because of the associated anatomic anomalous drainage of the right pulmonary veins.

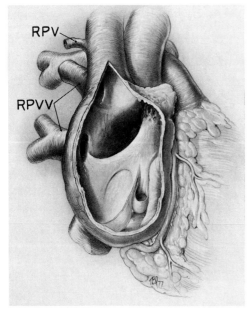

Fig. 65–5.—Sinus venosus defect in the characteristic superior portion of the atrial septum. The right pulmonary veins enter anomalously into the superior vena cava. *RPV* = right pulmonary vein, *RPVV* = right pulmonary veins.

ASSOCIATED DEFECTS.—An uncomplicated patent foramen ovale is seen by the cardiac surgeon most frequently in combination with other cardiac defects. The diagnosis of this lesion is established when cardiac catheterization is being performed for another major intracardiac defect, such as tetralogy of Fallot or ventricular septal defect. The most common associated defect with the other ostium secundum defects is anomalous drainage of the pulmonary veins. Since this is such an integral part of the pathologic anatomy, it, in general, is not considered as a separate defect. In older patients with secundum type atrial septal defects, the association of mitral valve insufficiency occurs with relative frequency.[12, 13] Until recently, this association had not been noted often; however, retrospective and prospective studies have established the importance of this relationship. Repair of the mitral valve should be considered when the insufficiency is of major significance and, in older patients, this combination provides a graver prognosis in the otherwise uncomplicated atrial septal defect.[14]

Symptomatology and Physiology

The majority of children presenting with secundum type atrial septal defects are entirely asymptomatic. The diagnosis is suggested by the presence of a soft systolic murmur and widely split second heart sounds over the base of the heart. Roentgenograms of the chest show cardiomegaly, with the enlargement confined to the right ventricular and right atrial components of the cardiac silhouette. There may be evidence of increased pulmonary blood flow. The diagnosis is confirmed by cardiac catheterization, which demonstrates left-to-right shunting at the atrial level, and the angiographic characteristics of a secundum type atrial septal defect. In the uncomplicated secundum type ASD, the shunt volume may be quite large and occurs primarily when the atrioventricular valves are open.[15] The shunt volumes can be ascribed to the location and size of the defect, as well as to the presence of anomalously draining pulmonary veins. With the low measurable pressure gradients between the right and left atria, however, the most significant factor allowing for left-to-right shunting is the low compliance of the right ventricle as compared to the left. Small but measurable amounts of right-to-left shunting occur with the standard ostium secundum defect. Generally this is attributed to streaming from the inferior vena cava.

In rare instances, ostium secundum type atrial septal defects will present in infancy with unrelenting congestive heart failure. This complex is relatively rare in our experience, but the possibility of secundum type atrial septal defects as a cause of progressive heart failure during infancy must be kept in mind. The lesion can be corrected safely in infants.[16]

Natural History

Except in the occasional case, such as just mentioned, the left-to-right shunting is remarkably well tolerated by most children. The shunt results in a significant volume overload of the right ventricle and pulmonary vasculature. This altered physiology is well tolerated until the third or fourth decade of life, at which time most of these patients become symptomatic. Symptomatology results from a slow increase in pulmonary vascular resistance secondary to changes in the pulmonary vascular bed. These changes, although slow to develop, usually are nonreversible. As the pressure in the pulmonary arterial bed and the right ventricle increases, the shunting at the atrial level reduces in volume and ultimately becomes bidirectional. The patient becomes progressively more fatigable and, ultimately, visibly cyanotic. The clinical course is progressively downhill. Patients so afflicted rarely survive the fourth decade of life.[17]

The indication for surgical closure of secundum type atrial septal defects is generally accepted as the demonstration of a significant shunt at the atrial level. Most surgeons believe that these defects should be closed electively as soon after diagnosis as is convenient. Because of the benign clinical course of most children with this defect, considerable counseling of the patient's family is necessary to ensure adequate understanding of the risks of the disease process if it is left untreated.

When patients with secundum type atrial septal defects present with increased pulmonary vascular resistance, the clinical indications for surgical intervention often are apparent to the patient and family. The surgical risk factor in this group of patients, however, now is elevated and in proportion to the increased pulmonary vascular resistance. In those patients in whom shunting is bidirectional as a result of increased pulmonary vascular resistance, the indications for operation become more complicated, and the increased operative mortality risk must be carefully considered as well as the reduced possibility of a totally successful outcome. When the pulmonary vascular resistance becomes greater than 75% of the systemic vascular resistance, the potential for benefit to the patient usually is outweighed by the risk. In some of these cases, the atrial septal defect may be successfully closed, only to have the pulmonary vascular changes continue to progress inexorably, with the ultimate demise of the patient.

Operative Technique

The closure of atrial septal defects today is routinely accomplished with the aid of cardiopulmonary bypass, to allow adequate exposure and time to repair the defect effectively. We use the pump oxygenator with hemodilution and varying degrees of hypothermia even in the smallest infants. The operation is conducted through a median sternotomy. Caval cannulation is through the right atrial wall (Fig. 65–6). In smaller children, the arterial return from the pump oxygenator usually is accomplished through the femoral artery. In larger children or adults, arterial return is into the ascending aorta. Hypothermia to levels of 25°C is used to afford myocardial protection if aortic cross-clamping is necessary to facilitate closure of the defect.

A longitudinal atriotomy is used to expose the atrial septum. We usually do not vent the left side of the heart. The patent foramen ovale and the standard ostium secundum type defect can be closed by direct suture. We use a running suture and reinforce the suture line with several interrupted sutures placed after the continuous suture has closed the defect (Fig. 65–7). In closing an ostium secundum defect, it is important to start the suture at the inferior limb of the defect so that one can clearly see that the inferior vena cava is not being transposed to the left side of the heart. Occasionally, a eustachian valve in this area is mistaken as the inferior margin of the defect. If this tissue is used to close the defect, the cava necessarily will be transposed.

Occasionally, a surgeon may wish to patch an ostium secundum type defect and this, of course, can be easily accomplished. We have not found this to be necessary unless the septum secundum is totally absent.

The sinus venosus defect presents more of a challenge for surgical closure. When this defect is suspected, one should

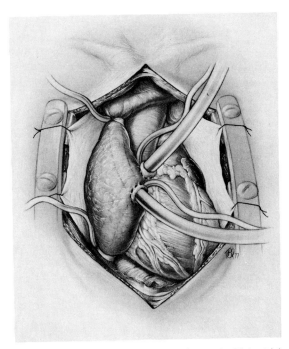

Fig. 65–6.—Surgical exposure of the heart for repair of interatrial septal defects. The caval cannulation is accomplished through purse strings in the wall of the right atrium.

cannulate the superior vena cava directly, or at least insert into it a cannula smaller than usual. By either of these techniques, the region of the junction of the superior vena cava with the right atrium is more easily visualized. The small sinus venosus defect can be closed with a running suture

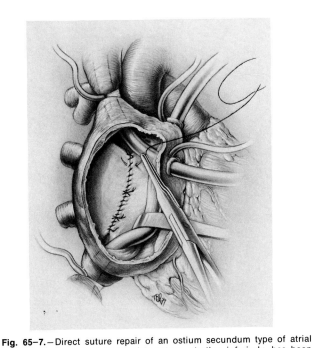

Fig. 65–7.—Direct suture repair of an ostium secundum type of atrial septal defect. A continuous running suture, starting inferiorly, has been completed and interrupted sutures are being placed to reinforce the suture line. The eustachian valve can be seen anterior to the inferior vena caval cannula and care has been exercised not to include this structure in the repair of the atrial defect.

TABLE 65–1.—SOME PUBLISHED RESULTS OF ASD CLOSURE USING CARDIOPULMONARY BYPASS

AUTHORS AND YEAR OF REPORT	YEARS REVIEWED	TYPES OF CASES	AGES	NO. OF CASES	HOSPITAL DEATHS	% MORTALITY	LATE DEATHS	COMMENT
Bircks, Reidemeister, 1971	1949–71	Ostium secundum	All ages	1125	35	3.1		
Cohn, Morrow, Braunwald, 1967		Ostium secundum 150 / Sinus venosus 25		175	6	3.4		All deaths secundum defects
Gerbode, Harkins, Ross, Osborn, 1960	1958–59	Ostium secundum		77	1	1.3		
Hallman, Cooley, 1975	1962–74	Ostium secundum / Sinus venosus		630 / 77	8 / 2	1.8 / 2.6		
Rahimtoola, Kirklin, Burchell, 1968	1954–65	Secundum 630 / Sinus venosus 66		696	22	3.2		All-inclusive experience of Mayo Clinic
	1954–60	No heart failure <45 yr		(279)	(2)	(0.7)		All had pulmonary pressure of 60 torr
Schrire, Beck, Barnard, 1966	1963–65 / 1958–65		All ages	(174) / 121	(0) / 0			No deaths in past 3 years
Sellers, Ferlic, Sterns, Lillehei, 1966	1955–65			275	10	3.6	4	Severe pulmonary hypertension in 2 deaths
Sloan, Morris, Mackenzie, Stern, 1962	1957–61	2°		84	2			Both severe pulmonary hypertension
Stansel, Talner, Deren, Van Heeckeren, Glenn, 1971	Pre 1970	Ostium secundum	All >5 yr	150	0	0		Consecutive cases

Bircks, W., and Reidemeister, Chr.: Results of surgical treatment of ventricular septal defect, Br. Heart J. 33:88, 1971.
Cohn, L. H., Morrow, A. G., and Braunwald, E.: Operative treatment of atrial septal defect. Clinical and haemodynamic assessments in 175 patients, Br. Heart J. 29:725, 1967.
Gerbode, F., Harkins, G. A., Ross, J. K., and Osborn, J. J.: Experience with atrial septal defects repaired with the aid of cardiopulmonary bypass, AMA Arch. Surg. 80:154, 1960.
Hallman, G. L., and Cooley, D. A.: *Surgical Treatment of Congenital Heart Disease* (2d ed.; Philadelphia: Lea & Febiger, 1975).
Rahimtoola, S. H., Kirklin, J. W., and Burchell, H. B.: Atrial septal defect, Circulation 37–38 (Supp. 5): 2, 1968.
Schrire, V., Beck, W., and Barnard, C. N.: An analysis of cardiac surgery at Groote Schuur and Red Cross War Memorial Children's Hospitals, Cape Town, for the 14 years April 1951–April 1965, S. Afr. Med. J. 40:461, 1966.
Sellers, R. D., Ferlic, R. M., Sterns, L. P., and Lillehei, C. W.: Secundum type atrial septal defects: Early and late results of surgical repair using extracorporeal circulation in 275 patients, Surgery 59: 155, 1966.
Sloan, H., Morris, J. D., Mackenzie, J., and Stern, A.: Open heart surgery: Results in 600 cases, Thorax 17:128, 1962.
Stansel, H. C., Talner, N. S., Deren, M. M., Van Heeckeren, D., and Glenn, W. W. L.: Surgical treatment of atrial septal defect. Analysis of 150 corrective operations, Am. J. Surg. 121:485, 1971.

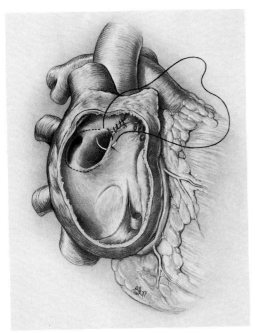

Fig. 65–8.—Direct suture closure of a small sinus venosus defect. Care must be exercised to ensure repositioning of the superior right pulmonary vein behind the closure into the left atrial chamber. This suture line frequently is reinforced with interrupted sutures.

(Fig. 65–8). The surgeon must be careful to reposition correctly any anomalously draining right pulmonary veins. Care also must be exercised to prevent compromise of the superior vena cava as it joins the right atrium. In larger sinus venosus defects we recommend the use of a patch, which can be placed so as to redirect the pulmonary veins and also prevent compromise of the superior vena caval orifice (Fig.

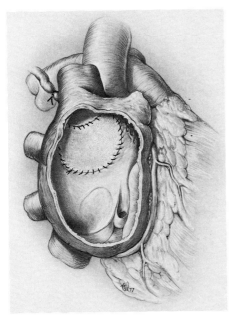

Fig. 65–9.—Patch closure of a larger sinus venosus defect. The superior right pulmonary vein now lies in the left atrium beneath the patch. Smaller pulmonary veins draining into the superior vena cava can be ligated individually without harmful effects.

65–9). When anomalous veins from the right lung drain into the superior vena cava in conjunction with a sinus venosus defect, the technical problem becomes more difficult. When such anomalous veins occur, the lung that they are draining should be inspected carefully. If one or more veins from the affected portion of lung can be appropriately redirected to the left atrium, residual veins can be ligated with impunity. If the anomalous veins are close to the caval atrial junction, the inferior portion of the cava may be divided by a pericardial patch, so that the anomalous veins drain beneath the patch through the defect to the left atrium.

Surgical Results

In uncomplicated secundum type atrial septal defects, the operative mortality should approach zero. Complete closure of the defect should be effected, and complications of significance should be less than 1%. The complication most frequently encountered is cardiac arrhythmia in the immediate postoperative period. These problems, in our experience, have been minimal and short lived. In closing sinus venosus defects, the risk of compromising the superior vena cava should be kept in mind and this complication avoided. The location of the sinoatrial node should be remembered when one is planning atrial incisions, and suture placement in the superior portion of the defect should be superficial in order to avoid injury to the arterial supply to the SA node.

In those patients with secundum type atrial septal defects complicated by other lesions or by the presence of pulmonary vascular disease, the risks, of course, are in proportion to the magnitude of the complicating problem. In general, the surgical repair of the secundum type atrial septal defect should be carried out with minimal or no mortality (Table 65–1), and the patient should anticipate a near-normal cardiovascular system as a result of the repair. These patients should be expected to return quickly to a normal life with no limitations on their physical activity.

REFERENCES

1. Gross, R. E., *et al.*: Surgical closure of defects of the interatrial septum by use of an atrial well, N. Engl. J. Med. 247: 455, 1952.
2. Sondergaard, T., *et al.*: Surgical closure of interatrial septal defect by circumclusion, Acta Chir. Scand. 109:188, 1955.
3. Bailey, C. P., *et al.*: Atrio-septo-pexy for interatrial septal defects, J. Thorac. Surg. 26:184, 1953.
4. Swan, H., and Stewart, B. D.: A modified button technique for the closure of experimental interauricular septal defects, J. Thorac. Surg. 25:397, 1953.
5. Murray, G.: Closure of defects in cardiac septa, Ann. Surg. 128: 843, 1948.
6. Bigelow, W. G., Mustard, W. T., and Evans, J. G.: Some physiologic concepts of hypothermia and their applications to cardiac surgery, J. Thorac. Surg. 28:463, 1954.
7. Lewis, F. J., and Taufic, M.: Closure of atrial septal defect with aid of hypothermia, Surgery 33:1, 1953.
8. Nadas, A. S., and Fyler, D. C.: *Pediatric Cardiology* (3d ed.; Philadelphia: W. B. Saunders Company, 1972).
9. Nora, J. J., McNamara, D. G., and Fraser, F. C.: Hereditary factors in atrial septal defect, Circulation 35:448, 1967.
10. Neill, C. A.: Genetic factors in congenital heart disease, Hosp. Practice 7:97, 1972.
11. Libshitz, H. I., and Barth, K. H.: Familial incidence of atrial septal defect. A report of four siblings and review of the literature, Chest 65:56, 1974.
12. Hynes, K. M., *et al.*: Atrial septal defect (secundum) associated with mitral regurgitation, Am. J. Cardiol. 34:333, 1974.
13. Murray, G. F., and Wilcox, B. R.: Secundum atrial septal defect and mitral valve incompetence, Ann. Thorac. Surg. 20:136, 1975.
14. Leachman, R. D., Cokkinos, D. V., and Cooley, D. A.: Associa-

tion of ostium secundum atrial septal defects with mitral valve prolapse, Am. J. Cardiol. 38:167, 1976.

15. Levin, A. R., *et al.*: Atrial pressure-flow dynamics in atrial septal defects (secundum type), Circulation 37:476, 1968.

16. Phillips, S. J., *et al.*: Complex of secundum atrial septal defect

and congestive heart failure in infants, J. Thorac. Cardiovasc. Surg. 70:696, 1975.

17. Lindesmith, G. G., *et al.*: Congenital Heart Disease, in Blades, B. (ed.), *Surgical Diseases of the Chest* (St. Louis: The C. V. Mosby Company, 1974).

66   GORDON K. DANIELSON

Endocardial Cushion Defects

DURING THE SIXTH WEEK of fetal life, when the embryo is approximately 10 mm in length, the dorsal and ventral endocardial cushions fuse to form a common mass dividing the primitive atrioventricular canal into right and left canals. The lower edge of the atrial septum then descends to join the fused cushions, thus completing cardiac septation except for the septum secundum portion of the atrial septum. Endocardial cushion defects are thought to be caused by failure of proper union of the endocardial cushions and lower edge of the atrial septum and involve both a variable deficiency of ventricular and atrial septa and also variable degrees of malformation of the mitral and tricuspid valves.

Septum primum atrial septal defect, also known as partial atrioventricular (AV) canal, occurs when the atrioventricular valves are fused to the crest of the underlying ventricular septum so that there is no interventricular communication. In the complete form of endocardial cushion defect (complete AV canal), the leaflets are connected to the septum only by chordae, or are free floating above the crest of the ventricular septum, allowing direct interventricular communication.

Associated findings in endocardial cushion defects occurring as a result of the central deficiency of ventricular and atrial septa include an abnormally caudally located position of the medial portions of both the tricuspid and mitral valves and an abnormally cephalad position of the aortic valve. These abnormalities cause the left ventricular outflow tract to be long and narrow and produce the characteristic "gooseneck" deformity seen on the anteroposterior projection of the left ventriculogram in both the partial and complete forms of AV canal.

Because the atrial and ventricular septa and both the atrioventricular valves are involved in the septation of the heart, defects in development of the endocardial cushions can result in many types of anomalies of these four structures. For example, ostium primum atrial septal defect usually is associated with a cleft in the mitral leaflet, but it can occur alone, or an isolated cleft in the mitral valve leaflet can occur with no atrial or ventricular septal defect. Similarly, a ventricular septal defect typical of AV canal defect can occur in isolation or it can be associated with a cleft mitral leaflet without atrial septal defect.

At our institution, the term "atrioventricular canal" has been considered to be more descriptive of the anomaly as it is found clinically, indicating that the anomaly involves both the atrioventricular septa as well as the atrioventricular valves.

In patients with AV canal defects, the abnormal physiology is related to the degree of insufficiency of the AV valves, particularly the mitral valve, and to the degree of left-to-right shunting allowed at the atrial and ventricular levels. When the patient has complete AV canal, the four chambers communicate and both ventricles function at systemic pressures. In the absence of coexistent pulmonary stenosis there is obligatory pulmonary hypertension with high pulmonary blood flows. With the development of pulmonary vascular disease, clinical signs of left-to-right shunting may diminish, and the patient actually may appear clinically improved. Because of the free communication of all chambers in the complete form, some right-to-left shunting may be detected at cardiac catheterization and there may be some arterial desaturation.

Diagnosis of Endocardial Cushion Defects

The diagnosis of atrioventricular canal can be suspected from the electrocardiographic abnormalities, which include first degree heart block, pronounced superior deviation of the mean QRS axis in the frontal plane, right ventricular overload and biventricular overload (especially in complete forms of the defect). In patients with congenital heart disease who have left-to-right shunts, the presence of a counterclockwise frontal plane loop with the initial vector directed inferiorly and to the right and with the major portion of the loop directed superiorly either to the left or to the right or in a figure-of-eight around the X axis is strong evidence for the diagnosis of AV canal. If the counterclockwise frontal plane loop is to the left and superior and the counterclockwise horizontal plane loop is to the left and posterior, the patient probably has partial AV canal whereas a counterclockwise frontal plane loop to the right and superior with a horizontal plane loop anterior and to the right indicates probable complete AV canal. The absence of such frontal plane QRS loops makes a diagnosis of AV canal very unlikely, but other congenital heart lesions may be accompanied by similar loops, so the electrocardiographic findings are not pathognomonic.

Specific and diagnostic echocardiographic observations have been reported in AV canal defect, and with the recently available vector echocardiogram, the diagnosis can be made in nearly every patient with a high degree of certainty as to whether the defect is partial or complete. Contrast echocardiography with indocyanine green dye injections adds to the specificity of the diagnosis.

The basic deficiency of the muscular ventricular septum

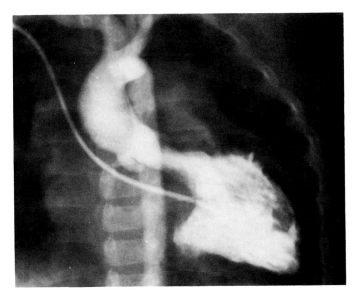

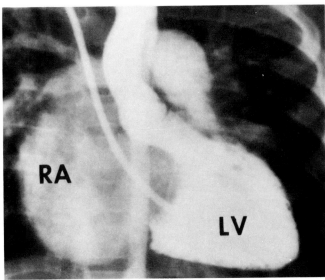

Fig. 66–1 (left).—Partial AV canal without mitral insufficiency. Antero-posterior left ventricular angiocardiogram. Note distorted and elongated left ventricular outflow tract (gooseneck deformity).

Fig. 66–2 (right).—Complete AV canal. Anteroposterior left ventricular angiocardiogram showing same gooseneck deformity of left ventricular outflow tract. Contrast material is also noted in enlarged right atrium (RA). LV = left ventricle.

and the abnormal attachment of the mitral valve that are typical of AV canal are demonstrated in the anteroposterior view of the left ventricular angiocardiogram (Figs. 66 – 1 and 66 – 2). The elongation and narrowing of the left ventricular outflow tract produce a gooseneck-like appearance that is diagnostic. These features are more evident in diastole than in systole, and the right border of the left ventricular silhouette is not smooth and vertical as it is in the normal left ventricular angiocardiogram but is concave as it outlines the edge of the scooped-out ventricular septum. This concave edge is serrated and scalloped, caused by the chordae tendineae that attach the anterior and posterior halves of the anterior leaflet of the mitral valve to the septum.

Operative repair is indicated at any age for cardiac failure not easily manageable by medical means. In the partial form, repair is performed electively at or before age 5. In the complete form, operation is advised before the onset of severe pulmonary vascular obstructive disease, usually before 2 years of age. Pulmonary artery banding no longer is advocated, even in infancy, because of the superior results achievable with total repair.

Partial AV Canal

Operative Technique

A median sternotomy is made and each cava cannulated separately through the right atrium. Arterial inflow from the pump is through an aortic cannula and the left heart is vented with a catheter inserted through the dome of the left atrium or the right superior pulmonary vein. An aortic tack vent on a suction line is placed to aid in prevention of air embolism. Bypass is instituted with the perfusate at 30° C, and after the left heart vent is inserted, the perfusate temperature is lowered to 25°C. The aorta is cross-clamped and cold cardioplegic solution is infused into the aortic root, allowing 30–40 minutes of safe ischemia time as the intracardiac repair is performed. Rewarming of the patient is timed so that no delay is encountered in discontinuing bypass at the conclusion of the repair.

The cleft in the anterior leaflet in the mitral valve is approximated with interrupted sutures placed through the thickened leaflet tissue present along each edge of the cleft (Fig. 66 – 3, B). The distal extent of the cleft at the free edge of the leaflet can be identified by the absence of chordae, which are present along the free edge of the mitral leaflets but which typically end where the cleft begins. It has not been demonstrated yet whether or not it is advisable to close the cleft when there is minimal or no incompetence of the valve. Certainly, if accurate orientation and alignment of the cleft do not seem possible, the cleft should not be sutured.

The suture at the apex of the cleft is not cut but is used to anchor the central portion of the atrial patch (knitted Teflon) (Fig. 66 – 3, C). Interrupted sutures are placed in the anterior (aortic) leaflet of the mitral valve 1.0 mm from the annulus, staying to the left side of the conduction bundle. The sutures then are placed through the patch, the patch is lowered into place and the sutures are tied. If there is any doubt about location of the conduction system, the heart may be allowed to beat during this portion of the repair. Continuous sutures are used when the free margins of the atrial septal defect are reached (Fig. 66 – 3, D).

Results of Operation

Between March of 1955 and September of 1972, 232 patients underwent correction of partial AV canal.[1, 2] There were 99 males and 133 females, whose ages ranged from 3 months to 50 years. Of the 232 patients, 184 (79%) had no symptoms or only mild symptoms, 33 (14%) had moderate symptoms of fatigue and dyspnea and 15 (7%) had severe symptoms, including congestive heart failure. Associated cardiovascular anomalies were present in 88 patients; some patients had more than one anomaly (Table 66 –1).

A total of 138 patients underwent cardiac catheterization prior to operation. Pulmonary blood flow was significantly elevated in all 138, averaging 2.8 times the systemic flow. Pulmonary vascular resistance seldom was significantly elevated and always was less than half the systemic resistance; the highest level was 7.5 units m². Assessment of mitral re-

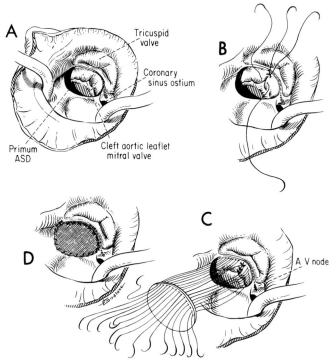

Fig. 66–3.—Partial AV canal (primum atrial septal defect) method of repair. The defect should be closed with a prosthetic patch. The cleft in the aortic leaflet of the mitral value is first approximated with interrupted sutures **(A and B).** Interrupted sutures are then placed in the aortic leaflet 1 mm from the annulus, staying to the left of the conduction bundle. The suture at the apex of the cleft is used as one of the interrupted sutures. The sutures are then placed through the patch, the patch is lowered into place and the sutures are tied **(C and D).** A continuous suture laterally and superiorly completes the closure **(D).**

gurgitation was typically inexact and estimates based on physical examination, left ventriculography and operation correlated poorly. Approximately one-half of the patients had no more than mild mitral incompetence, one-third moderate incompetence and about one-sixth severe incompetence. Only 1 patient underwent mitral valve replacement as a primary procedure.

Thirteen patients died in the hospital after operation (hospital mortality 6%). The risk was higher for patients who were less than 1 year of age, for those with severe preoperative disability and for those with larger hearts (cardiothoracic ratio >0.60).

Patients who survived operation numbered 219, and late follow-up data were available for 210 (96.8%).[2] In addition to 1 patient who required reoperation for mitral regurgitation and died, 8 of the 210 patients (3.8%) subsequently underwent mitral valve surgery 3 months to 14⅓ years after the initial procedure because of severe regurgitation that was residual or progressive or both. There was no demonstrable correlation between the need for late mitral valve replacement and symptom class, age, mitral regurgitation (as estimated by auscultation) or C/T ratio. Of this group of 8 patients, 2 died.

In addition to these 2 patients, 11 others died: 3 of unrelated trauma 10, 13 and 15 years after operation and 8 of factors related to cardiac dysfunction. Heart block was responsible for the deaths of 3 patients in the early experience, before the development of an implantable artificial pacemaker, all of whom died within 5 months of operation. The remaining patients died of congestive heart failure (2), arrhythmia (2) and unrecognized aortic stenosis (1).

In addition to the 3 patients who died of heart block, 2 patients having heart block are alive (Class II disability). Permanent complete heart block, however, has not occurred in the last 194 initial operations.

A computation of actuarial estimation of late survival was performed for all 210 patients on whom follow-up information was available. The estimated survival probabilities at 5, 10 and 15 years for patients recovering from operation were 96.5%, 95.3% and 93.8%, respectively (Fig. 66–4).

TABLE 66–1.—COMMON ASSOCIATED CARDIOVASCULAR ANOMALIES IN 88 OF 232
PATIENTS WITH PARTIAL AV CANAL

ANOMALY	NO. OF PATIENTS
Secundum atrial septal defect	47
Anomalous superior vena cava, including left superior vena cava	17
Pulmonary stenosis (>20 mm Hg peak systolic gradient)	15
Partial anomalous pulmonary venous connection	2
Coarctation of aorta	4
Common atrium	4
Patent ductus arteriosus	2

ACTUARIAL ESTIMATION OF SURVIVAL

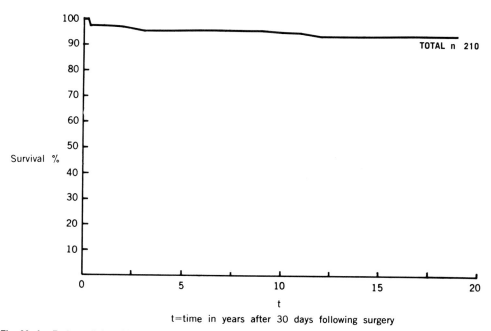

t=time in years after 30 days following surgery

Fig. 66–4.—Endocardial cushion defects. Actuarial estimation of survival for patients alive 30 days after operation for whom follow-up data were available.[2]

In an analysis of factors that might influence long-term survival, age, severity of preoperative symptoms and degree of mitral regurgitation as estimated by auscultation were not found to be statistically significant. There was a statistically significant difference in the survival curve for those patients with a cardiothoracic ratio ≥0.6 compared to those with a C/T ratio ≤0.5 (Fig. 66–5).

Evaluation of mitral regurgitation by auscultation at follow-up was available for 103 patients: 23 patients had no detectable murmur of regurgitation, in 54 it was mild, in 25 it was moderate and in 1 it was severe.

Of 60 patients whose heart size was measured on chest roentgenogram by C/T ratio before operation and at follow-up, 48 showed a decrease in heart size, 10 showed no change

HEART SIZE (C/T)
SERIES II

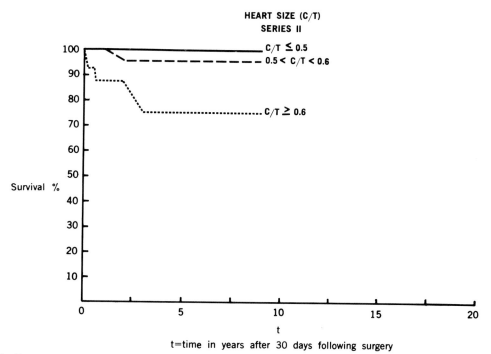

t=time in years after 30 days following surgery

Fig. 66–5.—Endocardial cushion defects. Actuarial estimation of survival, by preoperative cardiothoracic ratio (C/T). C/T curve ≥ 0.6 was significantly different (p = 0.05) from C/T curve ≤ 0.5.[2]

and 2 showed enlargement. In addition to this assessment, all 8 of those who later underwent operation on the mitral valve had evidence of progressive cardiomegaly.

Only 1 patient has required reoperation for late recurrence of the atrial septal defect. An Ivalon patch that had been used underwent dissolution 11 years later; reoperation was successful. Fourteen patients are known to have become pregnant and undergone successful delivery.

Comment: The main problem with respect to the operative management of patients with partial AV canal relates to the mitral deformity. Usually, accurate alignment of the anterior and posterior portions of the anterior (aortic) mitral leaflet reduces the degree of mitral regurgitation and only rarely is mitral valve replacement required as a primary procedure. However, it is necessary to recognize those instances in which deficient leaflet tissue and gross deformities of the valve preclude a successful repair so that mitral valve replacement can be performed at the time of the initial operation. Double sampling indocyanine green dye curves performed by injecting into the left ventricle and sampling simultaneously in the left atrium and ascending aorta are helpful in assessing the degree of mitral regurgitation.[3, 4] Despite the prevalence of an apical systolic murmur, most patients have an excellent late survival. Approximately 4% of the patients will have progression of mitral regurgitation and require reoperation, and this remains a possibility even into the second postoperative decade.

Complete AV Canal

Operative Technique

The operative approach is the same as described previously for partial AV canal, and the repair is carried out entirely through the right atrium. If the repair is not complete after 30 minutes of aortic cross-clamping, a second infusion of cold cardioplegic solution is given. After the anatomy of the anterior and posterior common leaflets is determined, the initial step in the repair is the approximation of their mitral components with a few interrupted sutures (Fig. 66–6, A). If the anterior common leaflet is attached to the septum by chordae (type A) but is incompletely divided, or is undivided and unattached to the ventricular septum (type C), the leaflet is incised to the anulus at the junction of mitral and tricuspid portions. A similar incision of the posterior common leaflet may be required, as shown by the dotted line, in patients with an interventricular communication beneath this leaflet.

A single Teflon patch is fashioned in an oval shape and of a size comparable to that of the over-all ventricular and atrial septal defect (Fig. 66–6, B). The inferior portion of the patch is sutured with interrupted or mattress sutures to the right side of the ventricular septum. All of the sutures are placed prior to lowering the patch into position. The aorta may be unclamped and the heart allowed to beat as the sutures are tied in the region of the conduction bundle.

The mitral margins of the naturally divided anterior common leaflet or the mitral and tricuspid margins of the incised leaflet then are sutured to the patch with interrupted horizontal mattress sutures at a level that corresponds to the plane of the normal mitral and tricuspid annuli (Fig. 66–6, C). The incised or naturally divided posterior common leaflet is attached to the patch in a similar manner. In infants with thin, friable leaflets, the mattress sutures may be buttressed with small pledgets of Teflon felt.

In those cases in which the posterior common leaflet is attached to the interventricular septum by a membrane or fused chordae, the patch shape is altered as shown in Figure 66–6, D and is sewn directly to the atrial surface of the leaflet.

The final step in the repair is closure of the atrial portion of the septal defect by suturing the most cephalad portion of the patch to the rim of the atrial septum (Fig. 66–6, E). The sutures must be placed very superficially, or omitted, in the area near the coronary sinus where the patch crosses over the conduction bundle. In the presence of associated pulmonary stenosis, valvotomy and infundibular resection are performed as indicated.

Recently, 2 patients have undergone successful repair of complete AV canal with anterior common leaflet attached to an abnormal papillary muscle arising in the right ventricle near the septum (type B). The repair of this variety is similar to that of type C.[6]

Results of Operation

Twenty-seven patients with complete AV canal were operated on between June of 1963 and December of 1971. Twenty had type A and 7 had type C anomalies. There were 15 females and 12 males with a mean age of 7 years in a range of 3–18 years. Associated cardiovascular anomalies included 9 instances of patent foramen ovale, 3 of left superior vena cava, 4 of pulmonary stenosis and 1 of patent ductus arteriosus. Roentgenographic examination of the chest showed an average preoperative C/T ratio of 0.63 (range 0.46–0.73).

Preoperative catheterization data were available in 25 of the 27 patients. The mean ratio of pulmonary to systemic flow (Qp/Qs) calculated in 16 patients without pulmonary stenosis or previous pulmonary arterial banding was 2.6, with a range of 1.5–4.6. The average pulmonary resistance was 6.3 units m² (range 1–14). Of 25 patients, the degree of mitral regurgitation was estimated by the surgeon at operation as none to mild in 15, moderate in 9 and severe in 1.

Two deaths occurred in this series, for a mortality of 7%. One death occurred in the type A group and the other in the type C group. Both deaths were related to technical factors, one to incomplete repair and the other to dehiscence of the anterior leaflet of the mitral valve from the patch. Teflon felt pledgets had not been used.

Eight patients developed dysrhythmias postoperatively, including supraventricular, nodal and atrial tachycardia and transient nodal rhythm. There were no instances of complete heart block.

Since the patients were not routinely catheterized postoperatively unless it was specifically required, the estimation of the degree of mitral regurgitation following operation was limited to evaluation by physical examination. A comparison of the preoperative physical examination with the postoperative examination showed some reduction in severity of mitral regurgitation in many patients, and no patient was thought to have severe mitral regurgitation postoperatively, either early or at the time of late follow-up.

Follow-up data were obtained for 23 of the 25 survivors. The duration of follow-up ranged from 3 months to 8¾ years, with a mean of 3.4 years. There were no late deaths and no patient required subsequent mitral valve replacement. Twenty-one of the patients were asymptomatic and in New York Heart Association Class I whereas 2 patients remained symptomatic with dyspnea on exertion and are in

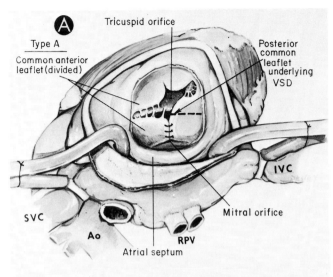

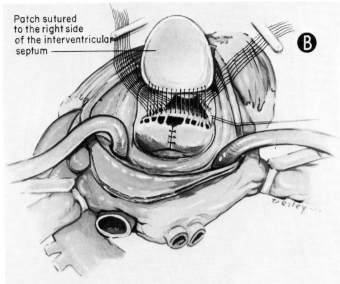

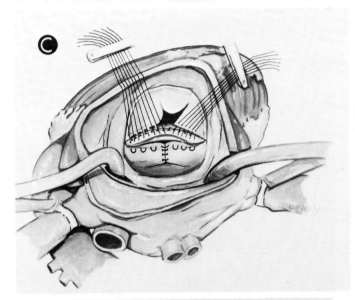

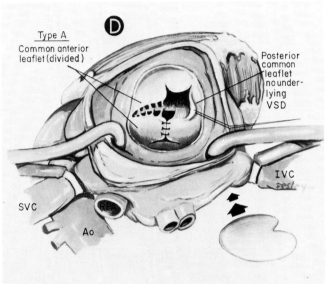

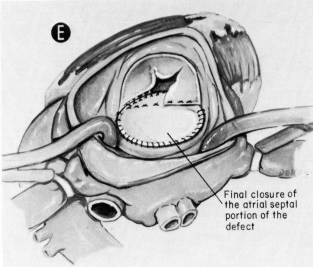

Fig. 66–6. — Repair of complete AV canal.[5] **A,** repair of mitral valve. **B,** insertion of oval, Teflon patch the size of the combined atrial and ventricular septal defects. All sutures to the right side of the septum are placed before the patch is lowered into position. **C,** the patch is sutured to the leaflets at a level that corresponds to that of the normal mitral and tricuspid anuli. **D,** if the posterior common leaflet is attached to the interventricular septum by a membrane or fused chordae, a patch of different shape is sewn to the atrial surface of the leaflet. **E,** the final step. The most cephalad portion of the patch is sutured to the rim of the atrial septum.

TABLE 66–2.—Repair Complete AV Canal
(1972 to May 1976)

	0–12 MO	1–2 YR	3–23 YR
Deaths/patients	1/7	5/12	1/30
Operative mortality = 14%			

Class II. This is in contrast to the preoperative status: 1 patient in Class I, 24 patients in Class II and 2 patients in Class III.

Comment: The low operative mortality of 7% achieved by this method of repair, as well as the gratifying quality of life achieved on long-term follow-up of these patients, all without resort to the use of prosthetic valves, establishes this as our technique of choice. Although occasional patients will require replacement of the mitral or even tricuspid valve, no such patients were encountered during this experience. We have had one case since these data were collected of a patient successfully operated on in whom it was necessary to replace both the mitral and tricuspid valves with prostheses. These results contradict the published recommendation and practice of others of replacing the mitral valve in many or most operations for complete AV canal because of alleged deficiency of leaflet tissue for reconstruction of the valve.[9] Until more perfect substitute mitral valves are developed, residual mild mitral regurgitation seems preferable to valve replacement, particularly since progression of the severity of the regurgitation is encountered infrequently.

Since this experience, the age limit for total repair has been lowered and now includes infants of all ages.[4] Table 66–2 shows our additional experience to May of 1976. These encouraging results and those being reported from other institutions for repair in infancy suggest that the most appropriate policy is to perform complete repair in infants who require early operative assistance rather than performing pulmonary arterial banding.[7, 8] The banding procedure, although occasionally beneficial, is least effective in patients who have mitral regurgitation as a prominent cause of cardiac failure.

As in the repair of partial AV canal, the surgeon must decide at the time of operation if the degree of residual mitral regurgitation is unsatisfactory so that he can proceed directly with replacement of the mitral valve with a prosthesis. In addition to assessment of the adequacy of leaflet tissue, it is helpful to perform intraoperative, double sampling, dye dilution curves as described under partial AV canal. If severe regurgitation is demonstrated, bypass is resumed, the left atrium is entered directly and a glutaraldehyde-preserved porcine heterograft valve is inserted. The plane of the mitral annulus lies at a level cephalad to the crest of the ventricular septum, so the mitral valve prosthesis must be attached in a special way to properly orient the valve and to avoid heart block. The prosthesis is attached to the mural aspect of the mitral annulus as usual, but on the septal aspect the line of attachment is carried across the patch in the plane of the anulus 1 or 2 cm cephalad from the crest of the midportion of the ventricular septum.

Mention should also be made of repair of complete AV canal associated with additional complex congenital cardiac lesions. Until recently, repair usually has been unsuccessful.[5] Several recent case reports of successful repair of complicated forms of complete AV canal now give encouragement to proceed with repair of such complex lesions, even in infants.[10, 11]

In summary, complete atrioventricular canal now can be repaired satisfactorily at all ages. We now prefer primary repair in infancy rather than a two-stage procedure. Many complex forms of complete atrioventricular canal are also amenable to total correction.

REFERENCES

1. Rastelli, G. C., Weidman, W. H., and Kirklin, J. W.: Surgical repair of the partial form of persistent common atrioventricular canal, with special reference to the problem of mitral valve incompetence, Circulation 31(Supp. 1):31, 1965.
2. McMullan, M. H., McGoon, D. C., Wallace, R. B., Danielson, G. K., and Weidman, W. H.: Surgical treatment of partial atrioventricular canal, Arch. Surg. 107:705, 1973.
3. Danielson, G. K., Exarhos, N. D., Weidman, W. H., and McGoon, D. C.: Pulmonic stenosis with intact ventricular septum: Surgical considerations and results of operation, J. Thorac. Cardiovasc. Surg. 61:228, 1971.
4. McGoon, D. C., McMullan, M. H., Mair, D. D., and Danielson, G. K.: Correction of complete atrioventricular canal in infants, Mayo Clin. Proc. 48:769, 1973.
5. McMullan, M. H., Wallace, R. B., Weidman, W. H., *et al.:* Surgical treatment of complete atrioventricular canal, Surgery 72:905, 1972.
6. Pacifico, A. D., and Kirklin, J. W.: Surgical repair of complete atrioventricular canal with anterior common leaflet attached to an anomalous right ventricular papillary muscle, J. Thorac. Cardiovasc. Surg. 65:727, 1973.
7. Culpepper, W., Kolff, J., Replogle, R., and Arcilla, R. A.: Correction of complete atrioventricular canal defect during infancy. Presented at the 26th Annual Scientific Session of the American College of Cardiology, Las Vegas, March 9, 1977.
8. Berger, T. J., Kirklin, J. W., Pacifico, A. D., and Kouchoukos, N. T.: Surgery for complete atrioventricular canal under two years of age. Presented at the 26th Annual Scientific Session of the American College of Cardiology, Las Vegas, March 9, 1977.
9. Castaneda, A. R., Nicoloff, D. M., Moller, J. H., and Lucas, R. V., Jr.: Surgical correction of complete atrioventricular canal utilizing ball-valve replacement of the mitral valve: Technical considerations and results, J. Thorac. Cardiovasc. Surg. 62:926, 1971.
10. Danielson, G. K., Giuliani, E. R., and Ritter, D. G.: Successful repair of common ventricle associated with complete atrioventricular canal, J. Thorac. Cardiovasc. Surg. 67:152, 1974.
11. Danielson, G. K., McMullan, M. H., Kinsley, R. H., and DuShane, J. W.: Successful repair of complete atrioventricular canal associated with dextroversion, common atrium, and total anomalous systemic venous return, J. Thorac. Cardiovasc. Surg. 66:817, 1973.

67 Aldo R. Castaneda / Gilbert A. Norwood

Obstruction to Pulmonary Venous Return, Including: Congenital Mitral Stenosis, Congenital Mitral Regurgitation, Cor Triatriatum and Pulmonary Vein Stenosis

SEVERAL anatomically diverse congenital cardiovascular anomalies share the common functional features of obstruction to pulmonary venous return. As early as 1715, Vieussens described a 30-year-old man with dyspnea and attributed the symptom to his calcified mitral valve, discovered at autopsy, and, in 1878, Welch recognized the relationship between left ventricular failure as a hindrance to pulmonary venous return and the subsequent development of pulmonary edema. Since then, the hemodynamic features and the clinical consequences of pulmonary venous obstruction secondary to acquired mitral stenosis and constrictive pericarditis have been further detailed. More recently, Lucas and coworkers have emphasized the occurrence of pulmonary venous obstruction in patients with congenital cardiac lesions, related the phenomenon to that of acquired mitral stenosis and defined the individual anatomic congenital causes of pulmonary venous obstruction. It is the common physiology and pulmonary pathology resultant from impeded pulmonary venous return that provides the basis for collectively considering these rare congenital cardiac anomalies: isolated pulmonary vein stenosis, cor triatriatum, congenital mitral stenosis and congenital mitral regurgitation.

Pathophysiology

Whatever the site of obstruction, increased pressure in the compartment proximal to the obstruction is transmitted to the pulmonary capillary bed and adjacent vasculature. As a consequence, physiologic and even anatomic alterations occur that produce the characteristic features of this group of lesions. As the intravascular hydrostatic pressure less the oncotic pressure in the pulmonary veins exceeds that in the interstitium surrounding the pulmonary capillary bed, the normal dynamic equilibrium of fluid leaving the vascular compartment at the pulmonary arterioles, percolating through the interstitial spaces to be resorbed at the pulmonary venules, is disturbed, with a resultant net movement of fluid into lung parenchyma. If such shifts are acute or large, frank pulmonary venous edema ensues. Less severe or more insidious obstruction to pulmonary venous return, on the other hand, induces physiologic and even anatomic compensations. Such compensations include: (1) increased capacity and drainage of the pulmonary lymphatic system, (2) the amplification of existing pulmonary to systemic venous communications (bronchopulmonary venous collaterals) and

(3) as in acquired mitral stenosis, reflux pulmonary arteriolar vasoconstriction, which reduces the amount of blood entering the pulmonary capillary bed. Pulmonary arterial pressure and resistance thus invariably are elevated by this group of lesions. During exercise, pulmonary arterial pressure rises inordinately whereas pulmonary blood flow increases little or not at all. Associated histologic findings in the pulmonary vasculature include medial hypertrophy of both pulmonary veins and arterioles. This sequence of changes is accompanied by the clinical picture of tachypnea, dyspnea, occasional cyanosis and roentgenographic findings of pulmonary edema, venous congestion, dilatation of the pulmonary veins and prominence of the pulmonary lymphatics. Eventually, the increased pulmonary arterial pressure and resistance result in right ventricular hypertrophy, detectable both roentgenographically and electrocardiographically.

Embryology

Isolated stenosis of individual pulmonary veins and cor triatriatum are believed to be embryologically related anomalies. The progenitor of the pulmonary vasculature is the splanchnic plexus, part of which enmeshes the lung bud from the foregut during pulmonary differentiation. Early in this development there is no direct connection between the pulmonary venous primordium and the heart, and communication with the cardinal veins and the umbilico-vitelline system provides the initial pulmonary venous drainage. As communication between the pulmonary portion of the splanchnic plexus and an evagination from the sinoatrial region of the heart (commonly pulmonary vein) is established, connections between the plexus and the cardinal and umbilico-vitelline veins markedly attenuate. At this point there generally are four major pulmonary veins draining into a common pulmonary vein, which, in turn, now empties into the common atrium. The common pulmonary vein, however, is also a transient structure and ultimately becomes incorporated into the left atrium following septation of the common atrium. Malabsorption of the common pulmonary vein into the posterior aspect of the heart is the cause of several congenital anomalies: stenosis of one or more of the individual pulmonary veins, total anomalous pulmonary venous connection (atresia of the common pulmonary vein) or cor triatriatum (stenosis of the common pulmonary vein).

Isolated Stenosis of the Pulmonary Veins

Pulmonary vein stenosis is an uncommon lesion that occurs in isolated form or in association with other cardiac anomalies. Even in isolated form, its infrequent occurrence leads to belated or missed diagnosis, and thus isolated pulmonary vein stenosis should be suspected in patients carrying the diagnosis of idiopathic or primary pulmonary hypertension. A feature that distinguishes this lesion from other causes of pulmonary venous obstruction is the angiocardiographic demonstration of delayed emptying of dilated pulmonary veins.

The technique of repair is dependent on the site and nature of the stenosis. Where the obstruction is membranous, excision of the diaphragm is effective whereas patch angioplasty may be required if a length of vein is hypoplastic. For segmental stenosis or atresia, direct anastomosis of the vein to the left atrium may be necessary. If the obstruction cannot be relieved and it is affecting only a limited amount of lung, resection of the undrained pulmonary tissue is recommended in order to avoid recurrent infections and hemoptysis.

Cor Triatriatum

Cor triatriatum is a rare cardiac anomaly that was initially described by Church in 1868. It is characterized by pulmonary venous drainage into a chamber that communicates with the left atrium via a small opening that embryologically represents the connection between the common pulmonary vein and the true left atrium.

Anatomy

The septum dividing the proximal accessory chamber from the true left atrium usually is fibromuscular and separates the pulmonary veins from the distal true left atrium containing the left atrial appendage, fossa ovale and a normal mitral valve. The associated clinical findings are all secondary to obstruction to pulmonary venous return, and the degree of these changes is directly related to the size of the opening between the accessory chamber and the true left atrium.

Pathophysiology and Natural History

It has been suggested that if atresia of the common pulmonary vein occurs prior to obliteration of the primitive venous channels, the resultant lesion is total anomalous pulmonary venous connection whereas, on the other hand, if the common pulmonary vein fails to communicate with the true left atrium following obliteration of the cardinal veins, type I cor triatriatum results. This is an uncommon form of cor triatriatum and those patients with this lesion are severely compromised; the majority die within the first month of life. With all types, the hemodynamic alterations, symptoms and natural history depend on the degree of restriction of pulmonary venous return. Most commonly, the hemodynamic and clinical picture is similar to that of severe mitral stenosis. Pulmonary arteriolar constriction and hypertrophy of the media of the pulmonary vasculature usually result in severe pulmonary hypertension and right ventricular failure in the first months of life. Pressure in the true left atrium, as well as left ventricle, is normal; thus, as the right atrial pressure rises, those patients with an atrial septal defect or patent foramen ovale will develop cyanosis from a right-to-left

shunt. Niwayana has reported a collected series of 36 patients with cor triatriatum in which 50% of the patients died before the age of 1 year and 64% within the first 5 years of life.

Clinical and Diagnostic Features

The clinical features of cor triatriatum are dyspnea, hyperpnea, failure to thrive and occasionally cyanosis occurring during the first year of life. Findings of cardiac enlargement and right ventricular hypertrophy usually are present. The first heart sound is normal whereas the second heart sound is markedly accentuated and is narrowly split or even single. Heart murmurs generally are absent but occasionally a diastolic murmur is audible at the left sternal border or the murmur of tricuspid insufficiency may be present. Generally, the electrocardiogram reveals varying degrees of right atrial enlargement and right ventricular hypertrophy with strain.

On chest roentgenogram, cardiac enlargement often is seen in conjunction with the characteristic findings of pulmonary venous obstruction; fine reticular markings extend out from each hilum, with dilated pulmonary lymphatics and pulmonary veins.

Recently, echocardiography has been increasingly helpful in distinguishing the anatomic variants resulting in obstruction to pulmonary venous return. An abnormal echo in the left atrium that is not closely associated with the mitral valve suggests cor triatriatum. Extraneous left atrial echoes are also seen with supravalvar stenosing ring but, in contradistinction to cor triatriatum, these almost always are contiguous with an abnormal mitral valve.

Given the multiplicity of anatomic anomalies leading to a common pathophysiology, angiocardiography is essential in delineating the site of obstruction of pulmonary venous return. Selective injections in the pulmonary artery are mandatory. In those instances in which the catheter can be manipulated across the atrial septum, the site of obstruction usually can be defined.

Surgical Management

Critical to an optimal outcome of surgical management is early diagnosis of the anatomic site of the obstruction, for, ultimately, the prognosis is dependent on the degree of irreversibility of alterations in the pulmonary vasculature and right ventricle. Having established the diagnosis of cor triatriatum, excision of the dividing septum and closure of the atrial communication generally is easily accomplished.

Congenital Mitral Stenosis

Congenital mitral stenosis is a rare cardiac malformation occurring in 1.2% of patients dying from congenital heart disease and 0.42% of all cardiac patients at Children's Hospital in Boston. Ferencz reports that approximately 4% of cardiac cases in her review had congenital mitral stenosis, and Bower and associates found that 7.5% of autopsied patients with congenital malformations of the heart had mitral stenosis or atresia. There is a male predominance in congenital mitral stenosis, as there is with other left-sided obstructive lesions. As with most other congenital cardiac anomalies, the etiology is not clear but patients with trisomy 18 frequently have stenotic and otherwise abnormal mitral valves. Unlike the other anatomic abnormalities resulting in obstruction to pulmonary venous return, mitral stenosis often is associated with other congenital cardiac lesions, complicating both its analysis and management.

Anatomy

Congenital mitral valve stenosis may result from the abnormal development of any portion of the valve apparatus: mitral valve leaflets, commissures, interchordal spaces, annulus or immediate supravalvar area and/or papillary muscles (Fig. 67–1). The left ventricle may be normal but in patients with severe mitral stenosis the ventricle usually is somewhat hypoplastic. In 1963, Shone recognized the association of parachute mitral valve with three other obstructing left-sided lesions: supravalvar ring, subaortic stenosis and coarctation of the aorta. Congenital mitral stenosis can also coexist with other combinations of left-sided obstructive lesions and it has even been found in association with right-sided obstructive lesions such as tetralogy of Fallot. In those patients in whom associated lesions are not dominant, the typical anatomic changes in the pulmonary vasculature and right ventricle of pulmonary venous obstruction are seen.

Pathophysiology and Natural History

The majority of patients with congenital mitral stenosis have moderate to severe obstruction. Pulmonary venous hypertension results and a compensatory rise in pulmonary vascular resistance secondary to reflex vasoconstriction results. Cardiac output is decreased at rest in critical mitral stenosis and the heart is unable to increase blood flow on demand without precipitating pulmonary edema. Tachycardia results in further decrease in cardiac output secondary to a shortened left ventricular filling time. Pulmonary venous congestion and pulmonary edema lead to decreased pulmonary compliance, with resultant tachypnea and dyspnea. The prognosis of patients with congenital mitral stenosis varies considerably, depending on the degree of stenosis and the associated cardiac lesions. Infants with severe stenosis usually die within the first months of life secondary to pulmonary edema and congestive heart failure. In Ferencz's collected series, almost 50% succumbed before 6 months of age. In our series at Children's Hospital, only 53% of all patients, both medically and surgically managed, are alive at 10 years of age.

Clinical and Diagnostic Features

Symptoms include shortness of breath, exertional dyspnea, syncope and repeated pulmonary infection within the first few months of life. Failure to thrive is a striking clinical feature. As with other lesions producing pulmonary venous obstruction, an accentuation of pulmonary valve closure almost invariably is present on auscultation. However, a loud first heart sound often distinguishes mitral stenosis from more proximal obstructing lesions. In addition, a mid-diastolic rumble is noted in all patients with significant mitral stenosis.

On chest roentgenogram, cardiac enlargement is present. About half of the patients demonstrate left atrial enlargement and usually there is redistribution of the pulmonary vasculature to the upper third of the lung field. The electrocardiogram reveals right ventricular hypertrophy, right axis deviation, spiked P waves or P mitrale.

Echocardiography has proved to be a useful tool in examining the mitral valve. The finding of anterior motion of the posterior leaflet of the mitral valve during diastole suggests chordal fusion, and a shortened diastolic closure rate of the mitral valve results from limited movement and prolonged filling through an obstructed mitral valve. At cardiac catheterization, patients with mitral stenosis have elevated pulmonary arterial and pulmonary capillary wedge pressures. The levo phase after right heart angiography may be helpful in outlining the size of the left atrium and demonstrating the presence or absence of a supravalvar ring. A selective left ventricular injection to determine the position and number of papillary muscles, assess the mobility of the leaflets and determine the existence and degree of mitral regurgitation is important for planning and timing surgical management. However, in the presence of associated cardiac lesions, severe congestive heart failure or a large intracardiac shunt, establishing the diagnosis of congenital mitral stenosis at catheterization alone may prove to be difficult.

The surgical treatment of congenital mitral stenosis is discussed with that for mitral regurgitation.

Mitral Regurgitation

Congenital mitral regurgitation is a rare cardiac anomaly. The most common cause of mitral regurgitation in infants and children is a defect of the atrioventricular canal, partial or complete (see Chap. 66). As with the valve lesions leading to mitral stenosis, mitral regurgitation often is associated with other left-sided anatomic defects, such as coarctation of the aorta, patent ductus arteriosus, ventricular septal defect and aortic stenosis. Anomalous origin of the coronary artery from the pulmonary artery may first manifest itself as mitral regurgitation (infarcted papillary muscles).

Anatomy

The anatomic defects that lead to mitral regurgitation are most conveniently classified according to the abnormalities of the various structural components of the mitral valve apparatus. We consider the classification recently advanced by Carpentier to be useful (Fig. 67–2). In association with the defects of the mitral valve apparatus there often is dilatation and hypertrophy of the left ventricle with a massively dilated left atrium. Occasionally, jet lesions are visible on the left atrial wall. As in other lesions resulting in obstruction to

I. Predominant valvar defect

A   B   C

II. Predominant subvalvar defect

D   E   F

Fig. 67–1.—Forms of mitral stenosis (according to Carpentier). *A,* annular hypoplasia. *B,* supravalvar ring. *C,* obliteration of interchordal spaces by endocardial cushion tissue. *D,* parachute mitral valve (often with single papillary muscle). *E,* hammock valve. *F,* fusion of papillary muscle to commissures.

I. Predominant valvar defect

A   **B**   **C**

II. Predominant subvalvar defect

D   **E**   **F**

Fig. 67–2.—Forms of mitral regurgitation (according to Carpentier). *A,* annular dilatation or deformation. *B,* cleft leaflet. *C,* double orifice or leaflet agenesis. *D,* leaflet prolapse from elongated chordae or abnormal papillary muscle. *E,* restricted leaflet motion from short or fused chordae. *F,* papillary muscle hypoplasia.

pulmonary venous return there are secondary changes of the pulmonary vasculature, dilatation of the main pulmonary artery and right ventricular hypertrophy.

Pathophysiology

During left ventricular systole, blood regurgitates into the left atrium. The increased pressure in the left atrium is transmitted to the pulmonary veins and ultimately to the pulmonary arteries. Pulmonary vascular resistance rises but seldom to the levels seen with the other lesions resulting in an obstruction to pulmonary venous return. The increased volume load on the left ventricle results in left ventricular dilatation and hypertrophy. Mild mitral incompetence is well tolerated without significant hemodynamic change, but if the regurgitation is moderate to severe, eventually the forward ejection fraction significantly decreases as the left ventricle continues to dilate. Because a large volume of blood is expelled early in systole into the relatively low-pressure left atrium, the myocardial wall tension, required to generate sufficient pressure to overcome the systemic after-load, is less than that for a comparably dilated ventricle secondary to aortic regurgitation. This may account for the observation that mitral regurgitation is tolerated much better than severe aortic regurgitation. Related to this phenomenon, it is important to bear in mind that surgical correction of longstanding mitral incompetence in patients with an extremely large dilated left ventricle and significantly decreased ejection fraction may initially aggravate left ventricular failure.

Clinical and Diagnostic Features

The severity of symptoms is determined by the degree of mitral regurgitation. Mild lesions cause no symptoms whereas patients with severe regurgitation have fatigue, weakness and dyspnea on exertion. Pulmonary edema and congestive heart failure are late sequelae. Cardiac enlargement is detectable on physical examination, along with a hyperdynamic left ventricular impulse. The first heart sound is normal whereas the second heart sound usually is widely split, with only moderate accentuation of the pulmonary component. Often a third heart sound is present as a result of the large volume of blood that fills the left ventricle. The classic murmur is high pitched, pansystolic, maximal at the

apex and radiates to the left axilla. A mid-diastolic murmur may be present. The electrocardiogram is normal in mild lesions but may show left ventricular hypertrophy in moderate and severe mitral regurgitation. The P wave usually is increased in duration and bifid (P mitrale). Signs of right ventricular hypertrophy can be found in the presence of pulmonary hypertension. On a chest film there usually is a prominence of the left atrial appendage, with elevation of the left main stem bronchus, cardiac enlargement and massive dilatation of the left atrium. Late sequelae produce prominence of the pulmonary artery and evidence of pulmonary edema.

Surgical Management of Congenital Mitral Valve Disease

The congenital anomalies of the mitral valve are uncommon, diverse and difficult to manage. Early attempts by Lillehei, Kay and Gross at closed mitral commissurotomy in the late 1950s often resulted in severe mitral insufficiency. In our experience, open valvotomy alone for relief from congenital mitral stenosis generally has not resulted in a complete reduction of the pressure gradient across the mitral valve (particularly in the infant group) because the contribution of the subvalvar component to obstruction usually is significant. However, valvotomy can provide palliation, reducing symptoms and allowing growth of the child. In those infants with supravalvar ring and associated mitral valve defects, resection of the supravalvar ring alone afforded some hemodynamic improvement and reduction of symptoms. On the other hand, repair of associated lesions while ignoring stenosis of the mitral valve proved to be uniformly unsatisfactory. Infants with mitral regurgitation and coarctation of the aorta have, in our experience, been improved or temporarily stabilized with resection of the coarctation alone.

The disadvantages inherent in the currently available prosthetic valves for infants and children have provided impetus for extensive surgical attempts at resculpturing of the mitral valve apparatus and subvalvar components. Carpentier and associates recently have reported excellent results with such surgical treatment of 47 children ages 4 months to 12 years (mean 6 years). Of these patients, 6 were less than 2 years of age and all but 1 of these 6 had some degree of mitral stenosis. Thirty-two of 47 patients had mitral regurgitation. Five of these ultimately required mitral valve replacement; the rest were managed by reconstruction of chordal and papillary muscle anatomy. Of the 15 patients with mitral stenosis, incision of fused commissures, fenestration of fused chordae with excision of hypertrophic papillary muscle mass was carried out in all but 4 patients who underwent valve replacement. The hospital mortality of the 38 patients undergoing valve repair was 8% (3 patients) whereas 33% (3 patients) died after valve replacement. Of the survivors, the clinical improvement was remarkable, despite the fact that minimal or moderate regurgitation or cardiomegaly frequently persisted.

Clearly, a detailed understanding of the pathology of congenital mitral valve disease is essential in carrying out the extensive resculpturing of the mitral valve, so impressively demonstrated by Carpentier. On the other hand, in the patient with extremely shortened chordae tendineae of an immature mitral valve, or agenesis of the mitral leaflets, it is difficult to avoid mitral valve replacement. Despite numerous reports of successful mitral valve replacement in infants and children, the ideal prosthetic valve is not yet available. The problems of valve replacement are compounded in infants and children by the limited size of the left ventricular cavity and mitral annulus, a potentially long life expectancy demanding durability of the prosthetic device and special problems of anticoagulation management in children. An additional problem in very small patients is that even valve prostheses of small annular dimensions tend to compromise the left ventricular outflow during systole. Recently, stented allograft dura mater valves have been constructed and studied by Nina Braunwald in sizes ranging from 12 mm to 18 mm for use in infants. These have excellent central flow characteristics and low thromboembolic potential. In our series, when an adequate mitral prosthesis could be placed, the hemodynamic and clinical improvement was excellent.

The indications for operation for congenital mitral valve lesions are congestive heart failure, pulmonary edema and severe pulmonary hypertension with failure to thrive. Our basic approach now is to attempt to reconstruct the mitral valve apparatus. In older children with a mitral annulus greater than 25 mm in diameter, if an excellent hemodynamic result is not achieved by reconstruction, the abnormal valve is replaced with a low-profile tissue valve. The problems of valve replacement in infants and smaller children, however, can be formidable and in this case we tend to accept some residual hemodynamic abnormality. Nevertheless, if the defect is not significantly improved, the mitral valve is replaced. We prefer a low-profile tissue valve in order to reduce the thromboembolic potential and to avoid the complications of anticoagulation in infants and children, despite the fact that extended durability of such valves is as yet uncertain.

REFERENCES

1. Berry, E., Ritter, D. G., Wallace, R. B., and Danielson, G. K.: Cardiac valve replacement in children, J. Thorac. Cardiovasc. Surg. 68:705, 1974.
2. Blieden, L. C., Castaneda, A. R., Nicoloff, D. M., Lillehei, C. W., and Moller, J. H.: Prosthetic valve replacement in children: Results in 44 patients, Ann. Surg. 14:545, 1972.
3. Braunwald, N. S., Brais, M., and Castaneda, A.: Considerations in the development of artificial heart valve substitutes for use in infants and small children, J. Thorac. Cardiovasc. Surg. 72:539, 1976.
4. Carpentier, A., Branchini, B., Cour, J. C., Asfaou, E., Villani, M., Deloche, A., Relland, J., D'Allaines, C., Blondeau, P., Piwnica, A., Parenzan, L., and Brom, G.: Congenital malformations of the mitral valve in children, J. Thorac. Cardiovasc. Surg. 72:854, 1976.
5. Carpentier, A., Deloche, A., Dauptain, J., Soyer, R., Blondeau, P., Piwnica, A., and Dubost, C.: A new reconstitutive operation for correction of mitral and tricuspid insufficiency, J. Thorac. Cardiovasc. Surg. 61:1, 1971.
6. Castaneda, A. R., Anderson, R. C., and Edwards, J. E.: Congenital mitral stenosis resulting from anomalous arcade and obstructing papillary muscles, Am. J. Cardiol. 24:237, 1969.
7. Collins-Nakai, R. L., Rosenthal, A., Castaneda, A. R., Bernhard, W. F., and Nadas, A. S.: Therapy and prognosis in congenital mitral stenosis, Am. J. Cardiol. 37:426, 1976.
8. Davachi, R., Moller, J. H., and Edwards, J. E.: Disease of mitral valve in infancy, Circulation 43:565, 1971.
9. Flege, J. B., Vlad, P., and Ehrenhaft, J. L.: Congenital mitral incompetence, J. Thorac. Cardiovasc. Surg. 53: 138, 1957.
10. Freed, M. D., and Bernhard, W. F.: Prosthetic valve replacement in children, Prog. Cardiovasc. Dis. 17:475, 1975.
11. Freed, M. D., Keane, J. F., Van Praagh, R., Castaneda, A. R., Bernhard, W. F., and Nadas, A. S.: Coarctation of the aorta with congenital mitral regurgitation, Circulation 49:1175, 1974.
12. Kaplan, S.: Cor Triatriatum, in Watson, H. (ed.), *Pediatric Cardiology* (St. Louis: The C. V. Mosby Company, 1968), p. 372.
13. Levy, M. J., Varco, R. L., Lillehei, C. W., and Edwards, J. E.: Mitral insufficiency in infants, children and adolescents: A review of etiologic, electrocardiographic, radiologic, and pathologic factors and surgical techniques, J. Thorac. Cardiovasc. Surg. 45:433, 1963.
14. Lucas, R. V., Anderson, R. C., Amplatz, K., Adams, P., and Edwards, J. E.: Congenital causes of pulmonary venous obstruction, Pediatr. Clin. North Am. 10:781, 1963.
15. Prado, S., Levy, M., and Varco, R. L.: Successful replacement of "parachute" mitral valve in a child, Circulation 32:213, 1965.
16. Sade, R. M., Freed, M. D., Matthews, E. C., and Castaneda, A. R.: Stenosis of individual pulmonary veins, J. Thorac. Cardiovasc. Surg. 67:953, 1974.
17. Shone, J., Sellers, R., Anderson, R., Adams, P., Lillehei, C. W., and Edwards, J. E.: The developmental complex of parachute mitral valve, Am. J. Cardiol. 11:714, 1963.

68 James R. Malm

Ventricular Septal Defects — Single Ventricle

HISTORY. — Steno, in 1671, first described the anatomy of ventricular septal defects (VSD). The first clinical description of this lesion was in 1879, when Roger[65] described 2 asymptomatic patients with harsh systolic murmurs. One was found at post mortem to have a small defect low in the interventricular septum. In 1891, Dupre presented the first case diagnosed during life and confirmed at autopsy.[32] This was believed to be a benign lesion and was termed the "maladie de Roger." Abbott,[1] in 1932, correlated the clinical and pathologic findings of ventricular septal defect. Taussig,[79] in the 1930s, contrasted the high, large VSDs to the small, low ones of Roger. Selzer,[67, 68] in 1949, emphasized that the main difference between the two types of defects was size, not location. The clinical and physiologic findings of this condition have been further considered by several authors.[29, 46, 67, 68]

In 1952, Muller and Dammann[59] reported clinical success with a palliative operation of wedging and banding of the pulmonary artery to diminish pulmonary blood flow. Albert,[3] in 1958, further modified this operation by constricting the pulmonary artery with a tape. In 1954, Lillehei and associates[55] successfully closed a VSD under direct vision using a cross circulation technique for cardiopulmonary bypass. Since that date, with the advances in cardiac surgery, VSD closure has been accomplished with increasing success in all age groups.

Incidence — Natural History — Pathophysiology

VSD is the most common congenital cardiac defect, occurring as an isolated lesion in 1.5 patients per 1000 live births,

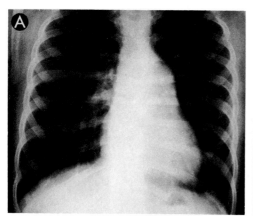
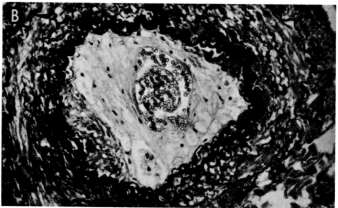

Fig. 68–1.—Ventricular septal defect, with pulmonary hypertension. **A,** anteroposterior roentgenogram of a 15-year-old boy with right ventricular pressure of 100/0. Note the small heart (cardiothoracic ratio 12.5: 240) and clear lung fields. He died suddenly 3 days after exploratory thora- cotomy. At autopsy, a large ventricular septal defect and vascular lung changes were found. **B,** photomicrograph of a small pulmonary artery from a section of this patient's lung. Note intimal proliferation and medial thickening of the vessel wall.

or in 25% of all infants with congenital heart disease.[20, 37, 38, 47] In addition, VSD occurs in approximately one-half of all patients with multiple cardiac anomalies.

An accurate prediction of the life span of a child with a VSD is difficult but depends on the size of the left-to-right shunt and the hemodynamic sequelae of the amount of pulmonary blood flow and subsequent changes in pulmonary vascular resistance.

The probability of spontaneous closure of small VSDs is estimated to be between 20% and 50% and such closure occurs, in most cases, before the age of 5 years.[20, 37, 38, 47] These defects, presumably less than 0.5 cm in diameter, are associated with small left-to-right shunts, normal or mildly elevated pulmonary artery pressure, normal pulmonary vasculature and pulmonary resistance. The mechanisms of spontaneous closure include sealing of the septal cusp of the tricuspid valve over the membranous septum, the formation of a fibrous patch over the defect or the development of right ventricular infundibular hypertrophy.

Ventricular septal defects measuring approximately 0.5–2.0 cm in diameter are associated with moderate left-to-right shunting with a pulmonary to systemic flow ratio of greater than 1.5 to 1 and with some degree of hyperkinetic pulmonary hypertension. These patients often are symptomatic in infancy when the elevated pulmonary vascular resistance present at birth decreases, allowing the increase in the dependent left-to-right shunt.

These infants often present with features of congestive heart failure, such as failure to thrive and frequent respiratory infections, but may respond to medical therapy and do fairly well for a time, perhaps due to a decrease in the size of the shunt. Approximately 35% of these defects become smaller, and spontaneous closure is thought to occur in about 5%.[20] The shunt may also be limited by the development of pulmonary infundibular hypertrophy. Improvement may also occur without diminution in the size of the shunt because of the development of left ventricular hypertrophy, with a resultant fall in left atrial pressure and main pulmonary artery pressure. If the child survives beyond the second year of life and still has high pulmonary arterial flow (greater than twice normal) and pressure (pulmonary artery systolic pressure 50% or more of aortic pressure), he is at risk for the development of pulmonary vascular disease. Those with normal pulmonary artery pressures and pulmonary flows of less than twice normal seldom, if ever, develop pulmonary vascular disease.

The sequence of development of changes of pulmonary vascular disease has been well defined.[34] There is initial medial hypertrophy (Grade I), which usually occurs at greater than 2 months of age and results from elevated pressures, and later intimal thickening and increased acellularity, as illustrated in Figure 68–1, resulting from increased velocities of flow (Grade II). This usually is seen after the age of 9–12 months but occasionally occurs earlier. Further increase in thickness and acellularity results in Grade III changes whereas angiomatoid formations and plexiform lesions develop with Grades IV and V. Extensive arteritis, usually resulting from a rapid rise in pressure, leads to Grade VI.

Defects larger than 2 cm often are associated with failure of involution of the pulmonary vascular bed and markedly elevated pulmonary vascular resistance. There is associated elevated left atrial pressure and left ventricular end-diastolic pressure, probably because of the immaturity of the left atrium and ventricle and reactive pulmonary arterial hypertension as manifest by medial thickening of the arteries. This limits the magnitude of the left-to-right shunting and there is a balance between the increased pulmonary blood flow and the ability of the left ventricle to handle the increased work load. Congestive heart failure results and death occurs despite intensive medical and often surgical treatment. A small percentage of these patients with very large defects have initial involution of vasculature, but evidence of rapidly progressive pulmonary vascular obstructive disease is seen with changes in the intimal layer of the small muscular arteries, with markedly narrowed lumina, obstruction and often pulmonary hemorrhage.

Approximately 10% of patients older than 2 years with VSD have pulmonary hypertension and pulmonary vascular resistance characteristic of Eisenmenger syndrome.[24] In these children, the left-to-right shunt remains only moderate and the children have relatively few symptoms despite grossly abnormal pulmonary vasculature with occlusive changes and obliterative lesions of the muscular arteries and arterioles in addition to medial hypertrophy. Because of progressive changes in the pulmonary vasculature, the disease becomes more pronounced, with cyanosis and right heart failure. The average life span of these patients usually is 25–35 years.

Anatomy

The ventricular septum is a partly fibrous and partly muscular structure separating the left and right ventricular cavities. A small portion of the upper membranous septum just inferior to the aortic valve also separates the left ventricle from the right atrium. The ventricular septum is formed by the atrioventricular endocardial cushions, the aortopulmonary conus septum and a ridge of ventricular wall. The location of ventricular septal defects is illustrated in Figure 68–2.

The largest number (approximately 70%) of ventricular septal defects arise from the failure of closure of the interventricular foramen by the posterior atrioventricular endocardial cushion and are located in the infracristal portion of the septum immediately beneath the right and noncoronary cusps of the aortic valve, to the left of the septal leaflet of the tricuspid valve and behind the crista supraventricularis. The defects may be oval, round or triangular and, although considered defects of the membranous septum, usually involve a large zone of muscular tissue adjacent to the membranous septum. The inferior margin is limited by the papillary muscle of the conus. A portion of the His bundle is located between the tricuspid valve and the conus and bifurcates into the right and left conduction bundles at the posterior and superior rim of the defect.

Imperfect fusion between the endocardial cushions and the primordial ventricular septum produces defects of the atrioventricular canal type. These defects are located posteriorly beneath the septal leaflet of the tricuspid valve at the upper or basal portion of the septum. Another feature is that the septal leaflet of the tricuspid valve is continuous with the anterior leaflet of the mitral valve at the posterior border of the defect.

Partial failure of development of the aorto-pulmonary conus septum leads to a supracristal defect related to the right ventricular outflow tract. These round defects are in close relationship to the pulmonary valve and lie immediately beneath the left aortic cusp.

Imperfect development of the ventricular ridges leads to defects in the muscular septum. These defects are located entirely in the muscular portion of the septum and are related to the inflow portion of the ventricles. They are located inferiorly in the septum toward the apex and frequently are multiple (Swiss cheese type).

Left ventricular to right atrial defects are the most uncommon types of VSD and occur in the interventricular portion of the membranous septum through a defect in the medial leaflet of the tricuspid valve or through a defect in the atrioventricular portion of the membranous septum superior to the annulus of the tricuspid valve.

Clinical Evaluation

The physical signs in a patient with VSD are related to the size of the left-to-right shunt and the status of the pulmonary vascular bed. There often is a paradoxic variation between the signs and symptoms. The murmur of VSD is loud, harsh, pansystolic and most prominent at the left sternal border in the third or fourth intercostal space with an associated thrill. The intensity of the murmur is related to the pressure differential between the ventricles. Smaller defects offer more resistance to flow and often are associated with louder murmurs. The intensity and length of the murmur also vary with the pulmonary vascular resistance and decrease with increasing pulmonary vascular resistance. Also, with rising pulmonary vascular resistance, the intensity of the pansystolic murmur diminishes toward the end of systole, giving the murmur an ejection quality and a shorter thrill. With markedly elevated pulmonary vascular resistance and small left-to-right shunt, the systolic murmur is short and soft and often preceded by a click caused by a high-pressure jet of blood striking the pulmonary artery. In large defects, the left ventricle is hyperkinetic and a mid-diastolic murmur is present at the apex because of the increased flow across the mitral valve. The murmur of pulmonic insufficiency occasionally is heard in patients with elevated pulmonary vascular resistance. The pulmonic component of the second heart sound (S2) also varies with the pulmonary vascular resistance, and with increasing resistance there is an increase in this sound, with narrow splitting of the second sound. S2 becomes single when the pulmonary artery pressure reaches systemic levels.

With signs and symptoms of congestive failure there is evidence of retarded growth and development. The precordium is hyperdynamic on inspection, and palpation reveals the presence of cardiomegaly. Chest deformity is seen commonly in these patients.

Chest radiographs may be entirely normal in patients with small VSDs whereas patients with large VSDs have cardiomegaly with evidence of biventricular hypertrophy, prominent pulmonary vasculature and enlargement of the left atrium, as illustrated in Figure 68–3. With increased pulmonary vascular resistance, peripheral vessels appear thin and tapered and the heart size may be normal.

The electrocardiogram in many patients with VSD is normal, but those with increased pulmonary blood flow have evidence of left ventricular enlargement. Patients with elevated pulmonary vascular resistance have evidence of right ventricular hypertrophy. Biventricular hypertrophy is seen in patients with both elevated pulmonary vascular resistance and large left-to-right shunts.

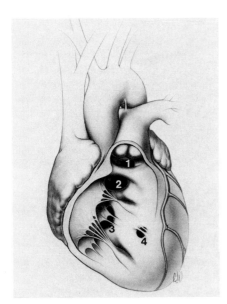

Fig. 68–2.—Illustration of types of ventricular septal defects. *1,* supracristal. *2,* infracristal. *3,* posterior or atrioventricular canal type. *4,* muscular.

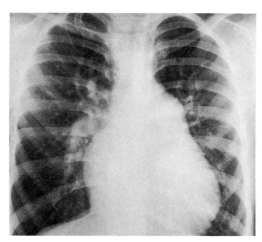

Fig. 68–3.—Ventricular septal defect; balanced shunt. Roentgenogram of a 6-year-old boy with catheter-proved isolated defect. Note prominence of pulmonary artery and increased vascular patterns in the lungs. Right ventricular pressure equaled systemic pressure on preoperative catheterization. Oxygen saturation rose 20% as the catheter passed from the right atrium to right ventricle. The ECG demonstrated a deep Q wave in V_6. The defect was closed and the postoperative course was smooth.

The diagnosis of VSD on catheterization is made by determining an increase in arterial partial pressure of oxygen between the right atrium and the right ventricle, indicating the presence of a left-to-right shunt at ventricular level. The calculation of the ratio between pulmonary blood flow and systemic blood flow indicates the size of the shunt and the level of pulmonary vascular resistance.

Angiography is used to identify the anatomic defects, the size of the ventricular cavities and the state of the atrioventricular valves. The localization of the septal defects is further elucidated by injection of contrast material into the left ventricle with the patient in the left lateral or left anterior oblique position to display the septum in profile.

Echocardiographic studies[66] are useful in the evaluation and management of infants with VSD. Anatomic defects can be defined and the presence of a shunt detected and quantitated by calculation of the ratio of left atrial to aortic root diameter in end systole and the mean velocity of circumferential fiber shortening.

Radionuclide angiocardiography[80] has been used in the evaluation of intracardiac shunts. In VSD, large recirculation is seen in the right ventricle and lung, and with numerical analysis of pulmonary time-activity curves, the pulmonary to systemic flow ratio (Qp/Qs) can be accurately measured when the pulmonary to systemic flow ratio is between 1.2 and 3.0.

Management

VSDs with pulmonary to systemic flow ratios of less than or equal to 2 to 1 and normal pulmonary artery pressures usually are asymptomatic. The hemodynamic consequences of this lesion are minimal and the risk of complication, especially bacterial endocarditis, is small; therefore, surgical intervention is not necessary.

Closure of VSD is recommended for all children with significant anatomic or hemodynamic abnormalities. The indications for operation include left-to-right shunt, with increased heart size, pulmonary to systemic flow ratio of greater than or equal to 2 to 1 with increased pulmonary artery pressure or only slightly increased pulmonary vascular resis-

tance and arterial oxygen saturation in the normal range. Correction is also indicated in the presence of left-to-right shunting with equal systemic pressure in the ventricles and pulmonary artery but with normal pulmonary vascular resistance. Supracristal or infracristal defects with associated aortic valvar insufficiency or sinus of Valsalva fistula require closure.

Most patients with VSD who survive the first year of life with mild symptoms or on a maximal medical regimen can undergo intracardiac repair on an elective basis. This must be undertaken before a marked elevation in pulmonary vascular resistance occurs, the factor that leads to failure of intervention. The optimal age for repair of large defects in patients with VSD and PVR of 4 units per square meter or less was 27 months.[9] Earlier intervention is necessary in those patients with elevated or rising levels of pulmonary vascular resistance. Those with pulmonary vascular resistance of 12 units per square meter should undergo early surgical repair if the pulmonary to systemic flow ratio is greater than or equal to 1.3 to 1.[9]

Infants with large VSDs and persistent congestive heart failure, failure to thrive and frequent respiratory infections despite maximal medical therapy require urgent surgical intervention. Associated defects such as patent ductus arteriosus and coarctation must be corrected, but often this is not enough to effect significant improvement. Some surgeons have preferred the palliative procedure of pulmonary artery banding to decrease the left-to-right shunt and, in turn, relieve congestive failure and protect the lungs from progressive changes of pulmonary vascular disease and then defer VSD closure until the patient is older. Others advocate definitive intracardiac repair for symptomatic infants and for those with elevated or rising pulmonary vascular resistance regardless of age.

Surgery is contraindicated in the presence of excessive pulmonary vascular resistance that approaches systemic levels and with Eisenmenger syndrome with negligible left-to-right shunt and arterial saturation of less than or equal to 85%.

Operative Considerations

Pulmonary Artery Banding

The objective of this palliative procedure is reduction of blood flow into the pulmonary circulation. The chest is entered through the third or fourth intercostal space on the left. After occlusion of the PDA or ligamentum arteriosum, the pericardium is incised longitudinally anterior to the phrenic nerve. The pulmonary artery is dissected free and constricted by a band of synthetic fabric sufficiently to reduce the pressure in the distal pulmonary artery to approximately one-third to one-half of its previous level, that is, 30–40 mm Hg. The band is secured in place with fine sutures to prevent migration and the pericardium loosely closed. A rise is noted in both ventricular pressures and a decrease in the left-to-right shunt with an increase in systemic pressure.

Intracardiac Repair of Ventricular Septal Defect

The intracardiac repair of VSD is accomplished using either standard cardiopulmonary bypass or deep hypothermia and circulatory arrest. Standard cardiopulmonary bypass is carried out using moderate core hypothermia with two venous and one aortic cannulas and a left ventricular vent. A right atriotomy is performed through which an atrial septal defect or patent foramen ovale is closed and the anatomy of the ventricular septum is evaluated by retraction of the tricuspid valve. Repair then is done either through the right atriotomy or a right ventriculotomy. Air is carefully evacuated from all chambers prior to termination of bypass.

For repair under deep hypothermia and circulatory arrest, the infant is intubated, thermistors applied and surface cooling accomplished with ice bags to body temperatures of 26–27°C. Through a median sternotomy, the ductus, if patent, is occluded. The aorta is cannulated after heparinization and a single venous cannula is placed in the right atrium. Bypass is instituted with the perfusate at 18° C and the venae cavae are encircled. The temperature is kept at 19° C for at least 2 minutes and 100% oxygen is administered for at least 1½ minutes prior to stopping cardiopulmonary bypass. The venous line is left open to drain, the aorta cross-clamped and the cavae occluded. The venous cannula is removed from the right atrium and the intracardiac repair carried out. The right atrium and left ventricle then are filled with saline, the venous line replaced and bypass restarted. The IVC and SVC snares are not released until the venous pressure is at least 15 mm Hg. Air is carefully evacuated from all chambers and an aortic needle vent is inserted prior to removal of the aortic cross-clamp. The patient is rewarmed to 37° C prior to discontinuing cardiopulmonary bypass.

VSDs less than 3mm in diameter, and not related to the membranous septum, can be directly sutured. Most defects from the left ventricle to the right atrium can be closed primarily. Large defects (usually greater than one-half the diameter of the aorta) are closed with synthetic patch material. The repair is illustrated in Figure 68–4. The conduction system is avoided and initial sutures are placed in the fibrous tissue parallel to the atrioventricular bundle. Sutures in the muscular rim usually are mattress sutures reinforced with pledgets. The right or noncoronary cusp of the aortic valve must be avoided in placing sutures in the superior aspect of the defect. In supracristal VSDs associated with aortic incompetence, simple closure, or patch closure, supplies the support afforded by the normal conus septum. This support on occasion is sufficient to prevent aortic insufficiency but more frequently aortic valvuloplasty is necessary because of the abnormalities in the commissures, elongation of one aortic cusp and the poor approximation of the free edges of the valve cusps.[60, 71]

To avoid right ventricular damage and valve dysfunction, the right ventriculotomy (transverse or vertical) should be as short as is feasible and major branches of the right coronary artery should be avoided. In cases of increased pulmonary vascular resistance or with lesions posteriorly placed in the septum, repair through the right atrium may be preferred using retraction of the tricuspid valve. Ventriculotomy is preferred for supracristal VSDs, trabeculated VSDs, infundibular VSDs and with associated infundibular stenosis. A combined approach through the atrium (closure of VSD) and the pulmonary artery (excision of infundibular stenosis) has been preferred by some but the advantages are not impressive. A combined right atrial and apical left ventricular approach has been used successfully in closure of multiple VSDs.

Associated lesions such as atrial septal defects, patent ductus arteriosus, aortic valve insufficiency, pulmonary valvar stenosis, infundibular stenosis or atrioventricular valve lesions must be corrected. If a pulmonary artery band is present, debanding is required. On occasion, simple release can be accomplished, whereas in other cases the task may be more formidable. The band and the area of the PA involved

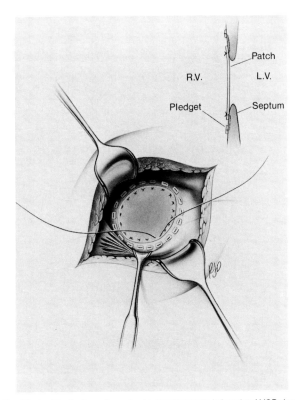

Fig. 68–4.—Illustration of repair of a membranous infracristal VSD demonstrating placement of initial sutures parallel to the conducting system in fibrous tissue. Sutures at the superior border are placed with care to avoid the left cusp of the aortic valve and sutures in the muscular portion of the rim are reinforced with pledgets.

may have to be excised and end-to-end anastomosis done. In other cases, the pulmonary artery is opened longitudinally across the band and, if possible, a portion of the band is removed. After ensuring the patency of the branch pulmonary arteries, the main pulmonary artery is reconstructed either by transverse closure of the arteriotomy or by inserting a patch of pericardium or prosthetic material. Peripheral pulmonary artery reconstruction may also be necessary, as may pulmonary valvotomy, infundibular resection or outflow tract reconstruction.

Results

Ventricular septal defects can be safely closed in children with an acceptable operative risk and with an ultimate result that is largely dependent on the degree of pulmonary vascular disease already present. Complications include a small incidence of heart block and residual shunts.

The palliative procedure of pulmonary artery banding is relatively simple and can be done with a low operative mortality rate (Table 68–1) but with significant morbidity, complications including cyanosis, supravalvar and valvar pulmonic stenosis, pulmonary artery branch stenosis or occlusion, supravalvar aortic stenosis and right ventricular infundibular hypertrophy. The band may also be ineffective in decreasing pulmonary blood flow and preventing the development or progress of pulmonary vascular disease. In any case, these children face a second operation for VSD closure and debanding, with its associated mortality (Table 68–2). The major operative complication is related to pulmonary artery reconstruction and often the total repair is suboptimal.

The alternative to this two-stage approach is primary clo-

TABLE 68–1.—HOSPITAL MORTALITY FOR BANDING FOR VENTRICULAR SEPTAL DEFECT IN INFANTS LESS THAN 12 MONTHS OF AGE

AUTHOR	YEARS	PUBLISHED	NUMBER		HOSPITAL DEATHS	
					Number	%
Hunt[41]	1960–1970	1970	Total	62	12	19.0
			Isolated VSD	40	2	5.0
Stark[72]	1957–1968	1969	Total	135	48	35.0
			Isolated VSD	55	4	7.3
Bernhard[7]	1964–1970	1972	Total	76	5	6.6
			Isolated VSD	50	0	
Menahem[58]	1960–1968	1972	Total	22	6	28.0
			Isolated VSD	15	3	25.0
Trusler[81]	1966–1971	1972	Total	29	9	31.0
			Isolated VSD	20	0	
Henry[35]	Through 1970	1973	Total	42	7	16.7
			Isolated VSD	24	5	21.0
Patel[62]	1966–1972	1973	Total	54	6	12.9
			Isolated VSD	32	3	9.4
Tatooles[78]	1969–1971	1973	Total	9	3	33.3
			Isolated VSD	4	0	0.0
Girod[30]	1968–1972	1974	Total	34	3	9.0
			Isolated VSD	34	3	9.0
McNicholas and Stark[57]	1971–1975		Total	21	3	14.0
			Isolated VSD	8	1	12.0
			TOTAL	484	102	21.0
			ISOLATED VSD	282	21	7.5

sure of the VSD in infancy. This has been accomplished in several centers, with results as listed in Table 68–3.

Recently we have reviewed our experience in the surgical management of ventricular septal defects in infants at the Babies Hospital of Columbia–Presbyterian Medical Center and the results are as presented in Table 68–4. Although pulmonary artery banding was done with a low operative mortality rate there were several late deaths, increasing the over-all mortality of the procedure. There were 3 operative deaths in the group of 40 children who underwent pulmo-nary artery debanding and VSD closure, for an operative mortality of 7.5%. One of these deaths was directly attributed to difficulty in reconstructing the pulmonary artery; another child had developed pulmonary hypertension despite a previously placed pulmonary artery band and died following VSD closure. During the same period, 30 infants with isolated VSD underwent intracardiac repair, with an operative mortality of 16.6%.

We believe that primary intracardiac repair of VSD is the treatment of choice for these infants.

TABLE 68–2.—HOSPITAL MORTALITY FOR REPAIR OF VENTRICULAR SEPTAL DEFECT AFTER PULMONARY ARTERY BANDING

AUTHOR	YEARS	PUBLISHED	NUMBER		HOSPITAL DEATHS	
					Number	%
Stark[75]	1966–1969	1970	Total	25	7	28.0
			Isolated	16	4	25.0
			Multiple	8	3	37.0
			Spontaneous closure	1	0	0.0
Hunt[41]	1960–1970	1970	Total	24	3	12.5
Coleman[15]	1963–1967	1972	Total	15	4	26.6
Patel[62]	1966–1972	1973	Total	20	6	30.0
			Isolated	18	6	33.3
Henry[35]	1961–1970	1973	Total	12	2	16.7
			Isolated	12	2	16.7
Girod[30]	1968–1972	1974	Total	32	1	3.1
			Isolated	32	1	3.1
Seybold-Epting[69]	1964–1974	1976	Total	90	8	9.0
McNicholas and Stark[57]	1971–1975		Total	50	4	8.0
			Isolated	24	2	8.0
			TOTAL	268	35	13.0
			ISOLATED	102	15	14.7

TABLE 68–3.—HOSPITAL MORTALITY FOR PRIMARY REPAIR OF VENTRICULAR
SEPTAL DEFECT IN PATIENTS UNDER 1 YEAR OF AGE

AUTHOR	YEARS	PUBLISHED	MAXIMAL AGE	NUMBER	HOSPITAL DEATHS	
					Number	%
Idriss[44]	1955–1970	1971	12 mo	6	0	0
Ching[14]	1955–1970	1971	12 mo	18	4	22
DuShane[20]	1967–1972	1972	12 mo	32	3	9.3
Rittenhouse[64]	1965–1972	1974	3–6 mo	9	3	33
Castaneda[13]	1969–1973	1974	3 mo	9	3	33
de Leval[18]		1974	3–9 mo	18	0	0
Subramanian[77]	1970–1972	1973	12 mo	15	0	0
Barratt-Boyes[4]	1969–1975	1976	12 mo	45	3	6.6
Kirklin[9]	1967–1976	1976	12 mo	27	4	14.8
McNicholas and Stark[57]	1971–1975		12 mo	28	1	3.5
				207	21	10.1

Single Ventricle

HISTORY.—Holmes,[4] in 1824, described a heart with one functioning ventricle. In 1936, Abbott,[1] in a study of 1000 cases of congenital heart disease, found single ventricle alone or with associated lesions in 27 patients. Until recently, the diagnosis was made only at autopsy, but with the development of biplane cineangiocardiography, clinical diagnosis has been possible and surgical correction performed.

Single ventricle has been defined by Van Praagh[83] as that anomaly in which a common or separate atrioventricular valve(s) opens into a ventricular chamber from which both great arterial trunks emerge.

Incidence—Natural History—Pathophysiology

Single ventricle is seen 3 times more commonly in males than in females and comprises approximately 3% of all congenital cardiac malformations. In Abbott's series based on autopsy data, the mean age at the time of death was 7¾ years, with a range from infancy to 35 years. In other reports, 20% of patients have survived into adulthood.

The pathophysiology of this lesion is dependent on outflow tract anatomy, which determines the predominance of the bidirectional shunt and the relative amounts of aortic and pulmonary blood flow.

Anatomy

Failure of development of one or both ventricular sinuses, with secondary involvement of the ventricular septum, results in a single ventricle. Van Praagh[83] has classified these lesions into four types, as illustrated in Figure 68–5. The classic and most common single ventricle, Type A, is composed of left ventricular sinus myocardium and has a rudimentary outflow chamber but no right ventricular sinus or inflow tract. The Type B ventricle is composed of right ventricular sinus myocardium whereas in Type C there are almost equal portions of right and left ventricular sinus myocardium with a rudimentary and apically located ventricular septum. In Type D there is absence of both ventricular sinuses. Further subclassifications are based on the relationship of the great arteries, the direction of the bulboventricular loop and the position of the atria with respect to the viscera.

Clinical Evaluation

Patients with single ventricle may present either with features of pulmonary undercirculation or with signs and symptoms of congestive heart failure resulting from pulmonary overcirculation. The auscultatory findings, chest radiographs and electrocardiograms are not specific for the diagnosis of single ventricle but are similar to those of ventricular septal defect with or without right ventricular outflow tract lesions. Abnormal relationship of the great vessels may be detected on chest x-ray and conduction defects noted on the electrocardiogram. At catheterization, equal pressures are found throughout the ventricle and an increase in oxygen saturation is noted at ventricular level.

The clinical diagnosis of single ventricle has only recently been made possible by the development of biplane ventricular angiocardiography, and this technique is the mainstay in the evaluation for surgical correction. Information is sought concerning the morphology of the ventricle, the presence or absence of an outflow chamber, the nature and function of the atrioventricular valve(s), relationship to the

TABLE 68–4.—PULMONARY ARTERY BANDING VERSUS PRIMARY REPAIR OF
VENTRICULAR SEPTAL DEFECT IN INFANCY, COLUMBIA–PRESBYTERIAN
MEDICAL CENTER, 1967–1976

OPERATION		NUMBER		MORTALITY	
				Number	%
Pulmonary artery banding		14	Hospital	1	7.1
			Over-all	4	28.5
Pulmonary artery debanding and VSD closure		40		3	7.5
Closure of VSD in infancy	Total	37		8	21.6
	Isolated VSD	30		5	16.6

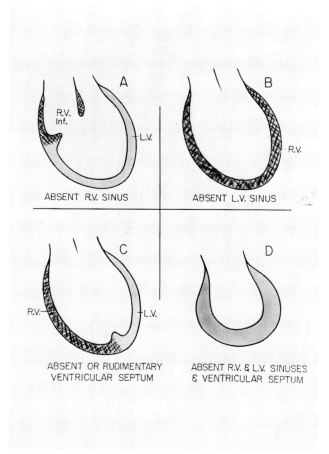

Fig. 68–5.—Classification of single ventricle Types A through D according to Van Praagh. Right ventricular myocardium is cross-hatched; left ventricular myocardium is solid. Type A contains a rudimentary right ventricular infundibulum. (Reprinted, with permission, from Edie *et al.*[22])

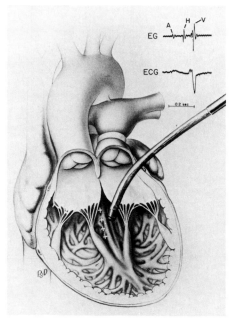

Fig. 68–6.—Illustration of the location of the bundle of His in a patient with single ventricle. The electric probe is used to record the operative electrogram *(EG)*. The characteristic His *(H)* spike is noted between the atrial *(A)* and ventricular *(V)* recordings. (Reprinted, with permission, from Edie *et al.*[22])

Operative Considerations

The conduction system must be carefully delineated and carefully avoided. An example of the location of the bundle of His is shown in Figure 68–6. The operative technique is illustrated in Figure 68–7. Stable fixation of the prosthetic septum must be achieved. Initial sutures are placed along

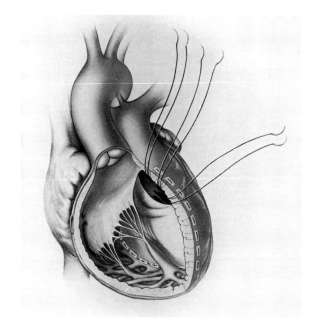

Fig. 68–7.—Single ventricle. The operative technique for reconstruction of the ventricular septum by placement of a prosthesis that separates the two atrioventricular valves. The anterior reinforced sutures are placed through the thickness of the ventricular wall. (Reprinted, with permission, from Edie *et al.*[22])

great arteries and outflow tract anatomy. The noninvasive technique of echocardiography[26] has been useful in the initial evaluation of patients with this lesion.

Management

In the past, total correction was not believed to be possible and only palliation was offered to these patients. Atrial septostomy was done in patients with a single ventricle, transposition of the great arteries, intact atrial septum and an elevated left atrial pressure, to improve the mixing and therefore increase arterial saturation. Pulmonary artery banding frequently is useful in reducing pulmonary blood flow in patients with pulmonary overcirculation and relieving symptoms of congestive heart failure. Those children with reduced pulmonary blood flow often are improved by systemic to pulmonary artery anastomoses.

Recent developments in the delineation of the bundle of His and in open heart surgical techniques have made possible total correction in certain selected cases. Precise preoperative definition of the number and position of the atrioventricular valves and the nature and severity of aorticopulmonary outflow tract obstruction are of utmost importance. Total correction is feasible if two atrioventricular valves are present.

the posterior wall between the AV valves and, if possible, through the annulus of the septal leaflet of the tricuspid valve. Sutures are continued between the semilunar valves and inferiorly toward the apex and the rudimentary septum if it is present. Anterior sutures are reinforced and are placed from the outside through the entire wall thickness. Successful repair is also dependent on relief from either pulmonary or outflow obstruction and complete correction of associated anomalies.

Results

In 1973, Edie et al.[22] described the total repair of 4 patients, 2 with Type A and 2 with Type C single ventricles. Since that time, encouraging results with that procedure of septation and with the use of valved conduits have been reported by several centers. This is accomplished in the relatively few patients with favorable anatomy. However, in the majority of patients, palliation still is the procedure of choice.

REFERENCES

1. Abbott, M. E.: *Atlas of Congenital Cardiac Disease* (New York: American Heart Association, 1936).
2. Agosti, J., and Subramanian, S.: Corrective treatment of isolated ventricular septal defect in infancy, J. Pediatr. Surg. 10:785, 1975.
3. Albert, H. M., Atik, M., and Fowler, R. L.: Production and release of pulmonary stenosis in dogs, Surgery 44:904, 1958.
4. Barratt-Boyes, B. G., Neutze, J. M., Clarkson, P. M., Shardey, G. C., and Brandt, P. W. T.: Repair of ventricular septal defect in the first two years of life using profound hypothermia-circulatory arrest techniques, Ann. Surg. 184:376, 1976.
5. Barratt-Boyes, B. G., Neutze, J. M., Seelye, E. R., and Simpson, M.: Complete correction of cardiovascular malformations in the first year of life, Prog. Cardiovasc. Dis. 3:229, 1973.
6. Becu, L. M., Fontana, R. P., DuShane, J. W., Kirklin, J. W., Burchell, H. G., and Edwards, J. E.: Anatomic and pathologic studies in ventricular septal defect, Circulation 14:349, 1956.
7. Bernhard, W. F., Litwin, S. B., Williams, W. W., Jones, J. E., and Gross, R. E.: Recent results of cardiovascular surgery in infants in the first year of life, Am. J. Surg. 123:451, 1972.
8. Berry, C. L.: Changes in the wall of the pulmonary artery after banding, J. Pathol. 99:29, 1969.
9. Blackstone, E. H., Kirklin, J. W., Bradley, E. L., DuShane, J. W., and Appelbaum, A.: Optimal age and results in repair of large ventricular septal defects, J. Thorac. Cardiovasc. Surg. 72:661, 1976.
10. Bloomfield, D. K.: Natural history of ventricular septal defect in patients surviving infancy, Circulation 29:914, 1964.
11. Breckenridge, I. M., Stark, J., Waterston, D. J., and Bonham-Carter, R. E.: Multiple ventricular septal defects, Ann. Thorac. Surg. 13:128, 1972.
12. Cartmill, T. B., DuShane, J. W., McGoon, D. C., and Kirklin, J. W.: Results of repair of ventricular septal defect, J. Thorac. Cardiovasc. Surg. 52:486, 1966.
13. Castaneda, A. R., Lamberti, J., Sade, R. M., Williams, R. G., and Nadas, A. S.: Open heart surgery during the first three months of life, J. Thorac. Cardiovasc. Surg. 68:719, 1974.
14. Ching, E., DuShane, J. W., McGoon, D. C., and Danielson, G. K.: Total correction of ventricular septal defects in infancy using extracorporeal circulation, Ann. Thorac. Surg. 12:1, 1971.
15. Coleman, E. N., Reid, J. M., Barclay, R. S., and Stevenson, J. G.: Ventricular septal defect repair after pulmonary artery banding, Br. Heart J. 34:134, 1972.
16. Cordell, A. R., and Suh, J. H.: The pulmonary artery lesion after banding, Ann. Surg. 179:805, 1974.
17. Dammann, J. F., Jr., McEachen, J. A., Thompson, W. M., Jr., Smith, R., and Muller, W. M., Jr.: The regression of pulmonary vascular disease, Surg. Gynecol. Obstet. 95:213, 1952.
18. de Leval, M., Taylor, J. F. N., and Stark, J.: Primary repair of ventricular septal defect in infancy (abstract), Br. Heart J. 36:400, 1974.
19. Dobell, A. R. C., Murphy, D. A., Poirier, N. L., and Gibbons, J. E.: The pulmonary artery after debanding, J. Thorac. Cardiovasc. Surg. 65:32, 1973.
20. DuShane, J. W., Weidman, W. M., and Ritter, D. C.: Influence of

21. Ebert, P. A., Canent, R. V., Jr., Spach, M. S., and Sabiston, D. C.: Late cardiodynamics following correction of ventricular septal defects with previous pulmonary artery banding, J. Thorac. Cardiovasc. Surg. 60:516, 1970.
22. Edie, R. N., Ellis, K., Gersony, W. M., Krongrad, E., Bowman, F. O., Jr., and Malm, J. R.: Surgical repair of single ventricle, J. Thorac. Cardiovasc. Surg. 66:350, 1973.
23. Edwards, J. E.: Congenital Malformation of the Heart and Great Vessels, in Gould, S. E. (ed.), *Pathology of the Heart and Blood Vessels* (Springfield, Ill.: Charles C Thomas, Publisher, 1968), p. 286.
24. Eisenmenger, V.: Die Angeborenen Defecte der Kammerscheiderwand des Herzens, Z. Klin. Med. 32:1, 1897.
25. Elliott, C. D., and Morgan, A. D.: Common Ventricle, in Moss, A. J., and Adams, F. H. (eds.), *Heart Disease in Infants, Children and Adolescents* (Baltimore: The Williams & Wilkins Company, 1968).
26. Feiner, J. N., Brewer, D. B., and Franch, R. H.: Echocardiographic manifestations of single ventricle, Am. J. Cardiol. 38:80, 1976.
27. Fontana, R. S., and Edwards, J. C.: *Congenital Cardiac Disease: A Review of 357 Cases Studied Pathologically* (Philadelphia: W. B. Saunders Company, 1962).
28. Freed, M. D., Rosenthal, A., Plantor, W. H., and Nadas, A. S.: Development of subaortic stenosis after pulmonary artery banding, Circulation 67–68 (Supp. III):III–7, 1973.
29. Fyler, D. C.: Ventricular septal defects in infants and children: A correlation of clinical, physiologic and autopsy data, Circulation 18:833, 1958.
30. Girod, D. A., Hurwitz, R. A., King, H., and Jolly, W.: Results of two-stage surgical treatment of large ventricular septal defects, Circulation 49–50 (Supp. II):II–9 1974.
31. Goldblatt, A., Bernhard, W. F., Nadas, A. S., and Gross, R. E.: Pulmonary artery banding: Indications and results in infants and children, Circulation 32:172, 1965.
32. Hallman, G. L., and Cooley, D. A.: *Surgical Treatment of Congenital Heart Disease* (Philadelphia: Lea & Febiger, 1975).
33. Hallman, G. L., Cooley, D. A., and Bloodwell, R. D.: Two-stage surgical treatment of ventricular septal defect. Results of pulmonary artery banding in infants and subsequent open-heart repair, J. Thorac. Cardiovasc. Surg. 52:476, 1966.
34. Heath, D., and Edwards, J. E.: The pathology of hypertensive pulmonary vascular disease. A description of six grades of structural changes in the pulmonary artery with reference to congenital cardiac septal defects, Circulation 18:533, 1958.
35. Henry, J., Kaplan, S., Helmsworth, J. A., and Schreiber, J. T.: Management of infants with large ventricular septal defects, Ann. Thorac. Surg. 15:109, 1973.
36. Hoffman, J. I. E.: Ventricular septal defect, indications for therapy in infants, Pediatr. Clin. North Am. 18:1091, 1971.
37. Hoffman, J. I. E.: Natural history of congenital heart disease. Problems in its assessment with special reference to ventricular septal defects, Circulation 37:97, 1968.
38. Hoffman, J. I. E., and Rudolph, A. M.: The natural history of ventricular septal defects in infancy, Am. J. Cardiol. 16:634, 1965.
39. Hoffman, J. I. E., and Rudolph, A. M.: Increasing pulmonary vascular resistance during infancy in association with ventricular septal defect, Pediatrics 38:220, 1966.
40. Holmes, W. F.: Case of malformation of the heart, Trans. Med. Chir. Soc., Edinb. 4:252, 1824. Reprinted in Abbott, M. E., Montreal Med. J. 30:522, 1901.
41. Hunt, C. E., Formanek, G., Castaneda, A. R., and Moller, J. H.: Closure of ventricular septal defect and removal of pulmonary arterial band, Am. J. Cardiol. 26:345, 1970.
42. Hunt, C. E., Formanek, G., Levine, M. A., Castaneda, A., and Moller, J. H.: Banding of the pulmonary artery. Results in 111 children, Circulation 43:395, 1971.
43. Ibach, J. R., Jr., Bartley, T. D., Daicoff, G. R., Wheat, M. W., Jr., Grossner, I. H., Van Mierop, C. H. J., Schriebler, G. L., and Miller, R. H.: Correction of ventricular septal defect in childhood, Ann. Thorac. Surg. 11:499, 1971.
44. Idriss, F. S., Nikaidoh, H., Paul, M. H., Blumerschein, S. D., and Riker, W.: Early repair of ventricular septal defect in infants and young children, Arch. Surg. 103:265, 1971.
45. Kaiser, G. A., Waldo, A. L., Beach, P. M., Bowman, F. O., Jr., Hoffman, B. F., and Malm, J. R.: Specialized cardiac conduction system: Infant electrophysiologic identification technique at surgery, Arch. Surg. 101:673, 1970.
46. Keith, J. D., Collins, G., Rose, V., and Kidd, L.: Course and

Prognosis in Ventricular Septal Defect, in *Symposium on Natural History of Congenital Heart Disease*, Toronto, Canada, December, 1969 (Springfield, Ill.: Charles C Thomas, Publisher, 1970).

47. Keith, J. D., Rose, V., Collins, G., and Kidd, B. S. L.: Ventricular septal defects. Incidence, morbidity, and mortality in various age groups, Br. Heart J. 33:81, 1971.

48. Keith, J. D., Rowe, R. D., and Vlad, P. (eds.): *Heart Disease in Infancy and Childhood* (New York: The Macmillan Company, 1958).

49. Kirklin, J. W.: Pulmonary arterial banding in babies with large ventricular septal defects, Circulation 43:321, 1971.

50. Kirklin, J. W., Appelbaum, A., and Bargeron, L. M. J.: Primary Repair vs. Banding for Ventricular Septal Defects in Infants, in *Proceedings of the International Symposium on Congenital Heart Disease in Children*, Toronto, Canada. (In press.)

51. Kirklin, J. W., Harshberger, H. G., Donald, D. E., and Edward, J. E.: Surgical correction of ventricular septal defect: Anatomic and technical considerations, J. Thorac. Cardiovasc. Surg. 33:45, 1957.

52. Kirklin, J. W., McGoon, D. C., and DuShane, J. W.: Surgical treatment of ventricular septal defect, J. Thorac. Cardiovasc. Surg. 40:763, 1960.

53. Levitsky, S., DuBrow, I. W., and Hastreiter, A. R.: Pulmonary artery banding in infants, Ann. Thorac. Surg. 17:492, 1974.

54. Lillehei, C. W., Anderson, R. C., Eliot, R. S., Wang, Y., and Fertic, R. M.: Pre- and post-operative cardiac constriction in 200 patients undergoing closure of ventricular septal defects, Surgery 63:69, 1968.

55. Lillehei, C. W., Cohen, M., Warden, H. E., Ziegler, N., and Varco, R. L.: The results of direct vision closure of ventricular septal defects in 8 patients by means of controlled cross circulation, Surg. Gynecol. Obstet. 101:446, 1955.

56. Lucas, R. V., Jr., Adams, P., Jr., Anderson, R. C., Meyne, N. G., Lillehei, C. W., and Varco, R. L.: The natural history of isolated ventricular septal defect. A serial physiologic study, Circulation 24:1372, 1961.

57. McNicholas, K. W., de Leval, M., and Stark, J.: Br. Heart J. (in press).

58. Menahem, J., and Venables, A. W.: Pulmonary artery banding in isolated or complicated ventricular septal defects. Results and effect on growth, Br. Heart J. 34:87, 1972.

59. Muller, W. H., Jr., and Dammann, J. F.: The treatment of certain congenital malformations of the heart by the creation of pulmonic stenosis to reduce pulmonary hypertension and excessive pulmonary blood flow, Surg. Gynecol. Obstet. 95:213, 1952.

60. Murphy, D. A., and Poirier, N.: A technique of aortic valvuloplasty for aortic insufficiency associated with ventricular septal defect, J. Thorac. Cardiovasc. Surg. 64:800, 1972.

61. Oldham, H. N., Kakos, G. J., Jarmakani, M. M., and Sabiston, D. C., Jr.: Pulmonary artery banding in infants with complex congenital heart defects, Ann. Thorac. Surg. 13:342, 1972.

62. Patel, R. G., Ihenouho, N. C., Abrams, L. D., Astley, R., Parsons, C. G., Roberts, K. D., and Singh, S. P.: Pulmonary artery banding and subsequent repair in ventricular septal defect, Br. Heart J. 35:651, 1973.

63. Pooley, R. W., Hayes, C. J., Edie, R. N., Gersony, W. M., Bowman, F. O., Jr., and Malm, J. R.: Open heart experience in infants utilizing normothermia and deep hypothermia, Ann. Thorac. Surg. 22:415, 1976.

64. Rittenhouse, E. A., Mohri, H., Dillard, D. H., and Merendino, K. A.: Deep hypothermia in cardiovascular surgery, Ann. Thorac. Surg. 17:63, 1974.

65. Roger, H.: Recherches cliniques sur la communication congenitale de deux coeurs, par inocclusion du septum interventriculaire, Bull. Acad. Med. 8:1074, 1879.

66. Sahn, D. J., Vaucher, Y., Williams, D. E., Allen, H. D., Goldberg, S. J., and Friedman, W. I.: Echocardiographic detection of large left to right shunts and cardiomyopathies in infants and children, Am. J. Cardiol. 38:73, 1976.

67. Selzer, A.: Defects of the ventricular system. Summary of twelve cases and review of the literature, Arch. Intern. Med. 84:798, 1949.

68. Selzer, A.: Defects of the cardiac septums, JAMA 154:129, 1954.

69. Seybold-Epting, W., Reul, G. J., Hallman, G. L., and Cooley, D. A.: Repair of ventricular septal defect after pulmonary artery banding, J. Thorac. Cardiovasc. Surg. 71:392, 1976.

70. Shah, P., Singh, W. S., Rose, V., and Keith, J. D.: Incidence of bacterial endocarditis in ventricular septal defects, Circulation 34:127, 1966.

71. Spencer, F. C., Bahnson, H. T., and Neill, C. A.: The treatment of aortic regurgitation associated with a ventricular septal defect, J. Thorac. Cardiovasc. Surg. 43:222, 1962.

72. Stark, J., Aberdeen, E., Waterston, D. J., Bonham-Carter, R. E., and Tynan, M.: Pulmonary artery constriction (banding): A report of 144 cases, Surgery 65:808, 1969.

73. Stark, J., Berry, C. L., and Silove, E. D.: The evaluation of materials used for pulmonary artery banding. Experimental study in piglets, Ann. Thorac. Surg. 13:163, 1972.

74. Stark, J., Hucin, B., Aberdeen, E., and Waterston, D. J.: Cardiac surgery in the first year of life: Experience with 1,049 operations, Surgery 69:483, 1971.

75. Stark, J., Tynan, M., Aberdeen, E., Waterston, D. J., Bonham-Carter, R. E., Graham, G. R., and Somerville, J.: Repair of intracardiac defects after previous constriction (banding) of the pulmonary artery, Surgery 67:536, 1970.

76. Steno, N.: Embryo monstro affinis Parisiis dissectus, Acta Medica & Philosophica Hafniencia 1:202, 1671–1672. Cited by Warburg, E.: Niels Steensens Beskrivelse af der forste publicerede Tilfaelde af "Fallots Tetrade," Nord. Med. 16:3550, 1942.

77. Subramanian, S.: Primary Definitive Intracardiac Operations in Infants: Ventrical Septal Defect, in Kirklin, J. W. (ed.), *Advances in Cardiovascular Surgery* (New York: Grune & Stratton, 1973).

78. Tatooles, C. J., and Miller, R. A.: Palliative surgery in infants with congenital heart disease, Prog. Cardiovasc. Dis. 15:331, 1973.

79. Taussig, H. B.: *Congenital Malformations of the Heart* (2d ed.; London: Oxford University Press, 1960), Vol. 2.

80. Treves, J., and Collins-Nakai, R. L.: Radioactive tracers in congenital heart disease, Am. J. Cardiol. 38:711, 1976.

81. Trusler, G. A., and Mustard, W. T.: A method of handling the pulmonary artery of a large isolated ventricular septal defect with and without transposition of the great arteries, Ann. Thorac. Surg. 13:351, 1972.

82. Van Praagh, R., and McNamara, J. J.: Anatomic types of ventricular septal defect with aortic insufficiency, Am. Heart J. 75:604, 1968.

83. Van Praagh, R., Van Praagh, S., Vlad, P., and Keith, J. D.: Diagnosis of the anatomic type of single or common ventricle, Am. J. Cardiol. 15:345, 1965.

84. Warden, H. E., Cohn, M., Read, R. C., and Lillehei, C. W.: Controlled cross circulation for open intracardiac surgery. Physiologic studies and results of creation and closure of ventricular septal defects, J. Thorac. Cardiovasc. Surg. 28:331, 1954.

85. Wood, P.: Posthumous papers. Cited by Bloomfield D. K.[10]

86. Wood, P.: Pulmonary hypertension, Mod. Concepts Cardiovasc. Dis. 28:513, 1959.

69 Aldo R. Castaneda / Gilbert A. Norwood

Tricuspid Atresia and Ebstein's Anomaly

Tricuspid Atresia

Tricuspid atresia is an uncommon congenital malformation that is characterized by absence of a direct communication between the right atrium and the right ventricle. In the total series of congenital heart defects at Children's Hospital Medical Center, Boston, the incidence of tricuspid atresia was 1.1%. Of congenital cardiac anomalies producing cyanosis, it follows in frequency only tetralogy of Fallot and transposition of the great arteries.

Tricuspid atresia is necessarily associated with additional anomalies, and the complex spectrum of clinical features, pathophysiology and natural history is related to the type and degree of the associated lesion.

Features common to all types of tricuspid atresia include: (i) an interatrial septal communication, (ii) enlargement of the mitral valve and of the left ventricle and (iii) hypoplasia of the right ventricle. Survival is dependent on the entire systemic venous return traversing the atrial septum and mixing with pulmonary venous return in the left atrium. This obligatory right-to-left shunt leads to systemic arterial desaturation and thus to the most constant clinical finding: cyanosis. However, the natural history and all other clinical features are dependent on the amount of pulmonary blood flow. About 70% of the patients with tricuspid atresia have obstruction to pulmonary blood flow, whereas the rest have either balanced or an increased pulmonary flow. Infants with either extremely high or extremely limited pulmonary blood flow usually die before the age of 3 months, whereas the average survival of patients with a more balanced pulmonary to systemic flow ratio is 7–8 years, with an occasional patient living several decades.

Anatomy

Van Praagh recognized three anatomic variants of the tricuspid valve region. The *muscular* form of atresia is the usual type (84%). Here, a central fibrotic umbilication commonly is present in the region where the tricuspid valve normally would be expected. The membranous type (8%) is composed of nonperforated fibrous tissue in the tricuspid region that transilluminates well. This type always is associated with juxtaposition of the atrial appendages. In the third type (8%), an Ebstein-like atrialized right ventricle forms a blind pouch beneath the right atrium and there is no opening in the tricuspid valve.

In all types, the right atrium invariably is enlarged, with thickened muscular walls, and the left atrium frequently is similarly affected. Usually the interatrial communication is by a patent foramen ovale, but either a true defect in the atrial septum or occasionally complete absence of the atrial septum may occur. The mitral valve usually is large, but normally located, and the left ventricle always is enlarged, with hypertrophic walls. The right ventricle, particularly the inflow portion, always is hypoplastic and if pulmonary atresia is present, the right ventricle may be undetectable by gross examination.

In 1949, Edwards and Burchell offered a classification of tricuspid atresia based on the position of the great arteries and degree of obstruction to the pulmonary blood flow. Type I is tricuspid atresia with normally related great arteries; type II is tricuspid atresia with transposition of the great arteries {S,D,D} (first recognized by Kuhne in 1906). This classification was later expanded by Keith, Rowe and Vlad and by Paul to include a small group of patients with congenitally corrected transposition of the great arteries {S,L,L}—type III.

The lesion is subclassified according to the degree of pulmonary blood flow.

Ia. This type has associated pulmonary atresia. The right ventricular cavity is either slit-like or entirely absent on gross inspection. The ductus arteriosus is patent but usually inadequate in size.

Ib. This is the most common type of tricuspid atresia. The VSD is small and the right ventricle is diminutive. The pulmonary annulus is narrow and the leaflets usually are thickened and bicuspid. The pulmonary artery is hypoplastic from its origin to its intrapulmonary branches. The ductus arteriosus is patent in about one-fourth of this group.

Ic. There is a medium-sized VSD with a pulmonary valve and main pulmonary artery that are either normal in size or enlarged.

IIa. The VSD is large and the right ventricular wall is thicker than it is in type I. There is pulmonary atresia and the aorta arises from the right ventricle. The ductus arteriosus is patent but, again, usually inadequate.

IIb. The VSD is large and high, extending to the semilunar valves. The aorta occasionally is overriding. The pulmonary stenosis is valvar, subpulmonary or both.

IIc. The VSD usually is large. Systemic blood flow frequently is reduced due to right ventricular infundibular stenosis, aortic coarctation, aortic atresia or relative hypoplasia of the aorta.

III. Tricuspid atresia in *l*-transposition is very rare. It has been described in association with both subpulmonary and subaortic stenosis.

Pathophysiology and Natural History

There are two distinct physiologic variants associated with the different anatomic types. The patients in the group (types Ia, Ib, IIa and IIb) representing the majority of patients (71%) have reduced pulmonary blood flow and therefore present with significant cyanosis; those in the other group (types Ic and IIC) with little or no obstruction to pulmonary blood flow have no clinical cyanosis but often present with congestive heart failure. Patients with type Ic tricuspid atresia frequently develop progressive cyanosis and decreasing congestive heart failure as the VSD becomes increasingly restrictive. Patients with type IIc tricuspid atresia have a high incidence of associated obstruction to systemic blood flow, and congestive heart failure may be severe, leading to death before the second or third month of life. Often, those who do not die develop pulmonary vascular obstructive disease.

Only 50% of patients with tricuspid atresia, allowed a natural course, live 6 months and only one-third survive beyond 1 year. By 10 years, 90% will be dead. The prognosis correlates with the degree of pulmonary blood flow. At the extremes, types Ia, IIa and IIc usually die before the age of 3 months. The average survival of patients with type Ib is 11 months. The oldest survivors are patients with type IIc; the oldest on record is 56 years.

Clinical and Diagnostic Features

Most patients with tricuspid atresia are cyanotic, and clubbing is present in patients over the age of 2 years. Severely limited pulmonary blood flow manifests as dyspnea, cyanosis and syncope (cyanotic spells). About three-quarters of patients with diminished pulmonary flow have a systolic murmur, whereas those with increased flow always have a relatively loud systolic murmur along the left sternal border or at the apex. The constellation of findings—hepatomegaly, peripheral edema and systemic venous congestion—usually suggests a small atrial septal defect but, of course, may occur with congestive heart failure.

On the electrocardiogram, left axis deviation is present in 90% of patients, and in a cyanotic child with decreased pulmonary vasculature on the chest roentgenogram this should raise the suspicion of tricuspid atresia. Left ventricular hypertrophy almost always is present and usually progresses with age. There is P-tricuspidale (notched P-wave with a taller initial peak) in 81% of patients. Patients with {S,D,D} transposition of the great arteries (d-TGA) have right axis deviation.

Although a characteristic configuration of the heart in tricuspid atresia has been described (a flattened right heart border and an abnormally rounded left heart border and concave pulmonary artery segment), the chest roentgenogram is variable and the cardiac silhouette may, for example, resemble that of tetralogy of Fallot or of d-TGA.

Angiocardiography is diagnostic for tricuspid atresia and the sequential appearance of contrast material in the left atrium, left ventricle and, finally, the great arteries following injection into the right atrium is typical. A triangular area within the cardiac silhouette that fails to fill with contrast medium early in the ventricular phase (the so-called right ventricular window), due to the absence of the inflow portion of the right ventricle, is also characteristic of tricuspid atresia.

Surgical Management

Until recently, the only surgical treatment for tricuspid atresia was palliative. There are, in general, three types of palliation available: (1) systemic-to-pulmonary shunts, (2) atrial septotomy or septectomy and (3) pulmonary artery banding. The most common indication for palliation is the presence of severe systemic arterial desaturation, and the therapeutic objective is to increase the delivery of blood to the pulmonary capillary bed. Although Alfred Blalock performed the first subclavian-to-pulmonary artery anastomosis (November 29, 1944) on a patient with tetralogy of Fallot, within a few months he applied this operation to a patient with tricuspid atresia. Although in the past the incidence of

shunt thrombosis and distortion of the pulmonary artery in patients under 6 months has been high, thanks to improvements in materials and technique there is renewed enthusiasm for the Blalock-Taussig anastomosis in infants requiring shunts.

A descending aorta-to-left pulmonary artery anastomosis (Potts, 1945) is relatively easy to construct and there is a low incidence of thrombosis even in very small infants. However, the difficulty in judging the appropriate size of the anastomosis often results in either persistent desaturation or the development of congestive heart failure. Also, the technical difficulties of obliteration at the time of definitive repair limit its acceptability as a palliative shunt. The Waterston anastomosis (aorta-to-right pulmonary artery shunt) reported in 1962 can also be done with relative ease in small infants, but it shares the major disadvantage of the Potts shunt in that there is a relatively high incidence of congestive heart failure, sometimes requiring reoperation. Kinking and obstruction of the right pulmonary artery is an additional complication. It is, however, easily closed at the time of repair.

In 1958, Glenn introduced the superior vena cava-right pulmonary artery anastomosis as a means of palliation for tricuspid atresia. Although it has a number of advantages, there are two major problems associated with this anastomosis: the development of superior vena cava syndrome (particularly when the operation is done in early infancy) and late deterioration of function of the shunt. A very high mortality during infancy has been attributed to high pulmonary artery pressure and the relatively small pulmonary artery. Increasing cyanosis with rising hematocrit and hemoglobin often appear 1– 10 years after the cavopulmonary shunt. This deterioration has been attributed to the development of collateral circulation between the superior and inferior vena cava, a persistent communication between a left superior vena cava and the right atrium and/or increasing pulmonary vascular resistance. The increasing resistance in the right lung sometimes is reversed after a Blalock-Taussig shunt and, consequently, it is speculated that at least part of the increased resistance is caused by hypoxic reflex vasospasm. Whatever the reasons for late deterioration, an additional operation often is necessary. In Glenn's series, only 22 of 56 long-term survivors (39%) had adequate arterial saturations with cavopulmonary shunt alone. Therefore, we no longer use the cavopulmonary shunt. For children under 3 months of age we have used a Waterston anastomosis but now prefer a Blalock-Taussig shunt regardless of age.

If the patient comes to cardiac catheterization in the neonatal period, we recommend a Rashkind balloon septotomy whether or not there is right-sided heart failure. In infants and children with evidence of a restrictive interatrial communication (pulsatile neck veins and a pulsatile liver) and a significant pressure gradient between the two atria (greater than 5 mm Hg), surgical creation of an atrial septal defect by the closed technique of Blalock and Hanlon is recommended. Almost all infants with tricuspid atresia of type IIc (18%) have excessive pulmonary blood flow and associated severe congestive heart failure. A reduction in the left-to-right shunt, improvement in the high-output congestive heart failure and protection of the pulmonary arterioles against the development of pulmonary vascular obstructive disease can be effected by pulmonary artery banding. Although patients without transposition of the great arteries but with a large VSD (type Ic) often have increased pulmonary blood flow early in life, they usually respond to medical management and rarely require pulmonary artery banding. In fact, these patients usually develop increasing cyanosis due to a closing VSD and may require a palliative shunt later.

The development of a definitive physiologic repair of tricuspid atresia awaited the conceptual advance that adequate pulmonary circulation can be maintained without a right ventricle. This notion was derived from the work of Warden (1954) and Robicsek (1966), who independently demonstrated that the function of the right ventricle is not mandatory for survival. The earliest clinical attempts at such repair were those of Hurwitt and co-workers and of Shumacker in 1955. Both anastomosed the right atrial appendage to the pulmonary artery; the patients did not survive the perioperative period. In 1962, Harrison reported a child who survived anastomosis of the right atrial appendage to the pulmonary artery at age 37 months. The child died, at age 44 months, after an attempt to close the atrial septal defect.

Finally, in 1966, Ross introduced the use of valve-bearing conduits in the repair of complex congenital lesions. From these foundations, Fontan was the first to successfully apply the concept of right atrium-to-pulmonary artery bypass for the physiologic repair of tricuspid atresia on April 25, 1968. For fear of causing splanchnic pooling, he believed it necessary to insert two allograft valves into the right heart circuit: one at the inferior vena caval junction with the right atrium and another in the atrium-to-pulmonary artery conduit. Originally, Fontan also included a Glenn shunt as part of the repair. The inferior vena caval return then was shunted into the left lung via the atrium-to-pulmonary artery conduit.

Since this original report, Fontan and others have described variations of the original operative technique (Fig 69–1). Ross and Somerville used an aortic allograft in the inferior vena cava and an aortic allograft conduit from the right atrium to the main pulmonary artery. One of their 2 patients survived. Miller and co-workers utilized Fontan's original technique in 12 patients, with 8 survivors, and Stanford and co-workers had 1 survivor in 2 patients. Because of the problem of allograft deterioration, Kreutzer and co-workers have utilized the native main pulmonary artery, including the pulmonary valve, anastomosed directly to the right atrium in 2 patients, with good results. The advantage here, of course, is the avoidance of a foreign graft and conceivably lends itself to use in small children with potential growth of the pulmonary valve and artery. We have used the principle of right atrium-to-main pulmonary artery shunt with a valved conduit (Hancock graft) without a second valve in the inferior vena cava. The patient has been fully saturated and asymptomatic since the operation.

Based on experimental studies published as early as 1971, Gago and co-workers recently repaired a patient with the more common type Ib tricuspid atresia with an external valved conduit from the right atrium to the right ventricular remnant in combination with patch enlargement of the right ventricular outflow tract. Such an approach has the theoretic advantage of recruiting any residual right ventricular impulse, thereby reducing the splanchnic pooling. Additionally, the potential hemodynamic hazard of atrial arrhythmias is lessened.

Fontan recently reported his total series, which now in-

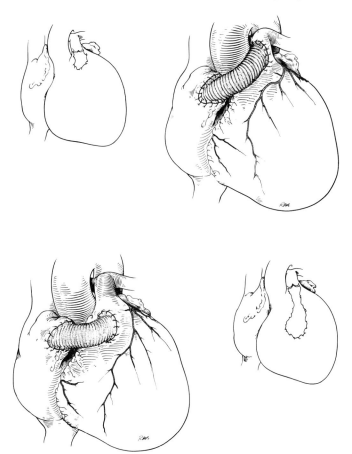

Fig. 69–1.—Modified Fontan procedure. Valved conduit from right atrial appendage to main pulmonary artery and ligation or division of proximal pulmonary artery. When right ventricular outflow chamber is adequate and the pulmonary valve is normal, placement of a valved or nonvalved conduit from right atrium to right ventricular outflow chamber is preferred.

cludes 33 patients, 25 of whom were children aged 27 months to 13.5 years (mean 7.5 years). Four of the first 8 patients died, primarily from elevated pulmonary vascular resistance (greater than 4 U/m²). However, in the last 19 patients, the operation has consisted of the interposition of a nonvalved Dacron conduit between the right atrium and right ventricular outlet chamber. There have been no deaths in the last 15 patients. Ten patients have been analyzed for late results 1–8 years following repair (mean 33 months). Cardiac arrhythmias occurred in 2 patients, permanent complete heart block immediately postoperatively in 1 and atrial fibrillation 4 years after operation, which was converted to sinus rhythm. The aortic saturation was above 90 % in all but 1 patient who had a residual right-to-left shunt at the atrial level. Right atrial pressure was elevated 7–22 mm Hg (mean 14 mm Hg), with a prominent A wave in all. Exercise was performed by 4 monitored patients. All were able to double their cardiac index.

Although most patients with tricuspid atresia can, in principle, be managed by these techniques (excepting only those with severely hypoplastic pulmonary arteries—types Ia and IIa), it is becoming increasingly obvious that survival may be anticipated only for those patients with normal pulmonary vascular resistance, left atrial pressure and left ventricular end-diastolic pressure. Analysis of large groups of patients with tricuspid atresia surviving palliative operations indicates that they have a very high likelihood of living at least 10–15 years after palliation. Thus, reparative operation should be considered between the ages of 5 and 8 years, or at any time the pulmonary resistance or left ventricular function begins to deteriorate. Despite many open questions, corrective surgery for tricuspid atresia has had promising early clinical results.

Ebstein's Anomaly

In 1866, Wilhelm Ebstein described the history and findings of a 19-year-old boy with dyspnea and palpitations since early childhood. The boy died with the clinical features of right heart failure, and at postmortem examination he was found to have dilatation of the right atrium and right ventricle, a patent foramen ovale and an inferiorly displaced and malformed tricuspid valve. Prior to 1949, this so-called Ebstein's anomaly of the tricuspid valve was diagnosed only after death, but along with the surge in interest in congenital heart disease soon after World War II, characteristic clinical, electrocardiographic and radiologic features of Ebstein's anomaly were delineated (Tournire 1949, Reynolds 1950, Engle 1950). Eventually, review of this lesion established its familial relationship (Gueron, 1966) and its frequent association with type B ventricular pre-excitation (Sodi-Pallares and Marsico, 1955).

Patients with Ebstein's malformation often survive into the second and third decades but arrhythmias, congestive heart failure, cerebral abscesses, paradoxic embolism and severe systemic desaturation secondary to right-to-left shunting at the atrial level result in death or lead to surgical intervention.

Anatomy

The essential anatomic features of Ebstein's anomaly include a downward displacement of the septal and posterior leaflets of the tricuspid valve to the level of the moderator band. The anterior leaflet forms a deep curtain-like structure extending from the annulus fibrosus to the papillary muscle of the right ventricle. Chordae are shortened or absent without interchordal spaces. The downward displacement of the valve apparatus partitions the right ventricle into a proximal portion (which has a thinned *atrialized* wall) and a small relatively inefficient distal pumping chamber. The malformed and inferiorly displaced leaflets result in variable degrees of obstruction and insufficiency. Consequently, the right atrium and the thin portion of the right ventricle often become extremely large. In severe cases, the chamber distal to the valve consists of little more than a right ventricular outflow tract. Review of pathologic specimens illustrates a broad spectrum in severity in this lesion.

The foramen ovale is patent in slightly more than half, and less commonly there may be a true atrial septal defect. Other associated lesions include ostium primum defect, ventricular septal defect, pulmonary atresia, pulmonary stenosis, a patent ductus arteriosus and hypoplastic aorta. A similar inferior displacement of the septal and posterior leaflets of the left AV valve has been reported in congenitally corrected transposition {S,L,L} of the great arteries.

Pathophysiology and Natural History

The incidence of this lesion is about 1 in 50,000 or 100,000 of the general population. This lesion is highly variable and the degree of tricuspid stenosis and/or insufficiency determines the severity of right-sided failure and when an atrial septal defect is also present, the severity of systemic desaturation secondary to a right-to-left shunt. Because of the wide spectrum of anatomic severity, it is difficult to generalize about the course and prognosis of the individual patient. In numerous series, however, the average age at death is remarkably constant: 20–25 years. Sudden death is common, presumably from arrhythmias, which occur frequently. Other complications include congestive heart failure, cerebral abscesses and paradoxic embolism. Subacute bacterial endocarditis appears to occur only rarely in this lesion.

Clinical and Diagnostic Features

The majority of infants with Ebstein's anomaly have no symptoms and go undetected save for paroxysmal tachycardia. At the one extreme there may be no symptoms referable to the cardiovascular system throughout life and the patient sustains a normal life expectancy. At the other extreme, death can occur from cardiac failure in the first weeks of life. In the newborn, who generally is not critically ill but has cyanosis, cardiac enlargement, systolic and diastolic murmurs, diminished pulmonary vascular markings and electrocardiographic features of right bundle-branch block, the diagnosis of Ebstein's anomaly should be suspected.

Fatigue, dyspnea and cyanosis are by far the most common clinical features. In patients with advanced degrees of this malformation, the precordial pulsations often are visible. Occasionally a characteristic rippling of pulsations across the left anterior chest wall toward the apex may be felt or seen. The heart sounds are not accentuated but the first sound may be widely split due to delayed closure of the anomalous tricuspid valve. A systolic blowing murmur commonly is heard along the lower left sternal border. Diastolic murmurs are less frequent.

The cardiac silhouette on chest roentgenogram reveals cardiomegaly in the most severe forms and a box-like silhouette due to the leftward deviation of the right ventricular outflow tract. The pulmonary vasculature usually is reduced, thus accentuating the outline of the cardiac silhouette. The electrocardiogram is diagnostically valuable, particularly in those patients with otherwise subtle findings. Characteristic features include prolonged PR interval, right bundle-branch block, tall wide P waves, low voltage rsr' complexes in the right precordial leads and frequent supraventricular tachycardia. About 10% of patients have preventricular pre-excitation, usually of type B. Arrhythmias occur in the normal course of events and may be precipitated by cardiac catheterization and/or induction of anesthesia. The most consistent finding at cardiac catheterization is an elevated right atrial pressure. The S wave may encroach on the V wave. On angiography, the displaced tricuspid valve sometimes can be identified.

Surgical Management

The primary indication for surgical intervention in patients with Ebstein's anomaly is functional limitation from low cardiac output, right-sided heart failure and/or systemic desaturation secondary to significant right-to-left shunting at the atrial level. In the early 1950s, patients, usually with the mistaken diagnosis of tetralogy of Fallot, were submitted to Blalock-Taussig and Potts-Smith operations with universally fatal results and these operations are contraindicated in Ebstein's anomaly. Primary closure of an associated patent foramen ovale alone generally has proved fatal. Lillehei and Hunter (1958) plicated the atrialized right ventricle by approximating the spiral line of attachment of the posterior and septal leaflets of the tricuspid valve to the true annulus fibrosus and concomitantly closed the atrial septal defect and defects in the valve leaflets. Their 2 patients died, and by 1963 Scott concluded that the Glenn shunt was the procedure of choice in patients with symptomatic Ebstein's anomaly. However, shortly thereafter, Barnard and Schrire replaced the severely deranged tricuspid apparatus with a prosthetic device with good results. They also suggested that surgically induced block, which is a risk during this procedure, could be avoided by deviating the valve suture line above the coronary sinus. Lillehei and Gannon, in 1965, also reported significant improvement in their patients following valve replacement. In addition, they closed the atrial septal defect with a Silastic flap valve, thus allowing a temporary right-to-left shunt until the right ventricle became a more proficient pump. In 1969, Hardy and Roe re-emphasized the importance of reduction in the aneurysmal atrialized portion of the right ventricle as part of the hemodynamic repair by anastomosing the spiral line of attachment of the posterior septal leaflets of the tricuspid valve to the true annulus fibrosus, thus plicating the aneurysmal right ventricle. In addition, they believed that, in the majority of patients, tricuspid valve function could be re-established by annuloplasty, thus avoiding a prosthetic device. More recently, several series have been reported championing the relative merits of tricuspid valve replacement, tricuspid annuloplasty and plication of the atrialized right ventricle.

Few patients with Ebstein's anomaly need operation. For those who do, however, our policy is to plicate the atrialized portion of the right ventricle if it is large and with paradoxic wall motion. This is combined with tricuspid annuloplasty. The ASD should be closed and the size of the right atrium may be reduced. If satisfactory tricuspid valve function is not achieved, we then proceed with tricuspid valve replacement with a low-profile tissue valve. The surgical management of this curious anomaly has had an interesting evolutionary course and today a generally satisfactory outcome may be anticipated.

REFERENCES

Tricuspid Atresia

1. Choussat, A., Fontan, F., Brom, A. G., Rohmer, J., Dupuis, C., and Chauve, A.: Late results after surgical repair of tricuspid atresia. Presented at the 7th Congress of the European Society of Cardiology, Amsterdam, June 20, 1976.
2. Dick, M., Fyler, D. C., and Nadas, A. S.: Tricuspid atresia: The clinical course in 96 patients, Am. J. Cardiol. 33:135, 1974.
3. Edwards, J. E., and Burchell, H. B.: Congenital tricuspid atresia: A classification, Med. Clin. North Am. 33:1177, 1949.
4. Fontan, F., and Baudet, E.: Surgical repair of tricuspid atresia, Thorax 26:240, 1971.
5. Fontan, F., Choussat, A., Brom, A. G., Chauve, A., Coqueran, J. E., and Locatelli, G.: Tricuspid atresia repair in childhood. Presented at the 7th Congress of the European Society of Cardiology, Amsterdam, June 20, 1976.
6. Gago, O., Salles, C. A., Stern, A. M., Spooner, E., Brandt, R. L., and Morris, J. D.: A different approach for the total correction of tricuspid atresia, J. Thorac. Cardiovasc. Surg. 72:209, 1976.
7. Kreutzer, G., Galindez, E., Bono, H., DePalma, D., and Laura, J. P.: An operation for the correction of tricuspid atresia, J. Thorac. Cardiovasc. Surg. 66:613, 1973.
8. Robicsek, F., Sanger, P. W., and Gallucci, V.: Long-term complete circulatory exclusion of the right side of the heart: Hemodynamic observations, Am. J. Cardiol. 18:867, 1966.
9. Ross, D. N., and Somerville, J.: Surgical correction of tricuspid atresia, Lancet 1:854, 1973.
10. Sade, R. M., and Castaneda, A. R.: Tricuspid Atresia, in Sabiston, D. C., and Spencer, F. C. (eds.), *Gibbon's Surgery of the Chest* (3d ed.; Philadelphia: W. B. Saunders Company, 1976), p. 1152.
11. Warden, H. E., DeWall, R. A., and Varco, R. L.: Use of the right auricle as a pump for the pulmonary circuit, Surg. Forum 5:16, 1954.

Ebstein's Anomaly

1. Barnard, C. N., and Schrire, V.: Surgical correction of Ebstein's malformation with a prosthetic tricuspid valve, Surgery 54:302, 1963.
2. Hardy, K. L., and Roe, B. B.: Ebstein's anomaly: Further experience with definitive repair, J. Thorac. Cardiovasc. Surg. 58:553, 1969.
3. Kitamura, S., Johnson, J. L., Redington, J. V., Mendez, A., Zubiate, P., and Kay, J. H.: Surgery for Ebstein's anomaly, Ann. Thorac. Surg. 11:320, 1971.
4. Kumar, A. E., Fyler, D. C., Miettinen, O. S., and Nadas, A. S.: Ebstein's anomaly: Clinical profile and natural history, Am. J. Cardiol. 28:84, 1971.
5. Lillehei, C. W., and Gannon, P. G.: Ebstein's malformation of

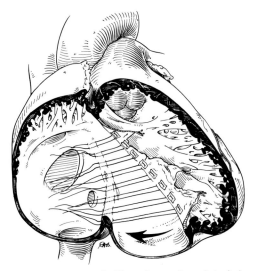

Fig. 69–2.—Ebstein's anomaly. The scheme of repair includes plication of the "atrialized" portion of ventricular wall and tricuspid valve replacement if required.

the tricuspid valve: Method of surgical correction utilizing a ball-valve prosthesis and delayed closure of atrial septal defect, Circulation 31–32 (supp. I): 1, 1965.
6. Lillehei, C. W., Kalke, B. R., and Carlson, R. G.: Evolution of corrective surgery for Ebstein's anomaly, Circulation 35–36 (supp. I): 1, 1967.
7. Lowe, K. G., and Watson, H.: Ebstein's Anomaly of the Tricus-

pid Valve, in Watson, H. (ed.), *Pediatric Cardiology* (St. Louis: The C. V. Mosby Company, 1968), Chap. 29, pp. 437–450.
8. Timmis, J. J., Hardy, J. D., and Watson, D. G.: The surgical management of Ebstein's anomaly: The combined use of tricuspid valve replacement, atrioventricular plication, and atrioplasty, J. Thorac. Cardiovasc. Surg. 53:385, 1969.

Special Conditions

70 Douglas M. Behrendt
Diverticula of the Heart

Congenital diverticula of the heart are rare anomalies that may involve any one of the four cardiac chambers. They may arise from the heart through a narrow neck or may be broad-based. Cardiac muscle fibers may be present or the wall may consist simply of fibrous tissue. Some authors have used the term "aneurysm" instead of "diverticulum," especially when discussing the broad-based variety. Whichever term is used, it is important to exclude acquired aneurysms such as left ventricular aneurysm from infarction or giant left atrium from mitral stenosis. Assigning a congenital etiology to these diverticula depends on ascertaining their presence at a young age, excluding other cardiac anomalies and finding no histologic evidence of a specific degenerative disease.

Diverticula of the Atria

Diverticula of the atria may involve either just the auricular appendage or the entire atrial wall. The condition is recognized because of: (1) an abnormality of the roentgenographic cardiac silhouette, (2) the occurrence of arrhythmias or (3) embolism. The symptoms and signs encountered are easily understood. Atrial arrhythmias are common, presumably either from ectopic foci in the diverticula or from circus movements established over the large surface area of the sac. This was dramatically demonstrated in one patient (Fig. 70–1) when the atrial arrhythmia was terminated at the precise moment when division of the aneurysmal sac was completed.[3] Atrial thrombi often are present, probably due to stasis of blood within the diverticulum.[4] A reduced cardiac output with resultant exercise intolerance may be caused by compression of the normal cardiac chambers by the diverticulum in a manner analogous to the more common restrictive or constrictive pericardial diseases.[3]

Because diverticulum of the atrium is not a benign condition, operative removal should be recommended.[6] Six of the 12 reported patients with left atrial diverticulum have had cerebral emboli. All of the 5 reported patients with right atrial and one-third of the reported patients with left atrial diverticula have had supraventricular tachyarrhythmias.[1]

Because clot is found so often at operation, the patient should be placed on cardiopulmonary bypass and the aorta clamped before the aneurysm is manipulated. The operative repair consists simply of excising the aneurysmal sac and suturing the resulting defect. The results of operation have been good, with no reported recurrence of emboli or arrhythmias.

Diverticula of the Ventricles

Diverticula of the left ventricle occur either as wide-based apical fibrous aneurysms similar to the acquired aneurysms that result from myocardial infarction or as narrow-necked diverticula, either muscular or fibrous, extending toward the midline (Fig. 70–2). The narrow muscular apical diverticula frequently are associated with midline defects in the chest or abdominal walls, both resulting presumably from failure of the embryonic mesoderm to fuse solidly in the midline.[10] Intracardiac defects are common in this group. The fibrous diverticula of the ventricle may be located at either the base or the apex, and they are not associated with midline somatic defects or with intracardiac anomalies. Most of the patients with fibrous sacs have been African, and these diverticula often have been calcified.[8] Mitral valve incompetence may occur with all types of left ventricle diverticula. Although one might reasonably assume this to be due to papillary muscle involvement, this relationship has not been noted in the reported patients. Diverticula of the right ventricle have also been reported.[5]

Midline left ventricular muscular diverticula usually are diagnosed in infancy because of a pulsating upper abdominal mass with associated omphalocele.[7] The risk of spontaneous rupture is high and operation should be performed. Other cardiac anomalies such as tricuspid atresia may be present, requiring additional operative therapy.

Patients with any of the other types of left or right ventricular diverticula may become symptomatic from endocarditis, congestive failure due to parodoxic pulsation or associated mitral valve incompetence.[2] Emboli and arrhythmias from ventricular diverticula are unusual, and many patients have been asymptomatic, the abnormality being recognized

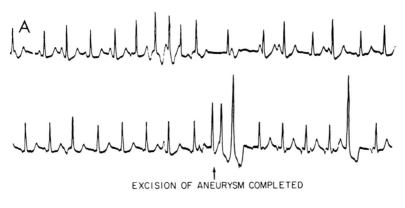

EXCISION OF ANEURYSM COMPLETED

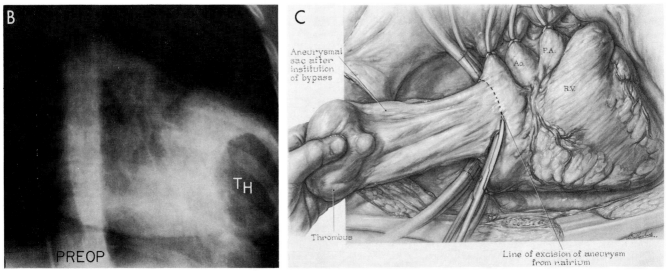

Fig. 70–1.—Atrial diverticulum. **A,** continuous recording of electrocardiogram during excision of right atrial diverticulum. A regular atrial rhythm appeared immediately after excision of diverticulum *(arrow)* and sinus rhythm developed shortly thereafter. **B,** angiocardiogram showing large thrombus in tip of massive right atrial diverticulum. **C,** operative excision of right atrial diverticulum under cardiopulmonary bypass. (From Morrow and Behrendt.[3])

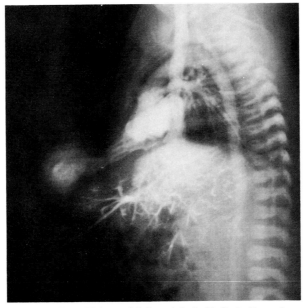

Fig. 70–2.—Midline diverticulum of left ventricle in an infant with Cantrell's syndrome (see Chap. 41). The aneurysm is in an omphalocele outside the body wall.

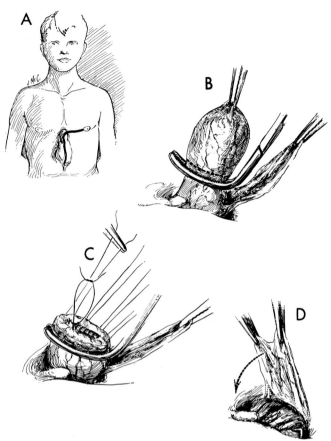

Fig. 70–3.—Ventricular diverticulum. Operative excision of midline left ventricular diverticulum. (From Potts *et al.*[9])

on chest roentgenogram. Operative removal seems desirable when the diverticulum is large or when the patient is symptomatic. In the reported cases, the sac has been uneventfully excised without cardiopulmonary bypass[9] (Fig. 70–3). However, resection on cardiopulmonary bypass might be preferable in some circumstances.

REFERENCES

1. Hougen, T. J., *et al.:* Aneurysm of the left atrium, Am. J. Cardiol. 33:557, 1974.
2. Gueron, M., *et al.:* Left ventricular diverticulum and mitral incompetence in asymptomatic children, Circulation 53:181, 1976.
3. Morrow, A. G., and Behrendt, D. M.: Congenital aneurysm (diverticulum) of the right atrium: Clinical manifestations and results of operative treatment, Circulation 38:124, 1968.
4. Behrendt, D. M., and Aberdeen, E.: Congenital aneurysm of the left atrium: Case report, Ann. Thorac. Surg. 13:54, 1972.
5. Copeland, J., *et al.:* Congenital diverticulum of the right ventricle, J. Thorac. Cardiovasc. Surg. 70:536, 1975.
6. Krueger, S. K., Fenlic, R. M., and Mooring, P. K.: Left atrial appendage aneurysm. Correlation of noninvasive with clinical and surgical findings: Report of a case, Circulation 52:732, 1975.
7. Taussig, H. B.: *Congenital Malformations of the Heart* (2d ed.; Cambridge, Mass.: Harvard University Press, 1960), p. 270.
8. Chester, E., Tucker, R. B. K., and Barlow, J. B.: Subvalvular and apical left ventricular aneurysms in the Bantu as a source of systemic emboli, Circulation 35:1156, 1967.
9. Potts, W. J., DeBoer, A., and Johnson, F. R.: Congenital diverticulum of the left ventricle. Case report, Surgery 33:301, 1953.
10. Cantrell, J. R., Haller, J. A., and Ravitch, M. M.: A syndrome of congenital defects involving the abdominal wall, sternum, diaphragm, pericardium, and heart, Surg. Gynecol. Obstet. 107:602, 1958.

71 WILLIAM G. WILLIAMS / GEORGE A. TRUSLER

Heart Block—Congenital and Acquired

Congenital Complete Heart Block

CONGENITAL HEART BLOCK is rare, occurring approximately once in 20,000 live births.[1] It accounts for less than 1% of congenital heart disease. Both sexes are affected equally.

The etiology of congenital heart block is varied.[2] Histologically, there may be complete agenesis of the AV node or His bundle or interruption of the conduction pathway by tumor,[3, 4] fetal endocarditis, endocardial fibroelastosis and localized fibrosis. The familial incidence of congenital heart block is similar to other forms of congenital heart disease.[5, 6]

Various malformations of the heart may be associated with congenital heart block, although in 70% of patients the cardiac anatomy is normal. Congenitally corrected transposition of the great arteries carries an increased risk of complete

heart block.[7] James *et al.*[8] recently have described the association of absent right superior vena cava with congenital heart block. The incidence of block with other malformations does not differ from that of the general population. In our series of 23 children requiring permanent pacing for congenital heart block, 13 have anatomically normal hearts and 8 have congenitally corrected transposition.

Natural History

Most children with congenital heart block are asymptomatic and have an excellent prognosis.[1, 9] However, infants in congestive heart failure,[1] children with Stokes-Adams attacks[10, 11] and with associated congenital heart malformations[12, 13] have an increased risk of sudden death. As in other forms of congenital heart disease, prognosis is worse if the problem is apparent in infancy. A slow ventricular rate (less than 55 beats per minute) associated with a rapid atrial rate (greater than 140 beats per minute) in the infant is a sign of a poor prognosis.[1]

A broad QRS (greater than 0.10 millisecond) is also associated with a poor outlook.[10, 14]

Treatment

Children with congenital complete heart block who are asymptomatic, have an anatomically normal heart and a QRS of less than 0.10 millisecond have a good prognosis. They can be followed by periodic physical examination and routine electrocardiogram.

INDICATIONS FOR PERMANENT PACEMAKER THERAPY. — *Absolute indications:* 1. Congestive heart failure in the infant in association with complete heart block should be treated promptly by temporary transvenous pacing and standard digitalis and diuretic therapy. When stabilized, the infant should undergo elective implantation of a permanent pacemaker (Fig. 71-1). All 8 infants in our series presented in congestive heart failure under 4 months of age and have had an excellent result from permanent pacing.

2. Stokes-Adams attacks are a serious event and sufficient indication for permanent pacing. These children tend to be older, averaging 11.4 years in our series, of whom 10 were paced for this indication.

Relative indications: Infants and children who are asymptomatic but have underlying congenital heart disease or a QRS width greater than 0.10 millisecond are at increased risk of developing congestive heart failure, Stokes-Adams attacks or sudden death. Serious consideration should be given to permanent pacing. If palliative or corrective operation for associated defects is contemplated, temporary pacing should be instituted prior to anesthesia and permanent pacing electrodes inserted following repair. Permanent pacing should be instituted at this time.

Postoperative Heart Block

Intracardiac repair of congenital or acquired defects may result in iatrogenic arrhythmias requiring permanent pacing. Injury of the conduction tissue or its blood supply can result in malfunction of sinoatrial node, interatrial tracts, atrioventricular node or bundle branches. The surgeon must have detailed knowledge of the conduction tissue anatomy in a normal and a malformed heart.[15-18]

Most intraoperative heart blocks occur in association with the repair of ventricular septal defect. In our series of 46 children requiring permanent pacing for heart block following intracardiac operations, 38 had undergone closure of a ventricular septal defect either alone (11 children) or in association with other defects (27 children). Repair of a primum atrial septal defect (5 children), mitral valve replacement (2 children) and a subaortic myectomy (1 child) accounted for the other lesions associated with iatrogenic complete heart block. The incidence of complete heart block following intracardiac repair in our experience is 1.5%. The malformation at greatest risk (6%) has been the primum atrial septal defect.

Postoperative complete heart block may be transient, resolving to sinus rhythm and subsequently recurring at a time remote from the operation. This sequence occurred in 11 of our 46 children who are being paced for iatrogenic block. The interval between initial operation and late onset of permanent complete block was as long as 7 years and averaged 3.3 years per child. This problem has been studied in detail.[19, 20] The child at risk of late-onset heart block will have a history of transient complete heart block at the time of operation. Complete block resolves to sinus rhythm with right bundle-branch block plus or minus left anterior hemiblock. Resolution to bifascicular block has been stressed as an indication of a high-risk category but we have encountered 2 children with late-onset complete block whose interval rhythm consisted of right bundle-branch block alone. The most important factor in late-onset block is the history of transient complete heart block at the time of operation. Conduction studies may unmask the presence of underlying disturbances if the H-V conduction time is prolonged[21] or if rapid atrial pacing produces fascicular block.[22]

Indications for Permanent Pacing

1. A child with complete heart block following intracardiac repair requires implantation of a permanent pacemaker. The routine use of temporary pacing wires intraoperatively allows the procedure to be done electively. An interval of up to 2 weeks will establish whether the block is permanent.

2. A child with transient complete heart block that resolves to sinus rhythm may not require permanent pacing. Electrophysiologic studies should be performed and if His bundle malfunction is present, permanent pacing should be recommended on a prophylactic basis. This opinion is not unanimous.[23]

Pacemaker Therapy in Children

Although there is considerable pacemaker experience in adults, very little has been written about pacing in children.[14, 24-26] There are important differences in managing the child. In discussing these problems, we rely on our experience in pacing 75 children, an average of 3.0 years per child.

Selection of a Pacemaker

SIZE. — The physical size of the pacing unit is extremely important. The technical problems of wound healing are proportional to the dose of foreign material and obviously the smaller the child the more critical this problem. Even the older child may not have adequate subcutaneous tissue to prevent superficial necrosis.

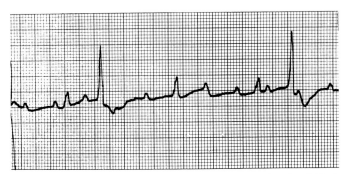

Fig. 71–1.—This electrocardiogram demonstrates complete heart block with a ventricular rate less than 50 and an atrial rate greater than 140 beats per minute. The patient is a newborn infant in severe congestive heart failure. Her heart is anatomically normal. She responded to temporary pacing and digitalization. A permanent pacemaker was implanted electively at 1 week of age and wound dehiscence required repair 9 days postoperatively. Elective pack replacement for battery depletion was performed at 2 years of age and a nuclear pacer inserted. Myocardial threshold at 2 years was 3.5 volts at 9.8 ma! At 3½ years of age, she is developing normally, not requiring medication and had no exercise limitations.

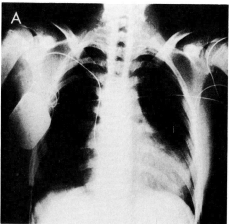 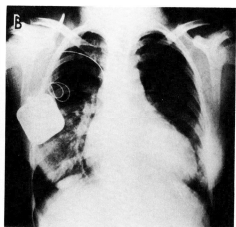

Fig. 71–2.—These chest x-rays are of a 14-year-old girl with recurrent dizzy spells due to lead retraction. She underwent surgical closure of a ventricular septal defect at 5½ years of age. The procedure was complicated by complete heart block, and epicardial pacing was begun in the early post-operative period. She had a succession of battery changes and lead repairs over the ensuing 4½ years. At age 10 years, her pacemaker wound became infected, necessitating conversion to a transvenous pacing system. The transvenous lead was advanced to accommodate her growth at ages 11½ years, 13 years and 14 years. Despite the elective lead advancement at 14 years of age **(A)**, the transvenous lead lost contact with the right ventricle 10 months later **(B)**, resulting in dizzy spells and necessitating lead replacement.

CIRCUIT.—Ideally, a circuit that re-establishes atrioventricular synchrony would be most appropriate in a child. This circuit should be demand for both atrial and ventricular contraction.

The ventricular demand pacemaker is most widely used. For infants we have selected the rate of 100 beats per minute; for older children 70 is appropriate. Where rate change may be required, such as overdrive suppression of ventricular arrhythmias, an externally programable pacemaker is preferred.

Fixed-rate pacemakers should not be used in children due to the high risk of pacer competition. Low-output circuits are also not recommended in children, as we have found that children tend to have higher thresholds.

POWER SOURCE.—The young child requires the most durable power source in the smallest possible package. Lithium iodide seems particularly suitable at present. Nuclear power may be useful for children, although one is aware of possible hazards of radiation. The relatively larger size and higher cost compared to lithium have made nuclear power less appropriate at present.

External power sources such as radiofrequency or rechargeable batteries are additional alternatives. Psychologic factors, reliance on patient performance, technical problems with leads and reliability have kept us from recommending such pacemakers.

In our series of patients, 37% of reoperations were required for battery failures.

Selection of a Pacemaker Lead

Pacemaker leads, a frequent cause of problems in children, accounted for 33% of reoperations in our experience. Fracture of the lead accounted for almost half of these complications. Displacement of transvenous electrodes can occur early, as in the adult patient, or late, due to growth of the child (Fig. 71-2). We electively advance transvenous leads at the time of battery replacement. We believe that transvenous leads should be used in the child only when there is a contraindication to epicardial leads. The transvenous lead also has obvious limitations in the presence of transposition. Outgrowth of transthoracic epicardial leads is a theoretic problem that we have not encountered.

A major difference in pacing children is a much higher stimulating threshold. Acute threshold averaged 1.4 volts at 2.6 ma in 25 children. Chronic thresholds were measured in 23 children and averaged 3.5 volts at 7.7 ma. The threshold may vary considerably between the left and right ventricles. In general, the more normal ventricle should be paced. One should also be aware of failure of sensing in leads placed near the apex of the right ventricle in patients with right bundle-branch block (and vice versa) as recently reported by Vera *et al.*[27]

Pacemaker Wound

Wound erosion by the pacemaker pack and/or wound infection accounted for 30% of reoperations in our series. As mentioned, the smallest possible pacemaker should be used. The wound should be made away from the pacer pocket, preferably higher than the pack, to avoid fluid accumulation under the incision. The pack should be placed under a protective muscle layer and on occasion we have placed it within the thorax as originally suggested by Escano *et al.*,[28] although we use an extrapleural pocket to facilitate replacement.

Successful implantation of a pacemaker must be followed by ongoing pacemaker surveillance. The child and his family also require continued assessment in addition to reassurance, to ensure complete rehabilitation of the child.

REFERENCES

1. Michaelsson, M., and Engle, M. A.: Congenital complete heart block: An international study of natural history, Cardiovasc. Clin. 4:86, 1972.
2. Lev, M.: Pathogenesis of congenital atrioventricular block, Prog. Cardiovasc. Dis. 15:145, 1972.
3. Linder, E., et al.: Congenital complete heart block. 11. Histology of the conduction system, Ann. Paediatr. Fenn. 11:11, 1965.
4. Kaminsky, N. I., et al.: Heart block and mesothelioma of the atrioventricular node, Am. J. Cardiol. 20:248, 1967.
5. Wendkos, M. H., and Study, R. S.: Familial congenital complete A-V heart block, Am. J. Cardiol. 34:138, 1947.
6. Wagner, C. W., and Hall, R. J.: Congenital familial atrioventricular dissociation, Am. J. Cardiol. 19:593, 1967.

7. Walker, W. J., *et al.:* Corrected transposition of the great vessels, atrioventricular heart block and ventricular septal defect. A clinical triad, Circulation 17:249, 1958.

8. James, T. N., Marshall, T. K., and Edwards, J. E.: Cardiac electrical instability in the presence of a left superior vena cava, Circulation 54:689, 1976.

9. Campbell, M., and Emanuel, R.: Six cases of congenital complete heart block followed for 34–40 years, Br. Heart J. 29:577, 1967.

10. Molthan, M. E., *et al.:* Congenital heart block with fatal Stokes-Adams attacks in childhood, Pediatrics 30:32, 1962.

11. Nakamura, F. F., and Nadas, A. S.: Complete heart block in infants and children, N. Engl. J. Med. 270:1261, 1964.

12. Kangos, J. J., Griffiths, S. P., and Blumenthal, S.: Congenital complete heart block, Am. J. Cardiol. 20:632, 1967.

13. Ayers, C. R., Boineau, J. P., and Spach, M. S.: Congenital complete heart block in children, Am. Heart J. 72:381, 1966.

14. Trusler, G. A., Mustard, W. T., and Keith, J. D.: The role of pacemaker therapy in congenital complete heart block, J. Thorac. Cardiovasc. Surg. 55:105, 1968.

15. Lev, M.: Conduction system in congenital heart disease, Am. J. Cardiol. 21:619, 1968.

16. Feldt, R. H., DuShane, J. W., and Titus, J. L.: The atrioventricular conduction system in persistent common atrioventricular canal defects: Correlations with electrocardiogram, Circulation 42:437, 1970.

17. Anderson, R. H., *et al.:* The conducting tissues in congenitally corrected transposition, Circulation 50:911, 1974.

18. Maloney, J. D., *et al.:* Identification of the conduction system in corrected transposition and common ventricle at operation, Mayo Clin. Proc. 50:387, 1975.

19. Godman, M. J., Roberts, N. K., and Izukawa, T.: Late postoperative conduction disturbances after repair of ventricular septal defect and tetralogy of Fallot, Circulation 49:214, 1974.

20. Sondheimer, H. M., *et al.:* Conduction disturbances after total correction of tetralogy of Fallot, Am. Heart J. 92:278, 1976.

21. Narula, O. S., and Samet, P.: Right bundle branch block with normal, left or right axis deviation, Am. J. Med. 51:432, 1971.

22. Fabergas, R. A., Tse, W. W., and Han, J.: Conduction disturbances of the bundle branches produced by lesions in the nonbranching portion of the His bundle, Am. Heart J. 92:356, 1976.

23. Yabek, S. M., Jarmakani, J. M., and Roberts, N. K.: Diagnosis of trifascicular damage following tetralogy of Fallot and ventricular septal defect repair, Circulation 55:23, 1977.

24. Liu, L., Griffiths, S. P., and Gerst, P. H.: Implanted cardiac pacemakers in children: A report of their application in five patients, Am. J. Cardiol. 20:639, 1967.

25. Benrey, J., *et al.:* Permanent pacemaker implantation in infants, children and adolescents: Long term follow-up, Circulation 53:245, 1976.

26. Glenn, W. W. L., *et al.:* Heart block in children: Treatment with a radiofrequency pacemaker, J. Thorac. Cardiovasc. Surg. 58:361, 1969.

27. Vera, Z., *et al.:* Lack of sensing by demand pacemakers due to intraventricular conduction defects, Circulation 51:815, 1975.

28. Escano, F. B., *et al.:* Intrapleural pacemaker generator in children, J. Thorac. Cardiovasc. Surg. 62:454, 1971.

72

HERBERT E. SLOAN, JR. / DOUGLAS M. BEHRENDT

Operative Treatment of Rheumatic Disease of the Mitral Valve

RHEUMATIC FEVER now is uncommon and rarely is severe in children in economically advanced countries where living conditions are less crowded and aggressive treatment of streptococcal infection with antibiotics has become standard practice.[1] Although one-half of all children with acute rheumatic fever have evidence of carditis, the majority recover from it without permanent cardiac damage. Only a few have severe enough involvement of a valve or of the myocardium to threaten life, and this valve damage often is not apparent for a decade or more following the attack. By contrast, in poorer countries, the disease is not only prevalent but also rapidly progressive, so that in India and Ceylon,[2, 3] for example, young patients often require operation for mitral valve disease.

In our experience, mitral insufficiency is the most common valve lesion requiring operation in children whereas mitral stenosis is seen rarely. Aortic insufficiency is the second most frequent valve abnormality resulting from rheumatic fever but this rarely produces symptoms in childhood.

Pathology

Rheumatic fever is a systemic disease that attacks many parts of the body but causes recognizable permanent damage only to the heart. The relationship between rheumatic fever and streptococcal infection now is clearly established. The rheumatic process may attack any or all of the cardiac structures. The basic changes consist of edema and proliferative inflammatory reactions in connective tissues. The microscopic appearance is one of edema of the ground substance in the heart valves, fragmentation of the collagen fibers and infiltration by round cells and scattered polymorphonuclear leukocytes. Scattered through the ground substance are deposits of granular eosinophilic material.

This initial reaction is followed by the proliferative phase, in which the characteristic Aschoff body of rheumatic fever develops. The Aschoff body is believed by many to be related to activity of the rheumatic process, although there seems to be little correlation between its presence in atrial biopsy specimens taken during operation and the results of correction of valve lesions. Finally, severe scarring and calcification of the valves may develop.

The mitral valve is damaged more often than the aortic valve and the aortic, in turn, is damaged more often than the tricuspid valve. This perhaps is related to the degree of pressure each valve must sustain in the closed position. The principal lesion is mitral insufficiency, which may occur early in the course of the disease. The mechanism producing this insufficiency is related to direct involvement of the valve structures and the annulus as well as to dilatation of the left atrium and left ventricle.

Mitral Insufficiency

Clinical Picture

Severe mitral insufficiency in children may cause a substantial increase in cardiac size, cough, dyspnea, poor weight gain and cardiac failure. The seriously ill child may be so orthopneic that he must sit upright to breathe. The signs of cardiac failure are present. There is gross cardiomegaly and the heart is hyperactive. A left ventricular heave may be present and a systolic thrill may be palpated over the apex. The major auscultatory finding is a loud, pansystolic apical murmur. An apical third heart sound or a short mid-diastolic murmur may be heard and is due to the increased volume of blood flowing across the mitral valve in diastole.

In severe mitral regurgitation, the electrocardiogram reflects enlargement of the left ventricle and left atrium. Chest roentgenograms show marked cardiac enlargement. The huge left atrium produces a double density along the right cardiac border, displaces the esophagus posteriorly and elevates the left main bronchus. The enlarged left ventricle increases the transverse diameter of the heart, with displacement of the apex downward and to the left. There is congestion in the lung fields.

The pulmonary wedge pressures are elevated and may show high V waves. Mild to moderate pulmonary hypertension usually is present. Left ventricular end-diastolic pressures may be elevated, depending on the severity of the cardiac failure. Contrast studies show marked reflux from the left ventricle into the huge left atrium through the incompetent mitral valve.

Most children with mitral insufficiency come to the attention of the surgeon after the initial attack of rheumatic fever has subsided and the rheumatic process no longer is in the acute phase. It is advisable to wait until active rheumatic myocarditis has subsided, only because the decrease in heart size that usually follows may lessen the severity of valvar incompetence and make operation unnecessary. Furthermore, the presence of active myocarditis greatly increases the risk of operation. However, mitral valvuloplasty may have to be attempted even in the presence of active carditis if it appears that the child may die otherwise.

Differentiating failure due to the mechanical effect of mitral insufficiency from failure due to myocarditis may be extremely difficult. Active rheumatic carditis may be suggested by fever, rash, elevated acute phase reactants, arthritis, subcutaneous nodules, changing murmurs and a friction rub. Anemia and an elevated white blood cell count may be present. Except in acute failure, the sedimentation rate usually is elevated.

Operation

The patients selected for operation should be those who have severe symptoms from overwhelming mitral insufficiency unresponsive to medical therapy. Operation is carried out with the aid of extracorporeal circulation. Although the mitral valve may be approached in several ways, we prefer a right thoracotomy through the fifth intercostal space with the patient in the lateral position. This approach provides excellent exposure and the opportunity to assess valve function after repair.

Because our early experience with the repair of congenital mitral insufficiency by annuloplasty was satisfactory,[4] we have used this technique to correct acquired mitral insufficiency. Annular dilatation is a major component of mitral insufficiency in children. The valve leaflets are thickened but scarring is not pronounced. There may be shortening and adherence of the chordae or they may appear grossly normal. The valve leaflets are mobile but do not approximate during ventricular systole. Satisfactory closure of the valve can be accomplished by placing annuloplastic sutures at each commissure so that the anulus is reduced in circumference enough to allow the anterior leaflet to fill the orifice. (Fig. 72–1). Competence of the valve can be tested by allowing the blood-filled ventricle to contract against it. Care must be taken to avoid trapping air in the ventricle, and it is advisable to aspirate the aortic root when the valve repair is completed. Insufficiency rarely is abolished but it is reduced to the point where it is physiologically unimportant and cardiac compensation is restored.

Other surgeons replace the regurgitant mitral valve with a prosthesis because they believe that correction of mitral insufficiency by annuloplasty has not resulted in long-term

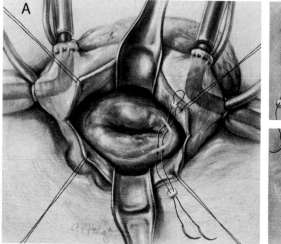
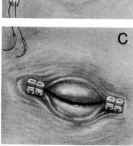

Fig. 72–1.—Technique of operation for rheumatic mitral insufficiency due to anular dilatation. One or more mattress sutures of 2-0 polyester with felt pledgets are placed across each commissure. The sutures are oriented so that most of the reduction in anulus size is accomplished posteriorly. Thus, the posterior leaflet is advanced toward the anterior and no stenosis is created.

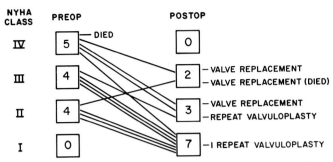

Fig. 72–2.—Rheumatic mitral insufficiency. Clinical course of children having valvuloplasty.

improvement. The hazards associated with the use of prostheses, despite their improvements, make the use of prosthetic appliances in children unwise if a more conservative repair, using the patient's own tissues, can be accomplished. Our own experience shows that long-term, satisfactory correction of acquired mitral insufficiency can be achieved with annuloplasty.

Operative Results

Thirteen children required correction of essentially pure rheumatic mitral insufficiency between 1960 and 1967 at The University of Michigan Medical Center, providing a follow-up period of 10 years or more.

One patient died in heart failure following operation. The decision in that patient to attempt repair of mitral insufficiency in the face of myocarditis reflected the severity of the uncontrolled failure. At postmortem examination, the heart of this desperately ill child showed the histologic stigmata of active rheumatic carditis.

The 12 of the 13 patients who survived have been followed for from 10 to 16 years. Seven are asymptomatic and 3 are improved (Fig. 72–2). Four require digitalis and 2 take diuretics. Four receive anticoagulants, 2 because of valve replacement and 2 because of embolic episodes. This clinical improvement has been accompanied by a reduction of cardiac size on chest roentgenograms in most (Fig. 72–3).

One patient has since been killed in an automobile accident 16 years after valvuloplasty. Two have required second valvuloplasties and now have Grade I systolic murmurs. Three patients required mitral valve replacements 2, 7 and 9 years after their original valvuloplasties. One of these died suddenly 1 month after the valve operation. All of the remaining 7 patients still have a murmur of mild mitral insufficiency that seems to be physiologically unimportant at present. Two of the 10 patients still alive have associated minimal aortic insufficiency.

These results are similar to those reported by Merendino and co-workers,[5] who have obtained excellent long-term results in 7 of 8 patients with acquired mitral insufficiency treated by annuloplasty. None of our patients has had recurrence of rheumatic fever. There is no evidence that operation increased the rate of progression of the valve lesions.

Repair of mitral insufficiency together with repair of major aortic or tricuspid insufficiency was attempted in 4 other patients. Three of these patients died, 2 with active rheumatic carditis. The presence of multiple valve lesions and active rheumatic carditis greatly increases the risk of operation.

Mitral Stenosis

Pathology

During the healing process of rheumatic valvulitis, the inflamed leaflet edges may adhere to each other at the commissures, resulting in stenosis. The chordae often are thickened, shortened and fused together and this may contribute to some associated insufficiency. In children, this process usually is not so severe that the valve cannot be repaired, and calcification of the valve is uncommon. For these reasons, acquired mitral stenosis in children usually is amenable to conservative repair and does not require valve replacement.

Clinical Picture

Like adult patients, children with mitral stenosis experience congestive failure, paroxysmal nocturnal dyspnea, cough, hemoptysis, precordial pain and palpitations. Signs of pulmonary hypertension are present in the majority of

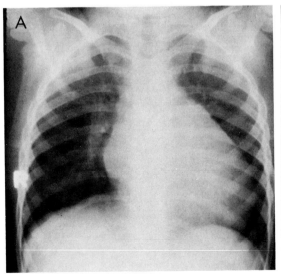
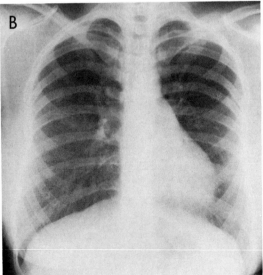

Fig. 72–3.—Mitral insufficiency. Chest roentgenograms before (A) and 10 years after (B) mitral annuloplasty.

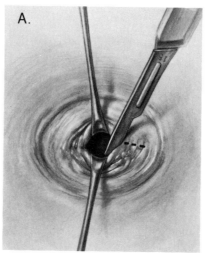 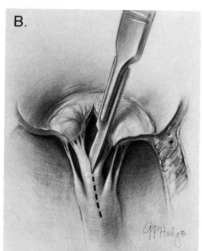

Fig. 72–4.—Technique of open mitral commissurotomy. The valve leaflets are held apart under tension, permitting identification and incision of each commissure. Then the underlying fused chordae and papillary muscles may be visualized. These may also be incised if necessary to achieve an adequate orifice.

these children, and there is evidence of tricuspid regurgitation in one-third of them. It is unusual for children to develop atrial fibrillation or peripheral emboli. There is a diastolic murmur with presystolic accentuation and the right ventricular heave characteristic of mitral stenosis.

The electrocardiogram usually shows normal sinus rhythm with left and right atrial enlargement and right ventricular hypertrophy. Pulmonary vascular congestion with right ventricular and left atrial enlargement is evident on chest roentgenogram.

At cardiac catheterization, elevation of left atrial and right-sided pressures is found. Thickening and immobility of the valve leaflets may be demonstrated by angiogram or echocardiogram.

Operation

In many centers, such as those in India, experience with closed mitral valvulotomy in children has been extensive and successful.[3] We have preferred open valvulotomy, believing that a more precise repair can be obtained with this method.

A right thoracotomy incision is made with the patient in the lateral position and cardiopulmonary bypass is established. The aorta is briefly clamped to prevent ejection of air until the mitral valve has been rendered incompetent. The mitral leaflets are brought into view with "valve lifters" or small right-angle clamps, permitting precise identification of the fused commissures. These then are sharply incised with a scalpel (Fig. 72–4). Often it is apparent that the underlying chordae are fused and foreshortened. If this is the case, the incision is carried between them, and the tip of the papillary muscle may be split for a few millimeters.

If there is associated mitral insufficiency, the annulus may be narrowed with annuloplastic sutures after the commissurotomy. The left ventricle then is allowed to fill with blood as the mitral leaflets are kept incompetent to evacuate air. Finally, the left atrium is allowed to fill with blood and is closed.

Results of Operation

The initial results from one closed and three open valvuloplasties for acquired mitral stenosis at The University of Michigan Medical Center in children between 9 and 18 years of age were excellent (Fig. 72–5).

Because stenosis recurred, 1 patient had an open valvuloplasty 5 years following the original closed valvuloplasty operation and then a valve replacement 4 years later. He now is in NYHA Class II. A second patient underwent valve replacement 11 years after valvuloplasty but did not survive this operation. The 2 other patients are asymptomatic and require no medications. Manabe and co-workers[6] recently have reviewed their excellent long-term results with closed mitral valvotomy in 29 children. Twenty were followed for an average of 10 years (6–20 years). Only 3 died and only 1 required mitral valve replacement during this interval.

Conclusions

We have achieved satisfactory long-term results in 14 of 17 patients with acquired mitral valve lesions using the techniques described above. Although such conservative measures may produce imperfect results, the palliation afforded often is long-lasting, delaying the necessity for valve replacement. All but 5 have been spared the hazard of long-term anticoagulation and risk of other complications to which they would have been subject had valve replacement been used. Furthermore, while children grow, prosthetic devices do not and may require one or more replacements before the children reach adulthood.

Thus, we continue to prefer repair of a child's own valve to prosthetic replacement whenever possible. When it is

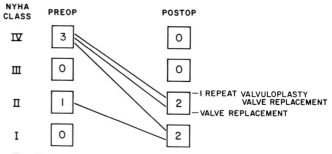

Fig. 72–5.—Clinical course of children having commissurotomy for rheumatic mitral stenosis.

necessary to replace a child's valve we presently use porcine xenografts, since it appears that they may be used with relative safety without anticoagulants, a major advantage in children.

REFERENCES

1. Selzer, A., and Cohn, K. E.: Natural history of mitral stenosis: A review, Circulation 45:878, 1972.
2. Reichek, N., Shelburne, J. C., and Perloff, J. K.: Clinical aspects of rheumatic valvular disease, Prog. Cardiovasc. Dis. 15:491, 1973.
3. Stanley, J., Krishnaswami, S., Jairaj, P. S., Cherian, G., Muralid-haran, S., Sukumar, I. P., and Cherian, G.: The profile and surgical management of mitral stenosis in young patients, J. Thorac. Cardiovasc. Surg. 69:631, 1975.
4. Kahn, D. R., Stern, A. M., Sigmann, J. M., Kirsh, M. M., Lennox, S. C., and Sloan, H.: Long-term results of valvuloplasty for mitral insufficiency in children, J. Thorac. Cardiovasc. Surg. 53:1, 1967.
5. Stevenson, J. G., Kawabori, I., Morgan, B. C., Dillard, D. H., Merendino, K. A., and Guntheroth, W. G.: Rheumatic mitral regurgitation. The case for annuloplasty in the pediatric age group, Circulation 51–52 (supp. I):1–49, 1975.
6. Manabe, H., Ohyama, C., Kitamura, S., and Kawashima, Y.: Valvotomy in young patients with rheumatic mitral stenosis, Ann. Thorac. Surg. 23:136, 1977.

The Pericardium

73 William G. Williams
Tumors of the Heart and Pericardium

PRIMARY TUMORS OF THE HEART are rare in adults and extremely rare in children. Fewer than 300 cases have been reported.[1-5] The majority of these tumors are histologically benign. Myxomas, which account for 50% of cardiac tumors in adults, are very rare in childhood. Rhabdomyoma, fibroma and teratoma are the most frequent tumors encountered in infants and children.

Rhabdomyoma

This tumor usually is multiple, deep within the wall and circumscribed. It consists of swollen muscle fibers containing glycogen.[6] The classic "spider cell" appearance is due to strands of cytoplasm extending from central masses to the cell periphery. They probably represent hamartomas rather than true tumors.[7] Rhabdomyomas account for approximately 60% of reported tumors in infancy and childhood. They commonly are associated with tuberous sclerosis. Although histologically benign, their deep location can produce intracardiac obstruction or conduction problems, accounting for the 80% mortality by 5 years of age.[8]

Successful resections of rhabdomyomas have been reported.[9, 10] Due to the multiplicity of the tumor, complete excision seldom is possible. We agree with the recommendation of Shaher to resect only those tumors producing significant obstruction. Prognosis may not always be unfavorable. Cases of spontaneous regression of rhabdomyoma as well as fibroma have been reported by Khattar *et al.*[11]

Intramural Fibroma

Intramural fibromas arise from the interventricular septum or the myocardium of the left and less frequently right ventricle. The tumor is firm, encapsulated and on cut section is white and composed of collagen-filled fibroblasts with scattered strands of cardiac muscle. Fibromas account for

about 25% of reported childhood cardiac tumors. Successful surgical resection has been reported by many authors.[12-15] Long-term results seem to be good, and our previously reported first patient now is very well 5 years after resection.

Miscellaneous Tumors

The remaining primary cardiac tumors in childhood are a mixture of histologic types. Intrapericardial teratomas usually present as pericardial effusions within the first 3 months of life. Successful resection was first reported by Beck[16] in 1942 but few cases have been described since.[4, 16]

Atrial myxomas are very rare in childhood; fewer than a dozen have been reported. They may have a familial occurrence.[18] They arise from the fossa ovalis, usually projecting into the left atrium. Surgical management should include resection of the adjacent atrial septum.[19, 20]

Sarcomas

Malignant tumors in childhood have been reported by Bigelow *et al.*[2] and Engle and Glenn.[21] Both children died and successful surgical intervention for a malignant cardiac tumor seems unlikely.

Secondary Tumors

Abdominal tumors may invade the lumen of the inferior vena cava and extend to the right heart chambers.[22] Cardiopulmonary bypass with circulatory arrest may extend resectability of these invasive tumors.[23-25] Wilms' tumor and adrenal carcinoma are the usual neoplasms.

Pericardial Tumors

Pericardial tumors, which may be mesotheliomas, teratomas, lipomas, fibromas or angiomas, often are malignant.

Successful resection was first reported by Beck and few cases have been reported since. Benign pericardial cysts are extremely rare, although they should be simple to resect.

REFERENCES

1. Pritchard, R. W.: Tumors of the heart. Review of the subject and review of one hundred and fifty cases, Arch. Pathol. 51:98, 1951.
2. Bigelow, N. H., Klinger, S., and Wright, A. W.: Primary tumors of the heart in infancy and early childhood, Cancer 7:549, 1954.
3. Nadar, A. S., and Ellison, R. C.: Cardiac tumors in infancy, Am. J. Cardiol. 21:363, 1968.
4. Van der Hauwaert, L.: Cardiac tumors in infancy and childhood. A joint research study of the Association of European Cardiologists Proceedings, Br. Heart J. 33:125, 1971.
5. Williams, W. G., et al.: Left ventricular myocardial fibroma: A case report and review of cardiac tumors in children, J. Pediatr. Surg. 7:324, 1972.
6. Heath, D.: Pathology of cardiac tumors, Am. J. Cardiol. 21:315, 1968.
7. Fenoglio, J. J., McAllister, H. A., and Ferrans, V. J.: Cardiac rhabdomyoma: A clinicopathologic and electron microscopic study, Am. J. Cardiol. 38:241, 1976.
8. Kidder, L. A.: Congenital glycogenic tumors of the heart, Arch. Pathol. 49:55, 1950.
9. Hudson, R. E. B.: *Cardiovascular Pathology 2* (London: Arnold, 1965), 1563.
10. Shaher, R. M., et al.: Clinical presentation of rhabdomyoma of the heart in infancy and childhood, Am. J. Cardiol. 30:95, 1972.
11. Khattar, H., et al.: Les tumeurs cardiaques chez l'enfant: Rapport de 3 observations avec evolution spontanee favorable, Arch. Mal. Coeur 68:419, 1975.
12. Geha, A. S., et al.: Intramural ventricular cardiac fibroma. Suc-

cessful removal in two cases and review of the literature, Circulation 36:427, 1967.
13. Kay, J. H., et al.: Successful excision of an intramural fibroma of the right ventricle and ventricular septum – four year follow-up, J. Cardiovasc. Surg. (Torino) 9:434, 1968.
14. Lincoln, J. C. R., Tynan, M. J., and Waterston, D. J.: Successful excision of an endocardial fibroma of the left ventricle in a 10 month old infant. J. Cardiovasc. Surg. (Torino) 56:63, 1968.
15. Bjork, V. O., et al.: Fibroma in the interventricular system of the heart. Successful removal in a 13-month-old infant. Scand. J. Thorac. Cardiovasc. Surg. I: 191, 1967.
16. Beck, C. S.: An intrapericardial teratoma and a tumor of the heart, both removed operatively, Am. Surg. 116:161, 1942.
17. White, J. J., Kaback, M. M., and Haller, J. A.: Diagnosis and excision of an intrapericardial teratoma in an infant, J. Thorac. Cardiovasc. Surg. 55:704, 1968.
18. Kylloen, K. E. J., et al.: Cardiac myxoma: A report of 8 cases, J. Cardiovasc. Surg. (Torino) 17:392, 1976.
19. Goldberg, H. P., et al.: Myxoma of the left atrium: Diagnosis made during life with operative and postmortem findings, Circulation 6:761, 1952.
20. Sanyal, S. K., et al.: Right atrial myxoma in infancy and childhood, Am. J. Cardiol. 20:263, 1967.
21. Engle, M. A., and Glenn, F.: Primary malignant tumor of the heart in infancy: Case report and review of the subject, Pediatrics 15:562, 1955.
22. Edwards, J. E.: Effects of malignant noncardiac tumors upon the cardiovascular system, Cardiovasc. Clin. 4:281, 1972.
23. Murphy, D. A., et al.: Wilms' tumor in the right atrium, Am. J. Dis. Child. 126:210, 1973.
24. Utley, J. R., et al.: Acute obstruction of tricuspid valve by Wilms' tumor, J. Thorac. Cardiovasc. Surg. 66:626, 1973.
25. Theman, T., et al.: Tumor invasion of the upper inferior vena cava: The use of profound hypothermia and circulation arrest as a surgical adjunct, J. Pediatr. Surg. 13: 331, 1978.

74

J. ALEX HALLER, JR. / JAMES S. DONAHOO

Pericarditis

HISTORY. — The pericardium was first described by Hippocrates in 460 B.C. Lower,[8] in the seventeenth century, first clearly defined pericardial tamponade and, in 1649, Riolan[13] suggested pericardiocentesis for its treatment. In 1896, Pick[10] described the clinical syndrome of constrictive pericarditis and, in 1913, Sauerbruch[16] and Rehn[12] independently performed pericardiectomy. More recently, Blalock,[1] McKusick[9] and Isaacs[7] have contributed to the understanding of the pathophysiology of pericardial compression and Roshe and Shumacker[14] have emphasized the importance of radical pericardiectomy to achieve dependable results.

Pathophysiology

In acute cardiac tamponade, filling of the heart during diastole is limited by increased intrapericardial pressure secondary to blood or fluid filling the pericardial space. Although the force of systolic contraction in acute tamponade usually is normal, the diastolic filling pressure is elevated and thus a greater venous pressure is required to fill the ventricles. Decreased stroke volume results in diminished cardiac output, hypotension and eventually a shock-like syndrome of clinical hypoperfusion at the capillary level. The clinical picture is one of shock. The patient has cool and moist skin, heart sounds are diminished, the pulse is rapid

and elevated venous pressure is manifested by distended veins. Classically, a paradoxic pulse is also present. The electrocardiogram may reveal low voltage, elevated ST segments or T wave inversion. The cardiac shadow on chest films frequently is of normal size and configuration in patients with acute tamponade. The pathophysiology of chronic constrictive pericarditis differs slightly from acute pericardial tamponade. A dense chronic inflammatory process has constricted the pericardium and epicardium, resulting in a limitation of diastolic ventricular filling and also an underlying myocardial fibrosis, which may restrict systolic ejection. The result of this dual pathology is an elevated venous pressure, diminished cardiac output and low systemic pressure. Reduced cardiac output results in diminished perfusion of liver and kidney and a tendency toward salt and water accumulation. The blood volume generally is increased due to chronic venous pooling and signs of both right- and left-sided heart failure often are present.

Clinically, the patient is easily fatigued, short of breath and may exhibit signs of peripheral edema and ascites. Classically, the patient exhibits increased venous pressure with prominent hepatojugular reflex, paradoxic pulse and an increase in venous pressure during inspiration (Kussmaul's sign). In a classic experimental preparation, Isaacs *et al.*[7] demonstrated the pathologic physiology of constrictive pericarditis and emphasized the importance of constriction about the ventricles. In contradistinction to acute pericardial tamponade, elevation of the filling pressure in constrictive pericarditis does not result in improvement of symptoms.

Acute Pericarditis

Acute pericarditis in infancy and childhood may occur as a primary disease process without systemic illness or it may be a secondary manifestation of systemic disease such as tuberculosis, rheumatic fever, rheumatoid arthritis, pneumonia, empyema and osteomyelitis. Usually the process is self limited, however, and surgical intervention is indicated only rarely.

The major exception to this is purulent pericarditis. Purulent pericarditis in infants and childhood is an infrequent but often fatal disease process unless it is recognized early and treated aggressively.[4, 16] In infancy, this disease has a reported mortality of 66%[4] and few infants less than 1 month of age have been documented to survive. Purulent pericarditis usually is secondary to a purulent process located else-where in the child's body. Pulmonary infection is the more common inciting condition, but osteomyelitis, meningitis, pyogenic liver abscess and other primary infectious disease processes have been associated with purulent pericarditis in children. Rarely has purulent pericarditis been reported as an isolated disease.

The differential diagnosis of purulent pericarditis is that of cardiac tamponade, hepatomegaly, distended neck veins, diminished heart sounds and a pericardial friction rub in a patient with systemic infection. The electrocardiogram usually shows ST-T wave changes, with ST-T wave elevation being the most common abnormality. The most reliable sign of cardiac tamponade appears to be a pulsus paradoxus with a pulse deficit of greater than 20 mm Hg.

Diagnosis of purulent pericarditis is suspected when an infant or small child has evidence of pericardial tamponade in the face of an infectious disease process. *Staphylococcus aureus* is the most common organism, accounting for about 50% of the patients with purulent pericarditis. Pneumococcus, *Hemophilus influenzae* and other organisms are indicted less frequently.

Occasionally the diagnosis of purulent pericarditis may be suspected by a classic history of systemic infection in the

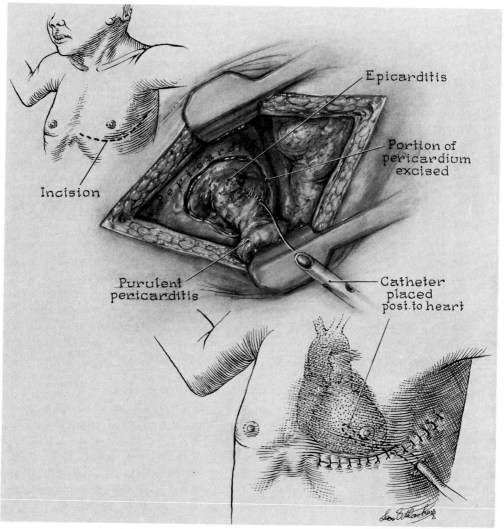

Fig. 74–1.—The pericardium is approached through an anterior thoracotomy.
The pericardium is incised and drained and a soft tube is left in the posterior pericardial space.

presence of pericardial friction rub. A pericardial effusion may be documented by echocardiography;[11] however, the definitive diagnosis of pericarditis can be made only by pericardiocentesis and culture.

Therapy for purulent pericarditis in infants and children has two components: pericardial drainage and antimicrobial agents. Gersony and MacCracken[4] reported no survivors of 17 patients treated with antibiotics alone and 14 of 17 survivors with antibiotics and pericardial drainage. At present, we prefer surgical pericardiostomy over the use of pericardiocentesis alone. Rare reported cases of acute purulent pericarditis[2, 15, 18] leading to constriction have been documented and we believe that effective pericardial drainage will help obviate this complication. The technique used for pericardiostomy is illustrated in Figure 74–1 (late cardiac tamponade: a potentially lethal complication of open heart surgery). Several surgical approaches can be used to drain the pericardium. Median sternotomy invites sternal osteomyelitis. A subxiphoid approach to the pericardium can be satisfactory. It allows a tube to be placed in the pericardial sac and affords dependent drainage. The most dependable approach is left anterior intercostal thoracotomy. This exposure allows exploration of the entire pericardial sac to ensure that no loculated areas of suppuration are left undrained. A generous segment of pericardial sac is removed and a large drain left in place. Despite pericardiostomy, an occasional patient with purulent pericarditis ultimately may require formal radical pericardiectomy because of chronic constriction.

Pericardial Effusion with Cardiac Tamponade

Pericardial effusion with cardiac tamponade is unusual in infants and children. However, it may require surgical intervention and pericardial resection. The etiology of chronic pericardial effusion may be viral, mycobacterial or associated with uremia in patients receiving chronic hemodialysis, and may follow mediastinal irradiation.[6] Frequently, massive pericardial effusion with cardiac tamponade is idiopathic in origin. The patient may present with a large heart shadow on x-ray (Fig. 74–2) and symptoms of congestive heart failure. Physical findings of distant heart sounds, ab-

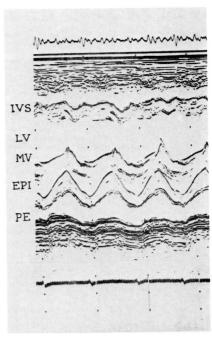

Fig. 74–3.—Echocardiogram demonstrating large posterior pericardial effusion. *IVS* = interventricular septum, *LV* = left ventricle, *MV* = mitral valve, *EPI* = epicardium, *PE* = pericardial effusion.

sence of murmurs and shifting intensity of heart sounds are found commonly in pericardial effusion. However, the physical findings and enlarged cardiac silhouette frequently make it difficult to distinguish this condition from cardiomegaly and congestive heart failure.

Recently, the echocardiogram has been used successfully to differentiate cardiomegaly from massive pericardial effusion. This is illustrated in Figure 74–3. The echocardiogram is a noninvasive study that requires little cooperation on the part of the child and frequently localizes the area of pericardial effusion.

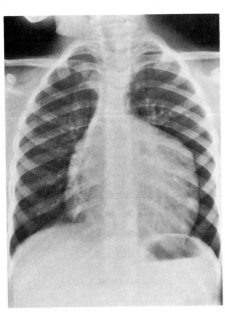

Fig. 74–2.—Large pericardial effusion of viral etiology in a 4-year-old child. "Epicardial fat pad" is a sign of pericardial effusion if present.

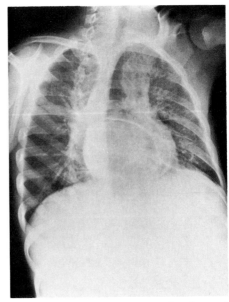

Fig. 74–4.—Oblique chest roentgenogram of a 6-year-old child with chronic constrictive pericarditis. Note dense calcifications in pericardium at area of atrioventricular groove.

Repeated pericardiocentesis may provide temporary relief from chronic pericardial effusion and tamponade. However, many patients require more extensive surgical procedures. At present, most surgeons prefer excision of the pericardium in cases of chronic effusion rather than creation of a pleural-pericardial window. Excellent results have been reported in children with chronic effusion and tamponade treated with pericardiectomy.[14]

Chronic Constrictive Pericarditis

Constrictive pericarditis is a relatively rare disease in infants and children but has an extraordinarily poor outcome if it is unrecognized.[3, 5, 17] The disease usually follows a chronic course characterized by ascites, shortness of breath and generalized failure to thrive. The symptoms may be confused with those of primary liver or kidney disease. In survey reports of pericarditis, the incidence of chronic constrictive pericarditis in children ranges from 1% to 13% of all cases.[3] Thus, although it is rare in the childhood age group, it occurs frequently enough that knowledge of its clinical presentation, cause and hemodynamic abnormalities is important. Usually of unknown origin, constrictive pericarditis has been reported to occur after purulent pericarditis, tuber-

culous pericarditis and viral pericardial effusion. Frequently, no specific etiology can be determined. Hemodynamic findings are the result of impaired ventricular filling and reduced stroke volume. Central venous pressure tracings demonstrate steep X and Y descents, and late diastolic pressures in the great veins and in the atria are increased. Ventricular pressure tracings demonstrate an early diastolic dip and a late diastolic plateau, the so-called square root sign. Almost all of these hemodynamic findings can be present, however. In patients with primary myocardiopathy, these two diseases frequently are difficult to distinguish from each other. The presence of concentric pericardial calcium on fluoroscopy or chest x-ray is a helpful sign (Fig. 74–4) but may not be present in all cases of constrictive pericarditis, especially in childhood.

After the diagnosis of constrictive pericarditis is made, treatment consisting of fluid restriction, digitalis and vigorous diuresis is instituted. The poor prognosis of untreated and medically treated patients without operation, however, underlines the necessity for urgent radical pericardiectomy. The operation can be performed through a bilateral anterior thoracotomy incision with division of the sternum. However, we prefer a median sternotomy incision, as illustrated in Figure 74–5. This affords excellent exposure to the

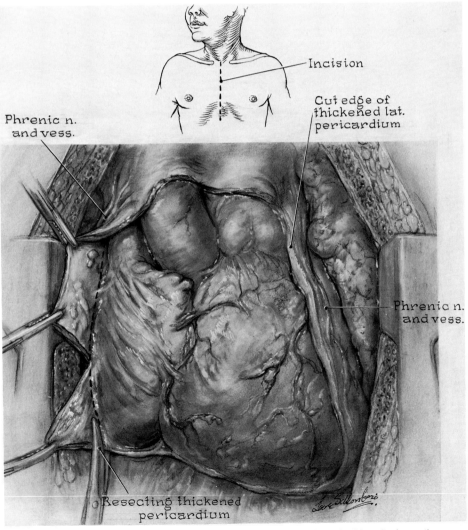

Fig. 74–5.—A sternotomy incision is used to expose the pericardium. A wide radical resection of both thickened pericardium and epicardium is necessary to ensure complete ventricular decortication.

pericardium and allows a wide resection of the pericardium, including removal of the pericardium from both ventricular surfaces, atrium and vena cava. Frequently it becomes necessary also to excise a thin layer of epicardium, which often is involved with the constrictive process. Radical pericardiectomy has resulted in markedly improved survival rates in children with chronic constrictive pericarditis. The determinant factors in survival and improvement appear to be the chronicity of disease and the degree of underlying myocardial fibrosis.

REFERENCES

1. Blalock, A., and Levy, S. E.: Tuberculous pericarditis, J. Thorac. Surg. 7:132, 1937.
2. Caird, R., *et al.:* Purulent pericarditis followed by early constriction in young children, Br. Heart J. 35:201, 1973.
3. DuShane, J. W., Kirklin, J. W., and Shea, D. W.: Chronic constrictive pericarditis in children. Report by a case and observation in seven others, Am. J. Dis. Child. 93:430, 1957.
4. Gersony, W. M., and MacCracken, G. H., Jr.: Purulent pericarditis in infancy, Pediatrics 40:224, 1967.
5. Goldring, D., Santa-Maria, M., and Strauss, A. W.: Constrictive pericarditis in children, Am. J. Dis. Child. 129:882, 1975.
6. Greenwood, R. D., *et al.:* Constrictive pericarditis in childhood due to mediastinal irradiation, Circulation 50:1033, 1974.
7. Isaacs, J. P., Carter, C. N., II, and Haller, J. A., Jr.: Pathology and physiology of constrictive pericarditis, Bull. Johns Hopkins Hosp. 90:259, 1952.
8. Lower, R.: *Fractatus de Corde* (Amsterdam, 1669), p. 104.
9. McKusick, V. A.: Chronic constrictive pericarditis; some clinical and laboratory observations, Bull. Johns Hopkins Hosp. 90:3, 1952.
10. Pick, F.: Über chronische unter dem Bilde der Lebercirrhose verlaufende Pericarditis (Pericarditische pseudolebercirrhose) nebst Bemerkungen über Zuckergussleber (Curschmann), Z. Klin. Med. 29:385, 1896.
11. Pieroni, D. R.: Echocardiographic diagnosis of septic pericarditis in infancy, J. Pediatr. 82:689, 1973.
12. Rehn, L.: Zu experimentellen Pathologic des Herzbeutels, Ges. Chir. 42:339, 1913.
13. Riolan, J.: Encheiridium Anatomicum et pathologicum Lugdini Batavorum ex Officina Adriani Wyngaerden, 1649, p. 206.
14. Roshe, J., and Shumacker, H. B, Jr.: Pericardiectomy for chronic cardiac tamponade in children, Surgery 46:1152, 1959.
15. Rubenstein, J. A., *et al.:* Acute constriction complicating purulent pericarditis in infancy, Am. J. Dis. Child. 124:591, 1972.
16. Sauerbruch, F.: *Die Chirurgie der Brustorgane* (Berlin, 1925), Vol. II.
17. Simcha, A., and Taylor, J. F. N.: Constrictive pericarditis in childhood, Arch. Dis. Child. 46:515, 1971.
18. Thomas, G. I., *et al.:* Pericardiectomy for acute constrictive staphylococcal pericarditis: Report of a case, N. Engl. J. Med. 267:440, 1962.
19. VanRecken, D., *et al.:* Infectious pericarditis in children, J. Pediatr. 85:109, 1974.

VOLUME TWO (pages 761–1622) of this work contains sections on the Abdomen, Genitourinary System, the Integument and Musculoskeletal Systems and the Nervous System. Since the pages are numbered consecutively throughout the two volumes, a complete index has been included in each volume and the inclusive page numbers in each volume have been shown on the spine of same.

Index

Index

(An asterisk following a page number indicates a reference to an illustration.)